HANDBUCH
DER EXPERIMENTELLEN
PHARMAKOLOGIE

BEGRÜNDET VON A. HEFFTER
FORTGEFÜHRT VON W. HEUBNER

ERGÄNZUNGSWERK

HERAUSGEGEBEN VON

O. EICHLER   UND   A. FARAH

PROFESSOR DER PHARMAKOLOGIE
AN DER UNIVERSITÄT HEIDELBERG

PROFESSOR DER PHARMAKOLOGIE
AN DER STATE UNIVERSITY OF NEW YORK

FÜNFZEHNTER BAND

CHOLINESTERASES AND
ANTICHOLINESTERASE AGENTS

SUB-EDITOR
GEORGE B. KOELLE

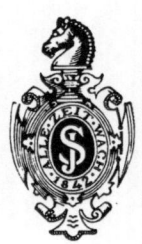

Springer-Verlag Berlin Heidelberg GmbH

1963

CHOLINESTERASES AND ANTICHOLINESTERASE AGENTS

CONTRIBUTORS

K. B. AUGUSTINSSON · L. E. CHADWICK · J. A. COHEN · H. CULLUMBINE · D. R. DAVIES · K. P. DuBOIS · D. GROB · C. O. HEBB · F. HOBBIGER · BO HOLMSTEDT · A. G. KARCZMAR · G. B. KOELLE · N. KRISHNA · A. S. KUPERMAN · I. H. LEOPOLD · J. P. LONG · X. MACHNE · L. A. MOUNTER · D. NACHMANSOHN · R. A. OOSTERBAAN · K. R. W. UNNA · G. WERNER · V. P. WHITTAKER · J. H. WILLS · E. ZAIMIS

SUB-EDITOR

GEORGE B. KOELLE

WITH 176 FIGURES

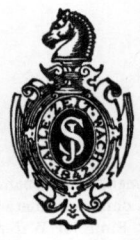

Springer-Verlag Berlin Heidelberg GmbH

1963

ISBN 978-3-642-99877-5   ISBN 978-3-642-99875-1 (eBook)
DOI 10. 1007/978-3-642-99875-1

Ursprünglich erschienen bei Springer-Verlag oHG. Berlin · Göttingen · Heidelberg 1963

Softcover reprint of the hardcover 1st edition 1963
Library of Congress Catalog Card Number Agr 25 — 699

Preface

Although the anticholinesterase (anti-ChE) agents have only limited applications in therapy, and from the viewpoint of practical significance they are more appropriately classified as toxic compounds or insecticides than as drugs, in their capacity of pharmacological tools they have few equals. The concept of neurohumoral transmission was originally established largely from experiments in which physostigmine, or eserine, was employed to protect acetylcholine (ACh), the transmitter of the cholinergic nerves, from rapid hydrolytic destruction by acetylcholinesterase (AChE) and other cholinesterases (ChE's). Since then, a great number of additional reversible and irreversible anti-ChE agents also have been indispensable in studies of synaptic and neuroeffector transmission, and of other physiological processes. At the same time, there is practically no other class of compounds for which a mechanism of pharmacological action can be described in such concrete biochemical and physiological terms. Consequently, it is not surprising that a huge literature has developed on these several closely interdependent topics. The assembling and proper correlation of this material for the present volume has taken the collaborative efforts of over two dozen investigators. It is believed that their contributions to this end will prove invaluable to future investigators in providing a ready, inclusive source of established information, in defining areas where further studies are indicated, and in preventing unnecessary duplication of past work. How well these aims have been accomplished will be for time and the reader to judge.

The volume is divided into four major sections. The first (I, Chapters 1 to 6) presents the biochemical and physiological background which is essential to an understanding of the primary mechanism of action of the anti-ChE agents. This includes the identification and distribution of ACh and other naturally occurring choline esters (Chapter 1), the known facts about the enzyme choline acetylase (ChAc), which catalyzes the final step in the synthesis of ACh (Chapter 2), and the current knowledge and hypotheses concerning the formation, storage, and liberation of ACh *in vivo* (Chapter 3). Chapter 4 presents a classification of the cholinesterases (ChE's) and the methods employed for their determination. The nomenclature and abbreviations used here are with few exceptions followed in the other chapters of the volume. The embryonic appearance and development of ChE's in various phyla are considered in relation to function in Chapter 5. Chapter 6 describes the cytological localizations of AChE and other ChE's throughout the body, and considers the possible functions of the enzymes and their known substrate, ACh, on the basis of these observations and pertinent data from physiological studies.

Section II is devoted to the chemistry of the anti-ChE agents. This includes the biochemical problems of the nature of the reactions between the various types of inhibitors and the enzymes (Chapter 7), and the pathways of metabolic degradation of the organophosphorus anti-ChE agents (Chapter 10), as well as the chemical classifications and relationships between structure and pharmacological actions of the reversible (Chapter 8) and organophosphorus (Chapter 9) anti-ChE agents.

The systematic pharmacology of the anti-ChE agents is covered in Section III. Here, the authors have attempted to distinguish as well as possible between effects due to inhibition or inactivation of ChE's and those which are more reasonably attributable to other mechanisms. The first four Chapters (11 to 14) of this Section discuss actions at sites where it is generally acknowledged that cholinergic transmission occurs, *i.e.*, at autonomic effector sites (11), autonomic ganglia (12), the neuromuscular junction of skeletal muscle (13), and certain regions of the central nervous system (14). The hypothesis that ACh and AChE are involved directly in the propagation of conducted axonal impulses is presented in Chapter 15; evidence to the contrary is considered in Chapter 6. The remaining two chapters here deal with the actions of anti-ChE agents on insects and other invertebrates (16), and on growth and development (17).

The final section (IV) treats the toxicological and therapeutic aspects of the anti-ChE agents. The general toxicological evaluation and the specific neurotoxic actions of the organophosphorus anti-ChE agents are presented in Chapters 18 and 19, respectively. Chapter 20 describes the pharmacology of the various types of antagonists of anti-ChE agents, with the exception of the compounds which reactivate alkylphosphorylated AChE; the latter are discussed in Chapter 21. The current clinical application of these findings to the treatment of intoxication with anti-ChE agents is presented in Chapter 22. Finally, the therapeutic uses of anti-ChE agents in myasthenia gravis (Chapter 23) and glaucoma (Chapter 24) are considered.

The Editor takes great pleasure in expressing to his collaborators in the preparation of this volume his deepest appreciation of their contributions and of their cooperative spirit and forbearance in bringing them into final form. He is most grateful for the invaluable editorial and secretarial help he has received from Miss CORNELIA GEESEY, Mrs. ZAROUG KABAKIAN, and Mrs. MARIAN SULLIVAN. For the accomplishment of this own investigative work, much of which is included in Chapter 6, he is deeply indebted to the stimulating participation of his past and present colleagues whose work is cited and acknowledged there. It is particularly appropriate to note the inspiration which he received from his early mentor, the late Dr. JONAS S. FRIEDENWALD, whose enthusiasm, genius, and kindly guidance first interested him in the application of histochemistry to pharmacological problems.

Finally, it is obviously not an Editor's prerogative to offer personal dedication of the work produced by his collaborators. However, his own efforts in assembling, contributing to, and editing this volume are dedicated with deepest affection to WIN, and to PETER, BILLY, and JONATHAN, who provided both constant inspiration and generous relinquishment of their rightful claims to the hours taken for its compilation.

Philadelphia. September, 1961   G. B. K.

List of Contributors

KLAS-BERTIL AUGUSTINSSON, Ph.D., Associate Professor, Institute of Organic Chemistry and Biochemistry, University of Stockholm, Stockholm 6, Sweden.

L. E. CHADWICK, Ph.D., Head, Department of Entomology, University of Illinois, Urbana, Ill., U.S.A.

J. A. COHEN, Ph.D., Professor of Applied Enzymology and Radiobiology, University of Leyden, and Director of the Medical Biological Laboratory, RVO-TNO, Rijswijk, Z.H., The Netherlands.

HARRY CULLUMBINE, M.D., Visiting Lecturer, Department of Pharmacology, Graduate School of Medicine, University of Pennsylvania, Philadelphia 4, Pa., U.S.A.

D. R. DAVIES, Senior Principal Scientific Officer, The Chemical Defence Experimental Establishment, Porton Down, Salisbury, England.

KENNETH P. DuBOIS, Ph.D., Professor of Pharmacology, University of Chicago, Chicago 37, Ill., U.S.A.

DAVID GROB, M.D., Professor of Medicine, State University of New York College of Medicine, and Director of Medical Services, Maimonides Hospital of Brooklyn, Brooklyn 19, N. Y., U.S.A.

CATHERINE O. HEBB, Ph.D., Head, Subdepartment of Chemical Physiology, Agricultural Research Council, Institute of Animal Physiology, Babraham, Cambridge, England.

F. HOBBIGER, M.D., D.Sc., Ph.D., Reader in Pharmacology, Middlesex Hospital Medical School, London, W. 1, England.

BO HOLMSTEDT, M.D., Associate Professor, Department of Pharmacology, Karolinska Institutet, Stockholm 60, Sweden.

ALEXANDER G. KARCZMAR, Ph.D., Professor and Chairman, Department of Pharmacology and Therapeutics, Stritch School of Medicine, University of Loyola, Chicago 12, Ill., U.S.A.

GEORGE B. KOELLE, Ph.D., M.D., Professor and Chairman, Department of Pharmacology, Schools of Medicine, University of Pennsylvania, Philadelphia 4, Pa., U.S.A.

NARENDRA KRISHNA, M.B.B.S., D.Sc. (Med.), Instructor in Ophthalmology, Graduate School of Medicine, University of Pennsylvania, and Research Associate, Wills Eye Hospital, Philadelphia 30, Pa., U.S.A.

ALBERT S. KUPERMAN, Ph.D., Assistant Professor of Pharmacology, Cornell University Medical College, New York 21, N. Y., U.S.A.

IRVING H. LEOPOLD, M.D., D.Sc. (Med.), Professor and Chairman, Department of Ophthalmology, Graduate School of Medicine, University of Pennsylvania, and Medical and Research Director, Wills Eye Hospital, Philadelphia 30, Pa., U.S.A.

J. P. LONG, Ph.D., Associate Professor, Department of Pharmacology, College of Medicine, State University of Iowa, Iowa City, Ia., U.S.A.

XENIA MACHNE, M.D., Assistant Professor of Pharmacology, University of Illinois College of Medicine, Chicago 12, Ill., U.S.A.

L. A. MOUNTER, Ph.D., Associate Professor, Department of Biophysics, Medical College of Virginia, Richmond 19, Va., U.S.A.

DAVID NACHMANSOHN, M.D., Professor of Biochemistry, College of Physicians and Surgeons, Columbia University, New York 32, N. Y., U.S.A.

R. A. OOSTERBAAN, Ph.D., Head of the Biochemical Department of the Medical Biological Laboratory, RVO-TNO, Rijswijk, Z.H., The Netherlands.

KLAUS R. W. UNNA, M.D., Professor and Head, Department of Pharmacology, University of Illinois College of Medicine, Chicago 12, Ill., U.S.A.

GERHARD WERNER, M.D., Associate Professor of Pharmacology, Cornell University Medical College. New York 21, N. Y., U.S.A.

V. P. WHITTAKER, D.Phil. (Oxon.), Member of the Scientific Staff, Biochemistry Department, Agricultural Research Council, Institute of Animal Physiology, Babraham, Cambridge, England.

J. H. WILLS, Ph.D., Chief, Physiology Division, Directorate of Medical Research, U.S. Army Chemical Research and Development Laboratories, Army Chemical Center, Maryland, U.S.A.

ELEANOR ZAIMIS, M.D., Professor of Pharmacology, University of London, Royal Free Hospital School of Medicine, London, W.C. 1, England.

Contents

Chapter 1

Identification of Acetylcholine and Related Esters of Biological Origin

By

V. P. WHITTAKER

With 6 Figures

Contents

D'autre part, la présence d'acétylcholine parmi les composants actifs de l'ergot de seigle, qui vient d'être signalée par Ewins, permet de supposer que, dans l'organisme animal, qui renferme, côte à côte, la choline et les acides gras supérieurs, et même certains dérivés contenant à la fois ces deux sortes de substances (lécithines), on pourra rencontrer un jour les homologues de l'acétylcholine, soit comme des constituants normaux des humeurs, soit comme les produits de certains états pathologiques.

(Fourneau and Page, 1914)

Introduction

Although acetylcholine (ACh) has been shown beyond reasonable doubt to be the transmitter substance at certain cholinergic nerve endings, there are several facts which warn us against attributing a too exclusive role to this compound. First, by analogy with other transmitters (e.g., the catecholamines) the transmitter role is likely to be subserved by a group of related substances rather than by a single compound. Second, ACh occurs in non-nervous tissue and is so widely distributed in nature as to suggest a non-nervous function for it. Third, several other carboxylic esters of choline possessing related or contrasting pharmacological properties are known to occur in nature. Though so far their presence in nervous tissue has not been unequivocally demonstrated, this tissue can undoubtedly synthesize homologues of ACh *in vitro* (Gardiner and Whittaker 1954, Frontali 1958, Berry and Whittaker 1959) and is well equipped, by its possession of two forms of cholinesterase (ChE), to destroy them rapidly. The possibility that ACh may not be the only transmitter substance at cholinergic nerve endings or that its function may be interfered with under pathological conditions by the appearance of similar compounds must be borne in mind when considering the mode of action of anti-cholinesterase (anti-ChE) agents and justifies the inclusion of a chapter on the identification of ACh and related esters in a monograph on this subject.

No one test is specific for ACh in the concentrations at which it is likely to be encountered in biological material. Pharmacological tests are the most sensitive and can be made specific if used in combination. One method is that of *parallel* or *differential assays*, introduced by Chang and Gaddum (1933), in which the unknown is quantitatively compared with a known ester in a series of pharmacological test systems which differ in their responsiveness to different esters. If the known and unknown esters are identical, the results of the assays should also be identical. Technical difficulties arise from the presence of interfering substances in tissue extracts, the relatively large error in biological assays, and the possible

Table 1. *Naturally occurring choline esters*

Ester	Species	Organ or tissue	References	Method of identification	Remarks
Esters of definite occurrence and known constitution					
Acetylcholine	rye ergot	extract	1	A	First identification as natural product; probably formed by bacteria in extract (1a)
	horse	spleen	2, 3	(2) A, (3) CbD	First isolation from mammalian tissue (2)
		small intestine	4	D	First use of parallel assay
	human	placenta	4, 5	(4) D, (5) CbD	
	cat	superior cervical ganglion (perfusate during nerve stimulation)	6	D	
	dog	stomach (perfusate during nerve stimulation)	7	D	
	ox	spleen	8, 3, 9, 10	(8) CaD, (3) CbD, (9) Ca, (10) CaCcD	First use of paper (8) and column (3) chromatography; this tissue also contains propionylcholine (q.v.)
		small intestine	5	CbD	
		blood	11	A	Much smaller amounts found by (12)
		brain	13, 5, 14, 15	(13) A, (5) CaCbD, (14) CaD, (15) ACaCcD	Formed *in vitro* (13). Tissue also stated to contain butyrylcholine (q.v.)
	sheep	small intestine	5	CbD	
	goat	brain	5	CbD	
		small intestine	5	CbD	
		abomasum	5	CbD	
		rumen	5	CbD	
		heart	5	CbD	
	rabbit	brain	5	CbD	
		small intestine	5	CbD	
		heart	5	CbD	
	Octopus vulgaris	nervous tissue	16	AD	First demonstration in nervous tissue and in marine organism
	Mytilus edulis	gill plates	17	CaD	
	Torpedo marmorata	electric organ	18	Ca	
	Thais lapillus	whole organism	19, 20	CbD	
	Urosalpinx cinereus	whole organism	19, 20	CbD	
	lobster	ventral nerve cord	20	CbD	
	Myxine glutinosa	heart	21	Ca	A second active component present, but not identified
	housefly	head	22	CaBCaCc	
	honey-bee	head	23	Ca	
		royal jelly	24	ACaCc	
		honey	25, 26	(25) ABCaD, (26) E	
	Vespa crabro	venom	26a	CaB	
	Pieris brassica	eggs	27	CbD	
	Arctia caja	silk gland	27a	CaD	

1*

Table 1. (cont.)

Ester	Species	Organ or tissue	References	Method of identification	Remarks
	Capsella bursae pastoris	—	28	A	
	Artocarpus integra	seeds and leaves	29	D	
	potato	tuber	30	ABCaD	
	Urtica urens	nettle hairs	31	D	
	Viscum album	—	32	A	
	Crataegus sp.	berries and leaves	33	CaD	
	Lactobacillus plantarum	whole organism	34	A	Earlier references to A identification in rotting vegetables given by (34)
	Lactarius blennius	press juice	1 a	D	Esters not present in 36 other species of fungus, yeast, or fresh ergot
	Trypanosoma rhodesiense	whole organism	34 a	D	
Propionyl-choline	ox	spleen	8, 3, 9, 10	(8) CaD, (3) BCbD, (9) Ca, (10)CaCcD	Not found in other tissues examined by (5). First identification of a naturally occurring, pharmacologically active homologue of acetylcholine (8)
Acrylylcholine (I, $R_1 = R_2$ = H)	*Buccinum undatum*	hypobranchial gland	35	BCaCb	
Senecioylcholine (I, $R_1 = R_2$ = Me)	*Thais floridana*	hypobranchial gland	36, 20, 37	(36, 20) BCaCb, (37) A	Pharmacology studied by (38, 39)
Sinapylcholine (sinapine) (I, $R_1 = 3:5$-dimethoxy-4-hydroxyphenyl, $R_2 = $ H)	*Sinapis alba*	seeds	40, 41	A	No reports of pharmacological activity
	Draba nemorosa	seeds	42	A	
	rape	seeds	42 a	A	
Urocanylcholine (murexine) (I, $R_1 = 4(5)$-imidazolyl-, $R_2 = $ H)	*Murex trunculus*	hypobranchial gland	43	AB	First isolated as a chemically unidentified base by (44); pharmacology studied by (45—48, 38)
	M. brandaris		44	A	
	Tritonalia erinacea		44	A	
	Urosalpinx cinereus		19, 20	BCaCb	
	Thais lapillus		19, 20	BCaCb	
	M. fulvescens		20	BCaCb	
γ-Aminobutyryl-choline	dog, pig	brain	49, 50	(49) Ca, (50) ABCa	Similar pharmacologically to fraction A of Factor I but not identical chromatographically (51). Has been studied pharmacologically by (52, 52 a)

Esters of doubtful occurrence, unknown constitution or incompletely characterized

Ester	Species	Organ or tissue	References	Method of identification	Remarks
Butyrylcholine	ox	brain	14	CaD	Found only in autolysing brain (15); can be synthesized by brain preparations *in vitro* (53) but acetylcholine only ester found in fresh brain (5, 15)

Table 1. (cont.)

Ester	Species	Organ or tissue	References	Method of identification	Remarks
Imidazolyl-acetylcholine	ox, horse, rat	brain	54	Ca	Results thought to be explained by presence of γ-aminobutyrylcholine (50)
Palmitylcholine	rat	liver	55	Cb	Synthesized *in vitro* by brain and liver (53)
Unidentified ester	honey-bee	head	23	Ca	
Unidentified ester	*Arctia caja*	cervical glands	56	Ca	Probably senecioylcholine
Unidentified ester	*Myxine glutinosa*	heart	57	Ca	
Unidentified ester	—	hypophysis	58	A	

Abbreviations: A, chemical; B, spectroscopic; Ca, by paper chromatography; Cb, by column chromatography; Cc, by paper electrophoresis; D, by parallel assay; E, enzymic; —, not stated.

References: (1) Ewins (1914), (1a) Oury and Bacq (1938), (2) Dale and Dudley (1929), (3) Gardiner and Whittaker (1954), (4) Chang and Gaddum (1933), (5) Keyl (1957), (6) Feldberg and Gaddum (1934), (7) Dale and Feldberg (1934), (8) Banister et al. (1951, 1953), (9) Augustinsson (1955), (10) Henschler (1957), (11) Kapfhammer and Bischoff (1930), (12) Dudley (1933), (13) Stedman and Stedman (1937), (14) Holtz and Schümann (1954), (15) Henschler (1956b), (16) Bacq and Mazza (1935), (17) Bülbring et al. (1953), (18) Woodin, personal communication, (19) Whittaker and Michaelson (1954), (20) Keyl et al. (1957), (21) Augustinsson et al. (1955), (22) Chefurka and Smallman (1956), (23) Augustinsson and Grahn (1954), (24) Henschler (1956a), (25) Marquardt and Vogg (1952a, b), (26) Goldschmidt and Burkert (1955), (26a) Bhoola et al. (1960), (27) David (1959), (27a) Morley and Schachter (1961), (28) Boruttau and Cappenberg (1921), (29) Lin (1955), (30) Marquardt, Schumacher and Vogg (1952), (31) Emmelin and Feldberg (1947), (32) Winterfeld (1942), (33) Fiedler et al. (1953), (34) Stephenson and Rowatt (1947), (34a) Bülbring et al. (1949), (35) Whittaker (1959a), (36) Whittaker (1957), (37) Whittaker (1959b), (38) Holmstedt and Whittaker (1958), (39) Erspamer and Glässer (1958), (40) Gadamer (1897), (41) Späth (1920), (42) Kung and Huang (1949), (42a) Schwarze (1949), (43) Erspamer and Benati (1953), (44) Erspamer and Dordoni (1947), (45) Erspamer and Glässer (1957), (46) Tabachnick and Roth (1957), (47) Quilliam (1957), (48) Keyl and Whittaker (1958), (49) Kuriaki et al. (1958), (50) Kewitz (1959), (51) McLennan (1959), (52) Takahashi et al. (1958, 1959), (52a) Holmstedt and Sjöqvist (1960), (53) Berry and Whittaker (1959), (54) Gruner and Kewitz (1955), (55) Kennedy (1956), (56) Bisset et al. (1960), (57) Augustinsson et al. (1955), (58) Freudenberg and Biller (1936).

existence of compounds which resemble each other in more than one test. Chromatographic methods, introduced by Whittaker and co-workers (Whittaker 1951b, Whittaker and Wijesundera 1951, 1952a, Banister, Whittaker and Wijesundera 1951, 1953, Gardiner and Whittaker 1954), have in recent years proved a valuable adjunct to purely pharmacological tests. If the compound in question fails to be identified with any known ester, identification can be achieved only by chemical methods which require the isolation of the active substance in milligram quantities or less.

The carboxylic esters of choline which are known or suspected in biological material are listed in Table 1. Some of them, e.g., propionylcholine, are intensely active substances: others, e.g., palmitylcholine, sinapine, are of doubtful physiological or pharmacological significance in the present context.

The ACh content of a very large number of different biological materials has been determined, usually by non-specific methods. In Table 1 the entries under ACh refer only to work in which at least some attempt was made to identify the active substance as ACh by parallel assay, chromatography, classical chemical, or physico-chemical techniques or a combination of these methods, and are intended to serve as a guide for future work of this kind. The relatively few materials to which these more rigorous methods have been applied and the wide range of different phyla which have been found to contain ACh will both be apparent. The high concentration of ACh in certain plants is noteworthy, but perhaps not surprising when we consider its close chemical relation to the plant alkaloids, particularly esters of straight chain or ali-cyclic hydroxyalkylamines like aconitine and atropine. It is perhaps more surprising that no other carboxylic ester of choline has been isolated from plant materials with the exception of sinapine (reviewed by KAHANE and LÉVY 1938), which has not been reported to be pharmacologically active. This compound, like the snail esters (q.v.) is a β-substituted acrylylcholine, and is historically interesting as the oldest known derivative of choline; the latter was prepared from it and called sincaline by BABO and HIRSCHBRUNN (1852), the discoverers of sinapine, ten years before STRECKER (1862) invented the name "choline".

Between 1930 and 1933, KAPFHAMMER and co-workers (KAPFHAMMER and BISCHOFF 1930, BISCHOFF, GRAB and KAPFHAMMER 1932), using apparently unexceptionable chemical methods, reported the isolation of ACh from a number of tissues in much larger amounts than could be confirmed by other workers (for a recent study see MARQUARDT and HIRSCH 1952); for this reason, most of this work has been omitted from Table 1. DUDLEY (1933) made a careful attempt to repeat part of the work in KAPFHAMMER's own laboratory and reported an "uncanny" sudden increase in the ACh content of an extract during the isolation procedure. To the author's knowledge, a full account of this curious episode in the history of ACh research has never been published, though many of the details must be known to persons still living. Also omitted from Table 1 is the identification of ACh in milk (cf. ALM and AUGUSTINSSON 1957), which could not be confirmed by WHITTAKER (1958).

The possibility that homologues of ACh might occur in animal tissues was envisaged soon after EWINS' (1914) pioneer isolation of ACh from extract of ergot, as is shown by the quotation at the head of this chapter. However, it was not until 1951 that FOURNEAU and PAGE's prediction was realised by the isolation of propionylcholine from ox spleen by BANISTER et al. (1951, 1953). Although a fairly extensive survey carried out in the author's laboratory by KEYL in 1953—1954 and so far reported only in thesis form (KEYL 1957) failed to reveal the presence of propionylcholine in other mammalian tissues, the work of BANISTER et al. has stimulated interest in the whole question of the natural occurrence of other pharmacologically active esters of choline, and several more have now been identified in animal tissues. These include acrylylcholine (cation as in I, $R_1 = R_2 = H$) and two β-substituted acrylylcholines,

$$\underset{R_2}{\overset{R_1}{\diagdown}}C = CHCO_2CH_2CH_2\overset{+}{N}Me_3$$

I

β,β-dimethylacrylylcholine (senecioylcholine) (I, $R_1 = R_2 = CH_3$) and β-imidazolyl-4(5)-acrylylcholine (urocanylcholine, murexine) (I, $R_1 = H$, $R_2 = C_3N_2H_3$), all present in the hypobranchial glands of different species of marine prosobranch gastropods of the division Rachiglossa, and γ-aminobutyrylcholine, present in mammalian brain.

Urocanylcholine was first isolated as far back as 1947 as a tissue base of unknown constitution by ERSPAMER and DORDONI, whose work is an excellent example of the value of parallel assays. They showed that the high ACh equivalence (for definition see section A. II p. 10) of the hypobranchial glands of species of the dye-secreting Muricidae, previously noted by VINCENT and JULLIEN (1938), could not be due to ACh because the pharmacological behaviour of the extracts differed from the latter in a series of tests. They succeeded in isolating the active substance as the crystalline styphnate and dipicrate and named it murexine. The compound was identified chemically by ERSPAMER and BENATI (1953), synthesized by PASINI, VERCELLONE and ERSPAMER (1953) and shown to have the *trans* configuration by PASINI and VERCELLONE (1955b). Murexine is present also in three other Muricidae not examined by ERSPAMER and co-workers, *Urosalpinx cinereus*, *Thais lapillus* and *Murex fulvescens* (WHITTAKER and MICHAELSON, 1954), but the related *Thais floridana* contains senecioylcholine (WHITTAKER 1957, 1959b, KEYL, MICHAELSON and WHITTAKER 1957); *Buccinum undatum*, a member of the same order but not of the same family and not a dye-secreting snail, contains acrylylcholine (WHITTAKER 1959a). The salivary gland of another of the Buccinidae, *Neptunea antiqua*, contains a high concentration of neurine (FÄNGE 1958, EMMELIN and FÄNGE 1958); the hypobranchial gland of this species has not been examined. Senecioylcholine has also been identified with fair certainty in the cervical glands of the moth, *Arctia caja* (BISSET et al. 1960).

The biogenesis and the function of these esters are alike obscure. The acid moieties have carbon skeletons identical with those of the amino-acids histidine (urocanylcholine), valine (senecioylcholine), and alanine (acrylylcholine) and could be derived from them by α-deamination; *Thais lapillus* has, indeed, been found to be a fairly rich source of histidine α-deaminase (KEYL et al. 1957). The esters are present in the snail glands in high concentration; urocanylcholine and senecioylcholine possess neuromuscular blocking action of the depolarizing variety (ERSPAMER and GLÄSSER 1957, 1958, KEYL and WHITTAKER 1958, HOLMSTEDT and WHITTAKER 1958), a property which could account both for the high toxicity and the paralysing action of glandular extracts noted by DUBOIS (1909) who regarded the glands as venom organs. Secretion of senecioylcholine in *Arctia caja* likewise appears as part of a defence reaction which includes a threatening display (BISSET et al. 1960). By contrast, acrylylcholine has only an extremely weak blocking action, and is intermediate in properties between ACh and propionyl-choline in a number of test systems (HOLMSTEDT, SUNDWALL and WHITTAKER unpublished). This raises the question as to whether the hypobranchial esters are paralysing toxins in all species. Invertebrate pharmacology and toxicology is still largely an unexplored field, and further work with the techniques now available might well bring to light many more choline esters.

The presence of γ-aminobutyrylcholine in brain, reported on somewhat slender evidence by KURIAKI et al. (1958), has been confirmed by KEWITZ (1959). There has been much discussion as to the relation of this ester and its parent acid to the inhibitory transmitter substance(s) assumed to be involved in central inhibition in the brain and spinal cord, and to Factor I, an inhibitory substance identified in brain by FLOREY and co-workers (FLOREY 1954, ELLIOTT and FLOREY 1956). According to the Japanese workers (KURIAKI et al. 1958, TAKAHASHI et al. 1958, TAKAHASHI et al. 1959), γ-aminobutyrylcholine has an intensely inhibitory action on the electrical activity of the cortex, about a thousand times more than γ-aminobutyric acid, but has otherwise little pharmacological activity of any kind. McLENNAN (1959) and HONOR and McLENNAN (1960) found that the ester resembles fraction A of Factor I in some respects but were unable to confirm its inhibitory action on cortical potentials. HOLMSTEDT and SJÖQVIST (1960) reported that it is largely inactive in a variety of peripheral test systems and is less active in some tests than the Japanese workers claimed. According to CURTIS, PHILLIS and WATKINS (1960), it resembles the free acid in depressing the ACh, glutamate, and synaptically evoked spikes of Renshaw cells, but differs from it in exerting no action on other spinal neurones. The depressant action on Renshaw cells is often followed by a prolonged excitation which appears to be an intrinsic property of the ester. However, the discovery of γ-aminobutyrylcholine undoubtedly opens up a

Table 2. *Methods available for the pharmacological assay of acetylcholine (ACh)
and other naturally occurring choline esters*

The sensitivity is defined by the approximate threshold dose of ACh in $\mu\mu$mole/ml bathing fluid (isolated organs) or kg body weight (animal preparation). The numbers in brackets refer to the references at the foot of the table.

Method	Sensi-tivity	Specificity		Remarks
		Choline esters	Interfering substances	
Frog rectus abdominus muscle (1, 2)	25	Responds to large numbers of esters some of which are more active than ACh	Choline, potassium, phosphate, and phosphate esters give contractions but only in high concentrations. They may also potentiate the response to ACh but this can be allowed for	Requires only simple equipment. Muscle contracts reproducibly and relaxes rapidly, permitting speedy, accurate assays. Sensitivity of $5\,\mu\,\mu$mole/ml attainable under favorable conditions with selected muscles
Guinea pig ileum (2)	10	Fairly specific for ACh	Histamine, substance P, 5-hydroxytryptamine also give contractions. Histamine response can be blocked by anti-histamines	Requires more elaborate equipment than frog rectus. More likely to be interfered with by other biological components. Muscle contracts and relaxes rapidly but response is not so reproducible as frog rectus
Cat blood pressure (2)	5 to 10	Low specificity	Tissue vasoactive substances	Simple, rapid method. More expensive in animals than above methods. The rat (3) can also be used
Venus heart (4, 5)	0.5	Highly specific for ACh	Tissue vasoactive substances	Extremely sensitive and discriminating, but test organ not generally available.
Leech dorsal muscle (2, 6)	5	Specificity similar to frog rectus		Contracts less reproducibly than frog rectus. Relaxes very slowly. Assays more time consuming and less accurate than frog rectus
Buccinum undatum radula muscle (7, 8)	50	Specificity not known	Neurine gives ACh-like contraction. Tryptamine or 5-hydroxytryptamine added with ACh cause rhythmical contraction	
Frog lung (9)	5×10^{-7}			
Stichopus regalis dorsal muscle (10)	0.05	Specificity not known	Relatively unaffected by pressor amines	
Cat sciatic-gastrocnemicus (11)	—	Assays esters (e.g., urocanylcholine) having neuromuscular blocking action		
Crayfish stretch receptor (12)	—	Assays γ-aminobutyrylcholine and other inhibitory substances	Also responds to γ-aminobutyric acid	
Sea urchin oesophagus (13, 14)	—	Assays γ-aminobutyrylcholine and other inhibitory substances, e.g., fraction A of Factor I		Unaffected by γ-aminobutyric acid

(1) CHANG and GADDUM (1933), (2) MacIntosh and PERRY (1950), (3) STRAUGHAN (1958), (4) WAIT (1943), (5) WELSH and TAUB (1948), (6) MINZ (1932), (7) FÄNGE (1958), (8) FÄNGE and MATTISSON (1958), (9) CORSTEN (1940), (10) BACQ (1939), (11) BURN, FINNEY and GOODWIN (1950), (12) FLOREY (1954), (13) FLOREY and McLENNAN (1959), (14) McLENNAN (1959).

new field for investigation in the pharmacology and biochemistry of choline esters; if it, or a related ester, turns out to be the much sought inhibitory transmitter, many facts concerning the specificity of the ChE's and choline acylases could be profitably re-examined.

The status of the remaining esters in Table 1 is less certain. A careful attempt to duplicate the work of HOLTZ and SCHÜMANN (1954) by KEYL (1957) failed to substantiate their claim to have identified butyrylcholine in ox brain; HENSCHLER (1956b) reported that this ester appears only in autolysing brain. The unidentified esters of bee brain (AUGUSTINSSON and GRAHN 1954) and *Myxine* heart (AUGUSTINSSON, FÄNGE, JOHNELS and ÖSTLUND 1955) might be chromatographic artifacts; this point is discussed in greater detail in Section B IV 2 c.

In the sections which follow, an account is first given of those properties of choline esters — pharmacological, chemical, spectroscopic and chromatographic — which are particularly useful for their identification and quantitative estimation. It is hoped that the fairly detailed treatment adopted will be useful not only to those working in the choline ester field but to all those who are interested in the identification of naturally occurring, pharmacologically active organic bases. With a few exceptions inserted for purposes of comparison, data are given only for known or suspected naturally occurring esters; for further information the reader is referred to the excellent monograph on biogenic amines by GUGGENHEIM (1951) and to the comprehensive survey of the pharmacology of synthetic drugs related to ACh by BOVET and BOVET-NITTI (1948). BARLOW's (1955) textbook also provides useful information. The chapter concludes with a section describing how the various properties of choline esters, as outlined in the previous sections, are utilized in their isolation and identification from biological material.

Properties of choline esters
A. Pharmacological properties
I. Introduction

It is not proposed to review in detail all the methods for the pharmacological assay of ACh as MACINTOSH and PERRY's (1950) account of the subject is still up-to-date. The main methods are summarized in Table 2. which indicates the sensitivity, specificity and general convenience of each. Also included are a few less well known methods the high sensitivity of which suggests that they would repay further investigation, and others which test properties possessed by some of the newer naturally occurring esters but not by ACh. It will suffice if in addition a few general points are mentioned concerning choice of materials and definition of terms.

No one method is specific for any one choline ester. This is not necessarily a disadvantage if it can be established by other means that the ester being assayed is the only one likely to be present or if the object is to determine the presence of unknown esters. More important than specificity are the stability of the preparation, the reproducibility and rapidity of its response, the degree of freedom from interference by adventitious substances, the simplicity of the equipment required, and the accessibility or cheapness of the test organism. By all these criteria the frog rectus assay method introduced by CHANG and GADDUM (1933) is probably the best. It is, however, somewhat less sensitive than other methods, and for the investigation of certain current problems there is a need for a really sensitive micro-assay method to complement the micro-pipette techniques which have been developed by the electrophysiologists. Possible methods include the isolated frog lung (CORSTEN 1940) and various invertebrate preparations (BACQ 1947) such as the smooth muscle of the sea cucumber, *Stichopus regalis* (BACQ 1939), and the heart of the clam, *Venus mercenaria* (SMITH and LEVINE 1938, WAIT 1943, WELSH and TAUB 1948). The microbath of less than 50 μl capacity devised by GADDUM and STEPHENSON (1958) should prove useful in conjunction with some of these preparations; unfortunately, attempts to scale down conventional assay methods by using small slips of muscle run into the difficulty that the response tends to become all-or-nothing.

It is possible that purely electrophysiological methods of assaying choline esters will eventually be developed, using characteristic changes in electric potentials in the C.N.S. or endplate regions.

II. Definitions

As pointed out in section B II. 1 below, choline esters are stable in acid solution and unstable in alkaline; many, but not all, are also rapidly hydrolysed by ChE's. These properties serve to distinguish them from choline, potassium, phosphate, nucleotides and many other substances which are present in biological extracts and which may simulate or modify the effect of choline esters on the frog rectus and other preparations. Any assay of a biological extract should thus include a demonstration that the activity being measured is alkali-labile, and when the extract is being matched against the standard, an amount of alkali-treated extract equivalent to the dose of the extract should be added with the standard to ensure that the latter is exerting its effect against the same background as the unknown (FELDBERG and HEBB 1947). Assayed in this way the activity of an extract

Table 3. *Relative molar potencies of some choline esters*

Choline ester	Fall in blood pressure uneserinized cat	Contraction of eserinized frog rectus	Contraction of eserinized leech	Contraction of guinea-pig intestine	Neuromuscular blockade (a)	Crayfish stretch receptor (b)
Acetyl	100	100	100	100	—	—
Propionyl . . .	20 (1) 1 (2)	160—200(3)	45(4)	5—10 (3) 1 (5)	—	—
Butyryl[1] . . .	0.8 (1)	90—100(3)	90(4)	0.1 (5)	—	—
Palmityl . . .	—	—	—	0.1 (6)	—	—
Acrylyl[2]. . . .	10 (2)	30—90 (2, 7)	—	1—20 (2,7)	0 (2)	—
Senecioyl . . .	rise (8)	20—70 (8, 9, 10c)	—	0.1 (8)	18 (8) 13 (10c)	—
Urocanyl[3] . . .	rise (8, 9, 10, 11)	10 (9, 11c)	—	0.02 (11c)	27 (8) 20 (11c)	—
γ-Aminobutyryl	0.1 (12)	0.025 (12c) 0.1 (13)	—	0 (12) 0.05 (13)	2.7 (13)	55(14cd)

References: (1) SIMONART (1932), (2) HOLMSTEDT, SUNDWALL and WHITTAKER, unpublished, (3) BANISTER et al. (1953), (4) CHANG and GADDUM (1933), (5) SCHNEIDER and TIMMS (1957), (6) ABDERHALDEN, PAFFRATH and SICKEL (1925), (7) WHITTAKER (1959a), (8) HOLMSTEDT and WHITTAKER (1958), (9) KEYL et al. (1957), (10) ERSPAMER and GLÄSSER (1958), (11) ERSPAMER and GLÄSSER (1957), (12) KURIAKI et al. (1958), (13) HOLMSTEDT and SJÖQVIST (1960), (14) McLENNAN (1959).

(a) Cat sciatic-gastrocnemius preparation (succinylcholine = 100). (b) γ-Aminobutyric acid = 100. (c) Calculated from authors' results, (d) on assumption that figures refer to free base.

[1] For higher homologues see BOVET and BOVET-NITTI (1948) and (5).
[2] For synthetic β-substituted acrylylcholines not included in table see (8).
[3] For synthetic heterocyclic choline esters not included in table see (10) and HOLMSTEDT, LARSSON and SUNDWALL (1960).

expressed as μg (or mμmole) ACh chloride (or other salt)/g tissue extracted gives the *ACh equivalence* of the tissue. The advantage of molar units is that the anion associated with the choline ester need not be specified.

When the ester assayed is not ACh, its actual concentration cannot be determined unless its *potency* relative to ACh is also known for the particular preparation and dose levels used. The *relative potency* of an ester is the amount of ACh giving a response equivalent to unit amount of the ester; if expressed as the moles of ACh equivalent to 100 moles of ester it becomes the *relative molar potency in percentage units*. Unfortunately this quantity may vary considerably with different preparations of the same test object and, since different esters may give dose-response curves of different slopes, with the dose level at which the comparison is made; interfering substances in the extracts may also alter the relative potency (GARDINER and WHITTAKER 1954). Some esters may show more than one kind of action on the test preparation and the nature of the action may differ in important respects from that of ACh. Examples of this are given in the next section. Thus, activity measurements of extracts containing unknown esters, if expressed in terms of ACh, are subject to considerable uncertainty; hence, the relative molar potencies recorded in Table 3 are intended merely as a guide.

III. Notes on individual methods

1. Frog rectus abdominis muscle

This preparation has a low specificity; it responds both to those esters having ganglion-stimulating properties (e.g., the lower homologues of ACh) and those producing the depolarizing type of neuromuscular blockade in mammals (e.g., succinylcholine). The most active ester so far discovered is β-4(5)-imidazolyl-propionylcholine (dihydromurexine) which has been reported to be 6 to 7 times more active than ACh (ERSPAMER and GLÄSER 1958); propionylcholine is 1.5 to 2 times more active (Table 3).

As used by the author, the procedure is essentially as described by MacIntosh and PERRY (1950) with the following modifications. Magnification is 16-fold, tension 1 g; 20 to 30 min are allowed for relaxation in frog Ringer solution (composition, NaCl, 0.65%; KCl, 0.016%; CaCl$_2$ anh., 0.012%; NaHCO$_3$, 0.01%, all w/v) before addition of physostigmine (eserine) sulphate (2 mg/l) to sensitize the muscle. Another 20 to 30 min is allowed for sensitization to become complete. The Ringer solution is conveniently made up just before use from stock solutions (stored at 4°) of the constituents 10 times (NaCl) or 100 times their final strength.

Neostigmine (Prostigmine) and tetraethylpyrophosphate (TEPP) may be used in place of physostigmine; they give more sensitive but less regular preparations. Pre-treatment of the frog with *p*-nitrophenyldiethylphosphate (Paraoxon, Mintacol, E 600), injected into the dorsal lymph sac, has been advocated by ROTSCHUH (1954) and HENSCHLER (1956b), and the use of other anti-ChE agents would probably repay study. The degree of sensitization with anti-ChE agents varies with different esters: this is a useful criterion of identity. The mechanism whereby anti-ChE agents cause sensitization of the frog rectus is not fully understood; they do not act merely by stabilizing added esters, since they also sensitize to non-esters such as choline and decamethonium; accumulation of sub-threshold amounts of endogenous ACh is probably involved (FLEISHER et al. 1960).

Contractions are allowed to take place for 90 sec; the drug is then washed out and the muscle allowed to relax; this is complete in $1^1/_2$ min. Electrical stimulation of the muscle has been used to achieve relaxation in an automatic cycle (GARDINER, personal communication). Doses are conveniently pipetted into a 10 ml measuring cylinder, made up to 3 ml with eserinized Ringer solution, and applied by emptying out the organ bath and pouring in the fresh medium containing the dose. The frog rectus is a robust preparation and can tolerate relatively large temporary deviations in the composition of the medium (as for example when assaying eluates in column chromatography) provided the pH and osmolarity of the latter are not changed. If pH adjustments are necessary, a drop of aqueous phenol red may be added when making up the dose to volume and the pH adjusted with 0.33 N HCl or NaOH. These concentrations when neutralized give isotonic saline solution. A bracketing or flanking procedure is used for accurate assay, but the response is usually sufficiently constant for this to be curtailed if large numbers of chromatographic fractions have to be assayed. It is convenient to plug the kymograph and tapper or buzzer (required to prevent the lever's sticking) into a simple timing device (Fig. 1) which turns on the drum for exactly 90 sec after the starting switch (A) is depressed. The stopping of the tapper gives auditory warning of the completion of the contraction. The spring loaded override switch (S_1, S_2), when depressed, allows a short length of baseline to be recorded before addition of the next dose without actuating the timing device.

A large number of substances including choline, potassium, and inorganic phosphate, besides giving a response themselves in sufficiently high concentrations, potentiate the action of ACh; this effect is additional to that of anti-ChE agents since it is seen in preparations already fully sensitized to eserine or TEPP. Thus, for accurate assays it is essential to use the Feldberg procedure as outlined in the previous section. SHEPPARD, COHN and MATHIAS (1953) have advocated the use of ion exchange resins to remove choline and potassium. The potentiating effect of these substances has been used by GARDINER (personal communication) to obtain a further 5-fold increase in sensitivity over that of the normal eserinized preparation. A predetermined amount of choline chloride in potassium phosphate buffer (4 mM in 0.04 M buffer, pH 7.4), equivalent to about 80% of a threshold dose, is added to each sample assayed. DAVIS (1950) and MORLEY and SCHACHTER (1961) have used acetone as a sensitizing agent.

The author has found recti from *Rana pipiens*, *R. clamatans*, and small *R. catesbiana*, all North American species, to be as sensitive as those of the common European species, *R. temporaria*; according to GOFFART (1939), *R. esculenta*, especially winter or spring females, gives more sensitive preparations. No attempt is made to separate the muscle from the rest of the abdominal wall. One rectus only is used per bath; the other may be stored in Ringer solution at 4° for use next day. Muscles which have been used all day can also be stored overnight at 4°, but their sensitivity soon declines when used the following day.

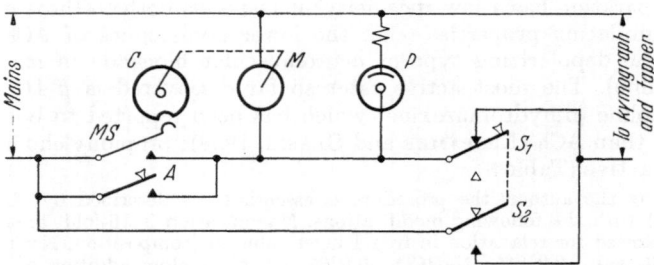

Fig. 1. Timer for kymograph. A is a spring-loaded, normally open, starting switch. When this is momentarily depressed, current from the mains starts the synchronous clock motor M which drives the cam C at $^1/_2$ rev./min. This closes the microswitch MS and supplies the kymograph and tapper with current until one revolution has been completed (90 sec). $S_1 S_2$ is a spring-loaded over-ride switch. It consists of two switches, one S_1, normally closed, the other, S_2, normally open. When depressed, S_2 closes to supply the kymograph while S_1 isolates M. A pilot light P is placed in parallel with M

Specific inhibitors. The action of ACh on the frog rectus is antagonized by neuromuscular blocking agents of the *d*-tubocurarine type. Depolarizing blocking agents (e.g. succinylcholine, BRITTAIN, CHESHER, COLLIER and GRIMSHAW 1959, senecioylcholine, WHITTAKER, unpublished observations), like ACh, give a contracture but also show the phenomenon, particularly in high doses, of self-inhibition or tachyphylaxis, i.e., the response to a dose declines as the dose is repeated. The response of the preparation to ACh may also be reduced. This effect may be connected with the finding of THESLEFF (1955) that the depolarizing type of blockade tends to become non-depolarising (competitive, curare-like) in the course of time.

Atropine antagonizes the action of acetylcholine on the frog rectus but only in much higher concentrations than on the guinea pig ileum, and reversibly.

A modification of the method using a superfusion technique has been described by AHMED and TAYLOR (1957).

2. Guinea-pig ileum

The guinea-pig ileum is a robust and sensitive preparation, but is not much used for assaying ACh because it responds to so many different substances, some of them likely constituents of tissue extracts. These include histamine, 5-hydroxytryptamine and substance P. However, preliminary precipitation as the reineckate in the presence of choline (BENTLEY and SHAW 1952, APRISON and NATHAN 1957) overcomes some of these difficulties.

Table 4. *Sites of action of drugs causing contraction of the guinea pig ileum*

Site of action[1]	Stimulation by	Inhibition by			
		Atropine	Hexa-methonium	GABA, morphine	Antihistamine
I	Acetylcholine	+	—	—	—
II	Butyrylcholine	+	+	—	—
III	Nicotine	+	+	+	—
IV	5-Hydroxytryptamine	—	—	+	—
V	Histamine	—	—	—	+
VI	Substance P	—	—	0	—

Symbols: +, inhibition; —, slight or no inhibition; 0, not tested; GABA, γ-aminobutyric acid.
    [1] See text.

The response of the preparation to different drugs has been analysed very fully by means of antagonists and a complex situation has been disclosed. At least six different sites of action must be postulated; these are listed in Table 4. Acetylcholine acts directly on the muscle (site I, Table 4); as is well known this effect resembles that of muscarine and is antagonized by atropine. Relatively few other esters are comparably active; acetyl-β-methylcholine (methacholine) and carbamylcholine (carbachol) are among these. The homologues of ACh (Table 3, col. 5) show a sharp decrease in activity with increasing chain length, and above propionylcholine their mode of action differs from that of ACh.

Above hexanoylcholine, spasmogenic activity disappears entirely and the esters show an atropine-like effect on the muscle (SCHNEIDER and TIMMS 1959). Unlike ACh and propionylcholine, the spasmogenic action of butyryl- and valerylcholine is antagonized by the ganglion blocking agent hexamethonium; maximum contractions may be impossible to evoke and the initial phase of contraction may be followed by a phase of rapidly fluctuating and gradually decreasing tone (SCHNEIDER and TIMMS 1959, WHITTAKER, unpublished observations). Nicotine shows somewhat similar effects. These are believed to indicate that the main site of action of these drugs is on ganglion cells rather than directly on the muscle. Nicotine contractions are, however, inhibited by morphine (KOSTERLITZ and ROBINSON 1958) and by γ-aminobutyric acid (HOBBIGER 1958), whereas butyrylcholine contractions are only partially inhibited (20 to 40%) even by high concentrations of these drugs (WHITTAKER, unpublished). This suggests that butyrylcholine and nicotine act mainly at different sites, the latter more centrally. These sites are denoted II and III in Table 4. 5-Hydroxytryptamine-induced contractions are also inhibited by morphine and γ-aminobutyric acid (GADDUM and PICARELLI 1957, KOSTERLITZ and ROBINSON 1958, HOBBIGER 1958), but since this drug is not blocked by hexamethonium and low concentrations of atropine, its site of action (IV in Table 4, equivalent to GADDUM and PICARELLI's M receptor) cannot be identical with that of nicotine. Both nicotine and 5-hydroxytryptamine are not completely antagonised by morphine and γ-aminobutyric acid; thus they probably act directly on the muscle also. The muscle sites at which 5-hydroxytryptamine acts are blocked by dibenzylamine (GADDUM and PICARELLI 1957) and have been referred to by these authors as D receptors; for simplicity, these have been omitted from Table 4.

The action of the acrylylcholines on the guinea pig ileum has recently been studied in some detail (WHITTAKER, unpublished). Senecioylcholine had a low potency and behaved like nicotine in all tests. Crotonylcholine was more active and resembled butyrylcholine; it was sensitive to hexamethonium but was even less affected by γ-aminobutyric acid or morphine than butyrylcholine. Acrylylcholine showed only partial inhibition by hexamethonium and by high concentrations of γ-aminobutyric acid; it thus probably has the direct site I (muscarinic) action of ACh together with some action on sites II and III. These varying patterns of behaviour of different choline esters should enable them to be characterized with some precision.

3. Cat blood pressure

This is a classical test object, sensitive, rapid, and suitable when large numbers of serial assays have to be made as, for example, in perfusion experiments. According to STRAUGHAN (1958), the rat makes an equally good preparation and requires smaller absolute doses. In the absence of atropine, ACh exerts its well known depressant effect by dilating the peripheral blood vessels; in its presence, the ganglion stimulating action is unmasked and a rise in blood pressure ensues. The homologues of ACh have mainly the ganglion stimulating action so that a pressor effect is seen even without atropine (Table 3).

4. Venus heart

This preparation is very sensitive and highly specific for ACh (WELSH and TAUB 1948), but responds, like others based on circulatory organs, to vaso-active substances other than choline esters; indeed, it has been used as much for the assay of 5-hydroxytryptamine as for ACh. Other molluscan hearts, e.g., those of *Mya arenaria* (HUGHES 1955, MEETER 1955), *Tapes turgida* (LADD and THORBURN 1955), and *Meretrix lusoria* (YOSHIHARA 1957) have also been proposed as test objects.

5. Leech dorsal muscle

This classical test object, superseded by other methods, shows signs of a revival. Its relaxation, the slowness of which has been its main disadvantage, may be greatly speeded by the use of morphine (MURNAGHAN 1958). Small strips of the muscle in a microbath have recently been used to provide a very sensitive assay method by SZERB (1961).

6. Other marine invertebrate preparations

The dorsal muscles of several holothurians are very sensitive to ACh, but that from *Stichopus regalis* has the advantages of stability and relative insensitivity to vasoactive amines (BACQ 1939). *Actinopyga agassiza* is another very sensitive species (FLOREY 1956). The specificity towards other choline esters of this preparation and the *Buccinum* radula muscle preparation described by FÄNGE (1958) has not been determined. The crayfish stretch receptor and sea urchin oesophagus preparations were introduced in connexion with work on the inhibitory substance, Factor I, from mammalian brain. McLENNAN (1959) has shown that γ-aminobutyrylcholine and a fraction (A) of crude Factor I preparations give similar responses in both these test systems. In the case of the stretch receptor, the response is a diminution in the electrical activity of the afferent (sensory) nerve induced by the application of a constant stretch to the end organ. In the sea urchin oesophagus preparation, the parameter measured is the reduction in the contraction of the smooth muscle of the organ in response to a fixed dose of ACh. This preparation is stated to be much more sensitive to γ-aminobutyrylcholine than the stretch receptor and unaffected by γ-aminobutyric acid and related compounds. It is not known what relation, if any, this inhibition of the response of the sea urchin oesophagus to ACh has to the inhibition by γ-aminobutyric acid of nicotine and 5-hydroxytryptamine induced contractions of mammalian smooth muscle, observed by HOBBIGER (1958).

B. Chemical and physical properties

I. General

Acetylcholine is present in such small quantities in the tissues and body fluids of the higher animals that chemical methods of identification and estimation are of strictly limited applicability. Its recognition as a transmitter would probably have taken much longer than it did if the synthetic compound had not already been known as a powerful parasympathomimetic drug. Nevertheless, the classical methods of organic chemistry, supplemented by the newer techniques of spectroscopy and chromatographic separation, remain the final basis for the identification of naturally occurring choline esters, and these must ultimately be obtained in sufficient quantity for such methods to be applied. A brief review of the principal chemical and physical properties of choline esters is therefore appropriate.

II. Chemical properties
1. Of the ester link

Acetylcholine and the other compounds falling within the scope of this chapter are all carboxylic esters and share the general chemical and biochemical properties of this class of compounds. Thus they are readily hydrolysed to the free acid and choline, a process catalysed by hydrogen and hydroxyl ions and also, to varying degrees, by the particular group of esterases known as the ChE's. They also form hydroxamates in alkaline solution, a reaction which is the basis of a convenient method of estimation.

a) Spontaneous hydrolysis

The pH of maximum stability of choline esters lies between 3.8 and 4.5. Within this range they are quite stable and can, for instance, be heated for several hours or stored for months in aqueous solution without appreciable breakdown. Stock solutions are conveniently made up in 0.1 M aqueous NaH_2PO_4 (pH 4.35). Since bound ACh is rapidly liberated below pH 4.5, heating tissue suspensions at these pH's is a convenient method of releasing bound ACh for assay (WHITTAKER 1959c). Outside this range, choline esters are unstable and are, for example, completely hydrolysed in a few minutes at 100° and pH 10, a fact which is made use of in FELDBERG's proce-

Table 5. *Rates of hydrolysis of some choline esters*
Entries for purely synthetic esters are in *italics*.

Choline ester	Rate of hydrolysis (as percentage of ACh rate) by	
	AChE	BuChE
Propionyl.	60 *a* (1)	150 *g* (1)
Butyryl	2 *a* (1)	225 *g* (1)
Palmityl.	0 *bcd* (2)	0 *f* (2)
Acrylyl.	1 *b* (3)	72 *f* (3)
Crotonyl	*1 b* (4)	*16 f* (4)
2-n-Pentenoyl . . .	*1 b* (4)	*12 f* (4)
Senecioyl.	0 *be* (4)	2 *f* (4)
Urocanyl.	0 *a* (5) *b* (6, 7)	6 *f* (5*) 8 *f* (6*) 7 *f* (7) 0 *h* (7)
Imidazolylpropionyl	*0 a* (5) *b* (6)	*100 f* (5) *200 f* (6*)
γ-Aminobutyryl. .	0 *b* (8)	10 *f* (8*)

* Calculated from results of author.

Sources of acetyl (AChE) and butyro- (BuChE) cholinesterases: '*a* human', '*b* bovine erythrocytes', '*c* pigeon', '*d* rat brain', '*e* Torpedo electric organ', '*f* human', '*g* horse', '*h* dog plasma'.

References: (1) WHITTAKER (1951a) and earlier references there cited; (2) BERRY and WHITTAKER (1959); (3) WHITTAKER, unpublished; (4) HOLMSTEDT and WHITTAKER (1958); (5) FOLDES, ERDÖS, BAART and SHANOR (1957); (6) GRELIS and TABACHNICK (1957); (7) KEYL and WHITTAKER (1958); (8) HOLMSTEDT and SJÖQVIST (1960).

dure for detecting interfering substances in pharmacological assays (see section A II, p. 10). TAMMELIN (1958) has summarized what is known of the kinetics, rate constants and pH-dependence of hydrolysis.

In addition to hydrolytic decomposition, urocanylcholine may undergo a variety of other chemical transformations on storage. These have been partly elucidated by PASINI and CODA (1957a, b).

b) Hydrolysis by cholinesterases

The rates of hydrolysis by ChE's of naturally occurring choline esters, established or putative, is given in Table 5. In general, they are consistent with what was previously known about the specificity of the ChE's (WHITTAKER 1951a). The low rate of hydrolysis of the β-substituted acrylylcholines, senecioyl- and urocanylcholine, with their relatively bulky acyl groups, is noteworthy, as is that of γ-aminobutyrylcholine with its potentially positively charged acyl group. The low rate of hydrolysis of the β-unsaturated esters relative to that of their saturated counterparts may be due to the greater molecular rigidity of the former. Palmitylcholine is also, as expected, hydrolysed at a negligible rate by both types of ChE. However, this ester is hydrolysed by an eserine-insensitive esterase, distinct from other ChE's, which is present in many tissues (BERRY and WHITTAKER 1959).

GOLDSCHMIDT and BURKERT (1955) used rates of hydrolysis by ChE as a means of characterizing ACh. The author has attempted to use similar enzyme methods for characterizing propionylcholine from ox spleen and hydroxytryptamine in brain, but has found them unreliable. It should be realised that at the concentrations of active substances likely to be present in tissue extracts, enzyme reactions are first order and therefore their rates are sensitive to small changes in both enzyme and substrate concentration.

c) Hydroxamate formation

Hydroxamate formation proceeds in alkaline solution according to the equation:

$$RCO_2CH_2CH_2\overset{+}{N}Me_3 + H_2NOH \rightarrow RCONHOH + HOCH_2CH_2\overset{+}{N}Me_3$$

Hydroxamates form complexes with ferric ion in acid solution with the structure II, which absorb in the range 500 to 520 mμ (FEIGL, ANGER and FREHDEN 1934, FEIGL 1947). This is the basis of a quantitative procedure which is useful for estimating choline esters in the 1 to 5 mM concentration range (HESTRIN 1949). The method is non-specific in that many other substances including non-choline esters, lactones, and thioesters give the same reaction. If used to follow choline ester synthesis by choline acetylase in the presence of cysteine, it may give spurious results due to the formation of the thioester, N,S-diacetylcysteine (BERRY and WHITTAKER 1959).

While the ferric hydroxamates of uni-functional carboxylic acids have almost identical absorption maxima and extinction coefficients, the presence of an α,β-double bond, as in acrylyl derivatives, causes a shift in the absorption maximum to lower wavelengths and a rise in the extinction coefficient (KEYL et al. 1957). The hydroxamates of long chain fatty acids are insoluble in water, and to estimate choline esters of such acids the procedure of LIPMANN and TUTTLE (1950) may be used (BERRY and WHITTAKER 1959). γ-Aminobutyrylcholine gives a very feeble hydroxamate reaction under the conditions used by HESTRIN (KEWITZ, personal communication); according to RAACKE (1958), amino acid hydroxamates are unstable at alkaline pH's and the reaction of their esters with hydroxylamine is often not complete; moreover, their ferric hydroxamates vary greatly in their molar extinction coefficients.

2. Of the acid moiety

Choline esters possess, except for the modifications imposed by the choline ester group, all the chemical properties of their parent acids, and apart from effects attributable to variations in the associated anion, any differences between them must obviously be referred to differences in their acid moiety. The identification of the free acid after hydrolysis is thus an essential step in the identification of an unknown choline ester. This may be rendered difficult if the free acid is unstable, as are acrylic and senecioic acids, under conditions which give complete hydrolysis (KEYL et al. 1957, WHITTAKER 1959a). Obviously no general rules can be given for the identification of the parent acids of choline esters, especially since those already found in nature vary so widely in their chemical constitution, but it may be mentioned that gas chromatography has proved an extremely useful method (KEYL et al. 1957, WHITTAKER 1957, 1959a).

3. Of the choline moiety

The presence of the choline moiety confers upon choline esters the properties of an organic base of a strength comparable to that of potassium hydroxide. They thus exist as positively charged cations in association with a negatively charged anion, even in the solid state. Since the ester link is highly labile at alkaline pH's, the hydroxides are virtually non-existent; indeed the greater rate of hydrolysis of choline esters compared to non-ionic esters under these conditions is probably due to the higher affinity of the hydroxyl ion for the positively charged ester.

a) Soluble salts

Choline esters are normally prepared as their halide salts which with few exceptions (e.g., sinapine iodide; SPÄTH 1920) are readily soluble in water. The chlorides are usually very hygroscopic, the bromides less so and the iodides hardly at all.

The perchlorates are less soluble in water than the halides and can be precipitated from strong aqueous solutions of the latter by the simple expedient of adding an excess of 60% (w/v) aqueous perchloric acid (BELL and CARR 1947). They are readily recrystallized as needles from ethanol in which they have a steep solubility curve. Since in addition to being readily prepared and purified they are non-hygroscopic and more stable than the iodides, they are the ideal salts for reference preparations.

The p-toluene sulphonates are also non-hygroscopic and crystallize in beautiful plates. The acid tartrate of ACh is non-hygroscopic and much more soluble in ethanol than the choline salt, a useful point of distinction (EWINS 1914).

b) Insoluble salts

Of importance in the isolation of ACh and related esters from biological material and in their subsequent characterization are the insoluble salts which they form with the reineckate, picrate, picrolonate, styphnate, flavianate, phosphotungstate, tetraphenylboride, mercurichloride, aurichloride, and platinichloride ions. Of these, the reineckates, picrates, and tetraphenylborides have most commonly been used to effect an initial precipitation of the esters (along with other tissue bases), the auri- and platinichlorides for final characterization. Some physical properties are summarized in Table 6.

Ammonium reineckate was first introduced as an ACh precipitant by KAPFHAMMER and BISCHOFF (1930); it has been extensively used by the author and co-workers in the isolation of propionylcholine (BANISTER et al. 1951, 1953)

Chemical properties

Base	Iodide	Perchlorate	Platinichloride	Aurichloride
Choline	readily forms periodides, (a) $+ I_5$, (a) $+ I_8$	(b) m.p. 273° s. aq. 3.4[15]	(c) o. from 50% aq.-et., r. from aq., d. 234 to 235° s. aq. 17[21]	(d) n. from hot et., o. from aq.-et. m.p. 243 to 244° s. aq. 1.33[21]
Acetylcholine	—	(b) n. from et., m.p. 116 to 117° s. aq., ac., hot et. (3)	(c) n. from 50% aq.-et., d. 242 to 244°; also readily forms choline double salt, (c) $+ (C_5H_{14}ON)_2PtCl_6$ o. from aq., m.p. 260 to 261° (4)	(d) p. or n. m.p. 166 to 168° (1)
Propionylcholine	(a) m.p. 130 to 132° (5)	—	(c) n. from aq., m.p. 244° d. (4)	(d) n., m.p. 131 to 133° (4)
Butyrylcholine	(a) m.p. 93 to 94° (5)	—	(c) n. from aq., m.p. 244° d. (4)	(d) t., m.p. 93 to 94°
Palmitylcholine	(a) m.p. 160 to 161° (5)	—	(c) n., m.p. 218°	(d) t., m.p. 110°
Acrylylcholine (6)	(a) m.p. 136°	—	—	—
Senecioylcholine	(a) m.p. 160° (7)	—	—	(d) from aq., m.p. 97° (7)
Sinapine (9)	(a) $+ 3 H_2O$, m.p. 185 to 186° sp. s. aq.	—	—	—
Urocanylcholine	—	—	—	—

Abbreviations.

Formulae: M, base; (a) MI, (b) $MClO_4$, (c) M_2PtCl_6, (d) $MAuCl_4$, (e) $M[(SCN)_4Cr(NH_3)_2]$, (f) $MC_6H_2O(NO_2)_3$, (g) $MC_{10}H_7O_5N_4$, (h) $MC_{10}H_5O_8N_2S$, (i) $MN[C_6H_2(NO_2)_3]_2$, (j) $MB(C_6H_5)_4$, (k) $MH(C_6H_2O_7N_3)_2$, (l) $M\{N[C_6H_2(NO_2)_3]_2\}_2$.

Crystal structure: o., octahedra; r., rhombs; n., needles; t., tablets; p., prisms.

Solvents: aq., water; et., ethanol; ac., acetone.

Solubility: s., solubility, soluble; sp., sparingly; all solubilities expressed as concentration in % w/v saturated solution at temperature given as superfix.

Other: m.p., melting point; d., decomposes.

References. (1) ACKERMANN and MAUER (1943), (2) MARQUARDT and VOGG (1952c), (3) BELL and CARR (1947), (4) DUDLEY (1931), (5) SCHNEIDER and TIMMS (1957), (6) ENANDER, unpublished, (7) WHITTAKER (1959b), (8) KEYL et al. (1957), (9) SPÄTH (1920), (10) ERSPAMER and BENATI (1953), (11) ACKERMANN and MENSSEN, personal communication.

and various snail esters (KEYL et al. 1957, WHITTAKER 1959a). BENTLEY and SHAW (1952) used precipitation with reineckate to separate ACh quantitatively from tissue extracts containing eserine, morphine, atropine, and other drugs as a preliminary to assay. The picrate, picrolonate, styphnate, and flavianate were used by ERSPAMER and DORDONI (1947) in the isolation of urocanylcholine. Sodium tetraphenylboride ("kalignost") was introduced as an ACh precipitant by MARQUARDT and VOGG (1952c); it has been used by FIEDLER, HILDEBRAND and NEU (1953) in the identification of ACh in *Crataegus* berries, by AUGUSTINSSON and GRAHN (1954) in their work on bee brain esters, and by KEWITZ (1959) in the isolation of γ-aminobutyrylcholine from pig brain. The use of dipicrylamine has been advocated by ACKERMANN and MAUER (1943) and HARRISON (1950).

soluble salts of naturally occurring choline esters
GUGGENHEIM (1951) unless otherwise stated.

Reineckate	Picrate	Picrolonate	Flavianate	Hexylate	Tetraphenyl boride	Styphnate
(e) t., s. aq. 0.02[18]	(f) m.p. 240° fairly s. aq., et.	(g) + H_2O, m.p. 158°, d. 241 to 245° s. aq., et.	(h) p., m.p. 162°	(i) n., d. 232 to 233° (1)	(j) m.p. 219 to 221° (2)	—
(e) r., m.p. 173° s. aq. 0.0183[21]	—	—	—	(i) t., m.p. 183° (1)	(j) m.p. 185 to 187° (2)	—
—	—	—	—	—	—	—
—	—	—	—	—	—	—
—	m.p. 101°	—	—	—	—	—
—	—	—	—	—	—	—
s. ac., sp. s. aq. (8)	—	—	—	(i) m.p. 111° (11)	—	—
—	—	—	—	—	—	—
amorphous m.p. 186 to 188° d. (10)	(k) t. or n., m.p. 221 to 222° (10)	t., m.p. 240 to 242° d. (10)	n., m.p. 320° d. (10)	(l) m.p. 101° (11)	—	m.p. 215 to 218° (10)

The mercuri-, auri-, and platinichlorides of choline esters are readily prepared by the addition of $HgCl_2$, $AuCl_3$, or $PtCl_4$ to the ester chloride. They were used in the first identification of ACh as a natural product by EWINS (1914). The particularly low solubility of the choline-ACh diplatinichloride is noteworthy and was utilized by DUDLEY (1931) for separation purposes. Auri- and platinichlorides crystallize well from ethanol or water [ACKERMANN (personal communication) found that decomposition of aurichlorides in the latter solvent may be prevented by the addition of HCl]; they are readily analysed by combustion to the free metal, and the anion does not interfere with infra-red determinations (see Section II. 1, p. 21); it is thus a pity that the expense of the reagents limits their use in the initial separation of choline esters from biological material.

Anions containing aromatic nitro-groups, heavy metals, or other reactive groups must be replaced before testing esters pharmacologically. The reineckate ion may be removed as the silver salt (KAPFHAMMER and BISCHOFF 1930), tetraphenylboride as the mercuric salt (MARQUARDT and VOGG 1952c), and picrate as the 4-octoxyphenyl-guanidine (PASINI and VERCELLONE 1954, 1955a) or 2, 4-diguanidinophenyl lauryl ether (PASINI et al. 1953). A more general and much more convenient method is the use of a strongly basic ion exchange resin such as De-Acidite FF (Permutit Co., Ltd., London) introduced by WHITTAKER and co-workers (KEYL et al. 1957, WHITTAKER 1958). The base salt (picrate, aurichloride, reineckate) is dissolved in a suitable solvent and passed through a small column of the resin in the chloride form. The anion is adsorbed as a coloured ring at the top of the column. The base is washed through with more solvent in close to

100% yield as the chloride; its emergence can be checked by suitable pharmacological, chemical, or spectroscopic procedures. Reineckates sometimes come to exchange equilibrium slowly in non-aqueous solvents; if so, pretreatment of the solution by stirring it with resin in a beaker may be an advantage.

4. Chemical estimation of acetylcholine

Several chemical methods have been described for ACh and related substances. As applied to biological extracts they are of limited value on account of their low sensitivity and specificity, and the relatively complicated procedures necessary to eliminate interfering substances. The ferric hydroxamate method has already been mentioned; it has been applied to brain tissue by STONE (1955b) and to bee-head extracts by AUGUSTINSSON and GRAHN (1954). In STONE's procedure, ACh is first precipitated by the addition of choline and phosphotungstic acid at pH 2.13 to 2.3; the method is stated to give results in fair agreement with bioassay. MARQUARDT and VOGG (1952c) and AUGUSTINSSON and GRAHN (1954) have applied the ferric hydroxamate reaction directly to the ester tetraphenylboride.

Other methods depend on the formation of coloured salts with complex ions such as enneaiodide, reineckate, hexylate or bromophenol blue. SHAW (1938) described a complex procedure making use of the differential solubilities of the phosphotungstates, reineckates and enneaiodides to remove choline and other interfering substances before estimating ACh as the enneaiodide. ACKERMANN and MAUER (1943) advocated the use of dipicrylamine. MITCHELL and CLARK (1952) made use of the solubility of the bromophenol blue complex of quaternary ammonium compounds in ethylene dichloride.

As applied to ACh in nervous tissue, 0.5 ml of the extract, deproteinized by the addition of an equal volume of 6% HPO_3, is shaken with 0.3 g K_2HPO_4, 0.3 g Na_2HPO_4, 0.5 ml freshly prepared 0.08% bromophenol blue in aqueous 30% K_2HPO_4 and 10 ml 4% *iso*amyl alcohol in ethylene dichloride for 10 min, the organic phase separated and the extinction read at 600 mμ against suitable standards. The limit of sensitivity is given as 1 μg/ml but no details of recoveries or specificity are given.

5. Methods of synthesis

As with other naturally occurring compounds, the identification of a choline ester ultimately involves its comparison with an authentic specimen obtained by chemical synthesis. The main methods of preparing choline esters are summarized in the following four reaction sequences:

$$RCOCl + HOCH_2CH_2\overset{+}{N}Me_3Cl^- \rightarrow RCO_2CH_2CH_2\overset{+}{N}Me_3Cl^- + HCl \tag{1}$$

$$RCO_2H + HOCH_2CH_2Br \rightarrow RCO_2CH_2CH_2Br \xrightarrow{NMe_3} RCO_2CH_2CH_2\overset{+}{N}Me_3Br^- \tag{2}$$

$$(RCO)_2O + HOCH_2CH_2NMe_2 \rightarrow RCO_2CH_2CH_2NMe_2 \xrightarrow{MeI} RCO_2CH_2CH_2\overset{+}{N}Me_3I^- \tag{3}$$

$$RCO_2Ag + BrCH_2CH_2\overset{+}{N}Me_3Br^- \rightarrow RCO_2CH_2CH_2\overset{+}{N}Me_3Br^- + AgBr. \tag{4}$$

Reaction 1 was the first method used for the synthesis of choline esters (BAEYER 1867, NOTHNAGEL 1894, HUNT and TAVEAU 1911). It goes smothly if R is aromatic in character (e.g., nicotinyl); the acid chloride and carefully dried choline chloride may be refluxed together under dry benzene or toluene for 12 to 15 hr (LÉVY and TCHOUBAR 1950; WHITTAKER, unpublished). The method is inferior to methods 2 and 3 when R is aliphatic.

The preparation of choline esters via the β-bromoethyl ester (reaction 2) was introduced by FOURNEAU and PAGE (1914) and is an excellent general method. The intermediate ester is often readily prepared by refluxing a mixture of the acid and β-bromoethanol in dry benzene in the presence of a suitable catalyst, using a water trapping device. It is then heated with anhydrous trimethylamine in dry benzene in a sealed tube; the choline ester crystallizes out as the reaction proceeds. A variant of this method was used by PASINI et al. (1953) to prepare urocanylcholine from the β-chloroethyl ester of α-chloro-β-imidazolylpropionic acid, itself readily prepared from histidine by diazotization; the formation of the choline ester was accompanied by the removal of HCl from the imidazole side chain, apparently by way of α-dimethylamino-β-imidazolylpropionylcholine chloride methochloride. A more general method of preparing β-substituted heterocyclic acrylic esters is via malonylmonocholine (PASINI and CODA 1957a).

In method 3, the choline ester is reached by way of the dimethylaminoethyl ester; this is also an excellent general method (KYI and WILSON in SCHNEIDER and TIMMS 1957) and avoids the use of anhydrous trimethylamine. The esterification of dimethylaminoethanol is usually best achieved by means of the acid anhydride (for review and references see TAM-MELIN 1958), but N-dimethylaminoethyl acrylate is obtained in better yield by transesterification between methyl acetate and dimethylaminoethanol (ENANDER, personal communication).

Method 4 was introduced by HORENSTEIN and PÄHLICKE (1938) and has been used *inter alia* for the preparation of γ-aminobutyrylcholine (KURIAKI *et al.* 1958, KEWITZ 1959).

III. Spectroscopic properties
1. Infra-red

Infra-red spectroscopy has been used in the identification of the following naturally occurring choline esters: ACh, as reineckate (MARQUARDT and VOGG 1952b) or tetraphenylboride (MARQUARDT and VOGG 1952c) in acetonitrile, and as perchlorate (WOOD 1954, CHEFURKA and SMALLMAN 1956); propionylcholine, as perchlorate (WOOD 1954, CHEFURKA and SMALLMAN 1956); urocanylcholine, as chloride hydrochloride (ERSPAMER and BENATI 1953); senecioylcholine, as aurichloride (WHITTAKER 1959b); γ-aminobutyrylcholine, as aurichloride (KEWITZ 1959). Probably the best way of examining choline esters isolated from biological material is as their aurichlorides using the potassium bromide window technique. The aurichlorides are readily prepared and crystallized in small amounts; they are non-hygroscopic and the anion is transparent to infra-red radiation in the relevant portion of the spectrum. The perchlorates and reineckates are less satisfactory; although non-hygroscopic, they show considerable absorption due to the anion. The use of a liquid cell is rendered difficult by the sparing solubility of choline esters in solvents which are transparent to infra-red radiation; however, acetonitrile has been used in spite of its strong C≡N absorption (MARQUARDT and VOGG 1952b). Normally, several milligrams of ester are required for spectroscopy but the use of a reflecting microscope attachment permits microgram quantities to be identified (WOOD 1954).

The infra-red spectra of choline and those carboxylic esters of choline of known or suspected natural occurrence are shown in Fig. 2 which includes unpublished work. The spectrum of choline (Fig. 2 A) shows a strong absorption maximum at 2.87 μ attributable to the stretching frequency of its free hydroxyl group; bands due to N-methyl and C—H deformations are in evidence between 6.75 and 7.2 μ, and are followed by others due to skeletal vibrations. On esterification, as in ACh (Fig. 2 B), the O—H band at 2.87 μ disappears, and C=O and C—O—C bands characteristic of the ester link make their appearance at 5.75 and 8.18 μ, respectively. At the same time, a band at 3.35 μ appears, which calls for some comment. It is a feature of all choline ester spectra so far examined including several not reproduced in Fig. 2; it is most likely due to C—H stretching frequencies of the acyl group superimposed on rather weak C—H absorptions of the choline moiety. X-ray crystallography of ACh bromide (SÖRUM 1959) has revealed the presence in the crystal lattice of a ring form of ACh (III), from which the existence of a strong hydrogen bond between a hydrogen atom of one of the N-methyl groups and the ester oxygen has been inferred. It is unlikely, however, that this bond is responsible for the band at 3.35 μ.

III

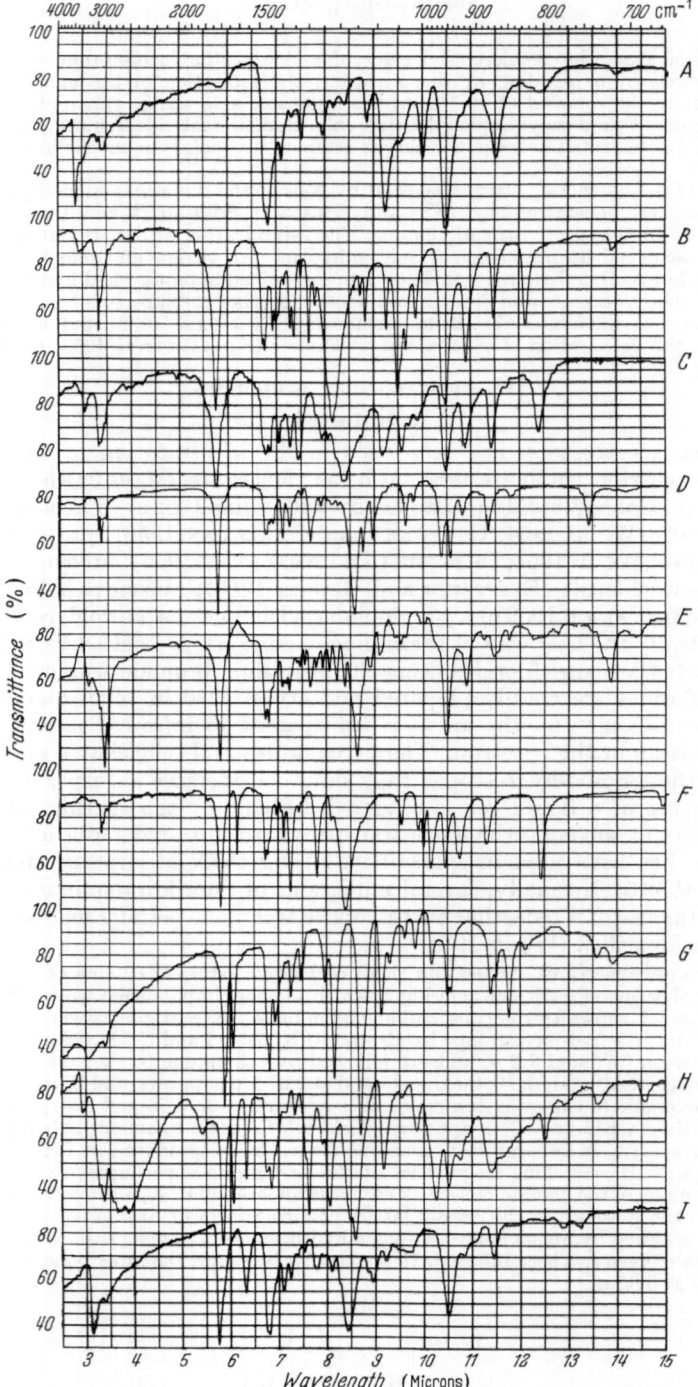

Fig. 2. Infra-red spectra of (*A*) choline aurichloride, (*B*) acetylcholine bromide, (*C*) propionylcholine iodide, (*D*) butyrylcholine iodide, (*E*) palmitylcholine bromide, (*F*) acrylylcholine bromide, (*G*) senecioylcholine auri-chloride, (*H*) urocanylcholine chloride hydrochloride, (*I*) γ-aminobutyrylcholine aurichloride. The spectra were recorded on a Perkin-Elmer Infracord using the potassium bromide window technique

The spectra of propionyl-, butyryl-, and palmitylcholine (Figs. 2 C, D, and E) resemble that of ACh except for the shifts and additional bands due to the longer carbon chains of the acid moieties. The bands at 13.45 μ (butyrylcholine) and 13.88 μ (palmitylcholine) are characteristic of compounds containing carbon chains of 4 or more atoms.

In acrylylcholine, (Fig. 2F) and its β-substituted derivatives, senecioylcholine (Fig. 2G) and urocanylcholine (Fig. 2H), a pair of bands attributable to a carbon-carbon double bond in conjugation with the ester carbonyl group is seen in the neighbourhood of 6 μ, in place of the single band at 5.75 to 5.8 μ in Figs. 2B to E. The spectrum of urocanylcholine (Fig. 2H) is complex and includes elements which can be referred to the imidazole ring.

The spectrum of γ-aminobutyrylcholine (Fig. 2I) resembles those of other saturated choline esters (cf. butyrylcholine, Fig. 2D) with the addition of a band attributable to the NH$_2$ group at 6.3 μ and the N—H bond at 3.15 μ.

2. Ultra-violet

In ACh and its simpler homologues, ultra-violet absorption occurs at wavelengths too short to be studied in the usual laboratory ultra-violet spectrophotometers. The conjugated C=C—C=O system of the snail esters gives rise to a band above 200 mμ which varies in intensity and position according to the β-substituent and the associated anion (WHITTAKER 1959b; Fig. 3 A—C). Urocanylcholine (Fig. 3 D, E) shows the characteristic absorption of the imidazole ring with a maximum at 275 mμ at pH 4.5, a shift of about 10 mμ to longer wavelengths as compared with urocanic acid (PASINI et al. 1953). Like other imidazoles, the absorption maximum is markedly dependent on pH, shifting from 285 to 295 mμ at pH 7.4 (Fig. 3 E). This has been explained, for urocanic acid, by MEHLER and TABOR (1953) in terms of the degree of protonation of the imidazole nitrogen. Care should be taken to minimize adsorption of esters on glassware which readily occurs with dilute solutions of unsaturated esters (Whittaker 1959b).

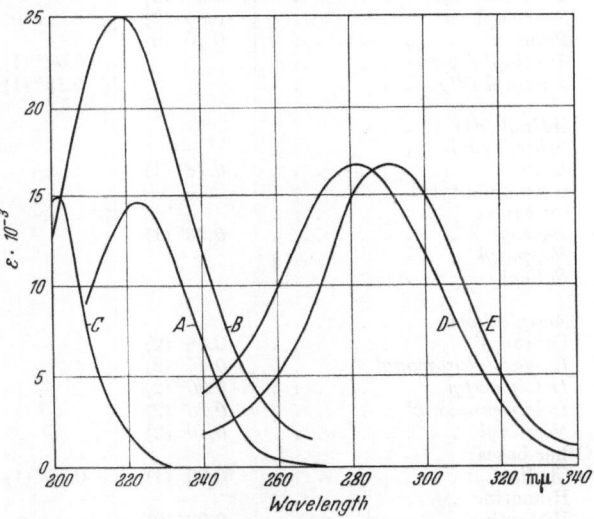

Fig. 3. Ultra-violet spectra of (A) senecioylcholine bromide ,(B) senecioylcholine aurichloride, (C) acrylylcholine bromide, (D) urocanylcholine chloride hydrochloride, pH 4.5, and (E) the same, pH 7.4

3. Nuclear magnetic resonance

There are no recorded instances of the use of this technique for identifying choline esters. It is, however, ideal for the purpose since it can be applied to aqueous solutions, requires only small quantities of materials, and gives readily interpretable spectra with aliphatic branched-chain molecules.

IV. Chromatographic properties

1. General

Chromatography in its various forms, and the allied techniques of paper and column electrophoresis, have been recognised for over a decade as an important

Table 7. R_F *values of some choline*

Entries for compounds not so far identified in nature are in *italics*. Values are for chlorides or

Substance	A	B	C	D
Choline esters[□]:				
Acetyl.	0.14 (1)	0.17 (1)	0.24 (1)	0.33 (1)
Acetyl-β-methyl	*0.19* (1)	*0.23* (1)	*0.35* (1)	*0.37* (1)
Propionyl	0.22 (1)	0.27 (1)	0.35 (1)	—
Butyryl	0.28 (1)	0.29 (1)	0.43 (1)	0.46 (1)
*Butyryl-β-methyl**	*0.49d* (1)	*0.59* (1)	*0.70* (1)	—
Valeryl	*0.31* (2)	*0.55* (1)	—	—
2-Methylbutyryl.	*0.36* (2)	—	—	—
iso*Valeryl*	*0.38* (2)	—	—	—
Hexanoyl	*0.36* (2)	—	—	—
Acrylyl	—	—	—	—
Crotonyl	*0.20* (2)	—	—	—
2-n-Pentenoyl.	*0.35* (2)	—	—	—
Senecioyl	*0.35* (2)	—	—	—
Palmityl	0.70 (5)	—	—	—
Succinyl (mono)	—	*0.04** (1)	—	*0.17** (1)
Succinyl (di).	—	*0.12** (1)	—	*0.30** (1)
Adipyl (di)	—	—	—	—
Sebacyl (di)	—	—	—	—
Lactyl	*0.18* (1)	—	—	—
γ-Aminobutyryl	—	—	—	—
Carbamyl	—	—	—	—
Benzoyl	*0.28* (1)	—	*0.43* (1)	*0.49* (1)
Hippuryl	—	—	—	—
Salicyl	—	—	—	—
Acetylsalicyl	—	—	—	—
Urocanyl[◊]	0.06 (2)	—	—	—
Imidazolylpropionyl	*0.15* (2)	—	—	—
Indolylacetyl	*0.20°* (2)	—	—	—
Indolylpropionyl	*0.26* (2)	—	—	—
Nicotinyl	*0.10* (2)	—	—	—
Other bases:				
Choline	0.09 (1)	0.13 (1)	0.24 (1)	0.25 (1)
Homarine	—	—	—	—
Histamine	0.03 (8)	—	—	—
Betaine	—	—	—	—

[□] For R_F values of thiocholine esters see HEILBRONN (1958). * Perchlorate. [△] Iodide. [○] Tailing. ( ) Double spotting. *d* Descending chromatography. [◊] For R_F values of urocanyl-choline derivatives see PASINI and CODA (1957 b) and PASINI and VERCELLONE (1955 b).

References: (1) WHITTAKER and WIJESUNDERA (1952a), (2) KEYL et al. (1957), (3) AUGUSTINSSON and GRAHN (1953), (4) MALYOTH and STEIN (1951), (5) BERRY and WHITTAKER (1959), (6) KEWITZ (1959), (7) AUGUSTINSSON (1955), (8) WHITTAKER, unpublished.

Papers used: (1) Whatman No. 4, (2, 4, 5, 8) Whatman No. 1, (3, 7) Munktell OB, Whatman No. 4, (6) Schleicher & Schüll, 2046 b washed in water.

Solvents: A, butanol saturated with water; B, butanol-propanol-water (4:2:1); C, propanol-water (9:1); D, propanol-benzyl alcohol-water (5:2:2); E, propanol-formic acid-water (8:1:1); F, propanol-0.1 N acetic acid (3:1); G, butanol-ethanol-acetic acid-water (8:2:1:3); H, butanol-acetic acid-water (78:5:17); I, butanol-propanol-ethanol-formic acid-water (6:2:1:1:2); J, ethyl acetate-pyridine-water (5:3:2); K, 20% KCl.

Other solvents: pyridine-, collidine-, lutidine-, phenol-, benzyl alcohol-, furfuryl alcohol- and dioxan-water mixtures all reported inferior to above (WHITTAKER and WIJESUNDERA, 1952a.)

esters and related substances
for chloride, hydrochlorides and for ascending chromatography unless otherwise stated.

E	F	G	H	I	J	K
0.46 (1)	0.65 (2)	0.46 (3)	—	—	0.36 (4)	—
0.56 (1)	—	*0.55* (3)	—	—	—	—
0.59 (1)	0.78 (2)	0.57 (3)	—	—	—	—
0.66 (1)	—	0.66 (3)	—	—	—	—
0.75 (1)	—	—	—	—	—	—
—	*0.78* (2)	*0.69* (2)	—	—	—	—
—	*0.80* (2)	*0.73* (2)	—	—	—	—
—	*0.82* (2)	*0.78* (2)	—	—	—	—
—	*0.79* (2)	*0.68* (2)	—	—	—	—
—	—	*0.78* (2)	—	—	—	—
—	*0.69* (2)	*0.50* (2)	—	—	—	—
—	*0.71* (2)	*0.71* (2)	—	—	—	—
—	*0.71* (2)	*0.70* (2)	—	—	—	—
0.62* (1)	—	—	—	—	—	—
0.30* (1)	—	*0.12△* (3)	—	—	—	—
—	—	*0.18△d* (3)	—	—	—	—
—	—	*0.22△d* (3)	—	—	—	—
—	—	*0.54△d* (3)	—	—	—	—
—	—	—	—	0.13 (6)	—	—
—	—	*0.30* (3)	—	—	*0.14* (4)	—
0.65 (1)	*0.71* (2)	*0.71* (2)	—	—	—	—
—	—	*0.50* (7)	—	—	—	—
—	—	*0.64* (3)	—	—	*0.97** (4)	—
					(0.69)* (4)	
—	—	*0.67* (3)	—	—	—	—
—	0.54 (2)	—	0.14 (2)	—	—	0.82 (2)
—	*0.29* (2)	*0.37* (2)	—	—	—	—
—	*0.73○* (2)	*0.63○* (2)	—	—	—	—
—	*0.73* (2)	*0.60* (2)	—	—	—	—
—	*0.58* (2)	*0.35* (2)	—	—	—	—
0.38 (1)	—	0.38 (3)	—	0.30 (6)	0.31 (4)	—
—	—	—	0.21 (2)	—	—	1.0 (2)
—	—	0.21 (3)	—	—	—	—
—	—	0.46 (3)	—	—	—	—

supplement to classical chemical methods for separating and identifying naturally occurring substances. They are particularly useful when these occur in relatively small amounts and as mixtures of closely related substances.

In view of its simplicity and popularity, it is not surprising that chromatography on paper was the first technique of this kind to be applied to the separation of choline esters. Although an R_F value for ACh was probably first recorded by BRANTE (1949), the technique was first applied to the separation of choline esters by WHITTAKER (1951 b) and WHITTAKER and WIJESUNDERA (1951, 1952 a). Publications by MALYOTH and STEIN (1951) and AUGUSTINSSON and GRAHN (1953) soon followed and the method was applied to the characterization of the products of enzyme reactions by WHITTAKER (1951 b), WHITTAKER and WIJESUNDERA (1952 b), LEWIS (1953), FRONTALI (1958), and BERRY and WHITTAKER (1959), and to biological extracts by BANISTER et al. (1951, 1953) and others, as listed in Table 1.

Paper chromatography has, however, serious limitations, especially when applied to the separation of trace components in the presence of a large

excess of interfering substances. For these reasons, GARDINER and WHIT-
TAKER (1954) turned to the use of ion-exchange resins and CHEFURKA and SMALL-
MAN (1956) and HENSCHLER (1956a) to paper electrophoresis. Many variants of
chromatography have never been applied to the separation of choline esters and
considerable improvements in technique may well be possible.

2. Paper chromatography

a) Choice of solvents

Table 7 shows the R_F values of ACh and related substances in a number of
different solvents. According to WHITTAKER and WIJESUNDERA (1952a), neutral
solvents containing a high proportion of the less water-soluble alcohols give the
best separations for the lower homologues of ACh. R_F values increase with molecular weight, with an increment of about 0.1 unit per C atom; isomers (e.g.,
propionylcholine, acetyl-β-methylcholine) have closely similar values. Solvents
containing a high proportion of water or water-miscible substances increase the
R_F values. Acidic solvents may give multiple spotting; this is related to the fact,
discussed below, that R_F values are influenced by the associated anion, and is
caused by partial replacement of this by the solvent anion. Alkaline and strongly
acid solvents cause hydrolysis of choline esters. The author has noted that prior
equilibration of papers with solvent vapour is not necessary for successful chromatography in Britain, but is essential in the warmer environmental temperature of
the Mid-Western United States.

b) Localization of esters on paper

Almost any of the chemical, physical, or pharmacological properties of choline
esters as outlined in previous sections can be utilized for localizing them on paper.
The main methods are listed in Table 8. The first group utilizes reagents which give
coloured products with choline and other organic bases. The iodine method is
particularly useful, as the colour fades rapidly, leaving the ester unaffected; other
methods can then be applied to the same strip. The mechanism is not understood
but may depend on differences in the water content of the paper brought about
by the presence or absence of organic material. The dipicrylamine method (0.2%
dipicrylamine in 50% aqueous acetone, applied as a spray) has also been widely
used, and gives stable spots with a few μg of ester.

Since choline esters rapidly diffuse in water, it is best to avoid aqueous reagents
as sprays or dips; colour reactions normally carried out in an aqueous medium
can usually be adapted to non-aqueous conditions. An example is the modification
of the ferric hydroxamate reaction described by WHITTAKER and WIJESUNDERA
(1952a).

In this, three stock solutions are used, A, 10% w/v hydroxylamine in 75% v/v ethanol,
B, 10% w/v ethanolic KOH, C, 2% w/v FeCl$_3$ in 0.66 N ethereal HCl. The paper is lightly
sprayed with an ethanolic alkaline hydroxylamine solution prepared by mixing equal parts
of A and B and filtering from precipitated KCl, dried, and then sprayed with C until the paper
is acid. Esters show up as purple spots on a yellow ground which are stable for many weeks.

In addition to the above general methods, particular esters may contain functional groups which can be detected in special ways. In the same category comes
the use of ultra-violet light. When inspected in ultra-violet light, esters which
absorb strongly in the ultra-violet show up as dark "quenching spots" against the
faintly fluorescent background of the paper.

Pharmacologically active esters of choline can be localized by the rather tedious
method of dividing the chromatogram up into a series of numbered areas, eluting
the ester from each one, and assaying the eluants. As even water-soluble sub-

Table 8. *Methods of localizing choline esters on paper*

Detection method	How applied	Appearance of spot	References
Colour reactions			
1. General reactions for organic bases			
Iodine	Vapour or spray	Dark brown on light brown background	BRANTE (1949); WHITTAKER and WIJESUNDERA (1952a)
Dipicrylamine	Spray	Dark yellow on light yellow background	MALYOTH and STEIN (1951)
Phosphomolybdic acid-SnCl$_2$	Spray, dip	Blue	WHITTAKER and WIJESUNDERA (1952a); CHEFURKA and SMALLMAN (1956)
Potassium bismuth iodide (Dragendorff's reagent)	Spray	Orange	BREGOFF et al. (1953); CHEFURKA and SMALLMAN (1956); FRONTALI (1958), KEWITZ (1959)
2. General reagent for ester link			
Hydroxylamine—FeCl$_3$	Spray	Purple on yellow	WHITTAKER and WIJESUNDERA (1952a)
3. Indicators	Spray	Indicator shows alkaline colour with basic, acid colour with acidic esters, e.g. succinylmonocholine	WHITTAKER and WIJESUNDERA (1952b); BERRY and WHITTAKER (1959)
4. Special reagents			
Pauly reagent (urocanylcholine)	Spray	Yellow	MICHAELSON (unpublished)
Ninhydrin (γ-aminobutyrylcholine)	Spray or dip	Blue	KEWITZ (1959)
U.V. quenching (acrylylcholines)	—	Dark on fluorescent background	KEYL et al. (1957)
Pharmacological assay			
Frog rectus	On extracts of successive areas	—	BANISTER et al. (1953)
Guinea pig ileum			WHITTAKER and WIJESUNDERA (1952a)

stances are often strongly adsorbed by paper, it is essential to make sure, by means of control experiments, that the extraction procedure adopted is quantitative. The author has not found dipping the paper sections directly in the organ bath satisfactory from this point of view (contrast AUGUSTINSSON and GRAHN 1954, AUGUSTINSSON et al. 1955; ALM and AUGUSTINSSON 1957, FRONTALI 1958).

c) Effect of associated anion on R_F value

As seen in Table 9, the associated anion has a considerable effect on the R_F value of choline esters. This means that great care must be taken,

Table 9. *Effect of associated anion on R_F values*

Anion	Choline	Acetylcholine	Propionylcholine	Butyrylcholine
SO$_4^=$	—	0.10	0.24	—
Cl$^-$	0.09	0.14	0.22	0.28
Br$^-$	0.12	0.16	—	—
I$^-$	0.18	—	0.43	0.45
ClO$_4^-$	0.21	0.30	0.42	0.39
p-CH$_3$C$_6$H$_4$SO$_3^-$	—	—	0.59	0.47

Results of HEILBRONN (1958), WHITTAKER and WIJESUNDERA (1952a) and WHITTAKER (unpublished). Ascending chromatography using butanol saturated with water.

before chromatographing biological extracts, to exclude all but one anion, otherwise multiple spotting may occur and spurious identifications be made. This is best done (BERRY and WHITTAKER 1959) by passing the extract through a strong basic resin in the chloride form (e.g., De-Acidite FF, The Permutit Co. Ltd. London, England, mesh $-16 + 50$), whereupon all other anions are replaced by chloride. The trichloracetate and reineckate ions are sometimes difficult to remove completely by other means and may give trouble. A similar situation is encountered with adrenaline and histamine (SHEPHERD and WEST 1952, WEST and RILEY 1954).

The KAPFHAMMER and BISCHOFF (1930) method of concentrating tissue bases from biological extracts by means of reineckate precipitation, followed by removal of reineckate with silver ions, does not eliminate zwitter-ions which may then form salts with ACh and other bases and cause double spotting. This effect was responsible for the false identification by BANISTER et al. (1953) and AUGUSTINSSON (1955) of a mixture of acetyl- and propionylcholine from ox spleen as a separate ester (WHITTAKER 1956, HENSCHLER 1957), and the unidentified active compounds in bee brain and *Myxine* heart described by AUGUSTINSSON and GRAHN (1954) and AUGUSTINSSON et al. (1955) may have a similar origin. Choline esters containing an ionizable group in the molecule in addition to the quaternary nitrogen of the choline moiety (e.g., urocanylcholine, succinylmonocholine) are liable to double spotting and tailing in some solvents due to the existence of more than one state of ionization of the molecule.

d) Limitations of paper chromatography

It will be realised from what has already been said that paper chromatography is not an ideal method of identifying choline esters in biological extracts. It is essential to effect a preliminary separation of the esters by reineckate precipitation or a similar method and rigorously to exclude all but one anion. Even then the presence of large amounts of somewhat hygroscopic impurities makes chromatography difficult; tailing, double spotting, and poorly localized horseshoe-shaped spots may occur. Chromatography on ion-exchange resins, described in the next section, avoids some of these difficulties.

3. Chromatography on weak acid ion exchange resins

a) Theory of ion exchange resins as applied to chromatography of organic cations

Since chromatography on ion exchange resins has been less used than paper chromatography for the separation and identification of pharmacologically active substances, a brief survey will be given of the theory involved, the terms used, and the advantages and disadvantages of the method.

A weak acid ion exchange resin such as Zeo-Carb 226 (The Permutit Co. Ltd., London, England), Amberlite IRC 50 or its fine grain modification, Amberlite XE-97 (Rohm & Haas Co., Philadelphia, Pa., U.S.A.) consists essentially of linear molecules of acrylic acid polymer held together in a three dimensional network by cross links derived from divinylbenzene, butadiene, or isoprene. The free carboxylic acid groups in the polymer (here represented as RCOOH) can be titrated with base to form salts. The cation M_1^+ of the salt form of the resin can be exchanged for another cation M_2^+ in solution according to the equation:

$$RCOO^- M_1^+ + M_2^+ \rightleftharpoons RCOO^- M_2^+ + M_1^+$$

The extent of this exchange will be determined by the relative affinities of the two ions and their relative concentrations in the non-resin phase. The affinity of a cation for the resin is determined by a number of factors including the following:

α) *Valency.* Multivalent cations (e.g., Ca^{++}, urocanylcholine) are more firmly bound than univalent cations (e.g., Na^+, ACh). Zwitterions (e.g., succinylmonocholine, aminoacids) have little or no affinity.

β) Permeability. Cations of large ionic radius may not penetrate the resin as readily as smaller ions. This is not an important factor in the low crosslinked resins normally used in biological work.

γ) Van der Waals and other intermolecular forces. An organic cation with a long aliphatic side chain, (e.g., butyrylcholine) may have a higher affinity than a lower molecular weight homologue (e.g., ACh).

δ) pH. A special situation arises with H^+ ion, due to its ability to combine with carboxylate groups to form undissociated carboxylic acid groups. This in effect confers upon it an extremely high affinity for the resin. As with any monomeric carboxylic acid, the proportion of carboxylic acid groups in ionized form, and therefore free to bind and exchange cations other than H^+, will depend on the pH. At low pH's (< 1) the resin will be almost entirely in the undissociated form and its capacity to exchange with most other ions will be negligible. At high pH's (> 10), the resin will be almost entirely in the ionized form and its capacity to exchange other cations will be maximal. Control of pH is thus of great importance in using weak acid exchange resins.

b) Some definitions

Normally the resin is used in column form and the exchange reaction may be displaced continuously to the right by elution with a solution containing the cation M_2^+. To separate two cations, M_1^+ and M_2^+, these are first adsorbed onto the resin by running them into the column, and are then exchanged for a third ion, M_3^+, by running a solution containing M_3^+ through the column. The cations with the lower affinity exchange more readily with M_3^+ and so will travel through the column more quickly. The ion M_3^+ may be the cation of a buffer with which the column has been equilibrated before use; the adsorption and elution of M_1^+ and M_2^+ take place at constant pH and ionic strength. This is known as *elution* chromatography and is the method of choice when M_1^+ and M_2^+ do not differ much in affinity (as with acetyl- and propionylcholine). If large differences in affinity exist, the ion with the lower affinity may be eluted at one concentration of M_3^+ and the other at a higher concentration. Under these circumstances M_3^+ is usually hydrogen ion; the cation of lower affinity is removed at one pH and the cation of higher affinity at a lower pH. This is termed *displacement* chromatography. Esters ionizing as uni- and bivalent cations, respectively, can be readily separated in this way (e.g., acetyl- and urocanylcholine).

It should be noted that the anions originally associated with M_1^+ and M_2^+ will have passed out of the column with the cations displaced from the column during the initial adsorption. The separated cations will emerge from the column with the anions of the eluting or displacing solution. The chromatographic behaviour of M_1^+ and M_2^+ is thus independent of their associated anions and also of any accompanying salts, unless present in such high concentrations as to overload the column. This is an important advantage over paper chromatography when dealing with biological extracts. On the other hand, the dilution of the product by relatively large amounts of the eluting or displacing solution is often a disadvantage; its separation from the latter may be difficult, and the sensitivity of the method correspondingly reduced.

The chromatographic behaviour of a substance on a column is defined by means of the *retention volume*. This is the volume of eluant required to attain a peak concentration of the substance being eluted. This quantity is dependent on the size of the column: accordingly its ratio to the volume of liquid held in the interstices of the resin (*free resin bed volume*), which is theoretically invariant with respect to column size, may be used instead; this is known as the *specific retention volume*. The reciprocal of the specific retention volume corresponds to the R_F value in paper chromatography, as may be seen in the following way.

Consider a column having a free resin bed column V. A substance having no affinity for the resin and travelling as a thin band would be eluted in a volume of eluant V. Its specific retention volume would therefore be unity, corresponding to an R_F of 1.0. A substance having some affinity for the resin would travel a fractional distance through the column, R. On elution with a second volume, V, it would travel a further distance, R, finally emerging after V/R volumes of eluant had passed through. Its specific retention volume would thus be $1/R$, the reciprocal of the quantity R corresponding to the R_F value.

c) Preparation of resin and columns

GARDINER and WHITTAKER (1954) give experimental details for preparing buffered Amberlite XE-97 for elution chromatography at pH 4.35. They found that cycling the resin through the hydrogen and sodium forms increased the sharpness of the separation but reduced the affinity of the esters for the resin, apparently by removing partially polymerized material.

As normally used, the resin ($-100 + 500$ mesh) is first freed from fines (i.e., particles less than about 200 mesh) by repeated suspension and sedimentation in water, transferred to columns, washed with N HCl until a flame-test on the effluent is negative, then with water to remove acid, and finally with 0.1 M NaH$_2$PO$_4$ until fully equilibrated (pH of influent and effluent identical). If large quantities of resin are being treated, 0.5 M NaH$_2$PO$_4$ may be used initially to speed up equilibration with buffer. For chromatography of esters, small columns 10 cm high and 0.6 cm in diameter, arranged as in Fig. 4, are convenient. Eluant is drawn in from the reservoir as the effluent leaves the column, thus maintaining the level of liquid on top of the column. In setting up the column, care must be taken to exclude air bubbles which cause "channelling" and poor separation; this is conveniently done by pipetting a slurry of resin and buffer into a column already partially filled with buffer. Time should be allowed for the resin to settle. The resin bed should never be allowed to run dry, but the surface of the liquid should be allowed to fall to the level of the top of the resin bed when running in esters or changing eluants, to avoid dilution effects.

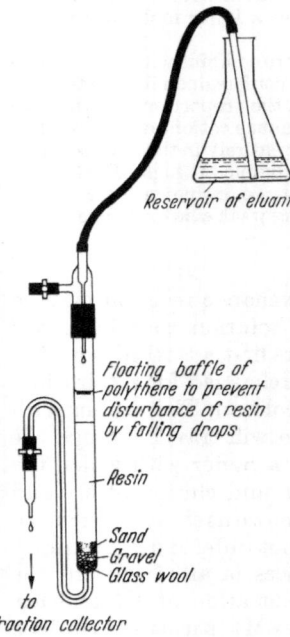

Reservoir of eluant

Floating baffle of polythene to prevent disturbance of resin by falling drops

Resin

Sand
Gravel
Glass wool

to fraction collector

Fig. 4. Arrangement for column chromatography of choline esters on carboxylic acid ion exchange resin

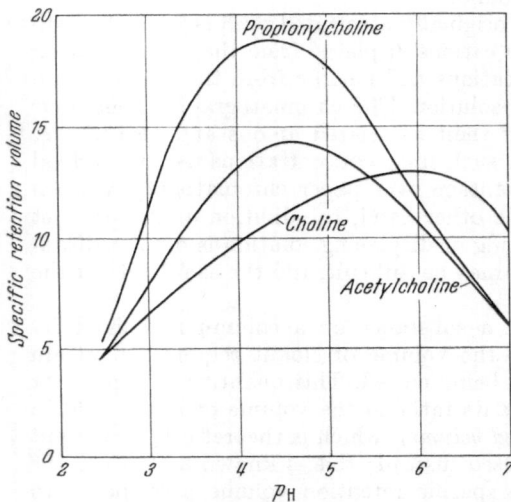

Fig. 5. Effect of pH on specific retention volumes of choline, acetylcholine, and propionylcholine on columns of buffered Amberlite XE-97 carboxylic acid ion-exchange resin. Eluants at pH 4.3 to 7.4, 0.1 M NaH$_2$PO$_4$—Na$_2$HPO$_4$ buffer; pH 2.5, 0.1 M glycine buffer. The resin was brought into equilibrium with the eluant before use

d) Effect of pH on retention volumes

Studies with columns buffered to different pH's showed (Fig. 5) that the best separation between ACh and its low homologues occurs at about pH 4.3 to 4.5, which is also close to the pH of optimum stability of the esters. At higher pH's, the retention volumes of the esters fall; at the same time the difference in retention volume becomes less. At lower pH's, the retention volumes of the esters fall as the exchange capacity of the resin decreases. Choline behaves similarly except that its retention volume-pH curve is shifted to the right, with the maximum falling at about pH 6.0; thus at pH 4.3, choline has little or no affinity for the resin and emerges ahead of its lower esters, whereas at pH 7.0 the order of elution is reversed.

e) Retention volumes of choline esters

Table 10 shows the specific retention volumes on columns of acid-washed XE-97, buffered to pH 4.35, of a number of choline esters and of a few other substances likely to be present in biological extracts. The table is divided into two sections, the left hand giving compounds which are more or less readily eluted at pH 4.35, the right, those which require displacement by 0.1 N HCl.

Table 10. *Specific retention volumes of choline esters and related compounds*
Entries for compounds not so far identified in nature are in *italics*.

Choline ester	Specific retention volume elution peak (0.1 M NaH$_2$PO$_4$)	Choline ester	Specific retention volume displacement peak (0.1 N HCl)	Other compounds	Specific retention volume elution peak(0.1 M NaH$_2$PO$_4$)
Succinyl (mono)	5	*Hexanoyl*	1	Homarine	5
Acetyl-β-methyl	15	*Succinyl (di)*	1	Choline	7
Acetyl	15	Urocanyl	1	5-Hydroxy-tryptamine	14
Propionyl	19	*Imidazolyl-propionyl*	1	Histamine	40
Butyryl	23	*Nicotinyl*	1	Senecioic acid	5
Valeryl	54	*Indolylacetyl*	4	Urocanic acid	11
iso *Valeryl*	48	*Indolylpropionyl*	12		
Hexanoyl	77				
Palmityl	77				
Acrylyl	17				
Crotonyl	34				
2-n-*Pentenoyl*	38				
Senecioyl	76				
Benzoyl	57				

Most values were determined on columns 12.0 cm high and 0.6 cm diameter having a free resin bed volume of 2.6 ml. The displacement peaks were measured from the point at which the effluent turned acid. Data calculated from KEYL et al. (1957), MICHAELSON (1955) and WHITTAKER (unpublished).

It will be seen that, in general, retention volumes increase with chain-length in both the saturated and αβ-unsaturated series; however, in the latter, the effect of chain branching is different and there is no predictable relationship between the retention volumes of a saturated ester and its αβ-unsaturated analogue. The higher saturated esters and the heterocyclic esters all have a high affinity for the resin, indolepropionylcholine having the highest. The former probably owe their high affinity to Van der Waals interactions between their paraffin side chains and the resin; the latter, to their ability to ionize as divalent cations, though exchange forces between the resin and the readily polarizable heterocyclic ring systems may be a contributory factor. The effect of a really long paraffin chain is seen in palmitylcholine, which cannot be removed from the resin even with 0.1 N HCl.

It will be noted that in contrast to the esters, which, with one exception, are all organic cations, anions and zwitterions (e.g., homarine, aminoacids) have a negligible affinity for the resin. Organic bases containing hydroxy groups (e.g., choline, 5-hydroxytryptamine) also have a low affinity, but that of bases such as histamine is fully comparable to those of the lower choline esters.

f) Effect of inorganic salts

MICHAELSON (1955) determined the effect of sodium chloride on the chromatographic behaviour of ACh. It will be seen, in Fig. 6, that sodium chloride in a 10-fold molecular excess has no effect on the ACh peak. A 100-fold excess slightly broadens the peak without altering the retention volume; not until there is a 500-fold excess is the running of the ester seriously interfered with. This relative freedom from the effects of a large excess of inorganic salts is in marked contrast to paper chromatography, and makes it possible to identify ACh directly in tissue extracts without preliminary reineckate precipitation (KEYL 1957).

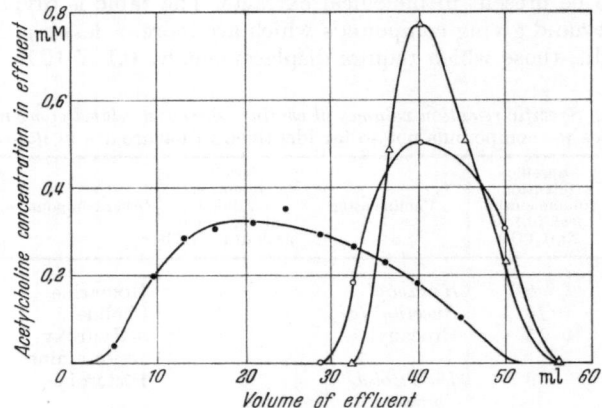

Fig. 6. Effect of sodium chloride on chromatography of acetylcholine on Amberlite XE-97 buffered to pH 4.3. Eluant, 0.1 M NaH₂PO₄; column size, 10 cm high, 0.8 cm diameter. Triangles, 10 μmole acetylcholine; open circles, the same with 1 m-mole sodium chloride; filled circles, the same with 10 m-mole sodium chloride

g) Application to biological extracts

Column chromatography was first applied to the identification of choline esters in biological extracts by GARDINER and WHITTAKER (1954). The identification of urocanylcholine and other acrylyl esters in marine gastropods (WHITTAKER and MICHAELSON 1954, KEYL et al. 1957, WHITTAKER 1957, 1959a) and that of ACh in mammalian tissues (KEYL 1957) and eggs of *Pieris brassica*, the cabbage white butterfly (DAVID 1959) are further examples of its use. It has also been used to characterize the products of enzymic synthesis by GARDINER and WHITTAKER (1954) and BERRY and WHITTAKER (1959).

4. Paper electrophoresis

CHEFURKA and SMALLMAN (1956) described the separation of ACh from choline on Whatman No. 3 MM paper soaked in lithium sulphate of ionic strength 0.1, using electrophoresis at potentials of 5 and 12.5 V/cm for 4 and 1 hr, respectively. The method was applied to the identification of ACh in fly head extracts. HENSCHLER (1956a) utilized Schleicher & Schüll 2043b paper, a triethylammonium acetic acid buffer of pH 4.6 and ionic strength 0.03, and a potential of 20 V/cm. This buffer has the advantage that it can be removed by volatilization in a vacuum. Choline, acetyl-, propionyl-, butyryl-, *iso*valeryl-, acetylthio-, benzoyl-, and carbamylcholine could all be separated from each other, but formylcholine ran with choline, and *iso*butyrylcholine with *n*-butyrylcholine. The method has been applied to the identification of choline esters in royal jelly and ox brain. FRONTALI (1958) used electrophoresis at 17 V/cm on Whatman No. 1 in 5% acetic acid for 30 min to identify acetyl- and propionylcholine in specificity studies on fly head choline acetylase.

Application to naturally occurring esters

The first step in the identification of naturally occurring choline esters, their extraction from tissues, may require some investigation before optimum conditions are found. Thus, although ACh chloride is extremely soluble in water, the ester in the form in which it is present in tissues is not readily extractable by water or neutral aqueous solutions. Estimates of the amount of ACh in tissues are subject to two kinds of error, (a) that resulting from incomplete extraction and (b) that resulting from post-mortem changes in ACh content due to the action of enzymes which catalyse its synthesis and breakdown. To extract ACh quantitatively from tissues it is therefore necessary to use extractants which will release ACh from its "bound" form and destroy enzymes which might otherwise alter its concentration. The usual methods involve the use of acid extractants and organic solvent, alone or in combination; they have been reviewed by MacIntosh and Perry (1950) and studied, *inter alia*, by Stone (1955a), Crossland (1951), and Fowler and Lewis (1958).

It would be out of place here to review the extensive literature on the subject of bound ACh and the various extraction procedures used by different authors. Hebb and Whittaker (1958) and Whittaker (1959c) have shown that bound ACh in brain is to be identified with that fraction of ACh which is sequestered in small particles. These particles have been isolated from homogenates of brain in isotonic sucrose; they are distinct from mitochondria and have been shown by Gray and Whittaker (1962) to consist of pinched-off nerve endings. Mildly disruptive procedures—freezing and thawing, hypotonic dilution, vigorous shaking, or treatment with cobra venom—release about 50% of the particulate ACh, which may represent a fraction in solution inside the particle. More drastic conditions, such as treatment with organic solvents or supersonic vibrations, keeping at 37° for 1 hr, or at 0° and pH 4.0 or less for a few minutes, release all the bound ACh, including a second more stable fraction which may be bound chemically to the matrix of the particle. While bound, ACh is not attacked even by high concentrations of purified ChE, and is not active pharmacologically. Little is known about the state of ACh and other esters in non-nervous tissues, but some form of binding is undoubtedly involved.

MacIntosh and Perry (1950) favour the use of cold 10% trichloroacetic acid as an extractant for whole tissue; this usually gives the highest value and may be regarded as the standard method; but extraction with dilute aqueous or ethanolic HCl gives similar results and is sometimes more convenient. For esters other than ACh, acetone (Erspamer and Benati 1953) and 2% perchloric acid (Kewitz 1959) have been used. Extracts made with organic solvents have the advantage that they contain less inorganic salts which may interfere with assays (e.g., K^+) and can be quickly concentrated by evaporation; on the other hand, they usually contain much lipid which may form troublesome emulsions and must be removed, e.g., by extraction into ether under acid conditions.

After extraction and removal or neutralization of substances (organic solvents, acids) which would interfere with biological assay, the active substance may be submitted to parallel assay, using the precautions already discussed in section A II (p. 10). If the results of parallel assays cannot be accounted for in terms of ACh, the most likely ester to be present, it will probably be necessary to have recourse to chromatographic and chemical methods of identification. Although the results of parallel assays can be expressed as simultaneous equations and solved for more than one component of a mixture (Banister et al. 1953), there are alway too many possible combinations of esters to permit of an identification solely by this means.

If the concentration of ester is high enough, identification may be made by chromatographing the unpurified extract directly on columns of ion-exchange resin; if low, or if paper chromatography is contemplated, it will be necessary to concentrate the ester along with other tissue bases by precipitation as the reineckate, tetraphenyl boride, or other complex salt as described in section B II 3b, pp. 17—19.

Further identification of the ester must be made by chemical means, and no general rules can be laid down. Much may be learnt from colour tests applied to chromatograms, and to the presence of absorption bands in the ultra-violet and infra-red characteristic of particular functional groups. The ultimate test of identity will come from a synthesis of the relevant ester and a demonstration that the properties of the synthetic and natural esters are identical.

Literature

ABDERHALDEN, E., H. PAFFRATH u. H. SICKEL: Beitrag zur Frage der Inkret-(Hormon-) Wirkung des Cholins auf die motorischen Funktionen des Verdauungskanales. II. Mitt. Pflügers Arch. ges. Physiol. 207, 241—253 (1925).

ACKERMANN, D., u. H. MAUER: Über einen empfindlichen Nachweis des Acetylcholins mit Hilfe von Dipikrylamin. Hoppe-Seylers Z. physiol. Chem. 279, 114—116 (1943).

AHMED, A., and N. R. W. TAYLOR: The assay of acetylcholine on the superfused frog rectus muscle. J. Pharm. (Lond.) 9, 536—540 (1957).

ALM, A., and K.-B. AUGUSTINSSON: The presence of acetylcholine in milk. Acta physiol. scand. 39, 203—208 (1957).

APRISON, M. H., and P. NATHAN: Determination of acetylcholine in small samples of fresh brain tissue. Arch. Biochem. Biophys. 66, 388—395 (1957).

AUGUSTINSSON, K.-B.: Hippurylcholine. Acta chem. scand. 9, 793—796 (1955).

—, R. FÄNGE, A. JOHNELS and E. ÖSTLUND: Histological, physiological and biochemical studies on the heart of two cyclostomes, hagfish (*Myxine*) and lamprey (*Lampetra*). J. Physiol. (Lond.) 131, 257—276 (1955).

—, and M. GRAHN: The separation of choline esters by paper chromatography. Acta chem. scand. 7, 906—912 (1953).

— — The occurrence of choline esters in the honey-bee. Acta physiol. scand. 32, 174—190 (1954).

BABO, L. VON, u. M. HIRSCHBRUNN: Über das Sinapin. Justus Liebigs Ann. Chem. 84, 10—32 (1852).

BACQ, Z. M.: L'acétylcholine et l'adrénaline chez les invertébrés. Biol. Rev. 22, 73—91 (1947).

— Un test marin pour l'acétylcholine. Arch. int. Physiol. 49, 20—24 (1939).

—, et F. P. MAZZA: Recherches sur la physiologie et la pharmacologie du système nerveux autonome. XVIII. Isolement de chloroaurate d'acétylcholine à partir d'un extrait de cellules nerveuses d'*Octopus vulgaris*. Arch. int. Physiol. 42, 43—46 (1935).

BAEYER, A.: Über das Neurin. Justus Liebigs Ann. Chem. 142, 322—326 (1867).

BANISTER, R. J., V. P. WHITTAKER and S. WIJESUNDERA: The chromatographic identification of propionylcholine in ox spleen. J. Physiol. (Lond.) 115, 55 P (1951).

— — — The occurrence of homologues of acetylcholine in ox spleen. J. Physiol. (Lond.) 121, 55—71 (1953).

BARLOW, R. B.: Introduction to Chemical Pharmacology. London: Methuen 1955.

BEILSTEIN, F. K.: Handbuch der Organischen Chemie. Berlin: Springer 1918—1957.

BELL, F. K., and J. C. CARR: The preparation and properties of the perchlorates of some choline esters. J. Amer. pharm. Ass. 36, 272—273 (1947).

BENTLEY, G. A., and F. H. SHAW: The separation and assay of acetylcholine in tissue extracts. J. Pharmacol. exp. Ther. 106, 193—199 (1952).

BERRY, J. F., and V. P. WHITTAKER: The acyl-group specificity of choline acetylase. Biochem. J. 73, 447—458 (1959).

BHOOLA, K. D., J. D. CALLE and M. SCHACHTER: The identification of acetylcholine, 5-hydroxytryptamine and other substances in hornet venom (*Vespa crabo*). J. Physiol. (Lond.) 151, 35—36 P (1960).

BISCHOFF, C., W. GRAB u. J. KAPFHAMMER: Acetylcholin im Warmblüter. 4. Mitteilung. Hoppe-Seylers Z. physiol. Chem. 207, 57—77 (1932).

BISSET, G. W., J. F. D. FRAZER, M. ROTSCHILD and M. SCHACHTER: A pharmacologically active choline ester and other substances in the Garden Tiger Moth, *Arctia caja* (L). Proc. roy. Soc. 152 B, 255—262 (1960).

BORUTTAU, H., u. H. CAPPENBERG: Beiträge zur Kenntnis der wirksamen Bestandteile des Hirtentäschelkrautes (Herba *Capsellae bursae pastoris*). Arch. Pharm. (Berl.) 259, 33—52 (1921).

BOVET, D., et F. BOVET-NITTI: Structure et Activité Pharmacodynamique des Médicaments du Système Nerveux Végétatif; Adrénaline, Acétylcholine, Histamine, et leurs Antagonistes. Bâle: Karger 1948.

BRANTE, G.: Iodine as a means of development in paper chromatography. Nature (Lond.) 163, 651—652 (1949).

BREGOFF, H. M., E. ROBERTS and C. C. DELWICHE: Paper chromatography of quaternary ammonium bases and related compounds. J. biol. Chem. 205, 565—574 (1953).

BRITTAIN, R. T., B. G. CHESHER, H. O. J. COLLIER and J. J. GRIMSHAW: Assay of suxamethonium and laudexium on the frog rectus abdominis. Brit. J. Pharmacol. 14, 158—163 (1959).

BÜLBRING, E., E. M. LOURIE and U. PARDOE: The presence of acetylcholine in Trypanosoma rhodesiense and its absence from Plasmodium gallinaceum. Brit. J. Pharmacol. 4, 290—294 (1949).

—, J. H. BURN and H. J. SHELLEY: Acetylcholine and ciliary movement in the gill plates of Mytilus edulis. Proc. roy. Soc. 141 B, 445—466 (1953).

BURN, H. J., D. J. FINNEY and L. G. GOODWIN: Biological Standardization. 2nd ed. London: Oxford University Press 1950.

CHANG, C. H., and J. H. GADDUM: Choline esters in tissue extracts. J. Physiol. (Lond.) 79, 255—285 (1933).

CHEFURKA, W., and B. N. SMALLMAN: The occurrence of acetylcholine in the housefly, Musca domestica L. Canad. J. Biochem. 34, 731—742 (1956).

CORSTEN, M.: Bestimmung kleinster Acetylcholinmengen am Lungenpräparat des Frosches. Pflügers Arch. ges. Physiol. 244, 281—291 (1940).

CROSSLAND, J.: The use of liquid air in the extraction of acetylcholine. J. Physiol. (Lond.) 142, 165—172 (1951).

CURTIS, D. R., J. W. PHILLIS and J. C. WATKINS: Cholinergic and non-cholinergic transmission in the mammalian spinal cord. J. Physiol. (Lond.) 158, 296—323 (1961).

DALE, H. H., and H. W. DUDLEY: The presence of histamine and acetylcholine in the spleen of the ox and the horse. J. Physiol. (Lond.) 68, 97—123 (1929).

—, and W. FELDBERG: The chemical transmitter of vagus effects to the stomach. J. Physiol. (Lond.) 81, 320—334 (1934).

DAVID, W. A. L.: The systemic insecticidal action of paraoxon on the eggs of Pieris brassicae (L). J. insect. Physiol. 3, 14—27 (1959).

DAVIS, J. E.: Acetylcholine estimation in body fluids by the acetone-sensitized frog rectus muscle test. Amer. J. Physiol. 162, 616—618 (1950).

DUBOIS, R.: Recherches sur la pourpre et sur quelques autres pigments animaux. Arch. Zool. exp. gén. (5) 2, 471—590 (1909).

DUDLEY, H. W.: Co-ordination compounds of the chloroplatinates of choline and its esters. J. chem. Soc. 763—769 (1931).

— The alleged occurrence of acetylcholine in ox blood. J. Physiol. (Lond.) 79, 249—254 (1933).

ELLIOTT, K. A. C., and E. FLOREY: Factor I — inhibitory factor from brain. J. Neurochem. 1, 181—191 (1956).

EMMELIN, N., and R. FÄNGE: Comparison between biological effects of neurine and a salivary gland extract of Neptunea antiqua. Acta zool. (Stockh.) 39, 47—52 (1958).

—, and W. FELDBERG: The mechanism of the sting of the common nettle (Urtica urens). J. Physiol. (Lond.) 106, 440—455 (1947).

ERSPAMER, V., u. O. BENATI: Isolierung des Murexins aus Hypobranchialdrusenextrakten von Murex trunculus und seine Identifizierung als β-[Imidazolyl-4(5)]-acryl-cholin. Biochem. Z. 324, 66—73 (1953).

—, e F. DORDONI: Chemical and pharmacological researches on extracts of the hypobranchial gland of Murex trunculus, M. brandaris and Tritonalia erinacea. III Presence in the extracts of a new derivative of choline or of a choline homologue: murexine (in Italian). Arch. int. Pharmacodyn. 74, 263—285 (1947).

—, and A. GLÄSSER: The pharmacological actions of murexine (urocanylcholine). Brit. J. Pharmacol. 12, 176—184 (1957).

— — The pharmacological actions of some murexine-like substances. Brit. J. Pharmacol. 13, 378—384 (1958).

EWINS, A. J.: Acetylcholine, a new active principle of ergot. Biochem. J. 8, 44—49 (1914).

FÄNGE, R.: Paper chromatography and biological effects of extracts of the salivary gland of Neptunea antiqua (Gastropoda). Acta zool. (Stockh.) 39, 39—46 (1958).

—, and A. MATISSON: Studies on the physiology of the radula-muscle of Buccinum undatum. Acta zool. (Stockh.) 39, 53—64 (1958).

FEIGL, F.: Qualitative Analysis by Spot Tests, Inorganic and Organic Applications. 3rd English ed. New York: Elsevier 1947.

—, V. ANGER u. O. FREHDEN: Über die Verwendung von Tüpfelreaktionen zum Nachweis von organischen Verbindungen (II). Mikrochemie 15, 12—24 (1934).

FELDBERG, W., and J. H. GADDUM: The chemical transmitter at synapses in a sympathetic ganglion. J. Physiol. (Lond.) 81, 305—319 (1934).

FELDBERG, W., and C. HEBB: The effect of magnesium ions and of creatine phosphate on the synthesis of acetylcholine. J. Physiol. (Lond.) 106, 8—17 (1947).

FIEDLER, U., G. HILDEBRAND u. R. NEU: Weitere Inhaltsstoffe des Weißdorns: der Nachweis von Cholin und Acetylcholin. Arzneimittel-Forsch. 3, 436—437 (1953).

FLEISHER, J. H., J. P. CORRIGAN and J. W. HOWARD: Reciprocal potentiating action of depolarizing drugs on the isolated frog rectus abdominis muscle. Brit. J. Pharmacol. 15, 23—28 (1960).

FLOREY, E.: An inhibitory and an excitatory factor of mammalian central nervous system, and their action on a single sensory neurone. Arch. int. Physiol. 62, 33—53 (1954).

— The action of Factor I on certain invertebrate organs. Canad. J. Biochem. Physiol. 34, 669—681 (1956).

—, and H. McLENNAN: The effects of Factor I and of gamma-aminobutyric acid on smooth muscle preparations. J. Physiol. (Lond.) 145, 66—76 (1959).

FOLDES, F. F., E. G. ERDÖS, N. BAART and S. P. SHANDOR: Interrelationship of murexine, dihydromurexine and human cholinesterases. Proc. Soc. exp. Biol. (N. Y.) 94, 500—503 (1957).

FOURNEAU, E., et H. J. PAGE: Sur les éthers de la choline. Bull. Soc. chim. Fr. (4) 15, 544—553 (1914).

FOWLER, K. S., and S. E. LEWIS: The extraction of acetylcholine from frozen insect tissue. J. Physiol. (Lond.) 142, 165—172 (1958).

FREUDENBERG, K., u. H. BILLER: Über Oxytocin. Naturwissenschaften 24, 523 (1936).

FRONTALI, N.: Acetylcholine synthesis in the housefly head. J. insect. Physiol. 1, 319—326 (1958).

GADAMER, I.: Über das Sinapin. Ber. dtsch. chem. Ges. 30, 2328—2330 (1897).

GADDUM, J. H., and Z. P. PICARELLI: Two kinds of tryptamine receptor. Brit. J. Pharmacol. 12, 323—328 (1957).

—, and R. P. STEPHENSON: A microbath. Brit. J. Parmacol. 13, 493—497 (1958).

GARDINER, J. E., and V. P. WHITTAKER: The identification of propionylcholine as a constituent of ox spleen. Biochem. J. 58, 24—29 (1954).

GOFFART, M.: Acétylcholine tissulaire du tube digestif chez le chien. Influence de l'énervation. Arch. int. Physiol. 49, 153—178 (1939).

GOLDSCHMIDT, S., u. H. BURKERT: Die Hydrolyse des cholinergischen Honigwirkstoffes und anderer Cholinester mittels Cholinesterasen und deren Hemmung im Honig. Hoppe-Seylers Z. physiol. Chem. 301, 78—89 (1955).

GRAY, E. G., and V. P. WHITTAKER: The isolation of nerve-endings from brain: an electron microscopic study of cell fragments derived by homogenization and centrifugation. J. Anat. (Lond.) 96, 79—88 (1962).

GRELIS, M. E., and I. A. A. TABACHNICK: The enzymatic hydrolysis of imidazoleacryloyl-choline (murexine) and imidazolepropionylcholine (dihydromurexine) by various cholin-esterases. Brit. J. Pharmacol. 12, 320—322 (1957).

GRUNER, G., u. H. KEWITZ: Das Vorkommen von Imidazyl-Essigsäure-Cholinester im Gehirn von Warmblütern. Naturwissenschaften 42, 628—629 (1955).

GUGGENHEIM, M.: Die biogenen Amine und ihre Bedeutung für die Physiologie und Pathologie des pflanzlichen und tierischen Stoffwechsels. 4te Aufl., Basel: Karger 1951.

HARRISON, K.: Isolation of acetylcholine from bacteria. Meth. med. Res. 3, 93—94 (1950).

HEBB, C. O., and V. P. WHITTAKER: Intracellular distributions of acetylcholine and choline acetylase. J. Physiol. (Lond.) 142, 187—196 (1958).

HEILBRONN, E.: Hydrolysis of carboxylic acid esters of thiocholine and its analogues. 1. Acid hydrolysis. Acta chem. scand. 12, 1481—1491 (1958).

HENSCHLER, D.: Zur Identifizierung von Cholinestern in biologischem Material, insbesondere von Acetylcholin in Bienenfuttersäften. Hoppe-Seylers Z. physiol. Chem. 305, 34—41 (1956a).

— Zur Frage des Vorkommens von Butyrylcholin im Rindergehirn. Hoppe-Seylers Z. physiol. Chem. 305, 97—104 (1956b).

— Die Cholinester der Rindermilz. Hoppe-Seylers Z. physiol. Chem. 309, 276—285 (1957).

HESTRIN, S.: The reaction of acetylcholine and other carboxylic acid derivatives with hy-droxylamine, and its analytical application. J. biol. Chem. 180, 249—261 (1949).

HOBBIGER, F.: Antagonism by γ-aminobutyric acid to the actions of 5-hydroxytryptamine and nicotine on isolated organs. J. Physiol. (Lond.) 144, 349—360 (1958).

HOLMSTEDT, B., L. LARSSON and A. SUNDWALL: Synthesis and pharmacology of nicotinyl-choline and three bisquaternary related derivatives. Biochem. Pharmacol. 3, 155—162 (1960).

—, and F. SJÖQVIST: Pharmalogical properties of γ-aminoburyrylcholine a supposed inhibitory neurotransmitter. Biochem. Pharmacol. 3, 297—304 (1960).

—, and V. P. WHITTAKER: Pharmacological properties of $\beta\beta$-dimethylacryloylcholine and some other β-substituted acryloylcholines. Brit. J. Pharmacol. 13, 308—314 (1958).

HOLTZ, P., u. H. J. SCHÜMANN: Butyrylcholin in Gehirnextrakten. Naturwissenschaften **41**, 306 (1954).

HONOR, A. J., and H. McLENNAN: The effects of γ-aminobutyric acid and other compounds on structures of the mammalian nervous system which are inhibited by factor I. J. Physiol. (Lond.) **150**, 306—318 (1960).

HORENSTEIN, H., u. H. PÄHLICKE: Über eine neue Umlagerungsreaktion und ihre Anwendung zur Darstellung von Estern der Aminoalkohole. Ber. dtsch. chem. Ges. **71**, 1644—1657 (1938).

HUGHES, B.: The isolated heart of *Mya arenaria* as a sensitive preparation for the assay of acetylcholine. Brit. J. Pharmacol. **10**, 36—38 (1955).

HUNT, R., and R. DE M. TAVEAU: The Effects of a Number of Derivatives of Choline and Analogous Compounds on the Blood Pressure. Bull. U.S. Publ. Hlth. Serv. (Hyg. Lab.), No. 73. Washington: Government Printing Office 1911.

KAHANE, E., et J. LÉVY: Biochimie de la Choline et de ses Dérivés. III. Colamine, Triméthyl-amine, Bétaïne, Carnitine, Muscarine, Bétaïnaldéhyde, Sinapine. Actualités scientifiques et industrielles, nr. 753. Paris: Hermann 1938.

KAPFHAMMER, J., u. C. BISCHOFF: Acetylcholin und Cholin aus tierischen Organen. I. Mitteilung. Darstellung aus Rinderblut. Hoppe-Seylers Z. physiol. Chem. **191**, 179—182 (1930).

KENNEDY, E. P.: The biological synthesis of phospholipids. Canad. J. Biochem. **34**, 334—347 (1956).

KEWITZ, H.: Nachweis von 4-Amino-n-butyrylcholin im Warmblütergehirn. Naunyn-Schmiede-berg's Arch. exp. Path. Pharmak. **237**, 308—318 (1959).

KEYL, M. J.: The distribution and some physiological properties of naturally occurring choline esters. Ph.D. Dissertation, University of Cincinnati, 1957.

—, I. A. MICHAELSON and V. P. WHITTAKER: Physiologically active choline esters in certain marine gastropods and other invertebrates. J. Physiol. (Lond.) **139**, 434—454 (1957).

—, and V. P. WHITTAKER: Some pharmacological properties of murexine (urocanoylcholine). Brit. J. Pharmacol. **13**, 103—106 (1958).

KOSTERLITZ, H. W., and J. A. ROBINSON: The inhibitory action of morphine on the contraction of the longitudinal muscle coat of the isolated guinea-pig ileum. Brit. J. Pharmacol. **13**, 296—303 (1958).

KUNG, H. P., and W.-Y. HUANG: Chemical investigation of *Draba nemorosa*, L. The isolation of sinapine iodide. J. Amer. chem. Soc. **71**, 1836—1837 (1949).

KURIAKI, K., T. YAKUSHIJI, T. NORO, T. SHIMIZU and SH. SAJI: Gamma-aminobutyryl-choline. Nature (Lond.) **181**, 1336—1337 (1958).

LADD, R. J., and G. D. THORBURN: New test animal for acetylcholine assay. Aust. J. exp. Biol. med. Sci. **33**, 207—213 (1955).

LÉVY, J., et B. TCHOUBAR: Relations entre la vitesse d'hydrolyse de divers esters de la choline par les cholinestérases et la constitution chimique des substrats. C.R. Acad. Sci. (Paris) **231**, 1262—1264 (1950).

LEWIS, S. E.: Acetylcholine in blowflies. Nature (Lond.) **172**, 1004—1005 (1953).

LIN, R. C. Y.: Presence of acetylcholine in the Malayan jack-fruit, *Artocarpus integra*. Brit. J. Pharmacol. **10**, 247—253 (1955).

LIPMANN, F., and L. C. TUTTLE: Lipase-catalysed condensation of fatty acids with hydroxyl-amine. Biochim. biophys. Acta **4**, 301—309 (1950).

MACINTOSH, F. C., and W. M. L. PERRY: Biological estimation of acetylcholine. Meth. med. Res. **3**, 78—92 (1950).

MALYOTH, G., u. H. W. STEIN: Beitrag zur Papierchromatographie der Cholinester und der Zucker. Biochem. Z. **322**, 165—167 (1951).

MARQUARDT, P., u. H. H. HIRSCH: Acetylcholin im Säugetierblut. Hoppe-Seylers Z. physiol. Chem. **289**, 131—153 (1952).

—, H. SCHUMACHER u. G. VOGG: Die chemische Konstitution des blutdrucksenkenden Faktors in der Kartoffel. Arzneimittel-Forsch. **2**, 301—304 (1952).

—, u. G. VOGG: Vorkommen, Eigenschaften und chemische Konstitution des cholinergischen Faktors im Honig, 1. Mitteilung. Arzneimittel-Forsch. **2**, 152—155 (1952a).

— — Vorkommen, Eigenschaften und chemische Konstitution des cholinergischen Faktors im Honig, 2. Mitteilung. Arzneimittel-Forsch. **2**, 205—211 (1952b).

— — Über einen empfindlichen Nachweis des Cholins und Acetylcholins mit Hilfe von Tetraphenyl-bor-natrium. Hoppe-Seylers Z. physiol. Chem. **291**, 143—147 (1952c).

McLENNAN, H.: The identification of one active component from brain extracts containing Factor I. J. Physiol. (Lond.) **146**, 358—368 (1959).

MEETER, E.: The heart of *Mya arenaria* as a test object for acetylcholine. Acta physiol. pharm. néerl. **4**, 233—242 (1955).

MEHLER, A. H., and H. TABOR: Deamination of histidine to form urocanic acid in liver. J. biol. Chem. **201**, 775—784 (1953).

MICHAELSON, I. A.: The chromatographic separation of choline esters with special reference to urocanylcholine, a constituent of certain marine invertebrates. M.S. Dissertation, University of Cincinnati, 1955.

MINZ, B.: Pharmakologische Untersuchungen am Blutegelpräparat, zugleich eine Methode zum biologischen Nachweis von Azetylcholin bei Anwesenheit anderer pharmakologisch wirksamer körpereigener Stoffe. Naunyn-Schmiedeberg's Arch. exp. Path. Pharmak. **168**, 292—304 (1932).

MITCHELL, R., and B. B. CLARK: Determination of quaternary ammonium compounds including acetylcholine, tetraethylammonium and hexamethonium. Proc. Soc. exp. Biol. (N. Y.) **81**, 105—109 (1952).

MORLEY, J., and M. SCHACHTER: Identification of acetylcholine in the silk gland of the caterpillar of *Arctia caja* (L.). J. Physiol. (Lond.) **151**, 1—2 P (1961).

MURNAGHAN, M. F.: The morphinized-eserinized leech muscle for the assay of acetylcholine. Nature (Lond.) **182**, 317 (1958).

NOTHNAGEL, G.: Über Cholin und verwandte Verbindungen, mit besonderer Berücksichtigung des Muscarins. Arch. Pharm. (Berl.) **232**, 261—306 (1894).

OURY, A., et Z. M. BACQ: Ester instable de la choline sans cholinestérase dans la pomme de terre et un champignon. Arch. int. Physiol. **47**, 92—101 (1938).

PASINI, C., e S. CODA: Murexine and related imidazole derivatives. Note I. On some routes of synthesis and on some properties of murexine. Isomurexine (in Italian). Gazz. chim. ital. **87**, 1440—1449 (1957a).

— — Murexine and related imidazole derivatives. Note II. Murexine and 4(5)-imidazolyl-carboxycholine:isomerization and demethylation (in Italian). Gazz. chim. ital. **87**, 1450 to 1463 (1957b).

—, u. A. VERCELLONE: Ein neues Reagens für die quantitative Bestimmung des Pikrat-Ions: das 4-Octoxy-phenyl-guanidiniumchlorid. Z. anal. Chem. **143**, 172—176 (1954).

— — Alkoxyphenylguanidinium salts. Their preparation and employment as precipitants of picric acid (in Italian). Farmaco **10**, 823—835 (1955a).

— — On the cis-trans isomerism of β-(4(5)-imidazole) acrylic acid (urocanic acid) and on murexine (in Italian). Gazz. chim. ital. **85**, 349—363 (1955b).

— — u. V. ERSPAMER: Synthese des Murexins (β-[Imidazolyl-4(5)]-acrylcholin. Justus Liebigs Ann. Chem. **578**, 6—10 (1953).

QUILLIAM, J. P.: The mechanism of action of murexine on neuromuscular transmission in the frog. Brit. J. Pharmacol. **12**, 388—392 (1957).

RAACKE, I. D.: On the reaction of hydroxylamine with esters of amino acids. Biochim. biophys. Acta **27**, 416 (1958).

ROTSCHUH, K. E.: Das herzmuskeleigene Acetylcholin. I. Mitteilung. Freisetzung und Bestimmungsmethodik. Pflügers Arch. ges. Physiol **258**, 406—414 (1954).

SCHNEIDER, R., and A. R. TIMMS: Some aspects of the pharmacology of an homologous series of choline esters of fatty acids. Brit. J. Pharmacol. **12**, 30—37 (1957).

SCHWARZE, P.: Über den Bitterstoff der Rapssamen. Naturwissenschaften **36**, 88—89 (1949).

SHAW, F. H.: The estimation of choline and acetylcholine. Biochem. J. **32**, 1002—1007 (1938).

SHEPHERD, D. M., and G. B. WEST: Effect of trichloracetic acid on adrenaline chromatograms. Nature (Lond.) **169**, 797 (1952).

SHEPPARD, C. W., W. E. COHN and P. J. MATHIAS: The estimation of choline esters by ion exchange. Arch. Biochem. Biophys. **47**, 475—477 (1953).

SIMONART, A.: On the action of certain derivatives of choline. J. Pharmacol. exp. Ther. **46**, 157—193 (1932).

SMITH, C. C., and L. LEVINE: The use of the clam heart as a test object for acetylcholine. Biol. Bull. Woods Hole **75**, 365 (1938).

SÖRUM, H.: The crystal and molecular structure of acetylcholine bromide. Acta chem. scand. **13**, 345—359 (1959).

SPÄTH, E.: Die Synthese des sinapins. Mh. Chem. **41**, 271—285 (1920).

STEDMAN, E., and E. STEDMAN: The mechanism of the biological synthesis of acetylcholine. I. The isolation of acetylcholine produced by brain tissue *in vitro*. Biochem. J. **31**, 817 to 827 (1937).

STEPHENSON, M., and E. ROWATT: The production of acetylcholine by a strain of *Lactobacillus plantarum*. J. gen. Microbiol. **1**, 279—298 (1947).

STONE, W. E.: Acetylcholine in the brain. 1. "Free", "bound" and total acetylcholine. Arch. Biochem. **59**, 181—192 (1955a).

— Acetylcholine in the brain. II. Chemical measurement of choline esters. Arch. Biochem. **59**, 193—198 (1955b).

STRAUGHAN, D. W.: Assay of acetylcholine on the rat blood pressure. J. Pharm. (Lond.) **10**, 783—784 (1958).

STRECKER, A.: Über einige neue Bestandteile der Schweinegalle. Justus Liebigs Ann. Chem. **123**, 353—360 (1862).

SZERB, J. C.: The estimation of acetylcholine, using leech muscle in a microbath. J. Physiol. (Lond.) **158**, 8—9 P (1961).

TABACHNICK, I. I. A., and F. E. ROTH: The potentiation of histamine by imidazoleacrylcholine (murexine) and imidazolepropionylcholine (dihydromurexine). J. Pharmacol. exp. Ther. **121**, 191—198 (1957).

TAKAHASHI, HIDEHIKO, A. NAJASHIMA and C. KOSHINO: Effect of γ-aminobutyrylcholine upon the electrical activity of the cerebral cortex. Nature (Lond.) **182**, 1443—1444 (1958).

— — — — and HISASHI TAKAHASHI: Effects of γ-aminobutyric acid (GABA), γ-aminobutyrylcholine (GABA-Ch) and their related substances on the cortical activity. Jap. J. Physiol. **9**, 257—265 (1959).

TAMMELIN, L.-E.: Choline esters: substrates and inhibitors of cholinesterases. Svensk kem. Tidskr. **70**, 157—181 (1958).

THESLEFF, S.: The mode of neuromuscular block caused by acetylcholine, nicotine, decamethonium and succinylcholine. Acta physiol. scand. **34**, 218—231 (1955).

VINCENT, D., et A. JULLIEN: Richesse de la glande à pourpre des *Murex* en esters de la choline. C. R. Soc. Biol. (Paris) **127**, 1506—1509 (1938).

WAIT, R. B.: The action of acetylcholine on the isolated heart of *Venus mercenaria*. Biol. Bull., Woods Hole **85**, 79—85 (1943).

WELSH, J. H., and R. TAUB: The action of choline and related compounds on the heart of *Venus mercenaria*. Biol. Bull., Woods Hole **95**, 346—353 (1948).

WEST, G. B., and J. F. RILEY: Chromatography of tissue histamine. Nature (Lond.) **174**, 882—883 (1954).

WHITTAKER, V. P.: Specificity, mode of action and distribution of cholinesterases. Physiol. Rev. **31**, 312—343 (1951a).

— Hydrolysis of succinylcholine by cholinesterases: simultaneous utilization of paper chromatography and the Warburg technique (in Italian). Experientia (Basel) **7**, 217—218 (1951b).

— Identification of the F component of ox spleen. Biochem. biophys. Acta **22**, 590 (1956).

— β,β-Dimethylacrylylcholine, a new naturally occurring, physiologically active ester of choline. Biochem. J. **66**, 35 P (1957).

— Acetylcholine in milk. Nature (Lond.) **181**, 856—857 (1958).

— Acrylylcholine: a new naturally occurring pharmacologically active choline ester from *Buccinum undatum*. Biochem. Pharmacol. **1**, 342—346 (1959a).

— The identity of natural and synthetic β,β-dimethylacrylylcholine. Biochem. J. **71**, 32—34 (1959b).

— The isolation and characterization of acetylcholine-containing particles from brain. Biochem. J. **72**, 694—706 (1959c).

—, and I. A. MICHAELSON: Studies on urocanylcholine. Biol. Bull., Woods Hole **107**, 304 (1954).

—, and S. WIJESUNDERA: The separation of esters of choline by paper chromatography. Biochem. J. **49**, xlv (1951).

— — The separation of esters of choline by filter-paper chromatography. Biochem. J. **51**, 348—351 (1952a).

— — The hydrolysis of succinyldicholine by cholinesterase. Biochem. J. **52**, 475—479 (1952b).

WINTERFELD, K.: Über die Inhaltsstoffe der Mistel. Pharm. Ind. **9**, 37—41 (1942).

WOOD, D. L.: The identification of spleen propionylcholine by infrared microspectroscopy. Biochem. J. **58**, 30—31 (1954).

YOSHIHARA, H.: Comparative studies in isolated molluscan hearts as biological assay material for various drugs. Nippon Yakurigaku Zasshi **53**, 393—399 (1957), abstracted in Chem. Abstr. **52**, 10406e (1958).

Chapter 2

Choline Acetylase[1]

By

David Nachmansohn

Contents

A. Historical background

The discovery of choline acetylase (ChAc) was the outcome of the theory that acetylcholine (ACh) is the specific operative substance in nerve activity. When the energy released by the breakdown of phosphocreatine during electrical activity of the electric organ of *Electrophorus* was found to be more than adequate to account for the electrical energy released, it was assumed that this energy was used as in muscle for the resynthesis of adenosine triphosphate (ATP) and that in the sequence of energy transformations the breakdown of ATP preceded that of phosphocreatine. Several characteristics of ATP breakdown make it unlikely that ATP is directly associated with the elementary process of bioelectrogenesis. In particular, the requirement of the high turnover time is not satisfied. If the theory that ACh was the trigger required in the elementary process was correct, then it appeared likely that the energy released by ATP breakdown should be used, at least partly, for the resynthesis of ACh. This assumption proved to be correct: on addition of ATP to cell-free extracts prepared from brain and electric organs, the first enzymatic acetylation of choline in a soluble system was achieved (NACH-MANSOHN and MACHADO 1943). The evidence that the energy of the breakdown of ATP may be used for a biosynthetic reaction outside the glycolytic cycle was rather unexpected. It opened the way for a detailed analysis of the mechanism of acetylation in general which at the time, in the early 1940's, began to attract increasingly the interest of many biochemists.

[1] The financial support of this work by the National Institutes of Health, by the National Science Foundation, and by the Muscular Dystrophy Associations of America, Inc., is gratefully acknowledged.

The importance of acetate in intermediary metabolism as a building stone of many cell constituents became apparent mainly through the application of isotope techniques. The first indication of the physiological importance of acetate goes back to the investigations of KNOOP (1905). He concluded that fatty acids were oxidized stepwise with the formation of a 2-carbon compound, presumably acetic acid, and postulated his well known β-oxidation theory. This concept was supported by the findings of DAKIN (1909) that the presumed intermediates in this oxidation gave similar yields of acetoacetic acid. There was for a long time little further progress, since no adequate methods for identifying and determining acetate in small amounts were available. The situation changed with the introduction of isotopes as a tool for intermediary metabolism. SCHOENHEIMER and RITTENBERG (1936) found in animals fed with D_2O, that about half of the fatty acid hydrogen was derived from the water. BERNHARD (1940) fed deuterium-labeled acetate together with sulfanilamide to rabbits and rats and recovered acetylsulfanilamide labeled with deuterium in the urine. The results indicate that acetate may be used directly for acetylation, although only a small fraction was labeled; the greater part was apparently derived from endogenously formed acetate. Experiments of RITTENBERG and BLOCH (1945) with doubly labeled acetate $(CD_3C^{13}OOH)$ fed to rats resulted in fatty acids with alternate $C^{13}H_2$ and CD_2 methylene groups and a terminal $-C^{13}OOH$. These observations further supported the incorporation of acetate into fatty acids. The results indicate that the acetic acid used in acetylation may be largely formed in intermediary metabolism; they also confirm BERNHARD's finding that part of the acetic acid fed was used directly for acetylation. In the following years, experiments with labeled acetate carried out in many laboratories have shown that many important cell constituents use this 2-carbon unit as a building stone.

Acetylation in tissue slices with added acetate was first demonstrated by KLEIN and HARRIS (1938) with guinea pig liver; they obtained acetylation of sulfanilamide in the presence of oxygen. No acetylation was observed in anaerobic conditions. The formation of ACh in brain slices in oxygen was observed by MANN et al. (1939). Both *in vivo* and *in vitro* observations indicated that acetate may be used directly for acetylation. The mechanism, however, remained obscure. Its exploration became possible by the discovery that the energy of ATP -hydrolysis is used in solution for the acetylation of choline.

B. Coenzyme A

Shortly after the discovery of ChAc, NACHMANSOHN and MACHADO observed that on dialysis the enzyme rapidly loses its activity. This finding suggested for the first time the presence of a coenzyme in the acetylating system. The observation was confirmed and extended by NACHMANSOHN, JOHN and WAELSCH (1943). In 1945 NACHMANSOHN and BERMAN (1946) obtained a purified preparation from *Kochsaft* of liver, heart, and brain of a coenzyme which reactivated completely a dialyzed ChAc solution prepared from acetone-dried powder of rat brain. In view of NACHMANSOHN's findings, LIPMANN (1945) tested the effect of ATP on the acetylation of sulfanilamide by liver extracts and confirmed that ATP provides the energy of acetylation. Simultaneously with Nachmansohn and Berman he prepared a coenzyme required for the sulfanilamide acetylating system. When the two findings were presented at a Symposium on "The Physico-Chemical Mechanism of Nerve Activity" in the New York Academy of Sciences, it became obvious that the formation of N- and O-acyl groups used a similar if not identical mechanism (NACHMANSOHN 1946, LIPMANN and KAPLAN 1946). Further developments have shown that the coenzyme is used in acylations in general, and Lipmann referred to it as coenzyme A (CoA).

In the following years Lipmann and his associates greatly contributed to elucidate the chemical structure of CoA. An important advance was the finding that CoA contains pantothenic acid linked to a nucleotide by phosphate groups (LIPMANN et al. 1947, LIPMANN 1950). SNELL and co-workers (1950) reported the requirements of a compound, referred to as the *Lactobacillus bulgaricus* factor, for bacterial growth; in this substance β-mercaptoethanolamine is bound to the β-alanine of pantothenic acid, giving N-pantothenyl-β-mercaptoethanolamine. This compound is referred to as pantetheine and may be obtained by the action of the intestinal phosphatase on CoA (BROWN et al. 1950). The exact position of the phosphate groups was studied by BADDILEY and THAIN (1951); they found that whereas two phosphate groups link the pantothenic acid to the ribose of the nucleotide, the third phosphate group must be attached to the second or to the third atom of the ribose. It was shown by SHUSTER and KAPLAN (1953) with the aid of a specific enzyme that it is the third carbon to which the phosphate is linked. NOVELLI and his associates confirmed the structure by enzymatic degradation and resynthesis (NOVELLI 1953; NOVELLI et al. 1954). The active group of CoA was elucidated by LYNEN et al. (1951). They found that acetate in the reaction with CoA forms an ester with an SH group. Thus, it became apparent that the SH group of the β-mercaptoethanolamine is the functional group of CoA and that the acetyl CoA is the thioester. On the basis of all these investigations the following structure of CoA has been established:

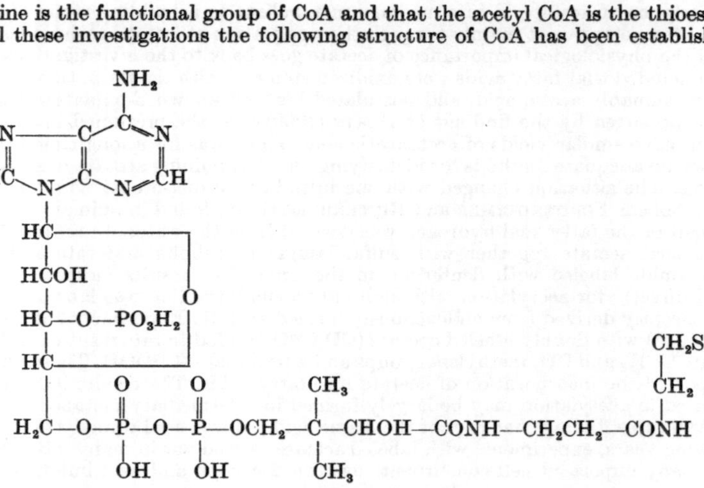

Coenzyme A

The change of the standard free energy of the acetyl CoA hydrolysis is large, as was found with the aid of various equilibrium reactions (STERN et al. 1952, STADTMAN 1952b). Thus, the thioester was shown to be a new type of a biologically important compound rich in energy. The ΔF° was estimated to be about $-10,000$ to $-12,000$ cal per mole.

C. Mechanisms of intermediary steps

Acetylation then takes place in at least two enzymatic steps. The first is the formation of acetyl CoA. In animal tissue and in yeast this step is catalyzed by an "acetate-activating" enzyme referred to as acetyl kinase. Thioacetate may replace ATP-acetate in the formation of acetyl CoA in the presence of the acetate-activating system prepared from pigeon liver or rabbit brain, although at a lower rate (NACHMANSOHN et al. 1952). Presumably, the reaction is:

$$CH_3\overset{O}{\overset{\|}{C}}\text{—SH} + \text{HS CoA} \rightleftharpoons H_2S + CH_3\overset{O}{\overset{\|}{C}}\text{—S CoA}$$

The formation of acetyl CoA in bacteria is catalyzed by an enzyme discovered and partially purified by STADTMAN (1950, 1952a and b). This enzyme is referred to as phosphotransacetylase. Acetylphosphate provides in this case the source of energy. The existence of this enzyme was suggested by observations of NOVELLI and LIPMANN (1950) and STERN and OCHOA (1951). An exception are the photosynthetic bacteria, *Rhodospirillum rubrum* (EISENBERG 1953, 1955). These bacterial cells use ATP for acetate activation.

The mechanism of the enzymatic formation of acetyl CoA from acetate and ATP, the acetate-activating reaction, is pictured as follows (BERG 1956a, b):

1. ATP + acetate ⇌ adenyl-acetate + P—P
2. Adenyl-acetate + CoA ⇌ acetyl-CoA + adenylic acid

BERG prepared synthetically adenylacetate and his data support the assumption of this compound as an intermediate.

There are two distinctly different types of activation of the acetyl group and their mechanism has been frequently discussed in recent years. Although ATP (or more generally nucleotide triphosphate) is the major source of energy in both types, in the one group activation results from the transfer of the terminal phosphate of ATP; a phosphoryl derivative is formed by the displacement and liberation of adenosine diphosphate (ADP). This mechanism is typical for all transphosphorylation reactions of the kinase type. In the second, quite different type, the group to be activated enters into reaction with the phosphate attached in 5'-position to the ribose of the nucleoside. Of this type there exist some varieties. In both types a nucleophilic attack of the carboxyl group on a P atom takes place, in an S_N2 reaction. The two processes may be pictured, according to LIPMANN (1957), as shown in reactions (1) and (2).

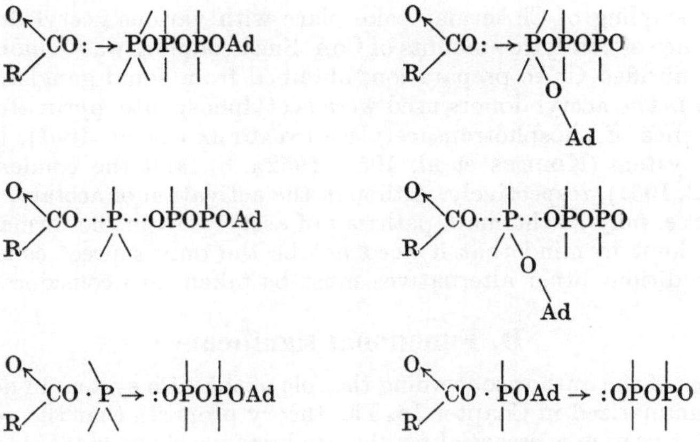

$$\begin{array}{l} \underset{R}{\overset{O}{\diagdown}} CO: \rightarrow POPOPOAd \\ \\ \underset{R}{\overset{O}{\diagdown}} CO \cdots P \cdots OPOPOAd \\ \\ \underset{R}{\overset{O}{\diagdown}} CO \cdot P \rightarrow :OPOPOAd \\ \\ \qquad (1) \end{array}$$

$$\begin{array}{l} \underset{R}{\overset{O}{\diagdown}} CO: \rightarrow POPOPO \\ \\ \underset{R}{\overset{O}{\diagdown}} CO \cdots P \cdots OPOPO \\ \\ \underset{R}{\overset{O}{\diagdown}} CO \cdot POAd \rightarrow :OPOPO \\ \\ \qquad (2) \end{array}$$

On the left (1) is shown the sequence of the reaction in which the terminal P is attacked by a carboxyl oxygen; the carboxyl group and ADP are connected to that phosphorus in the transition state, resulting in acyl phosphate and ADP. In the reactions shown on the right hand (2), the second type is shown in which the carboxyl group attacks the phosphorus linked to adenosine. In the transition state the carboxyl and pyrophosphate groups are linked to the P of adenosine monophosphate (AMP), yielding eventually AMP acylate by the displacement of pyrophosphate.

Once the acyl group is activated, a group transfer reaction to an acceptor takes place. In analogy to substitution reactions known from organic chemistry, KOSHLAND (1954) has proposed to refer to enzymatically catalyzed group transfer reactions, such as transacylation, transphosphorylation, etc., as enzymatic substitution reactions. In the reaction (3) between CoA and acyl-adenylate the break takes place between carbon and oxygen.

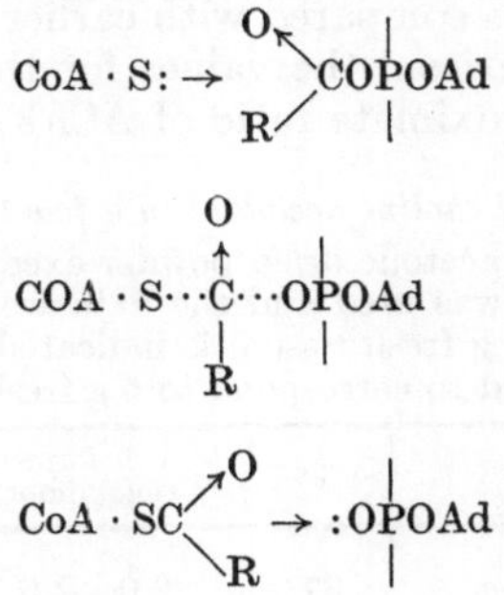

$$CoA \cdot S: \rightarrow \underset{R}{\overset{O}{\diagdown}} COPOAd$$

$$CoA \cdot S \cdots \underset{R}{\overset{\overset{O}{\uparrow}}{C}} \cdots OPOAd$$

$$CoA \cdot SC \underset{R}{\overset{\nearrow O}{\diagdown}} \rightarrow :OPOAd$$

$$(3)$$

Both activation and transfer reactions seem frequently to be catalyzed by the same enzyme.

When it became apparent that there are at least two enzymatic steps in the process of acetylation, choline acetylase (ChAc) was redefined as the enzyme which transfers the acetyl group from acetyl CoA to choline (KOREY et al. 1951). The specific reaction catalyzed by ChAc is then as follows:

$$\underset{\underset{CH_3}{|}}{\overset{\overset{CH_3}{|}}{CH_3-\overset{\oplus}{N}}}-CH_2CH_2OH + CH_3\overset{O}{\overset{\|}{C}}SCoA \rightleftharpoons \underset{\underset{CH_3}{|}}{\overset{\overset{CH_3}{|}}{CH_3-\overset{\oplus}{N}}}-CH_2CH_2O\overset{O}{\overset{\|}{C}}CH_3 + HSCoA$$

It is obvious from the discussion above that acetyl CoA may be derived in intact cells from various sources, since it is an intermediate form of many reactions.

Therefore, coupling of ChAc may take place with various acetyl donor systems in the presence of catalytic amounts of CoA. Such coupling was demonstrated with a partially purified ChAc preparation, obtained from squid ganglia, by KORKES et al. 1952a). The acetyl donors used were acetylphosphate, pyruvate, and citrate in the presence of phosphotransacetylase (STADTMAN et al. 1951), the pyruvate oxydation system (KORKES et al. 1951, 1952a, b), and the condensing system (STERN et al. 1951), respectively. Although the activation of acetate, with ATP as energy source, may be the main pathway of acetyl CoA in the formation of ACh, it must be kept in mind that it need not be the only source; especially under unusual conditions other alternatives must be taken into consideration.

D. Functional significance

The view of the author concerning the role of the ACh system in nerve activity has been summarized in Chapter 15. The theory proposes that the action of ACh on a receptor protein is essential for the conductance changes taking place during electrical activity within conducting membranes; acetylcholinesterase (AChE) rapidly removes the ester and restores the resting condition. The ability of conducting tissues to form ACh is then an obvious corollary to the postulate of its essential role in the elementary process. Following the discovery of ChAc in 1943, the author and his associates have tested its occurrence in a number of various types of conducting tissues, selecting those which offered from the physiological point of view some particular interest. In all conducting tissues tested, the enzyme was found to be present. At that time, however, the maximum rate may not have been achieved since the formation of acetyl CoA may have been inadequate and the rate-limiting factor for ChAc activity. Tests under optimal conditions carried out later in the author's laboratory by COHEN (1956) did, however, in most cases not show significant differences compared with earlier values. Table 1 summarizes the data obtained. For comparison, the values for the activity of AChE in these tissues is added, and the approximate ratio of AChE/ChAc is indicated.

Table 1. *Concentrations of choline acetylase in a few types of conducting tissue*

ChAc was tested in extracts of acetone dried powder except where the figures are marked by an asterisk; there fresh tissue was used and the data were calculated per g fresh tissue. The activity of AChE (referred to g fresh tissue) is indicated for comparison. One g powder is assumed to correspond to 5 g fresh tissue.

Tissue	Species	$t°$	ACh formed (mg/g/hour)	ACh split (mg/g/hour)	Ratio
brain	rat, guinea pig, rabbit	37	2.0—2.5	80—100	200
sciatic nerve	rabbit	37	1.0—1.3	12—15	50—80
ventral roots	ox	37	7.0—12.0	12—15	6—7
dorsal roots	ox	37	0.03—0.05	9	800—1000
dorsal roots	dog	37	0.015—0.02*	11—15	600—1000
optic nerve	rabbit	37	0.015—0.02*	18—25	800—1000
head ganglia	squid	25	10.0—15.0	3—4000	1000
abdominal chain . .	lobster	25	0.05—0.09*	20—30	300—400
electric tissue . . .	electric eel	25	0.3—0.5*	3—4000	1000
striated muscle . . .	pigeon	37	0.03—0.05	—	—
heart muscle[1] . . .	rabbit	37	0.02—0.04	5—7	1000
striated muscle . . .	goldfish	25	3.0—4.0	900	1000

[1] Apex only, free of nerve endings.

Studies as to the occurrence and concentration of ChAc carried out in the author's laboratory were, however, rather limited. Many additional data have been obtained in other laboratories, particularly, however, by the extensive investigations of HEBB and her associates, well summarized in her review on the "Evidence for the Neural Function of Acetylcholine" (HEBB 1957). This aspect will be discussed in Chapter 3. The information available about a number of biochemical aspects of ChAc is discussed in a lucid and competent way in her review. There is, however, a difference of opinion concerning the physiological role of the ACh system. Since most aspects of this question are described in Chapter 15, only the chief disagreement concerning the interpretation of the data on ChAc will be discussed in this chapter.

In describing the great differences of ChAc concentration encountered in different regions of the nervous system and in different types of nervous and non-nervous tissue, HEBB (l.c.) stresses the smallness of the enzyme activity in sensory fibers, leading frequently even to complete failure to discover any enzyme activity in some fibers, whereas in some others of the same type the amounts are small. As far as the facts are concerned the author agrees that the concentration of the enzyme in sensory fibers, such as for instance the dorsal roots of ox and dog, are small. Not in a single experiment, however, carried out in the reviewers laboratory by COHEN (1956) was the enzyme absent (Table 1). It is difficult to explain why in the experiments of HEBB, whose competence is not questioned, the results are irregular, varying, e.g., in dorsal roots from 0 to 30 $\mu g/g$ tissue. It must be remembered that the enzyme is quite unstable and the system is rather complex. If the concentrations of an unstable enzyme in a tissue are small and relatively large amounts of tissue must be used, many adverse factors may interfere which may be irrelevant in tissues with high activity because there they become too diluted for interference. There may be inhibitory components, there may be interference by other systems present, etc Even with a much more stable enzyme, such as AChE, which does not require for activity a complex system, quantitative evaluations become sometimes difficult if its activity in tissue is very low. HEBB is aware of these difficulties. She admits that small amounts of enzyme are probably present. Thus, the irregularity appears less pertinent for the evaluation of the functional significance of ChAc than the fact of the low concentration. The real disagreement becomes then a matter of interpretation. HEBB reasons as follows: assuming that sensory nerves are able to form 30 to 50 μg of ACh/g/hour, this would amount to only 0.003 $\mu g/g$/second (HEBB 1957). This rate would be far below that required for admitting a role of ACh in the conduction of these fibers and thus contradict the theory of the author. It is on this particular point where the views disagree sharply.

When the author initiated, in 1936, his studies on the distribution and concentration of cholinesterases (ChE's) in nerve tissues, he was impressed from the beginning by the remarkably great differences of concentrations encountered, particularly by the extraordinarily high concentration of the enzyme in the electric organ of *Torpedo* found in 1937. Although it became later apparent that part of the enzyme in some of the tissues is not AChE, the corrections required have not fundamentally changed the picture. Some of the early interpretations needed modification after the peculiar intracellular distribution of the enzyme became apparent (see Chapters 6 and 15).

However, the author has stressed time and again that no information is available at present to explain these remarkably great differences of enzyme concentrations in terms of function. Great quantitative differences of concentrations of many enzymes associated with special functions are commonly encountered without any apparent explanation. At present one can only speculate. Too little is known about the molecular organization of the various conducting membranes and many other factors which may be pertinent for the explanation of these differences.

Obviously, if ACh is required in axonal conduction, it must be present and formed in axons. The idea that AChE is present in the axon only on its way to the nerve endings is hard to reconcile with the evidence of its functional essentiality and has been recently contradicted by the observations of KOENIG and KOELLE (1960). So far, nobody has offered a satisfactory explanation for the extraordinarily high concentration of ChAc in ox ventral roots or in the nucleus caudate or squid head ganglia, or as to why ChAc is 40 to 60 times as high in the retina of birds and sheep as it is in the retina of dog and cat (HEBB 1957). There are also great and unexplained differences in the ratios of AChE to ChAc concentrations (see Table 1). It is pertinent to keep in mind the distinctly different character of the function of these two enzymes. The action of AChE must be extremely fast; it must act in milliseconds or less. No such speed is required for ChAc which acts during recovery and where the process may take seconds or minutes. The amount of ACh present in sensory fibers is small, but the ester is present there as has been demonstrated in many laboratories contrary to some early claims [for instance CHANG et al. (1939), and LISSAK and PASZTOR (1941)]. A synthesis of 30 to 50 μg ACh formed per hour per gram in sensory fibers, corresponding to 0.003 μg/g fresh tissue/second, is considered by HEBB as an activity being too small and incompatible with the theory.

The author is unable to agree with this view. Let us attempt an evaluation of these figures in terms of molecules formed per unit active surface area. The total surface area of the myelinated frog sciatic nerve fiber is estimated to be 1.6×10^3 cm² per gram (FENG 1936). Assuming a comparable surface area per gram of dorsal roots, which are also myelinated, an amount of 30 μg of ACh formed per gram per hour would correspond to about 4×10^{-14} mole per cm² per second. Even if the surface area in the dorsal roots would be 2 to 4 times as large, the figure would be 1 to 2×10^{-14} mole. However, only a very small fraction of the total surface area, particularly in myelinated fibers, is active. The order of magnitude of this fraction can be estimated. In the frog sciatic nerve fiber one Ranvier node, assumed to be the site of electrical activity, has a surface area of about 25 μ². The surface of the internodes, assuming a length of 2 mm and diameters of 3 to 15 μ on the average, amounts to about 0.2 to 0.8×10^5 μ². The active surface area would thus form somewhere between 0.02 and 0.1 % of the total. Let us assume a comparable ratio of active over total area in the dorsal roots and let us assume the active area to be 0.1 % of the total. If the formation of the ester does not take place evenly over the whole surface area but, as appears more likely, in the active area, from 1 to 4×10^{-14} mole would be formed per 10^5 μ². This corresponds to about 0.6 to 2.4×10^5 molecules per μ² active surface formed per second. Although the estimates of the active surface area are tentative and may have to be revised in either direction, up or down, when more information will be available, the corrections required are not likely to be verly large.

The period of time available for the formation of ACh required for unimpaired activity is unknown and even tentative estimates are not easy, since there are too many uncertain factors. However, the rate of formation per μ² area, even if some changes of the present estimates will be required, does not appear to justify HEBB's categorical rejection of the theory. It is known that 3 to 4 quanta of light may produce a stimulus in the retina. Is it then unreasonable to assume that 10^5 molecules of a substance formed per μ² of active surface area per second may be an order of magnitude adequate for the assumption that this substance is responsible for the changes of conductance in a membrane of less than 80 Å thickness ?

There are enzymic properties which are critical for the theory such as, for instance, the turnover time of AChE: if that value would have been 30 to 40 msec insted of 30 to 40 μsec, the theory would be untenable. But variations of concentration of either AChE or ChAc found in various types of tissue, although unexplained at present, cannot be construed as being incompatible with the theory. A much more pertinent feature than the absolute enzyme concentration is, in the author's view, the functional interdependence of two chief components of the chemical system and electrical activity, *viz.*, the evidence that specific inhibitors of the ACh receptor protein, such as local anesthetics, or of AChE, such as eserine, block electrical activity in sensory nerves in a way similar to that in motor nerves (see Chapter 15).

The presence of ChAc in some non-neural and even non-conducting tissue, such as placenta and spleen, offers another interesting and still unexplained problem. Obviously, this occurrence does not exclude the assumption of a specific role in nerve tissue. But is there perhaps some relationship with a related function ? At present, we can only speculate. An interesting working hypothesis appears to the author the possibility that the ACh system may have some role in control of some ion movements across cell membranes useful for the normal function of certain cells. Although this question has been repeatedly considered and discussed in relation to red blood cells, a satisfactory answer is still lacking (NACHMANSOHN 1959; see also Chapters 6 and 11). A role of the system in the control of ion movements may have been the original one which was then later developed on conducting cells for the propagation of electric currents. The hypothesis is accessible to experimental attack. Obviously, here again the mere presence of either ChAc or AChE or both is insufficient for providing a clue to their function.

Another problem of physiological interest may be briefly discussed, namely the relationship between the rate of disappearance of ChAc and of electrical activity in degenerating nerve fibers. When ChAc activity was first tested in rabbit sciatic nerve fibers, it was found that ACh was formed at a rate of about 100 μg/g fresh tissue/hour (NACHMANSOHN, JOHN and BERMAN 1945). Two days after section of the fiber, about 2/3 of the initial concentration was still present in the distal part of the fiber. Conduction usually ceases on the third day. Even at that time the enzyme activity was still about 1/3 of the normal. The absolute rates may be still higher than those found in these early experiments since the acetate activating system was probably not yet optimal. Using acetone dried powder prepared from normal sciatic nerve fibers, COHEN (1956) found that under optimal conditions more than one gram of ACh was formed per gram powder per hour. The improved conditions probably will not change the relative rates of disappearance in degenerating fibers (see also HEBB and WAITES 1956).

In contrast to the results obtained in the author's laboratory, FELDBERG (1943, 1945) claimed that in degenerating fibers the ability to form ACh ceases before that of conducting impulses. He considered this as an important argument against the role of ACh in conduction. FELDBERG used finely cut nerve fibers of sheep and cat in his experiments. Respiration in nerve fibers falls to low values when they are treated this way. Therefore, there was no source of energy available under the conditions of his experiments. FELDBERG found in the vagus nerve fibers of sheep and cat about 2 μg of ACh formed per g per hour. This is less than 1% of the actual activity. Even these values are open to question due to the difference of treatment of control and test. His failure to find ACh formation in degenerated fibers is, therefore, without significance.

An equally striking contrast to FELDBERG's data are those of BANISTER and SCRASE (1950) on ACh formation in normal and denervated sympathetic ganglia of the cat. BANISTER and SCRASE's values are more than one hundred times as high as those of FELDBERG. Moreover, their data show that 40 hours after denervation, 40% of the value of the control site was still present, and after 90 hours less than 20% (about 15%). Since electrical activity usually is hardly detectable after 70 hours, the results show that transmission fails before the disappearance of ChAc, whereas FELDBERG did not find any ACh formation on the second day. HEBB and WAITES (1956) investigated ChAc activity in the superior cervical ganglia of the cat and in the sympathetic nerve trunk with a still more complete system than that used by BANISTER and SCRASE, containing additional acetate activating enzyme. Some improvement of activity was found. Their data on the rate of disappearance of the enzyme in the ganglia are, however, in good agreement with those of BANISTER and SCRASE. In the nerve fibers, decrease of activity took place at the same rate as in the ganglia. Thus, in agreement with the data of this laboratory and in contrast to FELDBERG's data, ChAc was still present in significant amounts in the axons at the time when conduction ordinarily fails. There is apparently an excess of enzyme in normal fibers; this is in agreement with observations on AChE and on many other enzymes. In spite of the striking discrepancies as to absolute values as well as to functional relationships, both reports claimed, for reasons not apparent to the author, that the experiments essentially confirm those of FELDBERG.

E. Some properties of the enzyme

I. Partial purification of ChAc

In contrast to AChE, which does not depend for the hydrolytic process on either a coenzyme or any specific ions, ChAc requires for full activity a complex system. Some of the developments which led to the preparation of a partially purified enzyme, a prerequisite for studying enzyme properties, may be briefly described. Synthesis of ACh was first accomplished in cell-free extracts of brain and electric organ, i.e., in the supernatant of adequately centrifuged homogenized suspensions (NACHMANSOHN and MACHADO 1943). In view of the presence of adenosine triphosphatase, a satisfactory and reproducible rate of ACh formation was achieved only by the addition of sodium fluoride. Even under these conditions the enzyme was unstable and the rate of formation decreased rapidly and levelled off after 30 min. In the following year, however, extracts were prepared from acetone-dried powder of brains of rats and guinea pigs in which the enzyme system had a fair degree of stability (NACHMANSOHN and JOHN 1944, 1945). The amounts formed by this material were still rather small, even in the presence of an active coenzyme preparation; the specific activity was about 0.05 to 0.1 μmol/mg of protein/hour [2 to 3 mg of ACh per gram powder per hour (NACHMANSOHN and BERMAN 1946)]. The activity was tested by bioassay, which for many reasons is not satisfactory for studies of enzyme properties.

A suitable source for purification of the enzyme is provided by the head ganglia of squid. Extracts prepared from acetone-dried powder of this material were found to be quite active: per mg protein, about 5 to 10 μmol of ACh is formed per hour (NACHMANSOHN and WEISS 1948). The specific activity is thus 100 to 200 times as high as in the extracts prepared from acetone-dried powder of rat, rabbit, or guinea pig brain. Another advance, important for the studies with purified enzyme, was the elaboration of a simple and sensitive colorimetric method for the determination of ACh worked out by HESTRIN (1949). The procedure is based upon the reaction of hydroxylamine with O-acyl derivatives to form hydroxamic acids. All hydroxamic acids give in acid solution a red or red-purple color with ferric chloride with which a soluble inner complex salt is formed (FEIGL 1946). The method provides a convenient analytical procedure for testing ACh formation.

Once the two enzymatic steps of acetylation had been separated, it became possible to develop a satisfactory method of purification. Both the purified phosphotransacetylase obtained from *Escherichia coli* with acetylphosphate as energy source, and ATP plus the acetate activating enzyme purified from extracts of acetone-dried powder of pigeon liver proved to be active in forming ACh when added to CoA and ChAc (KORKES et al. 1952).

Due to these advances, a partial purification of the enzyme was accomplished. The degree of purity appeared to be adequate for the study of some properties of the protein (BERMAN et al. 1953). The usual purification procedures were applied: fractionation with ammonium sulfate, treatment with protamine sulfate, absorption by calcium gel, and subsequent elution. The enzyme preparation obtained had a specific activity of about 40 to 80 μmol/mg protein/hour. Although the degree of purity was not very high, the preparation proved to be satisfactory, especially after the removal of deacylase which interfered with some of the tests (BERMAN-REISBERG 1957).

Whereas the phosphotransacetylase system was used for the purification, for the study of specificity ChAc was the only active enzyme in the reaction mixture. The acetyl CoA added was prepared non-enzymatically (WILSON 1952; SIMON and SHEMIN 1953). While the rate of formation with the phosphotransacetylase system is linear, that with acetyl CoA is not, except for relatively short periods of time (BERMAN-REISBERG 1957). The reasons are not quite clear, but if the system is used for short periods of time only the rates remain fairly stable. The stability of the enzyme is quite satisfactory; it remains stable for 6 to 8 weeks when kept at -10 to $-20°$ C. The dissociation constant of the enzyme-choline complex was found to have a value of 5×10^{-4} M, and the value for acetyl CoA is 1.6×10^{-3} M. The dissociation constant between choline and ChAc is of the same order of magnitude as that between ACh and AChE.

The enzyme activity is readily blocked by compounds reacting with SH groups (BERMAN-REISBERG 1954, 1957). The sensititivity of the enzyme system towards compounds reacting with SH groups was observed in the very first observations (NACHMANSOHN and MACHADO 1943); however, after the functional group of CoA was identified as an SH group (LYNEN et al. 1951), a reexamination became necessary to ascertain whether the enzyme itself has an active SH group. The enzyme must be classified among the enzymes which have functional SH groups. Addition of ethylenediamine tetracetate and cysteine is necessary for optimal rates and enzyme stability.

II. Specificity

1. Substrates

The specificity of ChA has been tested with the purified enzyme preparation with respect both to various acyl derivatives of CoA and to ethanolamine, mono-, di-, and trimethyl ethanolamine, as substrates (BERMAN-REISBERG 1957). The question underlying these studies is whether the protein has some similarities with the active site and other characteristics of AChE.

The analysis of the reaction between the protein and small molecules has not been carried to the same extent as that of AChE, but some similar features have been found. Virtually no difference exists as to the rate of synthesis between acetyl and propionyl CoA sustrates; butyryl CoA, on the other hand, is very poor substrate; the rate of synthesis is only about 10% of that with acetyl CoA as substrate. The parallelism with AChE is apparent. It may be mentioned that butyrylcholine has been found in brain (HOLTZ and SCHUEMANN 1954), but HENSCHLER (1956) has stated that this compound appears only in autolyzing brain. Although the synthesis of this ester is markedly slower than that with acyl groups containing two and three carbons, it must be kept in mind, in considering possible functional relationships, that the rate of hydrolysis with purified AChE too is quite low, in fact less than 1% of that of ACh.

Of particular interest is the behavior of the protein towards the nitrogen group when the number of methyl groups is decreased. Studies of this kind with AChE have been discussed in Chapter 15. Dimethyl ethanolamine is acetylated at a rate which is only 8% of that of choline. Still lower is the rate of acetylation of the monomethyl derivative; in this case the rate of formation is only 2% compared with that of choline (BERMAN et al. 1953). The difference between the mono- and the dimethyl derivatives may possibly be attributed to better binding by VAN DER WAALS' forces, but the strong effect of the third methyl group requires another explanation. There again change of configuration of the protein appears to be a good possibility on the basis of the information obtained with AChE (see Chapter 15).

The specificity of ChAc towards the acyl group was recently tested also by BERRY and WHITTAKER (1959) with partially purified preparations obtained from mammalian brain. They found that ChAc from this source formed essentially only acetyl- and propionylcholine. The latter was formed at a rate about 30% of that of ACh. This is the same ratio as previously described by BERMAN et al. (1953). There was a different enzyme present in these extracts, referred to by the authors as choline acylase II, which was able to synthesize acyl cholines, probably from C_4 up to C_6. The optimal acyl group was not determined. A third enzyme, tentatively referred to as choline acylase III, synthesized palmitoylcholine. It may be noted, however, that the specific activity of the mammalian ChAc was much lower than that of the enzyme prepared from squid ganglia. Whereas the latter formed 40 to 80 μmol of ACh/mg protein/hr, the best preparation used by BERRY and WHITTAKER obtained from nucleus caudatus of sheep formed only about 0.15 μmol/mg protein/hr.

A very extensive study of the specificity of brain ChAc towards choline was carried out by BURGEN et al. (1953) with a partially purified enzyme prepared from rat brain. Acetyl CoA was added instead of acetate-activating enzyme systems. More than 20 alkanolamines were tested. If one methyl group on the N of the choline was substituted by an ethyl group, the activity increased by 40%. If two or three methyl groups were substituted by ethyl groups, the activity was essentially the same as with choline. With other substitutes the activity was either decreased or abolished. Replacement of one methyl group by increasingly longer chains had a relatively small decreasing effect until n-hexyl, which was not acetylated. Benzyl or *iso*propyl substitution reduced acetylation by one-third only. Increase in the hydroxyl-nitrogen separation by one carbon in γ-homocholine abolished acetylation, and side chain substitution, as in α-methylcholine and β-methylcholine, had the same effect. Increase in the hydroxyl-nitrogen separation to four carbon atoms in δ-hydroxybutyltrimethyl ammonium restored some acetylation. Of three bisquaternary molecules tested, only that with a C_{10} chain between the dimethylethanolamines was acetylated; those with a C_3 and C_5 chain were not. Ethanolamine and monomethylethanolamine were still acetylated at a rate 15% of that of choline. This is a much smaller decrease in activity than that obtained with these two compounds in experiments with squid ChAc. However, the specific activity of the brain enzyme preparation was very low compared with that of the squid enzyme: about 5 to 10 μmol ACh/gm powder/hr. Although the authors did not indicate the protein content of the solution used, the specific activity was probably not more than 0.01 μmol/mg protein/hr (~ 0.5 g protein/gm powder) or several thousand times lower than that of the preparation used by BERMAN et al. (1953).

2. Inhibitors

There are several reports on compounds having inhibitory effects on ACh formation in soluble enzyme systems. However, in the earlier investigations relatively crude preparations were used; both the acetate activating system and ChAc were present. Interpretation of effects with such multi-enzyme preparations is difficult. The data do not in general permit attributing the inhibition to a specific action. Whether some of these compounds inhibit ACh formation in living cells where the whole system is present, and by what mechanism, are again different questions which cannot be answered without much additional and presently not available information.

Shortly after the discovery of ChAc, NACHMANSOHN and JOHN (1944, 1945) observed an inhibitory action of α-keto acids on a crude enzyme preparation obtained from acetone dried powder of rat brains. The system was not yet fortified by addition of CoA. Pyruvic, phenylpyruvic, and hydroxyphenylpyruvic acids in 10^{-3} M concentration inhibited 30 to 50% of the activity, and α-ketoglutaric acid in 10^{-4} M. No inhibitory effect was observed with α-keto acids in the crude preparation, but only in the 15 times more active preparations obtained from squid head ganglia (NACHMANSOHN and WEISS 1948). On the other hand, several naphthoquinones inhibit the activity of the preparation obtained from squid ganglia as well as that of rat brain in 10^{-4} M concentration, and the K salt of 2-methyl-1,4-naphthoquinone-8-sulfonic acid inhibits even in 10^{-5} M (NACHMANSOHN and BERMAN 1946, NACHMANSOHN and WEISS 1948).

In a partially purified preparation obtained from extracts of acetone dried rabbit brains, FAHMY et al. (1954) observed an inhibition of ACh formation by nicotine. The acetate activating system was present in the preparation. Since nicotine had no effect on the rate of acetylation of sulfanilamide by extracts of acetone dried pigeon liver, the authors ascribed the inhibitory effect to the action on ChAc. This assumption appears reasonable. However, a 0.015 M concentration of nicotine was required for about 50% inhibition. In discussing the significance of their observation, the authors pointed out the possibility of additive effects of various actions of nicotine: the compound inhibits pyruvic dehydrogenase which forms active acetate from pyruvate; accumulation of pyruvate may contribute to the inhibitory action. On the other hand, brain cholinesterase is also inhibited by nicotine, even in much lower concentrations. Moreover, nicotine has a strong action on certain synaptic junctions, probably acting as a receptor activator. The concentration required for ChAc inhibition appears rather high, and the question remains open as to the significance of this effect. It is not inconceivable that in chronic nicotine poisoning, in addition to other effects, the enzyme may be affected.

Inhibitory effects of barbiturates on the acetylation of arylamines by pigeon liver enzyme were reported by MARKS (1956). Addition of extra CoA, but not of ATP, markedly decreased the inhibition. According to the author, the data support the idea that barbiturates may produce their effects by interfering with acetate activation and consequently with ACh formation. In addition to other difficulties confronting such an assumption, the high concentration required, 2 to 10×10^{-3} M, makes such an interpretation of the mode of action of barbiturates rather doubtful.

The observations on the inhibitory actions of ACh formation described so far were studied in multi-enzyme systems. Later, a test system was developed which permits measurement of ChAc activity in the absence of any acetate activating system; the enzyme preparation, obtained from squid head ganglia, had a relatively high specific activity, in that 40 to 80 μmol of ACh was formed/mg protein/hr (BERMAN et al. 1953). This preparation permitted direct measurements of specific inhibition of ChAc (BERMAN-REISBERG 1957).

Two types of inhibitors were tested, one presumably competing with choline, the other presumably competing with the acyl group. The inhibitory effects of the methylated nitrogen derivatives tested were found to be rather weak. Tetramethylammonium chloride, at 30 μmol/ml, blocked about 60% of the activity. The analogues tested were still weaker: at 80 μmol/ml, trimethylammonium hydrochloride (pK = 9.987) blocked about 30% of the activity, dimethylethanolamine about 20%, whereas dimethylamine hydrochloride did not inhibit at all. Acetylcholine, at 50 μmol/ml, inhibited 40% of the activity. The inhibitory power of neostigmine was even 2 to 3 times lower than that of the simple tetramethylammonium ion: 50% inhibition with 80 μmol/ml. This is strikingly different from the effect of neostigmine on AChE, which is inhibited at 10^{-7} M, i.e., at a concentration 10^5 times lower (*not* 10^{-5}). In contrast, the tertiary analogue of neostigmine, which is only about 1/100th as strong an inhibitor of AChE as neostigmine, in 5 μmol/ml inhibits 70% of ChAc activity. However, this relatively strong inhibition takes place only after preincubation for 15 to 30 minutes; this observation suggests that another interaction besides van der Waals' forces and electrostatic attraction to a negatively charged area on the enzyme may be involved. Moreover, if acetyl-CoA was present during the preincubation, the inhibition was reduced to less than half. Choline, on the other hand, did not protect the enzyme at all against this inhibitor. Thus, the mode of action of the tertiary analogue of neostigmine may involve another still undefined reaction with the protein.

Certain *bis*quaternary compounds are known to react more strongly with AChE and the ACh receptor protein than the corresponding monoquaternary compounds. This increased effect is generally attributed to the presence of a second negative group in the protein surface located at a proper distance from the anionic site. In contrast, in the case of ChAc no significant increase of inhibitory strength is observed with *bis*quaternary compounds. Decamethonium bromide inhibits 25% of the activity at a concentration of 25 μmol/ml, and succinylcholine 20% at 40 μmol/ml. Thus, there is so far no indication of the existence of a second negative group near the active site of ChAc, at least at a distance similar to that in the receptor and in the esterase proteins. *d*-Tubocurarine is relatively more potent, but again only after preincubation: whereas 5 μmol/ml inhibits only 5% of activity without pretreatment, the inhibition goes up to 60% after 15 minutes of pre-incubation.

Inhibition of ChAc by quaternary nitrogen derivatives in a preparation free of the acetate activating system was also tested by BURGEN et al. (1956). A partially purified preparation from acetone dried powder of rat brain was used; however, as mentioned before, the specific activity was more than 1000 times lower than that obtained from squid head ganglia. Three of the compounds tested produced at 5.5 μmol/ml a significant degree of inhibition: carboxymethyldimethyl-ethanolammonium inhibited 40% of the activity, betaine hydrazide 28%, and α-methylcholine 25%.

Among the inhibitors competing with the acyl group, benzoyl-CoA had a significant inhibitory effect: 0.4 μmol/ml inhibited 25%. No formation of benzoyl-choline could be detected. Sodium hippurate, at a much higher concentration, 70 μmol/ml, inhibits to the same extent but only after preincubation. Succinyl-Coenzyme A neither inhibited ACh formation nor was it utilized for the synthesis of succinylcholine (BERMAN-REISBERG 1957).

A really potent and specific inhibitor of ChAc has not been found as yet. Such a compound obviously would be of great interest.

Literature

BADDILEY, J., and E. M. THAIN: Coenzyme A. Part II. Evidence for its formulation as a derivative of pantothenic acid-4' phosphate. J. chem. Soc. 1951, 2253—2258.

BANISTER, J., and M. SCRASE: Acetylcholine synthesis in normal and denervated sympathetic ganglia of the cat. J. Physiol (Lond.) 3, 437—444, (1950).

BERG, P.: Acyl adenylates: An enzymatic mechanism of acetate activation. J. biol. Chem. 222, 991—1013 (1956a).

— Acyl adenylates: The synthesis and properties of adenyl acetate. J. biol. Chem. 222, 1015—1023 (1956b).

BERMAN, R., I. B. WILSON and D. NACHMANSOHN: Choline acetylase specificity in relation to biological function. Biochim. biophys. Acta 12, 315—324 (1953).

BERMAN-REISBERG, R.: Sulfhydryl groups of choline acetylase. Biochim. biophys. Acta 14, 442—443 (1954).

— Properties and biological significance of choline acetylase. Yale J. Biol. Med. 29, 403—435 (1957).

BERNHARD, K.: Über die Herkunft der Essigsäure bei den Acetylierungen in vivo. I. Die Acetylierung von Sulfanilamid and p-Aminobenzoesäure bei gleichzeitigen Gaben von Deutero-Essigsäure. Hoppe-Seylers Z. physiol. Chem. 267, 91—102 (1940).

BERRY, J. F., and V. P. WHITTAKER: The acyl-group specificity of choline acetylase. Biochem. J. 73, 447—458 (1959).

BROWN, G. M., J. A. CRAIG and E. E. SNELL: Relation of the Lactobacillus bulgaricus factor to pantothenic acid and coenzyme A. Arch. Biochem. 27, 473—475 (1950).

BURGEN, A. S. V., G. BURKE and MARIE-LOUISE DESBARATS-SCHONBAUM: The specificity of brain choline acetylase. Brit. J. Pharmacol. Chemother. 11, 308—312 (1956).

CHANG, H. C., W. M. HSIEH, L. Y. LEE, T. H. LI and R. K. S. LIM: Studies on tissue acetyl-choline. VII. Acetylcholine content of various nerve trunks and its synthesis in vitro. Chin. J. Physiol. 14, 27—38 (1939).

COHEN, M.: Concentration of choline acetylase in conducting tissue. Arch. Biochem. 60, 284—296 (1956).

DAKIN, H. D.: The mode of oxidation in the animal organism of phenyl derivatives of fatty acids. Part V. Studies on the fate of phenylvaleric acid and its derivatives. J. biol. Chem. 6, 221—243 (1909).

EISENBERG, M. A.: The tricarboxylic acid cycle in Rhodospirillum Rubrum. J. biol. Chem. 203, 815—836 (1953).

— The acetate-activating enzyme of Rhodospirillum Rubrum. Biochim. biophys. Acta 16, 58—65 (1955).

FAHMY, A. R., B. E. RYMAN and E. O'F. WALSH: The inhibition of choline acetylase by nicotine. J. Pharm. (Lond.) 6, 607—609 (1954).

FEIGL, F.: Qualitative analysis by spot tests. Amsterdam: Elsevier 1946.

FELDBERG, W.: Synthesis of acetylcholine in sympathetic ganglia and cholinergic nerves. J. Physiol. (Lond.) **101**, 432—445 (1943).
— Present views on the mode of action of acetylcholine in the central nervous system. Physiol. Rev. **25**, 596—642 (1945).
FENG, T. P.: The heat production of nerve. Erg. Physiol., Biol. Chemie und Exp. Pharm. **38**, 73—132 (1936).
HEBB, C. O.: Biochemical evidence for the neural function of acetylcholine. Physiol. Rev. **37**, 196—220 (1957).
—, and G. M. H. WAITES: Choline acetylase in antero- and retro-grade degeneration of a cholinergic nerve. J. Physiol. (Lond.) **132**, 667—671 (1956).
HENSCHLER, D.: Zur Frage des Vorkommens von Butyrylcholin im Rindergehirn. Hoppe-Seylers Z. physiol. Chem. **305**, 97—104 (1956).
HESTRIN, S.: The reaction of acetylcholine and other carboxylic acid derivatives with hydroxylamine and its analytical application. J. biol. Chem. **180**, 249—261 (1949).
HOLTZ, P., u. H. J. SCHUEMAN: Butyrylcholine in Gehirnextrakten. Naturwissenschaften **41**, 3C6 (1954).
KLEIN, J. R., and J. S. HARRIS: The acetylation of sulfanilamide in vitro. J. biol. Chem. **124**, 613—626 (1938).
KNOCP, F.: Der Abbau aromatischer Fettsäuren im Tierkörper. Beitr. chem. Physiol. Path. **6**, 150—162 (1905).
KOENIG, E., and G. B. KOELLE: Acetylcholinesterase regeneration in peripheral nerve after irreversible inactivation. Science **132**, 1249—1250 (1960).
KOREY, S. R., B. DE BRAGANZA and D. NACHMANSOHN: Choline acetylase V. Esterifications and transacetylations. J. biol. Chem. **189**, 705—715 (1951).
KORKES, S., A. DEL CAMPILLO, I. C. GUNSALUS and S. OCHOA: Enzymatic synthesis of citric acid IV. Pyruvate as acetyl donor. J. biol. Chem. **193**, 721—735 (1951).
— A. DEL CAMPILLO, S. R. KOREY, J. R. STERN, D. NACHMANSOHN and S. OCHOA: Coupling of acetyl donor systems with choline acetylase. J. biol. Chem. **198**, 215—220 (1952a).
— — and S. OCHOA: Pyruvate oxidation system of heart muscle. J. biol. Chem. **195**, 541—547 (1952b).
KOSHLAND, D. E.: Group transfer as an enzymatic substitution mechanism. In: The Mechanism of Enzyme Action, W. D. McELROY and B. GLASS, eds. p. 608. Baltimore: Johns Hopkins Press 1954.
LIPMANN, F.: Acetylation of sulfanilamide by liver homogenates and extracts. J. biol. Chem. **160**, 173—190 (1945).
— Biosynthetic mechanisms. Harvey Lect. 1948/1949, 99—123 (1950).
— Enzymatic group activation and transfer. In: Metabolism of the Nervous System, D. RICHTER, ed. pp. 329—340. Pergamon Press 1957.
—, and N. O. KAPLAN: A common factor in the enzymatic acetylation of sulfanilamide and of choline. J. biol. Chem. **162**, 743—744 (1946).
— — G. D. NOVELLI, L. C. TUTTLE and B. M. GUIRARD: Coenzyme for acetylation, a pantothenic acid derivative. J. biol. Chem. **167**, 869—870 (1947).
LISSAK, K., and J. PASZTOR: Azetylcholingehalt sensibler Nerven. Pflügers Arch. ges. Physiol. **244**, 120—124 (1941).
LYNEN, F., E. REICHERT and L. RUEFF: Zum biologischen Abbau der Essigsäure. VI. „Aktivierte Essigsäure", ihre Isolierung aus Hefe und ihre chemische Natur. Liebigs Ann. **574**, 1—32 (1951).
MANN, P. J. F., M. TENNEBAUM and J. H. QUASTEL: Acetylcholine metabolism in the central nervous system. The effects of potassium and other cations on acetylcholine liberation. Biochem. J. **33**, 823—835 (1939).
MARKS, B. H.: Effect of barbiturates on acetylation. Science **123**, 332—333 (1956).
NACHMANSOHN, D.: Chemical mechanism of nerve activity. Ann. N. Y. Acad. Sci. **47**, 395—428 (1946).
— Chemical and Molecular Basis of Nerve Activity. New York: Academic Press 1959.
—, and M. BERMAN: Studies on choline acetylase. III. On the preparation of the coenzyme and its effect on the enzyme. J. biol. Chem. **165**, 551—563 (1946).
—, and H. M. JOHN: Inhibition of choline acetylase by α-keto acids. Proc. Soc. exp. Biol. (N. Y.) **57**, 361—362 (1944).
— — Studies on choline acetylase. I. Effect of amino acids on the dialyzed enzyme. Inhibition by α-keto acids. J. biol. Chem. **158**, 157—171 (1945).
— — and M. BERMAN: Studies on choline acetylase. II. The formation of acetylcholine in the nerve axon. J. biol. Chem. **163**, 475—480 (1946).
— — and H. WAELSCH: Effect of glutamic acid on the formation of acetylcholine. J. biol. Chem. **150**, 485—486 (1943).

54 Literature

NACHMANSOHN, D., and A. L. MACHADO: The formation of acetylcholine. A new enzyme "choline acetylase." J. Neurophysiol. **6**, 397—044 (1943).
—, and M. S. WEISS: Studies on choline acetylase. IV. Effect of citric acid. J. biol. Chem. **172**, 677—697 (1948).
— I. B. WILSON, S. R. KOREY and R. BERMAN: Choline acetylase. VI. Substitution of ATP-acetate by thiolacetate. J. biol. Chem. **195**, 25—36 (1952).
NOVELLI, G. D.: Metabolic functions of pantothenic acid. Physiol. Rev. **33**, 525—543 (1953).
—, and F. LIPMANN: The catalytic function of coenzyme A in citric acid synthesis. J. biol. Chem. **182**, 213—228 (1950).
— F. J. SCHMETZ Jr. and N. O. KAPLAN: Enzymatic degradation and resynthesis of coenzyme A. J. biol. Chem. **206**, 533—545 (1954).
RITTENBERG, D., and K. BLOCH: The utilization of acetic acid for the synthesis of fatty acids. J. biol. Chem. **160**, 417—424 (1945).
SCHOENHEIMER, R., and D. RITTENBERG: Deuterium as an indicator in the study of intermediary metabolism. J. biol. Chem. **114**, 381—396 (1936).
SHUSTER, L., and N. O. KAPLAN: A specific b nucleotidase. J. biol. Chem. **201**, 535—546 (1953).
SIMON, E. J., and D. SHEMIN: The preparation of S-succinyl-coenzyme A. J. Amer. chem. Soc. **75**, 2520 (1953).
SNELL, E. E., G. M. BROWN, V. J. PETERS, J. A. CRAIG, E. L. WITTLE, J. A. MOORE, V. M. MCGLOHON and O. D. BIRD: Chemical nature and synthesis of the *Lactobacillus bulgaricus* factor. J. Amer. chem. Soc. **72**, 5349—5350 (1950).
STADTMAN, E. R.: Coenzyme A-dependent transacetylation and transphosphorylation. Fed. Proc. **9**, 233 (1950).
— The purification and properties of phosphotransacetylase. J. biol. Chem. **196**, 527—534 (1952a).
— The net enzymatic synthesis of acetyl coenzyme A. J. biol. Chem. **196**, 535—546 (1952b).
— G. D. NOVELLI and F. LIPMANN: Coenzyme A function in and acetyl transfer by the phosphotransacetylase system. J. biol. Chem. **191**, 365—376 (1951).
STERN, J. R., and S. OCHOA: Enzymatic synthesis of citric acid. I. Synthesis with soluble enzymes. J. biol. Chem. **191**, 161—172 (1951).
— — and F. LYNEN: Enzymatic synthesis of citric acid. V. Reaction of acetyl coenzyme A. J. biol. Chem. **198**, 313—321 (1952).
— B. SHAPIRO, E. R. STADTMAN and S. OCHOA: Enzymatic synthesis of citric acid. III. Reversibility and mechanism. J. biol. Chem. **193**, 703—720 (1951).
WILSON, I. B.: Preparation of acetylcoenzyme. J. Amer. chem. Soc. **74**, 3205—3206 (1952).

Chapter 3

Formation, Storage, and Liberation of Acetylcholine

By

CATHERINE HEBB

Contents

Introduction

To fulfil its function as a chemical transmitter, acetylcholine (ACh) must be held ready in the tissue so that it can be liberated on demand, and following its release be replaced rapidly enough for transmission to occur repetitively in response to successive nerve impulses. The question of how the ester is replaced at the release points of the synapse in available form is one which as yet can be answered only in the most general way. In tissue such as the superior cervical ganglion of mammals the amount of ACh liberated by a single volley of impulses is only a fraction of the total amount present, and one might suppose that replacement occurs from the existing store of ester; but experiment has shown that even at stimulation rates of 20 per sec the release of ACh may continue for an hour or more while the tissue stores remain normal or are increased (see BROWN and FELDBERG 1936b, MACINTOSH 1959). It is evident then that re-synthesis alone can account for the replacement of the ester at the synaptic release points. Evidently the situation is more complicated, however, since there are other experiments to show that when synthesis of ACh in the ganglion is prevented some release still occurs, and as much as 90% of the tissue store may be mobilized by stimulation of the preganglionic nerve continued for an hour or longer (MACINTOSH l.c.). It must be assumed therefore that both re-synthesis and translocation of ester are involved in its replacement at the release points at least over periods as long as this, although it can not be excluded that the immediate means of replacement is normally by re-synthesis. The probability of a close spatial relation between release and re-synthesis is strengthened by the evidence that whether resting or active the tissue store of ACh always remains nearly constant.

In recent years these problems have been placed in new perspective by the theory of quantal release of ACh evolved by KATZ and his co-workers (see FATT and KATZ 1952, CASTILLO and KATZ 1954 et seq.), by electron microscopy of synaptic structures, and by studies of the intracellular distribution of ACh and choline acetylase (ChAc), the enzyme which synthesizes ACh. These developments and their bearing on the release of ACh from cholinergic nerve endings form the main topic of discussion in the present chapter. Nevertheless it may appear that the discussion ranges rather far afield from the events which occur at the synapse or neuromuscular junction. It must be remembered, however, that these are not the only places where ACh is to be found. As is well known, ACh (MACINTOSH 1941) and ChAc (see FELDBERG 1945, HEBB 1955, COHEN 1956) are both present in the axons of cholinergic nerves. This has been thought by some (see NACHMANSOHN 1959) to show that ACh plays an essential part in the conduction of the nerve impulse along the axon. However, the evidence is now so overwhelmingly against that idea (CASTILLO and KATZ 1953, DALE 1955, FATT 1954, HEBB 1957a, FELDBERG 1957), but at the same time so fully in accord with the classical theory of its role as a transmitter, that some other explanation for its presence in the axon must be sought. The one that at present seems most promising is derived from a consideration of the mechanisms of protein synthesis in nerve cells, and the application of WEISS's (WEISS 1947, WEISS and HISCOE 1948) hypothesis of axonal flow to the particular case of ChAc.

Different aspects of the problem will first be considered separately. Formation of ACh in vivo and in vitro will be described, prefaced by methods of measurement, and evidence about the species and tissue distribution of the synthesizing system will then be considered. The storage of ACh and the question of the spatial relation between storage and synthesis follows, and this in turn will provide the basis for the discussion of the release of the ester at various synapses and neuro-effector junctions.

Terminology

The term *cholinergic* is here used in its original meaning as an adjective describing a nerve which transmits its effects by release of ACh from its endings; *adrenergic* has an analogous meaning; *cholinoceptive* denotes a nerve cell or effector cell which is specifically responsive to ACh. The word *conduction*, unless qualified, refers to the passage of impulses along the axon, i.e., within the boundries of a single cell; *transmission* is used to denote only the *inter*cellular passage of the impulse.

Methods of study

A. Estimation of ACh in organs

A crude measure of the capacity of a tissue to form ACh may be obtained by measuring how much ester it contains under certain experimental conditions. It must be remembered that the concentration of ACh is limited more by the capacity of a tissue to store it in the bound form than by the ability to synthesize it. Nevertheless, useful information about the normal rates of synthesis *in vivo* can be obtained by experiments of this kind. BROWN and FELDBERG (1936b), for example, were able to determine the amount of ACh formed by a sympathetic ganglion during stimulation in an experiment in which they estimated the ACh content of resting and stimulated perfused ganglia and also measured the amount released into the effluent during stimulation. By this method they found that the superior cervical ganglion of the cat could synthesize 4 to 5 times the amount of ACh originally present in the ganglion during 3 hours' stimulation. This gives an upper rate of synthesis of approximately 40 μg/g tissue per hr. More recently MACINTOSH (1959) has reported experiments on ganglia perfused with plasma in which the rate of synthesis was nearly 3 times as high as this.

Three steps are necessary in the measurement of ACh in the tissue or body fluids: (1) The sample is extracted in acid solution under suitable conditions to preserve the ACh from hydrolysis. Frequently an anticholinesterase (anti-ChE) agent is injected into the animal before death for this purpose. If this is done, however, there is the possibility that the injection itself will cause some release of ACh, and so increase the amount of free ACh recovered from the tissue. (2) The extract is treated to remove or neutralize the acid and to make it suitable for contact with the assay tissue. (3) The ACh present in the sample is estimated by biological assay.

The method which is used in the reviewer's laboratory is as follows. The tissue is rapidly weighed and placed in not less than 2 vol. of ice-cold 10% TCA (trichloroacetic acid), where it is minced finely with scissors. For organs as small as sympathetic ganglia the amount of TCA used should be at least 1 ml. When instead of a tissue sample, a solution or dilute suspension of minced tissue is to be examined, higher concentrations (approaching 100% W/V) of TCA are added in smaller volume, so that the final concentration is also 10%. The acid suspension is allowed to stand at room temperature (20°) with occasional stirring for 1½ hr; it is then filtered and the precipitate washed with further small additions of 10% TCA. The combined filtrates are shaken up with about 4 vol. of water-saturated ether 3 or 4 times, or until the extract is at pH 4 (just acid to Congo Red). The residual ether is blown off by aeration. The extract is neutralized and tested. For this purpose the reviewer prefers the eserinized frog rectus abdominis muscle, but as an alternative or additional method uses the eserinized leech muscle or the guinea pig ileum. The identity of the active principle is checked further by subjecting the samples to alkaline hydrolysis. (For further details see MACINTOSH 1950. Other biological and chemical assays are described in Chapter 1.)

The amount of ACh recovered in an acid extract represents the total of "free" and "bound" ACh. To determine the free ACh only, the tissue is macerated or homogenized in eserinized saline solution (or other suitable medium, such as Ringer solution or isotonic sucrose solution), centrifuged, and the ACh in the supernatant measured by bioassay. The bound ACh is taken to be the difference between the total and free fractions.

Assay controls

In all bioassays, the effects of bioactive substances other than ACh which may be present in tissue extracts or incubates must be controlled if an accurate estimate of the concentration of the ester is to be obtained. In the reviewer's laboratory, controls of two kinds are used: (1) in an aliquot of the solution to be tested, the ACh present is destroyed by adding alkali ($N/3$ NaOH) and boiling briefly. In the assay the responses to the test solution are compared with known amounts of ACh that are made up with addition of an equivalent amount of the boiled control, neutralized before use with $N/3$ HCl (see FELDBERG 1950). This method may be used as a control for assays of tissue extracts or incubation products. (2) In studies of ACh synthesis *in vitro*, an alternative control solution is obtained by incubating inactivated (boiled) material under the same conditions as the test material. This is more convenient for routine use than the alkaline-boiled control, but it is safer to check the identity of the bioactive substance obtained from time to time by alkaline hydrolysis. All incubates are routinely boiled in acid (pH 4), neutralized, and diluted before testing (see also Chapter 1).

B. Respiring tissue slices and homogenates

The tissue slice technique provides another way of studying ACh metabolism. With this method the rate of synthesis is estimated as the difference between the original content of the tissue and the final amount present in both the tissue and the incubate. The ACh is determined by bioassay methods similar to those described in the previous section. Yields up to 50 μg/g tissue/hr have been obtained by methods of this kind (see MANN et al. 1938, 1939).

The slices are incubated aerobically at 37° C (temperatures as low as 20° C may give greater yields over longer periods, however) in a medium containing KCl, NaCl. CaCl$_2$, buffer (either phosphate or bicarbonate) and glucose. Pyruvate, acetate, choline or coenzyme A (CoA) are other additions which may be made.

FELDBERG (1950) recommends a high concentration of K (5 mg KCl/ml), little or no Ca, a low glucose (50 μg/ml) content, and an incubation volume not exceeding 2 ml per g of tissue. He suggests addition of CoA if the volume of the incubation medium is higher than this.

QUASTEL and his colleagues (see BRAGANÇA et al. 1953) employ in some experiments 0.028 M bicarbonate-Locke solution in an atmosphere of 93% oxygen and 7% CO$_2$. They incubate their slices in a Warburg manometric apparatus which permits them to follow other biochemical changes that may accompany synthesis.

The slice technique has a number of important advantages because it reproduces fairly closely conditions which obtain *in vivo* and yet permits controlled biochemical analysis of metabolic changes that are concerned in ACh production. It should be kept in mind that in the intact tissue the activity of the enzyme, ChAc, is subject to rate-limitations imposed both by the supply of substrates, choline and acetyl-CoA, and the removal of the reaction product, ACh, from the vicinity of the enzyme. These conditions also obtain in the tissue slice so that it is a means of studying how they operate *in vivo*. An example of the way in which tissue slices may be used with great advantage is in the study of inhibitors. Almost all of the substances which block ACh production *in vivo* seem to do so by reducing the availability of the substrates, either by diminishing the formation of acetyl-CoA or by blocking access of choline to the enzyme, so a study of their effects on tissue slices may provide information about mechanisms which normally maintain the supply of substrates for the enzyme.

On the other hand the technique has the disadvantage that effects which are due to a direct action on the enzyme immediately responsible for synthesis, namely ChAc, cannot be distinguished from more remote effects such as those which influence the supply of substrates. Accumulation of ACh in the tissue can also slow down the rate of synthesis very considerably, and thus mask other significant events in the system. An analysis of the action of any substance, either stimulatory or inhibitory, on tissue slices may therefore be possible only by a study of its individual effects on isolated parts of the system as well.

Synthesis of ACh may be examined also in homogenates under conditions which are similar to those used for tissue slices and which preserve respiratory activity. Except that intracellular structures are more accessible to substrates and other agents, there is little difference in principle between such preparations and tissue slices or minces, and they will not be described further here. (For an example of the use of this method see BRAGANCA and QUASTEL 1952.)

C. Direct assay of choline acetylase activity in tissue extracts and homogenates

I. Incubation methods

In the methods previously described, the supply of one of the substrates that is required in the final step in the acetylation of choline, namely acetyl-CoA, depends upon its formation by other enzymes in the system through a number of intermediate steps, any of which may be rate-limiting on the next. The formation of adenosine triphosphate (ATP) is one necessary step, and it in turn must be maintained by the respiratory activity of the tissue; accordingly, a diminution in respiratory activity, by limiting ATP formation, also limits choline acetylase.

It is therefore not surprising that extracts of nervous tissues that normally have quite a high turnover of ACh should synthesize only very small amounts when incubated without provision for ATP formation. But as NACHMANSOHN and MACHADO (1943) were the first to show, the addition of ATP as a reagent to a non-respiring system *in vitro* (homogenates of nerve tissue) not only brings the ACh production up to the level of a respiring system but far above it. In the same way it has since been shown that if provision is made for a supply of acetyl-CoA independently of that formed by the test tissue, then the rate of ACh synthesis

Table 1. *Incubation systems for measurement of choline acetylase (ChAc)*

(1)	(2)
1. 0.05 ml containing 15—20 units of *coenzyme A*	1. *Coenzyme A* as in (1)
2. 0.08 ml containing 2% *choline Cl* and 15% *KCl*	2. 0.08 ml of a solution containing 2% *choline Cl*, 6.6% *KCl* and 0.05% *eserine sulphate*
3. 0.14 ml of 1% *acetylphosphate*	
4. 0.08 ml of *1.2% MgCl₂ · 6 H₂O*	3. 0.2 ml of 2% *K-ATP* (Pabst salt neutralized with KOH and made up to volume with water)
5. 0.12 ml of *l-cysteine* (60 mg *l-cysteine* HCl neutralized with KOH and made up to volume of 2 ml)	
	4. MgCl₂ as in (1)
	5. 0.08 ml 6.6% *Na citrate*
6. 0.1 ml of *PTA**: 2.5 mg in 1 ml 0.02 M KHCO₃ (Preparation obtained from dried cells of *Clostridium kluyverii* according to instructions given by suppliers: Sigma Chemical Co. St. Louis, U.S.A.)	6. 0.08 ml 1.36% *Na Acetate · 2 H₂O*
	7. 0.12 ml of *l-cysteine* [solution as given under (1)]
7. 0.1 ml of 0.1% *eserine sulphate*	8. 0.1—0.2 ml *PLE* (aged pigeon liver enzyme described by KAPLAN and LIPMANN 1948)
* phosphotransacetylase	

Both (1) and (2) are incubated for 5 to 20 min (as may be convenient) at 38° (mammalian tissues) before addition of test material containing choline acetylase. This is added in suitable volume to bring total incubation volume to 1 ml and incubation is then continued for 1 hr (see text). PTA is phosphotransacetylase.

in vitro is in general increased still further (HEBB 1955, COHEN 1956). Thus the formation of acetyl-CoA in the presence of ATP, CoA and substrate is rate-limiting (presumably because the extracts or homogenates have too little of the enzymes necessary for its production), so measurements of the ChAc concentration of a tissue will be valid only if the method of testing it ensures an adequate supply of acetyl-CoA. This is done by using a coupled enzyme system as originally described by KORKES et al. (1952). Two incubation systems of this kind, which are given in Table 1, are used in the reviewer's laboratory.

In the first system, the one which is more generally useful because it can be used over a wide temperature range, acetyl-CoA is generated from acetylphosphate and coenzyme A by phosphotransacetylase (PTA). The second depends upon its generation from citrate and co-enzyme A, in the presence of ATP, by pigeon liver enzyme (PLE). For this purpose, aged pigeon liver extract (KAPLAN and LIPMANN 1948) in 0.02 M KHCO$_3$ is generally satisfactory, but some preparations give poor results for reasons not yet determined. An alternative preparation is obtained by $(NH_4)_2SO_4$ fractionation of fresh pigeon liver extracts. The 20 to 30% (W/V) fraction contains most of the activity.

With both systems all ingredients except the test enzyme are incubated together for a preliminary period of 10 to 20 min. Then, after addition of the test material, incubation is continued generally for 1 hr, but this period may be varied from 10 min to 2 hrs over which time the rate of synthesis remains approximately constant. Shorter periods may be used but the amount of ACh formed in less than 10 min by even the most active mammalian tissues may be too small to estimate with accuracy.

When extracts of acetone-dried nervous tissue are tested in either of these incubation media it is found that over a wide range the ACh synthesized is proportional to the amount of enzyme, expressed in terms of the weight of acetone powder extracted, that is added to the system (0.5 to 10 mg powder/ml incubate). The same proportionality exists for homogenates of fresh tissue but within narrower limits (4 to 12.5 mg fresh tissue/ml). Some tissues (hen sciatic nerve is an example) contain substances which inhibit the enzyme and accurate estimates of its activity can then only be obtained by using the lowest permissible concentration of tissue extract.

II. Determination of ChAc concentration in extracts of acetone-dried tissue

Of the methods employed by the reviewer, acetone-drying followed by aqueous extraction of the enzyme is the most reliable for estimations of the ChAc concentration in mammalian and avian tissues. It is also used very generally as a first step in the extraction of ChAc in other classes of vertebrates and invertebrates. In the reviewer's experience, however, it has not given satisfactory results with frog or dogfish tissues; in both species considerably higher activities in proportion to the weight of tissue extracted have been obtained from fresh homogenates.

Acetone powders of tissues are made according to the following procedure: the tissue is weighed, cooled, then placed in a cold mortar sufficiently large so that it will easily accommodate 100 vol. or more of acetone. A large volume (at least 100 vol. per g of tissue) of cold acetone (sufficiently cold to reduce the temperature of the tissue to —10°, but not colder than this) is poured over the tissue which is then squeezed flat with the pestle. The acetone is decanted through a Buchner filter of appropriate size fitted with 2 sheets of No. 30 Whatman paper; more cold acetone (about half the volume of the first wash) is added to the tissue, which is macerated further, and the wash again filtered off. The whole process is repeated until the tissue is reduced to as fine a powder as possible. After drying for 5 min on the Buchner filter, the filter paper with its cake of powder is put in a desiccator containing P$_2$O$_5$ and evacuated. It is then left at 3 to 10° for 3 to 5 hrs, when the powder is removed, weighed, and suspended in freshly prepared neutral cysteine-saline solution (containing the equivalent of 3 mg *l*-cysteine HCl per ml of 0.9% NaCl) in a known concentration (10, 25, 50 or 100 mg/ml, depending upon the amount of material and its expected activity). The suspensions are frozen and stored at —15° until they are to be tested. Before incubation they are centrifuged and the supernatant is recovered for testing.

III. Choline acetylase activity of homogenates

When an homogenate of rabbit cerebrum is compared with an extract of acetone powder made from an equivalent weight of brain it is found that the ChAc activity of the homogenate is 50 to 70% lower than the activity of the extract. The reason for this is that part of the brain ChAc is in a bound form.

The simplest and quickest way of activating the homogenate is to dilute it 1:1 or 1:3 with NaCl solution containing enough salt so that the final concentration is at least 1%, then to shake it with ether, 0.25 ml per ml of diluted enzyme, allow it to stand in the cold with occasional shaking for 20 min, and finally to blow off the ether with N_2 gas. Homogenates of mammalian brain prepared in this way have the same activity as extracts made from acetone powder.

It was suggested by HEBB and SMALLMAN (1956) that the explanation of the activation by ether may be that it breaks down the lipid membrane of the subcellular particles which contain the largest fraction of the enzyme, and that acetone probably has a similar action. However, these two agents are not equally effective on all tissues of vertebrate species; in some cases they are unnecessary while in others they may inhibit the enzyme. For example, homogenates of the brain of wrasse (a teleost fish) are fully active without any treatment; most of the enzyme is in the particulate fractions, but these require no activation with ether and are inhibited by the presence of Na ions in the incubate. In the light of other evidence it seems probable that this inhibition is due to competition with choline for access to the enzyme.

D. Preparation and testing of subcellular fractions of tissue homogenates

The method of separation of subcellular fractions is too well-known to need description here. The procedure used in the reviewer's laboratory is summarized in Table 2. Although we have used several different concentrations of sucrose for the preparation of homogenates, we prefer 0.32 M for routine experiments.

The addition of sucrose to the incubate in relatively high concentrations (0.4 M) does not alter the rate of synthesis of ACh by ChAc, so suspension and extraction in sucrose solutions, even in concentrations used for density gradient separation, do not affect the recovery except by dilution.

Dilution is in fact a more serious danger. Certain tissues such as spinal motor nerves lose activity when they are much diluted, and in the course of procedures involving washing and re-centrifuging of separate fractions some may become very dilute; with separation of separate fractions over a density gradient this is inevitable. The loss of activity seems to be due to oxidation of -SH-groups. Incubation at 37° of dilute homogenates of motor roots in the absence of other reagents rapidly inactivates them, but if cysteine is added to the homogenates before incubation, inactivation is prevented. The inactivation occurring during preparation of the fractions may be nearly irreversible under some conditions; recently, some evidence has been obtained that within certain limits incubation with *l*-cysteine can restore the activity lost in this way.

The method of density-gradient separation of fractions as used in the reviewer's laboratory was described by HEBB and WHITTAKER (1958) and WHITTAKER (1959).

Table 2. *Separation and characterization of subcellular fractions of brain and other nervous tissues*

A. *Separation*

Homogenate: contains 50 or 100 mg tissue per ml of 0.32 M sucrose with or without eserine
$(5 \times 10^{-5}$ M)

Centrifuged at 1,200—2,000 × 5 (g × min)

Precipitate = P 1 resuspended[1]   Supernatant = S 1 (first part)

Centrifuged as before   → *Combined S 1*

P 1 retained   Supernatant = S 1 (2nd part)   centrifuged at 12,000—15,000 × 20—30

Precipitate = P 2 resuspended[1]   Supernatant = S 2 (first part)

Centrifuged as before   → *Combined S 2*

P 2 retained   Supernatant = S 2 (2nd part)   Centrifuged at 100,000 × 30—60

Precipitate = P 3 retained   *Final supernatant = S 3 retained*

[1] Resuspended in $^1/_4$ or $^1/_2$ the original volume, and rehomogenized before recentrifuging. P 1 may with advantage be resuspended and re-centrifuged a further time.

B. *Characterization of mammalian brain fractions*

Fraction	Type and size of particle present	Janus Green Reaction	Remarks
P 1 (nuclear)	Nuclei, some mitochondria, intact cells, cell and tissue fragments. (B. & B., H. & W.)	Positive (++)	High concentration DNA (B. & B.)
P 2 (mito-chondrial)	Mitochondria (0.6—4 μ in largest diameter), unidentified granular profiles, large and small vesicles, smallest are 0.02 μ in dia. (W)	Positive (++++)	Contains highest concentration of typical mitochondrial enzymes (see A. et al., B. & B., H. & W., W., G. et al.). Probably some AChE (T)
P 3	Microsomes, vesicles and granules less than 1 μ in dia. (B. & B.). A few mitochondria occasionally	Positive (+) occasionally	Contains high RNA associated with granular profiles in this fraction. AChE is associated with some of the vesicles (T)
S 3	No formed elements provided that centrifuging is for 60 min as shown under (A)		

The initials in brackets refer to authors as follows: A. et al. = ABOOD et al (1952); B. & B. = BRODY and BAIN (1952); G. et al. = GALLAGHER et al. (1956); H. & W. = HEBB and WHITTAKER (1958); T. = TOSCHI (1959); W. = WHITTAKER (1959).

Formation of ACh

A. Tissue and cellular distribution of choline acetylase

I. General considerations

The ability of a tissue or cell to synthesize ACh depends first and foremost on the presence of ChAc. Although the measurement of the enzyme or of the ester itself does not provide evidence about its rate of formation or turnover *in vivo*, it does provide an obvious means of identifying those cells which produce ACh, and in the analysis of the nervous system is as good a guide as any to what proportion cholinergic neurones contribute to the structure of any one part. If, for example, a mixed nerve, such as the sciatic, and its component roots are analysed, it is found that the highest concentration of ChAc is in the ventral roots; negligible amounts are in the dorsal roots, while the concentration in the mixed spinal roots is midway between the two. Further, the main trunk of the sciatic at a level above which it gives off branches to the thigh muscles has a higher concentration of enzyme than at more peripheral levels where motor fibres do not form such a large proportion of the total bulk of tissue. Similarly, the cervical sympathetic nerve, which probably contains only motor fibres most of which are preganglionic and so cholinergic, has the highest ChAc activity of all peripheral nerve trunks tested, approaching that of the ventral roots; in comparison, the cervical vagus, which has a large sensory component, has a rather a low concentration of enzyme.

It should be emphasized that quantitative comparison of tissues in this way is valid only if the system of incubation used is optimal for ChAc, and this requires that the enzyme be incubated in a coupled system of the kind already described (see Table 1). Even with such a system however, there are other possible dangers. The tissue being tested may contain an inhibitory component, possibly a rival enzyme system which competes effectively with ChAc for acetyl-CoA. It is therefore a useful check to incubate tissue extracts, the properties of which are in this respect unknown, with a standard preparation of ChAc. If there is no inhibition the synthesizing activities of the two should be additive. For this purpose the reviewer uses as a standard preparation the 16 to 32% $(NH_4)_2SO_4$ (W/V) fraction of a cysteine-saline extract of acetone-dried rabbit cerebrum; unfractionated aqueous extracts of brain may be used instead.

A second source of difficulty for quantitative investigation is partial inactivation of the acetylating enzyme. As mentioned earlier, aqueous dilution of homogenates of ventral root and sciatic nerve may result in lower yields of ACh on incubation, and there is in such cases the possible danger that some unrecognized loss of enzyme may have occurred during the preparation. However, it has been found that when the enzyme activity of acetone-dried tissue, instead of homogenates, is measured, this source of error is avoided; accordingly, for certain purposes the former method is to be preferred. Very fortunately there is no significant post-mortem loss of enzyme activity as long as the tissue is intact. In the reviewer's laboratory it has been found that brain or peripheral nerve after being dissected out may be left for as long as two days in a moist atmosphere at room temperature (17° C) and still retain normal ChAc activity.

In the interpretation of quantitative data about the distribution of ChAc it is important to consider what part of the neuron is involved. In mammals the ChAc activity of the ventral roots, which are composed of cholinergic axons, is generally of the same order as the activity of the superior cervical ganglion even though much of the total bulk of tissue in the ganglion is made up of non-cholinergic ganglion cells, and the choline acetylase activity is contributed practically solely by the preganglionic endings (HEBB and WAITES 1956). In contrast to this, sites from which cholinergic axons take their origin, such as the ventral horn of the spinal cord, have rather a low concentration of choline acetylase. It is evident then that the axonal terminals have a higher activity than the rest of the neuron. This may in part be due to loss of the myelin sheath, but it points also to accumulation of enzyme in this region (see MACINTOSH 1941). This is one consideration which suggests that a large proportion of the nerve fibres which reach the caudate nucleus from other centres are cholinergic, since the concentration of ChAc in this nucleus averages higher than its concentration in the ventral roots (HEBB and SILVER 1956) or elsewhere in the mammalian nervous system.

II. Comparative data

One organism without the animal or vegetable kingdom, *Lactobacillus plantarum*, has been found to synthesize ACh at a high rate, 16 μg/mg dried cells/hr (STEPHENSON and ROWATT 1947), but this is the only known instance of bacterial formation of ACh. Among plants reported to contain ACh are the fungus *Claviceps purpurea* (EWINS 1914), two varieties of nettles (EMMELIN and FELDBERG 1947, 1949), and most recently the Malayan Jack-fruit plant (LIN 1957). Except for two protozoa, *Paramecium* (BAYER and WENSE 1936) and *Trypanosoma rhodesiense* (BULBRING et al. 1949), only multicellular animals, and probably only those with specialized conducting tissue, can synthesize ACh. Among invertebrates, the highest rates of synthesis so far observed are in squid ganglia (KOREY et al. 1953) and in the nervous system of insects (SMALLMAN 1956, COLHOUN 1958b). Evidence of ACh synthesis, although at much lower rates, by non-nervous tissue of *Mytilus edulis* first reported by BULBRING et al. (1953) has recently been confirmed by MILTON (1959).

Among vertebrate species, very high rates of ACh synthesis are found among teleost fishes (COHEN 1956, MILTON 1958), birds (HEBB 1955) and mammals (HEBB 1955, COHEN 1956, HEBB and SILVER 1956). Unpublished experiments conducted in the reviewer's laboratory indicate that the rate of ACh synthesis may be lowest in elasmobranchs. It was found that the highest rates obtained on incubating nervous tissues of the dogfish were only about 2% of that observed with the brain of the teleost fish wrasse *(Labrus bergylta)*. The values observed for rates of synthesis in the frog, *Rana temporaria*, and the snake, *Natrix natrix*, were higher than this, but they too were low, particularly in the frog, in comparison with mammals, birds, and teleosts.

A number of instances of synthesis by non-nervous tissue of multicellular animals is recorded in the literature. In an earlier review (HEBB 1957a) to which the reader is referred for further information about this question it was concluded that the evidence for this occurrence was satisfactory for only relatively few tissues. Among these are the human placenta, the ungulate spleen, and the gill-plates of *Mytilus edulis*.

BULL et al. (1961) have recently reported very high rates of synthesis in immature human placentas. The rate of ACh production observed in some samples was higher than any found as yet in other vertebrate tissues.

III. Mammalian nervous system

1. Peripheral nerves

The distribution of ACh and ChAc have been more carefully studied in mammals than in other classes of animals. From the analysis of peripheral nerve trunks, two groups of neurons emerge: those which contain ACh and ChAc in relatively high concentrations and those which contain little or no ester or enzyme. The ability to form and store ACh appears to be confined to the cholinergic nerves (*i.e.*, the somatic motor nerves, all autonomic preganglionic trunks, and parasympathetic post-ganglionic fibres), but of these only the somatic motor and sympathetic preganglionic trunks have been examined under controlled conditions for either their ACh content (MacIntosh 1938, 1941) or their ChAc activity (Banister and Scrase 1950, Hebb 1955, Hebb and Waites 1956, Hebb and Silver 1956, Cohen 1956).

Table 3. *ACh and choline acetylase in some peripheral and central nervous tissues*

Tissue	ACh content		Choline acetylase	
	μg/g fresh tissue	(species)	μg ACh formed/g fresh tissue per hr	(species)

(a) *Peripheral*

Tissue	ACh content		Choline acetylase	
Ventral spinal roots . . .	9—18	(dog, cat)	2500, 4000, 5000 ‡	(goat, rabbit, dog)
—	—	—	2200, 4700*	(ox, dog)
Dorsal spinal roots . . .	0—0.25	(dog, cat)	0—6	(cat, dog, ox)
—	—	—	7—20*	(ox, dog)
Mixed spinal roots	6	(cat)	480—950, 2080 ‡	(goat, rabbit)
Sciatic N	4—6	(cat)	300—680, 1120 ‡	(goat, rabbit)
—	—	—	250*	(rabbit)
Superior cervical ganglion	18—44	(cat)	1600—2000‡	(sheep)

(b) *Central*

Tissue	ACh content		Choline acetylase	
Spinal cord, ventral horn of grey matter	1.5	(dog)	500 ‡	(goat)
Cerebellar cortex	0.1—0.3	(man, cat)	0—6	(man, dog, cat)
Retina	5—6	(ox, sheep)	1020, 3000—3500	(ox, sheep)
Optic N	0—0.3	(ox, cat)	0—6	(ox, cat, rabbit)
—	—	—	15—20*	(rabbit)
Sup. colliculus	1.7	(cat)	400	(cat)
Basal ganglia	7	(cat)	—	—
Caudate nucleus	—	—	3000—4000 ‡	(sheep, goat)
Occipital lobe cortex . . .	2.2	(cat)	175	(cat)
Frontal lobe cortex . . .	4.5	(cat)	270	(cat)
Olfactory bulb	1.3	(cat)	440	(cat)

Notes: (1) Values for ACh content are from MacIntosh (1941) and Feldberg (1945).
(2) Most of the values for choline acetylase are from Hebb and Silver (1956) recalculated for fresh tissue on the assumption that 1 g acetone powder is equivalent to 5 g fresh tissue, but those marked * are from Cohen (1946), while those marked ‡ are unpublished values obtained in the reviewer's laboratory.

The evidence that postganglionic adrenergic fibres do not contain ACh or the synthesizing enzyme is derived mainly from experiments in which the superior cervical ganglion and the proximal part of its postganglionic fibres have been analysed after chronic preganglionic denervation of the ganglion. Evidence that ACh and ChAc are not present in peripheral sensory nerves is derived from analysis of predominantly sensory nerves (MacIntosh 1941) and dorsal roots (MacIntosh 1941, Hebb 1955, Wolfgram 1954, Hebb and Silver 1956, Cohen 1956). Whether ACh and the synthesizing enzyme are absent from all first order sensory fibres is not so certain as that it must be absent from most. Their concentrations in the dorsal roots are so small that they cannot be detected with certainty (see Table 3). Cohen, however, obtained rates of synthesis of ACh by dorsal roots of ox of 7 to 49 μg/g acetone powder per hr; that might suggest that the dorsal roots of this species contain at least a small number of cholinergic fibres. Obviously, however, not all can be cholinergic since in the corresponding ventral roots the rate of synthesis is about 300 times greater.

In the reviewer's laboratory, we have never found rates of synthesis in dorsal roots of any species, including the ox, exceeding 25 μg/g acetone powder per hr except when the roots were dissected out in such a way as to include part of the ganglion, and so possibly to contaminate the preparation with some ventral root fibres; at the level of the ganglion there is no longer a clear demarcation between motor and sensory fibres. It is just possible, therefore, that the higher values reported by COHEN for the dorsal roots were due to contamination with ventral root fibres.

Nevertheless, our results do not exclude absolutely the possibility that a very small proportion of fibres may contain choline acetylase, but by extrapolation from results on other mixed nerves this could not amount to more than 10% at most. The difficulty is that the sensitivity of the method is not sufficient to detect such small amounts, and any values from 0 to 25 μg (which are those we have reported) can be taken as evidence only that they are below the values we are able to detect with certainty. In this connection it is perhaps worth pointing out that apparently higher values can be obtained if the assays are done without the kind of controls indicated in the first section of this chapter; this danger becomes greater as higher concentrations of tissues are used in the incubation (see HEBB 1955).

Since about 10 to 15% of the dorsal root ganglion cells contain relatively high concentrations of acetylcholinesterase (AChE) in their cytoplasm, as GIACOBINI (1956) originally reported and we have confirmed (unpublished histochemical data), it is conceivable that these cells also contain ChAc and give rise to fibres that contain the enzyme. This suggestion is put forward as a possibility rather than a probability. Apart from the unreliability of measurements of ChAc activity in this tissue, already referred to, there is as yet no other independent evidence to suggest the presence of such fibres in the dorsal roots.

MACINTOSH's (1941) finding, based on two experiments on cats, that after aseptic section of the vagus nerve above the nodose ganglion ACh disappears more slowly from the cervical portion of the nerve than would be expected if all the cholinergic fibres in the trunk had been separated from their cells of origin, should also be mentioned here. He thought that the result might be attributable to the presence of cells in the nodose ganglion that give rise to efferent cholinergic fibres running downwards in the vagus. HOWEVER, choline acetylase disappears almost completely from the nodose ganglion itself when denervated in this way (BANISTER and SCRASE 1950) so MACINTOSH's explanation seems unlikely; and for the same reason it is equally unlikely that the fibres responsible could be derived from sensory cells belonging to the ganglion. What is more probable is that in MACINTOSH's experiments the vagal trunk which he analyzed contained aberrant fascicles of fibres properly belonging to the cervical sympathetic trunk since dissection of the two nerve trunks quite frequently reveals communicating branches between them, especially near the level of the middle cervical ganglion (see DALY and MOUNT 1951).

To summarize then, there is at present no certain evidence to show that any first order sensory or adrenergic neurons contain either ACh or the enzyme system which synthesizes it. On the other hand, it is probable that the majority of such fibres are virtually devoid of both.

2. Central nervous system

Turning now to the central nervous system (CNS) the position is somewhat different, since here it is more difficult to relate the analytical data for ACh and ChAc to specific groups of neurons. However, it can be shown, as in the periphery, that there are some central neurons which contain neither enzyme nor ester and equally there are others which do. The optic nerve and exterior layers of the cerebellar cortex are both tissues that are devoid of significant amounts of ACh (MACINTOSH 1941, FELDBERG 1945) and ChAc (HEBB 1955, HEBB and SILVER 1956). Other tissues of the CNS sampled by MACINTOSH, contain amounts of ACh varying from less than 0.02 μg/g fresh tissue (less than significant) in some tracts to as much as 7 μg/g in the basal ganglia. There are even larger variations in the ChAc content, for which the ratio of highest to lowest value (taken as 25 μg/g fresh tissue) is of the order of 700:1 in most mammals.

None of the centres, however, has such high concentrations of ACh as have the majority of peripheral ganglia and motor nerve trunks. For this reason one might suspect that the proportion of cholinergic neurons contributing to any one part of the brain is always lower. However, it is possible that the lower concentrations may simply reflect a lower storage capacity in a tissue which has an equally high turnover rate of the ester. This view is to some extent borne out by the results of analyses of ChAc concentration in different parts of the brain.

These shown that in some parts of the CNS, notably the caudate nucleus, olfactory trigone, and retina, the enzyme concentration may be higher than it is in most peripheral nerves and ganglia. Furthermore while tissues in the CNS which do not contain significant amounts of the enzyme are also devoid of ACh, in other respects their distributions are not so well correlated. For example, the occipital lobe cortex of the cat has an ACh content about 70% higher than that of the olfactory bulb, while the ChAc concentration in the same region of the cortex is less than one-half that of the bulb.

These are differences which can at least in part be related to differences in the parts of the neuron which contribute the highest proportion of enzyme and ACh to the tissue being sampled. Where these are nerve endings, as in ganglia, the total ACh tends to be higher in proportion to the ChAc content than it is when cholinergic axons make up the bulk of the tissue. The difference is referred to again in a later part of this chapter.

Table 3 gives some representative values of ACh and ChAc concentrations in the mammalian nervous system. The original papers quoted should be consulted for other values.

FELDBERG and VOGT (1948) originally put forward the interesting idea that in the CNS cholinergic may alternate with non-cholinergic neurons somewhat as they do in sympathetic pathways. In support of this idea they cited evidence showing that in two sensory pathways, auditory and visual, the second and fourth order neurons are probably cholinergic, while the first and third are not. Since then evidence for a similar alternation involving at least the first two neurons has been found in the olfactory pathway (HEBB and SILVER 1956), but except in the sensory pathways the rule generally breaks down. For example, when the proprioceptive pathways are followed into the cerebellum it appears that a second order cholinergic neuron is followed by several non-cholinergic neurons in succession to one another (HEBB 1957b and unpublished experiments).

TOWER and ELLIOTT (1952) carried out a series of measurements on the cortical tissue of 9 species of mammals of varying brain weights that enabled them to compare the relations of cholinesterase (ChE) activity, ACh content, and free and bound ACh synthesis (in tissue slices) with the relation of cell density, or number of neurons per mm³, to brain weight, which varied in the species chosen from 0.4 g (the mouse) to 1320 g (man). Their results showed that both the parameters of the ACh system and the density of the cell population declined with increasing brain size. Moreover, there was an approximately linear relation between the log brain weight and the log of each ACh component, as well as the log of the cell counts; and the slopes of all these lines were roughly parallel. They therefore drew the conclusion that the "decrease in values for components of the ACh system with increasing brain mass may be associated with or reflected in the decrease in neuron density of the cortex". That in turn might be interpreted to mean that the proportion of cholinergic to non-cholinergic neurons remains constant during the evolutionary enlargement of the cerebral cortex in the higher mammals.

On the other hand HEBB and SILVER (1956) concluded from a comparative study of ChAc that the great decline in enzyme concentration of the neocortex which is associated with its evolutionary development implies a relative increase in the numbers of non-cholinergic neurons. Part of this enzyme change must be attributed to change in cell density, however, as ELLIOTT (personal communication) has pointed out; but if the logs of the values for ChAc concentration for a given area of the cortex, such as area 17, are plotted against the logs of brain weight and superimposed on the curve relating cell density to brain weight, we find that the values for man fall significantly below the curve while those for certain species, e.g., the horse, ox, sheep, dog, guinea-pig, and rabbit, are considerably above it, so it would appear to be true that in man, at least as compared with these other mammals, the decline in ChAc is proportionately greater than the decline in cell numbers.

The fact that the ACh content, tissue slice synthesis, and ChE values appear to be more closely related to the cell density (numbers per unit volume) than is the ChAc concentration is not perhaps surprising. As mentioned earlier the ratio between ChAc and ACh content tends to be lower in synaptic tissue than it is in axonal tissue; that is, ACh is relatively higher in synapses probably because the endings are structurally adapted for ACh storage. The correlation observed by TOWER and ELLIOTT may therefore mean that the volume of synaptic tissue to which cholinergic endings contribute is a function of the total number of cells present even though the proportion of cholinergic neurons decreases. In that case it would appear that increasing branching and arborization of the axon terminals compensates in part for a decrease in numbers of cholinergic neurons that give rise to them. It would also suggest that the proportion of cholinoceptive cells remains constant from one species to another.

B. Intracellular distribution of choline acetylase and ACh

I. In brain

By the method of differential centrifugation HEBB and SMALLMAN (1956) showed that 70 to 90% of the ChAc present is attached to the particulate cell structure; the balance is in the soluble cytoplasmic fraction recovered as the final supernatant; of all particulate fractions, the one which exhibits most enzyme activity is the large granule fraction which also contains the mitochondria. Fifty to 70% of the enzyme is present in this fraction. By the normal methods of preparation, however, the fraction has only about 20% of its true ChAc activity; its full activity can be realised *in vitro* by treatment with ether or by some other organic solvents. The activating effect of the ether was thought to be due to the destruction of a lipid membrane which might act as a barrier preventing contact of the substrates (particularly choline) with the enzyme. Since mitochondria have selectively permeable membranes it seemed possible then that the enzyme might be held within these cell organelles. Later, however, this was shown to be incorrect by HEBB and WHITTAKER (1958) who found that the particles containing ChAc could be separated from the mitochondria by centrifuging over a density gradient column (0.8 to 1.6 M sucrose). The ChAc particles found between the 0.8 and 1.2 M layers were lighter than the mitochondria, the bulk of which were recovered between the 1.2 and 1.6 M layers.

In these experiments it was shown also that the intracellular distribution of ACh in brain tissue is similar to that of ChAc. In the same way that 70 to 90% of ChAc is attached to the particulate fractions so the same proportion of ACh is 'bound' to the particulate, while the balance, corresponding to the "free" ACh, is recoverable as a dissolved constituent of the cytoplasm in the final supernatant. Again, the largest proportion of the bound ACh is in the large granule fraction and when this is analyzed further by the density gradient technique the activity appears in the same layers (between 0.8 and 1.2 M sucrose) as does the ChAc. From these experiments it is possible to equate the classical 'free' ACh with the dissolved fraction, and 'bound' ACh with the particulate fractions; correspondingly, all the dissolved enzyme is fully active, while that which is attached to the particulate is only partially active. These analogies in the binding of enzyme and ester suggested that in the particulate fractions they are both held together within the same particles, an idea that was to same extent supported by additional evidence showing that agents such as ether which fully activate the enzyme also release all the ACh from the particulate, while other procedures, such as freezing and thawing, which partially activate the enzyme release a proportionate amount of ACh.

The question next considered by WHITTAKER (1959) was whether these particles, which may carry 50% or more of the brain ACh and ChAc, are synonomous with the synaptic vesicles that have been identified by electron microscopy and are thought by some to be carriers of neurohumours, such as ACh and "sympathin" (see DE ROBERTIS and BENNETT 1955, PALAY and PALADE 1955, CASTILLO and KATZ 1956, FERNANDÉZ-MORÁN 1957). WHITTAKER examined the particulate fraction containing the highest concentrations of ACh and ChAc, under the electron microscope. This fraction, which had a density lying between 0.8 M and 1.2 M sucrose, he found to contain particles 0.02 to 0.3 μ in diameter; over 60% had a diameter of between 0.02 and 0.08 μ, and so corresponded in size to the synaptic vesicles which have a diameter ranging between 0.02 to 0.06 μ. WHITTAKER showed also that this same fraction contains most of the brain 5-hydroxytryptamine. Finally, from his analysis of the binding of ACh present in this fraction he suggested that the bound ester present at the synapse is held with ChAc in vesicles, which contain some ACh in simple solution and some attached to the matrix. The presence of two fractions of 'bound' ACh was postulated to account for the fact that mildly disruptive procedures liberate part but not all of the ACh, and that the bound ester still remaining after such procedures is protected from hydrolysis by ChE (see Chapter 1 of this volume). It has been suggested elsewhere (HEBB 1959) that this evidence may be accounted for by the alternative hypothesis that some vesicles in the total population are more labile than others. According to this view, all the ACh within each particle is in solution in a concentration governed by the equilibrium between substrate supply and the ester accumulated by the activity of the ChAc present.

II. In the peripheral nervous system

The subcellular distribution of ChAc in the ventral roots has been studied in detail by HEBB et al. (1959 and unpublished experiments). One of the objectives of this work was to find out whether the distribution revealed by centrifugation of brain homogenates is representative of the distribution in all parts of the neurons containing the enzyme, or whether it is an average distribution for material to which nerve endings may have contributed the largest proportion of enzyme. If this second alternative is right and the enzyme is not similarly bound in all parts of the cell, then centrifugal analysis of the motor roots may be expected to reveal a distribution different from that of brain.

The results of the centrifugal analysis of the motor roots seem to fulfil this expectation. In the first place it was found that the fraction with the greatest activity is the microsomal or small granule fraction. This contains only 5 to 15% of the enzyme of brain tissue, but is the most active of the ventral root fractions, containing up to 50% of the total enzyme. The percentage distribution of activity in the separate fractions is shown in Table 4. Another difference between the ventral root and brain homogenates is that ether treatment does not have the same effect. Treatment of the whole homogenate of the roots with ether in the presence of NaCl increases its activity by about 25 to 50%, but there is little or no activating effect on the larger particulate fractions, nuclear or mitochondrial, while the microsomal fraction is activated to about the same extent as the whole homogenate. The addition of NaCl in concentrations of 0.25% is essential to the activating effect of ether on nerve homogenates; it is not essential for activation of brain homogenates.

The axonal enzyme differs also from the brain enzyme in being less stable. As already mentioned under "*Methods*", some inactivation of the enzyme may occur during the separation of the different fractions. Accordingly, it is difficult to obtain a reliable balance sheet to show how the original activity is distributed in the different fractions, although in general the recovery is of the order of 70 to 90%, so the error is not large (see Table 4). All the fractions tend to show some loss but the most stable is the microsomal fraction which, as already stated, is the most active. However, attempts to refractionate microsomal preparations over a density gradient have failed to yield more than 33% recovery to date, apparently due to losses of activity associated with dilution of the material. Of the activity recovered, 90% was found in a narrow band in the region corresponding in density to 0.8 M sucrose.

Table 4. *Intracellular distribution of choline acetylase in central and peripheral nervous tissue of some vertebrates*

Species	Tissue	% of recovered activity in particulate and supernatant fractions				% recovery
		P 1	P 2	P 3	S	
Sheep, goat, rabbit guinea-pig	*Cerebrum and caudate nucleus*	13—30	**46—49**	3—14	5—30	93—100
Dog, rabbit, goat	*Ventral spinal roots*	18—30	4—21	**45—55**	5—15	70—90
Goat, rabbit	*Sciatic N*	35—40	2—15	28—45	15—20	70—80
Sheep (2 expts)	*Superior cervical ganglion*	**67—79**	14—16	3—5	2—14	85—94
Pigeon and chicken	*Cerebrum*	7—13	**43—47**	7—9	32—42	94—104
Chicken (1 expt)	*Sciatic N*	6	5	8	81	83
Wrasse (1 expt)	*Brain*	49	44	7	—	108

Notes: (1) The fractions, P 1—P 3 and S correspond approximately to those in Table 2; the recoveries given in the last column refer to the sum of the activities in the fractions expressed as a percentage of the activity in the whole homogenate.

(2) Figures in heavier type indicate the fraction which for a given tissue is regularly found to have the highest activity. In birds the supernatant (*S*) has the highest activity for tissues other than the cerebrum, including optic lobes, hindbrain, spinal cord, and sciatic nerves. This may reflect a greater fragility of subcellular structures. See text.

(3) The values given in this table are taken from HEBB and SMALLMAN (1956), HEBB and WHITTAKER (1958) and other experiments carried out in the reviewer's laboratory not yet published.

The smaller effect of ether, the greater instability of the enzyme, and the fact that most of it is in the microsomal fraction were all differences suggesting that in the axon the enzyme is bound differently from the way in which it is bound in the brain. There appears to be a difference also between the brain and spinal roots in the way in which ACh is bound.

In two unpublished experiments, WHITTAKER and HEBB found that most of the ACh which could be recovered from homogenized ventral roots was free; since then, two further experiments have given a similar result, and in this tissue it would appear that the correlation between the intracellular distributions of ACh and ChAc does not obtain. This result is not altogether unexpected however if it is considered in terms of the vesicular hypothesis. It has already been suggested that the effect of ether in activating ChAc and releasing ACh is due to the disruption of vesicles containing both enzyme and ester; but the fact that the activating effect of ether on the enzyme is relatively slight would suggest either that in the axon ChAc is not so completely protected by a vesicular membrane as it is in the brain, or that in the axon the vesicles are less stable structures. In either case one would expect to find in the axon by the usual methods of extraction less bound ACh associated with the enzyme.

These results do not show that the distribution of ChAc in ventral roots is typical of axons as such. It may be typical of peripheral as opposed to central nervous tissues. For this reason it is of interest to consider the distribution in cholinergic nerves nearer to their terminations, and at the terminations themselves. The values given in Table 4 show how the distribution in the sciatic nerves and in the superior cervical ganglia compares with the distribution of the enzyme in the brain and spinal roots. The higher enzyme activity in Pl (the nuclear fraction) of the sciatic nerve trunk is probably due to the presence of incompletely homogenized tissue in this fraction. Tissues of this kind are extremely tough and it is not possible to break them up completely in an homogenizer. However, that explanation does not apply to the superior cervical ganglia. The ganglia were considerably easier to homogenize then the sciatic nerves; microscopic examination of Pl indicated that the proportion of intact tissue in it was about the same as in the same fraction of ventral root or brain homogenates. Nevertheless it contained 65 to 80% of all the enzyme recovered.

A possible explanation is that at the subcellular level the ganglion does have a greater mechanical resistance and that this is sufficient to prevent complete separation of the ChAc particles. This might be due to protection afforded to the synaptic terminals by the satellite cells (see CAUSEY and HOFFMAN 1956). Because of this an assembly of vesicles in an axon terminal might precipitate as a single particle of nuclear dimensions. In this connection it is of interest that ANDERSSON-CEDERGREN (1959) has described the grouping together of vesicles in peripheral axon terminals in what she has termed "X" components. In these it appears that relatively large numbers of vesicles are held together within a much larger vesicular type of structure. Possibly structures such as these sediment with the nuclear fraction of the ganglionic homogenates and so account for its high ChAc activity.

These considerations suggest the further possibility that the relatively small particles recovered in the large granule fraction of brain, which apparently contain ACh and ChAc, are present in that fraction because they too are held together in aggregates which precipitate more readily than the constituent particles would do. PALAY (1956 and 1958) has emphasized that the vesicles in the *boutons terminaux* of the CNS are arranged in clusters; these might be held together in such a way that they would precipitate in the same fraction as the mitochondria since the clusters are about that order of size. This idea is to some extent born out by the results recently obtained by GREY and WHITTAKER (1960).

It is possible then that differences in the distribution of ChAc in the particulate fractions of brain, ventral roots, and peripheral nerve endings are related not to differences in the size of the individual particles bearing the enzyme but to differences in their grouping. It may be that it is only in the axon that the particles can be separated from one another experimentally with the consequence that they precipitate, as would be expected from their size, in the microsomal fraction. It may also be that it is due to their isolation that their enzyme is more unstable and apparently in a more exposed position.

III. Comparative data

The subcellular distributions of ACh and ChAc have not been studied extensively in species other than mammals, but data have been published for the pigeon (HEBB and WHITTAKER 1958, BELLAMY 1959) and for the locust, *Schistocerca gregaria* (BELLAMY 1958). COLHOUN (1958b) has indicated that in the cockroach, *Periplaneta americana L.*, ChAc and ACh have a similar subcellular distribution, but he gave no details. In unpublished experiments HEBB and MILTON studied the ChAc distribution in particulate fractions of the brain of a teleost fish, *Labrus bergylta*. The particulate enzyme of this species differed from its mammalian counterpart in that it required no activation by ether, was inhibited by as little as 0.1% NaCl, and was osmotically more sensitive. In 0.3 M sucrose, for example, much of the enzyme was apparently freed from the particulate fraction, but in 0.5 M sucrose all the enzyme was distributed among the particulate fractions, as shown in Table 4. This table and the next summarize some of the comparative data about the distribution of ACh and the enzyme.

Significance of ChAc and ACh in the proximal part of the axon

Two explanations for the presence of ACh and ChAc in the axon have been suggested. According to the first, ACh has a function in the conduction of the nerve impulse (NACHMANSOHN 1959). However, in the reviewer's opinion, there is as yet no critical evidence to substantiate this theory, while against it there is a great deal of evidence to show that ACh and the synthesizing enzyme are not present in all types of nerve fibres although conduction in them appears to be dependent on similar mechanisms. Moreover, BRADY et al. (1958) have recently shown that injection of a number of potent inhibitors of ACh synthesis as well as other substances, including AChE, into the squid giant axon has no effect on conduction, although ACh is normally found in these fibres.

A second explanation is based on the theory of axoplasmic flow, as outlined experimentally by WEISS in 1947 and more fully stated by WEISS and HISCOE (1948) the following year. In some ways this theory is an elaboration of the doctrine of continuity, according to which the growth or regeneration of the axon is dependent upon its continuity with the perikaryon and upon the trophic influence exerted by the Nissl bodies and nucleus (see CAJAL 1928). But neither CAJAL nor his predecessors who had helped to develop this concept were able to say precisely how the trophic influence of the neuronal cell body is exerted; because WEISS's experiments seemed to offer the first concrete explanation of this relation, they immediately attracted a great deal of interest.

In his first experiments WEISS (1947) showed that ligature of a nerve permanently reduces the diameter of the constituent nerve fibres on the distal side, while causing them to swell on the proximal side, and that subsequent release of the ligature allows the dammed-up material to advance distally at about 1 mm or more per day. From these and subsequent experiments it was concluded that the growth of a nerve fibre depends upon the production by the perikaryon of new axoplasm which is siphoned into the axon by an "axomotile" mechanism, and that the column of axoplasm originating in this way is maintained in constant proximo-distal motion. Thus, the trophic influence of the cell is defined as a material supply line that maintains the structure of the axon as a whole, and the somewhat vague ideas of earlier workers about the nutritive function of the cell-body are given a more precise meaning that accords well with modern ideas about the role of the Nissl bodies and nucleus in protein synthesis (see CASPERSSON 1941, HYDÉN 1943, CAUSEY and STRATMANN 1956).

In 1948, FELDBERG and VOGT suggested that the presence of ChAc in the axon might be most simply accounted for in terms of this hypothesis by assuming that it is in transit between the cell body, where it is manufactured, and the nerve endings where it has its function. Subsequently, HEBB and WAITES (1956) verified this idea experimentally when they showed that ligation or section of the cervical sympathetic nerve causes ChAc to accumulate on the proximal side, rising to a maximum some 7 days after section, and to decrease on the distal side. On the distal side almost all of the enzyme disappears in 3 to 4 weeks. Its sole provenance therefore appears to be the cell-bodies of the neurons.

Section of the nerve produces similar changes in other axonal constituents, namely AChE (SAWYER 1946), lipolytic esterase (LUMSDEN 1952) and substance P (HOLTON 1959), but while each of these falls to about 40% of its original level in the distal segment in the first stages of degeneration, there is little or no further loss in the later stages. This argues that these moieties are in part attached to the neurilemma or some associated tissue which is not destroyed by sectioning. Whatever the reason, however, the fact they that do not wholly disappear from the distal segment leaves open the possibility that they are derived originally not only from the neurons but from other elements, such as the cells of Schwann or the connective tissue cells, as well.

Nevertheless it should be pointed out that of the enzymes concerned in ACh metabolism, it is only AChE which has been identified with certainty in the cell bodies of cholinergic neurons. Moreover, any doubts that may exist about its manufacture at this site should now be dispelled by the recent, very elegant experiments of FUKUDA and KOELLE (1959), who have shown that after poisoning with di*iso*propylphosphorofluoridate (DFP), AChE first reappears in the perikaryon, and within so short a period that it must be assumed to be new enzyme (for a fuller account of these experiments see Chapter 6).

All evidence therefore implicates the cell body as the sole or chief site of *de novo* protein synthesis within the neuron; and if this is accepted it follows that the ChAc found at the nerve terminals must previously have traversed the whole length of the nerve fibre; hence its presence is to be expected in all parts of those neurons in which it has a function. There is still little evidence, however, to show how transport of the enzyme is effected. One possibility is that it forms a static part of the moving column of axoplasm, *i.e.*, that the enzyme is a fixed constituent of the continuously growing axon. In that case its movement distad should be equal to the axonal growth rate, which may be as high as 3 mm a day according to WEISS and HISCOE (*l.c.*). The alternative is that there is centrifugal flow or transport of individual substances independently of the growth of the axon as a whole. WEISS and HISCOE seem to have envisaged this as a possibility, and it appears to be implied in discussions by MACINTOSH (1959) and by FUKUDA and KOELLE (*l.c.*).

In some recent experiments done in the reviewer's laboratory (some of which have been published by HEBB et al. 1959) an attempt has been made to decide between these alternatives by investigating further the effect of section of cholinergic nerves on their ChAc and protein contents. The nerve sectioned was the sciatic (in goats) and the information sought was: (1) what change, if any, would occur in the binding or intracellular position of ChAc in the ventral roots contributing to the sciatic nerve, 4 to 7 days after section, the time when the enzyme concentration in the proximal segment is at a maximum, and (2) what part of the proximal segment is involved in the enzyme change.

The results showed that after section there was no significant difference in the particulate distribution of the enzyme in the ventral roots, or apparently in the proximal segment of the sciatic itself, although as expected this had a higher enzyme content than the control unsectioned nerve. Protein, as well as ChAc concentration per unit length of nerve, was greatly increased in the proximal segment, but there were no significant differences in the concentration of either in the mixed or in the ventral spinal roots. By analysis of shorter lengths of nerve it was found that the rise in enzyme was in fact confined to a segment between 2 and 2.5 cm in length, immediately proximal to the section. These are preliminary results, but they suggest that the accumulation of protein is related to the rate of growth of the axon as a whole. In regenerating nerves this may reach 4 mm per day. We are here implying, of course, that when the axon is prevented by ligature from going forward its growth will continue for a time at least but be reflected backwards to the same extent. In ligated nerves axon sprouts do indeed grow back parallel to the remaining nerve fibres (CAJAL 1928), but from WEISS and HISCOE's (l.c.) experiments it is more probable that the additional axoplasm is accommodated by mechanical distortion, including ballooning, intussusception or telescoping, and spiralling. It is doubtful, however, that these changes go back as for as the distances we have observed; WEISS and HISCOE speak of a few mm in describing the mechanical distortion produced by incomplete compression of a nerve, and it may be relevant that in the earlier experiments of HEBB and WAITES (1956) the damming effect of ligation on ChAc began to subside after 7 days.

The evidence therefore seems to indicate that the proximo-distal movement of the enzyme is related to the growth of the axon, and we have provisionally come to the conclusion that ChAc is attached to some part of the axon structure, such as the endoplasmic reticulum, and is kept in transit by the growth of this structure. It may be surmised that as it reaches the nerve terminals the enzyme-carrying membrane breaks up or is budded off to form the synaptic vesicles, which, as has already been suggested, may be the carriers of the synaptic transmitter. Elastic recoil of the cut nerve fibres may account for some of the distortions of fibre structure described by WEISS and HISCOE (*l.c.*) and should be taken into consideration when seeking the reason for the rise in ChAc in the proximal segment. However, it appears that the recoil affects the cut fibres for only a few mm above the section, whereas the enzyme change occupies a stretch of nerve 5 to 6 times longer. It is probable, however, that contraction or recoil following section of the fibres contributes some of the increase in enzyme observed.

Storage of ACh: The meaning of bound ACh

A. In mammals

Early evidence about the tissue storage of ACh was reviewed by FELDBERG (1945), who reached certain general conclusions both about the conditions of storage and its relation to the synthetic mechanism. It was evident first that the ester is in some way bound to the tissue structure since it remains attached to the particulate fraction obtained on grinding up nervous tissues; further it could be shown that any losses from the particulate fraction are made up by synthesis, and that in its bound state the ester is protected against the hydrolytic action of cholinesterases (ChE's). Another important point made was that 'free' ACh must be treated as released ACh, and that it is the level of 'bound' ACh which tends to remain constant and represents the balance between production and utilization.

FELDBERG rejected altogether the idea that ACh is released from an inactive precursor substance; subsequent evidence has supported his alternative suggestion that the tissue ACh is inactive because of binding to some tissue component or granule. It is of interest to note in this connection the evidence that lipids apparently confer upon the tissue stores of ACh their immunity from attack by the ChE's. This fits in with WHITTAKER's (1959) recent experiments showing that the ester in the ACh-rich particles separated by centrifugation is immune to the action of ChE's until released by ether or a similar agent.

The nature of the tissue component to which ACh is bound was not specifically discussed by FELDBERG; BODIAN (1942) and later BRODKIN and ELLIOTT (1953) thought that it might be some particle akin to, or possibly the mitochondrion itself. As we have already seen, ACh is not in the mitochondria, but is instead in smaller, lighter particles.

For the present it seems simplest to regard the ACh-rich particles isolated from brain as vesicles, corresponding in size to the synaptic vesicles identified by electron microscopy (see PALAY and PALADE 1955, DE ROBERTIS and BENNETT 1955, CASTILLO and KATZ 1956). If this is the storage particle, then it may not be necessary to assume any chemical linkage to explain the binding of the ester to the tissue. It would be simpler to assume that in the resting condition the vesicle is a diffusion-tight compartment with a solution of ACh inside it; the release of ACh then would depend upon disruption or a reversible change in the permeability of the vesicular membrane. This of course would have to coincide with a permeability change of the presynaptic membrane, as CASTILLO and KATZ (1956) have pointed out. A possible solution to this problem may be suggested on the basis of PALAY's description, referred to previously, of the synaptic vesicles in the *boutons terminaux* of the CNS.

According to PALAY (1956), clusters of small circular profiles of 200 to 650 Å in diameter may take up almost all of the available space in the axonal end-feet not occupied by the mitochondria. Frequently, groups of these vesicles seem to lie against the presynaptic membrane at points where it is thickened and roughened, and in some of his sections it was possible to see that some of them opened into the intrasynaptic space. It is possible then that the synaptic vesicles abutting on these specialized areas or patches actually form part of the presynaptic membrane, and in this way are already oriented so that only one membrane separates them from the intrasynaptic space. These vesicles would then be regarded as functional units in contradistinction to those further back in the axon terminal which would be in the nature of a reserve force, and which, according to the theory of continuous axonal growth, would eventually replace those at the synaptic border. It may be objected that the lack of regenerative capacity by central neurons is at variance with the idea that they grow continuously in the same way as peripheral axons may do. However, the evidence reviewed by CAJAL (1928) shows that neural sprouting occurs from severed cerebral axons; the failure to reestablish normal connections is apparently due to the absence of certain sheath elements, rather than to inability of the neuron to produce new axoplasm.

This argument also provides an explanation for HEBB and WHITTAKER's finding, mentioned earlier, that bound ACh of brain is in two fractions, one which is relatively labile and released by mildly disruptive procedures, and a more firmly bound fraction which is dislodged only by more drastic procedures. The distinction applies as well to ChAc, about 50% of which is more easy to activate than the remainder. These findings could all be explained if the vesicles containing the ester and enzyme are not all equally labile; for example, those on the synaptic border might constitute the more labile population, while those in reserve, which are the newer vesicles, might be less labile. From this view, it would be expected that vesicles bordering on the synaptic cleft would each eventually be disrupted spontaneously and liberate its transmitter substance into the synaptic cleft. This could account for the spontaneous release of quanta of ACh postulated by FATT and KATZ (1952).

If, as many workers have urged, the synaptic vesicles are the carriers of neurohumors such as ACh, a number of other problems is immediately raised. Biochemical evidence suggests strongly that the enzyme which synthesizes ACh is present in the same vesicle; if this is so, the constancy of the tissue storage of ACh may be most simply explained by the fact of its confinement in a small, diffusion-tight particle in which the accumulation of ACh will have a braking action on the catalytic activity of ChAc. However, it is then necessary to assume that the particle which stores ACh must also have the means of making the substrates, choline and acetyl-CoA, or be selectively permeable to them.

So far as acetyl-CoA is concerned, there is as yet no evidence to show how mobile it is between one cell organelle and another — the obvious source of supply is the mitochondria which are another feature of the axon terminals — or whether it can be formed by the particles in which ACh is concentrated. Against this, there is some indirect evidence about the relation of choline to ACh synthesis in whole tissue which indicates that choline must cross a membrane barrier in order to maintain the normal production of ACh.

Much of this evidence has been obtained by MacINTOSH and his colleagues (for a review of this work see MacINTOSH 1959) in a study of the action of one of the hemicholiniums, HC-3, on the synthesis and release of ACh from the perfused superior cervical ganglion. The effects of this agent on the ganglion are (1) to reduce the output of ACh obtained with continued intermittent stimulation of the preganglionic nerve and (2) to reduce as well the store of ACh in the tissue to 15 to 20% of the control level. The differences due to HC-3 are largest when the ganglion is perfused with plasma. The results clearly point to a reduction by HC-3 in the synthesis of ACh. However, HC-3 does not inhibit significantly ChAc or the formation of acetyl-CoA, although it does inhibit ACh synthesis by brain slices and brain homogenates which have not been ether-treated (GARDINER 1957). Further, MacINTOSH's group has shown that HC-3 inhibits the renal excretion of choline in the chicken in a manner which suggests that it may be competitive for sites normally occupied by choline. This and other evidence, including experiments by SHELLEY (1956) showing that eserine can compete with choline to reduce ACh synthesis in tissue slices although it does not inhibit ChAc, indicate that to gain access to ChAc *in vivo*, choline must cross a selectively permeable membrane. This then would fit with other evidence suggesting that the enzyme is in an enclosed structure, together with the ACh which it produces, and relies on the entry of choline from the outside.

Another problem to consider is the genesis of the synaptic vesicles. One possibility is that the enzyme which is in the axon is a fixed component of the axoplasmic structure, attached to the endoplasmic reticulum, and that as this continues to grow downwards it becomes pinched off at the axonal terminals to form the separate vesicles. Or, it may be that these are already formed in the axon, although part of the growing structure, and are represented by the microsomal fraction of the axons already described, but are modified structurally as they reach the endings.

To what extent the axonal particles store ACh is another question related to this problem. Our evidence, admittedly from only a few experiments, suggests that they do not store very much and that the high values for ACh in the ventral roots, for example (MacINTOSH 1941), may include a large proportion of free ACh. In tissue with such a high ChAc activity this might form post-mortem, and so be an artifact. On the other hand, if the bound ACh in the ventral roots should prove to be higher than we have judged it to be, such evidence might go far towards showing that the vesicles found at the nerve endings are formed in or near the cell body of the axon.

At present it is a great disadvantage to any arguments of this sort that there are still too few data about the differences in ChAc and ACh distributions in the peripheral and central nervous systems. It is infinitely easier to study their particulate storage in central structures because these are easier to homogenize than are peripheral nerves. On the other hand, more is known about conduction and transmission in the periphery. It is obviously desirable that the data of more than one disciplinary approach to this problem should be related to one and the same tissue.

B. In other species

The proportion of free to bound ACh which is observed experimentally shows large species variations which are due to a number of factors. In some insects measurements on homogenates of tissue are complicated by the rapid synthesis and release of ACh into the suspending medium. In a study of two species of blowfly, LEWIS (1953) found that ACh was higher in eserinized Ringer homogenates than in comparable acidified homogenates that had been boiled before assay. Thus, there was the anomalous situation that the "free" ACh appeared to be higher than the total. There is no doubt, however, that the proportion of free ACh tends to be higher in homogenates of insect nervous tissue than in many other species because of factors other than the synthesis of new ester. COLHOUN (personal communication) has found, for example, that in homogenates of the cockroach nervous system release of ACh from the particulate fraction is affected both by the pH and the tonicity of the suspending medium. Under certain conditions as much as 55% was found in the particulate fraction, but under other conditions it was considerably less (see Table 5). This suggests that the subcellular structure may be easily broken down during homogenizing. BELLAMY

(1958), however, has found a high concentration of ACh in particles of locust (*Schistocerca gregaria*) nervous tissue which were precipitated by centrifuging at 10,200, for 10 min. These particles, which probably correspond to the mitochondrial or large granule fraction of mammals, were also able to synthesize ACh (see Table 5).

A preliminary study of the binding of ACh in the dogfish brain has been made in the reviewer's laboratory. No ACh was detected in eserinized homogenates (in NaCl or sucrose) before acid extraction, but in acidified homogenates there was a small amount of activity equivalent at most to 1 μg ACh/g fresh tissue. The low ACh values could be due to a paucity of cholinergic neurons; on the other hand, we think it possible that more ester is present in the tissue but remains inaccessible because of the resistance of the cellular particles to damage.

Table 5. *Particulate binding of ACh in different species*

Species	Tissue	Bound ACh (% of total recovered)	ACh in large granule fraction (% of total bound ACh)	References
Cockroach	Thoracic nerve cord.	16—55	not stated	COLHOUN (unpublished)
Desert locust	Head	(no E)	56	BELLAMY (1958)
Pigeon	Brain	(no E)	54	BELLAMY (1959)
Pigeon	Cerebrum	67	75	HEBB and WHITTAKER (1958)
Pigeon	Optic lobes	56	64	HEBB and WHITTAKER (1958)
Rat	Brain	(no E)	70	BELLAMY (1959)
Guinea pig, rabbit	Cerebrum	70—90	60—80	HEBB and WHITTAKER (1958)
Sheep	Caudate nucleus	100	64	HEBB and WHITTAKER (1958)

Notes: (1) The large granule fraction is equivalent to the mitochondrial or P 2 fraction (see Table 2).

(2) The entry "no E" in the table indicates that in BELLAMY's experiments he did not add eserine during extraction of the tissue, and so the values he has reported represent only the bound fraction of ACh.

(3) WELSH and HYDE (1944) stated that in rat brain (extracted in cold eserinized Ringer solution) the proportion of total to free ACh is between 1.5:1, and 4:1, a figure in agreement with ratios obtained by other investigators whose work they quoted. This means that the amount of bound ACh is between 33 and 75% of the total, a result which by contrast with the data given above for mammals strongly suggests that liberation of ester from the particulate must have occurred in some of their experiments. This may have been due to the extraction medium. (For relevant evidence see BRODKIN and ELLIOTT 1953, STONE 1955 and WHITTAKER 1959.)

As shown in Table 5 there is little difficulty in recovering ACh from pigeon brain homogenates, and it may be because the particles are more than ordinarily labile that in this species the proportion of free to bound ACh was found to be very high by HEBB and WHITTAKER (1958; unpublished protocol referred to by the authors in the text). BELLAMY (1959) on the other hand did not find any ACh in the supernatant; all that he recovered was in the particulate fraction, but as indicated in the note in Table 5 this is because his extractant did not contain eserine or other anti-ChE agent.

The release of ACh

A. The nerve impulse as the required stimulus

So far as is known, release of ACh in amounts necessary for transmission occurs only through stimulation of the presynaptic nerve. While perfusion of a sympathetic ganglion with excess K (BROWN and FELDBERG 1936a) or with Rb, Cs, or NH$_4$ ions will release ACh from the preganglionic endings, their effect is apparently due to depolarization and stimulation of the preganglionic fibres. They also stimulate the ganglion cells directly. Leakage of ACh from cholinergic endings is known to occur in the absence of specific stimuli and is probably a normal physiological event. However, as will appear from later discussion, the amounts involved are very much less than the amounts necessary for transmission of the nerve impulse.

As a whole, evidence obtained in studies of the release of ACh from brain slices and minces or homogenates tends to confirm experiments *in vivo* which suggest that the sole physiological stimulus for the release of ACh in effective quantities is the nerve impulse. Applied electrical pulses increase the ACh of the system in the presence of eserine (ROUSSEL 1954), while release by K, Rb, and Cs ions has also been demonstrated (see FELDBERG 1945). Ammonium ions apparently inhibit the release of ACh from respiring brain slices, but this appears to be an indirect metabolic effect due to inhibition of ACh synthesis (BRAGANCA et al. 1953).

Another way in which ACh may be released from tissue slices or homogenates is by the action of certain agents which are thought to break down the tissue storage particles. The effects of ether, and of freezing and thawing, have been mentioned earlier in this chapter. Another agent which seems to have a similar effect is the lecithinase of cobra venom (GAUTRELET and CORTEGGIANI 1939, BRAGANCA and QUASTEL 1952). In the experiments of BRAGANCA and QUASTEL this increased the ACh produced by respiring brain slices, and at the same time caused a release of much of the bound ACh, so that the end effect was a sharp rise in the proportion of free to bound ester. This evidence is in agreement with that obtained by HEBB and WHITTAKER (*l.c.*) that ChAc and ACh reside in the same storage particles.

The quantity of ACh released by a single nerve impulse at a single receptor has generally been estimated by measuring the amount released by stimulation at a known rate of a large number of nerve fibres, such as a preganglionic trunk of the sympathetic nervous system, or the motor nerve to a muscle for which an estimate of the number of endplates can be obtained (see ACHESON 1948, ROSENBLUETH 1950, EMMELIN and MACINTOSH 1956, MACINTOSH 1959). ACHESON concluded that the amount of ACh released near a single ending is of the order of 1.5×10^{-16} g, while figures which are quoted by MACINTOSH from work by EMMELIN and MACINTOSH for the tibialis anticus muscle of the cat indicate that the rate of liberation is about one-half of this. However, as the authors originally pointed out, these are average figures for release per volley and may be far below the true values. Thus the amount liberated in the superior cervical ganglion with repetitive stimulation may average out at an amount per impulse of about one-fourth of the rate of release at the outset of stimulation. It is therefore probable that the value for tibialis anticus should be four or more times the average calculated. Furthermore, even this may be an underestimate since there is the danger that under the conditions of these and other similar experiments the nerve fibres may not all have been active.

On the other hand, there is some evidence for the view that the amount of ACh released at cholinergic endings far exceeds the amount required for transmission. Thus, BROWN (1954) found that in a "cold" ganglion, perfused with eserinized Locke solution at 20° C, the output of ACh in response to maximal stimulation was about one-tenth of the output at 39° C, although the response of the indicator organ, the nictitating membrane, was about the same at the two temperatures; he suggested that this meant that the amount of ACh liberated at normal body temperature is in considerable excess of transmission requirements. This would appear to be the most reasonable interpretation; nevertheless, there are certain difficulties in accepting this conclusion. One of the difficulties is that the response of the nictitating membrane does not provide a reliable guide for judging the number of ganglion cells excited. In the first place, the membrane is innervated by a relatively small proportion of all the cells present in the ganglion and it is conceivable that the preganglionic fibres in synaptic relation to these have more resistance to cold or fatigue than the others. Secondly, the contraction of the nictitating membrane as it is usually recorded does not provide a very sensitive assessment of the number of impulses reaching it; and failure of a small proportion of the fibres concerned might escape observation. What is required is some record of the response at the synapse itself, and even more important, some independent means of testing the sensitivity of the receptor cells to ACh under similar experimental conditions.

As ACHESON (1948) has pointed out, however, there are large discrepancies between the amounts of ACh recovered from release at nerve endings and the amounts which it is necessary to inject in order to mimic the neuronal response to nerve stimulation. This is attributable to two factors: one, as already suggested, is that presynaptic failure may prevent the release of ACh from some of the endings of a nerve trunk when this is maximally stimulated either for too long a period or at too high a rate; the other is that the distance between the receptors, either endplate or ganglion cell, and the site of injection is always longer than the distance (probably less than 200 Å) between the receptors and the points at which ACh is released by nerve stimulation. Therefore diffusion losses make an injection relatively less effective. In addition, the important factor of tissue barriers must be considered (see chapter 6).

This difficulty has been partly overcome in experiments on muscle by applying ACh electrophoretically from a micropipette inserted into the tissue close to an endplate (NASTUK 1953, CASTILLO and KATZ 1955, KRNJEVIC and MILEDI 1958a). Even with this method the potentials elicited by injection have a slower time-course than those arising from nerve stimulation. However, KRNJEVIC and MILEDI have been able to demonstrate an endplate potential (e.p.p.) on the rat diaphragm in response to 10^{-15} g ACh, with an amplitude and time-course, except for a slower rise time, closely approximating to an e.p.p. produced in another diaphragm in response to nerve stimulation. This amount is approximately twenty times the average amount of ACh recovered from release at the neuromuscular junction by EMMELIN and MACINTOSH (1956), but it appears to be a fairly accurate estimate not only of the amount required to stimulate the endplate but of the amount released from the presynaptic endings in the region of one endplate, because KRNJEVIC and MITCHELL (unpublished experiments) have since been able to recover from the rat phrenic-diaphragm preparation at low rates of stimulation amounts of ACh equivalent to 1 to 5×10^{-15} g per impulse per endplate. This is about the same as the largest amount of ACh found to be liberated per cell in the superior cervical ganglion with one preganglionic volley (EMMELIN and MACINTOSH, l.c.).

B. Quantal release of ACh

In 1952, FATT and KATZ advanced the suggestion that the miniature endplate potentials (m.e.p.p.'s) which occur spontaneously in resting muscle are due to the spontaneous release of "multimolecular" quanta of ACh from the terminals of the presynaptic axons. Much of the evidence which led them to identify ACh as the 'micro-transmitter' was pharmacological. The effects of curare in reducing and of neostigmine in enlarging and prolonging them are similar to their effects on the normal e.p.p. Further evidence was that the m.e.p.p.'s are reduced in muscle denervated for two weeks, a result which was to be expected if ACh is responsible for them, because as is well known ACh and ChAc both fall in the distal part of a degenerating nerve at a rate such that probably little ester would be present in the terminals 2 weeks after the section. (but see later papers by KATZ and his colleagues; and HEBB 1962). The authors found also that in the presence of reduced Ca the e.p.p. is reduced stepwise, although the amplitude (0.5 mV) and possibly the frequency of the m.e.p.p.'s are unaffected. The inference that suggests itself from the observations is that the e.p.p. is made up of a group of m.e.p.p.'s, possibly one hundred or more, and that these correspond in size to the unit discharge of ACh. Calculations showed that the amount present in such units must be much more than a single molecule and is probably between one-hundredth and one-thousandth of the amount normally released at a motor endplate by a single nerve impulse (see earlier discussion). Subsequently CASTILLO and KATZ (1956) suggested that the carriers for ACh may be the synaptic vesicles of the axonal terminal, and that spontaneous release from these may account for the m.e.p.p.'s; the synchronous discharge of a large number of vesicles would account for the e.p.p.

A possibility which has already been discussed is that the release occurs by disruption of the vesicles; alternatively, it may be that the ester is released in response to a nerve impulse by a reversible change in permeability of all the vesicles concerned, and that the occasional disruption of individual carriers accounts for the miniature responses. Evidence that the mechanisms governing the release of ACh in the two different events may not be the same is given by CASTILLO and KATZ (1954) who found that Mg ions have no effect on the frequency of the miniature potentials although they affect the quantum content of the e.p.p. (see also BOYD and MARTIN 1956, LILEY 1956b).

While FATT and KATZ's conclusions were drawn from experiments on frog muscle, BO D and MARTIN (1956a and b) and LILEY (1956a and b) were able to confirm them in all important respects in experiments on mammalian muscle. BOYD and MARTIN found some quantitative differences but concluded that, as in the frog, the mammalian e.p.p. is built up of unit responses corresponding in amplitude and time course with the m.e.p.p.'s. In the cat's tenuissimus muscle the frequency of the m.e.p.p.'s at 37° C varies from 0.5 to 5/sec, with an average of 1.5/sec, and for any given fibre tends to remain nearly constant over long periods. LILEY found that the frequency of the m.e.p.p.'s was 1 to 2/sec. in rat muscle. In this respect mammalian muscle exhibits greater stability than does frog muscle. Another difference from frog muscle is that the frequency of the m.e.p.p.'s increases with Ca concentration, whereas, as already indicated, there is no obvious relation between Ca concentration and frequency of m.e.p.p.'s in the frog, but the difference may well have been due to the greater instability of the frog preparation as shown by greater variability in the frequency of the m.e.p.p.'s under control conditions.

Various attempts have been made to estimate the amount of ACh constituting a single quantum but these have been hampered by uncertainties both about the number of quanta making up the full-sized e.p.p. and the amount of ACh discharged at a receptor by one impulse. The rate of leakage of ACh in the superior cervical ganglion reported by MACINTOSH (1959) is 0.3 mμg/min, and from this one might hope to calculate the amount of ACh per quantum, but in this tissue it is not known what the frequency of quantal release is. Assuming that the ganglion contains about 100,000 cells, then about 20,000 molecules of ACh could be released per second per cell. If the frequency of release is of the same order as for tenuissimus this would mean a quantal discharge of 4,000 to 40,000 molecules.

From calculations already referred to, BIRKS (personal communication to MACINTOSH 1959) reached the conclusion that in muscle the synaptic carriers, which he took to be the vesicles, contain about 900 molecules of ACh each. In this calculation he assumed, on the basis of MARTIN's (1955) work, that about 300 quanta are released by a single impulse at one motor endplate, and related this result to the figures given by EMMELIN and MACINTOSH (l.c.) for the total amount of ACh released in the muscle by one volley. The evidence already given, however, suggests that the amount of ACh released per volley is likely to be much higher than the figure quoted. From KRNJEVIC and MITCHELL's (l.c.) work it may be even 20 to 100 times higher. In that case the amount of ACh per vesicle would work out to be more than 15,000 molecules.

BIRKS estimated also what the concentration of ACh would be in one vesicle with a diameter of 400 Å if i accommodates 1 quantum of ester. He found this to be 0.11 M, but if the quantum is equivalent not to 400 molecules of ACh, as he reckoned it to be, but 20 to 100 times more than this, as other data suggest, then the concentration would be between 2 and 10 M. This is of importance because it raises a serious difficulty for the vesicular hypothesis. Other evidence mentioned earlier suggests that the synthesizing enzyme is in close association with the store of ester it produces, probably existing within the same subcellular particle, and there is a strong probability that its activity *in vivo* is limited by the concentration of ACh in its immediate vicinity. Experiments *in vitro* show that this inhibition amounts to 40% at an ACh concentration of 0.05 M (REISBERG 1957), so it seems probable that the concentration of ester in the immediate vicinity of the enzyme *in vivo*, in the active state at least, would be even lower than this.

One way in which higher concentrations of ACh might exist in the vesicle together with ChAc is suggested by WHITTAKER's (*l.c.*) proposal that about half the intravesicular ACh is bound to the containing structure. In this case the concentration of ACh present in simple solution in the vesicle, and free to exert a restraining influence upon the enzyme, would be half of the estimated concentration for the vesicle as a whole. But even so this is still too high, and it is difficult to see how the more firmly bound fraction of ACh could be mobilized rapidly enough so that its discharge would be synchronized with the discharge of the more labile store.

Another possibility is that the quantity of ACh which elicits a miniature potential corresponds with the quantity not in a single vesicle but in a group of vesicles. That is the m.e.p.p. may itself be a compound rather than a unitary event, although in that case it would be necessary to postulate some structural grouping of the vesicles at the presynaptic membrane so that a multiple of vesicles would function effectively as a unit. One way in which this might be achieved is suggested by PALAY's description (PALAY 1956, 1958) of the arrangement of vesicles along the axonal margin of the synaptolemma in central synapses. The vesicles are throughout the terminal grouped in clusters but those which are ranged along the margin are in close relation to denser patches of membrane, and these may be the points of transmitter discharge. It is possible then to imagine that the membrane in any of these areas is sufficiently unstable so that discharge from the vesicles which abut upon it will occur spontaneously from time to time.

Clearly there are still many problems to resolve about the mechanism of the quantal discharge of ACh. There can be little doubt, however, that the basic concept of quantal release, as first put forward by KATZ and his co-workers, is correct. The work has been substantiated and confirmed for a number of species by many workers and there has been no evidence to oppose it. Perhaps what is more convincing is the fact that as a consequence of this new concept of ACh release it is possible to explain many odd findings about neurohumoral transmission which were not previously understood at all.

C. Conditions modifying ACh release

Failure of the nerve endings to release ACh can arise from a number of causes. These can be divided as follows: (1) failure of the stimulus to invade the endings and/or failure to mobilize the ACh stores, (2) failure of ACh synthesis, and (3) failure of the release mechanism itself. This is a rather arbitrary classification but, as will appear, there is an experimental basis for making distinctions between these three situations.

I. Failure of the stimulus

KRNJEVIC and MILEDI (1958b) in an analysis of neuromuscular fatigue have obtained evidence of presynaptic failure of transmission, and have concluded that

at high rates of stimulation presynaptic failure of propagation, probably in the
fine terminal branches of the motor axon, can be one of the factors that set
a limit upon the frequency at which nerve impulses reach the neuromuscular
junction. Failure of ACh supply in these experiments was eliminated by the finding that spontaneous m.e.p.p.'s continued at a time when the stimuli failed to
evoke e.p.p.'s. It is possible that the situation is similar to that in magnesium
block of transmission. BOYD and MARTIN (1956) have found, in confirmation of
CASTILLO and KATZ (1954), that m.e.p.p.'s still occur spontaneously when, in the
presence of a high concentration of Mg ions, e.p.p.'s are no longer evoked by nerve
stimulation. But in the latter case it may be that the failure is more peripheral,
and that the point of attack is the mechanism which enables the nerve impulse
to mobilize the ACh at the storage sites. In contrast to Mg block, the effect of
low Ca which reduces the e.p.p. does not appear independently of changes in the
m.e.p.p.'s; as already mentioned, BOYD and MARTIN found that the frequency of
the miniature potentials was reduced by reducing Ca. It is therefore possible that
the blocking effect of low Ca is due to an action on the membrane.

II. Failure of ACh synthesis

The most convincing example of failure of ACh release due to a reduction of
synthesis is the inhibition of synaptic and neuromuscular transmission by the
hemicholinium, HC-3 (see MACINTOSH 1959). MACINTOSH's work has shown that
the failure to release ACh in the superior cervical ganglion poisoned with HC-3
is associated with a reduction of 85 to 90% of the normal ACh content of the
ganglion; as shown by evidence reviewed in an earlier part of this chapter, this
loss of ACh is clearly related to a failure of synthesis. Similarly, eserine in high
concentrations may also reduce synthesis *in vivo*, and so reduce to some extent
the capacity of the ganglion to release ACh.

Other work by MACINTOSH and his colleagues on the action of HC-3 makes
it probable that many if not all the prominent features of HC-3 poisoning are
derived from this single effect on ACh synthesis; this is confirmed by the work
of DESMEDT (1958) and of LONGO (1959), both of whom studied the effect of
the drug on neuromuscular transmission. From DESMEDT's experiments it appears that the blocking action observed is proximal to the endplate; that is,
it is not due to a curare-like effect; on the other hand, LONGO was able to show
that there is no interference in conduction of the impulse to the nerve endings
(see also WILSON and LONG 1959). [The reader should also consult the Recent
Symposium on hemicholiniums (SCHUELER 1961)].

It is possible, although not yet certain, that the failure of ACh release in tick paralysis
(see EMMONS and MCLENNAN 1959) may also be due to an inhibition of synthesis. However,
MURNAGHAN (1959) has recently found that ACh synthesis is unaltered in dogs paralyzed by
this parasite. Similarly the action of tetrodotoxin, the active principle responsible for the
poisonous effects of the roe of the *Fugu* fish in blocking synaptic transmission, may be in
part due to inhibition of ACh synthesis (KURIAKI and NAGANO 1957), but pure tetrodotoxin
has no inhibitory effect on choline acetylase (personal observation). The method by which
the Japanese workers demonstrated inhibition of ACh synthesis did not show whether
it acted directly or indirectly by inhibition of coenzyme A acetylation.

III. Failure of the release mechanisms

In an analysis of the action of botulinum toxin on the neuromuscular junction,
BROOKS (1956) has shown that the onset of block is preceded by a decrease in
miniature endplate potential frequency, a result which strongly suggests that the
failure of transmission is due to inability of the nerve terminals to liberate ACh.
Whilst this might be ascribed in turn to a reduced synthesis of the ester, such an

explanation seems less likely in view of the further observation that it is possible to restore the m.e.p.p.'s to their normal frequency, and reverse the block at least temporarily, by tetanic stimulation of the nerve.

Similarly it seems probable that reduced Ca blocks ACh release independently of any effect on synthesis (see MacINTOSH 1959). There is a danger here that too fine a distinction may be made between blocking of release and the ability of the nerve impulse to mobilize ACh; but if we accept BOYD and MARTIN's evidence that the frequency of the miniature potentials is reduced with reduced Ca, then it seems to be clear that there is some change in the state in which the ester is held so that it does become less labile.

In conclusion, it is perhaps worthwhile drawing attention to the possibility that some agents might have more than one effect by which they can influence the release of ACh. The work of BRAGANCA and QUASTEL quoted earlier is evidence of such a possibility, since the effects of lecithinase which they observed were an increase in the release of ACh, due to a reduced storage capacity, coupled with an increased synthesis rate. These events are not likely to occur under normal conditions *in vivo* but the experiment illustrates some of the problems of analyzing the action of individual agents and the use which can be made of studies *in vitro* in determining their mechanism.

Summary

The evidence and ideas outlined in this chapter focus attention on the synapses and neuro-effector junctions of the vertebrate as sites of ACh function. It is here that the ester is released to transmit to the postsynaptic structure, either nerve cell or muscle, the excitatory disturbances arising at the terminals of the presynaptic cell. The question posed at the beginning of the discussion was how can the synaptic mechanism for release of the ester be set, and reset after use, so that transmission is enabled to occur at the high frequencies observed experimentally. The answer suggested is that the enzyme for the synthesis of ACh may reside in the same particle, possibly the synaptic vesicle, as the ester itself; that the resynthesis of ACh will occur the moment the vesicles have discharged their load into the synaptic cleft; and that these vesicles may be the functional units of neurohumoral transmission.

It has also been proposed that the vesicles which are immediately active in transmission are only those in the front line abutting on the synaptic membrane and possibly constituting part of the membrane in the particular areas where the vesicles are clustered behind it. The storage of ACh in vesicles, a number of which can release their content of ester simultaneously, provides a mechanism which could account for the quantal release of ester in response to the nerve impulse. This concept of the motor endplate response as the sum of a number of separate events, depending upon the synchronous release of numerous 'packets' of ACh, since it was first proposed by FATT and KATZ, has provided a new understanding of the events at the neuromuscular junction and other synapses; while it may require modification in detail it now seems likely to be a true picture of an important part of the transmission process.

Another aspect of this problem is the continued maintenance of the axoplasmic structure. Modern research indicates that the axoplasm is continuously growing, and it now seems probable that some of the proteins which have been identified at the axon terminals are manufactured in the cell body. Among these is choline acetylase (ChAc). Degeneration experiments show that without replacement from above the enzyme and the ester almost disappear from the axon and, although this may be in part a pathological event, it does fit in with other evidence that a slow replacement of ChAc at the endings is going on nearly continuously. On that basis it has been suggested here that the miniature endplate potentials which occur spontaneously at the neuromuscular junction may be associated with the breakdown or catabolism of the most terminal parts of the presynaptic structure, although it may only be that the spontaneous release of ACh is an index of greater instability of the membrane. But perhaps greater instability is the condition which foreshadows the final breakdown of the membrane at any one point.

It has been mainly the mammalian and frog nervous systems that have furnished the evidence about the release of ACh which has been reviewed here. The sections dealing with the distribution of ACh and ChAc have shown, however, that the ester must have equal importance in many invertebrate species. Indeed it may be of greater importance. The record for the ability of nervous tissue to synthesize ACh is now held by the cockroach, as COLHOUN (1958b) has shown. The reason why the role of ACh in invertebrate nerves has not been dealt with more fully here is that its study has not yet provided sufficient detailed information about its distribution at the intracellular level, nor how it is released from the tissues containing it. Furthermore, it is still very difficult to obtain a clear picture of the action of anticholinesterase (anti-ChE) agents on the insect, although this property is evidently very important in many insecticides. One of the difficulties may be provided by the peculiarly effective compartmentation of the insect nervous system which makes it less accessible to outside interference and study. This may account for the fact that substances such as TEPP, Malathion, and Parathion increase the ACh content of the insect nervous system in proportion to their anti-ChE action (SMALLMAN and FISHER 1958, COLHOUN 1958a). Some ACh is released into the haemolymph by anti-ChE agents but the greater part is retained in the nerve cord, the total increase being related to greater activity of the nerves (COLHOUN, l.c.). A puzzling finding is that DFP produces only a slight increase in ACh, a result which has been attributed to inhibition of synthesis of ACh (WINTERINGHAM et al. 1957), but the mode of action is not clear since DFP does not inhibit ACh synthesis in vitro. An additional effect of DFP on houseflies is a shift of ACh from the head to the trunk (LEWIS and FOWLER 1956, SMALLMAN and FISHER, l.c.). The original papers should be consulted for more information about this interesting problem (see also FRONTALI 1956, and LEWIS and SMALLMAN 1956 for further evidence about the storage and synthesis of ACh in insects). These subjects are discussed in Chapters 16 and 17 of the present volume.

Literature

ABOOD, L. G., R. W. GERARD, J. BANKS and R. D. TSCHIRGI: Substrate and enzyme distribution in cells and cell fractions of the nervous system. Amer. J. Physiol. **168**, 728—738 (1952).
ACHESON, G.: Physiology of neuromuscular junctions. Chemical aspects. Fed. Proc. **7**, 447 — 457 (1948).
ANDERSSON-CEDERGREN, E.: Ultrastructure of motor endplate and sarcoplasmic components of mouse skeletal muscle fibre as revealed by three-dimensional reconstructions from serial sections. J. Ultrastruct. Res. Suppl. 1. New York and London: Acad. Press. 1959.
BANISTER, R. J., and M. SCRASE: Acetylcholine synthesis in normal and denervated sympathetic ganglia of the cat. J. Physiol. (Lond.) **111**, 437—444 (1950).
BAYER, G., and T. WENSE: Über den Nachweis von Hormonen in einzelligen Tieren. I. Mitteilung. Cholin und Acetylcholin in Paramecium. Pflügers Arch. ges. Physiol. **237**, 417 bis 422 (1936).
BELLAMY, D.: The structure and metabolic properties of tissue from Schistocerca gregaria (desert locust). Biochem. J. **70**, 580—589 (1958).

BELLAMY, D.: The distribution of bound acetylcholine and choline acetylase in rat and pigeon brain. Biochem. J. **72**, 165—168 (1959).

BODIAN, D.: Cytological aspects of synaptic function. Physiol. Rev. **42**, 140—162 (1942).

BOYD, I. A., and A. R. MARTIN: Spontaneous subthreshold activity at mammalian neuromuscular junctions. J. Physiol. (Lond.) **132**, 61—73 (1956a).

— — The endplate potential in mammalian muscle. J. Physiol. (Lond.) **132**, 74—91 (1956b).

BRADY, R. O., C. A. SPYROPOULOS and I. TASAKI: Intra-axonal injection of biologically active materials. Amer. J. Physiol. **194**, 207—213 (1958).

BRAGANCA, B. M., and J. H. QUASTEL: Action of snake venom on acetylcholine synthesis in brain. Nature (Lond.) **169**, 695—703 (1952).

— P. FAULKNER and J. H. QUASTEL: Effects of inhibitors of glutamine synthesis on the inhibition of acetylcholine synthesis in brain slices by ammonium ions. Biochim. biophys. Acta **10**, 83—88 (1953).

BRODKIN, E., and K. A. C. ELLIOTT: Binding of acetylcholine. Amer. J. Physiol. **173**, 437 — 442 (1953).

BRODY, T. M., and J. A. BAIN: A mitochondrial preparation from mammalian brain. J. biol. Chem. **195**, 685—696 (1952).

BROOKS, V. B.: An intracellular study of the action of repetitive nerve volleys and of botulinum toxin on miniature end-plate potentials. J. Physiol. (Lond.) **134**, 264—277 (1956).

BROWN, G. L.: The effect of temperature on the release of acetylcholine from sympathetic ganglia. J. Physiol. (Lond.) **124**, 26 P (1954).

— and W. FELDBERG: The action of potassium on the superior cervical ganglion of the cat. J. Physiol. (Lond.) **86**, 290—305 (1936a).

— — The acetylcholine metabolism of a sympathetic ganglion. J. Physiol. (Lond.) **88**, 265 bis 283 (1936b).

BULBRING, E., J. H. BURN and H. J. SHELLEY: Acetylcholine and ciliary movement in the gill plates of *Mytilus edulis*. Proc. roy. Soc. B. **141**, 445—466((1953).

— E. M. LOURIE and U. PARDOE: The presence of acetylcholine in *Trypanosoma Rhodesiense* and its absence from *Plasmodium gallinaceum*. Brit. J. Pharmacol. **4**, 290—294 (1949).

BULL, G. B., C. O. HEBB and D. RATKOVIĆ (1962). Nature (Lond.), in press.

CAJAL, S., and Y. RAMON: Degeneration and Regeneration of the Nervous System. London: Oxford University Press 1928.

CASPERSSON, T.: The protein metabolism of the cell. Naturwissenschaften **29**, 33—43 (1941).

DEL CASTILLO, J., and B. KATZ: The failure of local circuit transmission at the nerve-muscle junction. J. Physiol. (Lond.) **123**, 7—8 P (1953).

— — The effect of magnesium on the activity of motor nerve endings. J. Physiol. (Lond.) **124**, 553—559 (1954).

— — On the localization of acetylcholine receptors. J. Physiol. (Lond.) **128**, 157—181 (1955).

— — Biophysical aspects of neuromuscular transmission. In: J. A. V. BUTLER, Ed., Progr. in Biophys. and Biophys. Chem. **6**, 122—160. London: Pergamon Press 1956.

CAUSEY, G., and H. HOFFMAN: The ultrastructure of the synaptic area in the superior cervical ganglion. J. Anat. **90**, 502—507 (1956).

— and C. J. STRATMANN: Changes in the nucleic acid content of ganglion cells during chromatolosis and after stimulation. Biochem. J. **64**, 29—32 (1956).

COHEN, M.: Concentration of choline acetylase in conducting tissue. Arch. Biochem. **60**, 284 — 296 (1956).

COLHOUN, E. H.: Tetraethyl pyrophosphate and acetylcholine in *Periplaneta americana*. Science **127**, 25 (1958a).

— Distribution of choline acetylase in insect conductive tissue. Nature (Lond.) **182**, 1378 (1958b).

DALE, H. H.: Junctional transmission of nervous effects by chemical agents. Proc. Mayo Clin. **30**, 5—20 (1955).

DALY, M. DE B., and L. E. MOUNT: The origin, course and nature of bronchomotor fibres in the cervical sympathetic nerve of the cat. J. Physiol. (Lond.) **113**, 43—62 (1951).

DESMEDT, J. E.: Myasthenic-like features of neuromuscular transmission after administration of an inhibitor of acetylcholine synthesis. Nature (Lond.) **182**, 1673—1674 (1958).

EMMELIN, N., and W. FELDBERG: Pharmacologically active substances in the fluid of nettle hairs (*Urtica urens*). J. Physiol. (Lond.) **106**, 14 P (1947).

— — Distribution of acetylcholine and histamine in nettle plants. New Phytol. **48**, 143 — 148 (1949).

— and F. C. MACINTOSH: The release of acetylcholine from perfused sympathetic ganglia and skeletal muscles. J. Physiol. (Lond.) **131**, 477—496 (1956).

EMMONS, P., and H. MCLENNAN: Failure of acetylcholine release in tick paralysis. Nature (Lond.) **183**, 474—475 (1959).

EWINS, A. J.: Acetylcholine, a new active principle of ergot. Biochem. J. 8, 44—49 (1914).

FATT, P.: Biophysics of junctional transmission. Physiol. Rev. 34, 674—710 (1954).

— and B. KATZ: Spontaneous subthreshold activity at motor nerve endings. J. Physiol. (Lond.) 117, 109—128 (1952).

FELDBERG, W.: Present views on the mode of action of acetylcholine in the central nervous system. Physiol. Rev. 25, 596—642 (1945).

FELDBERG, W.: Synthesis of acetylcholine (choline acetylase). In: R. W. GERARD, Ed., Methods in Medical Research, vol. 3, 95—106. Chicago: Year Book Publishers 1950.

— Cholinergic and non-cholinergic transmission. In: D. RICHTER, Ed., Metabolism of the Nervous System, 493—509. London: Pergamon Press 1957.

— and M. VOGT: Acetylcholine synthesis in different regions of the central nervous system. J. Physiol. (Lond.) 107, 372—381 (1948).

FERNÁNDEZ-MORÁN, H.: Electron microscopy of nervous tissue. In: D. RICHTER, Ed., Metabolism of the Nervous System, 1—34. London: Pergamon Press 1957.

FRONTALI, N.: Synthesis of acetylcholine in the head of Musca domestica (Ital.). Boll. Soc. ital. Biol. sper. 32, 1062—1063 (1956).

FUKUDA, T., and G. B. KOELLE: The cytological localization of intracellular neuronal acetylcholinesterase. J. biophys. biochem. Cytol. 5, 433—439 (1959).

GALLAGHER, C. H., J. D. JUDAH and K. R. REES: Glucose oxidation by brain mitochondria. Biochem. J. 62, 436—440 (1956).

GARDINER, J. E.: Experiments on the site of action of a choline acetylase inhibitor. J. Physiol. (Lond.) 138, 13—14 P (1957).

GAUTRELET, J., and E. CORTEGGIANI: Étude comparative de la libération de l'acétylcholine du tissu cérébral in vitro par les venins de Cobra ou de Vipera aspis, la lysocithine et la saponine. C. R. Soc. Biol. (Paris) 131, 951—954 (1939).

GIACOBINI, E.: Histochemical demonstration of AChE activity in isolated nerve cells. Acta physiol. scand. 36, 276—290 (1956).

GREY, E. G., and V. P. WHITTAKER: The isolation of synaptic vesicles from the central nervous system. J. Physiol. (Lond.). 153, 35—37 (1960).

HEBB, C. O.: Choline acetylase in mammalian and avian sensory systems. Quart. J. exp. Physiol. 40, 176—186 (1955).

— Biochemical evidence for the neural function of acetylcholine. Physiol. Rev. 37, 196—220 (1957a).

— Chemical transmission of nerve impulses in vertebrates and invertebrates. Nature (Lond.) 180, 627—628 (1957b).

— Chemical agents of the nervous system. In: C. C. PFEIFFER and J. R. SMYTHIES, Eds. Int. Rev. Neurobiol. 1, 165—193 (1959).

— Acetylcholine content of the rabbit plantaris muscle after denervation. J. Physiol. (Lond.). In press (1962).

— M. KRAUSE and A. SILVER: Intracellular binding of choline acetylase in the ventral spinal roots. J. Physiol. (Lond.) 148, 69—70 P (1959).

— and A. SILVER: Choline acetylase in the central nervous system of man and some other mammals. J. Physiol. (Lond.) 134, 718—728 (1956).

— and B. N. SMALLMAN: Intracellular distribution of choline acetylase. J. Physiol. (Lond.) 134, 385—392 (1956).

— and G. M. WAITES: Choline acetylase in antero- and retro-grade degeneration of a cholinergic neuron. J. Physiol. (Lond.) 132, 667—671 (1956).

— and V. P. WHITTAKER: Intracellular distributions of acetylcholine and choline acetylase. J. Physiol. (Lond.) 142, 187—196 (1958).

HOLTON, P.: Further observations on substance P in degenerating nerve. J. Physiol. (Lond.) 149, 35—36 P (1959).

HYDÉN, H.: Protein metabolism in the nerve cell during growth and function. Acta physiol. scand. 6, Suppl. 17 (1943).

KAPLAN, N. O., and F. LIPMANN: The assay and distribution of coenzyme A. J. biol. Chem. 174, 37—44 (1948).

KOREY, S. R., B. DE BRAGANZA and D. NACHMANSOHN: Choline acetylase. V Esterifications and transacetylations. J. biol. Chem. 189, 705—715 (1953).

KORKES, S., A. DEL CAMPILLO, S. R. KOREY, J. R. STERN, D. NACHMANSOHN and S. OCHOA: Coupling of acetyl donor systems with choline acetylase. J. biol. Chem. 198, 215—220 (1952).

KRNJEVIC, K., and R. MILEDI: Acetylcholine in mammalian neuromuscular transmission. Nature (Lond.) 182, 805—806 (1958a).

— — Failure of neuromuscular propagation in rats. J. Physiol. (Lond.) 140, 440—461 (1958b).

KURIAKI, K., and H. NAGANO: Susceptibility of certain enzymes of the central nervous system to tetrodotoxin. Brit. J. Pharmacol. 12, 393—396 (1957).

LEWIS, S. E.: Acetylcholine in blowflies. Nature (Lond.) 172, 1004—1005 (1953).
— and K. S. FOWLER: Effect of diisopropylphosphorofluoridate on the acetylcholine content of flies. Nature (Lond.) 178, 919—920 (1956).
— and B. N. SMALLMAN: The estimation of acetylcholine in insects. J. Physiol. (Lond.) 134, 241—256 (1956).
LILEY, A. W.: An investigation of spontaneous activity at the neuromuscular junction of the rat. J. Physiol. (Lond.) 132, 650—656 (1956a).
— The quantal components of the mammalian end-plate potential. J. Physiol. (Lond.) 133, 571—587 (1956b).
LIN, R. C. Y.: The distribution of acetylcholine in the Malayan jack-fruit plant, Artocarpus integra. Brit. J. Pharmacol. 12, 265—269 (1957).
LONGO, V. G.: Action of hemicholinium no. 3 on phrenic nerve action potentials. Arch. int. Pharmacodyn. 119, 1—9 (1959).
LUMSDEN, C. E.: Quantitative studies on lipolytic enzyme activity in degenerating and regenerating nerve. Quart. J. exp. Physiol. 37, 45—57 (1952).
MacINTOSH, F. C.: L'effet de la section des fibres préganglionnaires sur la teneur en acetyl-choline du ganglion sympathique. Arch. int. Physiol. 47, 321—324 (1938).
— The distribution of acetylcholine in the peripheral and central nervous system. J. Physiol. (Lond.) 99, 436—442 (1941).
— Biological estimation of acetylcholine. In: R. W. GERARD, Ed., Methods in Medical Research, vol. 3, 78—92. Chicago: The Year Book Publishers 1950.
— Formation, storage and release of acetylcholine at nerve endings. Canad. J. Biochem. 37, 343—356 (1959).
MANN, P. J. G., M. TENNENBAUM and J. H. QUASTEL: On the mechanism of acetylcholine formation in brain in vitro. Biochem. J. 32, 243—261 (1938).
— — — Acetylcholine metabolism in the central nervous system. The effects of potassium and other cations on acetylcholine liberation. Biochem. J. 33, 822—835 (1939).
MARTIN, A. R.: A further study of the statistical composition of the end-plate potential. J. Physiol. (Lond.) 130, 114—122 (1955).
MILTON, A. S.: The effect of temperature on the synthesis of acetylcholine by the enzyme choline acetylase from mammalian and fish brain. J. Physiol. (Lond.) 142, 25 P (1958).
— Choline acetylase in the gill plates of Mytilus edulis. J. Physiol. (Lond.) 145, 33—34 P (1959).
MURNAGHAN, M. F.: A defect in the release mechanism of acetylcholine caused by tick paralysis. Can. Fed. Proc. 2, 48—49 (1959).
NACHMANSOHN, D.: Chemical and Molecular Basis of Nerve Activity. New York: Academic Press 1959.
— and A. L. MACHADO: The formation of acetylcholine. A new enzyme: "Choline acetylase". J. Neurophysiol. 6. 397—403 (1943).
NASTUK, W. L.: Membrane potential changes at a single muscle end-plate produced by transitory application of acetylcholine with an electrically controlled microjet. Fed. Proc. 12, 102 (1953).
PALAY, S. L.: Synapses in the central nervous system. J. biophys. biochem. Cytol. Suppl. 2, 193—202 (1956).
— The morphology of synapses in the central nervous system. Exp. Cell. Res. Suppl. 5, 275 — 293 (1958).
— and G. E. PALADE: The fine structure of neurons. J. biophys. biochem. Cytol. 1, 69—88 (1955).
REISBERG, R. B.: Properties and biological significance of choline acetylase. Yale J. biol. Med. 29, 403—435 (1957).
DE ROBERTIS, E. D. P., and H. S. BENNETT: Some features of the submicroscopic morphology of synapses in frog and earthworm. J. biophys. biochem. Cytol. 1, 47—58 (1955).
ROSENBLUETH, A.: The transmission of Nerve Impulses at Neuroeffector Junctions and Peripheral Synapses. New York: John Wiley and Sons 1950.
ROUSELL, E. V.: Applied electrical pulses and the ammonia and acetylcholine of isolated cerebral cortex slices. Biochem. J. 57, 666—673 (1954).
SAWYER, C. H.: Cholinesterases in degenerating and regenerating peripheral nerves. Amer. J. Physiol. 146, 246—253 (1946).
SCHUELER, F. W., and others: The Hemicholiniums (symposium). Fed. Proc. 20, 561—599 (1961).
SHELLEY, H.: The inhibition of acetylcholine synthesis in guinea-pig brain slices by eserine and neostigmine. J. Physiol. (Lond.) 131, 329—340 (1956).
SMALLMAN, B. N.: Mechanisms of acetylcholine synthesis in the blowfly. J. Physiol. (Lond.) 132, 343—357 (1956).
— and R. W. FISHER: Effect of anticholinesterases on acetylcholine levels in insects. Can. J. Biochem. 36, 575—586 (1958).

STEPHENSON, M., and E. ROWATT: The production of acetylcholine by a strain of *Lactobacillus plantarum*. J. gen. Microbiol. 1, 280—298 (1947).

STONE, W. E.: Acetylcholine in the brain: I. "Free", "bound" and total acetylcholine. Arch. Biochem. 59, 181—192 (1955).

TOSCHI, G.: A biochemical study of brain microsomes. Exp. Cell. Res. 16, 232—255 (1959).

TOWER, D. B., and K. A. C. ELLIOTT: Activity of acetylcholine system in cerebral cortex of various unanaesthetized mammals. Amer. J. Physiol. 168, 747—759 (1952).

WEISS, P.: Protoplasm synthesis and substance transfer in neurons. Abstr. XVII Int. Physiol. Congress. Oxford, 101, 1947.

— and H. B. HISCOE: Experiments on the mechanism of nerve growth. J. exp. Zool. 107, 315—395 (1948).

WELSH, J. H., and J. E. HYDE: The distribution of acetylcholine in brains of rats of different ages. J. Neurophysiol. 7, 41—49 (1944).

WHITTAKER, V. P.: The isolation and characterization of acetylcholine containing particles from brain. Biochem. J. 72, 694—706 (1959).

WILSON, H., and J. P. LONG: The effect of hemicholinium (HC-3) at various peripheral cholinergic transmitting sites. Arch. int. Pharmacodyn. 120, 343—352 (1959).

WINTERINGHAM, F. P. W., A. HARRISON, M. A. McKAY and A. WEATHERLEY: Biochemistry of di*iso*propylphosphorofluoridate poisoning in the adult housefly. Biochem. J. 66, 49 P (1957).

WOLFGRAM, F. J.: Relative amounts of choline acetylase and cholinesterases in dorsal and ventral roots of cattle. Amer. J. Physiol. 176, 505—507 (1954).

Chapter 4

Classification and Comparative Enzymology of the Cholinesterases and Methods for their Determination

By

Klas-Bertil Augustinsson

With 1 Figure

Contents

Introduction

Cholinesterases (ChE's) are defined simply as enzymes which catalyze the hydrolysis of choline esters. There has been considerable discussion during the last 20 years on the specificity of these enzymes, their role in physiological systems, and the pharmacological importance of cholinesterase inhibitors. Everybody taking part in this discussion on the biochemical level will probably agree with the following: There are enzymes present in the animal body which split acetylcholine (ACh) and other choline esters at a very high rate. None of these enzymes so far studied splits only esters of choline; non-choline esters are also hydrolyzed, but at a lower rate. The specificity of cholinesterases therefore is not absolute, and "true" cholinesterases do not exist as far as the specificity is concerned.

In the following presentation, the esterases which have ACh as their natural substrate, according to a general (although not universal) agreement, are referred to as *acetylcholinesterases* (AChE). Other esterases, which according to their specificity and other characteristics are defined as cholinesterases, are termed *butyrocholinesterases* (BuChE), *propionocholinesterases* (PrChE), etc., referring to the substrates hydrolyzed at the highest rate. Such terms, however, carry no implications as to their physiological substrates, which are unknown for these enzymes.

The various aspects of ChE have been reviewed by AUGUSTINSSON (1948, 1950a), and the literature cited in his monograph of 1948 is fairly completely covered up to that date. WHITTAKER (1951) has reviewed critically the specificity, mode of action and distribution. The work of NACHMANSOHN and his collaborators has been compiled in a number of reviews, of which his paper published with

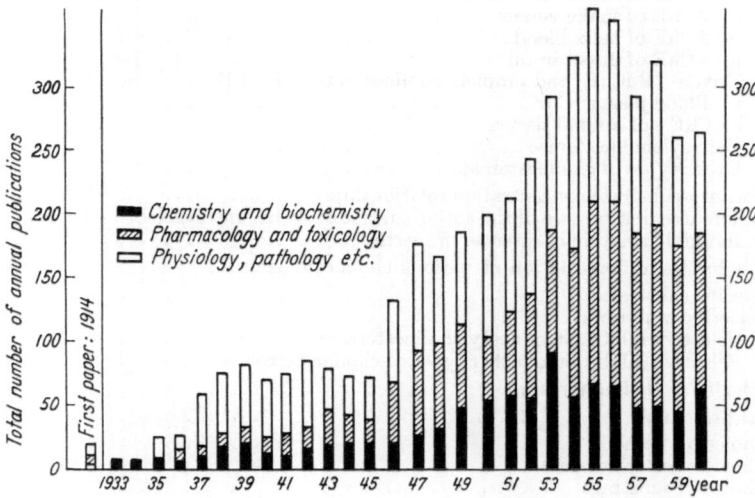

Fig. 1. Number of publications on cholinesterases and cholinesterase inhibitors

WILSON (1951), his comprehensive German article (1955) and particularly his fine recent monograph (1959) are the most notable. Less comprehensive surveys and discussions on special aspects of these enzymes have been made by THOMPSON (1953, 1954), DAVIES (1954), AUGUSTINSSON (1954), VINCENT (1955), and ARVY (1958). WILSON (1960) and AUGUSTINSSON (1960) are the authors of the chapters on these enzymes in the second edition of "The Enzymes". The fine papers by

DAVIES and GREEN (1958) and BERGMANN (1958) discuss the various aspects of the mechanism of action of ChE.

The number of annual publications on ChE's and ChE-inhibitors is illustrated in Fig. 1. There were only a few papers published up to 1934. Between 1937 and 1945 the number of papers was fairly constant, and the subject was characterized by studies on the relationship between esterase activity and physiological and pathological conditions and on the specificity of these enzymes. After World War II, when the organophosphorus compounds were made available for free scientific studies, there appeared an ever increasing number of annual publications on various aspects of these enzymes. The maximum number of publications seems to have been reached at about 1955. Still 250 to 300 papers on this subject are published each year.

Various types of cholinesterases

A. Historical

As early as 1914, Dale suggested that an enzyme is present in the blood which brings about the destruction (hydrolysis) of ACh. Such an enzyme was shown to exist in nearly all animal tissues (PLATTNER and HINTNER 1930), but has not been found in the plant kingdom. STEDMAN et al. (1932) prepared from horse serum an enzyme, called choline-esterase, which was considered to be a specific esterase for ACh and other choline esters. During the following years, a great number of papers appeared which dealt with the ACh-splitting activity of various animal tissues, vertebrate as well as invertebrate. One of the problems involved was the question of the existence of an esterase specific for ACh, a question of considerable interest in view of the physiological function of this ester.

STEDMAN et al. (1932) and SIMONART (1933) considered that the enzyme from blood serum is specific for choline esters, although not for ACh since it splits butyrylcholine and propionylcholine at a higher rate than ACh. Later experiments, however, have indicated that the ChE's present in some sera are not specific for choline esters, although they split them faster than non-choline esters (VAHLQUIST 1935; GLICK 1938b, 1939, 1941). ALLES and HAWES (1940) were the first to demonstrate that human serum ChE differs markedly from the esterase present in human erythrocytes; the latter enzyme is inhibited by high concentrations of ACh and, in contrast to the serum esterase, hydrolyzes acetyl-β-methylcholine (methacholine, Mecholyl). These observations were confirmed and added to by a number of investigators. RICHTER and CROFT (1942) pointed out that the ChE's are differentiated from other "simple" esterases *(aliesterases)* by being sensitive to 10^{-5} M eserine (physostigmine). MENDEL and RUDNEY (1943a, b, 1944) proposed benzoylcholine as a selective substrate for the serum ChE (MENDEL et al. 1943) and designated the two types of eserine-sensitive esterases as "true" and "pseudo" ChE. ZELLER and BISSEGGER (1943) proposed tentative models for the active surface of the two types of ChE, and AUGUSTINSSON (1944) separated electrophoretically the serum and erythrocyte ChE of horse. NACHMANSOHN and ROTHENBERG (1945) demonstrated that the ChE in nerve and muscle tissues and in erythrocytes, in contrast to serum esterase, splits propionylcholine at the same or at a lower rate than ACh, whereas butyrylcholine and non-choline esters are split at a very low rate or not at all. A comprehensive kinetic study of human serum and erythrocyte ChE was performed by SCHAEFER (1947).

These and subsequent investigations indicated the existence of two types of choline ester-splitting enzymes for which various names have been proposed

(Table 1). The "specific (true) ChE" of brain and erythrocytes was found not to be specific for choline esters (BODANSKY 1946; AUGUSTINSSON 1948, 1949; ZELLER et al. 1949) and the importance of a careful consideration of the substrate concentration when following the enzymatic hydrolysis of various esters was emphasized (AUGUSTINSSON 1948). In view of the fact that this esterase has a higher affinity for ACh than for any other ester so far tested, and ACh most probably is its physiological substrate, AUGUSTINSSON and NACHMANSOHN (1948) proposed the term *acetylcholinesterase* (AChE) which has been widely accepted among enzyme chemists.

Table 1. *Names in general use to designate various types of cholinesterase (ChE)*

Authors	Designation	
Present article	acetylcholinesterase (AChE)	butyrocholinesterase (BuChE) propionocholinesterase (PrChE) benzoylcholinesterase (BzChE)[1]
STEDMAN et al. 1932	not studied	choline-esterase
Most of the authors 1933—1942	cholinesterase	cholinesterase
MENDEL and RUDNEY 1943a, b; MENDEL et al. 1943, and subsequent publications, including those by MYERS and the British investigators of Sir HENRY DALE's school	true cholinesterase (specific cholinesterase)	pseudo-cholinesterase
ZELLER and BISSEGGER 1943 and subsequent publications	e-type cholinesterase[2]	s-type cholinesterase
NACHMANSOHN and ROTHENBERG 1945 and subsequent publications until 1949	cholinesterase	unspecified esterase
GLICK 1945	specific cholinesterase	non-specific cholin-esterase
AUGUSTINSSON 1948, BURGEN and HOBBIGER 1951	cholinesterase I	cholinesterase II
AUGUSTINSSON and NACHMANSOHN 1949 and subsequent publications by both authors and those by most American investigators	acetylcholinesterase	cholinesterase
KOELLE and GILMAN 1949; KOELLE 1950 and subsequent publications by KOELLE until 1955	specific cholinesterase	non-specific cholin-esterase
RICHTER, cited by STURGE and WHITTAKER 1950, WHITTAKER 1951	acetocholinesterase	butyrocholinesterase
KARCZMAR et al. 1953	acetylcholinesterase	pseudocholinesterase (cholinesterase)
JACOB 1954	acetylcholinesterase	XChE

[1] The existence of a "benzoylcholinesterase" (SAWYER 1945) is still controversal.
[2] The ChE of colubrine venoms was considered by ZELLER (1948) as a separate class and was called by him ophio-cholinesterase or c-type cholinesterase. BOVET-NITTI (1947) proposed the name "acetylase" for this enzyme.

WHITTAKER (1951) and his collaborators (ADAMS 1949, ADAMS and WHITTAKER 1949, MOUNTER and WHITTAKER 1950, WHITTAKER 1953) demonstrated in a fine series of papers that the ChE's of erythrocytes and brain are most active towards those choline and non-choline esters, the structure of which approaches closely that of ACh; the serum ChE's, on the other hand, exhibit highest activity towards those esters which resemble butyrylcholine in their structure (ADAMS and WHITTAKER 1949, STURGE and WHITTAKER 1950). RICHTER (cited by WHITTAKER 1951) therefore suggested that the two types of ChE should be designated as *aceto-cholinesterase* and *butyrocholinesterase*. AChE present in rat heart, and hydrolysing propionylcholine most rapidly, was demonstrated by ORD and THOMPSON (1951) and should consequently be classified as *propionocholinesterase*.

From a more extensive investigation of ChE's present in mammalian and avian sera, MYERS (1953) concluded that there is no clear distinction between BuChE and PrChE. Results obtained with various tissues indicated that these esterase appear to be species-specific, and not organ-specific. A comprehensive study of the ChE's of vertebrate plasma, separated electrophoretically from other esterases present, confirmed and enlarged upon these ideas (AUGUSTINSSON 1959a, b, c). It was demonstrated that an *"acetocholinesterase"* (AcChE) probably exists in the plasma of lower vertebrates and that no clearly cut classification of ChE's present in plasma and in various animal tissues can be made because types intermediate between "specific" ChE, as BuChE, PrChE, and AcChE, also exist.

B. Cholinesterases as a separate group of esterases

Cholinesterases constitute a group of esterases which hydrolyze choline esters at a higher rate than other esters, when hydrolysis rates are compared at optimum conditions regarding substrate concentration, pH, ionic strength, etc., using preparations free from other esterases. All esterases which show this specificity are inhibited by 10^{-5} M eserine or the same concentration of neostigmine (Prostigmine), and are also much more sensitive to quaternary ammonium ions than are other esterases. This outstanding affinity of ChE's for cationic substrates and inhibitors is the most characteristic feature of these enzymes, and suggests that the active center of ChE's, in contrast to other esterases, includes a negative group ("anionic site") in addition to the ester-binding group ("esteratic site"). The existence of an anionic site in ChE's seems to be the structural characteristic of these enzymes, and determines in many cases the *action specificity* of the enzymes. The hydrolysis of esters of choline and structurally analogous alcohols, in addition to the inhibition by cationic compounds, depends on the existence of this site in the active surface. These compounds are therefore not hydrolyzed by, and do not inhibit, respectively, other esterases. The importance of the anionic site for the formation of enzyme-substrate or enzyme-inhibitor complexes differs from one type of ChE to an other, as will be discussed in Section C. III. On the other hand, there is no evidence presented so far that the structure of the esteratic site of ChE's is much different from that in other esterases, especially those which are sensitive to organophosphorus compounds. Consequently, cholinesterases *a priori* can hydrolyze any ester, irrespective of the presence of a positively charged group in the substrate molecule. In contrast to the anionic site, the esteratic site primarily determines the *substrate specificity*, particularly regarding the acid radical of the ester.

Cholinesterases belong to a wider group of esterases which are readily inhibited by a variety of organophosphorus compounds; such esterases were called *B-esterases* by ALDRIDGE (1953b) and include also the so-called *aliesterases*. All these enzymes probably exhibit an essentially similar reaction mechanism (WILSON 1954, DAVIES and GREEN 1958), i.e., the esterase reacts with the ester to produce an intermediary acyl-enzyme complex which can react with a variety of acyl acceptors, including water. An analogous mechanism is used to explain the inhibition of these esterases by certain phosphoryl, carbamyl, and sulphonyl derivatives. Further details of this mechanism are found in COHEN's chapter (7) in the present volume.

Aliesterases differ from ChE's in being unable to hydrolyze choline esters and in being resistant to 10^{-5} M eserine. The latter agent, however, is not an absolutely selective inhibitor of ChE's, because aliesterases exist (e.g., in the plasma of duck, frog, pike) which are sensitive to eserine in comparatively low concentrations (pI_{50} 5.5 to 4.5), although they do not hydrolyze choline esters (AUGUSTINSSON 1959 b). This is indicative of a close relation between the ChE's and aliesterases. The turtle plasma esterase displays the characteristic of both an aliesterase and a ChE, being highly sensitive to eserine (pI_{50} 6.3) and certain organosphosphorus compounds. This esterase is the first example of an eserine-sensitive esterase which hydrolyzes non-choline esters (e.g., tripropionin, phenylpropionate, *iso*amyl-propionate) more rapidly than choline esters (e.g., propionylcholine). It may represent an intermediate stage in the phylogenetic evolution of plasma esterases, of which the aliesterases are suggested to represent a more primitive stage, and the ChE's (and also the arylesterases, see below) may be regarded as specialized forms (AUGUSTINSSON 1959 b, c).

Esterases which differ from ChE's and aliesterases in being resistant to organo-phosphorus compounds were designated by ALDRIDGE (1953 b) as *A-esterases*. Like the aliesterases (B-esterases), they hydrolyze carboxylic esters other than choline esters; since aromatic esters are hydrolyzed at particularly high rates, these enzymes are also called *arylesterases* (AUGUSTINSSON 1959 a). Some of them are probably responsible also for the hydrolysis of organophosphorus compounds (e.g., DFP, Paraoxon). In contrast to the ChE's and aliesterases, the arylesterases are inhibited by chelating agents and activated by Ca^{++} (MOUNTER 1955), which suggests that the mechanism of action of arylesterases may differ from that of the other esterases. Arylesterases are typical SH-enzymes (AUGUSTINSSON, unpublished) in contrast to other esterases including the *"C-esterases"* (BERGMANN et al. 1957).

In conclusion, the ChE's may be regarded as a group of esterases with certain characteristics, of which the high affinity to cationic substrates and inhibitors, and the sensitivity to low concentrations of eserine are the most important. Other esterases, such as arylesterases, aliesterases and certain proteolytic enzymes (e.g., trypsin, chymotrypsin, thrombin) cannot hydrolyze esters of choline. All types of ChE, however, can act on esters other than those of choline.

C. Comparison of properties of various types of cholinesterases

As stated in the historical introduction to this chapter, various types of ChE exist. One type is called *acetylcholinesterase* (AChE) and has rather well defined properties, which differentiate it from other ChE's (BuChE, PrChE, etc.). The properties of the latter differ more strikingly from animal to animal (MYERS 1953; AUGUSTINSSON 1958 a, 1959 c) than do those of AChE. Therefore, designation must always be made according to the source of enzyme.

I. Substrate specificity

1. Acetylcholinesterases (AChE)

Acetylcholinesterases isolated from the mammalian brain (grey substance), erythrocytes, or electric tissue of certain fish show much the same substrate specificity, with only a few exceptions. Other types of AChE, present in high concentration in colubrine venoms, *Helix* blood, and insect brain, show specificity and other properties which differ slightly from those of mammalian AChE.

a) AChE of nerve tissues and erythrocytes

These enzymes split choline esters or thiocholine esters at decreasing velocity in the following order: ACh > PrCh > BuCh, the latter ester being hydrolyzed at a very low rate or not at all (NACHMANSOHN and ROTHENBERG 1945, AUGUSTINSSON 1949, WHITTAKER 1951). The relative hydrolysis rates of ACh and PrCh differ from tissue to tissue; in some cases, e.g., chicken brain, the rate with PrCh can exceed that with ACh. Acetyl-β-methylcholine (ALLES and HAWES 1940, MENDEL and RUDNEY 1943 b, AUGUSTINSSON and ISACHSEN 1957, HEILBRONN 1959) is hydrolyzed, but not benzoylcholine (MENDEL et al. 1943, ADAMS and WHITTAKER 1949).

Acetylcholinesterases can hydrolyze many non-choline esters. As for choline esters, the optimum acyl group is acetate for aliphatic esters (ADAMS and WHITTAKER 1949, ADAMS 1949); butyrates are split only very slowly. The configuration of the alkyl group also determines the hydrolysis rate of an ester. It is a general characteristic of these enzymes that they hydrolyze the carbon analogue of ACh (3,3-dimethylbutyl acetate) at a high rate. This property shows that interaction with the active center of the enzyme and activation of an ester link can occur in the absence of a positively charged group in the substrate, and that molecular shape is an important factor governing the rate of hydrolysis by AChE. Systematic studies of this kind have been made with human erythrocytes (ADAMS 1949), horse erythrocytes (MOUNTER and WHITTAKER 1950), and pigeon brain (WHITTAKER 1949).

Minor differences in specificity properties among AChE in various tissues have been reported (BERGMANN and SEGAL 1955).

b) AChE of snake venom

A systematic study of the specificity of the cobra venom AChE (MOUNTER 1951) revealed that this esterase is a typical AChE, differing only in detail from other members of this group of esterases. ZELLER's (1948) first conclusion that this esterase is of a separate type (ophio-ChE or c-type ChE) was later withdrawn (ZELLER 1949; ZELLER and UTZ 1949). Among choline esters, the acetate is hydrolyzed at the highest rate and other relative hydrolysis rates for this esterase are similar to those of mammalian AChE (AUGUSTINSSON 1949, 1951 a, b; MOUNTER 1951). The acetate link of acetylsalicylcholine is split at even a higher rate than that in ACh (AUGUSTINSSON 1951 b). The earlier observed fact that water-soluble aliphatic esters (e.g., ethyl and propyl acetates) are hydrolyzed in contradistinction to sparingly soluble esters (e.g., amylacetate) (BOVET-NITTI 1947) was probably due to a non-specific inactivation by oily substances (MOUNTER 1951). Aliphatic esters, including triglycerides, show the same relative hydrolysis rates as for mammalian AChE, the high hydrolysis rate for 3,3-dimethylbutyl acetate being typical also for this enzyme. Acetylaneurin is hydrolyzed at a comparatively high rate (AUGUSTINSSON 1951 b). Haloesters (e.g., β-chloroethyl acetate) (ZELLER et al. 1949; ZELLER and UTZ 1949) and phenol esters (ZELLER et al. 1949, MOUNTER and WHITTAKER 1953) are also split. The observation that cobra venom, in contrast to the venoms of other elapids, hydrolyzes tributyrin (GHOSH and SARKAR 1956) has not been confirmed. Acetylcholinesterase is probably the only esterase present in colubrine venoms.

c) AChE of Helix blood

This invertebrate blood is serveral times more active towards ACh than the blood of vertebrates (AUGUSTINSSON 1946, 1948, 1949). The substrate pattern for this esterase is similar to those of AChE from other sources. The affinity of acetyl-β-methylcholine for the snail blood esterase is much lower than that for the erythrocyte AChE. Acetylaneurin is split at a comparatively high rate (AUGUSTINS-SON 1951 b) and so also are procaine and other esters of p-aminobenzoic acid (BASTIDE and DASTUGUE 1953).

Other tissues of *Helix* (BASTIDE 1954) have not been studied in sufficient detail to allow a definition of the ChE present, but the AChE type in the blood probably also exists in other tissues. The dart sac is especially active and contains, in addition to an AChE, a ChE of unknown type (AUGUSTINSSON 1948).

d) AChE of insect brain

The substrate specificity patterns among insect esterases differ greatly (CASIDA 1955). The activity of insect-head breis toward choline esters can be differentiated into at least two types of AChE with regard to their behavior toward ACh and acetyl-β-methylcholine (METCALF and MARCH 1950, BABERS and PRATT 1951, METCALF et al. 1955, WOLFE and SMALLMAN 1956). The house-fly head enzyme is responsible for the hydrolysis of both these esters, but the bee-head appears to contain an esterase which hydrolyzes acetyl-β-methylcholine (cf., RICHARDS and CUTKOMP 1945), but not ACh, butyrylcholine, or phenyl acetate. Acetyl-β-methylcholine, however, is not present as a natural substrate in the bee brain (AUGUSTINS-SON and GRAHN 1954), as was suggested by TOBIAS et al. (1946). The high hydrolysis rate of acetyl-β-methylcholine compared with that of ACh, especially at high substrate concentration, is also characteristic of the AChE present in the CNS of other insects (TOBIAS et al. 1946; CHADWICK and HILL 1947; KOOISTRA 1950; STEGWEE 1950, 1951; BABERS and PRATT 1951; ROAN and MAEDA 1953, 1954). These esterases are all similar to that present in house fly, the substrate specificity of which is otherwise similar to mammalian AChE (WOLFE and SMALL-MANN 1956). Fly and bee AChE also hydrolyze aliphatic esters at different rates, fly AChE having maximum rate with 3,3-dimethylbutyl acetate and bee AChE a maximum rate with *iso*amyl propionate (METCALF et al. 1955). Insect CNS also contains other esterases, e.g., arylesterase (LORD and POTTER 1954; METCALF et al. 1955).

It will be noted that the specificity properties of AChE present in other invertebrate species also differ from those of mammalian AChE and those of the other types presented above (AUGUSTINSSON 1946, 1948; WALOP 1951; WALOP and BOOT 1950).

2. Butyro- (BuChE) and propionocholinesterases (PrChE)

Cholinesterases which hydrolyze butyrylcholine or propionylcholine at a higher rate than ACh show much divergence in specificity toward various choline and non-choline esters. It is therefore not possible to apply results obtained with enzyme preparations (pure or crude) of one species to those of any other species. The idea that these esterases have less claim to be regarded as ChE's than has AChE receives no support from their specificity properties and sensitivity to esterase inhibitors.

a) Blood plasma ChE

In addition to the properties in common, such as high affinity to choline esters and cationic inhibitors, the electrophoretic mobility relative to other plasma proteins, including other types of esterases, is practically the same (between the α_2- and β-globulins) for most ChE's present in mammalian plasma (TOGNI and MEIER 1953; COHEN and WARRINGA 1957; AUGUSTINSSON 1958a, 1959a). The presence of a BuChE is characteristic of the plasma of man, dog, cat, horse, and guinea-pig. Although they all hydrolyze butyrylcholine at a higher rate than lower homologues, the enzymes of this type differ in their capacity to split non-choline esters (AUGUSTINSSON 1959) and in certain other respects (KALOW 1952a). For horse and human plasma BuChE the optimum acyl group is butyrate, for both aliphatic and choline esters (GLICK 1941, ADAMS and WHITTAKER 1949, STURGE and WHITTAKER 1950). The relationship between alkyl group configuration and rate of hydrolysis with these esterases is similar to that of AChE. The high rate of hydrolysis of esters of 3,3-dimethylbutanol, compared with other aliphatic esters, is also characteristic of BuChE. Substitution in position "1" of the alkyl chain, giving esters of secondary alcohols, lowers the hydrolysis rate of both choline (e.g., acetyl-β-methylcholine) and aliphatic derivatives (ADAMS and WHITTAKER 1949). This effect does not occur with thioesters (KOELLE 1950, AUGUSTINSSON and ISACHSEN 1957, HEILBRONN 1959). Due to the absence of an aliesterase (lipase) from human and dog plasma, present in the other vertebrate plasma, the BuChE of the former is alone responsible for the hydrolysis of aliphatic esters, including triglycerides. On the other hand, aromatic esters, e.g., phenyl acetate, are hydrolyzed mainly by an arylesterase present in these plasma (WHITTAKER 1951, AUGUSTINSSON 1959a). There is no evidence for the presence of a specific "procaine-esterase" in human plasma; BuChE is responsible for this activity (HUC 1950; KALOW 1952a, b; AUGUSTINSSON 1952).

The ruminant plasmas have very low ChE activity (GUNTER 1946, MENDEL and MYERS 1955) and the specificity of the esterases present varies considerably from species to species, but in no case has a typical BuChE been detected (MYERS 1953, TOGNI and MEIER 1953, HARDWICK 1956, AUGUSTINSSON 1959a). A BuChE with a substrate specificity pattern differing from those of all other ChE's is present in low concentration in swine plasma (LEVINE and SURAN 1950, 1951; MYERS 1953; AUGUSTINSSON 1958b, AUGUSTINSSON and OLSSON 1959). This enzyme hydrolyzes phenyl acetate at a rate which is only slightly lower than that of butyrylcholine. The same BuChE is present in sow's milk in 20 to 25 times higher concentration (HINES and MC CANCE 1953, AUGUSTINSSON 1958b, AUGUSTINSSON and OLSSON 1959).

Rat (LÉVY 1951c, MYERS 1953), rabbit (LÉVY 1951b, KOELLE 1953), and chicken (EARL and THOMPSON 1952, AUSTIN and BERRY 1953, PAULESU 1956, FERRARI 1957) are characterized by PrChE, the properties of which differ in various respects (BLUMENTHAL and WOODARD 1957, AUGUSTINSSON 1959a, b). For instance, chicken plasma PrChE hydrolyzes acetyl-β-methylcholine considerably more rapidly than other PrChE's and ChE's of mammalian plasma (MYERS 1953). The single esterase present in turtle plasma has also the properties of a PrChE, but differs from all other ChE's so far studied in hydrolyzing choline esters at a rate lower than that for the corresponding non-choline esters (e.g., tripropionin) (AUGUSTINSSON 1959b); see further Section B. Diacetylmorphine (heroin) is also split at a very high rate by this enzyme (ELLIS 1948).

Plasma ChE's are regarded as a group of esterases with many divergent properties, not only with regard to specificity for various choline and non-choline esters, but also to sensitivity to inhibitors and to activity-substrate concentration relationship. No clearly defined classification can therefore be made, and in most vertebrate plasmas the ChE present seems to be characteristic of the species.

b) ChE's of animal tissues

Species differences of ChE's present in various tissues also exist, but have not been so thoroughly investigated as those of plasma ChE's. Some authors are of the opinion (GOLDSTEIN 1951, MYERS 1953) that the specificity pattern of a particular ChE is species specific but not organ specific. However, a variation in the specificity pattern of the ChE's from one tissue to another within the same animal has been reported (SAWYER and EVERETT 1947; KOELLE 1950, 1951; DAVIES et al. 1953; BERGMANN and SEGAL 1955). Noticeable are the extensive studies of rat tissues by ORD and THOMPSON (1950). These authors (ORD and THOMPSON 1951) demonstrated that rat heart ChE hydrolyzes propionylcholine more rapidly than either ACh or butyrylcholine. This PrChE is probably identical with the esterase present in rat serum (MYERS 1953). The different opinions as to the specificity problem may be due to the fact that the experiments were carried out with crude preparations in which disturbing proteins, including various types of other hydrolyzing enzymes, may be limiting factors.

Evidence has also been accumulated that all types of ChE are widespread in different mammalian tissues and that this is particularly true for BuChE and PrChE. These enzymes occur, for instance, in the central nervous system, particularly in white fiber tracts (ORD and THOMPSON 1952), in other nerve tissues (KOELLE 1951, 1954; BERNSOHN and POSSLEY 1958), striated muscle (BECKETT and BOURNE 1957) and other tissues, together with AChE. ORD and THOMPSON (1950) classified rat tissues into three groups depending on the relative concentrations of AChE and PrChE: A: tissues containing chiefly AChE (brain, skeletal mucsle, adrenal glands); B: tissues containing both AChE and PrChE (stomach, liver, lung, salivary glands); C: tissues containing chiefly PrChE (heart, intestinal muscle and mucosa, skin). The occurrence of these enzymes in cat tissues has been investigated histochemically by KOELLE (1950, 1951) who gives a more detailed presentation of his results in this volume (Chapter 6).

In lower forms of animals, the ChE patterns differ greatly from those of vertebrates. Enzymes similar to the BuChE or PrChE of mammalian plasma have not been detected in any invertebrate species so far studied. In most cases, the eserine-sensitive esterases are similar to the AChE of mammals. Some of these enzymes, however, seem to have pronounced resistance to eserine, e.g., an esterase of *Planaria* (HAWKINS and MENDEL 1946), but have not been further investigated.

3. Benzoylcholinesterase

The existence of a benzoylcholinesterase which hydrolyzes benzoylcholine at a higher rate than other esters is questionable (MENDEL and MYERS 1955). It was observed first by SAWYER (1945) that an esterase is present in the guinea-pig liver and to a lesser extent in the rabbit liver which splits benzoylcholine but is not concerned with ACh hydrolysis. Evidence of a similar esterase has been noted in guinea-pig kidney (NACHMANSOHN and ROTHENBERG 1944), ox kidney (GUNTER 1946, BLASCHKO et al. 1947) and the plasma of certain rabbits (ELLIS 1947, LÉVY 1951d, KOELLE 1953). The properties of this enzyme, which is different from BuChE (LÉVY and TCHOUBAR 1952) and splits certain derivatives of benzoylcholine and phenylacetylcholine at relatively high rates (ORMEROD 1953, ROSNATI and BOVET-NITTI 1955), have not been investigated further. The activity may well be due to an eserine-resistant esterase of the arylesterase type. This does not exclude, however, the possibility that ChE's of this or other types exist and may be more widespread than previously considered (KOELLE 1953).

4. Other types of cholinesterases

It is an open question whether still other types of ChE exist. An "acetocholinesterase" is probably present in low concentration in the plasma of goat and sheep and in that of certain teleostian fish (AUGUSTINSSON 1959b). The hydrolysis of palmitoylcholine by certain pigeon and rat tissues with liver as most active (BERRY and WHITTAKER 1959) is not due to a ChE but to an eserine-resistant esterase, the relation of which to tissue lipases and other esterases has not been established. In many cases, there is probably no reason for suggesting new types of ChE; the fundamental properties are mostly similar, differing only slightly from species to species.

II. Activity-substrate concentration relationship

Extensive studies have been presented on the relationship between ChE activity and substrate concentration, due mainly to the observation (ALLES and HAWES 1940; ZELLER and BISSEGGER 1943; AUGUSTINSSON 1948) that this relationship differentiates between AChE and most other types of ChE. Studies of this relationship must be carried out with esterase preparations free from disturbing proteins. Mixtures of esterases, as found in crude tissue homogenates (BERGMANN and SEGAL 1955), are not suitable and the results obtained will, accordingly, be difficult to interpret.

It is characteristic of the activity of AChE (demonstrated with erythrocytes and nervous tissue from various species, and with electric tissue) that it is inhibited by a high concentration of ACh, in contrast to the BuChE activity of human serum and most of the ChE's which show substrate preference for butyryl-choline and other butyrate esters. When the hydrolysis rates obtained with pure AChE enzymes are plotted against the logarithms of substrate concentration (pS), bell-shaped curves are obtained. The optimum substrate concentration is at about 3×10^{-3} M ACh and the dissociation constant (K_s) of the AChE-ACh-complex is about 5×10^{-4}. In most instances, this relationship between activity and substrate concentration is the same with ACh and propionylcholine (AUGUSTINSSON 1949); minor differences, however, have been observed, especially in cases of asymmetrical bell-shaped curves (MYERS 1952) which are also obtained with the corresponding thiocholine esters (HEILBRONN 1959). When other substrates are used this relationship may be completely different. Therefore, in studying substrate specificity, the effect of substrate concentration on the rate of hydrolysis is of importance (AUGUSTINSSON 1948, 1949). Thus, it is characteristic of AChE's that acetyl-β-methylcholine is hydrolyzed at a lower rate than ACh at low substrate concentration, but at a higher rate when the concentrations of substrates are high, i.e., the optimum substrate concentration is not the same with ACh and its β-methyl derivative. Other esters, especially non-choline esters, e.g., triacetin, do not inhibit esterase activity at high substrate concentration. These esters, therefore, are hydrolyzed more rapidly than ACh at high concentrations. Various AChE's from a number of sources have been shown to behave similarly in this respect, e.g., mammalian erythrocytes and brain (HOLTON 1948, AUGUSTINSSON 1950b), fish muscle (LUNDIN 1959), electric tissue (AUGUSTINSSON 1949), cobra venom (HOLTON 1948, AUGUSTINSSON 1951b), insect brain (KOOISTRA 1950, BABER and PRATT 1951, ROAN and MAEDA 1954, METCALF et al. 1955, WOLFE and SMALLMAN 1956).

All ChE's so far studied which split butyrylcholine at a higher rate than other esters of choline (i.e., those present in human, horse and dog plasma) give the usual dissociation curves $(K_s = 2 \times 10^{-3})$ with butyrylcholine, propionylcholine, and ACh, and esterase activity is therefore not inhibited by high concentrations of these substrates. This property studied with ACh has been used extensively to characterize the type of esterase present (MENDEL and RUDNEY 1943; AUGUSTINSSON 1948, 1949; GRÉGOIRE et al. 1955b) and is still useful in differentiating AChE from other types of ChE. It is, however, not recommended for differentiating these enzymes in mixtures. Moreover, the MICHAELIS constant as judged from the

7*

activity-pS curve is dependent on the concentration of certain salts (e.g., KCl) (MYERS 1952; SMALLMAN and WOLFE 1955; GRÉGOIRE et al. 1955 b, 1956).

No difference between the activity-pS curves for AChE and BuChE is obtained when substrates other than those mentioned are employed. Thus, certain aromatic esters, as for instance benzoylcholine (AUGUSTINSSON 1948; TODRICK et al. 1951; KALOW et al. 1956), acetylsalicylcholine (AUGUSTINSSON 1948), furfuroylcholine (LÉVY 1951 a), and procaine (KALOW 1952 b), produce inhibition of human serum BuChE with excess of substrate. The similarity between the systems ACh-AChE and benzoylcholine-BuChE has been considered, especially by KALOW et al. (1956). An equation (SCHAEFER 1947), which differs from the classical one of MICHAELIS and MENTEN and which is independent of whether the enzyme is inhibited by excess substrate or not (HARDEGG and SCHAEFER 1952), predicts that in addition to hydrolysis, other reactions occur between substrate and enzyme which give rise to inhibition of the catalytic activity; the latter reactions have been called "Autokatastase" by HARDEGG and POCHE (1952). This phenomenon is common to both AChE and plasma BuChE, and the specificity of the esterases is consequently determined by both the rate constant for the time-dependent hydrolysis reaction and the specificity of "Autokatastase", which in its turn is dependent on the affinity of the substrate for the inhibitory group(s) of the enzyme (HARDEGG et al. 1956).

The PrChE's behave similarly to the BuChE's as far as the activity-substrate concentration relationship is concerned.

III. Differences in structure of the active surface of AChE and BuChE

In contrast to AChE, which is available as highly purified and stable preparations with high specific activity and constant substrate specificity pattern, few of the other types of ChE have been obtained pure enough to allow detailed studies of the structure of the active surface. The few studies described, such as those involving degradation of phosphorylated enzymes and kinetic analysis, have been performed with partly purified human or horse plasma BuChE, the structures of which differ in certain details from that of AChE. Other ChE's have not been studied in this respect.

Like most animal carboxylic esterases, none of the different types of ChE contains nor requires any specific prosthetic group or metal for activity. Various cations (e.g., Ca^{++}, Mg^{++}) have been found to increase the activity, but it is improbable that any of these are essential for ChE activity. The activity of these esterases must therefore be a function of their amino-acid sequence. The exact structure of the "active center" of any of these enzymes, discussed in detail by COHEN and OOSTERBAAN in this volume (Chapter 7), is still controversial, and tentative models proposed are, with a few exceptions, hypothetical.

The great affinity of ChE for cationic substrates and inhibitors suggests, as was pointed out in Section B, that the active center is composed of a negative group ("negative nitrogen-attracting group", ADAMS and WHITTAKER 1950; "anionic site", WILSON 1951, 1954, 1955) in addition to the ester-binding group ("esteratic site"). The phenomenon of inhibition by excess acetylcholine (cf. Section C. II), characteristic of the AChE's and explained by the existence of two active sites, is, however, not shown by many of the other cholinesterases. It is partly because of this difference that the existence of an anionic site in BuChE and related enzymes has been the subject of much argument. Evidence has been presented for a variety of hydrolyzing enzymes, including AChE and BuChE, that inhibition by organophosphorus compounds occurs by irreversible phosphorylation of a single group at or near the active center (see Chapter 7). It has been demonstrated that the phosphorus is always bound eventually to the hydroxyl group of serine, and, therefore, it has been suggested that one of these amino acid residues in the molecules of both AChE and BuChE might be responsible for the catalytic activity. As far as this phosphorylation mechanism is concerned, there is probably no fundamental difference between various types of ChE.

However, the pH-dependence of the esterase activity is inconsistent with the view that the serine-hydroxyl is the active group. It has been claimed (WILSON 1954, 1955; BERGMANN et al. 1956, 1958) that the esteratic site contains one basic (nucleophilic) group (pK_a 5.8 to 7.0) and one acidic (electrophilic) group (pK_a 8.9 to 9.5). The imidazole ring in histidine is the only group in proteins with a pK_a (5.6 to 7.1) in the range exhibited by the basic group. However, the hypothesis that imidazol is a constituent of the esteratic site is based on indirect evidence obtained by kinetic studies, and also on observations that the pH-activity relationship may be influenced by several independent ionizable groups in the substrate (DAVIES and GREEN 1958). The acidic group with $pK_2 \approx 9$ is not so easily explained. From comparative studies with oxy- and thiol-esters, BERGMANN (1958) concluded that the acidic group (perhaps the phenolic hydroxyl of tyrosine) forms a hydrogen bridge with the ethereal oxygen of an oxy-ester, but not with thiol-esters. This idea was extended recently by HEILBRONN in her studies on spontaneous (1958) and enzymatic hydrolysis (1959) of the β-methyl derivatives of acetylcholine and its thiol analogue. In plasma BuChE, in contrast to AChE, the hydrolysis rates of the thiocholine esters were independent of a shielding β-methyl group, and therefore, a binding to the sulfur might not be essential for enzymatic hydrolysis by the former esterase. This finding was used to explain why the β-methyl thiol-ester, but not the oxy-ester, is hydrolyzed by the plasma enzyme (AUGUSTINSSON and ISACHSEN 1957). The minor importance of an acidic group in the esteratic site of the plasma BuChE, in contrast to the fairly well established importance of such a group in AChE, is suggested by these studies, but needs further support.

There has been much argument as to the presence of a negative group ("anionic site") in the plasma BuChE and other types of ChE which do not show inhibition by excess cationic substrate. In order to explain this property and other differences, such as the specificity against homologous choline esters, two hypotheses have been advanced: AChE alone contains an anionic site (ZELLER and BISSEGGER 1953, ADAMS and WHITTAKER 1950), and the number of anionic sites is different, 2 for AChE and 1 for the others (BERGMANN 1955, 1958). Several experimental data have been presented to show which of these views is the more likely, but they are controversial in many points.

From studies on the inhibitory effect of quaternary ammonium ions (e.g., tetraethylammonium) as a function of pH, it has been concluded (BERGMANN 1955, 1958; BERGMANN et al. 1956) that human plasma BuChE possesses an anionic site. The inhibition of this enzyme by bis-quaternary ammonium salts was similar to that produced by mono-quaternary compounds, in contrast to the behavior of AChE which was more sensitive to molecules having two quaternary groups. This difference between the two types of esterases was assumed by BERGMANN et al. to be due to the presence of one anionic site in plasma BuChE and two anionic sites in AChE. The existence of an anionic site in the plasma enzyme was further supported by the observation (BERGMANN and WURZEL 1954) that quaternary ammonium ions inhibit the hydrolysis of acetylcholine more than that of neutral substrates (e.g., n-propyl fluoroacetate). The presence of an anionic site in plasma BuChE was also used as an explanation for the findings that tertiary amino compounds (e.g., diethyl-aminoethyl acetate) as substrates were hydrolysed at a higher rate, and that eserine was a stronger inhibitor in acid solution, where these compounds are protonated to give cations, than in neutral solution (WILSON and BERGMANN 1950, WILSON 1954, BERGMANN and WURZEL 1954).

Several arguments against this view have been presented. In contrast to the large difference in hydrolysis rates of ACh and its uncharged carbon analogue, $(CH_3)_3 C-CH_2-CH_2-O-COCH_3$, by AChE, the ratio of affinities for the two substrates to plasma BuChE is only 1.29. ADAMS and WHITTAKER (1950) therefore concluded that for plasma BuChE it makes no difference whether a quaternary nitrogen or carbon combines with the active surface. Consequently, it was concluded that this esterase probably does not possess a negatively charged group. If it existed, it would have to exert less than 7% of the potential of the corresponding group in AChE.

The difference in the inhibitory effects of diquaternary ammonium salts on AChE and plasma BuChE was attributed by BERNHARD (1955) to VAN DER WAALS' forces. Other forces, such as ion-induced dipole interaction, may also be involved (ADAMS and WHITTAKER 1950). BERGMANN (1958) argued that in the absence of a negative charge the binding of quaternary ions to the enzyme becomes negligible, and that VAN DER WAALS' forces cannot contribute much to this binding, because of the spherical structure of the cation. Recent observations made with phosphoryl-cholines (FREDRIKSSON and TIBBLING 1960) strongly suggests that an anionic site does not play the same important role in plasma BuChE as it does in AChE.

Another explanation, although not very convincing, is that the activation energy for the hydrolysis of ACh by plasma ChE is of the same order of magnitude as for the hydrolysis of neutral esters by "unspecific" esterases. Therefore, ELEY and STONE (1951) concluded that electrostatic forces are unimportant for plasma ChE, and that the main point of attack of this enzyme is on the ester group. However, the problem must be regarded as unsolved, until more direct evidence is presented.

IV. Individual variation of esterase properties

Individual variation of ChE activity is appreciable in both plasma and tissues, due to physiological factors (such as age, sex, nutritional status) and genetic factors (LEHMANN and RYAN 1956, LEHMANN et al. 1958) which regulate esterase synthesis, particularly in the liver. Especially interesting is the observation, first made by KALOW et al. (with LINDSAY 1956, with GENEST 1957, with STARON 1957) that individual variation of esterase properties also exists. It was demonstrated that the susceptibility to dibucaine (2-butoxy-N-(2-diethylaminoethyl) cinchonin-amide, Nupercaine, a local anestetic drug produced by CIBA), as an inhibitor of human serum ChE, varies from person to person. By testing a large population, it was possible to divide the sera into three groups according to degree of inhibition: usual, intermediate and atypical. Familial studies revealed that this division was genetically determined. It was suggested that there exist two autosomal alleles without dominance, and that these are responsible for the synthesis of two types of serum ChE. The homozygotes appeared to have either the normal or the atypical ChE in their serum, while the heterozygotes possessed a mixture of these two enzymes (KALOW and DAVIES 1958). This concept was supported by studies with a number of other inhibitors, mostly of the cationic type. The two types of esterase could also be correlated with the effects of succinyl-choline; the response of a person to this muscle-relaxant compound is prolonged if the serum contains atypical BuChE (KALOW and GUNN 1957; see also LEHMANN and SIMMONS 1958). However, no direct measurements were made of succinylcholine hydrolysis by sera of the two groups. The frequency of the gene for atypical BuChE in the healthy population (2000 persons examined) was estimated by KALOW and GUNN (1959) to be 0.019 ± 0.002.

The fact that the more frequently used inhibitors, e.g., eserine, are equally strong inhibitors of the two types of esterases, may explain why this observation has not been made earlier. In studies with extracts of potato peel, which contains a comparatively strong inhibitor (ORGELL et al. 1958), this material was shown to discriminate between the three phenotypes as sharply as does dibucaine (HARRIS and WHITTAKER 1959). The esterase of the homozygous normal (usual) group was more sensitive to the inhibitor than the esterase of the homozygous atypical group, while the heterozygotes, having the two esterases in equal amounts, were intermediate. Attempts to separate the two types of cholinesterase by electrophoresis or other techniques have failed so far (KALOW and GUNN 1959). The difference between the types appears to be due to subtle structural differences between the active sites, presumably the anionic site, of otherwise identical or very similar enzyme proteins.

D. Methods for the differentiation of various cholinesterases

Methods for differentiating various types of ChE have been the subject of many studies. Irrespective of the technique employed for activity measurement (see Section E), the best way to assay one type of ChE in a mixture of various esterases is the use of a combination of "specific" substrates and "selective" inhibitors. It should be pointed out, however, that the results obtained with various substrates, as well as with various inhibitors, are dependent on the enzyme preparations used; both species and organ specificity are of importance, as well as the presence of interfering compounds in crude preparations.

I. Specific substrates

The early proposal (MENDEL et al. 1943) to use "specific" substrates (acetyl-β-methylcholine for AChE, and benzoyl-, butyryl-, or propionylcholine for other types of ChE) to differentiate between ChE's will not give a complete picture of the presence of various types of active proteins in crude tissue homogenates (ORD and THOMPSON 1950, MYERS 1954, MENDEL and MYERS 1955, AUGUSTINSSON 1959c). When tissues contain AChE in excess, the assay of other ChE's in these tissues by means of selective substrates (benzoyl- or butyrylcholine) leads to falsely high activity values, because AChE is partly responsible for the hydrolysis. Moreover, an ester which is a suitable substrate for one type of esterase may inhibit another. Eserine-resistant esterases may also interfere. In some special cases, however, certain "specific" substrates may be useful, e.g., in the routine assay of the two types of ChE's present in human blood.

II. Selective inhibitors

The introduction of selective esterase inhibitors has been of value, not only for differentiating ChE's from other esterases, but also for differentiating various types of ChE. A fine, comprehensive study on such inhibitors has been published by MYERS (1954). The most useful of the selective ChE inhibitors are listed in Table 2. Only the most pertinent data will be mentioned in the following.

1. Selective inhibition of acetylcholinesterase

The selective inhibition of AChE was first demonstrated for the methyl-hydroxy purines (e.g., caffeine) (ZELLER and BISSEGGER 1943, NACHMANSOHN and

Table 2. *Selective inhibitors used to differentiate between various cholinesterases*

Selective inhibitor for		Inhibition		References
Chemical name	Code name	ChE's compared	Inhibition ratio	
Acetylcholinesterases				
1,5-*Bis*(4-allyldimethylammoniumphenyl) pentane-3-one diiodide	297C50 (284C51)	a	217,000	Austin and Berry 1953, Fulton and Mogey 1954, Todrick 1954. Bayliss and Todrick 1956
Bis(3-dimethylamino-5-hydroxyphenoxy)-1,3-propane dimethiodide	3116CT	b	250,000	Funke et al. 1954, De-pierre and Funke 1954
Bis-(piperidino-methyl coumaranyl-5) ketone dimethiodide	3318CT	c	10,000	Funke et al. 1953, Jacob 1955, 1956; Paulesu et al. 1955
N,N'-*Bis*(diethyl-2-chlorobenzylammoniumethyl)oxamide dichloride	WIN 8077, Ambenonium	b	2,000	Arnold et al. 1954, Lands et al. 1958, Holmstedt (personal communication)
Butyrocholinesterases and others				
Di*iso*propyl phosphorofluoridate	DFP	b	270	Hawkins and Mendel 1947, Aldridge 1953a, Davison 1953
N,N'-Di*iso*propylphosphorodiamidic fluoride	Mipafox	b	56	Aldridge 1953a, Davison 1953
		d	4,200	
		e	30,000	
Tetramono*iso*propyl pyrophosphortetramide	*iso*-OMPA	b	56	Austin and Berry 1953, Aldridge 1953a, Davison 1953
		d	11,200	
		e	41	
10-(2-Diethylamino-1-propyl) phenothiazine hydrochloride	Lysivane	f	2,800	Todrick 1954; cf., Gordon 1948
10-(1-Diethylaminopropionyl) phenothiazine hydrochloride	Astra 1397	b	10,000	Augustinsson 1955b

a Rat brain/horse plasma. b Human erythrocyte/human plasma. c Dog erythrocyte/dog plasma. d Horse erythrocyte/horse plasma. e Chicken brain/chicken plasma. f Rat brain/rat intestinal mucosa.

Schneemann 1945, Vincent and Lagreu 1950), nitrogen mustards (Adams and Thompson 1948, Bullock 1955) and the N-*p*-chlorophenyl-N-methyl carbamate of *m*-hydroxyphenyltrimethylammonium bromide (Nu-1250) (Hawkins and Mendel 1949, Casier and de Vleeschhouwer 1952). Much greater selectivity for AChE vis-à-vis other ChE's has been obtained with recently synthesized compounds (Table 2). Compounds containing two quaternary nitrogen groups separated by 12 to 15 Å are generally more effective as inhibitors of AChE than are monoquaternary ammonium bases and stronger inhibitors of AChE than of other types of ChE; a list of the best-known *bis*-quaternary ammonium compounds in this respect has been published by Holmstedt (1959). One group of these compounds has the general formula

$$R-\langle\!\!\bigcirc\!\!\rangle-CH_2-CH_2-CO-CH_2-CH_2-\langle\!\!\bigcirc\!\!\rangle-R$$

where the R's are substituted quaternary nitrogens. The most useful selective inhibitors have the following substituents: $(CH_3)_3\overset{+}{N}$- (62C47), $C_2H_5(CH_3)_2\overset{+}{N}$- (25C48), $(CH_2=CH-CH_2)_3\overset{+}{N}$- (297C50 or 284C51), and n-$C_3H_7(CH_3)_2\overset{+}{N}$- (298C50).

They are almost as active as neostigmine or eserine in inhibiting AChE, but have low activity against other ChE's (e.g., human serum BuChE).

Other groups of selective AChE inhibitors also contain two quaternary nitrogens, but the chain of atoms linking these is more complex, as for instance, in 3116CT and WIN 8077 (ambenonium) (see Table 2 for references):

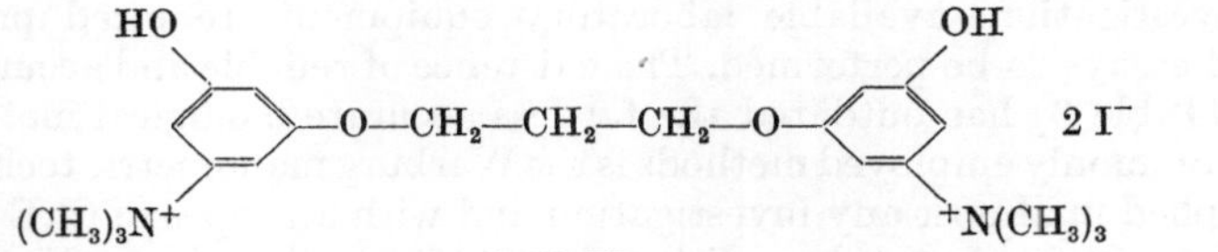

HO — O—CH₂—CH₂—CH₂—O— OH 2 I⁻

(CH₃)₃N⁺ ⁺N(CH₃)₃

3116 CT

Cl C₂H₅ C₂H₅ Cl
—CH₂—N⁺—CH₂—CH₂—NH—CO—CO—NH—CH₂—CH₂—N⁺—CH₂— 2 Cl⁻
C₂H₅ C₂H₅

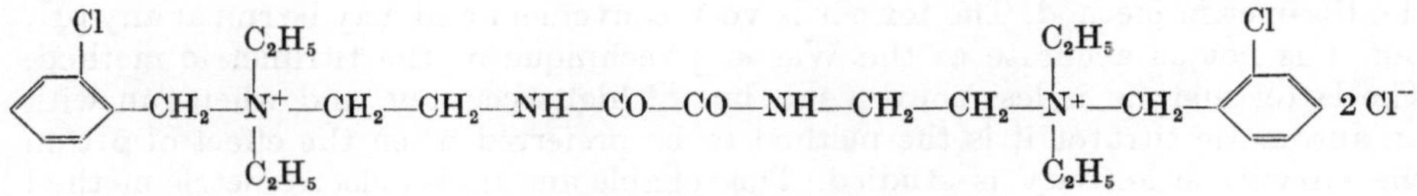

WIN 8077

The specific activity of these compounds is similar to that of those mentioned above, and they are also recommended as selective inhibitors of AChE. All these compounds are characterized by reversible enzyme inhibition, although with ambenonium reversal occurs extremely slowly excepting in the presence of relatively high concentrations of certain cations, e.g., Mg^{++} (KOELLE 1957). Some of the phosphorylcholines (e.g., methyl-fluorophosphoryl choline and methyl-ethoxy-phosphoryltiocholine) are stronger inhibitors of AChE than of human serum BuChE. The inhibitory mechanism of these latter compounds, however, is more complex (TAMMELIN 1958).

2. Selective inhibition of other types of cholinesterase

One of the first useful selective inhibitors of human BuChE was the dimethyl-carbamate of *m*-hydroxyphenylbenzyltrimethyl ammonium bromide (Nu-683) (HAWKINS and GUNTER 1946, BLASCHKO et al. 1949, MYERS 1952). Among the many compounds tested later as selective inhibitors of human serum ChE and similar esterases, the most active ones belong to two quite different groups of compounds. One group is a number of organophosphorus compounds characterized by inactivating ChE more or less irreversibly (see further, Chapter 9). D*iso*propyl phosphorofluoridate (DFP) has a selective inhibiting effect on the serum BuChE, but its specificity in this respect is greatly surpassed by *iso*-OMPA and Mipafox (see Table 2). When these compounds are used as selective inhibitors, the progressive and irreversible nature of the inhibition must be remembered, as well as the protective effect of the substrate (ACh) against inhibition, i.e., the inhibitor has to be in contact with the enzyme prior to the substrate in order to realize the full effect of the inhibitor (AUGUSTINSSON and NACHMANSOHN 1949).

To the other group of selective inhibitors of serum BuChE belong derivatives of phenothiazine. Two such derivatives, the 10-(2-diethylaminopropyl) (Lysivane) and the 10-(1-diethylaminopropionyl) (Astra 1397) derivatives, have recently been found to be as good selective inhibitors as the organophosphorus compounds. In contradistinction to the latter, the phenothiazine derivatives are reversible inhibitors and therefore more useful in particular cases.

Assay Methods for Cholinesterases

A. General principles

I. Choice of method

The choice of assay methods for the ChE's is dependent mainly on the purpose of the investigation, available laboratory equipment, required precision, and number of assays to be performed. The existence of reliable and accurate chemical methods (Table 3) has outdated the far less accurate biological methods. One of the most commonly employed methods is the Warburg manometric technique, which can be applied in almost any investigation and with all types of ChE preparations under different experimental conditions, except in studies where pH of the medium is varied. Other all-round methods are the hydroxylamine-ferric chloride test and the titrimetric method. The former is very convenient and may be run at any pH, but it is not as accurate as the Warburg technique or the titrimetric method. The latter method is less convenient, but of high accuracy, and when run with an automatic titrator it is the method to be preferred when the effect of pH on the enzymatic activity is studied. The reliable and useful electrometric method makes use of the change in pH during ester hydrolysis. The colorimetric modification of this technique is also recommended, either in a form useful in standard laboratories or in a form found to be satisfactory and rapid as a screening test. The experimental temperature of choice for any of the methods preferred is 25° or 37.5°, the former generally being the more convenient.

Review articles with details of various assay methods have recently been published by POCHET (1955), STUMPF (1956), BARNES et al. (1957) and AUGUSTINSSON (1957).

References to Table 3

a GOLDSTEIN 1944, 1949; AUGUSTINSSON 1948, 1955a; METCALF and MARCH 1949, MENDEL and HAWKINS 1950, HARDEGG and SCHAEFER 1952, MYERS 1954.

b Results directly comparable with those obtained by Michel: GIANG and HALL 1951, HAMBLIN and MARCHAND 1951, MARCHAND 1952, ALDRIDGE and DAVIES 1952, WOLFSIE and WINTER 1952, WOLFSIE 1957, FRYER et al. 1955. Results not directly comparable with those obtained by Michel: ALCALDE 1950, MACDONALD et al. 1952, FRAWLEY et al. 1952, SHIBATA and TAKAHASHI 1953, MOLANDER et al. 1954, GRÉGOIRE et al. 1955a, GREENBERG and CALVERT 1957; calibrated pH meter: TAMMELIN 1953, TAMMELIN and LÖW 1951, TAMMELIN and STRINDBERG 1952, EINSEL et al. 1956.

c Indicator used, m-nitrophenol: RAPPAPORT et al. 1959.

d Indicator used, phenol red: TAKAHASHI and SHIBATA 1951, TAKAHASHI 1956, GRÉGOIRE and COTTE 1952, GRÉGOIRE et al. 1955a, b, 1956, MOLANDER et al. 1954, LOWRY et al. 1954, LALLI and CASCINO 1956, CARAWAY 1956, PRIBILLA 1957.

e WOLFSIE and WINTER 1954, DAVIES and NICHOLLS 1955, HERZFELD and STUMPF 1955, FLEISHER et al. 1956, BIGGS et al. 1958, SAILER and BRAUNSTEINER 1959.

f ALLES and HAWES 1940, SANZ 1944, SCHÜMMELFEDER 1947, DELAUNOIS and CASIER 1948, MOMMAERTS et al. 1953, SMALLMAN and WOLFE 1955, HARGREAVES 1953, HARGREAVES and DA SILVA 1959; automatic devises: NEILANDS and CANNON 1955, LARSSON and HANSEN 1956, JENSEN-Holm et al. 1959.

g PIGHINI 1939, JACOBSOHN and TAPADINHAS 1943, SACK and ZELLER 1943, VINCENT 1944, MORAND and LABORIT 1947, PAGET and DHELLEMMES 1947, BROCA 1948, COHEN et al. 1948, CERVINI 1950, SNYDER et al. 1951, ARELLANO CELIS and VILLASANTE 1953, HARDERS and VAN MULKEN 1954, ZAVALETA 1955, LUNA PÉREZ 1956.

h METCALF 1951, FLEISHER and POPE 1954, FLEISHER et al. 1955, SABINE 1955, BELLI and ZAZO 1955, BONTING and FEATHERSTONE 1956, AUGUSTINSSON 1957, WETSTONE et al. 1957, VINCENT and SEGONZAC 1958, PILZ 1958, KURODA et al. 1959.

Table 3. *Methods recommended for the assay of cholinesterases*

Method (Principle)	Technique	Special equipment needed	Medium	Particularly suitable studies	Precision	Expression of units of ChE commonly used	Reference to Sectn. in this vol.	First employment	References to modifications of general techn.
CO₂ production	Manometric	Warburg app.	Bicarbonate buffer, pH 7.4	Routine assays; kinetic and other studies with great possibility for variation of exptl. conditions at fixed pH	High (2 to 3%)	μl CO₂/30min	B.I.1	AMMON 1933	a
Change in pH	Electrometric	pH meter, preferably calibrated	Barbital buffer, initial pH 8	Routine assays, especially in clinical work with blood	High to moderate	Δ pH/hr (or μmol. of acetic acid)	B.II.1	MICHEL 1949	b
"	Color change of indicator	Colorimeter, preferably calibrated	"	"	High to moderate	"	B.II.2	CROXATTO et al. 1939	c
"	Color change of indicator	None	No buffer	Field studies of human whole blood ChE	Low	Time for fixed color to occur	B.II.2	REINHOLD et al. 1953	d
"	"							LIMPEROS and RANTA 1953	e
Continuous titration to fixed pH	Electrometric	Automatic recording devises recommended	Little or no buffer required	Rapid detn. with a variety of substrates and enzyme prepns., at various pH and other exptl. conditions	High	ml of 0.01 M NaOH/20min	B.III.2	GLICK 1937, SCOZ and CATTANEO 1937	f
"	Indicator	Colorimeter	"	"	Moderate	"	B.III.1	STEDMAN et al. 1932, 1933; HALL and LUCAS 1937	g
Formation of hydroxamic acid from un-reacted ACh	Colorimetric	Colorimeter	Phosphate buffer, pH 7.2	Convenient under widely different exptl. conditions	Moderate	μmol. of ACh/hr	D	HESTRIN 1949	h

II. Choice of esterase units

Direct comparisons of the results obtained with various methods are not possible, primarily because of the different experimental conditions used in each method (temperature, pH, composition of medium, substrate concentration). The activity should always be expressed in absolute values, such as μmoles of ACh hydrolyzed or μl CO_2 evolved, rather than in artificial units. Whenever possible, the initial reaction velocity should be used in any quantitative assay of ChE. Specific ChE activity is expressed best as μmoles of ACh hydrolysed in one hour per mg of protein, or in other absolute units per ml enzyme solution (e.g., blood plasma) or per mg dry weight (after dialysis of enzyme preparation used).

III. Choice of substrate

In order to be sure that the activity measured is due to a ChE, activity measurements should always be made with a choline ester, and the eserine-sensitivity of the esterase has to be proved. If the activity is measured irrespective of type of ChE, ACh is the substrate of choice; any of its available water-soluble salts can be used, but the iodide, bromide or perchlorate is to be preferred because each of these is non-hygroscopic. The ACh concentration should be close to the optimum concentration (1 to 10 mM) when the enzyme is an AChE; when other types of ChE are studied (e.g., human serum BuChE) a higher concentration (> 10 mM) is recommended (to obtain maximum activity).

The choice of substrate, except ACh, is dependent on the purpose of the study. Butyrylcholine is the best substrate for human serum ChE, and esterases with similar properties when these enzymes are mixed with other esterases (including AChE), e.g., whole human blood. Benzoylcholine has to be used with care because it is hydrolysed by both Bu ChE and eserine-resistant esterases (MENDEL and MYERS 1955). Acetyl-β-methylcholine can be used to measure AChE in crude preparations containing various esterases, but should not be regarded uncritically as a "specific" substrate for AChE.

The use of non-choline esters as substrates for ChE should be avoided. The main problem in this connection is to determine whether an ester is actually split by a ChE alone, or in addition by another esterase. However, any ester can be used as substrate for ChE activity assuming the preparation studied contains only ChE, and the specificity of the esterase activity is known in detail. In special cases, certain non-choline esters may be the choice, for instance in histochemical detection of ChE, or when a ChE preparation is used in the detection of specific ChE inhibitors (e.g., the organophosphorus compounds). Esters are known which on hydrolysis give reaction products with characteristic colors useful in tissue-staining (CHESSICK 1954) or testing enzyme inactivation (actually, non-inactivation); such esters are, for instance, indoxyl esters (BARRNETT 1952, HOLT 1956, HOBBIGER 1957, UNDERHAY 1957), naphthyl esters (GOMORI 1952, 1955; RAVIN et al. 1953), and indophenylacetate (KRAMER and GAMSON 1958).

IV. Enzyme preparations

1. Crude preparations

a) Tissue homogenates

Whole homogenates of fresh tissue can be used and prepared by generally accepted procedures. If not used immediately, an organ may be stored after rapid freezing (in solid CO_2) without loss of ChE activity. The choice of medium for the homogenates depends on the intended uses, the method to be used for esterase assay, and stability and solubility of the enzyme. The buffer solution recommended for the assay method is to be preferred as medium for the homogenate. Whole tissue homogenates should be used if the solubility of the esterase studied is unknown or questionable. Many ChE's, especially the erythrocyte and nerve tissue AChE's, are very difficult to take up into solution. They may be extracted first after disruption of the cell membrane and dissociation of the protein (lipoprotein) complex with which the enzymes seem to be associated. A number of procedures for extracting AChE from such cell material have been described, e.g., extraction with ammonia (MENTHA et al. 1947), lysolecithin (AUGUSTINSSON 1948, MARPLES et al. 1959), chlorophyllin (INAGAKI et al. 1953), butanol (MORTON 1955), and surface-active agents (TOSCHI 1958). Other ChE's, e.g., those of vertebrate blood plasma, cobra venom, and *Helix* blood, are in natural solution.

The presence of endogenous salts in tissue homogenates is of importance for ChE activity. When comparing the activities of various homogenates, the salt concentration must therefore be known. The homogenates are preferably dialyzed against the buffer solution used in the assay procedure

b) Blood sampling

Whole blood of mammals is best taken up in heparinized tubes. Citrate, oxalate, and fluoride must be avoided since these ions form complexes with certain divalent metallic ions (e.g., Ca^{++}) which activate ChE activity. Serum and heparinized plasma show the same ChE activity, since the enzymes are not influenced by heparin (see, however, SKOŘEPA 1956). The blood is centrifuged and the red cells washed three times with saline; the cells are then hemolyzed with distilled water.

Special techniques for blood sampling have been reported, mainly for use in clinical studies. Micro sample methods are described by HAMBLIN and MARCHAND (1951), by WOLFSIE and WINTER (1952) and HAGAN et al. (1953). Blood samples dried on filter paper have been used successfully in routine determinations (AUGUSTINSSON and HEIMBÜRGER 1953; AUGUSTINSSON 1955a; DYBING and HJELLE 1957; GOLZ 1958).

c) Stable preparations

Partly purified preparations can be stabilized by mixing with certain albumins, bovine serum albumin being especially favorable. The technique has been described for electric tissue AChE (AUGUSTINSSON 1955c; SCAIFE 1959) and erythrocyte AChE (FLEISHER et al. 1955). Gelatine has also been used as stabilizer for partly purified preparations (NACHMANSOHN and WILSON 1955).

2. Purified preparations

a) Acetylcholinesterases

Among favorable sources for highly active and purified AChE preparations (see Table 4 for references) the electric organs are the most important (AUGUSTINSSON 1955c). *Electrophorus electricus* (from the Amazon and Orinoco rivers) and *Torpedo marmorata* and *T. oscellata* (from the Mediterranean and the Atlantic coast of U.S.A.) are the most suitable species. Actually, the most active and purest AChE preparation obtained so far is that prepared by ROTHENBERG and NACHMANSOHN (1947). They used mucin-free preparations of *Electrophorus* electric organ, which were fractionated with ammonium sulfate at various pH values. Modifications of the original method have been described. Of those preparations described, the best had a specific activity of about 400 mmol. ACh (split per hr per mg of protein).

Table 4. *References to selected methods used for purifying cholinesterases from various sources*

Starting material — Tissue	Starting material — Animal	Type of ChE present in the original material	Principle of method used for purification	Degree of purification X-fold	Yield %	Sp. activity μmol. ACh split per hr per mg protein[1]	References
Erythrocytes	Man, horse, sheep, ox	AChE	Adsorption on infusorial earth	20—30	—	—	MENDEL and RUDNEY 1943a, MOUNTERandWHITTAKER1950
,,	Man	AChE	Extn. with NH_3 soln., pH 8.3	100	—	—	MENTHA et al. 1947
,,	Man	AChE	Extn. with $CHCl_3$; adsorption on $Ca_3(PO_4)_2$, elution with NH_4OH	80	—	—	ARRAGON and SALA 1948
,,	Man, ox	AChE	Pptn. of stroma with HAc, fractionation with $(NH_4)_2SO_4$. Stabilization with serum or egg white	—	—	—	LESUK 1949
,,	Man, horse	AChE	Extn. with lysolecithin	—	—	—	AUGUSTINSSON 1948, GREIG and GIBBONS 1956, MARPLES et al. 1959
,,	Man	AChE	Pptn. with Cd acetate, solubilization with Tween 20 and toluene, etc.	100	10—20	440	ZITTLE et al. 1954, 1955
,,	Ox	AChE and others	Extn. with butanol, etc.	250—400	—	250	COHEN and WARRINGA 1953, WARRINGA and COHEN 1955
Brain	Rat	AChE and others	Fractionation with $(NH_4)_2SO_4$, use of surface active agents	10	25	—	ORD and THOMPSON 1951
,,	Pig	AChE and others	Stable fractions described	3—4	—	—	TAUBER 1953, TOSCHI 1959,
,,	Ox	AChE and others	Differential centrifugations	—	—	—	ALDRIDGE and JOHNSSON 1959
Electric organ	Electrophorus	AChE	Mucin free preps. fractionated with $(NH_4)_2SO_4$ at various pH	75	15	120,000—400,000	ROTHENBERG and NACHMANSOHN 1947, NACHMANSOHN and WILSON 1955, LAWLER 1959
,,	,,	AChE	Mucins not removed, otherwise according to ROTHENBERG and NACHMANSOHN 1947	20	—	6,000	HARGREAVES and LOBO 1953, HARGREAVES et al. 1959
Snake venom	Cobra	AChE	Fractionation with sulfates; electrophoresis and adsorption	20	24	(1,540)	CHAUDHURI 1944, 1946
Plasma (Serum)	Horse	BuChE	Fractionation with $(NH_4)_2SO_4$	5,000	5	12,000	STRELITZ 1944, AUGUSTINSSON 1948
,,	Man	BuChE	Ether fractionation	48	—	2,100	KEKWICK et al. 1953
,,	Man	BuChE	Ethanol fractionation at low temp.	3,400	7	9,000	SURGENOR et al. 1949, SURGENOR and ELLIS 1954
,,	Man	BuChE	Ethanol fractionation and combined chromatography on $Ca_3(PO_4)_3$ and Dowex 2	—	—	20,000	MALMSTRÖM et al. 1956
Pancreas	Dog	BuChE	Fractionation with $(NH_4)_2SO_4$, adsorption on infusorial earth	2,000	20	20,000	MENDEL and MUNDELL 1943

[1] Specific activity values have to be taken with precaution because activity was measured at various pS, temperature, and by methods not comparable.

The nucleus caudatus in the brain of mammals has a very high AChE activity and is therefore useful as starting material for purification by various techniques. The main problem is to get the esterase into solution. By differential centrifugation AChE is recovered in the mitochondrial and microsomal fractions. To obtain it in soluble form, this material can be treated with surface-active agents (ORD and THOMPSON 1951, TAUBER 1953, TOSCHI 1959), lipolytic enzymes (TOSCHI 1959), lysolecithin (MARPLES et al. 1959) or organic solvents (TOSCHI 1959). Proteolytic enzymes (e.g., trypsin, chymotrypsin) inactivate brain AChE (ORD and THOMPSON 1951, BERGMANN and SEGAL 1955, TOSCHI 1959). TOSCHI (1958) reported on the chromatographic and electrophoretic separation of ChE's present in nerve tissue.

A variety of methods has been reported for purifying AChE from the erythrocytes. The most successful procedure is probably that described by COHEN and WARRINGA (1953), who used extraction with butanol in the cold or with a pancreatic extract, ammonium sulfate and ethanol fractionations. Various other techniques have been employed (Table 4), as for instance extraction with ammonia, chloroform, or lysolecithin, adsorption on infusorial earth or calcium phosphate, precipitation with ammonium sulfate or cadmium acetate. Stable preparations as standard were described by FLEISHER et al. (1955).

b) Other cholinesterases

The most active preparations of human or horse serum (plasma) BuChE are those obtained by fractionation with ammonium sulfate (especially that described by STRELITZ 1944) or with ethanol fractionation at low temperature (see Table 4 for references). The latter preparation, available from blood-plasma fractionation laboratories (e.g., Kabi AB, Stockholm, Sweden), is most suitable as starting material for further purification by electrophoresis (GLICK et al. 1942; GOUTIER 1956; PINTÉR 1957; AUGUSTINSSON 1959a) and chromatographic techniques (MALMSTRÖM et al. 1956). Enzyme purified by the latter procedure has a high specific activity. Ether fractionation has also been employed in this connection. A crystalline serum muco-protein with high ChE activity (BADER et al. 1944) has not been further investigated.

Active ChE preparations from pancreas (MENDEL and MUNDELL 1943), heart (ORD and THOMPSON 1951), and liver (TAMAI 1950) have also been described. The high ChE activity of ceratin myosin preparations obtained from striated muscle (VARGA et al. 1954, KÖVÉR et al. 1957, KÖVÉR and KOVÁCS 1957) needs to be further studied, especially regarding the presence in these preparations of ChE, known to be present in muscle tissue. It is probable that the preparation used by the Hungarian workers contained a mixture of active proteins.

B. Methods based upon acid production from choline esters

I. Gasometric methods

Enzymatic hydrolysis of the ester proceeds in a bicarbonate-CO_2 buffered system, and through acid production, CO_2 is evolved in equivalent amounts and estimated manometrically.

1. Warburg technique

This manometric method is most frequently used, and is probably the most reliable for assaying ChE activity. In most methods described, the medium (pH 7.5) contains not only bicarbonate but also Ca^{++} or Mg^{++} as activator, and Na^+ or K^+, depending on the type of esterase studied (MYERS 1952; SMALLMAN and WOLFE 1955). This medium is used to dissolve the substrate and dilute (and/or dissolve) the enzyme preparation. The method is useful in all types of experiments, including those involving inhibitors and activators. The only disadvantage of the technique is that the pH of the medium cannot be altered. The variation in pH over a relatively small range, made possible by altering the bicarbonate concentration and the partial pressure of CO_2, is not recommended in studies on the pH-dependence of ChE activity; in these cases other methods must be used.

Details of the method are found in publications, among others, those listed in Table 3. A modification of the general technique, a "free manometer" technique, in which both pressure and volume are allowed to vary, was described by GOLDSTEIN (1949).

2. Cartesian diver technique

This ultramicro manometric method, extensively investigated by LINDERSTRØM-LANG, HOLTER, and ZEUTHEN, was applied for the first time by LINDERSTRØM-LANG and GLICK (1938) to the assay of serum ChE and later by BOELL and SHEN (1944) in their study of ChE in developing *Amblystoma*. The method was improved considerably by ZAJICEK and ZEUTHEN (1956) for ChE determinations with single cells (e.g., nerve cells, megakaryocytes) and later used by GIACOBINI (1959) in his studies on isolated ganglion cells and even their constituent organelles (i.e., nucleus, nucleolus).

3. Other techniques

The manometric gas analyzer of VAN SLYKE and NEILL was used by STRAUS and GOLDSTEIN (1943) in their important study of the "zone behavior" of human serum ChE and also by others (e.g., FRIEND and KRAYER 1941). An adaptation of the BARCROFT differential apparatus for ChE was described by STEDMAN and STEDMAN (1935) in one of their classical papers, and AMMON and ZAPP (1955, ZAPP 1957) constructed recently a simpler gasometric apparatus, the usefulness of which can be better judged after further experience.

II. Change in pH

The change in pH due to the production of acid is either measured electrometrically with a pH meter or determined by the change in color of an indicator.

1. Electrometric measurement

The enzyme is allowed to act on ACh in a standard buffer solution for a definite period of time (usually 1 to 2 hr). The pH of the mixture is measured using a glass electrode at the beginning and at the end of this period. The rate of change in pH (Δ pH/hr) is a measure of enzymatic activity. This principle was first employed by MICHEL (1949), and his original method has been frequently used since then, minor modifications having been made regarding the equipment for pH measurements and micro sample methods for collecting blood. The direct proportionality between the fall in pH and time has been established (DAVIES and RUTLAND 1950) using various enzyme preparations. The sources of error and the margin of error have been studied experimentally (STREHLER and MEYER 1952).

Modifications of MICHEL's method have been proposed, but the results thus obtained are not directly comparable with those obtained using the original method. In the first place, certain modifications of the buffer solutions and enzyme dilutions have been employed. The method has also been applied to animal blood ChE (WILLIAMS et al. 1957; FRAWLEY and FUYAT 1957). A calibration procedure making use of a recorder was described by TAMMELIN (1953). This convenient apparatus, which is able to register simultaneously six enzyme reactions, is a considerable improvement on the original method. TAMMELIN's method was modified by EINSEL et al. (1956) who maintained constant pH by removing H^+, using an automatic electrolytic titrator. The method described by COURVILLE and LEDINGTON (1951) is based on an accurate measurement of the time required for a given sample of enzyme to change the pH of a standard substrate solution over a definite pH range (8.200 to 7.800). This accuracy, and the rapidity with which the determinations are carried out, suggest that the method may be useful for routine analysis.

2. Change in color of an indicator

Change in pH resulting from the liberation of acid can be estimated by the change in color of an indicator, using a photometer, rather than with a pH meter. Methods using phenol red, which otherwise adhere closely to the conditions established by MICHEL, and are recommended as useful modifications of the original method, were worked out by REINHOLD et al. (1953) and by GRÉGOIRE et al. (1955a, b, 1956). The principle of these methods was used by LIMPEROS and RANTA (1953) for the development of a screening test, in which the color of a solution containing bromthymol blue was used to assay the approximate ChE activity of human blood. This screening test was later simplified by WOLFSIE and WINTER (1954) who matched the indicator color with the corresponding ΔpH/hr and per cent of normal ChE activity values. Other modifications have also been proposed (Table 3). Such a screening test can be carried out in the field. The same principle has been used for a spot test for locating ChE inhibiting organophosphorus compounds on paper chromatograms (COOK 1955).

3. Nephelometric method

Production of acid during the hydrolysis of acetylcholine can be estimated quantitatively by making use of the opacity produced in dilute protein solutions, such as diluted milk (GAL 1940, 1948; GAL and VEGH 1948; ADLER et al. 1949) or casein solution (POLONOVSKI et al. 1953). The opalescence is directly proportional to the amount of acetic acid produced. The method is simple, rapid, and does not require special apparatus. It is, however, not very accurate. The protein indicator may influence the enzyme activity and the course of enzyme reaction; each enzyme solution needs a special standard curve, and the conditions for direct proportionality between enzyme concentration and activity are difficult to determine.

III. Titrimetric methods

The principle of this method is to determine the acetic acid, liberated during the hydrolysis of acetylcholine, by titration with alkali at constant pH, using either an indicator or a potentiometer, or employing conductometric titration.

1. Indicator methods

The indicator is added to an aqueous solution of ACh, and alkali is then added to give the solution a certain fixed color. This solution is then mixed with the enzyme solution. By adding alkali continuously, the color of the buffer-free solution is kept constant, or alkali is added after a certain period of time to restore that color. The total amount of alkali added to neutralize the liberated acid is used as the unit of esterase activity. STEDMAN et al. (1932, 1933) employed this technique in their classical papers on blood serum ChE, bromthymol blue or cresol red being the indicators used. Since then a number of investigators have described methods, the details of which vary only slightly from each other. The best-known method in the English literature is that of HALL and LUCAS (1937); in the French, on the other hand, reference is usually made to a method described by MORAND and LABORIT (1947). The two methods, however, are almost identical and cresol red is used as indicator. The MORAND-LABORIT method in its turn is identical with a method described earlier by VINCENT et al. (1944) and later discussed in detail by BROCA (1948). PIGHINI (1939) also, in his many papers published during the early 1940's, used a titrimetric method with phenolphthalein as indicator. The results cannot be compared with those obtained with other methods (MENGHI et al. 1953). BUCKLES and BULLOCK (1956) made use of the principle of this technique for a method of assaying pharmaceutical preparations containing small quantities of certain ChE inhibiting drugs (e.g., neostigmine). A micro-titration method was developed by GLICK (1938a). SERLIN and COTZIAS (1955) used CONWAY's micro-diffusion technique.

The use of indicators in the titrimetric assay of ChE has certain shortcomings. It is often difficult to observe the color change of the reaction mixture, and the indicator may influence the enzyme. Moreover, when studies are carried out with enzyme inhibitors or activators, these additional components of the system may influence the development of the color.

2. Electrometric methods

The first to use an electrometric technique at constant pH were GLICK (1937), who used a glass electrode, and SCOZ and CATTANEO (1937), who used a quinhydrone electrode. Various modifications of this principle have been described, many with illustrations of special apparatus required. Notable are the micromethods (RA-DOUCO et al. 1952, SABINE 1953) and the methods used for routine assay of serum ChE (BROWN and BUSH 1950, KAUFMAN 1954, CHOUTEAU et al. 1956). Fully automatic instrumentation for following enzyme reactions as a function of time at constant pH is an excellent tool for ChE studies (NEILANDS and CANNON 1955, LARSSON and HANSEN 1956, JENSEN-HOLM et al. 1959).

3. Conductometric methods

There is a possibility of carrying out the titration by following changes in conductivity during the enzyme reaction (Dutch Pat. 73307, Sept. 15, 1953). However, more convenient and reliable methods are preferable.

IV. Colorimetric methods

1. Ferric chloride test for acetic acid

When ferric chloride is added to a solution of acetic acid or an acetate, a brownish-red colored complex is formed. ABDON and UVNÄS (1937) used this reaction for assaying the acetic acid formed during the hydrolysis of ACh by human blood serum. Only a few investigators have employed this method.

2. Carbonaphthoxycholine as substrate

β-Carbonaphthoxycholine iodide is a specific substrate for serum ChE and was used for a colorimetric assay method by RAVIN et al. (1951). During the hydrolysis, β-naphthylcarbonic acid is released, which decarboxylates spontaneously to yield β-naphthol. The latter is coupled with a suitable diazonium salt to give an azo dye which is extractable with ethyl acetate and can be determined in a colorimeter. This method is simple, reliable, and specific for serum ChE. It has been used, mostly in its original version, in clinical studies on liver diseases (SLEISENGER et al. 1953, DELCOURT and VAN DER HOEDEN 1954) and on the diagnostic significance of serum ChE in children (BLEISCH and SHWACHMAN 1954). By using naphthyl acetate as a substrate, the total esterase activity of human serum (ChE plus arylesterase, AUGUSTINSSON 1959c) can be assayed in the same way.

V. Ultraviolet spectrophotometric method

The ultraviolet absorption spectra of certain aromatic esters are displaced towards longer wave lengths, and have high extinction coefficients compared to the absorption spectra of their hydrolysis products. This principle was introduced by HOFSTEE (1951) for investigating the hydrolysis by serum ChE of acetylsalicylic acid, and by KALOW (1952b) for the hydrolysis of local anesthetics. The method was described in detail by KALOW and LINDSAY (1955) for assaying human serum esterase activity, using benzoylcholine as a substrate. The method does not seem to have many advantages over other methods described. It is not very convenient for routine analysis, and is not useful for other than very dilute enzyme solutions. Moreover, it is by no means certain that the activity measured with benzoylcholine or other aromatic esters of choline is due wholly to ChE; other esterases, more or less specific for aromatic esters, are known to be present in serum as well as in other tissues.

C. Methods based upon choline (thiocholine) production

The determination of choline produced during the hydrolysis of ACh or other choline esters is not convenient, because it is difficult to determine choline in mixtures with its esters. The use of thiocholine esters might be expected to give improved results since it is comparatively easy to determine the free SH groups produced during the reaction. Such thioesters have been used with great success in the histochemical detection of ChE (see Chapter 6). The idea of using these substrates for blood ChE assay was first proposed by MEYER and WILBRANDT (1954). A modification of this method was published later (AUGUSTINSSON 1955b) making use of whole blood applied on filter paper, butyrylthiocholine as a substrate for plasma ChE activity, and acetylthiocholine in the presence of a specific plasma ChE inhibitor when the erythrocyte AChE was assayed. The free SH groups produced during the substrate hydrolysis were titrated iodometrically. Acetyl-β-methylthiocholine is not as specific for the human erythrocyte AChE as its oxygen analogue, and therefore cannot be used (KOELLE 1950, AUGUSTINSSON and ISACHSEN 1957, HEILBRONN 1959). It is also possible to measure the SH-production with the nitroprusside reaction (MCOSKER and DANIEL 1959) or with 2,6-dichlorophenol indophenol as an indicator (MEYER and WILBRANDT 1954). The accuracy of these methods is not as good as that of other methods described.

A more promising modification of the thiocholine method is to measure changes in optical density (at 250 mμ) during the hydrolysis of thioesters (TABACHNICK 1956, RUBIN et al. 1957, TABACHNICK et al. 1958, GAL and ROTH 1957).

D. Methods based upon chemical determination of unreacted acetylcholine

The residual ACh from a known amount incubated with the enzyme preparation for a certain period of time can be estimated pharmacologically on isolated organs by comparing its action with that of known amounts of ACh. These

8*

biological methods, however, are less accurate and more cumbersome than the chemical methods, and are therefore not recommended.

A sensitive chemical method for the determination of ACh was introduced by HESTRIN (1949) and is based upon reactions previously used as spot tests for carboxylic acids, esters and anhydrides. The ester reacts with hydroxylamine to form acethydroxamic acid, which forms a soluble red-purple complex with ferric ions in acid solution. The intensity of the color is proportional to the concentration of ACh present. Various minor modifications of HESTRIN's original method have been proposed, especially to make the method suitable for routine assay of blood ChE. The use of benzoylcholine instead of ACh as substrate (HUERGA et al. 1952, PASQUALIN and MOSCOVICI 1953) is of no advantage.

This method is very convenient and can be used with a small amount of enzyme. It can be employed under widely different experimental conditions, including wide ranges of pH, substrate and enzyme concentrations, in almost any buffer solution and in systems in which acid or alkali is formed by a concomitant side reaction. The upper limit of measurement exceeds 5 μmol. and the lower limit is about 0.04 μmol. of ester per ml of final solution. The accuracy is less than for mano-metric, electrometric, or titrimetric methods, since the remaining ester is measured, and the activity is obtained by difference; generally, about 30% of the ester must be hydrolyzed.

The principles of this method were recommended by the Association of Official Agricultural Chemists (COOK 1954) to be used for the determination of organophosphate insecticides in food products. A similar method was used earlier by DIGGLE and GAGE (1951) for the same purpose, and later employed by KATSH (1955) for assaying the anticholinesterase activity of drugs.

A modification of the original method for ACh determination has been made by WHITTAKER and WIJESUNDERA (1952) for tracing ACh (and other esters) on paper chromatograms. If used at a quantitative level, such a chromatographic procedure should be applicable for following ACh hydrolysis (HOMANN 1955).

Literature

ABDON, N.-O., and B. UVNÄS: A step-photometric method for determining the activity of acetylcholine esterase in blood plasma. Skand. Arch. Physiol. 76, 1—14 (1937).

ADAMS, D. H.: The specificity of the human erythrocyte cholinesterase. Biochim. biophys. Acta 3, 1—14 (1949).

— and R. H. S. THOMPSON: The selective inhibition of cholinesterases. Biochem. J. 42, 170 to 175 (1948).

— and V. P. WHITTAKER: The cholinesterases of human blood. I. The specificity of the plasma enzyme and its relation to the erythrocyte cholinesterase. Biochim. biophys. Acta 3, 358 to 366 (1949).

— — The cholinesterases of human blood. II. The forces acting between enzyme and substrate. Biochim. biophys. Acta 4, 543—558 (1950).

ADLER, P., I. GÁL u. L. VÉGH: Der Einfluß von Lokalanästhetika verschiedener Struktur auf die Cholinesterase-Aktivität im menschlichen Serum. Z. Vitamin-, Hormon- u. Ferment-forsch. 3, 236—243 (1949).

ALCALDE, J. M. O.: Serum cholinesterase determination in the differential diagnosis of jaundice. J. Lab. clin. Med. 36, 391—398 (1950).

ALDRIDGE, W. N.: The differentiation of true and pseudo cholinesterase by organophosphorus compounds. Biochem. J. 53, 62—67 (1953a).

— Serum esterases. I. Two types of esterase (A and B) hydrolysing p-nitrophenyl acetate, propionate and butyrate, and a method for their determination. Biochem. J. 53, 110—117 (1953b).

— and D. R. DAVIES: Determination of cholinesterase activity in human blood. Brit. med. J. 1952 I, 945—947.

— and M. K. JOHNSSON: Cholinesterase, succinic dehydrogenase, nucleic acids, esterase and glutathione reductase in sub-cellular fractions from rat brain. Biochem. J. 73, 270—276 (1959).

ALLES, G. A., and R. C. HAWES: Cholinesterases in the blood of man. J. biol. Chem. 133, 375—390 (1940).

AMMON, R.: Die fermentative Spaltung des Acetylcholins. Pflügers Arch. ges. Physiol. 233, 486—491 (1933).

— u. F. J. ZAPP: Eine einfache klinisch-chemische Methode zum Nachweis der Cholinesterase im Serum. Klin. Wschr. 33, 759—762 (1955).

ARELLANO CELIS, H., and J. G. VILLASANTE: The practical usefulness of the method of Morand and Laborit for the determination of cholinesterase activity in exploration of liver function (Spanish). Rev. clin. esp. 50, 22—24 (1953).

ARNOLD, A., A. E. SORIA and F. K. KIRCHNER: A new anticholinesterase oxamide. Proc. Soc. exp. Biol. (N. Y.) 87, 393—394 (1954).

ARRAGON, G., et E. SALA: Recherches sur la cholinestérase. II. Extraction à partir des hématies. Bull. Soc. Chim. biol. (Paris) 30, 51—54 (1948).

ARVY, L.: Les techniques actuelles d'histoenzymologie. Les estérases carboxyliques. Biol. méd. (Paris) 47, 12—160 (1958).

AUGUSTINSSON, K.-B.: Studies on blood choline esterase. Ark. Kemi, Miner. Geol. 18 A, No. 24, 1—16 (1944).

— Cholinesterases in some marine invertebrates. Acta physiol. scand. 11, 141—150 (1946a).

— Studies on the specificity of choline esterase in Helix pomatia. Biochem. J. 40, 343—349 (1946b).

— Cholinesterases. A study in comparative enzymology. Acta physiol. scand. 15, Suppl. 52, 1—182 (1948).

— Substrate concentration and specificity of choline ester splitting enzymes. Arch. Biochem. 23, 111—126 (1949).

— Acetylcholine-esterase and cholinesterase. In: J. B. SUMNER and K. MYRBÄCK, Eds., The Enzymes, vol. I, Part 1, 443—472. New York: Academic Press 1950a.

— The hydrolysis of non-choline esters by acetylcholine-esterase from human erythrocytes. Acta chem. scand. 4, 948—956 (1950b).

— Comparison between the acetylcholinesterases of Helix blood and cobra venom. I. The hydrolysis of acetylcholine and its inhibition by various compounds. Acta chem. scand. 5, 699—711 (1951a).

— Comparison between the acetylcholinesterases of Helix blood and cobra venom. II. The hydrolysis of certain choline and non-choline esters. Acta chem. scand. 5, 712—723 (1951b).

— Protection of cholinesterases by procaine against inactivation by Tabun in vitro. Acta physiol. scand. 27, 10—17 (1952).

— Neuere Ergebnisse auf dem Gebiet der Cholinesterases und ihre Bedeutung für Pharmakologie und Toxikologie. Arzneimittel-Forsch. 4, 242—249 (1954).

— The normal variation of human blood cholinesterase activity. Acta physiol. scand. 35, 40—52 (1955a).

— A titrimetric method for the determination of plasma and red blood cell cholinesterase activity using thiocholine esters as substrates. Scand. J. clin. Lab. Invest. 7, 284—290 (1955b).

— The electric organs and their cholinesterase activity. Pubbl. Staz. zool. Napoli 27, 189—198 (1955c).

— Assay methods for cholinesterases. Meth. biochem. Anal. 5, 1—63 (1957).

— Electrophoretic separation and classification of blood plasma esterases. Nature (Lond.) 181, 1786—1789 (1958a).

— A new type of cholinesterase in sow's milk. Acta chem. scand. 12, 1150—1152 (1958b).

— Electrophoresis studies on blood plasma esterases. I. Mammalian plasmata. Acta chem. scand. 13, 571—592 (1959a).

— Electrophoresis studies on blood plasma esterases. II. Avian, reptilian, amphibian and piscine plasmata. Acta chem. scand. 13, 1081—1096 (1959b).

— Electrophoresis studies on blood plasma esterases. III. Conclusions. Acta chem. scand. 13, 1097—1105 (1959c).

— Butyryl- and propionylcholinesterases and related types of eserine-sensitive esterases. In: P. D. BOYER, H. LARDY and K. MYRBÄCK, Eds., The Enzymes, 2nd ed., vol. 4, 521—540. New York: Academic Press 1960.

— and G. HEIMBÜRGER: The determination of cholinesterase activity in blood samples absorbed on filter paper. Acta physiol. scand. 30, 45—54 (1953).

— and T. ISACHSEN: The enzymic hydrolysis of the β-methyl derivatives of acetylcholine and acetylthiocholine. Acta chem. scand. 11, 750—751 (1957).

— and D. NACHMANSOHN: Distinction between acetylcholine-esterase and other choline ester-splitting enzymes. Science 110, 98—99 (1949).

— and B. OLSSON: Esterases in the milk and blood plasma of swine. 1. Substrate specificity and electrophoresis studies. Biochem. J. 71, 477—484 (1959).

AUSTIN, L., and W. K. BERRY: Two selective inhibitors of cholinesterase. Biochem. J. **54**, 695—700 (1953).

BABERS, F. H., and J. J. PRATT jr.: A comparison of the cholinesterase in the heads of the house fly, the cockroach, and the honey bee. Physiol. Zool. **24**, 127—131 (1951).

BADER, R., F. SCHÜTZ and M. STACEY: A crystalline serum mucoprotein with high choline-esterase activity. Nature (Lond.) **154**, 183 (1944).

BARNES, J. M., W. J. HAYES and K. KAY: Control of health hazards likely to arise from the use of organophosphorus insecticides in vector control. Annex: Blood-cholinesterase determinations. Bull. Wld Hlth Org. **16**, 41—61 (1957).

BARRNETT, R. J.: The distribution of esterolytic activity in the tissues of the albino rat as demonstrated with indoxyl acetate. Anat. Rec. **114**, 577—600 (1952).

BASTIDE, P.: Contribution à l'étude de la richesse enzymatique des humeurs et des tissus chez les *Helix*. Clermont-Ferrand: Imp. G. de Bussac 1954.

— et G. DASTUGUE: Sur l'hydrolyse enzymatique de quelques anesthésiques locaux (procaïne et autres esters para-aminobenzoïques) par les humeurs et les organes d'*Helix pomatia* L. Thérapie **8**, 744—748 (1953).

BAYLISS, B. J., and A. TODRICK: The use of a selective acetylcholinesterase inhibitor in the estimation of pseudocholinesterase activity in rat brain. Biochem. J. **62**, 62—67 (1956).

BECKETT, E. B., and G. H. BOURNE: Histochemical demonstration of cholinesterase and 5-nucleotidase in normal and diseased human muscle. Nature (Lond.) **179**, 771—772 (1957).

BELLI, R., and S. ZAZO: Micromethod for the determination of serum cholinesterase (Italian). Rif. med. **69**, 1076—1080 (1955).

BERGMANN, F.: Fine structure of the active surface of cholinesterases and the mechanism of enzymatic ester hydrolysis. Disc. Faraday. Soc. **20**, 126—134 (1955).

— The structure of the active surface of cholinesterases and the mechanism of their catalytic action in ester hydrolysis. Advanc. Catalysis **10**, 130—164 (1958).

— S. RIMON and R. SEGAL: Effect of pH on the activity of eel esterase towards different substrates. Biochem. J. **68**, 493—499 (1958).

— and R. SEGAL: The characterization of tissue cholinesterases. Biochim. biophys. Acta **16**, 513—519 (1955).

— — and S. RIMON: A new type of esterase in hog-kidney extract. Biochem. J. **67**, 481—486 (1957).

— — A. SHIMONI and M. WURZEL: The pH-dependence of enzymic ester hydrolysis. Biochem. J. **63**, 684—690 (1956).

— and M. WURZEL: The structure of the active surface of serum cholinesterase. Biochim. biophys. Acta **13**, 251—259 (1954).

BERNHARD, S. A.: A simple model of molecular specificity in enzyme-substrate systems. I. Theory and applications to the system acetylcholinesterase-substrate. II. The correlation of the Michaelis constant with the inhibition constant. J. Amer. chem. Soc. **77**, 1966—1972, 1973—1974 (1955).

BERNSOHN, J., and L. POSSLEY: Butyrylcholinesterase in human and ruminant nervous tissue. Neurology **8**, Suppl. 1, 94—95 (1958).

BERRY, J. F., and V. P. WHITTAKER: The acyl-group specificity of choline acetylase. Biochem. J. **73**, 447—458 (1959).

BIGGS, H. G., S. CAREY and D. B. MORRISON: A simple colorimetric method for measuring activities of cellular and plasma cholinesterase. Amer. J. clin. Path. **30**, 181—186 (1958); Techn. Bull. Registry med. Techn. **28**, 137—142 (1958).

BLASCHKO, H., E. BÜLBRING and T. C. CHOU: Tubocurarine antagonism and inhibition of cholinesterases. Brit. J. Pharmacol. **4**, 29—32 (1949).

— T. C. CHOU and I. WAJDA: The affinity of atropine-like esters for esterases. Brit. J. Pharmacol. **2**, 108—115 (1947).

BLEISCH, V. R., and H. SHWACHMAN: Serum cholinesterase values in childhood in health and disease. Pediatrics **13**, 426—438 (1954).

BLUMENTHAL, H., and G. WOODARD: Comparison of plasma triglyceride esterases and cholinesterases in various species. Fed. Proc. **16**, 283 (1957).

BODANSKY, O.: Cholinesterase. Ann. N. Y. Acad. Sci. **47**, 521—547 (1946).

BOELL, E. J., and S.-C. SHEN: Functional differentiation in embryonic development. I. Cholinesterase activity of induced neural structures in *Amblystoma punctatum*. J. exp. Zool. **97**, 21—41 (1944).

BONTING, S. L., and R. M. FEATHERSTONE: Ultramicro assay of the cholinesterases. Arch. Biochem. **61**, 89—98 (1956).

BOVET-NITTI, F.: Sur la nature de l'estérase contenue dans le venin de cobra. Experientia (Basel) **3**, 283 (1947).

BROCA, J.: Le dosage de la cholinestérase comme test de diagnose du sérum de cheval et de son état de conservation. Montauban: Imprimerie Forestié 1948.

Brown, H. V., and A. F. Bush: Parathion inhibition of cholinesterase. Arch. indust. Hyg. 1, 633—636 (1950).

Buckles, J., and K. Bullock: The application of enzyme inhibition to the estimation of small quantities of drugs possessing anticholinesterase activity. The assay of injection of neostigmine methylsulphate. J. Pharm. (Lond.) 8, 946—955 (1956).

Bullock, K.: The anticholinesterase activity of certain cytotoxic substances. Chem. Indust. 1955, 36—38.

Burgen, A. S. V., and F. Hobbiger: The inhibition of cholinesterases by alkylphosphates and alkylphenolphosphates. Brit. J. Pharmacol. 6, 593—605 (1951).

Caraway, W. T.: Photometric determination of serum cholinesterase activity. Amer. J. clin. Path. 26, 945—955 (1956).

Casida, J. E.: Comparative enzymology of certain insect acetylesterases in relation to poisoning by organophosphorus insecticides. Biochem. J. 60, 487—496 (1955).

Casier, H., et G. R. de Vleeschhouwer: Sur les propriétés anti-cholinestérasiques et pharmacologiques du bromure de N-p-chloro-phenyl-méthyl-carbamate de m-hydroxy-phényl-triméthylammonium (Nu-1250). Arch. int. Pharmacodyn. 90, 412—420 (1952).

Cervini, C.: Simple alcalimetric method for the determination of serum cholinesterase activity (Italian). Minerva med. (Torino) 41, I, 456—458 (1950).

Chadwick, L. E., and D. L. Hill: Inhibition of cholinesterase by di-isopropyl fluorophosphate, physostigmine and hexaethyl tetraphosphate in the roach. J. Neurophysiol. 10, 235—246 (1947).

Chaudhuri, D. K.: Studies on cholinesterase. Ann. Biochem. exp. Med. 4, 77—86 (1944); 6, 91—94 (1946).

Chessick, R. D.: The histochemical specificity of cholinesterases. J. Histochem. Cytochem. 2, 258—273 (1954).

Chouteau, J., P. Rancien et A. Karamanian: Recherches sur les estérases du sérum sanguin. I. Méthode de détermination des activités cholinestérasique et tributyrinasique sérique. Bull. Soc. Chim. biol. (Paris) 38, 1329—1336 (1956).

Cohen, J. A., F. Kalsbeek and M. G. P. J. Warringa: Reversibility of the inhibition of true cholinesterase by physostigmine. Biochim. biophys. Acta 2, 549—560 (1948).

— and M. G. P. J. Warringa: Purification of cholinesterase from ox red cells. Biochim. biophys. Acta 10, 195—196 (1953).

— — The labelling of human serum by ^{32}P-diisopropylphosphorofluoridate (DF^{32}P). Biochim. biophys. Acta 25, 600—607 (1957).

Cook, J. W.: Report on determination of insecticides by enzymatic methods. J. Ass. agric. Chem. (Wash.) 37, 561—564 (1954).

— Paper chromatography of some organic phosphate insecticides. IV. Spot test for in vitro cholinesterase inhibitors. J. Ass. agric. Chem. (Wash.) 38, 150—153 (1955).

Courville, D. A., and W. Ledington: A new method of assay for serum esterase. J. biol. Chem. 190, 575—584 (1951).

Croxatto, H., R. Croxatto and F. Huidobro: New photometric method for determination of cholinesterase activity of serum (Portuguese). An. Acad. Biol. Univ. Chile 3, 55—65 (1939).

Dale, H. H.: The action of certain esters and ethers of choline and their relation to muscarine. J. Pharmacol. exp. Ther. 6, 147—190 (1914).

Davies, D. R.: Cholinesterases and the mode of action of some anticholinesterases. J. Pharm. (Lond.) 6, 1—26 (1954).

— and A. L. Green: The mechanism of hydrolysis by cholinesterase and related enzymes. Advanc. Enzymol. 20, 283—318 (1958).

— and J. D. Nicholls: A field test for the assay of human whole-blood cholinesterase. Brit. med. J. 1955 I, 1373—1375.

— J. E. Risley and J. P. Rutland: The hydrolysis of choline esters by tissues of the ruminant. Biochem. J. 53, P 15 (1953).

— and J. P. Rutland: The electrometric method of Michel for the estimation of cholinesterases. Biochem. J. 47, P 22—P 23 (1950).

Davison, A. N.: The reactions of rabbits to poisoning by p-nitrophenyldiethylphosphate (E 600). Brit. J. Pharmacol. 8, 208—211 (1953).

Delaunois, A. L., et H. Casier: Micro-méthode potentiométrique pour la détermination de l'activité des cholinestérases. Arch. int. Pharmacodyn. 75, 371—381 (1948).

Delcourt, A., et R. Hoeden: Pseudocholinestérase et affections hépatiques: à propos d'une nouvelle technique de détermination. Acta gastro-ent. belg. 17, 102—109 (1954).

Depierre, F., et A. Funke: Anticholinestérasiques. II. Dérivés analogues à la prostigmine. Influence de la structure chimique sur l'intensité et la sélectivité de l'action antiacétyl-cholinestérasique. C. R. Acad. Sci. (Paris) 239, 370—372 (1954).

Diggle, W. M., and J. C. Gage: Cholinesterase inhibition in vitro by 0,0-diethyl 0-p-nitrophenyl thiophosphate (Parathion, E 605). Biochem. J. 49, 491—494 (1951).

DYBING, O., and A. HJELLE: Cholinesterase activity in blood of cattle (Norwegian). Nord. Vet.-Med. 9, 41—48 (1957).

EARL, C. J., and R. H. S. THOMPSON: Cholinesterase levels in the nervous system in tri-ortho-cresyl phosphate poisoning. Brit. J. Pharmacol. 7, 685—694 (1952).

EINSEL, D. W. jr., H. J. TRURNIT, S. D. SILVER and E. C. STEINER: Self-equilibrating electrolytic method for determination of acid production rates. Anal. Chem. 28, 408—410 (1956).

ELEY, D. D., and G. S. STONE: Kinetic investigations on pseudo-cholinesterase. Biochem. J. 49, P 30 (1951).

ELLIS, S.: Benzoylcholine and atropine esterase. J. Pharmacol. exp. Ther. 91, 370—378 (1947).
— Enzymic hydrolysis of morphine esters. J. Pharmacol. exp. Ther. 94, 130—135 (1948).

FERRARI, W.: Insensitivity of chicken cholinesterase to specific inhibitors of true- and pseudo-enzyme. Nature (Lond.) 180, 144 (1957).

FLEISHER, J. H., and E. J. POPE: Colorimetric method for determination of red blood cell cholinesterase activity in whole blood. Arch. indust. Hyg. 9, 323—334 (1954).
— — and S. F. SPEAR: Determination of red blood cell cholinesterase activity in whole blood. An application of the colorimetric method to the blood of the rabbit, rat, pig, dog, goat, and monkey. Arch. indust. Hlth 11, 332—337 (1955).
— S. SPEAR and E. J. POPE: Stable cholinesterase preparations as laboratory standards of activity. Anal. Chem. 27, 1080—1083 (1955).
— G. S. WOODSON and L. SIMET: A visual method for estimating blood cholinesterase activity. Arch. indust. Hlth 14, 510—520 (1956).

FRAWLEY, J. P., and H. N. FUYAT: Effect of low dietary levels of parathion and systox on blood cholinesterase of dogs. J. Agric. Food Chem. 5, 346—348 (1957).
— E. C. HAGAN and O. G. FITZHUGH: A comparative pharmacological and toxicological study of organic phosphate-anticholinesterase compounds. J. Pharmacol. exp. Ther. 105, 156 to 165 (1952).

FREDRIKSSON, T., and G. TIBBLING: Inhibition of cholinesterase with methylfluorophosphoryl-choline and -carbocholine. Spontaneous return of activity. Biochem. Pharmacol. 3, 184 to 189 (1960).

FRIEND, D. G., and O. KRAYER: The estimation by a manometric method of the activity of cholinesterase in lymph. J. Pharmacol. exp. Ther. 71, 246—252 (1941).

FRYER, J. H., R. G. D. STEEL and H. H. WILLIAMS: Cholinesterase activity levels in normal human subjects. A statistical evaluation with reference to the detection of minimal absorption of the organic phosphate insecticides. Arch. indust. Hlth 12, 406—411 (1955).

FULTON, M. P., and G. A. MOGEY: Some selective inhibitors of true cholinesterase. Brit. J. Pharmacol. 9, 138—144 (1954).

FUNKE, A., J. BAGOT et F. DEPIERRE: Anticholinestérasiques. I. Synthèse de diphénoxyalcanes porteurs d'une ou deux fonctions phénoliques libres. C. R. Acad. Sci. (Paris) 239, 329—331 (1954).
— J. JACOB et K. VON DÄNIKEN: Propriétés analgésiques et anticholinestérasiques du dichlor-hydrate et du diiodométhylate de la bis-(pipéridinométhyl-coumaranyl-5) cétone. C. R. Acad. Sci. (Paris) 236, 149—151 (1953).

GAL, E. M., and E. ROTH: Spectrophotometric methods for determination of cholinesterase activity. Clin. chim. Acta 2, 316—326 (1957).

GAL, I.: Choline-esterase and vegetative nervous system; new method for determination of choline-esterase activity of blood. Budap. Orv. Ujság 37, 391—394 (1939).
— Une nouvelle technique de dosage de l'activité cholinestérasique du sérum sanguin. Ann. Biol. clin. 6, 363—365 (1948).
— and L. VEGH: Etude de l'activité cholinestérasique du sérum sanguin par la méthode néphélometrique. Ann. Biol. clin. 6, 366—367 (1948).

GHOSH, B. N., and N. K. SARKAR: Active principles of snake venoms. Amer. Ass. Advanc. Sci. 44, 189—196 (1956).

GIACOBINI, E.: The distribution and localization of cholinesterases in nerve cells. Acta physiol. scand. 45, Suppl. 156, 1—45 (1959).

GIANG, P. A., and S. A. HALL: Enzymatic determination of organic phosphorus insecticides. Anal. Chem. 23, 1830—1834 (1951).

GLICK, D.: Properties of choline esterase in human serum. Biochem. J. 31, 521—525 (1937).
— Studies on enzymatic histochemistry. XXV. A micro method for the determination of choline esterase and the activity-pH relationship of this enzyme. J. gen. Physiol. 21, 289—295 (1938a).
— Studies on the specificity of choline esterase. J. biol. Chem. 125, 729—739 (1938b).
— Further studies on the specificity of choline esterase. J. biol. Chem. 130, 527—534 (1939).
— Some additional observations on the specificity of choline esterase. J. biol. Chem. 137, 357—362 (1941).
— The controversy on cholinesterase. Science 102, 100 (1945).

GLICK, D., S. GLAUBACH and D. H. MOORE: Azolesterase activities of electrophoretically separated proteins of serum. J. biol. Chem. 144, 525—528 (1942).

GOLDSTEIN, A.: The mechanism of enzyme-inhibitor-substrate reactions. Illustrated by the cholinesterase-physostigmine-acetylcholine system. J. gen. Physiol. 27, 529—580 (1944).

— A "free manometer" technique for use with the Warburg apparatus. Proc. Amer. Acad. Arts Sci. 77, 235—253 (1949).

— Cholinesterase specificity patterns in the tissues of man, cat, and teleost fish. J. Pharmacol. exp. Ther. 101, 13 (1951).

GOLZ, H. H.: Anticholinesterase activity. Recognition and detection in the field and hospital. Arch. indust. Hlth 18, 138—141 (1958).

GOMORI, G.: The histochemistry of esterases. Int. Rev. Cytol. 1, 323—335 (1952).

— Histochemistry of human esterases. J. Histochem. Cytochem. 3, 479—484 (1955).

GORDON, J. J.: N-Diethylaminoethylphenothiazine: a specific inhibitor of pseudocholinesterase. Nature (Lond.) 162, 146 (1948).

GOUTIER, R.: Etude électrophoretique des estérases sériques et de la fixation du $DF^{32}P$ dans le sérum, chez le lapin et le cobaye. Biochim. biophys. Acta 19, 524—534 (1956).

GREENBERG, S., and C. CALVERT: Modification of Michel method for cholinesterase determination. Med. Techn. Bull. 8, 59—64 (1957).

GRÉGOIRE, J., et M. COTTE: Test spectrophotométrique des cholinestérases sériques. C.R. Soc. Biol. (Paris) 146, 741—744 (1952).

— J. GRÉGOIRE et N. LIMOZIN: Sur l'activité des cholinestérases. I. Méthode de dosage spectrophotométrique de l'activité des cholinestérases. Bull. Soc. Chim. biol. (Paris) 37, 65—79 (1955 a).

— — — Sur l'activité des cholinestérases. II. Application de la méthode spectrophotométrique à l'étude cinétique de l'activité des cholinestérases purifiées aux très faibles concentrations en substrat. Bull. Soc. Chim. biol. (Paris) 37, 81—87 (1955 b).

— N. LIMOZIN et J. GRÉGOIRE: Sur l'activité des cholinestérases. III. Application de la méthode spectrophotométrique à l'influence des concentrations salines sur l'affinité des cholinestérases purifiées vis-à-vis de l'acétylcholine. Bull. Soc. Chim. biol. (Paris) 38, 147 to 163 (1956).

GREIG, M. E., and A. J. GIBBONS: Cation transport in erythrocytes treated with lecithinase A. Arch. Biochem. 61, 343—347 (1956).

GUNTER, J. M.: Absence of pseudo-cholinesterase from the tissues of ruminants. Nature (Lond.) 157, 369 (1946).

HAGAN, E. C., P. M. JENNER, W. I. JONES and O. G. FITZHUGH: Blood withdrawal and processing preparatory to plasma and cell cholinesterase determinations in rats. J. Ass. agric. Chem. (Wash.) 41, 899 (1958).

HALL, G. E., and C. C. LUCAS: Choline esterase activity of normal and pathological human sera. J. Pharmacol. exp. Ther. 59, 34—42 (1937).

HAMBLIN, D. O., and J. F. MARCHAND: Cholinesterase tests and their applicability in the field. Amer. Cyanamid Co., New York, March 1951.

HARDEGG, W., D. BECHINGER u. R. DOHRMANN: Zur Bedeutung der Gleichung von Schaefer für unsere Auffassung über die Kinetik bei Cholinesterasen. Pflügers Arch. ges. Physiol. 263, 33—47 (1956).

— u. R. POCHE: Bemerkungen zur Kinetik und Substratspezifität der Cholinesterasen (Vorläufige Mitteilung). Klin. Wschr. 30, 799—800 (1952).

— u. H. SCHAEFER: Zur Kinetik der Cholinesterases. Mit einer Verbesserung der Warburgschen Apparatur. Pflügers Arch. ges. Physiol. 255, 136—153 (1952).

HARDERS, C. L., and J. M. VAN MULKEN: Simple determination of pseudocholinesterase activity in blood serum (Dutch). Pharm. Weekblad 89, 845—848 (1954).

HARDWICK, D. C.: Cholinesterases in bovine plasma. Biochem. J. 64, P 1 (1956).

HARGREAVES, A. B.: Action of acetate ion on hydrolysis of acetylcholine and its application to the titrimetric determination of cholinesterase (Spanish). An. Acad. bras. cienc. 25, 291—301 (1953).

— C. CALMON LEMME and L. LUDMILA LIEPIN: Experiments on the acetylcholinesterase of the electric organ of the Electrophorus electricus. An. Acad. bras. cienc. 31, 59—66 (1959).

— and L. C. G. LOBO: An improved step in the method of Rothenberg and Nachmansohn for the purification of acetylcholinesterase from electric tissue. Arch. Biochem. 46, 481 to 482 (1953).

— Titrimetric determination of cholinesterase in blood serum (Spanish). Hospital (Rio de J.) 55, 99—106 (1959).

HARRIS, H., and M. WHITTAKER: Differential response of human serum cholinesterase types to an inhibitor in potato. Nature (Lond.) 183, 1808 (1959).

HAWKINS, R. D., and J. M. GUNTER: Studies on cholinesterase. 5. The selective inhibition of pseudo-cholinesterase in vivo. Biochem. J. 40, 192—197 (1946).

HAWKINS, R. D., and B. MENDEL: True cholinesterases with pronounced resistance to eserine. J. Cell. comp. Physiol. **27**, 69—85 (1946).
— — Selective inhibition of pseudo-cholinesterase by di*iso*propyl fluorophosphonate. Brit. J. Pharmacol. **2**, 173—180 (1947).
— — Studies on cholinesterase. 6. The selective inhibition of true cholinesterase *in vivo*. Biochem. J. **44**, 260—264 (1949).
HEILBRONN, E.: Hydrolysis of carboxylic acid esters of thiocholine and its analogues. 1 and 2. Acta chem. scand. **12**, 1481—1491, 1492—1506 (1958).
— Hydrolysis of carboxylic acid esters of thiocholine and its analogues. 3. Hydrolysis catalysed by acetylcholine esterase and butyrylcholine esterase. Acta chem. scand. **13**, 1547—1560 (1959).
HERZFELD, E., u. C. STUMPF: Ein neuer Kurztest zur Bestimmung der Serumcholinesterase-aktivität. Wien. klin. Wschr. **67**, 874—876 (1955).
HESTRIN, S.: The reaction of acetylcholine and carboxylic acid derivatives with hydroxyl-amine, and its analytical application. J. biol. Chem. **180**, 249—261 (1949).
HINES, B. E., and R. A. McCANCE: Pseudo-cholinesterase activity in secretions and organs of piglets and pigs. J. Physiol. (Lond.) **122**, 188—192 (1953).
HOBBIGGER, E. E.: The hydrolysis of indoxyl esters by rat esterases. Biochem. J. **67**, 600—607 (1957).
HOFSTEE, B. H. J.: Spectrophotometric determinations of esterases. Science **114**, 128—130 (1951).
HOLMSTEDT, B.: Pharmacology of organophosphorus cholinesterase inhibitors. Pharmacol. Rev. **11**, 567—688 (1959).
HOLT, S. J.: The value of fundamental studies of staining reactions in enzyme histochemistry, with reference to indoxyl methods for esterases. J. Histochem. Cytochem. **4**, 541—554 (1956).
HOLTON, P.: The enzymic hydrolysis of triacetin. Biochem. J. **43**, P 13 (1948).
HOMANN, W.: Eine papierchromatographische Methode zur Messung der Cholinesterase-aktivität. Naunyn-Schmiedeberg's Arch. exp. Path. Pharmak. **224**, 176—178 (1955).
HUC, M.: Recherches sur la détermination et la signification de l'activité procainestérasique du sérum humain. Lille: Douriez-Bataille 1950.
HUERGA, J. DE LA, C. YESINICK and H. POPPER: Colorimetric method for the determination of serum cholinesterase. Amer. J. clin. Path. **22**, 1126—1133 (1952).
INAGAKI, K., M. MORITA, M. IGUCHI and S. TSUDA: The extraction of erythrocyte cholin-esterase with chlorophyllin solution. Yokohama med. Bull. **4**, 358—364 (1953).
JACOB, J.: Sur l'inhibition sélective des acétylcholinestérases *in vivo* chez le chien. Experientia (Basel) **10**, 33—34 (1954).
— Propriétés antiacétylcholinestérasiques spécifiques du di-iodo-méthylate de la bis-(piper-idinométhylcoumaranyl-5) cétone (3318 CT). I—II. Arch. int. Pharmacodyn. **101**, 446—468 (1955); **106**, 395—436 (1956).
JACOBSOHN, K. P., et J. TAPADINHAS: Action des métaux lourds sur la cholinestérase. Bull. Soc. port. Sci. nat. **14**, 103—106 (1943).
JENSEN-HOLM, J., H. H. LAUSEN, K. MILTHERS and K. O. MØLLER: Determination of the cholinesterase activity in blood and organs by automatic titration. With some observations of serious errors of the method and remarks of the photometric determination. Acta pharmacol. (Kbh.) **15**, 384—394 (1959).
KALOW, W.: Zur Kenntnis der Butyrylcholin-Esterase im Serum von Mensch und Pferd. Naunyn-Schmiedeberg's Arch. exp. Path. Pharmak. **215**, 370—377 (1952a).
— Hydrolysis of local anesthetics by human serum cholinesterase. J. Pharmacol. exp. Ther. **104**, 122—134 (1952).
— and R. O. DAVIES: The activity of various esterase inhibitors towards atypical human serum cholinesterase. Biochem. Pharmacol. **1**, 183—192 (1958).
— and K. GENEST: A method for the detection of atypical forms of human serum cholin-esterase. Determination of Dibucaine Numbers. Canad. J. Biochem. **35**, 339—346 (1957).
— — and N. STARON: Kinetic studies on the hydrolysis of benzolcholine by human serum cholinesterase. Canad. J. Biochem. **34**, 637—653 (1956).
— and D. R. GUNN: The relation between dose of succinylcholine and duration of apnea in man. J. Pharmacol. exp. Ther. **120**, 203—214 (1957).
— — Some statistical data on atypical cholinesterase of human serum. Ann. human. Genet. **23**, 239—250 (1959).
— and H. A. LINDSAY: A comparison of optical and manometric methods for the assay of human serum cholinesterase. Canad. J. Biochem. **33**, 568—574 (1955).
— — Abnormal behavior of human serum cholinesterase. J. Pharmacol. exp. Ther. **116**, 34 (1956).
— and N. STARON: On distribution and inheritance of atypical forms of human serum cholin-esterase, as indicated by dibucaine numbers. Canad. J. Biochem. **35**, 1305—1320 (1957).

KARCZMAR, A. G., T. KOPPANYI and G. C. SHEATZ: Further studies on intravenously injected cholinesterase preparations. J. Pharmacol. exp. Ther. **107**, 501—518 (1953).

KATSH, S.: Anticholinesterase activity of drugs assayed by a rapid colorimetric method. J. appl. Physiol. **8**, 215—219 (1955).

KAUFMAN, K.: Serum cholinesterase activity in the normal individual and in people with liver disease. Ann. intern. Med. **41**, 533—545 (1954).

KEKWICK, R. G. O., M. E. MACKAY and N. H. MARTIN: The preliminary isolation and characterization of human serum cholinesterase. Biochem. J. **53**, P 36—P 37 (1953).

KOELLE, G. B.: The histochemical differentiation of types of cholinesterases and their localizations in tissues of the cat. J. Pharmacol. exp. Ther. **100**, 158—179 (1950).

— The elimination of enzymatic diffusion artifacts in the histochemical localization of cholinesterases and a survey of their cellular distributions. J. Pharmacol. exp. Ther. **103**, 153 to 171 (1951).

— Cholinesterases of the tissues and sera of rabbits. Biochem. J. **53**, 217—226 (1953).

— The histochemical localization of cholinesterases in the central nervous system of the rat. J. comp. Neurol. **100**, 211—235 (1954).

— Histochemical demonstration of reversible anticholinesterase action at selective cellular sizes *in vivo*. J. Pharmacol. exp. Ther. **120**, 488—503 (1957).

— and A. GILMAN: Anticholinesterase drugs. J. Pharmacol. exp. Ther. **95** (Part II, Pharmacol. Rev.), 166—216 (1949).

KÖVER, A., and T. KOVÁCS: On the specificity of myosincholinesterase. Acta physiol. Acad. Sci. hung. **11**, 259—265 (1957).

— — and T. KÖNIG: On the properties of myosincholinesterase. Acta physiol. Acad. Sci. hung. **11**, 253—258 (1957).

KOOISTRA, G.: Contribution to the knowledge of the action of acetylcholine in the intestine of *Periplaneta americana* L. Physiol. comp. oecol. **2**, 75—80 (1949).

KRAMER, D. N., and R. M. GAMSON: Colorimetric determination of acetylcholinesterase activity. Anal. Chem. **30**, 251—254 (1958).

KURODA, K., M. FUJINO and K. IRINO: A portable micromethod of the determination of cholinesterase activity in blood serum. Tokushima J. exp. Med. **6**, 73—80 (1959).

LALLI, G., and L. CASCINO: Colorimetric method for the determination of cholinesterase activity in plasma and red blood cells (Italian). Riv. Med. aero. **19**, 103—137 (1956).

LANDS, A. M., J. O. HOPPE, A. ARNOLD and F. K. KIRCHNER: An investigation of the structure-activity correlations within a series of ambenonium analogs. J. Pharmacol. **123**, 121—127 (1958).

LARSSON, L., and B. HANSEN: An automatic recording titrator. Svensk kem. T. **68**, 521—527 (1956).

LAWLER, H. C.: A simplified procedure for the partial purification of acetylcholinesterase from electric tissue. J. biol. Chem. **234**, 799—801 (1959).

LEHMANN, H., V. PATSTON and E. RYAN: The inheritance of an idiopathic low plasma pseudocholinesterase level. J. clin. Path. **11**, 554 (1958).

— and E. RYAN: The familial incidence of low pseudocholinesterase level. Lancet **1956 II**, 124.

— and P. H. SIMMONS: Sensitivity to suxamethonium. Apnoe in two brothers. Lancet **1958 II**, 981—982.

LESUK, A.: Stabilized cholinesterase. U.S. Pat. 2,475,792—2,475,793, July 12, 1949.

LEVINE, M. G., and A. A. SURAN: A new cholinesterase in swine serum. Nature (Lond.) **166**, 698 (1950).

— — A survey of some mammalian serum cholinesterases. Enzymologia **15**, 17—20 (1951).

LÉVY, J.: Sur les estérases du sérum humain. J. Physiol. (Paris) **43**, 103—125 (1951 a).

— Sur les estérases du sérum de lapin. J. Physiol. (Paris) **43**, 127—138 (1951 b).

— Sur les estérases du sang de rat. J. Physiol. (Paris) **43**, 217—222 (1951 c).

— Sur la benzoylcholinestérase. J. Physiol. (Paris) **43**, 783—784 (1951 d).

— et B. TCHOUBAR: Relations entre la vitesse d'hydrolyse de divers esters de la choline par la benzoylcholinestérase et la constitution chimique des substrats. J. Physiol. (Paris) **44**, 95—97 (1952).

LIMPEROS, G., and K. E. RANTA: A rapid screening test for the determination of the approximate cholinesterase activity of human blood. Science **117**, 453—455 (1953).

LINDERSTRØM-LANG, K., and D. GLICK: Micromethod for determination of choline esterase activity. C. R. Lab. Carlsberg, Sér. chim. **22**, 300—306 (1938).

LORD, K. A., and C. POTTER: Differences in esterases from insect species: toxicity of organophosphorus compounds and *in vitro* anti-esterase activity. J. Sci. Food Agric. **5**, 490—498 (1954).

LOWRY, O. H., N. R. ROBERTS, M.-L. WU, W. S. HIXON and E. J. CRAWFORD: The quantitative histochemistry of brain. II. Enzyme measurements. J. biol. Chem. **207**, 19—37 (1954).

LUNA PÉREZ, J. L.: A new method for determination of serum cholinesterase (Spanish). Rev. clín. esp. **61**, 245—247 (1956).

LUNDIN, S. J.: Acetylcholinesterase in goldfish muscles. Studies on some substrates and inhibitors. Biochem. J. **72**, 210—214 (1959).

MACDONALD, W. E., C. B. POLLARD and A. H. GROPP: A rapid micromethod for electrometric determination of red cell cholinesterase activity in whole blood. Arch. indust. Hyg. **6**, 271—275 (1952).

MALMSTRÖM, B. G., Ö. LEVIN and H. G. BOMAN: Chromatography of human serum cholinesterase. Acta chem. scand. **10**, 1077—1082 (1956).

MARCHAND, J. F.: Microtest for cholinesterase. Interpretation after nerve gas or agricultural insecticide exposures. J. Amer. med. Ass. **149**, 738—740 (1952).

MARPLES, E. A., R. H. S. THOMPSON and G. R. WEBSTER: The liberation of active enzymes from brain tissue by lysolecithin. J. Neurochem. **4**, 62—70 (1959).

McOSKER, D. E., and L. J. DANIEL: A colorimetric micro method for the determination of cholinesterase. Arch. Biochem. **79**, 1—7 (1959).

MENDEL, B., and R. D. HAWKINS: Estimation of the cholinesterases. Meth. med. Res. **3**, 107—115 (1950).

— and D. B. MUNDELL: Studies on cholinesterase. 2. A method for the purification of a pseudo-cholinesterase from dog pancreas. Biochem. J. **37**, 64—66 (1943).

— — and H. RUDNEY: Cholinesterase. III. Specific tests for true cholinesterase and pseudo-cholinesterase. Biochem. J. **37**, 473—476 (1943).

— and D. K. MYERS: Identification of pseudocholinesterase in the tissues of ruminants. Nature (Lond.) **176**, 783 (1955).

— and H. RUDNEY: Studies on cholinesterase. 1. Cholinesterase and pseudo-cholinesterase. Biochem. J. **37**, 59—63 (1943a).

— — On the type of cholinesterase present in brain tissue. Science **98**, 201—202 (1943b).

— — The cholinesterases in the light of recent findings. Science **100**, 499—500 (1944).

MENGHI, P., E. GRASSO and V. QUINTÉ: Methods for the determination of cholinesterase activity. Minerva pediat. (Torino) **5**, 1039—1043 (1953).

MENTHA, J., H. SPRINZ and R. BARNARD: Rapid extraction of human erythrocyte cholinesterase by alkali pseudoagglutination. J. biol. Chem. **167**, 623 (1947).

METCALF, R. L.: The colorimetric microestimation of human blood cholinesterases and its application to poisoning by organic phosphate insecticides. J. econ. Ent. **44**, 883—890 (1951).

— and R. B. MARCH: Studies of the mode of action of parathion and its derivatives and their toxicity to insects. J. econ. Ent. **42**, 721—728 (1949).

— — Properties of acetylcholine esterases from the bee, the fly and the mouse and their relation to insecticide action. J. econ. Ent. **43**, 670—677 (1950).

— — and M. G. MAXON: Substrate preferences of insect cholinesterases. Ann. ent. Soc. Amer. **48**, 222—228 (1955).

MEYER, A., u. W. WILBRANDT: Zur Bestimmung der Aktivität der Cholinesterasen im menschlichen Blute. Helv. physiol. pharmacol. Acta **12**, 206—216 (1954).

MICHEL, H. O.: An electrometric method for the determination of red blood cell and plasma cholinesterase activity. J. Lab. clin. Med. **34**, 1564—1568 (1949).

MOLANDER, D. W., M. M. FRIEDMAN and J. S. LaDUE: Serum cholinesterase in hepatic and neoplastic diseases: a preliminary report. Ann. intern. Med. **41**, 1139—1151 (1954).

MOMMAERTS, W. F. H. M., P. A. KHAIRALLAH and M. F. DICKENS: Acetylcholinesterase in the conductive tissue of the heart. Circulat. Res. **1**, 460—465 (1953).

MORAND, P., et H. LABORIT: La mesure de l'activité cholinestérasique du sérum. Mise au point d'une méthode applicable à la clinique. Presse méd. **55**, 131—132, 251 (1947).

MORTON, R. K.: Methods of extraction of enzymes from animal tissues. In: S. P. COLOWICK and N. O. KAPLAN, Eds., Methods in Enzymology, vol. I, 25—51. New York: Academic Press 1955.

MOUNTER, L. A.: The specificity of cobra-venom cholinesterase. Biochem. J. **50**, 122—128 (1951).

— The complex nature of dialkylfluorophosphatases of hog and rat liver and kidney. J. biol. Chem. **215**, 705—711 (1955).

— and V. P. WHITTAKER: The esterases of horse blood: 2. The specificity of horse erythrocyte cholinesterase. Biochem. J. **47**, 525—530 (1950).

— — The hydrolysis of esters of phenol by cholinesterases and other esterases. Biochem. J. **54**, 551—559 (1953).

MYERS, D. K.: Effect of salt on the hydrolysis of acetylcholine by cholinesterases. Arch. Biochem. **37**, 469—487 (1952).

— Studies on cholinesterase. 9. Species variation in the specificity pattern of the pseudo cholinesterase. Biochem. J. **55**, 67—79 (1953).

— Studies on Selective Esterase Inhibitors. 's-Gravenhage: Uitgeverij Excelsior 1954.

NACHMANSOHN, D.: Die Rolle des Acetylcholins in den Elementarvorgängen der Nerven-leitung. Ergebn. Physiol. 48, 575—683 (1955).
— Chemical and Molecular Basis of Nerve Activity. New York: Academic Press 1959.
— and M. A. ROTHENBERG: On the specificity of choline esterase in nervous tissue. Science 100, 454 (1944).
— — Studies on cholinesterase. I. On the specificity of the enzyme in nerve tissue. J. biol. Chem. 158, 653—666 (1945).
— and H. SCHNEEMANN: On the effect of drugs on cholinesterase. J. biol. Chem. 159, 239 to 240 (1945).
— and I. B. WILSON: The enzymic hydrolysis and synthesis of acethylcholine. Advanc. Enzymol. 12, 259—339 (1951).
— — Acetylcholinesterase. In: S. P. COLOWICK and N. O. KAPLAN, Eds., Methods in Enzymology, vol. I, 642—651. New York: Academic Press 1955.
NEILANDS, J. B., and M. D. CANNON: Automatic recording pH instrumentation. Anal. Chem. 27, 29—33 (1955).
ORD, M. G., and R. H. S. THOMPSON: The distribution of cholinesterase types in mammalian tissues. Biochem. J. 46, 346—352 (1950).
— — The preparation of soluble cholinesterases from mammalian heart and brain. Biochem. J. 49, 191—199 (1951).
— — Pseudo-cholinesterase activity in the central nervous system. Biochem. J. 51, 245—251 (1952).
ORGELL, W. H., K. A. VAIDYA and P. A. DAHM: Inhibition of human plasma cholinesterase in vitro by extracts of Solanaceous plants. Science 128, 1136 (1958).
ORMEROD, W. E.: Hydrolysis of benzoylcholine derivatives by cholinesterase in serum. Bio-chem. J. 54, 701—704 (1953).
PAGET, M., et G. DHELLEMMES: Sur le dosage de la pseudocholinestérase du sérum humain. Technique personelle. Ann. Biol. clin. 5, 380—385 (1947).
PASQUALIN, R., and R. MOSCOVICI: Colorimetric determination of cholinesterase in blood serum (Portuguese). Arch. Biol. (S. Paulo) 37, 59—65 (1953).
PAULESU, F.: Differences in cholinesterase activity of various biological material. III. A new type of cholinesterase resistant to CT 3318 and eucupine (Italian). Arch. int. Pharmacodyn. 105, 366—380 (1956).
— L. VARGIU e G. GIBERTONI: Differences in cholinesterase activity of various biological material. II. Inhibitory effect of CT 3318 (Italian). Arch. int. Pharmacodyn. 104, 11—18 (1955).
PIGHINI, G.: Cholinesterase in various parts of the nervous system (Italian). Biochim. Terap. sper. 26, 157—159 (1939); also: Boll. Soc. ital. Biol. sper. 15, 237—238 (1940).
PILZ, W.: Untersuchungen über Fermente des menschlichen Blutes. I. Die photometrische Mikrobestimmung der Acetylcholinesterase in Serum und Erythrocyten. Klin. Wschr. 36, 1017—1021 (1958).
PINTÉR, I.: Esterase activity of serum protein fractions. Acta physiol. Acad. Sci. hung. 11, 39—44 (1957).
PLATTNER, F., u. H. HINTNER: Die Spaltung von Acetylcholin durch Organextrakte und Körperflüssigkeiten. Pflügers Arch. ges. Physiol. 225, 19—25 (1930).
POCHET, A.: Mesures de l'activité cholinestérasique. J. Pharm. Belg. 10, 339—357 (1955).
POLONOVSKI, M., I. IZZAT and M. ROBERT: Méthode turbidimétrique pour le dosage de l'activité des estérases. Bull. Soc. Chim. biol. (Paris) 35, 225—230 (1953).
PRIBILLA, O.: Die Bestimmung der Serumcholinesterase an der Leiche. Dtsch. Z. ges. gerichtl. Med. 46, 79—92 (1957).
RADOUCO, C., et E. FROMMEL: Microméthode électrométrique pour la mesure de l'activité des cholinestérases. Helv. physiol. pharmacol. Acta 10, C 39 (1952).
RAPPAPORT, F., J. FISCHL and N. PINTO: An improved method for the estimation of cholin-esterase activity in serum. Clin. chin. Acta 4, 227—230 (1959).
RAVIN, H. A., K.-C. TSOU and A. M. SELIGMAN: Colorimetric estimation and histochemical demonstration of serum cholinesterase. J. biol. Chem. 191, 843—857 (1951).
— S. I. ZACKS and A. M. SELIGMAN: The histochemical localization of acetylcholinesterase in nervous tissue. J. Pharmacol. exp. Ther. 107, 37—53 (1953).
REINHOLD, J. G., L. G. TOURIGNY and V. L. YONAN: Measurement of serum cholinesterase activity by a photometric indicator method. Together with a study of the influence of sex and race. Amer. J. clin. Path. 23, 645—653 (1953).
RICHARDS, A. G., and L. CUTKOMP: Cholinesterase of insect nerves. J. cell. comp. Physiol. 26, 57—61 (1945).
RICHTER, D., and P. G. CROFT: Blood esterases. Biochem. J. 36, 746—757 (1942).
ROAN, C. C., and S. MAEDA: The cholinesterase of the oriental fruit fly and its in vitro reactions with various insecticidal compounds. J. econ. Ent. 46, 775—779 (1953).

ROAN, C. C., and S. MAEDA: The cholinesterase systems of three species of fruit flies and the effects of certain insecticidal compounds on these enzymes. J. econ. Ent. 47, 507 to 514 (1954).

ROSNATI, V., and F. BOVET-NITTI: Pharmacological properties and sensibility of esterases to various derivatives of benzoylcholine and phenylacetylcholine (Italian). R. C. Ist. sup. Sanità 18, 971—982 (1955).

ROTHENBERG, M. A., and D. NACHMANSOHN: Studies on cholinesterase. III. Purification of the enzyme from electric tissue by fractional ammonium sulfate precipitation. J. biol. Chem. 168, 223—231 (1947).

RUBIN, A. A., J. MERSHON, M. E. GRELIS and I. I. A. TABACHNICK: A spectrophotometric method for assaying anticholinesterase activity. Fed. Proc. 16, 333 (1957).

SABINE, J. C.: The clinical significance of erythrocyte cholinesterase titers. I. A method suitable for routine clinical use, and the distribution of normal values. Blood 10, 1132—1138 (1955).

SACK, A., and E. A. ZELLER: New method of determination of the choline-esterase activity. Science 97, 449 (1943).

SAILER, S., u. H. BRAUNSTEINER: Über eine neue, sehr einfache Methode zur Bestimmung der Serumcholinesteraseaktivität und ihre klinische Bedeutung. Klin. Wschr. 37, 986—990 (1959).

SANZ, M. C.: Bestimmung der Cholinesterase-Aktivität mit Glaselektrode. Helv. physiol. pharmacol. Acta 2, C 29—C 32 (1944).

SAWYER, C. H.: Hydrolysis of choline esters by liver. Science 101, 385 (1945).

— and J. W. EVERETT: Cholinesterases in rat tissues and the site of serum non-specific cholinesterase production. Amer. J. Physiol 148, 675—683 (1947).

SCAIFE, J. F.: Stability of cholinesterase of the electric eel. Nature (Lond.) 183, 541 (1959).

SCHAEFER, H.: Über das normale Verhalten der Cholinesterase im Blut. Pflügers Arch. ges. Physiol. 249, 405—430 (1947).

SCHÜMMELFEDER, N.: Untersuchungen über Cholinesterase im Blut nach experimentellen Schädigungen. I. Mitteilung. Bestimmungsmethode und Einfluß von Narkose, operativen Eingriffen und Blutentnahmen. Naunyn-Schmiedeberg's Arch. exp. Path. Pharmak. 204, 454—465 (1947).

SCOZ, G., and C. CATTANEO: Determination of cholinesterase activity in blood with electrometric titration (Italian). Enzymologia 4, 157—162 (1937).

SERLIN, I., and G. C. COTZIAS: Microdiffusion of acetic acid as an assay for acetylcholinesterase. J. biol. Chem. 215, 263—268 (1955).

SHIBATA, S., and H. TAKAHASHI: A simple procedure for the estimation of serum cholinesterase by means of comparator with phenol red as indicator. Bull. Yamaguchi med. School 1, 188—197 (1953).

SKOREPA, J.: Electrophoretic mobility of plasma esterase after injection of heparin. Clin. chim. Acta 1, 499—500 (1956).

SIMONART, A.: Contribution à l'étude des propriétés pharmacologique des dérivés de la choline. Rev. belge Sci. méd. 5, 73—112 (1933).

SLEISENGER, M. H., T. P. ALMY, H. GILDER and G. PERLE: Colorimetric determination of serum cholinesterase: its value in hepatic and biliary tract diseases. J. clin. Invest. 32, 466—472 (1953).

SMALLMAN, B. N., and L. S. WOLFE: The effect of salts on the estimation of cholinesterase activity. Enzymologia 17, 133—144 (1955).

SNYDER, H. H., C. D. SNYDER and L. D. BUNCH: Serum cholinesterase levels in surgical patients. A preliminary report. Amer. Surg. 17, 959—980 (1951).

STEDMAN, E., and E. STEDMAN: The relative choline-esterase activities of serum and corpuscles from the blood of certain species. Biochem. J. 29, 2107—2111 (1935).

— — and L. H. EASSON: Choline-esterase. An enzyme present in the blood-serum of the horse. Biochem. J. 26, 2056—2066 (1932).

— and A. C. WHITE: A comparison of the choline-esterase activities of the blood-sera from various species. Biochem. J. 27, 1055—1060 (1933).

STEGWEE, D.: Properties of insect cholinesterase. Acta physiol. pharmacol. neerl. 1, 336—337 (1950).

— Studies on cholinesterase in insects. Physiol. comp. oecol. 2, 241—247 (1951).

STRAUS, O. H., and A. GOLDSTEIN: Zone behavior of enzymes. Illustrated by the effect of dissociation constant and dilution on the system cholinesterase-physostigmine. J. gen. Physiol. 26, 559—585 (1943).

STREHLER, E., u. H. MEYER: Die Plasma-Cholinesterase bei Gesunden und Kranken. Helv. med. Acta 19, 555—577 (1952).

STRELITZ, F.: Studies on cholinesterase. 4. Purification of pseudo-cholinesterase from horse serum. Biochem. J. 38, 86—88 (1944).

STUMPF, C.: Methoden zur Bestimmung der Cholinesteraseaktivität im Blut. Z. Vitamin-, Hormon- u. Fermentforsch. 8, 36—48 (1956).

STURGE, L. M., and V. P. WHITTAKER: The esterases of horse blood. 1. The specificity of horse plasma cholinesterase and ali-esterase. Biochem. J. 47, 518—525 (1950).

SURGENOR, D. M., and D. ELLIS: Preparation and properties of serum and plasma proteins. Plasma cholinesterase. J. Amer. chem. Soc. 76, 6049—6051 (1954).

— L. E. STRONG, H. L. TAYLOR, R. S. GORDON and D. M. GIBSON: The separation of choline esterase, mucoprotein, and metal-combining protein into subfractions of human plasma. J. Amer. chem. Soc. 71, 1223—1229 (1949).

TABACHNICK, I. I. A.: A rapid, spectrophotometric assay of purified cholinesterase. Biochim. biophys. Acta 21, 580—581 (1956).

— J. MERSHON, M. E. GRELIS and A. A. RUBIN: A rapid spectrophotometric assay of cholinesterase inhibitors. Arch. int. Pharmacodyn. 114, 351—353 (1958).

TAKAHASHI, H.: Studies on serum cholinesterase. I. A method for the estimation of serum cholinesterase activity which is useful in the routine work of clinical laboratory. Bull. Yamaguchi med. School 3, 155—165 (1956).

— and S. SHIBATA: A simple method for the serum cholinesterase determination applicable to routine examination (Japanese). Igaku to Seibutsugaku 20, 96—98 (1951); Chem. Abstr. 46, 9647 (1953).

TAMAI, A.: On the cholinesterase of dog liver. J. Japan. biochem. Soc. 22, 29—32 (1950); J. Biochem. (Tokyo) 38, June, III (1951).

TAMMELIN, L.-E.: An electrometric method for the determination of cholinesterase activity. I. Apparatus and cholinesterase in human blood. Scand. J. clin. Lab. Invest. 5, 267—270 (1953).

— Choline esters. Substrates and inhibitors of cholinesterases. Svensk kem. T. 70, 157—181 (1958).

— and H. LÖW: Calibration of an electrometric method for the determination of cholinesterase activity. Acta chem. scand. 5, 322—323 (1951).

— and B. STRINDBERG: Cholinesterase activity determined with an electrometric method. Acta chem. scand. 6, 1041—1047 (1952).

TAUBER, H.: A method for the preparation of a stable brain fraction containing acetylcholinesterase. J. Amer. chem. Soc. 75, 326—328 (1953).

THOMPSON, R. H. S.: Cholinesterases. Brit. med. Bull. 9, 138—141 (1953).

— Cholinesterases and anti-cholinesterases. In: Lectures on the Scientific Basis of Medicine, vol. II, 165—180. London: The Athlone Press 1954.

TOBIAS, J. M., J. J. KOLLROS and J. SAVIT: Acetylcholine and related substances in the cockroach, fly, and crayfish and the effect of DDT. J. cell. comp. Physiol. 28, 159—182 (1946).

TODRICK, A.: The inhibition of cholinesterases by antagonists of acetylcholine and histamine. Brit. J. Pharmacol. 9, 76—83 (1954).

— K. P. FELLOWES and J. P. RUTLAND: The effect of alcohols on cholinesterase. Biochem. J. 48, 360—368 (1951).

TOGNI, G. P., u. O. MEIER: Über das Verhalten der Serumcholinesterase des Pferdes bei der Papierelektrophorese. Experientia (Basel) 9, 106—107 (1953).

TOSCHI, G.: Chromatographic and electrophoretic studies on cholinesterases of nerve tissue (Italian). R. C. Ist. sup. Sanità 21, 1077—1096 (1958).

— Biochemical study of brain microsomes. Exp. Cell. Res. 16, 232—255 (1959).

UNDERHAY, E. E.: The hydrolysis of indoxyl esters by esterases of human blood. Biochem. J. 66, 383—390 (1957).

VAHLQUIST, B.: On the esterase activity of human blood plasma. Skand. Arch. Physiol. 72, 133—160 (1935).

VARGA, E., J. SZIGETI u. E. KISS: Hydrolyse des Azetylcholins in Gegenwart von gereinigtem Myosin. Acta physiol. Acad. Sci. hung. 5, 383—392 (1954).

VINCENT, D.: Acétylcholine, cholinestérases et anticholinestérases. Prod. pharm. 10, 17—24, 85—97 (1955).

— et R. LAGREU: Action comparée de qulques dérivés alcaloidiques puriques (caféine, théobromine, théophylline et théophylline-éthylène-diamine) sur les cholinestérases. C. R. Soc. Biol. (Paris) 144, 925—927 (1950).

— et G. SEGONZAC: Adaptation pratique de la méthode de Hestrin au dosage de la pseudo-cholinestérase sérique. Ann. Biol. clin. 16, 227—232 (1958).

— — et J. DE PRAT: La cholinestérase du sérum, son dosage. Intérêt clinique de son étude. Ann. Biol. clin. 2, 35 (1944).

WALOP, J. N.: Studies on acetylcholine in the crustacean central nervous system. Arch. int. Pharmacodyn. 59, 145—156 (1951).

— and L. M. BOOT: Studies on cholinesterase in Carcinus maenas. Biochim. biophys. Acta 4, 566—571 (1950).

WARRINGA, M. G. P. J., and J. A. COHEN: Purification of cholinesterase from ox red cells. Biochim. biophys. Acta **16**, 300 (1955).

WETSTONE, H. J., R. TENNANT and B. V. WHITE: Studies of cholinesterase activity. I. Serum cholinesterase, methods and normal values. Gastroenterology **33**, 41—49 (1957).

WHITTAKER, V. P.: The specificity of pigeon-brain cholinesterase. Biochem. J. **44**, P 46—P 47 (1949).

— Specificity, mode of action and distribution of cholinesterases. Physiol. Rev. **31**, 312—343 (1951).

— The specificity of pigeon brain aceto-cholinesterase. Biochem. J. **54**, 660—664 (1953).

— and S. WIJESUNDERA: The separation of esters of choline by filter-paper chromatography. Biochem. J. **51**, 348—351 (1952).

WILLIAMS, M. W., J. P. FRAWLEY, H. N. FUYAT and J. R. BLAKE: Modification of the Michel electrometric technique for dog and rat blood cholinesterase. J. Ass. agric. Chem. (Wash.) **40**, 1118—1120 (1957).

WILSON, I. B.: Mechanism of enzymic hydrolysis. I. Role of the acide group in the esteratic site of acetylcholinesterase. Biochim. biophys. Acta **7**, 466—470 (1951).

— The mechanism of enzyme hydrolysis studies with acetylcholinesterase. In: W. D. MCELROY and B. GLASS, Eds., The Mechanism of Enzyme Action, 642—657. Baltimore: Johns Hopkins Press 1954.

— Promotion of acetylcholinesterase activity by the anionic site. Disc. Faraday Soc. **20**, 119—125 (1955).

— Acetylcholinesterase. In: P. D. BOYER, H. LARDY and K. MYRBÄCK, Eds., The Enzymes, 2nd ed., vol. 4, 501—520. New York: Academic Press 1960.

— and F. BERGMANN: Acetylcholinesterase. VIII. Dissociation constants of the active groups. J. biol. Chem. **186**, 683—692 (1950).

WOLFE, L. S., and B. N. SMALLMAN: The properties of cholinesterase from insects. J. cell. comp. Physiol. **48**, 215—235 (1956).

WOLFSIE, J. H.: Blood cholinesterase activity. Practical consideration in routine testing programs. Arch. indust. Hlth **16**, 403—410 (1957).

— and G. D. WINTER: Statistical analysis of normal human red blood cell and plasma cholinesterase activity values. Arch. indust. Hyg. **6**, 43—49 (1952); **7**, 352 (1953).

— — Bromothymol blue screening test. Value for determination of blood cholinesterase activity. Arch. indust. Hyg. **9**, 396—401 (1954).

ZAJICEK, J., and E. ZEUTHEN: Quantitative determination of cholinesterase activity in individual cells. Exp. Cell. Res. **11**, 568—579 (1956).

ZAPP, F. J.: Eine modifizierte Warburg-Apparatus. Hoppe-Seylers Z. physiol. Chem. **307**, 36—41 (1957).

ZAVALETA ZAVALETA, O.: Blood cholinesterase in apparently healthy subjects. Laboratorio (Granada) **20**, 301—324 (1955).

ZELLER, E. A.: Enzymes of snake venoms and their biological significance. Advanc. Enzymol. **8**, 459—495 (1948).

— Über die Cholinesterase der Schlangengifte. 5. Mitteilung über die Biochemie der tierischen Gifte. Helv. chim. Acta **32**, 94—105 (1949).

— u. A. BISSEGGER: Über die Cholinesterase des Gehirns und der Erythrocyten. 3. Mitteilung über die Beeinflussung von Fermentreaktionen durch Chemotherapeutica und Pharmaka. Helv. chim. Acta **26**, 1619—1630 (1943).

— G. A. FLEISHER u. R. A. MCNAUGHTON: Non-choline esters as substrates of e-cholinesterase ("true" cholinesterase). Fed. Proc. **8**, 268 (1949).

— — and J. S. SCHWEPPE: New substrates for cholinesterases. Proc. Soc. exp. Biol. (N. Y.) **71**, 526—529 (1949).

— u. D. C. UTZ: Über die Spezifität der Cholinesterase der Schlangengifte. 6. Mitteilung über über die Biochemie tierischer Gifte. Helv. chim. Acta **32**, 338—347 (1949).

ZITTLE, C. A., E. S. DELLAMONICA and J. H. CUSTER: Purification of human red cell acetylcholinesterase. Arch. Biochem. **48**, 43—49 (1954).

— — — and R. KRIKORIAN: Purification of human red cell acetylcholinesterase by electrophoresis, ultracentrifugation and gradient extraction. Arch. Biochem. **56**, 469—475 (1955).

Chapter 5

Ontogenesis of Cholinesterases

By

Alexander G. Karczmar

With 7 figures

Contents

Introduction

I. Significance of phylogenesis and ontogenesis of cholinesterases

Cholinesterases (ChE's) and particularly acetylcholinesterase (AChE) were early (LOEWI and NAVRATIL 1926) associated with rapidly occurring events of neurohumoral or synaptic transmission and with function and motility (BACQ 1935a). Thus, together with enzymes concerned with adrenergic function, ChE's are dramatically different from enzymes concerned with relatively sluggish phenomena of growth or energetics, and their full significance can be suitably explored by neurophysiological and biophysical means applied to isolated or localized structures.

Yet, it was realized almost equally early (BACQ o.c.; YOUNGSTROM 1938a, 1938b; NACHMANSOHN 1938b) that the physiological significance of ChE's may be pinpointed by demonstrating that in evolution or in ontogenesis the appearance of these enzymes coincides with the emergence of a distinct morphological apparatus and of function. When the difficulties of the neurophysiological analysis became better known, phylogenetic or ontogenetic approaches were employed frequently (NACHMANSOHN 1939—1940; SAWYER 1943a, 1943b). The phylogenetic approach seemed particularly rewarding when applied to protozoan, bacterial, and invertebrate forms, where transmission systems, when present, are comparatively uncomplicated and easily related to function and to ChE's; in fact, in this case certain complications characteristic of embryologic investigations do not arise. And yet, unexpected difficulties and problems were encountered in the course of investigations on phylogenesis of ChE's.

While the ontogenetic approach is the special concern of this review, the philosophically akin phylogenetic approach illustrates, all the more clearly because of its simplicity, the problems which will be encountered in the analysis of embryologic data. The section which follows will serve then the purpose of illustrating and enumerating those problems; altogether, it will bring forward the viewpoint frequently adopted in this review of the tentative rather than final nature of concepts that can be formulated today with regard to the ontogenetic significance of ChE's.

Finally, it should be stated that our understanding of the ontogenic and phylogenetic significance of ChE should be improved by our knowledge of pertinent effects of anticholinesterase (anti-ChE) agents. Indeed, at crucial moments of embryonic or phylogenetic development but not earlier, anti-ChE agents should produce functional abnormalities, and this was realized (SAWYER 1943a) after BROWN et al. (1936) demonstrated the usefulness of these agents in the analysis of cholinergic neuroeffectors. Yet again, investigations of effects of anti-ChE agents in early evolution or ontogenesis proved fraught with technical difficulties and the data obtained equivocal. These questions are discussed in Chapter 17.

II. Comparative physiology of ChE's of certain invertebrates

Subsequently to NACHMANSOHN's earlier work (cf. NACHMANSOHN 1940a), BULLOCK and NACHMANSOHN (1942) proposed that the nervous system requires ChE for its functioning and that therefore the phylogenetic appearance of ChE should coincide with that of the nervous system. This was actually a more conscious formulation of an earlier postulate of BACQ (1935a). It appeared that this was indeed the case, since no enzyme was found in a protozoan, *Paramecium multi-micronucleolatum*, or in the sponge, *Scypha*, while significant amounts were found in the *Hydrozoa* "coinciding with the first appearance of a differentiated nervous system" (BULLOCK and NACHMANSOHN o.c., p. 242).

Five-mg (dry weight) tissue samples were assayed for ChE by means of the Warburg technique and Q_{ChE} (mg of acetylcholine split per mg dry weight per hour) values of 0.01 could be reliably measured.

Although those data agree insofar as *Paramecium* is concerned with the results of MITROPOLITANSKAYA (1941), both acetylcholine (ACh) and ChE were found previously in *Paramecium* by BEYER and WENSE in 1936 and this was confirmed by SEAMAN and HOULIHAN (1951) with regard to still another protozoan, *Tetrahymena*.

Homogenates of concentrated *Tetrahymena gelii* cells, 100 to 170 mg dry weight per sample, were exposed to ACh-containing medium; the residual ACh was measured by HESTRIN's (1949) chemical method. The homogenates were incapable of hydrolyzing butyrylcholine (BuCh). Q_{ChE} Values were expressed as above. It was found that the enzyme splits 0.08 mg of ACh per hour per mg of dry weight of cells. Thus, the activity was within the range of sensitivity of the method used by BULLOCK and NACHMANSOHN, o.c.

The hypothesis of BULLOCK and NACHMANSOHN taken in its restricted sense of an absolute correlation between the phylogenetic presence of AChE and that of the nervous system seems thus refuted. However, the nervous system can be understood as a special type of conductile tissue. Ample evidence is available (for references cf. TAYLOR 1941) that the fibrillar structure connecting bases of the cilia is actually a primitive conducting and coordinating organ analogous to the nervous system. Thus, the presence of ChE in *Tetrahymena* could be correlated both with its primitive conductile system and with its motility. Evidence for this relationship was provided when BÜLBRING, LOURIE and PARDOE (1949) showed that the highly motile, ciliated *Trypanosoma rhodesiense* but not the ameboid blood form of *Plasmodium gallinaceum* contained ACh as well as choline acetylase (cf. also Chapter 1).

Thus, it is tempting to generalize that the appearance of ChE and of the cholinergic system coincides in evolution with the establishment of the nervous system and of nervous function in one phylogenetic series which begins with *Tubularia*, and with that of the fibrillar conductile system in another evolutionary series initiated by the ciliated *Protozoa*. Yet, important exceptions to this generalization exist. First of all, it is difficult to correlate the phylogenetic and anatomic position of the nervous system of various forms with their enzymic activity. This is true on the species or phyletic level. BULLOCK and NACHMANSOHN (1942) stated that "judging from its behavior and musculature, *Tubularia* should present not only a poorly developed neuro-muscular system, among coelenterates, but a very small amount of nerve and muscle tissue. But surprisingly, its Q_{ChE} is the highest of any of the coelenterates tested" (o.c., p. 240). In fact, *Cyanea capillata*, a jellyfish with the neuromuscular system much further developed than that of the polyp *Tubularia*, was found to have no ChE (o.c.). Flat worms were found to have "prodigious" (o.c., p. 240) quantities of the enzyme; whole animals as well as the dorsal longitudinal muscle had a higher Q value than the vertebrate cerebral cortex (cf. also SMITH et al. 1940). On the other hand the tunicate, *Ciona intestinalis*, free swimming and exhibiting a nervous system as a larva (cf. pp. 134—135) and motile and ciliated as an adult, exhibited no ChE in its larval nervous system (DURANTE 1956, 1957) and seemed to lack it altogether after metamorphosis (BACQ 1935b).

Secondly, non-motile forms apparently devoid of conductive or transmitive systems were found to possess at least some components of the cholinergic system; for instance STEPHENSON and ROWATT (1947; cf. also ROWATT 1948) found ACh in *Lactobacillus planatarum*. However, ROWATT and STEPHENSON demonstrated dependance of both growth and ACh synthesis of *Lactobacillus* on pantothenic acid, a coenzyme concerned with acetylation. Thus, ACh may be a metabolite involved in growth processes of *Lactobacillus*. Altogether, the significance of the data of ROWATT (1948) requires further investigation.

The last paragraph illustrates a problem to be confronted throughout this review. Can ontogenetic appearance of either ChE or ACh be taken as a proof of the presence of cholinergic transmission or of cholinergic function? Earlier work of NACHMANSOHN implied that the presence of ChE suffices alone for such an indentification (cf. however NACHMANSOHN 1959) and this lead was frequently followed. The uncertainty of such an identification will be stressed subsequently (v. *Conclusions*). Moreover, the data of ROWATT and STEPHENSON indicate that the presence of ACh may have sometimes a significance entirely unrelated to transmission. While joint consideration of ACh and ChE should be therefore preferred, the meaning of their presence cannot be taken for granted in the absence of other evidence of the existence of cholinergic transmission.

Thus, correlation of motility or transmission with ChE in the course of phylogenesis while very suggestive is not perfect; in fact, certain forms seem to remain outside of such a correlation. As will be seen, the studies of the relation between ontogenesis of ChE's, neurogenesis, and development of function similarly present hopeful indications of correlation, but at the same time many exceptions and difficulties of interpretation.

Cholinesterases in invertebrate embryonic development

A. ChE's in echinoderm and ascidian development

I. Ontogenesis of AChE, functional development, and morphogenesis in echinoderms

AUGUSTINSSON, GUSTAFSON and their associates studied ontogenesis of ChE's in the development of the sea urchin *(Paracentrotus lividus)*.

Fifty-mg samples of egg powder were obtained (AUGUSTINSSON and GUSTAFSON 1949) by the freeze-dry technique. Activity of ChE's was measured manometrically with ACh and BuCh as substrates and expressed in b_{30} values (AUGUSTINSSON 1948). The enzyme could be identified as AChE by its activity-substrate concentration curve; it was inhibited by physostigmine, 3.36×10^{-6} M, but not by lithium (0.1 M; for the significance of this finding, v. infra, p. 134).

Echinoderm development and its experimental modification should be reviewed briefly at this point. At the 16-cell stage (Fig. 1) the embryo consists of mesomeres, macromeres, and micromeres. During subsequent divisions, mesomeres and macromeres give rise to "animal" (an_1 and an_2) and "vegetative" (veg_1 and veg_2) cells (Fig. 1). "Animal" cells form the ciliary apparatus of the blastula and of the later stages (Fig. 1), and, together with some veg_1 cells, the endoderm. Veg_2 invaginates during gastrulation, forming endoderm; finally, cells originating from micromeres migrate at gastrulation into the blastocoele and give rise to the skeleton. The free-swimming, ciliated pluteus metamorphoses into the familiar star-shaped adult *Paracentrotus*. While the nervous system is absent from the young larvae, a dorsal ganglion is found in older plutei (MACBRIDE 1903); the adult has a rather advanced nervous system composed of plexuses and rings of nerves and nerve cells which branch off to the tube feet and spines.

This normal pattern of development was changed experimentally in classical researches which led to the postulate that the regional determination of endodermal parts depends upon gradients of two metabolically different fields, animal and vegetal (RUNNSTRÖM 1928; LINDAHL 1942; HÖRSTADIUS 1949; for review, cf. NEEDHAM 1942). When the relationship of the two fields was changed chemically or surgically, either a "vegetalized" or an "animalized" pluteus resulted. For instance, lithium produced a "vegetalized" embryo consisting of a small vesicle

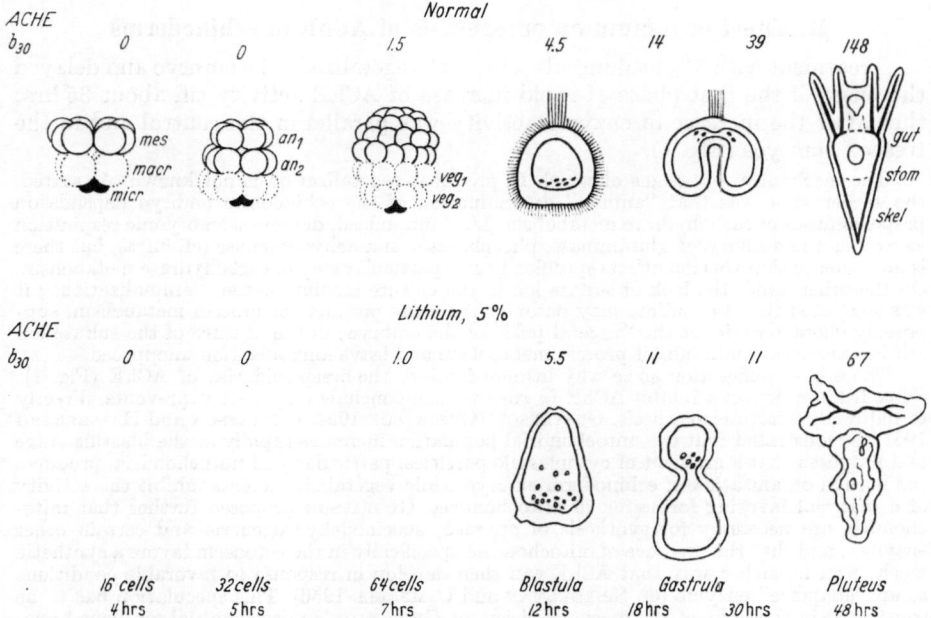

Fig. 1. Normal and lithium-inhibited echinoderm development. AChE activities expressed in b_{30} values (AUGUSTINSSON and GUSTAFSON 1949). Development stages and times of their occurrence at the bottom of the figure. Sixteen-cell stage: mes — mesomeres; macr — macromeres; micr — micromeres. Thirty-two-cell stage: an_1, an_2 — animal$_1$ and animal$_2$ mesomeres. Sixty-four-cell stage: veg$_1$, veg$_2$ — vegetal$_1$ and vegetal$_2$ macromeres. Pluteus exhibtis the gut, stomodaeum (stom), and the skeleton (skel)

of ectoderm attached to a hypertrophic, exogastrulated endoderm (Fig. 1). It was also proposed that "animalizing" and "vegetalizing" determinations should be associated with carbohydrate metabolism and with protein breakdown, respectively (for complete analysis and references, cf. NEEDHAM 1942 and SHAVER 1957).

Unfertilized eggs showed no hydrolytic activity with regard to AChE; a butyro-cholinesterase (BuChE) was present however. Acetylcholinesterase appeared 7 hrs after fertilization (64-cell stage; $b_{30} = 1.5$). Increase of enzyme activity progressed slowly till after gastrulation. Thereafter the increase was more rapid and ChE activity reached the b_{30} value of 148 in the pluteus (Fig. 1). This increase occurred therefore in the absence of neurogenesis. Yet, even the blastula shows good motility while the pluteus exhibits complex locomotion and precise coordination of the ciliary activity; even reflexes can be demonstrated in the case of oral cilia (RUNNSTRÖM 1917). RUNNSTRÖM hypothesized that the motility depends on plasma-bridge conduction; AChE, a synaptic and neurotropic enzyme, should not be required for this type of "conduction". However, coordinated ciliary and reflex movement may depend on the fibrillar conductive system described for ciliated Protozoa, which seems to require ChE (cf. p. 131 and Chapter 17).

The increase of ChE activity levelled off subsequently, but a second peak occurred during morphogenesis of the alimentary canal and development of intestinal contractility. GUSTAFSON, in the discussion of his and AUGUSTINSSON's data (1949), correlated this second peak of AChE activity with the emergence of intestinal function; it is of interest that in mammals intestinal motility may depend to a large extent on the BuChE (KOELLE et al. 1950). Further increase of AChE activity was correlated by GUSTAFSON with further ectodermization, including the formation of the dorsal ganglion in the advanced pluteus.

II. Effect of lithium on ontogenesis of AChE in echinoderms

Treatment with 5% lithium salt solution "vegetalized" the embryo and delayed the onset of the first phase of rapid increase of AChE activity till about 35 hrs; thereafter the increase of enzyme activity was parallel in the control and in the treated embryos (Fig. 1).

The mechanism by means of which Li produces vegetalization is not known. As stated, the earlier view was that "animal" determination of the echinoderm embryo depends on preponderance of carbohydrate metabolism. Lithium, indeed, depresses embryonic respiration as well as the activity of glutaminase, phosphatase, and dehydrogenase (cf. infra), but there is no evidence that this ion affects specifically any particular step in carbohydrate metabolism. On the other hand, the lack of sulfate ion in the culture medium causes "animalization"; it was suggested that the sulfate may detoxify the toxic products of protein metabolism, supposedly characteristic for the "vegetal pole" of the embryo; in the absence of the sulfate ion self-intoxication would inhibit protein metabolism and leave animalization unopposed.

There is no suggestion as to why lithium inhibits the first rapid rise of AChE (Fig. 1). Since lithium does not inhibit AChE *in vitro* we can conclude only that it prevents, directly or indirectly, enzymic synthesis. GUSTAFSON (GUSTAFSON 1954, GUSTAFSON and HASSELBERG 1951) demonstrated that the mitochondrial population increases rapidly at the blastula stage and proposed that a gradient of cytoplasmic particles, particularly of mitochondria, produces the normal organization of echinoderm embryo while vegetalizing agents inhibit the activity of a material favoring formation of mitochondria. GUSTAFSON proposed further that mitochondria are necessary for synthesis of apyrase, succinodehydrogenase, and certain other enzymes, and that the presence of mitochondria specifically in the ectoderm favors a synthetic mechanism in such a way that AChE can then develop in response to favorable conditions as an "adaptive" enzyme (cf. SPIEGELMAN and CAMPBELL 1956). This speculation has to be considered in the light of the recent criticism of GUSTAFSON's mitochondrial gradient hypothesis (cf. SHAVER 1957).

It is of interest to compare the pattern of biogenesis of AChE in echinoderm development with that of other enzymes (GUSTAFSON and HASSELBERG 1951). A number of phosphatases and esterases show constant activity throughout development. On the other hand, the activity of glutaminase, cathepsin II, and succinic and malic dehydrogenases increases in the course of development; this occurs, however, at the late gastrula, some 12 hrs before the phase of rapid biogenesis of AChE. However, these enzymes share with AChE the characteristic of being inhibited by lithium-caused "vegetalization".

III. ChE's in tunicate development

DURANTE (1956, 1957) suggested a lack of correlation between neurogenesis and ontogenesis of ChE's in the case of the urochordate (tunicate) *Ciona*, which, like the echinoderms, exhibits two distinct "animalizing" and "vegetalizing" metabolisms during ontogenesis.

Apart from profound differences between the development of echinoderms on one hand and of the urochordate *Ciona* on the other, there is a general similarity of the organization of the two eggs, since in both cases an animal-vegetal or dorso-ventral gradient controls ontogenesis. In tunicates this organization is indicated already in the unfertilized egg by pigmentation differences; anterior and posterior "vegetal" blastomeres control the formation of the medulla by the "animal" blastomeres; the anterior stimulate and the posterior blastomeres inhibit the development of neural tissue[1]. In addition, the posterior blastomeres give

---

[1] The neural tissue develops ultimately into a prominent chordate-like nervous system of the ascidian tadpole. However, after metamorphosis, only a single ganglion is present in the adult which thus resembles the chordates less than does the larva.

rise to most of the muscle tissue. Posterior "vegetal" blastomeres, analogous to "vegetalizing" macromeres and micromeres of the echinoderms, are characterized by a high concentration of mitochondrial materials containing cytochrome oxidase, succinic dehydrogenase, adenosine triphosphatase, and RNA (cf. NEEDHAM 1942 and BRACHET 1960). Since posterior blastomeres are concerned with controlling "animalization" and neurogenesis, and as the inhibition of their enzymes affects differentiation of the muscle rather than that of the head, brain and of sensorial organs, one would expect that ChE's would be associated with the anterior, "animal," blastomeres. Actually, the available data indicate that the opposite holds true. DURANTE (1956), who used the GOMORI (1952) modification of KOELLE's (1951) histochemical method, found that AChE appeared already at gastrulation and that subsequently it was localized in the mesoderm and in the muscle cells originating from the posterior blastomeres. No AChE could be found in the neural tissue. DURANTE subsequently (1957) separated anterior from posterior blastomeres. The former gave rise to a hemiembryo composed of ectoderm and nervous tissue and never showing AChE staining; the hemiembryo derived from posterior blastomeres and containing muscle and mesenchyme, exhibited good enzymic activity. Similarly, tails isolated from the tadpoles until degeneration of their neural elements was complete, showed AChE staining in the muscle cells. It should be stressed that 80% ethanol was used as fixative and may have inhibited neural AChE. It should be added that the adult *Ciona* with its simple nervous system was not adequately studied. AUGUSTINSSON (1948) stated briefly that muscles of adult tunicates contain ChE's but did not mention neural tissues. On the other hand, BACQ (1935b) found no ChE in adult *Ciona*.

B. ChE's in insect development[1]

Anticholinesterase agents play an important role in the control of insects as pests and parasites. Their ovicidal effect and their ability to prevent hatching and to affect larval pupal forms aroused early the interest in the ontogenesis of insect ChE's, as evidenced by the wide literature in this area. It should be stressed also that these enzymes must be of particular importance to the insect, since AChE is as concentrated in its nervous system as it is in the electric organs of *Torpedo* and *Electrophorus* (cf. Chapters 6, 13, 16, and METCALF et al., 1955).

Insect neurogenesis will be briefly described. The ectoderm of the early insect embryo is formed around the yolk after the daughter nuclei migrate peripherad and form cell walls (Stage A, Fig. 2). The neural groove with its mesodermal roof is formed subsequently, and within two days neuroblasts of ectodermal origin appear at either side of the groove (Stage C). Daughter cells of the neuroblasts form neurospongium and ganglion cells, and still later, connectives and commissures (Stage F, Fig. 2).

In the case of insect eggs with much yolk (eggs of the grasshopper and the silkworm), blastokinesis occurs now, i.e., a few days before hatching: the embryo rotates until its head, which faced the posterior end of the egg, turns toward its anterior pole. Next, longitudinal connectives may form between ganglia so that two nerve cords or a single fused one develop, or connectives are absent but left and right ganglia fuse to a varying extent. Within one week of ontogenesis a complex dorsal brain consisting of three pairs of fused ganglia is formed. Segmental transverse commissures are well developed, although sometimes visible only in sections. The inner and outer neurilemmas are formed and the nervous system is similar to the one found in the fully developed embryo. Only mouth parts, appendages, the gut, and the muscle bands continue differentiating until the hatching time.

The subsequent development differs from order to order. The hatched form, an instar or a nymph, may differ very little from the adult, as in the case of the grasshopper. On the other hand, metamorphosis occurs in the bugs where it is incomplete, and in the holometabolar flies, moths, and butterflies where it is complete and involves a succession of molts and instars, leading to the pupa, from which the adult ultimately emerges.

At almost any point, the development can come to a standstill, the diapause. In the grasshopper this occurs in the egg after 21 days of development; after several months of diapause, growth is resumed and takes another 3 weeks. Subsequently, the central nervous system reactivates the growth and final metamorphosis, as considered later in detail (v. pp. 139—140).

Part of the problem of the interpretation of the results dealing with insects is due to the diversity of the methods employed for the measurement of ChE's, ACh, and ACh synthesis. Cholinesterase assay was carried out manometrically in the Warburg apparatus (POTTER et al.

---

[1] Of necessity, some overlapping exists between this Chapter and Chapter 16.

1957; STAUDENMAYER 1955 and 1957 and others) or by means of Cartesian microdiver technique (POULSON and BOELL 1946); titrimetrically (TAHMISIAN 1943); colorimetrically (LORD and POTTER 1951); or by the bioassay or chemical determination of residual substrate (YUSHIMA and CHINO 1953a and 1953b). Methods of extraction of ACh and of ChE as well as the substrates employed also differed widely. These technical details cannot be described at length here (cf. also Chapter 2).

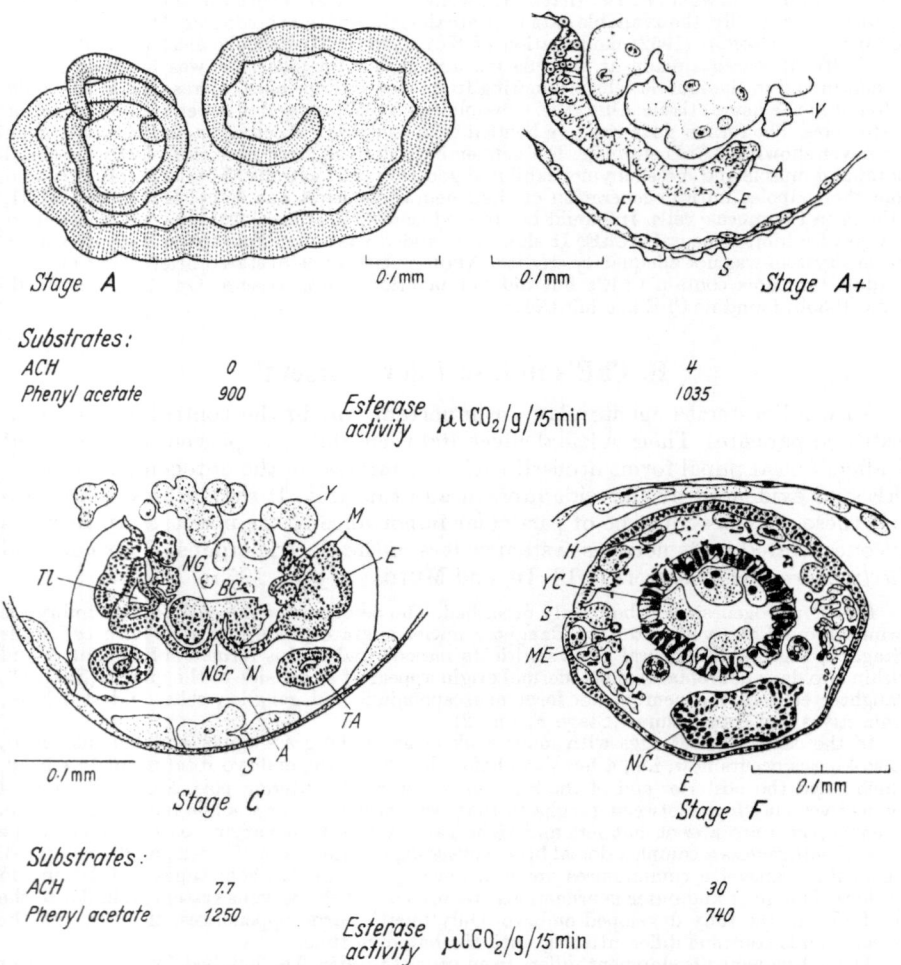

Fig. 2. Characteristic stages of development and of ontogenesis of ChE's in *Pieris brassicae* (after POTTER et al. 1957). ChE (ACh substrate, 2.75 × 10⁻³ M) and arylesterase (phenyl acetate substrate, 3.66 × 10⁻³ M) activities in $\mu l/CO_2/g$ of eggs/15 min (from POTTER et al., o.c.). *Stages A* and *A +*, first day of incubation: Y — yolk, S — serosa, A — amnion, E — ectoderm, Fl — future inner layer. *Stage C*, fourth day of incubation: Y, S, A and E — as above; N — neuroblast; NG — nerve ganglion; Tl — tracheal invagination; TA — thoracic appendage; BC — blood cells. *Stage F*, one week of incubation (after blastokinesis): H — heart; YC — yolk cells; S — spiracle; ME — midgut epithelium; NC — nerve cord; E — ectoderm

The exact moment of the first appearance of both ACh and ChE in insect development is uncertain; the difference in the results may depend upon the sensitivity of the method or on the species investigated. It must be stressed that ACh was identified in insects, whether adult or embryonic, only relatively recently (LEWIS 1953; CHERFURKA and SMALLMAN 1956).

Exceptionally, ChE's could be found very early in development, i.e. before the formation of neuroblasts.

POULSON and BOELL (1946), using the sensitive Cartesian microdiver technique, found ChE in unfertilized eggs of *Drosophila melanogaster*. POTTER et al. (1957) found trace amounts of ChE in one out of three tests on *Pieris* eggs, stage A; ChE was present more consistently but still in small amounts (5.0 to 8.5 μl of CO_2 per g per 15 min) at stage C, that is, in the 3 to 4-day old embryo (Fig. 2). Also, although SMITH and WAGENKNECHT (1956) did not find any ChE in untreated milkweed bug eggs till relatively late in development (4th day), they found some depression of CO_2 production in the 1 and 2-day old eggs treated with Parathion when evolution of CO_2 was corrected for both brei and substrate blank readings; these data may suggest slight ChE activity early in development. A somewhat similar finding, possibly subject to analogous interpretation, was reported by STAUDENMAYER (1957, p. 417).

Generally, ChE's, or the phase of rapid increase of their activity, appear approximately toward the midpoint of embryonic development; this is also true of ACh (TAHMISIAN 1943; LORD and POTTER 1951; CHINO 1957; CHINO and YUSHIMA 1953; STAUDENMAYER 1955; SMITH and WAGENKNECHT, 1956). This may occur before blastokinesis; it may either precede (cf. above), follow, or coincide with neuroblastogenesis.

CHINO and YUSHIMA (1953, 1954) reported the presence of ChE's in the rice-stem borer, *Chilo simplex*, and cabbage army worm, *Barathra brassicae*, at 40 and 70 hours, respectively. In both these forms neuroblast formation occurs at 24 hours. It is of interest that in these two forms ACh and ACh-synthesizing capacity appeared at about 20 hours of development, i.e., 20 to 50 hours before the appearance of ChE activity. That ChE appears relatively late is indicated also by the fact that the measurement of ACh content of the supernatant of the homogenate was affected by eserine beginning at 36 hrs in the borer and, somewhat less markedly, at 70 hrs in the army worm. Another indication of this is the occurrence of very high levels of ACh, many times higher than those encountered in the vertebrates, before the appearance of ChE (1.2 to 1.3 mg of ACh per g of eggs). The synthetic activity increased till blastokinesis at 70 hrs in the borer, and at 90 hrs in the army worm, respectively. A decrease in ACh content began at 120 hrs in the borer and at 90 hrs in the army worm; ACh ceased to be detectable several hours before hatching in both species (YUSHIMA 1956a, b; YUSHIMA 1957; YUSHIMA and CHINO 1953a, b).

Similarly late in development appeared the enzyme of the peach tree borer (*Sanninoidea exitosa*) and the milkweed bug (*Oncopeltus fasciatus*); in both these forms AChE activity was first recorded about the 4th day of incubation and increased thereafter until hatching at 8.5 and 6.1 days, respectively (SMITH and WAGENKNECHT 1956). In the housefly (*Musca domestica*, incubation time 12 hr) ChE activity could be first measured at 7 hr. It is of interest that in this form ACh appeared after ChE (at 9 hr of incubation). While both ACh and ChE went up from the 9th hour until hatching, the increase of the former was two-fold, and of the latter 100-fold (MEHROTRA and SMALLMAN 1957). Similarly, POTTER et al. (1957) reported "definite" appearance of ChE for stage E (5 to 6 days) of *Pieris brassicae* (incubation of 8 to 10 days); subsequently, the enzymic activity increased rapidly.

Thus, in the rice-stem borer and in the army worm ChE appeared some 20 to 40 hrs *after*, and ACh was detectable just at the time (24 hrs) of neuroblast formation; in the white butterfly ChE may appear 2 to 3 days after neuroblastogenesis. On the other hand, in the grasshopper (TAHMISIAN 1943) and in the silkworm (STAUDENMAYER 1955; CHINO 1957), the appearance of ChE seemed to coincide with neuroblast formation, and the subsequent pattern of ontogenesis of the enzyme with neurogenesis. In the grasshopper, no ChE activity could be detected till the seventh day of embryonic development; ACh could not be found till much later (17 days after diapause). Subsequently, the enzyme activity increased rather slowly till a peak was reached on the 21st day; thereafter, the enzymic activity was maintained unchanged through diapause, which begins on the 28th day of development. Six days after a 3-month diapause the activity increased steeply and the increase did not level off till hatching. This agrees with the results obtained in the silkworm, *Bombyx mori*, by STAUDENMAYER (1955) and CHINO (1957). In this form the appearance of ACh and of ACh-synthesizing capacity coincided with that of AChE (STAUDENMAYER 1957); all three components of the cholinergic system appeared simultaneously immediately after blastokinesis and at about the time of neuroblastogenesis. Their levels increased first slowly and then rapidly till a maximal level was reached 1 day before hatching. The activities of choline acetylase (ChAc) and the content of ACh in *Bombyx* were 3 to 4 times higher than those found in the rice-stem borer and cabbage army worm. It is interest that a similar pattern of ontogenesis of ACh and ChAc was noticed in *Bombyx* eggs in which diapause was prevented artifically, although it was said that such eggs showed higher synthetic activity than diapausing eggs (CHINO 1957).

Finally, while in *Drosophila* enzyme activity did not change much during the first 15 hrs of incubation, it increased rapidly thereafter in parallel with neurogenesis (POULSON and BOELL 1946). The same investigators ingeniously related ChE to the nervous system in this form. They compared the enzyme activity of Notch[8] mutant embryos, characterized by a hypertrophic nervous system, with that of normal embryos, and showed that the activity ratio was the same as the ratio of sizes of the respective nerve tissues; moreover, in the larva the enzyme was concentrated in the nervous system.

I. Types of ChE's during insect ontogenesis

In the adult insect AChE is the characteristic enzyme of the central nervous system (METCALF et al. 1955; cf. also Chapter 16). It may differ in the housefly and the bee from mammalian AChE in that it can split benzoylcholine (BzCh), although a separate enzyme may be involved (cf. METCALF et al. o.c., and Chapter 4). Also in the embryo, AChE may predominate. Butyrocholinesterase, or pseudo-ChE, and ali- and aryl-esterases are found in some early embryos, as they are in the adult (v. Chapter 16). In some forms, the activity of AChE is higher than that of other esterases throughout development; in other insects there is a shift from ali- or aryl-esterases in the early embryo to AChE or other ChE's in the later stages.

While in the case of the milkweed bug eggs no hydrolysis of BzCh could be demonstrated and the activity curves with ACh and methacholine (MeCh) as substrates were similar throughout embryonic development (SMITH and WAGENKNECHT 1956 and 1959), a shift in pattern was evident in the housefly (CASIDA 1954, 1955). Using mixed substrates as well as inhibitors, CASIDA (o.c.) showed that the egg contained two enzymes, each capable of hydrolysing both ACh and o-nitrophenyl acetate; AChE activity increased greatly between the embryonic and the larval stages and beyond, and finally replaced the other enzyme entirely, so that the adult head contained only one enzyme. Also, there may be a shift in the waxmoth enzymes during development (CASIDA 1954). The fact that an enzyme capable of hydrolyzing o-nitrophenyl acetate is present early in development was shown also by LORD and POTTER (1951 and 1953) and by POTTER et al. (1957). Using ethanol extraction, LORD and POTTER (1951) found aryl-esterase but no ChE activity in eggs of *Tribolium castaneum* and of *Tenebrio molitor*. O'BRIEN (1953) found a ChE in the larvae of these forms and suggested that ethanol inhibited ChE in the case of the experiments of LORD et al. (1951; cf. however LORD and POTTER 1953, and Chapters 16 and 17).

Arylesterase was present in the eggs of two moths, *Diataraxia oleracea* and *Ephestia kuhniella*, and of the white butterfly *Pieris brassicae* (LORD and POTTER 1951); in the case of *Diataraxia* and *Pieris* its activity was already high in eggs devoid of any embryonic rudiments (Fig. 2). While in *Pieris* the activity did not increase much till stage G or hatching, it was always many times higher than that of ChE which appeared "definitely" at stage E. In this case, POTTER et al. (1957) extracted the enzymes with water, not with ethyl alcohol, and presumably recorded ChE activity accurately.

It must be stressed that enzymes capable of splitting phenyl acetate were present in adult heads of many insects and again their activity was substantially higher than that of ChE (METCALF et al. 1955). Finally, an enzyme capable of hydrolyzing ethyl butyrate was demonstrated in the larva of *Tenebrio molitor* (o.c.); this does not signify that there was a shift from these esterases to AChE, since adult bees and flies have enzymes which can split a number of aliphatic esters including acetylbutyrate (METCALF et al. 1955).

II. Evidence for relationship between ChE's and neurogenesis in insect development

It is striking that data can be provided for, as well as against, the notion of a correlation between ChE's and insect neurogenesis; when ACh is considered also, the problem becomes even more complicated. Lack of such a correlation (SMITH and WAGENKNECHT 1959) is indicated by the precocious appearance of ChE in *Drosophila* (POULSON and BOELL 1946) and perhaps in the white butterfly eggs (POTTER et al. 1957), and by its delayed appearance with regard to neuroblast formation in the rice-stem borer and cabbage army worm (CHINO and YUSHIMA 1953).

However, while in *Pieris* and *Drosophila* ChE appeared precociously, the phase of the rapid increase of its activity coincided with neurogenesis. Also, in other forms such as the silkworm and the grasshopper the appearance of ChE correlates well with neurogenesis. Indeed, in these two forms, in which diapause and blastokinesis occur with relation to neurogenesis at widely different periods of development, ontogenesis of ChE's depends only on neurogenesis. In the silkworm, neuroblasto-genesis and blastokinesis occur after diapause; in the grasshopper neuroblastogenesis precedes diapause by 3 weeks and hatching occurs 30 days after a 3-month diapausal standstill. However, in both forms the appearance of ChE coincides with that of neuroblasts and the increase of its activity with their proliferation and the differentiation of ganglia and of commissures (TAHMISIAN 1943; STAUDENMAYER 1957).

This positive correlation between neurogenesis and ChE's may or may not extend to ACh. Such a triple correlation exists in the silkworm. However, in the fly the appearance of ACh is delayed with respect to that of ChE and to neuroblasto-genesis. Finally, ACh may appear before the enzyme, and in certain forms (rice-stem borer and cabbage army worm) it serves better as a correlate of neuroblast formation than ChE.

The comment of TAHMISIAN (1943) that ontogenically ACh rather than ChE is indicative of the appearance of a cholinergic system is well taken; by this criterion, this system seems present at the very onset of the differentiation of the nervous system in the silkworm, rice-stem borer, and army worm, and only at later stages of neurogenesis in the grasshopper and in the fly. It must be remembered, however, that as pointed out by CHINO and YUSHIMA (1953) technical improvements in testing for ACh as well as for ChE may change our estimates of the first ontogenetic moment of their appearance.

Altogether, the data available at present do not allow us to decide whether function and transmission depend on ACh, on ChE, or perhaps upon other factors. However, certain dapausal events point to the functional importance of ChE.

III. ChE's and diapause

A most interesting parallelism between ChE and brain-controlled onset of diapausal cessation of growth and activity was demonstrated by VAN DER KLOOT (1955) in the silkworm, *Platysamia cecropia*.

Cholinesterase was measured both colorimetrically and manometrically. VAN DER KLOOT measured also ACh, which he extracted conventionally and bioassayed on the *Venus mercenaria* heart. He used lysergic acid diethylamide (LSD-25) to mask substances such as 5-hydroxytrypt-amine which might be present in the extract, and additionally identified the active principle by blocking it by benzoquinonium (WELSH 1954; WELSH and TAUB 1953). Spontaneous and induced electrical activity of the brain was recorded by means of bipolar macro- and micro-electrodes, placed by means of a micromanipulator.

In *P. cecropia* twenty-six neurosecretory cells of the brain release a hormone which activates the secretion of the prothoracic gland. When the secretion of the brain hormone ceases just prior to pupation, pupal diapause ensues. Five to 6 months later, the neurosecretory cells start to release the neurohormone again and the prothoracic gland activates growth and development (WILLIAMS 1952, 1954). Brain neurosecretory cells may be triggered by en-vironmental temperature changes and, probably, by nerve impulses which can arise reflexly.

VAN DER KLOOT demonstrated that the larval brain shows high ChE and ChAc titer, as well as both spontaneous and evoked electric activity. Cholinesterase activity of the brain remained constant in the fourth and fifth instar and then slowly increased to the high titer characteristic of the brains of spinning caterpillars. Activity remained high for 6 days after completion of the cocoon before falling precipitously 2 days before pupal molt; it was undetectable at pupation. The electric activity of the brain ceased, and both the electric silence and absence of ChE persisted throughout diapause. It is of interest that throughout diapause ChE and both evoked and spontaneous electric activity of the ganglia and of the nerve cord retained their larval, prediapausal levels.

When adult development was initiated by restoring chilled pupae to room temperature, ChE activity became detectable on the fifth day and increased thereafter. This, parenthetically, did not require the presence of prothoracic glands. Electric activity reappeared on the 6th or 7th day at the time when the ChE level reached was about 1/3 that of the adult; growth and development were resumed on the 9th day.

Traces of ACh were present in the brains of newly pupated animals, and ACh increased steadily throughout diapause. The extracts did not, on the other hand, contain adrenergic substances. The ACh level decreased at the termination of diapause, coincidentally with the reappearance of ChE. Low levels of ACh persisted until the emergence of the young adult and then increased 5-fold to the high level characteristic of the adult. These changes were peculiar to the brain and were not encountered in the ganglia. To the contrary, ChAC did not vary throughout diapause, its termination, or the onset of development; it seemed to increase thereafter, however.

VAN DER KLOOT, in discussing these data, suggested that the ChE level determines whether or not the brain is electrically and neurohormonally active; he pointed out that that these three variables run parallel before and at the termination of the diapause, and that a non-diapausing lepidopteran showed no changes in either electric or ChE activity during the stages prior to and following the pupal molt. He suggested that accumulation of ACh causes the reappearance of ChE which then behaves as an adaptive enzyme. The effect on diapause of the only anti-ChE agent that has been tested (cf. Chapters 16 and 17) is consistent with these views.

IV. Levels of ChE's after emergence and during aging

In the honeybee, ChE activity increased after emergence to a peak reached at nine days of age (3.8 to 4.5 μmol of ACh/hr/brain; ROCKSTEIN 1950). Similarly, in the flour beetle, the waxmoth, and the housefly the ChE activity in the adult was higher than that found at emergence (O'BRIEN 1953). In the honeybee, there was no further change in ChE activity with age. Yet, in a 73-day old honeybee the number of brain cells decreased by about 38%. This decrease of cell number which was also reported by others in insects and mammals, including man (v. ROCKSTEIN 1950, 1953 for further references), implies that ChE activity expressed per cell actually increased somewhat (by 18%) with age; ROCKSTEIN suggested that this increase is due to the progress of synaptic arborisation, to a rise in the number of synaptic afferents, or to a differential increase of ChE-rich neuron areas.

In subsequent work ROCKSTEIN (1953) reported that acid β-glycerophosphatase also increased during the first 9 days after emergence and remained constant thereafter. To the contrary, alkaline β-glycerophosphatase decreased during the early adult life and remained constant subsequently. The reciprocal relationship between the two phosphatases may signify a transfer of energy of intermediate metabolism from embryonic differentiation to adult processes (MOOG 1946; KARCZMAR and BERG 1951). Since cytochrome oxidase also increases in insects during the first days after emergence (SACKTOR 1950; cf. however WATANATE and WILLIAMS, 1951), ROCKSTEIN suggested that the interrelationship between the two phosphatases, cytochrome oxidase, and ChE in the early post-emergence insect life characterizes the specialization of the neuromotor mechanism for intensive flying; he pointed out that the adult honeybee is relatively quiet for the first 3 to 5 days after emergence and does not exhibit the adult flying pattern till 7 to 10 days after emergence, i.e., at the time of the peak ChE activity.

Correlation between ontogenesis of ChE and of cytochrome oxidase in the honeybee should be contrasted with the absence of such a correlation in amphibians (v. infra, p. 149) and in echinoderms (v. p. 134). However, these enzymes were studied in the early adult life in the case of the honeybee, and during embryogenesis in that of echinoderms and amphibians. In adult life the changes in the activity of both these enzymes may constitute functional adaptations, as suggested by ROCKSTEIN, while during embryogenesis cytochrome oxidase may be concerned with energetics, and ChE with nerve function and motility.

C. Comment

No correlation between ChE on the one hand and neurogenesis on the other could be shown during embryogenesis of echinoderms and ascidians.

Acetylcholinesterase may appear prior to and independently of neurogenesis, but its appearance may be correlated with that of motility and of coordinated ciliary activity. During subsequent development both in echinoderms and in ascidians, ChE's were associated apparently with muscle rather than with nerve function. Altogether, ascidians present a peculiar case of seemingly complete dissociation between neurogenesis and ontogenesis of ChE.

In the case of insect ontogenesis, in some forms a relationship can be established between ChE on the one hand and the nervous system and its function on the other. In fact, insects afford the opportunity of studying this relationship in either direction, since the diapause, an anti-developmental event so to speak, occurs in parallel with the ontogenic disappearance of the enzyme, while in certain forms, a three-fold correlation can be found between ACh, ChE, and neurogenesis. However, the latter correlation does not obtain in all forms, and both precocious and delayed appearance of ChE, with respect to neurogenesis, was noticed, while ACh may also appear early or late in neurogenesis. It has to be kept in mind that, with few exceptions, the data deal with ChE or ACh of whole eggs or embryos rather than with the enzyme of the nervous system, let alone with that of restricted synaptic or conductile areas, and much additional evidence will be required before establishing specific correlations between emergence of the cholinergic system, ACh, ChE's, and function.

GUSTAFSON and HASSELBERG (1951) speculated that ChE's are adaptive enzymes depending on a metabolism coupled with mitochondria and favoring formation of ectoderm and "animalization" in echinoderms. It is unfortunate that data on the emergence of ACh in echinoderms are lacking, since in insects, where frequently the appearance of the substrate precedes that of ChE, the adaptation mechnism may depend on ACh; this was suggested as the mechanism underlying the reappearance of ChE and the termination of diapause (VAN DER KLOOT 1955).

Cholinesterases in vertebrate embryogenesis

A. ChE's in the vertebrate central nervous system and development of function

I. Amphibia and fishes

The development of function, behavior, and simple reflexes was thoroughly correlated in a series of classical studies in *Amblystoma* and in certain fishes with neuro- and synapto-genesis (COGHILL 1929; HERRICK 1948; DETWILER 1946 and 1948; HARRIS and WHITING 1954; WHITING 1955; v. Table 1).

This animal material offers many advantages for such a study. In *Amblystoma*, jelly-enclosed clusters of 100 to 200 eggs can be easily found in nature or obtained from a single female; eggs of many fishes are equally easily accessible (for breeding and experimental techniques, v. RUGH 1948). Moreover, in both these forms the embryos and the subsequently motile and swimming larvae can be easily studied and discrete steps in the development of "overt behavior" (HOOKER 1944) readily observed.

There is no doubt that the relative completeness of such correlations in these forms attracted the attention of YOUNGSTROM (1938a) and SAWYER (1940—1942) to the possibility of extending them to ChE; these investigators were also motivated by the definite formulation at that time (DALE 1937) of the neurotransmitter function of ACh, and by the early work of Nachmansohn (1938—1940) on young mammals (v. infra, p. 160).

The earlier work of both Youngstrom (1938a) and Sawyer (1940, 1943a) was concerned with ChE of whole embryos; the results encouraged hypothesizing that the biogenesis of ChE is correlated with neurogenesis and development of function, and this hypothesis was further tested by measuring ChE in the neuroeffectors themselves. The results obtained in whole embryos and larvae will be discussed first.

Table 1. *Neurogenesis and ontogenesis of overt behavior[1] and of ChE in* Amblystoma

Stage (after HARRISON)	Behavior	Neurophysiological correlates	ChE of the central nervous system
0—31	Nonmotile	—	Present in neural tissues and ectoderm; not in entoderm
32—33	Slow myotonic response to direct stimulation	Few motor fibers reach anterior myotomes; motor and internuncial systems not in contact	Slow increase in activity
34	*Early flexure:* bending of body away from stimulus; rapid relaxation	Sensori-motor internuncials are complete; sensory system of one side linked with opposite motor system (cf. Fig. 6)	Slow increase in activity
36	*Coil:* contralateral response to stimulation; more myotomes included in a faster movement	Complete arc composed of motor tract, commissural floor plate cells, and motor cells of the opposite motor tract (cf. Fig. 6)	Slow increase in activity
36—37	*S-flexure:* wave of contraction passes down stimulated side before relaxation of original contralateral contraction	Development of ipsilateral reflex arcs and of inhibitory collaterals	More rapid increase in activity. Caudocephalad direction of ontogenesis
37—38	*Early swimming:* repeated S-flexures cause some forward progress	Integration of sensori-motor, commisural, and inhibitory pathways which embrace finally limb and jaw movements	Continued rapid increase in activity
38—39	*"Strong"* and *"late" swimming* (progression through > 3 and > 10 body lengths, respectively)	Further development of antagonist and agonist pattern and individuation of limb and gill movement from control by axial muscles. Mesencephalic control of swimming	Continued rapid increase in activity. Appearance of ChE in the brain (Stage 42)

[1] Data from Dushane and Hutchinson (1941), Rugh (1948), Whiting (1955) and Sawyer (1943a).

1. Whole embryos

Both investigators found ChE in the premotile stages of the *Amphibia* studied. This agrees with later results obtained with concentrated extracts of *Amblystoma punctatum* by means of Cartesian microdiver techniques by Boell and Shen (1944).

Sawyer (1940, 1943a) found the enzyme in the premotile stages (Table 1; Harrison's stages 13 to 27) of *A. punctatum*; Youngstrom found small amounts of ChE as early as in the 2 to 4-cell stages of *A. punctatum* and *Bufo terestris*, and relatively large amounts at similar stages of *Rana sphenocephala*. In *Rana*, the enzymic activity decreased through the gastrula and neurula (96 hrs of development), remained low at early motility (120 hrs), increased thereafter at early swimming stages (196 hrs), but still remained at that time below the levels recorded at the 2-cell stage (Youngstrom 1938b).

Generally, these early activities did not change much until transition from early to advanced swimming, when increases of activity ranging from 4 to 13-fold were recorded (YOUNGSTROM 1938a, 1938b; SAWYER 1943a).

In *A. punctatum*, for instance, there was little change of the low initial enzyme level during early motility (early flexure and coil stages, Table 1), but a sharp, approximately 4-fold increase coincided with non-tetanic S-flexure. Thereupon the activity increased steeply and continually throughout the functional stages of development, including the "swimming" and "strong swimming" stages. SAWYER's illustration of the correlation of functional with enzymic development (Fig. 3) is today a classic.

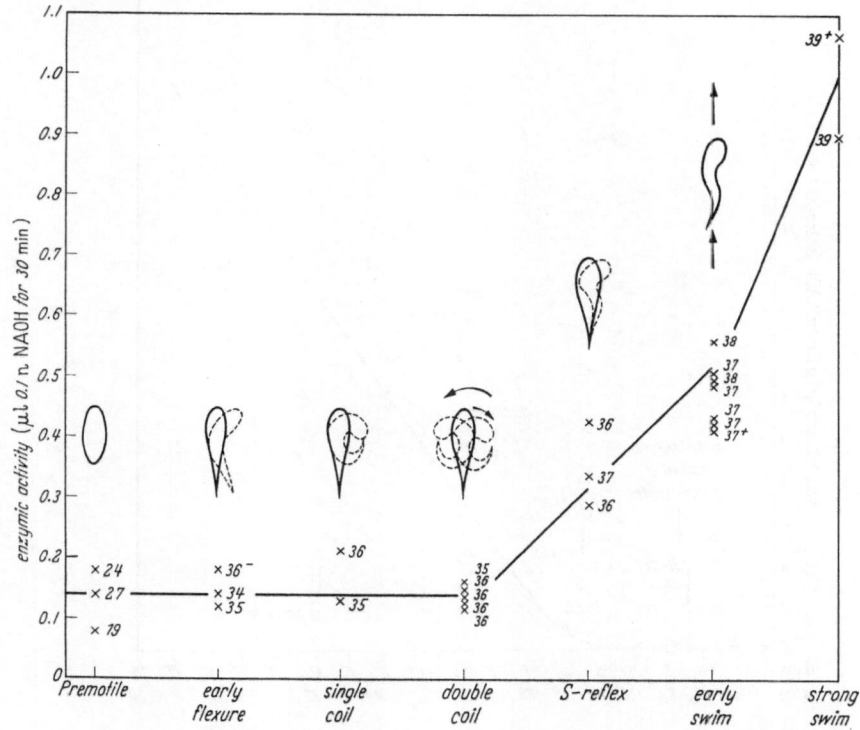

Fig. 3. Relationship between function and cholinesterase activity during development of *Amblystoma punctatum* (from SAWYER 1943a). Numerals opposite points indicate morphological stages. At room temperature, approximately 10 days of development separated stages 19 and 39+ (cf. also Table 1). For measurement of enzymic activity, cf. text

On the other hand, the early fish embryo showed "no demonstrable cholinesterase" (SAWYER 1944, p. 11). Actual readings were approximately 0.02 μl 0.1N NaOH/animal per 30 min, and thus some 5 times less than the readings at premotile stages of *Amblystoma* (v. infra). However, shortly after the onset of early motility the fate of ChE in the *Fundulus* embryo resembled that in *Amblystoma*. A significant amount of the enzyme was found first on the 3rd developmental day, i.e., one stage after the appearance of spontaneous somatic movements (Fig. 4). Enzymic activity increased rapidly thereafter, coinciding with the appearance of the true reflex response to compression of the fourth ventricle; the animals capable of responding to this stimulus had four times as high a ChE content as those capable of only the somatic response. The activity increased rapidly during the rest of development; no particular breaks in the curve characterized the appearance of swimming and hatching, and the steep increase continued after hatching (Fig. 4).

ARTEMOV (1941) could not find any ChE in the frog between the 16-cell blasto-
mere and the tail bud stages, although at the latter stage the brain is well differentiated. Acetylcholine was present in the frog tadpole (o.c.).

In discussing the significance of the presence of the enzyme during the early, premotile
stages, it is important to ascertain the sensitivity of the method and to calculate insofar as
possible the actual quantities of the enzyme that we are dealing with. YOUNGSTROM (1938a)
assayed the enzyme by exposing a medium containing ACh to embryonic homogenates (1.25 to
5 embryos per assay) and bioassaying the residual ACh on the guinea pig ileum. The method

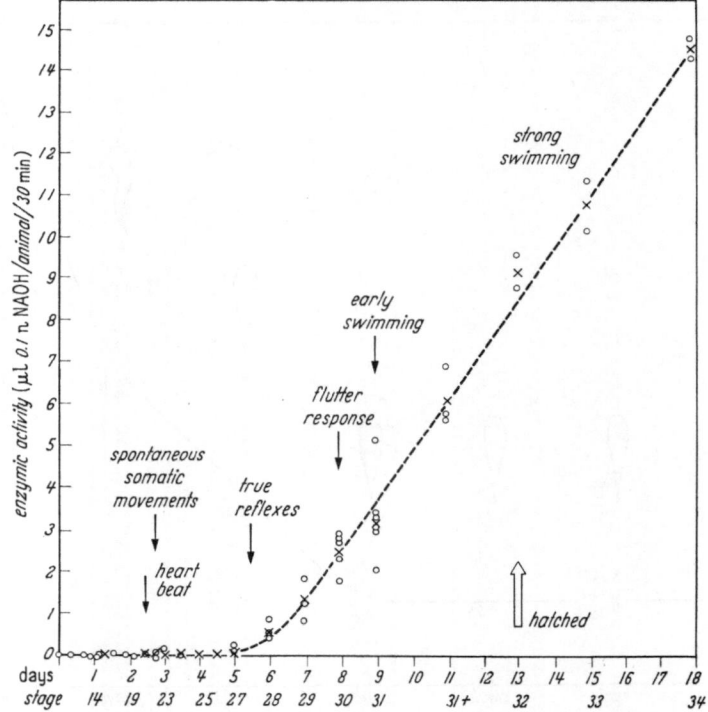

Fig. 4. Relationship between function and ChE activity during development of *Fundulus heteroclitus* (from SAW-
YER 1944). The animals are classified according to stages of OPPENHEIMER (1937) and the approximate time of
onset of various movements is listed. The mean ChE level for each stage is represented by an "x". Spontaneous
movements occur while there is as yet very little enzyme present. For measurement of enzymic activity, cf. text

was sensitive to concentrations of 1 : 7,500,000 of ACh iodide, and ChE was detected at the
2- to 4-cell stage of *R. sphenocephala*, which could hydrolyze approximately 10^{-9} mol of ACh
per embryo per minute. ARTEMOV (1941) used a similar method but exposed ACh to extracts
rather than homogenates of the embryonic material; the extraction was carried out for a short
time, which may account for the apparently low sensitivity of the method.

Finally, SAWYER (1943a and 1944; v. also SAWYER and HOLLINSHEAD 1945) ground single
Amblystoma and *Fundulus* embryos and extracted them for 24 hrs with glycerine; the supernatant was incubated with ACh and the liberated acetic acid microtitrated alkalimetrically for
2 to 3 hrs. The method would detect 0.9 μg or 5×10^{-9} mol of ACh chloride.

The figures for sensitivity of SAWYER and YOUNGSTROM are not too far apart, but indicate
a sensitivity some 20 and 50 times less, respectively, than that of the Cartesian microdiver
technique employed by BOELL and SHEN (1944). In view of the great efficiency of AChE
(ROTHENBERG and NACHMANSOHN 1947) we must assume that hydrolysis of 10^{-9} mol of ACh
per min per few mg of embryonic tissue (YOUNGSTROM, o.c.) corresponds to a very low concentration of ChE (perhaps of the order of 10^{-12} M) in the early amphibian egg. Similarly, the
figure of SAWYER (1944) of 0.019 $\pm$ 0.007 μl 0.1 N NaOH/animal per 30 min indicates a "trace"

of, rather than "no demonstrable cholinesterase" (o.c., pp. 73 and 77, respectively) in the early, premotile *Fundulus* embryo.

While the techniques employed in these early papers did not allow a differentiation between AChE and ChE, SAWYER showed more recently (1955) that the enzyme present in *Amblystoma* is probably AChE, since it is inhibited by excess of ACh and since it hydrolyzes MeCh; the *Fundulus* enzyme also may have been an AChE (SAWYER 1944). The rate of hydrolysis of BzCh was from 1/20th to 1/5th that of MeCh in various urodele species, and did not change in the course of development.

In *A. punctatum*, but not in other larval urodeles, the rate of hydrolysis of MeCh was found to be as high as that for ACh. This is unusual for vertebrates, but was reported in other forms. SAWYER (1955) showed that the enzyme in question is not a separate methacholinesterase, but an AChE endowed with somewhat unusual properties with respect to MeCh. Parenthetically, there seems to be a difference of 2 to 3 anatomical stages between the onset of the rapid phase of increase of enzyme activity in the case of SAWYER's 1943a and 1955 data. Functional rather than anatomical stages (cf. Fig. 3) are pertinent for the enzyme levels, according to SAWYER (1943a), and these unfortunately were not recorded in the 1955 investigation.

The pattern of the ontogenesis of the enzyme as measured in the whole larva and the fact that it is an AChE agree with the pattern of the development and the nature of the enzyme of *Amblystoma* central nervous system and muscle (cf. infra); in view of the paucity of the enzyme outside of muscle and nervous tissue (SAWYER 1943b), it seems that the increase of the enzyme of the whole larva can be attributed chiefly to its increase in these tissues.

2. Neuroeffector ChE's

a) Central nervous system

SAWYER (1943b) should be credited with the first demonstration of a differential increase in the ChE content in the isolated, developing central nervous system.

In fact, the enzyme was already present in small quantities in the skin ectoderm and presumptive neural tissue as early as at stages 12 to 14; neural tissues showed higher activity than the rest of the ectoderm only at the time of formation of the neural folds (stage 19); to the contrary, ventral ectoderm and yolk showed no enzyme activity. At stages 31 to 35 (primitive motility, Table 1 and Fig. 3) both skin and nerve tissue showed an increase in activity, but the difference between their respective activities was maintained. A more rapid phase of increase of the activity of the enzyme of the central nervous system was noted at stage 37, and the increase was particularly steep during the transition in "overt behavior" from double coil to swimming (Fig. 3). The maximal level was reached a few days after the feeding stage. Of particular interest was the subsequent decrease of enzyme activity beginning at metamorphosis and continuing during growth into adulthood. A similar decrease was noticed in *Amblystoma* muscle during and past metamorphosis (v. p. 168), and it is comparable to that noticed by NACHMANSOHN (1940a) in chick muscle (but not in chick brain).

When brain and spinal cord were assayed separately after the beginning of feeding stages, it was noticed that the decline was localized in the spinal region, while the brain suffered no fall. This was interpreted by SAWYER as being due to the "dilution" of the enzyme-rich material of the central nervous system by enzymically inactive myelin and glia cells. Due to the decrease in the activity of the spinal cord, the ratio between the brain and the spinal enzyme changed from 1 : 2 during feeding stages to 1 : 1 and 1.3 : 1 in the metamorphosed animal and in the adult, respectively. In the brain of the adult, ChE activity was highest in the hindbrain, intermediate in the midbrain and lowest in the forebrain; the hindbrain activity was about twice as high as that of the spinal cord.

These results were confirmed and extended by BOELL, SHEN and their associates. BOELL and SHEN (1950), using in this case a less sensitive variant of the Cartesian diver method, noted the first appearance of the enzyme in the central nervous system of *Amblystoma* at stage 36 (Fig.3 and Table 1; double coil stage); this agrees rather well with the data of SAWYER (1943b).

At that time the enzyme was demonstrated in the spinal cord only. Later, it appeared in progressively higher areas of the central nervous system, and reached the forebrain at stage 42 (Fig. 3, Table 1). In each region the increase followed a similar curve. This and the earlier publication of BOELL and SHEN (1944) indicate that both the presumptive skin and the young and mature central nervous system contain predominantly AChE.

Subsequently BOELL, GREENFIELD and SHEN (1955) used the Cartesian microdiver technique for a study of the development of cholinesterase of the optic lobes of the frog. Between the 10th day and the completion of metamorphosis (192nd day), the optic lobe nitrogen increased 32-fold and the Q value of ChE 18 times;

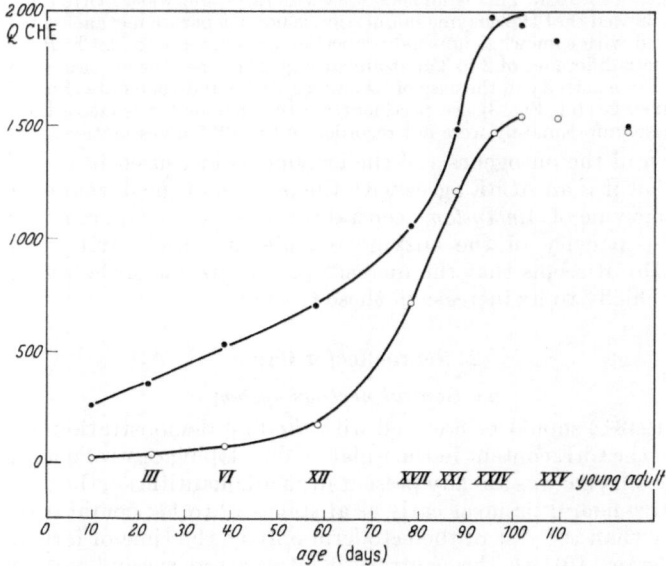

Fig. 5. ChE activity in the anterior and the posterior halves of the optic lobe during normal development of *Rana pipiens* (from BOELL et al. 1955). Abscissa: developmental age in days and stages (III—XXV) after TAYLOR and KOLLROS (1946); ordinate: ChE activity in Q values (full and open circles — activity of the anterior and posterior lobe, respectively)

an additional three-fold increase of nitrogen occurred between metamorphosis and adulthood, while the Q value of ChE remained stationary during this period. Since the Q values express enzyme activity per mg of nitrogen, these figures indicate that cholinesterase activity increased during premetamorphic stages many times faster than the weight of neural tissues; the most drastic differential increase occurred at stage 36 and tapered off thereafter.

The increase was localized mostly in the anterior part of the lobe; analysis of posterior and anterior parts showed that in the former ChE appeared only at stage VI (40 days), i.e., 30 days after the appearance of the anterior lobe enzyme, and started increasing exponentially at stages VI to XII (55 days); between stages XII and XXV it increased 35 times, in contrast to a 2 to 3-fold increase of the enzyme of the anterior lobe during that time (Fig. 5). While the ChE of the anterior lobe fell off somewhat after metamorphosis, that of the posterior lobe remained unchanged; consequently, both lobes had similar amounts of the enzyme in the adult.

It is of interest that the very rapid increase of the enzyme content of the whole *Amblystoma* larvae noted by SAWYER (1943a; v. Fig. 3) at the onset of early swimming does not show up as clearly in the subsequent work of SAWYER (1943b, SAWYER's Fig. 1) and in the work of BOELL and SHEN (1944 and 1950). It appears rather that there is a relatively constant rate of increase of the enzyme activity from the single coil to the "strong" swimming stage (Table 1). This, however, may be due to the fact that the time scale used by SAWYER and by BOELL and his associates is arbitrary, each stage, either physiological (SAWYER 1943a) or anatomical (SAWYER o.c.; BOELL and SHEN o.c.), being assigned the same magnitude.

The data of SAWYER and of BOELL and SHEN indicate that each level of anatomical development of the central nervous system is characterized by a specific level of enzyme activity; the nervous system thus matures both anatomically and biochemically. Accordingly, the neural cord inductor (SPEMANN 1938) which can organize as yet undetermined tissue in the direction of neurogenesis could be expected to change the biochemical development in the same direction. BOELL and SHEN (1944) showed that a piece of chorda-mesoderm implanted at stage $10^1/_4$ caused both chemical and anatomical induction; in fact, the Q values of central nervous tissue of the host on one hand, and of the secondary, induced neural tube on the other were similar in the case of successful induction, and different when faulty induction led to incomplete differentiation of the secondary neural structures.

b) Optic pathways

These data were extended by means of histochemical techniques by BOELL, GREENFIELD and SHEN (1955) in the frog central nervous system, particularly its optic pathways; the effect of enucleation also was studied.

BOELL et al. (o.c.) used Cartesian microdiver techniques as well as the third (1951) version of the histochemical method of KOELLE; their data refer to AChE. In histochemical preparations the diffusion of the enzyme was prevented by "fixing" the enzyme with high concentration of Na_2SO_4 (cf. KOELLE 1950 and 1951; Chapter 6). BOELL et al. (o.c.; cf. also SHEN and GREENFIELD with SIPPEL 1952 and with BOELL 1955) used paraffin embedding of lyophilized tissues and xylene deceration rather than freezing fresh tissues as recommended by KOELLE. Earlier, they followed xylene with acetone and found that this procedure leads to enzyme inactivation; however, xylene treatment alone may have a similar effect. The problem of the reliability of the histochemical procedure with regard to fixation and other factors cannot be minimized (cf. also infra, p. 151) and the interested reader should consult KOELLE (1955) and HOLMSTEDT (1959) for its detailed discussion.

SHUMWAY (1940; arabic numbers) and TAYLOR-KOLLROS (1946; roman numerals) staging of frog development was employed.

α) ChE of intact optic pathways. Acetylcholinesterase, as determined histochemically, makes its first appearance in the central nervous system at stage 20 of the developing frog, when it can be shown in the spinal cord, particularly at the roots of spinal nerves (BOELL et al. 1955). This particular localization was confirmed by LEWIS and HUGHES (1937) who, however, used formalin-fixed tissues. Immediately thereafter (stage 21) cranial nuclei, optic pathways, and neuroretina begin to exhibit AChE staining. Increase of enzymic activity in these areas, and differentiation of AChE layers in the optic tectum (corresponding with but somewhat delayed as regards its histological stratification), progresses through stages 25 and XII.

Habenular nuclei begin to stain for AChE at stage 21; in fact, they can be listed among the heaviest staining areas in the adult frog as well. Staining for AChE next appears in the basal optic nuclei, IIIrd nerve nuclei, isthmal nuclei, and motor nuclei of the cranial nerves; this occurs shortly after optic fibers connect with the tectum (stage 23). At stage 25, stratification of the optic tectum is not as yet accompanied by differentiation of AChE-staining, which is uniformly distributed in the optic layer. At stage III the tectum differentiates into a thin surface layer and an inner one, which divides again and stains heavily along a narrow band. This is presumably a synaptic focus where optic fibers arborize with neurons (RAMON's 12th layer). Acetylcholinesterase staining of the tectum progresses then caudally (stages XI—XII). The deeper tectal layers are enzyme-poor and do not show stratification. Thus, both histochemical and manometric (cf. supra) data support the anatomical notion (KOLLROS 1953) of an antero-posterior differentiation sequence of the frog eye.

At about this time, the interpeduncular neuropil stains also, but not the cells in the nucleus itself; likewise stained is the tractus retroflexus which emerges from the ventrolateral base of the habenular nuclei and extends to the interpeduncular neuropil. Further delineation of AChE-staining in the neuropil accompanies formation of the pretectal nucleus. At stage X, diffuse enzymatic staining is present at the dorso-anterior head, and forms spindles late during metamorphosis, at which time there is also condensation of staining in the antero-lateral portion of the isthmal nucleus, the site of the principal synaptic field.

With regard to the neuroretina, AChE-staining appears first in its innermost layer at the time when the future ganglion cells of this layer enlarge and send axons into the eye stalk (stage 21). Additional AChE-staining appears at stage 22 in the inner plexiform layer, which forms between the ganglionic and nuclear layers. This staining becomes more intense peripherad till stage III, and stratifies into two or more layers, which are never as distinct as those of avian retina (cf. infra, p. 157). The thin outer plexiform layer appears at the time of differentiation of primary neurons (stage 24) and stains very faintly, although quite distinctly. Staining is present also in the ganglion cells and in some amacrine cells.

β) **Effects of enucleation.** The enucleation experiment carried out by BOELL and his associates throws additional light on the relationship between ChE, anatomical differentiation, and function, particularly since it showed that non-optical structures and enzymes of the eye other than ChE remained unaffected by enucleation. This is revealed most clearly in histochemical studies of the tectum and of the cranial and spinal neuropils.

Unilateral removal of the frog eye at stages 21 to 23 slows the growth of the contralateral lobe some 10 days later (at stage V); the growth is slow between that stage and stage XII, and ceases altogether thereafter; at stage XXV the affected lobe is about one-half as large as the control. On the other hand, the first difference between Q values of AChE of the lobes appears at stage II, that is, before enucleation affects growth. By stage XII the affected side shows on the average a Q value of 340 against a value of 535 for the controls. However, between stages XII and XXV the Q values increase at the same rate in both lobes; actually, AChE of the posterior lobe, which appears only by stage XII, increases thereafter at a similar rate for the control and experimental sides. Ultimately, the two lobes never reach the same Q value; the *total* ChE of the affected side is about 45% of that of the control side.

As will be remembered, histochemical studies showed that in the normal tectum ChE is still equidistributed throughout the tectum at stage 25; thereafter, it stratifies in the antero-posterior sequence into the outer thin (RAMON's) and broader inner layer. Following enucleation the enzyme is missing at the affected side by stage 25; it appears first as one thin surface layer only at stage III. There is never any stratification on the affected side and particularly the staining of the 12th layer is missing. The diffuse, unstratified staining of the deeper tectum (optic layer) is not affected; this staining is probably located at the arborisations of bulbar and spinal afferent fibers.

Outside of the tectum, the normal development of the enzyme involves enzyme-rich neuropils which subsequently differentiate into more definite synaptic fields, extending caudad from the basal optic and IIIrd nerve nuclei to the spinal motor nuclei. The ChE-rich neuropils are affected to very different degrees by enucleation. The basal optic nucleus and pretectal nucleus disappear. The heavy enzymic staining of the antero-lateral portion of the isthmal nucleus, which normally receives tecto-isthmic fibers, is greatly reduced, while the rest of the nucleus continues to stain diffusely. In all affected areas, particularly in the isthmal nucleus, the number and the size of the neurons may be unaffected but arborisation is lacking in parallel with the lack of AChE-staining. This is of great interest since LARSELL (1924) could not conclude on the basis of his neurohistological studies whether or not the isthmal nuclei are synaptically connected with optic fibers. BOELL and his associates suggested the existence of such connections in antero-lateral portions of the isthmal nuclei where the stain disappears after enucleation. Finally, motor centers of the cranial nerves suffer no reduction in size or in enzymic staining.

3. Amphibian regeneration

An interesting growth process in the course of which a change in ChE and ACh content was recently reported (SINGER et al. 1960a) is that of regeneration of the amphibian limb after its amputation. HESTRIN's (1949) and AMMON's (1933) methods were used to measure ChE; AChE and ChE were also studied histochemically by means of the 1950 version of KOELLE's method. Acetylcholine was bioassayed on the heart of the clam (WELSH and TAUB 1948).

In *Triturus viridescens*, ChE activity of the regenerate was many times below that of control limbs or of the stump. It stayed low during the early stages of dedifferentiation and blastema formation. Increase first occurred at about 13 days of regeneration within the differentiating new muscle and the cut, healing muscle; ChE activity reached normal values about the 25th day, i.e., 10 days before completion of regeneration. The ACh content of the regenerate was from the beginning of regeneration higher than that of control limbs; it increased further (from 7.5 to 11.0 microgm/gm) between the 9th and 20th day of regeneration. Thus, ACh was higher in the amputated limb than in controls during dedifferentiation, blastematization, and early differentiation, when it began to fall off.

These data are of interest, as it has been long known (RUBIN 1903; SCHOTTÉ 1922) that nerves are necessary for regeneration. It was postulated (SCHOTTÉ 1926; KARCZMAR 1946) that the nerve influence is due to a transmitter. This, jointly with data of SINGER (1960) may suggest a "trophic" (KARCZMAR o. c.) effect of ACh. In fact, SINGER et al. (1960b) stopped regeneration by the infusion of atropine into the regenerate. However, the concentrations required were very high and in fact "atropine blisters" developed; thus, the effects of atropine may have been due to a non-specific antigrowth action of this compound (SINGER o.c.; cf. also Chapter 17). Also, ACh levels did not predicate regenerative capacity when the latter was varied experimentally (SINGER 1960). Finally, nerves are necessary for regeneration in terms of their quantity (KARCZMAR, o.c.) rather than type, and they do not have to be cholinergic (for refs., v. SINGER 1960). Thus, the role in regeneration of changes in ChE and ACh levels cannot be stated at present.

It is of interest that the cells of the early regenerate showed no ChE's. At that time the tissues of the amputation area dedifferentiate and their cells become generalized and morphologically embryonic (BUTLER and SCHOTTÉ 1941). This morphological change corresponds then to the biochemical one, since muscle cells lose ChE as well as certain other enzymes (KARCZMAR and BERG 1951) during dedifferentiation. Behavior of ACh, however, seems to constitute an exception to this "law" of biochemical dedifferentiation.

4. Comment

The data on ontogenesis of ChE's of the amphibian and fish central nervous system will be now summarized and related to neurogenesis and development of function.

In amphibians, ChE's appear anywhere between 2- to 4-cell and premotile stages. Emergence of ChE's prior to neurogenesis was already described in the case of certain invertebrates and will be shown to occur also in the chick embryo. This perhaps unexpected appearance of ChE's in certain tissues, both embryonic and adult, as well as their presence in non-motile unicellular organisms illustrates the incompleteness of our knowledge of the functional meaning of ChE's.

Interpretation of subsequent ontogenesis of ChE may be easier. It must be of functional and behavioral significance that the development of ChE differs from that of enzymes concerned with growth and general cellular energetics. For instance, in the developing central nervous system, ChE's on the one hand, and respiratory enzymes on the other differ in several respects. The activity of cytochrome oxidase and of succinic dehydrogenase increases at a steady rate throughout development, while ChE's at first maintain a constant low level during premotile stages and then increase rapidly. Moreover, the distribution of the three enzymes differs for various parts of the brain: the sequence of concentrations of AChE in the hind-, mid- and fore-brain of the larval *Amblystoma* is opposite to that of the respiratory enzymes (BOELL and SHEN 1950; SHEN 1958). Enucleation of the optic lobe affects AChE but not succinoxidase (BOELL et al. 1955). Since synthesis of AChE oustrips growth of the central nervous system (BOELL 1948; BOELL et al. 1955) as well as that of respiratory enzymes, during certain developmental periods and in certain parts of the amphibian brain, there must be a shift in the pattern of protein synthesis with development.

Patterns of ontogenesis of ChE's after the onset of motility can be correlated to a certain extent with neurogenetic events and with functionalization (Table 1). Earliest correlation of this type might be established for the neuromyal junction and for spontaneous somatic movement.

When spontaneous somatic movement and myotonic response to stimulation appear first in the fish and in amphibians (Table 1), *Amblystoma* but not *Fundulus* exhibits significant amounts of AChE. This may then substantiate COGHILL's (1933) view that this activity is, in the case of *Fundulus*, myogenic rather than neurogenic (see also SAWYER 1944); indeed, in both forms motor innervation is incomplete at this time. However, this movement may be neurogenic and mediated by ACh diffusing from an axon terminating at a distance from the muscle. In an analogous situation described for the embryonic rat (v. infra, p. 171) it was suggested that the lack of close association between the transmitter and the effector and the paucity of AChE may explain the slow, tetanic character of its early movement; the same explanation may hold for *Fundulus*. If the early activity in *Amblystoma* should be similarly mediated, it might be expected that it would be rapid in view of the presence of AChE; since the movement is slow, early *Amblystoma* activity may be purely myogenic (cf. however, YOUNGSTROM 1938 a and b, and infra, p. 171).

The subsequent rapid increase of AChE content in *Amblystoma* and in *Fundulus* probably can be linked firstly with the beginning of neurogenic reponse, possibly resulting from direct stimulation of the motoneurone and dependent upon establishment of the muscle innervation, and secondly, with the appearance of "coil" and swimming motion (Figs. 3 and 4) dependent upon the progress of synaptization.

Sensori-internuncial arcs are completed in *Amblystoma* by stage 34; synaptization of motor tracts via commisural plates is present by stage 36; ipsilateral reflex arcs mediated possibly via inhibitory collaterals (for further explanation, cf. Fig. 6) are completed by the swimming stages (Table 1). Whether or not in amphibians and in the fish, as in the mammals (ECCLES et al. 1956), motor fiber collaterals set up cholinergic volleys upon interneurones causing motoneurone inhibition, the pathways in question are multineuronic and some of the synapses can be expected to be cholinergic (FELDBERG 1957). These possibilities are further discussed (cf. Chapter 17) with reference to the effects of anti-ChE agents in *Amblystoma* and in the fish.

Further correlation between function, neurogenesis, and ChE's may be suggested for stages 40 to 42. At that stage, motor capacity of *Amblystoma* larvae can be affected for the first time by the removal of the midbrain (DETWILER 1946 and 1948). Thus, at this stage the swimming mechanism, previously spinal, autonomous and clumsy, becomes skillful and subservient to mesencephalic control, probably concommitantly with the development of the midbrain (stages 40 to 41) and the tectobulbar and tecto-spinal tracts (Table 1).

More specifically than the data analyzed above, histochemical studies of AChE mark out areas of synaptization within the neuroretina and the cholinergic centers of the optic pathways. In the neuroretina, synaptic areas are probably represented by one or more strata of the inner plexiform layer, more easily observable in the retina of the bird

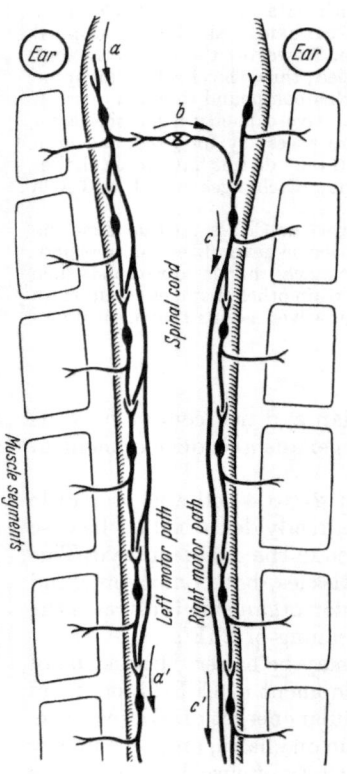

x = *Floor plate cell*

Fig. 6. A diagram of the neuromotor mechanism of swimming in *Amblystoma punctatum* (from COGHILL 1929). Sensory mechanism omitted. The arrows indicate direction of conduction. Arrow *a* represents the initial impulse which passes tailward to *a'* and beyond and excites muscle segments to a wave of contraction progressing caudad. At swimming stages, motor tract neurons in the anterior region develop collaterals which grow towards the median plane to synapse with commissural cells of the floor plate; at *b*, an impulse crosses to contralateral motor system and passes caudad (*c* and *c'*). The impulse excited by collaterals may be inhibitory (cf. COGHILL, o.c. and text)

(SHEN, GREENFIELD and BOELL 1956; v. infra). Ganglionic cells, which also show AChE in the case of the amphibian neuroretina, synapse in the chick with axonal processes of bipolar cells (o.c.). Other faintly staining synaptic layers, such as the outer layer which in the avian retina does not exhibit AChE at all (v. infra, p. 158), may be non-cholinergic (FELDBERG and VOGT 1948). Finally, AChE staining in habenular nuclei, certain areas of isthmal and pretectal nuclei and of the optic lobe, and certain layers of the tectum, probably indicates cholinergic synapses important for visual transmission.

This is suggested by the effects of enucleation. In these areas both AChE and the anatomical integrity depend upon incoming optic fibers and their synaptic contribution to the area in question; in the tectum, the 12th layer, most richly stained and identifiable with the principal synaptic field of the area (SHEN et al. 1955) is most strongly affected by enucleation. Finally, as the areas in question carry other than optic tracts, AChE activity is not lost completely upon enucleation; parts of several nuclei such as tectal as well as cranial motor centers are not affected in their AChE staining or in arborisation by enucleation. Altogether, loss of stain can be associated with loss of synaptic fields rather than with that of neurons.

It should be said that the above correlations have to remain speculative since the ontogenic appearance of ACh in fish and amphibians is unknown; thus, little can be said on the emergence of cholinergic synapses in these forms. Also, it is impossible to relate the distinct steps in neuro- and synaptogenesis illustrated in Table 1 to the essentially smooth rise of AChE activity recorded titrimetrically during development (cf. Figs. 3 and 4). Thus, while nothing more than general correlation of AChE with neurogenesis and development of function can be proposed at present, nevertheless the significance of AChE as an enzyme characteristic of ontogenesis of synaptic arborisations and of certain optic areas of the frog is clearly borne out.

II. Chick embryo

Ontogenesis of ChE was studied in the chick in the extraembryonic membranes, the central nervous system, and in the retina; the data obtained acquired added significance as a result of the availability of precise staging of chick development (HAMBURGER 1948; HAMBURGER and HAMILTON 1951) and because its neurogenesis was well correlated with the development of function (TELLO 1923; WINDLE and ORR 1934; WINDLE and AUSTIN 1936; KUO 1932a, b and 1938; v. Table 2).

1. Central nervous system and extraembryonic membranes

a) Histochemical data

ZACKS (1954; v. also RAVIN, ZACKS and SELIGMAN 1953) employed the 6-brom-2-naphthyl acetate and diazo blue B (tetrazotized di-ortho-ansidine) method (v. Chapter 6 for details). This substrate is hydrolyzed by lipase and esterases in addition to AChE and other ChE's. Carbo-naphthoxycholine iodide, which is hydrolyzed by BuChE but not by AChE, as well as various selective inhibitors and activators were used for additional identification of the enzyme. An acetone and physostigmine-sensitive enzyme which hydrolyzes 6-brom-2-naphthylacetate, but not carbo-naphthoxycholine, was regarded by ZACKS as AChE; this identification may be open to criticism (v. Chapter 6). GEREBTZOFF (1953; 1955) and BONICHON (1957a, b; 1958) used a modification of the method of KOELLE (1950 and 1951; cf. also KOELLE et al. 1950, FUKUDA and KOELLE 1959). They used tissues fixed for 4 to 6 hrs in formalin instead of fresh frozen sections, and eliminated magnesium from the incubation medium. Acetylthiocholine, which is hydrolyzed by both AChE and BuChE, and butyrylthiocholine, which is hydrolyzed more repidly by BuChE, were the substrates used also by KOELLE. Diisopropylphosphoro-fluoridate (DFP), 10^{-7} M, served additionally to differentiate AChE from BuChE. More recently (1955) KOELLE introduced the dimethyl carbamate of (2-hydroxy-5-phenylbenzyl)-trimethyl-ammonium bromide (Nu 683) on the one hand, and 1—5-bis (4-allyl dimetylammonium phenyl) pentan-3-one dibromide (B.W. 284) on the other as specific inhibitors of AChE and BuChE, respectively, to obtain best resolution of the two enzymes histochemically. GEREBTZOFF (1953) stated that fixing the tissues and omitting magnesium creates conditions unfavorable for maximal enzyme activity, thus reducing diffusion artefact. Since the latter was largely eliminated by KOELLE and his group (o.c.), the criticism of HOLMSTEDT (1959) that the use of formalin transforms a histochemical method into a histological one, seems valid. Indeed, formalin inhibition of ChE's was noticed as early as in 1935 by AMMON and SCHÜTTE. Thus, the results by GEREBTZOFF reported in this section and also elsewhere (pp. 161, 163) may not be taken as precise indications of the physiological activity of the enzyme *in vivo*.

Histochemical methods allowed earlier identification of the enzyme than the manometric techniques (cf. infra). In fact, ZACKS (o.c.) demonstrated it at the primitive streak stage (15 hrs), i.e. 3 to 4 days before onset of motility; the enzyme appeared subsequently in the neural folds and in the spinal neuroblasts (BONICHON o.c.).

At its earliest appearance, the staining due to AChE was particularly dense in the area of Hensen's node and of the anterior crescent. It appeared subsequently at the surfaces of the neural folds in the form of scattered granules in the 21 hrs embryo and in the form of denser deposits 2 hrs later (4-somite stage). At that time, the sinus region stained also. Three hours later (8-somite stage) there was high activity in pros- and mesencephalon and at the line of closure; the sinus rhomboidalis, intersomite furrows, and dorsal somite surface stained less intensely; the somites adjacent to the neural tube stained most intensively.

This situation did not change much till the 48 to 52 hrs embryo was examined. At this time, enzymatic activity decreased in the brain, which then stained less than the spinal cord. ZACKS explained this by the dilution of AChE due to the appearance of enzyme-poor cells; while a similar explanation for apparent decrease of ChE activity was given by SAWYER (1943b) and by NACHMANSOHN (1938c), it referred to much later developmental stages of Amblystoma and to the postembryonic chick. In fact, an increase of the stain could be expected in the case of the chick neural fold at 48 to 52 hrs, since this is the time of intense neurogenesis, culminating with histogenesis of neuroblasts (Table 2). This paradox might be resolved as follows: the areas of early enzymic activity described by ZACKS — Hensen's node, head, and neural folds — are rich in cytochrome oxidase and phosphatases (MOOG 1946 and 1952). Thus, contrary to what happens later in development, the early enzymic activity ascribed by ZACKS to ChE's is parallel to that of enzymes concerned with the respiratory and carbohydrate metabolism. The areas in question show a high affinity for several oxidation-reduction indicators which also stain ChE-rich areas of adult tissues, such as endplates and mitochondria (WELSH and ZACKS 1949; ZACKS and WELSH 1951). Therefore, it may be that the stain used may exhibit affinity for areas of high metabolism, which later in development become rich in ChE's.

Well staining notochord appeared between 52 and 72 hrs; clusters of granules appeared in the metencephalon, in the region of the Vth nerve nucleus, in the retina, the lens, and in the posterior regions of the neural tube (ZACKS 1954). At this time, BONICHON (1957a, 1958) found AChE in the neuroblasts, particularly of the medullary and optic lobe region.

After 96 hr, staining of neuroblasts was particularly pronounced in the anterior horn region (BONICHON 1957a, 1958). The staining as well as that of certain intraspinal fibers increased between $4^1/_2$ and 8 to 9 days, and decreased subsequently.

The increase of the neuroblast staining followed a spino-cephalad sequence (GEREBTZOFF 1959). Toward the end of this period the staining, previously cytoplasmic, tended to concentrate at the peripheries of the cells. The fibers of the posterior funiculus exhibited AChE at 5 days (stage 26), the staining increasing till the 8th day and being always more intense than that of the anterior horn neuroblasts. On the 9th day it appeared that the Lissauer zone of the posterior funiculus stained more than the medial part of the posterior funiculus. A little later, the posterior (stage 27) and anterior (stage 30) roots appeared; they stained weakly at first, and progressively more intensely till the 8th day (GEREBTZOFF 1959).

AChE activity decreased and disappeared subsequently in the anterior root, posterior root, and posterior funiculus; it persisted at a low level into adulthood in the zone of Lissauer and in certain parts of the posterior root. GEREBTZOFF correlated this disappearance with myelination (10 days, stage 36) and he pointed out that myelination is absent or limited in the case of Lissauer fibers and lateral part of the posterior root. He suggested that loss of AChE from certain sites is due to the "transfer" or "migration" of the enzyme.

b) Manometric estimations

The subsequent fate of ChE following stage 20 or 21 of development (Table 2) was studied manometrically by AMMON and SCHÜTTE (1935) and by NACHMANSOHN (1938a, b, c, d; 1939b). While NACHMANSOHN was particularly concerned with the enzyme of the central nervous system, AMMON and SCHÜTTE studied also ChE's and related enzymes of the chick extraembryonic materials.

In the brain, no distinct activity of ChE could be demonstrated by the Warburg technique before the sixth day of development (NACHMANSOHN 1938a, b); this agrees with the data of AMMON and SCHÜTTE on the whole embryo, where rather high activity (392 micromol of ACh per hr/ml of extract) appeared at the 110-hr stage.

This is a considerably older stage than that at which ChE was found histochemically in the rudiments of the central nervous system. A difference of opinion arises also with reference to the appearance of the extra-embryonic enzyme. AMMON and SCHÜTTE reported rather high levels of ChE in the egg yolk endoderm $2^1/_2$ days after fertilization. The same enzyme appeared in the yolk sac on the 6th, and in the allantois on the 10th day after fertilization. In addition, AMMON and SCHÜTTE found an extraembryonic lipase, simple esterase, and tributyrase; the two latter were found even in unfertilized egg. To the contrary, ZACKS (o.c.), using his histochemical method, did not find any extraembryonic ChE, although he confirmed the presence of a lipase or ali-esterase. The latter was identified by being only slightly sensitive to cold acetone and physostigmine; it appeared first in the area opaca of the 21 hrs embryo. It was subsequently localized in the yolk sac endoderm where it was intimately associated with yolk globules. During the third and fourth day of development, this enzyme was found in the fore- and mid-gut, hepatic and pancreatic rudiments, and stomach glands, as well as in mesenchyme. ZACKS (o.c.) pointed out that the appearance of this esterolytic activity coincided with the completion of the vascular system, and thus might be concerned with providing the vascular carrier with the products of yolk digestion; utilization of lipids may indeed become important after 4 days of development, following the phase of the utilization of carbohydrates (SPRATT 1949).

According to AMMON and SCHÜTTE, extraembryonic ChE increased 2 to 6 times between the 6th and 15th day, tributyrase increased much faster, while the esterase (methylbutyrate esterase) of the yolk, allantois, and the yolk sac increased very little. It is of interest that during this time both ChE and esterase increased faster in the embryo than in the extraembryonic membranes; the opposite was true in the case of tributyrinase.

Cholinesterase activity of the central nervous system began to increase roughly geometrically 4 to 5 days before hatching, that is, after 15 days of incubation (NACHMANSOHN 1938a, c, d; 1939b; Table 2). This rapid increase continued through hatching but stopped abruptly around the 7th day after hatching; the enzyme content was at that time identical with that of the adult (NACHMANSOHN 1939b).

The weight of the chick brain increases logarithmically between the 6th day of incubation and hatching (Table 2); it begins increasing again at the 7th or 8th post-embryonic day, i.e., when the Q_{ChE} has reached its maximal value (NACHMANSOHN 1938a); thus, general growth of the chick brain and ontogenesis of ChE follow two different patterns. The 6-day old brain could hydrolyze 6, the adult brain 950 mg of ACh per hour. This last figure corresponds to about 10^{15} molecules of ACh per millisecond. NACHMANSOHN (o.c.) showed also that the Q_{ChE} increases, between the 15th developmental day and adulthood, 5 to 6 times in the telencephalon, 10 times in the optic lobes and cerebellum, and 3 times in the rest of the brain. At the 15th day, Q_{ChE} values were higher in the rest of the brain than in the optic lobes and in the cerebellum; the situation was reversed in the adult. There was, then, a postero-anterior sequence of ChE ontogenesis in the chick central nervous system similar to that reported for many other forms, including mammals. This is substantiated by the data of WENGER (1951) showing relatively early onset and early rapid increase in the ChE of the spinal cord of the $5^1/_2$- to 11-day old (stages 28 to 37 of HAMBURGER and HAMILTON) chick embryos, and particularly a 5-fold increase at the onset of spontaneous and reflex activity. Brachial and lumbosacral enlargements had generally more enzyme than spinal levels not corresponding to limbs; at $7^1/_2$ to $8^1/_2$ days (stages 33—34) the increase of enzyme at the thoracic level was higher than that at other levels.

NACHMANSOHN commented (1938d) that the increase of the Q value of ChE just prior to hatching coincides with the onset of synaptic arborisation. Subsequently, the ratio of synapses to the non-synaptic material does not change, contrary to the situation in the case of avian and amphibian muscle (cf. infra, p. 168); in other words, the neuron density increases in the young adult at a rate corresponding to that of the synthesis of ChE, and the Q value remains unchanged. On the other hand, TORDA (1938) claimed to have found a decrease of spinal cord ChE a few days after hatching.

Before discussing the biogenesis of ChE with reference to neurogenesis and development of function, it is of interest to review the few data available with respect to another component of the cholinergic system, ACh.

KUO (1939) found ACh (0.33 μg/g, or 0.0044 μg/embryo) after $2^1/_2$ days. It increased rapidly thereafter, reaching the value of 0.94 μg/g, or 0.17 μg/embryo, on the 5th day of incubation. Thereupon the values calculated on the per g basis did not change, although the ACh/embryo

Table 2. *Neurogenesis and ontogenesis of*

| Incubation | | Stage | | Maximal weight, gm | | General |
Hours	Days	(Hamburger)	(Hamburger-Hamilton)	Head	Total	
0—24	1		1—6			Primitive streak and headfold formation
24—26	1		7			Neural folds; one to two somites
26—29	1		8			Four somites
29—33	1 +		9			Seven somites
33—38	$1^1/_2$		10			Ten somites
39—45	2 —		11			Thirteen somites
46—53	2 +		12—14			Sixteen-22 somites; auditory pit
54—64	$2^1/_2$	3 n 3	15—17			Formation of limb buds, epiphysis and visceral arches
65—84	3 — 3 +		18—21			Formation of limbs, tail, mandible and maxilla; eye pigment
85—108	3 + — 4	4 n 2	22—25	0.070	0.103	Formation of joints and digits
109—144	4 + — 6	5 n 4	26—29	0.20	0.31	Beak formation
	6 + — 7 +	6 n 12	30—32	0.67	1.15	Formation of feather-germs and scleral papillae
	$7^1/_2$—9		33—35	0.84	1.49	Phalanges; nictitating membrane
	10—13		36—39	1.45	8.23	Maturation of scales and eyelids
	14—20		40—45			Elongation of beak and toes
	20—21		46	4.77	26.1	

[1] Data from WINDLE and ORR 1934, HAMBURGER 1948, HAMBURGER and HAMILTON 1948,

Central nervous system	Function and Motility	ChE's and ACh
		Enzyme in Hensen's node (histochemical technique)
Neural folds meet at mid-brain level		Enzyme in neural folds (histochemical technique)
Primary optic vesicles		
Three primary brain vesicles; beginning of neuro-fibrillar differentiation; reticulo-spinal tract appears (intersegm. neurones)	Some embryos show heart beat	Enzyme in prosen- and metencephalon (histochemical technique)
Five hindbrain neuromeres; medial longitudinal fascicle		
Telencephalon; spino-, tecto-, and thalamo-bulbar tracts; optic tract; IIIrd, Vth, VIIth, and IXth to XIIth nuclei present		ACh present in the whole embryo and in the spinal cord
Lateral and ventrolateral funiculus; IVth, VIth and spinal ventral and dorsal nuclei present		ACh content increases rapidly
Tractus solitarius, spinal neuroblasts; peak of mitotic activity of spinal basal plate	66 hrs — head vibrations; 68 hrs — body vibrations; 70 hrs — embryos lift heads; 72 hrs — embryos bend heads;	Enzyme in primitive neuroblasts (histochemical technique)
Motor column; dorso-lateral funiculus; olfactory tracts	85—95 hrs — trunk movement 88—90 hrs — swinging and turning of head; movement of tail and limbs	Enzyme in the Vth nerve nucleus (histochemical technique)
Dorso-spinal funiculus; stria medullares; collaterals betw. ventral plate and motor neurones	5 d. — beak and toe movement 6 d. — response to pressure and electricity; eyelid movement; local reflexes; swimming movement; spontaneous flexions	Enzyme in the spinal cord (titrimetric technique); it increases 5-fold at reflexogenic stages. Ganglion cells stain in neuroretina. Manometric demonstration of enzyme in the brain. ACh present in midbrain
Peak of mitotic activity of spinal alar plate, wing level; collaterals from the posterior funiculus (sensory pathway); dorsal column	Eyeball movement	Arithmetic increases of brain ChE
End of intense mitotic activity of spinal cord	8 d. — swallowing, leg folding, fixation of body position, bill clapping 9 d. — response to touch; limbs and wings move independently 11 d. — wriggling 13 d. — turning of body 16 d. — neck protrusion, respiratory movements 17—18 d. — rotation, response to light, sound and vibration, breaking of shell 21 d. — hatching	Arithmetic increase of brain ChE Arithmetic increase of brain ChE 15 d. — logarithmic increase of brain enzyme 19 d. — cholinergic maturation of the retina (by AChE stain and high level of ACh)

WENGER 1951, ZACKS 1954, BONICHON 1957a and others (cf. Text).

value increased further to 3.75 μg on the 12th day of incubation. SZEPSENVOL and CARETTI (1942a and b) reported the presence of an ACh-like agent in the spinal cord and rhombencephalon on the 2nd day, in the di- and mesencephalon on the 5th day of incubation, and later in the cerebellum and in the telencephalon; it increased in all these structures till hatching. On the other hand they noticed a decrease of the spinal cord ACh between the 6th and 20th day of incubation. Since the values for ACh reported by KUO on one hand, and by SZEPSENVOL and CARETTI on the other, refer to the embryonic and central nervous system extracts, respectively, their data cannot be compared directly.

c) Comment

Cholinesterase was reported to be present in the 15 hr chick embryo 1 to 2 days prior to the formation of neuroblasts and neurofibrillar differentiation, 2 to 3 days before the onset of spontaneous movement, and 5 days before that of reflex activity (Table 2). This then is analogous to the precocious appearance of ChE in *Amphibia*, in echinoderm larvae, and in certain insects. Obviously, such an early appearance of the enzyme cannot be related to transmission. It may be suggested that biochemical maturation precedes anatomical differentiation and functionalisation, or that ACh and ChE serve as embryonic inductors of nervous tissue. Finally, they could be related to functions other than transmission; this must be true for ChE's of the extraembryonic tissues.

The appearance, subsequently, of ChE in the chick brain may be naturally of significance for transmission. Histochemical evidence for the presence of ChE in the 1-day old brain and subsequently in the neuroblasts, as well as the demonstration of ACh on the 3rd day of incubation, are not inconsistent with neurogenetic and functional events.

Collaterals of the ventral spinal column and motor and sensory neurones are established between the 3rd and 5th day. The olfactory reflex tract and muscle movement are present by the 5th day (ORR and WINDLE 1934; WINDLE and AUSTIN 1936); unilateral and ventral flexion and integrated, smooth movement and reflex activity occur by 5$^1/_2$ days of incubation (Table 2). This differentiation includes that of afferent pathways and is not consistent with the speculation of GEREBTZOFF (1959), that the sensory and visceral afferent impulses, carried into the cord via the Lissauer zone and lateral posterior roots, depend functionally on AChE which appears within these structures by the 9th day only.

In view of this considerable neurogenetic and functional development, results of determinations by manometric methods, according to which ChE could not be determined till the 6th day of development, are open to question. On the other hand, manometric determination of the onset of the logarithmic increase of ChE activity on the 15th day may be related to certain neurogenetic and functional events.

The diencephalon is differentiated on the 12th day (KUHLENBECK 1937); pentylenetetrazol (Metrazol) induces electric responses at 9, and typical spiking at 12 days; spontaneous EEG activity is present on the 15th day of development (PETERS et al. 1956). PETERS et al. (o.c.) suggested the following chronological sequence of functionalization of the chick nervous system: medulla, spinal cord and midbrain, diencephalon, and cerebral lobes. The sequence of ontogenesis of ChE, whether estimated histochemically or manometrically, is consistent with that of functionalization. This is, however, an agreement only in general terms, since quantitative manometric measurement of ChE ontogenesis shows no discontinuities during that time, and the curves for several parts of the brain run parallel; the same seems to be true for ACh.

2. Chick retina

LINDEMAN (1947) attempted to correlate ontogenesis of retinal ChE and ACh with development of optic function as determined by the appearance of the pupillary constrictor reflex.

Presence of the pupillary constrictor reflex was tested by flashing a strong light on chick embryos deprived of eyelids, as well as by electric stimulation of the brain. Electric stimulation led to pupillary constriction by the 14th day of incubation, although the true reflex occurred only on the 19th day. Cholinesterase was extracted by means of glycine-NaOH buffer and measured microtitrimetrically; ACh was extracted conventionally after 2 min boiling, and bioassayed.

Cholinesterase and ACh were found in the retina on the 8th day of development and their concentration increased till hatching (20th day). LINDEMAN stated that a peak in the rate of increment was noticeable between the 18th and 20th days of development, coincidentally with the appearance of a true constrictor reflex (19th day); this does not appear too clearly from his data, particularly with regard to ChE activity.

Histochemically (SHEN, GREENFIELD and BOELL 1956), ChE was demonstrated some 4 days earlier than it could be done by LINDEMAN.

The histochemical technique used was that of KOELLE (1951), modified by the present investigators (1955; see above, p. 147). Eyes were removed from the embryo in chick Ringer, frozen in an ether-solid CO_2 mixture, and lyophilized; to facilitate this, the lens was removed from older retinae. For histological studies, tissues fixed in formalin-alcohol-acetic acid or in Zenker-formalin proved least distorted for phase microscopy. Golgi preparations fixed (14 to 18 days) in several changes of 2% potassium dichromate and 1% osmium tetraoxide and impregnated (2 days) in 0.75% $AgNO_3$, were used for tracing of terminal processes of individual neurons.

Prospective ganglion cells were the first structures to stain for AChE at stage 24 ($4^1/_2$ days); by stage 29 (6 days), all ganglion cells of the prospective innermost retinal layer stained for the enzyme (Fig. 7. I). Amacrine cells, immediately external to the ganglion cells, showed AChE shortly thereafter (Fig. 7. II). The enzyme was probably concentrated on the cell surface.

In the case of the optic lobe, neuroblasts migrating peripherad from its germinal layer began to show faint AChE staining by stage 24 or 25 (BONICHON et al. 1958; GEREBTZOFF 1959). Migration was ended by the 12th day, at which time several layers of the optic lobe stained for AChE, the intensity of the stain increasing till hatching (GEREBZOFF 1959).

In the retina, the ganglion cells move away from the external layer at stage 33 or 34, and leave a cell-free zone, the prospective inner plexiform layer (SHEN et al. 1956), which stains diffusely and intensely. One stage later, the enzyme is concentrated in a dark band which soon resolves into two bands, a and d. At this time, phase contrast microscopy and silver staining show that layer d arises from dendrites of ganglion cells, particularly the flask shaped g'' cells which are detached from the main ganglion cell layer, and from branches of axons of small amacrine cells, a' and a''. Cells a' have single processes extending to one of the four AChE-rich bands, or terminating on the ganglion cells; cells a'', located only between the inner nuclear and inner plexiform layer, send collaterals to all 4 bands. In turn, "centrifugal" terminations, originating in the brain, impinge upon the amacrine cells. Therefore, the enzyme accumulates at the surface of the ganglion and amacrine cells *prior* to the arrival at their surface of the synaptic terminals. Silver impregnation indicates that the short dendrites of ganglion cells of the innermost layers do not reach layer d. Layer a arises shortly thereafter from the dendrites of ganglion cells g and ganglion cells g' (Fig. 7. III, IV) which are displaced into the innermost zone of the inner nuclear layer, as well as from the dendrites of the unipolar amacrine terminals; both these types of terminals form a distinct band on silver impregnation.

After gradual increase of the activity of the enzyme in bands a and d and their extension throughout the retina marginad from the fundus, additional weaker bands, b and c, appear by stage 42 (16 days); it can be shown histologically that at that time processes of the amacrine cells (a') terminate in one of the bands as well as on the surface of the ganglion cells. By the 14th or 15th day of incubation, bipolar cells of three distinct types, which do not stain and which occupy zones extending from the outer plexiform layer to the inner nuclear layer, contribute centripetally by some of their terminals to the four AChE-rich zones as well as to the ganglion cells. In addition, giant amacrine cells a, heavily impregnated with silver by the 10th day and located at the internal border of the inner nuclear layer in line with the displaced ganglion cells g', send thick dendrites spreading between the nuclear and inner plexiform layers; this dendritic layer does not stain for AChE.

Faint but definite AChE staining appears within the horizontal cells by the 14th day; histologically, these cells form synapses with visual elements. Moreover, a zone peripherad to the external limiting membrane becomes enzymatically active by the 15th day (stage 41); this is the future location of the myoids of rods and cones (Fig. 7. V).

a) Comment

SHEN, GREENFIELD and BOELL applied their findings to two propositions, firstly that AChE is confined to the sites of synaptic connections of cholinergic

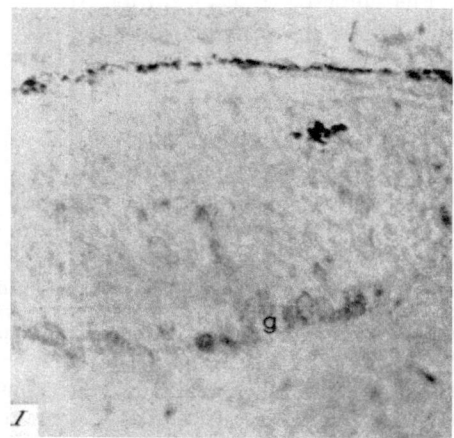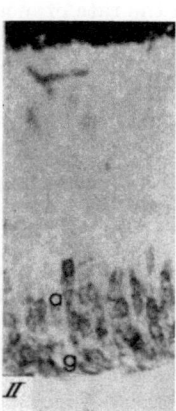

Fig. 7. Histochemical localization of AChE in the chick retina at various stages of embryonic development (from SHEN et al. 1956). Stages according to HAMBURGER and HAMILTON (1951)
7 — *I, II, III*: Transverse sections, 10 μ, uncounterstained. × 350
I. 4½ days (stage 25): only a few ganglion cells (g) in the fundus show definite enzyme activity
II. 8 to 9 days (stage 35): ganglion and amacrine (a) cells stain near the fundus prior to the formation of the inner plexiform layer (IPL)

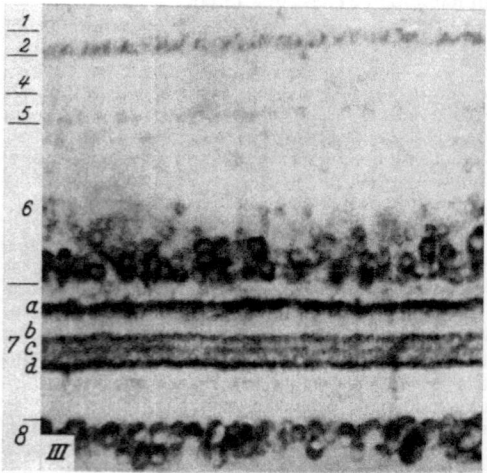

Fig. 7. *III*. At hatching: AChE localization has attained the adult appearance. The enzyme is concentrated in the ganglion cells, 4 bands (a — d) in the IPL, the amacrine cells and the myoids of the visual elements; very slight activity is present in the horizontal cells lining the inner border of the outer plexiform layer (5); other legends: 1 — pigment layer; 2 — rods and cones; 4,5 — outer nuclear and plexiform layers; 6,7 — inner nuclear layer and IPL; 8 — ganglion cell layer.

neurons, and secondly, that secondary neurons (bipolar cells) are cholinergic while primary (cones and rods) and tertiary (ganglion cells) neurons are not, insuring alternation of cholinergic and non-cholinergic synapses in the optic pathways (cf. FELDBERG and VOGT 1948).

It can be said with regard to the first preposition that in the chick no less than in the frog (cf. above p. 147) AChE emerges frequently at the time of arborization and synaptization, as for instance in the case of the formation of the inner plexiform layer. Yet, the enzyme also may arise in the absence of, or prior to, synaptization: ganglion cells stain in transplanted optic vesicles differentiating in the absence of central connections (SHEN 1958); the enzyme of the inner plexiform layer precedes the differentiation of the bipolar cells and the arrival of their terminals.

Localization of AChE in the inner, and its absence from the outer plexiform layer (Fig. 7) agree with the postulate of alternation in the retina of cholinergic and non-cholinergic neurons. Yet, cholinergic neurons cannot be identified by AChE staining alone. Acetylcholinesterase appears in assumedly non-cholinergic tertiary neurons early in retinogenesis and, toward its end, in similarly non-cholinergic visual elements and horizontal cells.

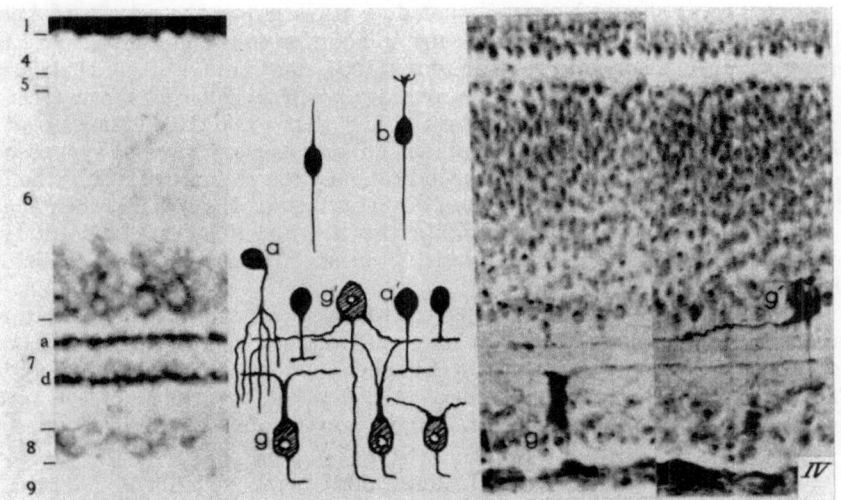

7 — IV, V: Composite of AChE localization, semi-schematic drawings of Golgi preparations and de Castro preparations illustrating synaptic terminals in the inner plexiform layer in relation to enzyme localization

Fig. 7. IV. 12 days (stage 38): axons of bipolar cells (b) do not extend into IPL. Although some amacrine cells terminate in the zone between bands a and d, a conspicuous synaptic band is not present. g′ — displaced ganglion cell; a′ — simple amacrine cell. Other legends as above. x 420

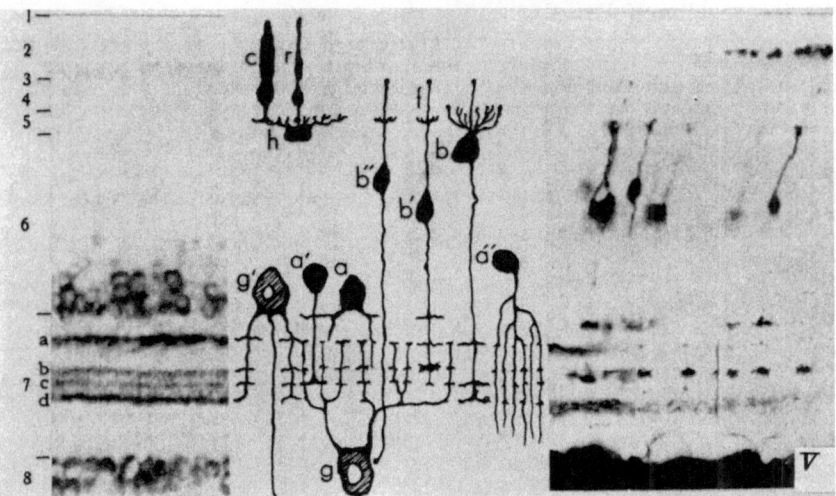

Fig. 7. V. Newly hatched chick. The enzyme appears to be localized in the four synaptic bands in the IPL, in the amacrine and ganglion cells. The bipolar cells and the outer plexiform layer exhibit no enzyme activity. c — cone; r — rod; h — horizontal cell; f — fiber of Landolt; b — b″ various types of bipolar cells. Other legends as above. x 400

Nor can it be stated that cholinergic neurons are the only source of AChE. The enzyme is present at the synapses of primary neurons with the horizontal cells; in Amphibia (see p. 148) the outer layer stains faintly but distinctly at the time of differentiation of primary neurons; finally, the earliest AChE staining of the inner plexiform layer seemed to originate in the dendrites of assumably non-cholinergic ganglion cells.

Altogether, it should be stated that demonstration of the release of ACh, as well as functional analysis are necessary, in addition to the presence of AChE, to identify a neuron as cholinergic (FELDBERG 1957 and Chapter 6). On this basis, it may be suggested that cholinergic neurons synapse in the inner plexiform layer just before hatching. This is suggested by the fact that while ACh is present in the retina from the 12th day of development on, and primary neurons synapse with the horizontal cells by the 15th day, as indicated by the presence of AChE, the light reflex is not established until the 19th day (LINDEMAN 1947). This, then, should be the moment of synaptization within the AChE-rich inner plexiform layer. However, this information is not available on strictly histochemical or histological grounds.

Altogether, it appears clearly that AChE, assayed at strategic sites, can be related to synaptization although it may not characterize all synapses; secondly, when AChE is considered jointly with the other member of the cholinergic system, ACh, as well as with function, it may predicate the occurrence of the specific biochemical and anatomical steps leading to functionalization.

III. Mammals

1. Ontogenesis of mammalian ChE's in the nervous system

NACHMANSOHN tried early (1938—1940; cf. also YOUNGSTROM 1941) to pinpoint the physiological significance of ChE by associating its ontogenesis or early postnatal development in various mammals with the development of function and behavior, two lines followed since by many investigators.

Also at that time NACHMANSOHN (1939b) presented data on the differential distribution of the enzyme in various parts of adult mammalian brain. Cholinesterase was found to be more concentrated in the diencephalon, corpora quadrigemina, and cerebellum than in telencephalon and olfactory bulbs; it was found also to be quite concentrated in the "rest of the brain" (o.c.), and this may be today ascribed to the high concentration of the enzyme in the medulla and the mesencephalon. The same distribution was found in the brains of all mammalian species investigated, as well as in those of the fetus or of the infant; on the other hand, the adult showed relatively more ChE in the brain than in the spinal cord, while the reverse was true in the fetus (cf. infra).

NACHMANSOHN used manometric techniques (p. 131); his Q and T values for ChE activity correspond to mg of ACh hydrolyzed per hour per 100 mg of fresh tissue, and by the whole organ, respectively. KAVALER and KIMEL (1952) similarly used the manometric technique and employed the differential substrates, MeCh and BzCh, to distinguish between AChE and BuChE. Manometric techniques and several differential substrates were also used by RISLEY and DAVIES (1953b), ELKES, EAYRS and TODRICK (1955) and by BAYLIS and TODRICK (1953b); the last mentioned authors employed also the specific inhibitors, 1,5-bis (4′trimethylammonium-phenyl) pentan-3-one diiodide (Wellcome 62-C 47) and ethopropazine methosulphate (Lysivane, cf. BAYLIS and TODRICK 1953a) to differentiate between BuChE and AChE. METZLER and HUMM (1951) used the technique of SAWYER (1943a and b, cf. p. 144). Manometric techniques and ACh substrate were employed by HIMWICH and his associates (v. HIMWICH and APRISON 1955). In his work on the human embryo, YOUNGSTROM (1941) used a bioassay already described (cf. p. 144). He reported enzymic activity in mg of ACh iodide hydrolyzed by 100 g of tissue (dry weight) per hour. Fetuses were obtained from therapeutic abortions.

a) Prenatal development

In the *sheep*, gestation period 147 days, NACHMANSOHN (1940b) found relatively high levels of the spinal cord enzyme in the 60-day fetus, which was the earliest specimen examined. The Q values were 11.6 and 12.9 in the second cervical and eighth dorsal segment, respectively. In the former, the enzyme activity decreased steadily till on the 136th day — the last investigated — the Q value was 5.6. In the dorsal segment enzymic activity first increased and a peak (Q value of about 16) was reached on the 80th day; it decreased subsequently to a Q value of 5.0 recorded on the 136th day. In the 60-day brain the Q values were lower, and varied from 1.3 in the cortex to 5.1 in the corpora quadrigemina; they started increasing at about the 75th to 80th day of gestation, the increase being more rapid in the caudate nucleus than in the corpora quadrigemina, cerebellum, and the cortex (Q values at 136th day were: 32.6, 15.5, 13.3, and 3.4 respectively; the differences are even more pronounced when expressed in terms of T values). Thus, while 90 days before birth enzymic activity was lower in the brain than in the spinal cord, 14 days before birth most parts of the brain except for cortex were richer in the enzyme than the spinal cord.

The decrease of enzymic activity in the spinal cord during this period was explained by NACHMANSOHN as being due to the dilution in the course of development of enzyme-rich spinal grey matter by enzyme-poor myelin sheaths. Similarly, he thought that the Q value for the 8th dorsal segment was higher than that of other spinal segments because the 8th segment has a higher ratio of cell bodies.

Using whole brain of the *rat*, METZLER and HUMM (o.c.) found the earliest indication of the enzyme on the 14th or 16th day of gestation, i.e., about one week before birth; the increase of the enzymic activity was slow till birth. In the cerebral cortex of the *guinea pig*, KAVALER and KIMEL (1952) found the first measurable AChE activity on the 28th day of gestation, i.e., some 40 days prior to parturition. The enzyme remained constant till the 35th day of gestation and thereafter increased rapidly, reaching its peak at birth. Finally, in the case of the *rabbit*, HIMWICH and APRISON (1955) found ChE activity in the brain of a 20-day old embryo — the youngest investigated — 12 days before parturition. As in the adult, the highest enzymic levels were found in the medulla and caudate nucleus, and lowest in the frontal cortex; the increase during fetal life was also slowest in the latter.

Similarly, KAKUSHKINA and ARKHIPOVA (1941) found at 15 days relatively low levels of ChE's in whole embryos of the rabbit; the activity increased till parturition.

Similar data were obtained in the *human* fetus (YOUNGSTROM 1941). In the central nervous system of the fifty-six-day embryo — the earliest studied — the highest values were found in the spinal cord, midbrain and medulla (values of 3 to 4), and the lowest in the cerebral hemispheres (less than 1). Incidentally, the highest ChE activity (value of 9) was found in the liver. Subsequently, the enzymic activity increased, first in the midbrain and then in succession in the spinal cord, diencephalon, basal ganglia, and cerebral hemispheres. The first three areas showed a particularly rapid rate of increase of enzymic activity; in the spinal cord, a particularly rapid rate was encountered between the 80th and 120th day of development. The cerebellum was first assayed on the 102nd day; the value of 10 found at that time doubled by the 189th day.

KALOW (personal communication) found manometrically (BzCh substrate) that between the 5th and 9th month BuChE activity decreased when measured on the dry weight basis, and increased when calculated on the wet weight basis.

While all these data indicate the appearance of ChE during the prenatal development of various mammals, GEREBTZOFF (1955) using his modification of the histochemical method, found no enzyme in the brain or in the spinal cord of the fetal *mouse*. While the mouse seems thus to differ from other mammalian species investigated, this aberrant result may be attributable to technical drawbacks of GEREBTZOFF's method (cf. above, p. 151).

b) Postnatal rat

In the rat, the spinal cord is at birth richer in AChE and BuChE than the brain (BAYLIS and TODRICK 1953 b; ELKES and TODRICK 1955). This situation is reversed about two weeks later, since in the cord the enzyme activity and the ratio between the true and pseudo enzyme (15 : 1) remained constant between the 1st and 4th week of postnatal development while AChE activity of the brain increased; immediately after birth this increase was particularly rapid (300 units per day; BAYLIS and TODRICK o.c., METZLER and HUMM 1951). Subsequently, the activity of the spinal cord enzyme decreased to values 1/3 of those recorded at birth (RISLEY and DAVIES 1953).

There seems to be a divergence of opinion as to the subsequent fate of the AChE. Several investigators have reported a continued increase of the enzymic activity in the postnatal rat, extending into adulthood; other workers recorded a decrease, although they differ as to the moment of the onset of this decrease. ELKES, EAYRS and TODRICK (1955) reported an increase between the 1st and 77th postnatal day, and RISLEY and DAVIES (1953) a 4-fold increase between birth and adulthood. ELKES and TODRICK (1955) confined this increase within two reference periods, one extending from the 8th to the 22nd day, and another from the 22nd to 77th day of postnatal development. Acetylcholinesterase increases rapidly during both periods in the caudate nucleus (reaching there the highest activity value recorded — 23,700 μl of CO_2 per g of wet weight per hr), rhinencephalon, olfactory bulb, and cerebral cortex, and slowly in the thalamus; the increases are more rapid during the first than during the second period. The enzymic activity increases during the first period only in the medulla, midbrain, and cerebellum. Similarly, NACHMANSOHN (1939 b) reported continuous increases between the 10th and 110th days of rat postnatal development in the telencephalon, diencephalon, olfactory lobes, corpora quadrigemina, and cerebellum; a slight decrease may have occurred during the end of this period in "the rest of the brain". Finally, RISLEY and DAVIES (1953) reported a 4-fold increase between birth and adulthood of enzymes splitting ACh, MeCh, BzCh, BuCh, and propionyl-choline; this agrees with the data of FREEDMAN and HIMWICH (1948).

On the other hand, BAYLIS and TODRICK (o.c.) and METZLER and HUMM (o.c.) found a peak of AChE activity at 20 or 22 days, and a subsequent decrease of activity to a level half as high as that at the peak. Thereafter, beginning with the 100th to 120th day of postnatal development the activity remained more or less constant. While ROSENZWEIG and his collaborators (1958a, 1958b) also reported a decrease of ChE's in the rat cortex beginning at 108 days, they found that the decrease of activity never levelled off, but continued through adulthood till the 401st day of age, the total decrease amounting to 15% (for methods used by ROSEN-ZWEIG et al., o.c., and their reliability, cf. infra p. 166).

It is generally agreed that BuChE of the rat brain increases during postnatal development.

ELKES and TODRICK (o.c.) found increases between the 8th and 77th days in the midbrain, thalamus, caudate nucleus, and cerebral cortex, and during the earlier part of this period (8th and 22nd postnatal days) in the medulla and cerebellum; there was no increase in the olfactory bulb. Thus, except for the olfactory bulb, the patterns and the rates of increase of AChE and BuChE activities were similar. In the olfactory bulb, the AChE/BuChE ratio increased from 0.9 at 9 days to 4.2 at 77 days; elsewhere it varied little with time, but considerably from area to area, being less than 2 in the cerebellum and between 13.8 (8th day) and 19.1 (77th day) in the caudate nucleus. The activity of BuChE toward BzCh was reported by ELKES and TODRICK to be much less than that of AChE toward MeCh. It was suggested by the writers that the rise of brain BuChE between the 10th and 23rd postnatal days may be related to the rapid increase of brain capillaries at that time (HORNE CRAIGIE 1955); in fact, KOELLE (1954) suggested that BuChE is located in the walls of the capillaries and of the muscle fibers of the arterioles and venules, and in the glia. A four-fold increase of the activity of an enzyme splitting BuCh and BzCh between birth and adulthood was reported by RISLEY and DAVIES (1953).

A quantitative difference exists between these data and those of BAYLIS and TODRICK (1953b). BAYLIS and TODRICK (o.c.) also noted the increase in the activity of rat brain BuChE beginning with the 10th postnatal day, but they reported a peak on the 23rd day. At birth, the activities were 150 and 200 μl CO_2/hr for BuChE and AChE, respectively; by the 23rd postnatal day the value for BuChE was as high as that for AChE. This high level of the pseudoenzyme in the central nervous system is somewhat surprising; since pertinent data were reported only in an abstract it is difficult to evaluate them critically. However, it appears from the subsequent review paper of ELKES and TODRICK (1955) that BuCh, the substrate split preferentially by BuChE but also to some extent by AChE, was used in conjunction with an AChE inhibitor,

1,5-bis (4'-trimethylammonium-phenyl) pentan-3-one diiodide (WELLCOME 62-C47) at a concentration of 10^{-6} M. Data of COPP (1953), to which ELKES and TODRICK refer, are insufficient to ascertain whether or not this concentration of the inhibitor was sufficient to block all AChE activity and permit readings of the pseudoenzyme alone; the allyl congener of WELLCOME 62-C47, B.W. 284, inhibits AChE completely only at levels of about 10^{-5} M (KOELLE 1955).

α) ACh in the central nervous system of the postnatal rat. It is of interest that in the rat the changes in the concentration of free and bound ACh of the developing brain and in the spinal cord are parallel with those of AChE (WELSH and HYDE 1944).

At birth, rat medulla contained from two to four times more ACh than the brainstem (0.6 and 0.28 μg/g respectively), pallium or cerebellum. While between the 1st and 21st to 26th day of postnatal development, the ACh content increased relatively little in the medulla and in the pallium and even decreased during this period in the cerebellum, it rose 3-fold in the brainstem. After the 26th day, the ACh content decreased in the brainstem and in the medulla. On the basis of the brain as a whole, the level of ACh increased from infancy to adulthood.

c) Postnatal ChE in other species

The detailed data presented for the rat may serve as a framework of reference for other mammalian species studied. Postnatal increase of the brain enzymes were recorded in the *rabbit* (NACHMANSOHN 1939 b; KAKUSHKINA and ARKHIPOVA 1941; HIMWICH and APRISON 1955) and in the *mouse* (GEREBTZOFF 1955). The pattern in the rabbit resembled on the whole that described for the postnatal rat.

While the activity increased in all parts of the brain except in the medulla and the cortex (i.e., in the telencephalon, diencephalon, corpora striata and quadrigemina, nucleus caudatus and superior colliculus; cerebellum), the increase did not persist in all these parts from birth to adulthood and the final levels were different. Generally, the increase terminated between the 20th and 31st days (NACHMANSOHN o.c.) or even earlier (HIMWICH and APRISON o.c.); as in the rat, the highest values seem to be reached in the caudate nucleus and corpora quadrigemina. No decrease was noticed up to 4 years of age except in the medulla, where the adult activity is about 2/3 of that reached on the 20th day.

While GEREBTZOFF (1955), using his modification of the thiocholine histochemical technique, recorded a similar increase in the brain of *mice*, particularly in the corpora striata and in the amygdaloid nucleus, and found this increase to be especially pronounced between the 13th and 15th days of postnatal development, he recorded also rapid increases in the spinal cord. This result is different from those recorded for the spinal cord of the rat and the rabbit medulla by many investigators.

The method (v. p. 151) was designed to demonstrate AChE. In the spinal cord, the staining increased rapidly between the 1st and 28th postnatal days; a particularly rapid increase occurred between the 13th and 15th days. On the 28th day the intensity of staining reached peak (adult) levels and was as heavy in the cord as in the brain. The increase was particularly rapid in the anterior horn motoneurones. Moreover, the vicinity of the ependymal cells and the surface of the neighboring neuroblasts stained well during the 2nd postnatal day; this staining weakened subsequently till it disappeared between the 7th and 30th days. Parenthetically, the ependyma of the brain did not stain.

GEREBTZOFF suggested that the ependymal enzyme may have a role unrelated to transmission processes. He suggested also that the particularly rapid rise noticed on the 13th to 15th postnatal days might be related to the fact that at this time the mouse opens its eyes. It is difficult to see from GEREBETZOFF's tables (o.c.) how his qualitative method could distinguish changes in the rate of increase of enzyme activity. As interesting as his two comments are, they should be considered in the light of certain limitation of his method, considered more fully earlier (cf. p. 151).

This pattern of postnatal increase of the activity of cerebral AChE in the rabbit, mouse, and rat, and of the brain levels' overtaking the initially higher spinal cord or medullary levels is not repeated in the guinea pig and the cat. NACHMANSOHN (1939 b and 1940 a) showed that in the *guinea pig* there is, between the 1st and the 19th postnatal days, a slight decrease of the enzyme activity in the telencephalon, diencephalon, and cerebellum, and a striking four-fold lowering in the anterior corpora quadrigemina. Similarly, KAVALER and KIMEL (o.c.) found that the motor

11*

cortex of the guinea pig shows at term AChE activity a little lower than that of the adult cortex. Parenthetically, while in the *guinea pig* the telencephalic enzyme was as active as that of the diencephalon, the diencephalic enzyme was much more active in the *rabbit, mouse,* and *rat.*

It is possible that, insofar as BuChE is concerned, the human brain resembles that of the guinea pig. KALOW (personal communication) found between the 6th and 80th years of life a continual decrease in the activity of human cerebral BuChE, whether calculated on wet or dry weight basis; the decrease over this span amounted to about 2/3.

In the *cat* there is little enzymic increase between the newborn and the 21-day old animal in the case of telencephalon, diencephalon, and cerebellum, although in the corpora quadrigemina the enzyme activity increases two-fold.

2. Comment

Many investigators attempted to correlate rather categorically ontogenesis of ChE of the mammalian central nervous system with neurogenesis and function. It can be listed as an argument in favor of this that, as in the case of Amphibia (p. 149), ontogenesis of enzymes concerned with cellular respiration and energetics differs from that of ChE.

In the *guinea pig* cortex (FLEXNER 1952, 1955a, 1955b), apyrase and cytochrome oxidase appear some 4 weeks after ChE; acid phosphatase and succinic oxidase, while coincidental with ChE, do not show rapid increases in activity till parturition.

In the postnatal *rat* dephosphorylation does not increase till about 10 days (JORDAN and MARCH 1955), and cerebrosides not till 20 days after birth; (cf. NEEDHAM 1931); glucose-6-phosphate dehydrogenase, phosphorus, cholesterol, and phosphatides remain constant between birth and adulthood. In the *human*, postnatal development of cerebrosides, phosphorus, cholesterol, and phosphatides occurs relatively late, while oxygen consumption probably does not change much during fetal life, and increases rapidly postnatally (RAIHA 1954). Again, these patterns do not resemble that of ChE.

Another argument in favor of functional significance of central ChE was advanced by NACHMANSOHN (1939b and 1940a). He pointed out that while the *guinea pig* is born fairly mature, has at birth synaptically differentiated central neurons, and exhibits postnatally no increase of Q values of brain ChE, the opposite is true of the rat, mouse, and rabbit.

The related suggestion (o.c.; KAVALER and KIMMEL 1952) that brains of species immature at birth should have low Q values cannot be substantiated (Table 3). This may be due to the fact that ChE activities reported by various investigators (Table 3) differ considerably, even when referring to one and the same species, perhaps because of differences in the substrates or substrate concentrations used. Uncertainties involved in comparing Q values at birth in various species may be contrasted with the apparent validity of comparing postnatal patterns of ChE of the rat and of the guinea pig. While ChE activity of various parts of the guinea pig brain is not necessarily higher than that of corresponding areas of the rat brain, it increases postnatally only slightly as compared to a rapid increase of the rat brain enzyme lasting for at least 22 days (Table 3). Concomitantly, the rat is born very immature after only 21 days of gestation; the young has its eyes shut and for some 4 days postnatally is capable of only simple reflexes and movements, such as sucking, squeaking, and flexing the body and tail, while the piglet, born after a gestation of 66 days, can walk and see almost as soon as it is born (cf. NEEDHAM 1931).

Finally, in certain species some degree of relationship could be established between ChE and specific neurogenetic and behavioral phenomena. In the *guinea pig* the first appearance of cortical AChE on the 28th day of gestation antedates the first responses to cortical stimulation by 3 days (CARMICHAEL 1934; KAVALER and KIMMEL 1952), while its rapid growth coincides with the critical period of electrical (JASPER et al. 1937) and cytological (PETERS and FLEXNER 1950; FLEXNER 1955b) maturation of the cortex. This agrees rather well with the thesis of KAVALER and KIMEL (1952) that a certain level of AChE activity is essential for cortical function.

Table 3. *Cholinesterase activity and maturity at birth in various mammalian species*

Species	Length of gestation (days)	Maturity at parturition	Cholinesterase activity at or about parturition in Q values[1]		Postnatal increase of ChE	Substrate and concentration
			Spinal cord	Brain level (as indicated)		
Guinea pig	66	Mature		9.1 Diencephalon 4.2 Telencephalon 8.2 Corp.quadrigem. (NACHMANSOHN 1939b) 3.7 Cortex (KAVALER and KIMEL 1952)	Little increase in all areas investigated	ACh; 0.014 M (NACHMANSOHN 1939b) ACh; 0.045 M (KAVALER and KIMEL 1952)
Sheep	147	Relatively Mature	5.0—5.6	3.4 Cortex 35.5 Nu.caudat. (at 138 days NACHMANSOHN 1940b) 13.5 Corp. quadrigem.		ACh; 0.014 M
Rat	21	Immature		5.4 Diencephalon 2.7 Telencephalon 5.0 Corp. quadrigem. (NACHMANSOHN 1939b) 0.9 Caudate nu. (ELKES et al. 1955)	Four-fold increase in telencephalon and corp. quadrigem. Four-fold increase in caudate nu.	ACh; 0.014 M (NACHMANSOHN 1939b) MeCh; 0.03 M (ELKES et al. 1955)
Rabbit	32	Immature		9.1 Diencephalon 2.3 Telencephalon 8.9 Corp. quadrigem. (NACHMANSOHN1939b) 2.6 Cortex 15.6 Caudate nu. (HIMWICH and APRISON 1955)	2.5-fold increase in corp. quadrigem. and telenceph. almost 2-fold increase in diencephalon 2—2.5-fold increase in both areas	ACh; 0.014 M (NACHMANSOHN 1939b) ACh; 0.005 M (HIMWICH and APRISON 1955)
Cat	62—63	Relatively immature		2.3 Telencephalon 6.7 Diencephalon 8.9 Corp. quadrigem. (NACHMANSOHN 1939b)	Almost 2-fold increase in telenceph. and corp. quadrigem., less elsewhere	ACh; 0.014 M (NACHMANSOHN 1939b)

[1] In the cases of data of HIMWICH and APRISON (1955), ELKES et al. (1955), and KAVALER and KIMEL (1952), ChE activity recalculated and expressed in Q values.

Glial cells which are rich in BuChE (KOELLE 1954) might have to be considered also; McILWAIN (1955) pointed out between the 43rd and 46th days of gestation, glial cells, rather than neurons, multiply and differentiate.

Spinal motility (flexion) of the guinea pig embryo precedes cortical responsiveness and maturation; while pertinent data are not available, it is likely also that the enzyme appeared in subcortical areas earlier than in the cortex.

On the other hand, in other species function correlates with ChE less well or not at all. METZLER and HUMM (o.c.) suggested that a relationship exists for the *rat*. They quoted ANGULO Y GONZALES (1932) as finding that from the 14th day of gestation, at which time the fetus is immobile, to parturition there is only "a slight increase in ability to respond," and correlated this with the appearance of ChE on the 16th day of development, its slow increase until birth, and rapid increase subsequently. However, they interpreted the findings of ANGULO Y GONZALES incorrectly; in fact, he described well established spontaneous and reflex activity in the rat fetus at the time of the first finding of ChE; also, rapid progress of integration and of complexity of behavior, and appearance of spontaneous movement occur long before the postnatal phase of rapid increase of enzymic activity.

It should be added that the micrometric technique employed by METZLER and HUMM could measure enzyme activity corresponding to the hydrolysis of 0.9 μg of ACh chloride (SAWYER 1943; cf. p. 144) and was some 10 times more sensitive than the manometric method by means of which KAVALER and KIMMEL (1952) established to an extent parallelism between cortical function and ChE in the guinea pig.

In the case of the *sheep*, correlation is difficult, since the earliest fetus studied for ChE (NACHMANSOHN 1940 b) was 60 days old, i.e., exhibited extero- and proprioceptive reflex movements for 25, and complex, generalized motility for 16 days (BARCROFT and BARRON 1939; BARRON 1941; for review, v. HOOKER 1952). The activity of the brain enzyme did not increase rapidly till the 75th or 80th day of gestation; at that time systems located in the midbrain and the intercalated neurons (inter- and intra-segmental internuncial cells) had been mature functionally and morphologically for about a month. Thus, while the caudo-cephalad sequence of ontogenesis of sheep ChE agrees in the general sense with that of neurogenesis and function, the statement of NACHMANSOHN that there is "a close relationship between the time when the synapses begin to function and the appearance of a high concentration of choline esterase" (1940a, p. 580) may be unduly optimistic.

The earliest *human* fetus in which ChE was measured (56 days, YOUNGSTROM 1941) was, in contradistinction to the sheep embryo, just exhibiting the first reflexes (contralateral flexion of the neck and uppermost trunk upon exteroceptive stimulation; HOOKER 1952). Subsequent rapid increase of the midbrain and spinal enzyme (11th—17th week) may be related to the extension of the pattern of response from the neck to the trunk and limbs. Yet, it is impossible to relate this increase specifically to the rapid increase and "totalization" of the response pattern between the 13th and 14th weeks. Nor it is clear why a high level of enzyme activity was encountered very early in the spinal cord and why it increased so notably at this site; indeed, trunk and lower limbs are not included in the behavior pattern till considerably later (HOOKER, o.c.). The role of BuChE in the relatively young brain (KALOW 1960) is also obscure.

3. AChE, aging, and "adaptive" behavior of rats

ROSENZWEIG et al. (1948a and b) tried to relate levels of AChE activity to a pattern of rat behavior which they throught characterizes a flexible (intelligent?) animal.

These findings are unusual and warrant a rather detailed description of methods. Three strains of rats of CASTLE and TRYON breeds were used; it was stated that they differ significantly in the levels of cortical ChE activity. Samples were obtained from the visual and somaesthetic cortex and from the subcortical brain. They were analyzed fresh, or quick-frozen and stored till the day of measurement. Samples were homogenized and 7.5 to 12.0 mg aliquots brought up to volume of 12 ml with saline. After an initial equilibration period of 10 minutes, the hydrolysis of 0.1 M ACh was titrated with 0.005 M NaOH over a 10 to 12 minute period in a Nielands-Cannon automatic titrator. After correction for "blank" hydrolysis of ACh, the results were expressed as mol of $ACh \times 10^{10}$ per minute per mg of tissue. ROSENZWEIG et al. used 1,5-bis (4'-trimethyl-ammonium-phenyl) pentan-3-one diiodide (Wellcome 62-C47), a selective inhibitor of AChE, to show that less than 5% of the activity of their homogenates could be attributed to pseudocholinesterase. It may be assumed (v. ROSENZWEIG et al. 1958a, p. 344) that they used Wellcome 62-C47 at the concentration employed by ELKES and TODRICK 1955; if so, this method of differentiation between the two enzymes may be open to criticism.

Psychological experiments were carried out in a Hypothesis Apparatus, which is a maze that cannot be solved by the rat, and in which alleys of choice are labeled by light and darkness, and, of course, by spatial orientation (left and right). In this maze, most rats show at first light orientation. Those animals which subsequently follow spatial directions were considered as "adaptive" because they ceased to persist in light preference as they learned that this behavior is not rewarded, and tended instead to "test other hypotheses." When the maze was then arranged so as to become progressively soluble with regard to space orientation, the adaptive, "spatial" rats took advantage of this situation. When, to the contrary, light cues, first meaningless, became progressively correct, "adaptive" rats were penalized since they abandoned "light hypothesis" when it was originally proven incorrect, while "light oriented" animals, which retained their "hypothesis" longer and developed stereotypic behavior, were rewarded under these circumstances.

ROSENZWEIG et al. (o.c.) claimed first of all that "spatial" rats show a significantly higher level of AChE in the cortical areas than "light-directed", less adaptive rats. Moreover, while they found in all rats that AChE decreases between the 108th and 401st day of age, as already described (v. supra, p. 162), they claimed that this decrease is slower in "adaptive" than in "non-adaptive" rats. They found also that relative rather than absolute enzyme activities are pertinent: "spatial" rats of a strain characterized by a low inherent enzyme activity are richer in AChE than the "light-oriented" rats of the same strain, although they may have less enzyme than "light oriented" rats of a strain characterized by a high AChE activity.

They found also that strains characterized by considerable heterogeneity of cortical enzymic activity can be bred selectively for high and low AChE titers, and that the differences become significant by the third generation.

It should be stated that the differences in question are small, although ROSENZWEIG et al. considered them statistically significant. For instance, the difference in AChE activity between enzymically rich and poor strains amounted to about 12%; differences between "adaptive" and "non-adaptive" rats at the age for which the greatest divergence was claimed were less than 5%. In fact, in the former case the difference would have been much smaller if the authors had considered subcortical rather than cortical enzyme.

Variability of AChE measurement was not stated. While the statistical treatment of data by ROSENZWEIG et al. cannot be fully considered here, it should be mentioned that some of the analysis is based on the χ^2 test and on Fisher's r to z transformation; in this analysis, AChE levels were not averaged but classified in two categories as being above or below the strain mean, and correlated with spatial or light preference.

It is also most surprising that the "adaptive" and "non-adaptive" rats did not exhibit the difference in the levels of enzyme activity at the time of the behavioral test, but only 30 days later. Finally, the criterion which the authors used in evaluation of the adaptive behavior has been criticized (KLÜVER 1958). Altogether, it cannot be easily accepted at present that levels of "intelligence" or "adaptivity" of behavior can be related to small differences of AChE levels. In fact, DFP and eserine, injected into the visual or somatic cortex in subconvulsive or even convulsive doses (2 to 7 μg per animal), did not affect hypothesis behavior of rats (CHOW and JOHN 1958).

B. Ontogenesis of ChE's in the vertebrate muscle and heart

I. Striated muscle and neuromyal junction

1. Time of appearance of ChE's and their ontogenetic pattern

Manometric methods were used by NACHMANSOHN (1938—1940; v. p. 131), RISLEY and DAVIES (1953; v. p. 160); TORDA (1938), DOMINI (1938), and KUPFER and KOELLE (1951). NACHMANSOHN on one hand and TORDA and DOMINI on the other reported drastically different Q values although they all worked on the same chick tissue. SAWYER's (1943b) microtitrimetric method and YOUNGSTROM's (1941) bioassay technique were already described (p. 144).

For histochemical methods used by KUPFER and KOELLE (1951) and by GEREBTZOFF (1954) see p. 147 and p. 151. LEWIS and HUGHES (1957) fixed the tissues in formalin and stained for ChE by the β-naphthylacetate method of ZACKS (1954; v. p. 151). BONICHON (1957b) used basically the method of GEREBTZOFF with prolonged formalin fixation.

The first appearance of ChE generally preceded that of innervation. In the *rat*, AChE appeared at 16 days of development, i.e., some 4 days before muscle becomes innervated, but more or less coincidentally with function (KUPFER and KOELLE 1951). In the *sheep*, NACHMANSOHN (1940b) found ChE in the intercostal and extrinsic eye muscles at about the 100th day of development, i.e., 7 weeks prior to birth and before the appearance of the endplates at 137 days (DICKSON 1940). In the *human* embryo of 56 days — the earliest investigated — the Q value of the skeletal muscle was already higher than that of the spinal cord, and as high as that of the midbrain and of the medulla (YOUNGSTROM 1941); it is thus likely that the appearance of the enzyme preceded the innervation of the muscle and onset of motility which take place at $7^1/_2$ weeks (v. p. 166). In the *guinea pig* (GEREBTZOFF 1954, 1959) AChE was present in the noninnervated myoblast at 19 days. In *Amblystoma* the enzyme was present in the muscle already at stage 13 (SAWYER 1943b); in fact, till stage 36, its activity was higher than that of the nervous system. SHEN (1958) however, using the Cartesian microdiver as well as histochemical techniques, claimed that ChE appeared at the time of innervation of axial musculature (stage 36). This information is available from a review and the data, to the best of this reviewer's knowledge, are not described in detail elsewhere. Finally, in the *chick*, ChE could be demonstrated histochemically (BONICHON 1957b) and manometrically (TORDA 1938; DOMINI 1938) at 100 hrs of development; this is the time of the first movement and precedes innervation by some 2 days (GEREBTZOFF 1959).

On the other hand, in the *toad, Xenopus laevis*, LEWIS and HUGHES found no ChE before the appearance of innervation in the muscle and the onset of tail movement. Cholinesterase staining was localized at the end of muscle fibers where the Bodian stain indicated the presence of the myoneural junctions. It is likely, however, that formalin fixation interfered with earlier localization of the enzyme.

It seems also generally true that enzyme activity increased rapidly after its first appearance, reaching a peak at either birth or hatching, or, in *Amblystoma*, at the onset of feeding stages. Subsequently, the activity diminished to descend to a relatively low adult level. This was true in the rat (KUPFER and KOELLE 1951; RISLEY and DAVIES 1953), rabbit (TORDA, 1938; LEIBSON 1939; RYABINOWSKAJA 1940), chick (NACHMANSOHN o.c.; TORDA o.c.; DOMINI 1938), and, finally, in *Amblystoma*, where the activity was at its lowest after metamorphosis, i.e., when *Amblystoma* acquires a terrestrial habitat.

Manometric data agreed with histochemical ones; in the latter case, staining reached its maximum intensity and concentration at the endplate (v. infra) at or about birth; this was described for the rat (KUPFER and KOELLE 1951), cat, dog, and chick (GEREBTZOFF et al. 1954). The changes in enzymic activity of the muscle were conspicuous. In the chick, a 10-fold increase of Q value occurred between the 5th and 11th day of development (TORDA, o.c.), and a 20-fold decrease was noticed between hatching and adulthood (NACHMANSOHN, 1938b, c). In the human, the increase between 8 and 11 weeks of development was about 60-fold; it was as rapid as, and parallel with that of the brain enzyme, although it occurred later than the increase of spinal cord ChE's (YOUNGSTROM 1941). It is possible that these changes affect AChE and BuChE differentially; in the rat, the AChE/BuChE ratio may increase from birth to adulthood (RISLEY et al. o.c.).

2. Cytological pattern of ontogenesis

In several species, ChE appeared first in the form of scattered granules in the sarcoplasm of the as yet non-innervated myoblasts; subsequently, it aggregated and concentrated about the prospective endplate. However, in the chick, rat, and other species, ChE's accumulated also at the point of tendon insertion, where early in development ChE staining appeared to be more intense than at the region of the future endplate (GEREBTZOFF 1959; BONICHON 1957 b). At the peak of enzymic activity, staining appeared particularly compact within a small endplate area of the rat, dog, and chick (KUPFER and KOELLE 1951; GEREBTZOFF et al. 1954); in the chick and rat, staining at the tendon insertion point decreased at that time (o.c.).

LEWIS and HUGHES were of the opinion that in the toad, *Xenopus laevis*, innervation determined the distribution of the enzyme (cf. supra). In muscles in which the nerves run lengthwise, ChE staining appeared along the path of the nerve at intervals of 30 to 40 μ, or it was found at the sites where the nerve fiber crossed the muscle fibers. Finally, in the abdominal musculature the nerve sent off a fine, short twig, making a single contact in the shape of the synaptic knob, with the muscle fiber.

In the albino *rat* (KUPFER and KOELLE 1951) and in the *guinea pig* (GEREBTZOFF 1954, 1959) scattered granules of AChE staining appeared first in the uninnervated myoblast on the 16th and 19th day, respectively, and aggregated into large bodies subsequently. Another staining appeared in the vicinity of the tendon insertion and rapidly became intense; this was true also of the cat (GEREBTZOFF o.c.). In the *rat*, these bodies could be later identified as muscle nuclei oriented along the fiber axis; still later, the enzyme concentrated at the nuclear surface. At 19 days the nuclei came together. Weaker-staining nuclei aggregated peripherally immediately beneath the sarcolemma to serve as satellite nuclei about the site of the future endplate; deeper-staining nuclei remained in the center and formed a soleplate-like structure resembling that of the guinea pig (GEREBTZOFF o.c.). Throughout these processes myofibrils increased in number, and the muscle fibers grew more rapidly than the future endplate. At birth, the darker-staining nuclei formed a horseshoe-shaped structure of a diameter up to 80 μ, with lighter satellite and still lighter fusiform nuclei at the periphery. There was no AChE beyond this area.

Extreme localization of the enzyme occurred shortly after birth; at 9 days of age AChE activity concentrated in granules at the surface of approximately 4 nuclei. At about this time the endplate staining caught up with that of the musculo-tendinous apparatus. GEREBTZOFF et al. found, however, that in the young rat the difference in staining between the muscle and the endplate was not as pronounced as in the adult. Subsequently, the endplate of the rat as well as those of the cat and dog may increase in size (GEREBTZOFF o.c.).

Although between the 9th and the 16th postnatal day the nerve endings abound and arborize within the muscle cell, there seemed to be no significant enzyme in nerve fibers or Schwann cells (KUPFER and KOELLE o.c.); in the adult endplate, the "beads" of muscle cells leading to the endplate may be mistaken for staining nerve fiber or Schwann cell.

This cytological picture of differentiation of mammalian muscle ChE resembled that in the chick. Sarcoplasmic, scattered granules appeared on the 4th day (BONICHON 1957 b); they began to concentrate at the ends of the myoblast at the time when the nerve fibers reached the myotome (6th day). Staining concentrated and intensified further through the 7th day, forming at that time spherical structures at tendon insertion points. The tendon staining increased subsequently, while that of the sarcoplasm diminished. On the 10th day a few fibers stained at the equatorial endplate region. While both the tendon and the endplate stained more intensely subsequently, activity of the endplate enzyme caught up with that of the tendon at the 21st day, i.e., at hatching.

3. Origin of ChE of the neuromyal junction

The above results, with the exception perhaps of the data of LEWIS and HUGHES, indicate that the enzyme appears in the muscle of various vertebrates before the contact of the nerve with the muscle cells. KUPFER and KOELLE (o.c.) pointed out that even after innervation the enzyme does not seem to be present in significant concentrations in the nerve fibers or Schwann cells. Experiments with nerveless muscle and tissue culture data support on the whole the notion that at least some ChE originates in non-neural elements.

To produce *Amblystoma* embryo with a nerveless muscle, the spinal cord and the neural crest were removed prior to the outgrowth of nerve fibers (stages 23—27; SAWYER 1943b and SHEN 1958). The absence of nerves in older larvae was verified by BODIAN's protargol stain. Muscles of the nerveless larvae showed usually a deficiency of myo-fibrils; they responded by contraction to direct stimulation and to eserine at stages 30 to 40, but not later. It is to be stressed that we are dealing here not with a denervated muscle, usually studied by pharmacologists, but with a muscle which never became innervated.

Until stage 39, the enzyme activity of the nerveless muscle was either somewhat lower (SAWYER o.c.) or as high as that of the control musculature (SHEN 1958). Both investigators agreed that following stage 39 the enzyme activity of the nerveless muscle increased only slightly and, since this is the period of very rapid increment of enzyme activity in the normal muscle, the former exhibited 30% of control activity at stage 46 (SAWYER o.c.). SAWYER concluded that the nerve endings or end organs are instrumental in the ontogenesis of the bulk of the enzyme. He stressed that his operating procedure deprived the larva of branching nerve endings as well as of the soleplate (Schwann's sheath cells, peripheral neuroglia), and favored the hypothesis of the sheath cells as the source of the enzyme.

Since ChE was present in the nerveless muscle and since its activity actually increased somewhat in the absence of neuronal apparatus, SHEN favored some non-neural or post synaptic elements — not necessarily muscle cells, but possibly connective tissue or sarcolemma — as the source of ChE. However, he suggested that its continued accumulation may depend on the participation of neural or presynaptic elements.

The problem was also attacked by using the tissue culture approach. Mesodermal cells morphogenizing *in vitro* into the muscle developed ChE; due to cellular disorientation occurring in culture conditions, SHEN (1958) could not localize ChE with regard to its site within the muscle cell. In fact, he had the impression that the enzyme was synthesized not by muscle cells but by the connective fibers becoming later part of the specialized region of the sarcolemma.

These data on skeletal muscle should be compared with those of THOMAS and NACHMANSOHN (1938) on the chick heart. Innervated and contracting 8-day heart had a Q value of 1.0 which gradually decreased in tissue culture. After 12 days the neuronal elements of the heart disappeared and the Q value remained constant at the level of about 0.45. Chick embryo heart of corresponding age should have a Q value of at least 20 (SIPPEL 1955; cf. p. 173). Thus, a distinct ChE activity which is, however, only a small fraction of that of the normal adult heart is maintained by the nerveless heart; this is then similar to what occurs in the nerveless amphibian muscle and in mesoderm cultured *in vitro*. THOMAS and NACHMANSOHN commented that the Q value of the nerveless, tissue-cultured heart is comparable to that of certain aneural tissues, such as vitelline entoblast or ectoblast; since it is, however, somewhat lower than that of nerveless parts of innervated tissues, THOMAS et al. speculated that the latter require some ChE for protection against traces of ACh diffusing away from innervated areas.

Incidentally, it appears that while weak ChE activity persists in cultured chick hearts, ACh may disappear entirely. However, experiments dealing with ChE on one hand and ACh on the other, cannot be easily compared: while THOMAS and NACHMANSOHN cultured 8-day old chick hearts for some two weeks, LLSSAK, TORO and PASZTOR (1942) isolated 13 to 16-day old hearts and grew them *in vitro* for up to 3 weeks before the disappearance of ACh.

When discussing muscle or some non-neuronal tissue as a source of ChE, it should be remembered that COUTEAUX (1947) suggested that ChE may be located chiefly in the muscular portion of the sole plate and concentrate at the level of the subneural apparatus. Finally, recent data derived from electron microscopy (ROBERTSON 1955) combined with cytochemistry (GIACOBINI 1959) indicate that in the adult neuromyal junction the enzyme concentrates in complex multimembranous foldings to which muscle nuclei and both neural and muscle mitochondria and cytoplasmic granules seem to contribute. Thus, it is difficult to trace the origin of any particular entity, including ChE, to either muscle or nerve. (For further discussion, see Chapter 6.)

4. Comment

It might be expected that the triple correlation between ChE, neurogenesis, and function could be more easily established in the case of this monosynaptic and admittedly cholinergic junction than in that of the central nervous system. Yet, it seems that there is a divorce between these three entities. First of all, early muscle movement seems to be concomitant with the appearance ChE rather than with innervation of the muscle or maturation of the endplate.

In *Amblystoma*, some enzyme was present prior to the first movement but the rapid increase of its activity coincided with the latter (v. Table 1 and Fig. 3). In the rat, human, guinea pig, and possibly in the chick (cf. TORDA 1938) no enzyme could be detected, manometrically or histochemically, till the first muscle movement; innervation and formation of the endplate followed several days later (ORR and WINDLE 1934; STRAUS and WEDDELL 1940; BONICHON 1957b). In the sheep, ChE was first assayed (at 100 days) some time after function set in; the endplates did not appear till 137 days (DICKSON 1940). The toad may be an exception (vide supra, p. 168). LEWIS and HUGHES suggested that in this form ChE is first synthesized in the motor cells of the cord, and subsequently transported down the motor axons; the first muscle movement would then coincide with the appearance of ChE and of the motor fibers in myocommata (septa). The data on which this suggestion is based may be, however, criticized on technical grounds (vide supra).

Since ChE seems generally to be associated with earliest muscle activity, it may be that the latter is not purely myogenic in nature. In fact, KUPFER and KOELLE (o.c.) suggested that in the young rat the muscle contraction may be mediated by transmitter released at a distance from and diffusing toward the muscle cell. This mechanism is consistent with the high threshold, long latent period, and rapid fatigue of the early muscle. Cholinesterase would be then necessary to terminate the effect of the transmitter, even though the enzyme could not be very efficient prior to its concentration at the synapse. Teleologically, this explains the aneuronal origin of ChE indicated by evidence already reviewed.

On the other hand, it seems that while the development of ChE can be initiated aneuronally, its high level cannot be achieved in the absence of innervation. In several forms, more rapid increment of ChE activity occurred at the time of ramification of the nerves in the muscle; this was true for instance, in *Amblystoma* (SAWYER 1943b) and in the rat (KUPFER and KOELLE 1951). Accordingly, the peak of ChE activity generally coincided with birth, maturation of the endplate, and concomitant increase of muscular activity[1]. In fact, NACHMANSOHN (1939c) suggested that the increase of Q value in the course of embryonic development of the muscle is due solely to the increased synthesis of ChE in the endplate region.

The sheep may be an exception to this rule. In this form the Q value decreased by one-half between the 100th and 137th day of development (NACHMANSOHN 1940b), even though the endplates did not appear till the end of that period.

Altogether, it may be suggested that while initiation of early muscle activity may be associated with the appearance of ChE, its effective functioning depends both upon a relatively high level of ChE and a close relationship of several anatomical systems.

---

[1] In *Amblystoma* it coincided with increased activity at reaching the feeding stage.

Toward the end of neuromyal development, i.e., postnatally, the Q value generally began to decrease. This does not mean that the decrease occurs at the endplate. Actually, the enzyme concentrates in the endplate during development, particularly postnatally (MARNAY and NACHMANSOHN, 1937; NACHMANSOHN 1939c; KUPFER and KOELLE 1951; GEREBTZOFF et al. 1954), and the decrease of the Q value must be due to dilution, subsequent to the maturation of the endplate, of ChE-rich material by ChE-poor fibers (NACHMANSOHN, o.c.; SAWYER 1943b).

Postnatally, muscle fibers continue to grow after the endplate has reached its final size (COUTEAUX 1938). Moreover, SAWYER (1943b) provided experimental evidence for NACHMAN-SOHN's suggestion. When stage 46 *Amblystoma* larvae were left unfed, the muscle atrophied. As a result, the endplate: muscle fiber weight ratio increased and the starved muscle exhibited a higher Q value than that of control larvae, which showed the usual decline of enzyme activity with age.

Thus, the full maturation and functionalization of the neuromyal junction coincides with concentration and high activity of AChE within the endplate, while the rest of the muscle begins to exhibit a "baseline" ChE activity, resembling that of aneural or denervated tissues.

II. Vertebrate heart

SIPPEL (1955) provided interesting data on the development of ChE's during cardiac ontogenesis of *Amblystoma* and of the rat; he further compared ChE's on one hand and succinoxidase on the other with regard to their importance for cardiac function and cardiac efficiency.

With chick and rats, isolated atria and ventricles were homogenized separately; entire hearts were used in the case of *Amblystoma*. AMMON's (1933) method or the Cartesian microdiver (cf. BOELL and SHEN 1949) was employed according to the suitability of the material. The substrates were chlorides of ACh, 0.01 M, BzCh, 0.01 M, and MeCh, 0.02 M. For Kjeldahl and succinoxidase determinations, v. SIPPEL 1954. Q values of ChE were expressed in terms of μl CO_2/mg N/hr.

Amblystoma hearts do not hydrolyze BzCh, and hydrolyze MeCh at a rate about 74% that of hydrolysis of ACh. This and other evidence (SIPPEL 1955) indicate that *Amblystoma* heart contains only AChE. The enzyme is first measurable at stage 39; at stage 45 (hatching) it is about 1/3 as active as at the maximum reached a few days later. There is no visible change in the rate of development of AChE at the time of the innervation of the heart, at which time the enzyme exhibits considerable activity (Table 4).

Table 4. *AChE and cardiac function in* Amblystoma

Harrison-Sippel stages	Cardiac cytology and physiology	AChE
34	Cardiac beat present.	None
36	Circulation present.	None
38	Pacemaker shifted to its definitive caudal position in the sinus venosus (COPENHAVER 1939a)	None
37—40	Cross-striations and myofibrils (COPENHAVER 1939b)	First appreciable activity of the enzyme (earlier activity possibly obscured by massive yolk)
44	Preganglionic vagal fibers at the sinus	$Q = 13$
45	Post-ganglionic fibers in the sinus wall	$Q = 20$
45—46	Reflex vagal inhibition present (COPENHAVER 1939b)	$Q = 26$ at stage 46
54		$Q = 75$

In the *rat*, non-specific ChE is present besides AChE: BzCh is split at relatively high rates, particularly in the atrium, and this activity is not inhibited by excess of ACh; by comparing the extent of DFP (10^{-6} M) inhibition of total enzymic activity on one hand and of that of AChE on the other, SIPPEL (1955) calculated that AChE constitutes only one-fifth of the total ChE activity. Other considerations allowed SIPPEL to calculate separately Q values for AChE and non-specific ChE throughout development. The earliest values (10th day) reported for either enzyme were relatively high and the enzymes must have appeared earlier. After the 10th day of development, AChE activity increased faster than that of non-specific ChE, both in the atrium and in the ventricle; it reached the peak in the ventricle and in the atrium at the 12th and $16^1/_2$ day, respectively, and subsequently declined in both sites (Table 5). The activity of non-specific ChE increased slightly in early development of the ventricle, to remain essentially constant following the 16th to 18th day of development; in the atrium it increased between the 10th and 18th day of development, somewhat more slowly than the activity of AChE.

Few data are available for other forms. In the rabbit, the enzyme was first measured at the 18th to 19th day, that is, at about the 1/3 mark of gestation (SHAMARINA 1939, 1940). On the 28th to 30th day, the concentration of the enzyme in the atria was only slightly lower than that in the adult, but it fell immediately after birth to reach a low on the 4th to 6th postnatal day. A subsequent rise led to adult values in the 9 to 10-day old atrium. SHAMARINA also reported briefly that ChE activity of the embryonic atrium of the guinea pig increases from an intial low value to reach a peak on the last prenatal day. She used a rather crude method of bioassaying ACh after prolonged exposure of the substrate to extracts of auricles of rabbits and guinea pigs. The method seemed rather insensitive and did not differentiate between AChE and non-specific ChE. Finally, in the chick, ZACKS (1954) found AChE histochemically (v. p. 151) in the 4-day heart while LISSAK et al. (1942) found ACh one day earlier. Manometrically, THOMAS and NACHMANSOHN (1938) reported a Q value of 1.02 for the 8-day old chick heart ChE (youngest heart assayed).

Table 5. *ChE's and cardiac function in the rat*

Day of gestation	Cardiovascular cytology and physiology	Cholinesterase activity			
		Atria		Ventricle	
		Q_{AChE}	Q_{ChE}	Q_{AChE}	Q_{ChE}
$9^1/_2$	Contractions (Goss 1938); myofibrils present	no values			
$10^1/_2$	Circulation; cross-striations present (Goss 1940)	no values		40	60
12		45	55	145	70(?)
$14^1/_2$	Branches of vagus in the sinus venosus (HALL 1951)	160	120	155	90
$15^1/_2$	Ganglion cells in atrial wall (HALL 1951)	200	145	140	100
21	Birth; shortly before, vagal reflex becomes functional	155	200	95	115

a) Comment

Cholinesterases seem to appear some time after the onset of cardiac contractility in *Amblystoma* and perhaps in the chick, but may coincide with the latter in the rat (Tables 4 and 5). In all these forms the pattern of ontogenesis of the enzyme does not run parallel to embryogenesis of the innervation of the heart or to the establishment of the vagal reflex. In fact, in the case of the chick heart it is possible that two components of the cholinergic system, ChE and ACh, appear before the onset of vagal innervation of the heart on the 5th day of development (KRAMER 1950).

SIPPEL (1955) pointed out that the initial phase of development of succinoxidase coincides with that of ChE's. In the rat ventricle, succinoxidase activity increased much more rapidly than that of AChE and reached the plateau at just about the time of the onset of vagal innervation of the heart. This, plus other signs of cardiac biochemical and physiological maturation (v. SIPPEL 1955) suggest that ChE's as well as succinoxidase are related to the metabolic and physiological functions rather than to the vagal control of the heart, contrary to the view of SHAMARINA (1940). These functions may be concerned with contractility (cf. also BÜLBRING and BURN 1949) and conduction. This is particularly suggested for non-specific ChE, characteristic for the homoiothermic heart of the embryonic chicken and the rat (SIPPEL o.c.), and which concentrates in the intraventricular septum of the adult rat (ZAMBOTTI and PINNOTTI 1949). The importance of ChE's in these processes is also indicated by the effects of anti-ChE agents on the cardiac rhythm in the adult heart (BÜLBRING and BURN 1949; BÜLBRING et al. 1954; BURN and WALKER 1958). Whether or not AChE, which apparently predominates in the heart of *Amblystoma* and of the frog (SIPPEL o.c.), plays a similar role in the poikilotermic heart cannot be answered at present.

C. Ontogenesis of cholinesterases in other tissues

There are only a few data on the activity of ChE's during development in tissues other than those already referred to.

I. Extraembryonic tissues

Two extraembryonic tissues will be considered briefly at present. The amnion is composed solely of foetal tissues, while the placenta receives contributions from embryonic and maternal tissues; both structures share the important characteristic of being ephemeral and non-innervated.

a) Amnion

Acetylcholinesterase could be demonstrated in the amnion of a 7 to 9-day old chick embryo (KUSCHINSKY et al. 1954). At that time the amnion consists of an epithelial layer, an intermediate membrane, a double layer of smooth muscle cells and mesenchyme, and is not innervated (BAUTZMANN and SCHRÖDER 1953a and 1953b). When a histochemical technique was applied to the amnion of 5 to 11-day old chick embryos, the muscle cells showed weak activity intracellularly (HOEFKE and LULLMANN 1956). The authors could not conclude on the basis of their data whether the enzyme in question was AChE or non-specific ChE.

KUSCHINSKY et al. (1954) employed the micromanometric technique of LINDERSTRØM-LANG (1943). The substrates used were BzCh, ACh, and MeCh; since only the two latter were hydrolyzed, the authors thought that the enzyme in question was AChE. HOEFKE and LULLMANN (1956) used the histochemical technique of GEREBTZOFF (1953, v. p. 151), and employed butyryl- and acetylthiocholine as substrates. Staining was obtained with both substrates after 2 hrs of incubation. HOEFKE and LULLMANN (o.c.) stated that AChE can be expected to split only acetylthiocholine, while BuChE can hydrolyze both substrates (o.c.). This would indicate that the activity was due either to a mixture of enzymes, or to BuChE alone; however, AChE can hydrolyze butyrylthiocholine as well, although slowly (HOLMSTEDT 1959). The staining was suppressed to a similar degree with either substrate by eserine, about 0.5×10^{-6} M. This concentration is much lower (0.3×10^{-4} M) than that used by KOELLE (1955) to inhibit both enzymes; the effectiveness of eserine merely suggests that we are dealing here with ChE's rather than with other esterases. To complicate matters further, it may be added that EARL and THOMPSON (1952) suggested, on the basis of their own criteria, that the chick enzyme is an atypical non-specific ChE. Finally, the histochemical technique used by HOEFKE and LULLMANN can be criticized, since formalin-fixed tissues were used. Altogether, the original view held earlier by KUSCHINSKY et al. (1954), that the chick amnion contains AChE, may be correct.

The amnion is thus an organ which is relatively rich in ChE's, shows coordinated spontaneous movement, and is not innervated (PIERCE 1933; VERZAR 1941). Thus, its response to anti-ChE agents and to cholinomimetic drugs may throw light on the question of the possibility of the existence of a cholinergic mechanism or cholinergic receptor in an organ which is never innervated.

Anticholinesterase agents were so employed in the case of a developing heart prior to innervation, or in a heart prevented experimentally from becoming innervated, in developing denervated muscle, and finally in non-innervated amphibian melanophores (Chapter 17). Unfortunately, only cholinomimetic agents, but not anti-ChE agents were employed in the case of the chick (KUSCHINSKY et al. 1954; v. Chapter 17).

These data supplement the earlier results of AMMON and SCHÜTTE (1935, v. p. 152) with regard to the extraembryonic membranes of the chick. Altogether, an ACh-hydrolyzing, eserine-inhibited enzyme can be found in the yolk, yolk-sac, allantois, and amnion from the fifth day of incubation on; while it remains constant between the 5th and 15th day in the yolk-sac and allantois, it increases in the yolk as it does in the embryo itself.

b) Placenta

GEREBTZOFF (1957, 1959) studied ChE's of developing guinea-pig placenta histochemically (p. 151) and manometrically. As in the human (ORD and THOMPSON 1950), the guinea-pig placenta was stated to contain mainly AChE. On the basis of his results GEREBTZOFF concluded that AChE of the placenta originates primarily in the maternal blood vessels and is synthesized only secondarily in the fetal portions of the placental syncytium.

The mesometrial portion of the uterus was devoid of ChE's until the 14th day of gestation, at which time AChE staining appeared in the walls of the mesometrial capillaries; a weak AChE reaction was noticed also in the vicinity of the capillaries in the tissues which would form later the placental syncytium of the foetus. At 19 days, AChE staining reached the base of the fetal portion of the placenta (the trophoderm or the "syncytial cords" of GEREBTZOFF) surrounding the maternal capillaries and blood sinuses. The vascularisation of the chorionic part of the placenta occurred between the 20th and the 26th days of gestation. While AChE of the maternal portions of the placenta increased slightly during that period, it did not appear in the fetal placenta till the last days of gestation. It increased rapidly between the 39th and 40th day till it became more active than in the maternal portion of the placenta, in which it actually decreased; a small increase was noticed also in the case of fetal erythrocytes. At birth, AChE activity of the placenta decreased as indicated both by histochemical and manometric studies; this loss was accompanied by that of AChE of fetal erythrocyctes.

GEREBTZOFF suggested also the maternal origin of AChE of fetal blood, although he agreed that AChE would have difficulty in migrating from maternal blood into fetal placenta. Finally, the finding of AChE in the capillary wall is unexpected, since KOELLE (1954) found only BuChE in walls of the brain capillaries of the rabbit. Decidual cells also stained for AChE at 19 days (GEREBTZOFF 1959); the staining was found to spread and gain in intensity, and to move toward chorionic portions of the placenta till it occupied the zone of the giant cells of Duval. Altogether, further verification is desirable of the blood vessel wall as the site of origin of placental AChE.

It is unfortunate that there are no data on ChE's of human extra-embryonic membranes, particularly the placenta where very high concentrations of ACh (28 μg/g) were found by CHANG and GADDUM (1933); it seems derived from the villous tissue of the foetal trophoblast (for review of literature, v. NEEDHAM 1942). The presence of the enzyme at strategic extra-embryonic sites which may be exposed to ACh could be expected, since these sites are sensitive to ACh; uterine musculature may be one of such sites.

II. Miscellaneous results

Sporadic developmental data are available on blood ChE's of the newborn as compared to the adult mammal (MCCANCE et al. 1949; JONES et al. 1956; JONES and MCCANCE 1949), and on ChE's of the embryonic mammalian kidney (RISLEY and DAVIES 1953) and liver (YOUNGSTROM 1941). Acetylcholinesterase was measured in the suprarenal gland of young and old rats and dogs (MEHES and DECSI 1958). In view of the paucity of the data, as well as of the interspecies variability, their further description or interpretation is not warranted. (For analysis of ChE's in erythropoiesis, v. Chapter 6).

Unusual data were provided by M. JONES et al. (1956). These investigators utilized chick embryo intestine cultured *in vitro*. Intestine grew, or barely maintained viability, depending on whether it was cultivated in embryonic extract or in synthetic medium. In either case, there was a 50% loss of ChE activity, and this loss could be prevented by the single addition of ACh, 0.02 M final concentration, to the medium.

M. JONES et al. interpreted their data as indicating enzymic induction (SPIEGEL-MAN et al. 1956), although they stated that "enzyme stabilization", i.e., ACh protection of the enzyme from breakdown, could also explain their data. In the past, ChE induction was speculated upon when the enzyme appeared prior to neurogenesis (p. 156) or prior to the appearance of ACh; only this last case — a response to the presence of a substrate — qualifies theoretically as that of enzyme induction (COHN et al. 1953).

It must be stated, however, that the enzymic loss noticed by M. JONES et al. in the absence of exogenous ACh, has been recorded before (THOMAS and NACHMAN-SOHN 1938; LISSAK et al. 1942; cf. however SHEN 1958; vide supra, p. 170) in tissues containing endogenous ACh (LISSAK et al. o.c.). While M. JONES et al. did not analyze their tissues for ACh, it can be asked why endogenous transmitter cannot protect as well as added ACh.

It is finally of interest that M. JONES et al. characterized the enzyme of the embryonic chick intestine as AChE, since in the mammalian adult intestine the chief functional enzyme seems to be BuChE (KOELLE et al. 1950).

Final conclusions

A. Techniques and scope

Certain limitations, whether of techniques or of scope, characteristic for much of the research reviewed here should be stated first. Sensitivity of the methods employed in measurement of activity of ChE's varied widely; the same was true in the less frequent cases of measurement of ACh. This may explain why investigators frequently differed in their estimations of first ontogenetic appearances of ChE even when working with the same species, as in the case of insects, and also as to the important matter of whether the enzyme appeared precociously with regard to substrate or vice versa.

Obviously, data obtained by the Cartesian microdiver, capable to measure approximately 10^{-12} mol of the enzyme per few mg of tissue (cf. p. 144) cannot be compared with results obtained by the Warburg (AMMON 1933) technique which is 100-fold less sensitive. The sensitivity of manometric methods is affected by substrate concentration (cf. Table 3) and the absence or presence of activators, such as magnesium; all this varied from one investigator to another. In the case of histochemical methods, some investigators used fixed preparations as well as other measures leading to enzymic inactivation (cf. p. 151); while this may preserve structural detail and limit the diffusion artifact, it also limits the sensitivity of the method. It was also generally difficult to ascertain which ChE was actually measured. In earlier investigations ACh was used as the only substrate. Subsequently, particularly in the case of histochemical methods, differential substrates were employed; however, the use of differential inhibitors varied among investigators. Frequently, the term "ChE" had to be used in this review to denote total cholinesterase activity, and only rarely could it be dependably stated that onto-genesis of AChE or BuChE was actually studied.

Furthermore, in certain areas, limited evidence precludes further generalization. Little study has been done on tissues other than the nervous system, the heart, or muscle; data concerned with the liver, pancreas, blood, and smooth muscle are sporadic. This omission will be stressed subsequently. The related problem is that our knowledge of specific ontogenesis of BuChE, AChE, and other esterases, particularly in tissues other than the nervous system, is very incomplete. Finally, ontogenesis of ChE's should be considered in relation to that of other components of cholinergic systems; unfortunately, data on ACh and ChAC are quite scanty.

B. Significance of early ontogenetic appearance of ChE's

There is no doubt that generally ChE's appear during very early embryonic stages. This occurs so long before differentiation and functionalization of various organs that the suggestion of BODINE and BOELL (1935) that certain enzymes are precocious because biochemical mechanisms must appear in anticipation of future function does not seem to provide an adequate explanation. This phenomenon is, however, baffling only if ChE's are considered as purely neurotropic enzymes concerned only with nerve transmission. Yet, the problem of their precocious appearance is akin to that of their presence in both adult and embryonic aneural tissues such as amnion, placenta, and blood. Thus, the rationale of the precocious ontogenetic appearance of ChE's would be vindicated if they could be traced subsequently to aneural tissues; unfortunately, pertinent data are lacking. Also, in these as well as certain innervated tissues ChE's may be related to energetics and functional efficiency as proposed for the heart (BÜLBRING and BURN 1949). In this context, it is of interest that in the heart and skeletal muscle, ChE's appear in most species considerably prior to innervation. Acetylcholine on the other hand may play a role in bacterial (ROWATT 1948) or regenerative (SINGER 1960) growth. This possibility will be analyzed later (v. Chapter 17) in the light of effects of anticholinesterase agents on growth.

C. Relationship between ChE's, neurogenesis, and function

Many investigators have considered that the best evidence for the physiological significance of the ChE's is their relationship to neurogenesis and ontogenesis of function and of motility. Ontogenesis of ChE's is indeed an expression of biochemical differentiation characteristic of the nervous system (BOELL 1948), and it differs from that of cellular respiration. It may be expected that the same should be true of other enzymes implicated in the function of the nervous system such as monoamine oxidase; unfortunately, no data on this point are available. Moreover, a *general* correlation can be made out for ontogenesis of ChE's on one hand and development of function and neurogenesis on the other; in fact, sometimes a case can be made for a *specific* correlation between ChE's and the appearance of a neurogenetic or functional event. This is true for instance for synaptization within optic pathways and perhaps, when the correlation is extended to ACh, also for functionalization of the light reflex in the chick. Similarly, the appearance of ChE's predicates cytological maturity and electric activity of the guinea pig cortex; conversely, their disappearance is concomitant with diapause and electric silence of the brain in the insect.

Yet, the correlations break down in many specific instances, as in the tunicates or in echinoderms, where ChE's appear to be associated with endodermal rather than with neural determination, or in the rat where considerable neurogenesis and functional development take place before the first appearance of the enzyme or before the phase of rapid increase of its activity. Even when some correlation can be established, it cannot be applied in most cases to specific neurogenetic and functional steps; generally, a rather smooth pattern of ontogenesis of ChE's of various parts of the brain coincides with important functional events.

The difficulty may lie partially in the general inappropriateness of methods used for ChE measurement for the solution of the problem at hand. It seems quite likely that improvements in methodology or the introduction of new techniques may provide for a better of correlation between ChE's, neurogenesis, and development of function. Analysis of large areas of the central nervous system which include millions of neurons, most likely of mixed nature with regard to their transmitters, should be replaced by microanalysis, Cartesian microdiver technique, and more general than heretofore application of histochemical methods, perhaps in conjunction with electron microscopy.

In the second place, general rather than specific correlation between ChE's and neurogenesis may be all that should be expected. Indeed, ACh rather than ChE's should be considered as the identifying marker of cholinergic transmission (FELD-BERG 1957) and as the ultimate correlate of maturation of cholinergic synapses. In fact, ACh and ACh synthesis appear in some species, as for instance in certain insects, to be a better indicator of neurogenesis and function than ChE's. Unfortunately, in view of the paucity of data on ontogenesis of ACh, even a preliminary estimate of the status of ACh as a correlate of function and neurogenesis is impossible.

Yet, this is an important point not only from the viewpoint of the relationship of ontogenesis of the cholinergic system to that of function but also for the understanding of the role of ChE's. If ACh and the cholinergic receptor appear in development before ChE's, as seems to be the case in many forms or organs, the necessity of these enzymes for the protection of synapses (KOPPANYI and KARCZ-MAR 1951; KOELLE and KOELLE 1959) rather than for their functionalization may be borne out. Such a sequence of appearance may suggest also that ChE appears in ontogenesis as an "adaptive" enzyme by means of a mechanism suggested by SPIEGELMAN (cf. SPIEGELMAN and CAMBELL 1956). In turn, it may be that the cholinergic system or its components not only condition transmission and function, but also induce anatomic substrates of these processes and act as inductors or evocators (SPEMANN 1938); in this case their appearance should precede that of certain structures of the nervous system.

Finally, cholinergic transmission should not be considered purely biochemically, but also from the viewpoint of the structural aspect of its ontogenesis (KARCZMAR 1955). It suffices to use here as illustration the development of the neuromyal junction, where functionalization depends not only on biogenesis of the pertinent enzymes and substrates, but also upon anatomical juxtaposition and developmental synchronization of probably two cholinergic systems, one originating in the muscle and the other about the motor nerve terminal (KUPFER and KOELLE 1951).

The questions raised at present as to the role of ChE's in transmission as well as to the possibility of their other functions should be considered again in the light of the studies of the effects of anti-ChE agents during development (Chapter 17).

References

AMMON, R.: Die fermentative Spaltung des Acetylcholins. Pflügers Arch. ges. Physiol. **233**, 486—491 (1933).
—, and E. SCHÜTTE: Über das Verhalten von Enzymen im Hühnerei während der Bebrütung. Biochem. Z. **275**, 216—233 (1935).
ANGULO Y GONZÁLEZ, A. W.: The prenatal development of behavior in the albino rat. J. comp. Neurol. **65**, 395—442 (1932).
ARTEMOV, N. M.: The content of cholinesterase and acetylcholine in developing eggs of amphibians. Bull. Acad. Sci. U.R.S.S. Ser. Biol. 272—276 (1941).
AUGUSTINSSON, K. B.: Cholinesterases; study in comparative enzymology. Acta physiol. scand. Suppl. **52**, 1—182 (1948).
—, and T. GUSTAFSON: Cholinesterase in developing sea-urchin eggs. J. cell. comp. Physiol. **34**, 311—321 (1948).
BACQ, Z. M.: Recherches sur la physiologie et la pharmacologie du système nerveux autonome. Arch. int. Physiol. **42**, 24—60 (1935a).
— Observations physiologiques sur le coeur, les muscles et le système nerveux d'une Ascidie (Ciona intestinalis). Arch. int. Physiol. **40**, 357—373 (1935b).

BARCROFT, J., and D. H. BARRON: Movement in the mammalian foetus. Ergebn. Physiol. 42, 107—152 (1939).

BARRON, D. H.: The functional development of some mammalian neuromuscular mechanisms. Biol. Rev. 16, 1—33 (1941).

BAYLISS, B. J., and A. TODRICK: The use of specific inhibitors in the estimation of the pseudo-cholinesterase in nervous tissue. Biochem. J. 54, XXIX (1953a).

— — The development of the cholinesterase in the brain and spinal cord of the young rat. Biochem. J. 54, XXIX (1953b).

BAUTZMANN, H., and R. SCHRÖDER: Amnionstudien zur vergleichenden Histogenese, Struktur und Funktion des Amnions beim Hühnchen und beim Menschen. Anat. Anz. (Erg. Heft) 100, 135—140 (1935a).

— — Studien zur funktionellen Histologie und Histogenese des Amnions beim Hühnchen und beim Menschen. Z. Anat. Entwickl.-Gesch. 117, 166—214 (1953b).

BEYER, G., and T. WENSE: Über den Nachweis von Hormonen in einzelligen Tieren. I. Cholin und Acetylcholin im Paramecium. Arch. ges. Physiol. 237, 417—422 (1936).

BODINE, J. H., and E. J. BOELL: Enzyme in ontogenesis (Orthoptera). I. Tyrosinase. J. cell. comp. Physiol. 6, 263—275 (1935).

BOELL, E. J.: Biochemical differentiation during amphibian development. Ann. N. Y. Acad. Sci. 49, 773—800 (1948).

— Energy exchange and enzyme development during embryogenesis. In: B. H. WILLIER, P. A. WEISS and V. HAMBURGER, Eds., Analysis of Development, 520—535. Philadelphia: W. B. SAUNDERS 1955.

— P. GREENFIELD and S. C. SHEN: Localization of cholinesterase in the optic lobes of the frog (Rana pipiens). J. exp. Zool. 129, 415—452 (1955).

—, and S. C. SHEN: Functional differentiation in embryonic development. I. Cholinesterase activity of induced neural structures in Amblystoma punctatum. J. exp. Zool. 97, 21—41 (1944).

— — Experimental modification of cholinesterase development in the midbrain of Amblystoma punctatum. Anat. Rec. 105, 490 (only) (1949).

— — Development of cholinesterase in the central nervous system of Amblystoma punctatum. J. exp. Zool. 113, 583—600 (1950).

—, and R. WEBER: Cytochrome oxidase activity in mitochondria during amphibian development. Exp. Cell. Res. 9, 559—567 (1955).

BONICHON, A.: Evolution de l'activité de l'acétylcholinestérase au niveau des lobes optiques chez l'embryon de poulet. C. R. Acad. Sci. (Paris) 245, 1345—1347 (1957a).

— Localisation de l'acétylcholinestérase dans les muscles striés au cours du développement chez l'embryon de poulet. Ann. Histochim. 2, 301—309 (1957b).

— L'acétylcholinestérase dans la cellule et la fibre nerveuse au cours du développement. Ann. Ann. Histochim. 3, 85—93 (1958).

BRACHET, J.: The biochemistry of development. New York: Pergamon Press 1960.

BROWN, G. L., B. D. BURNS and W. FELDBERG: Reactions of the normal mammalian muscle to acetylcholine and to eserine. J. Physiol. 87, 394—424 (1936).

BÜLBRING, E., and J. H. BURN: Action of acetylcholine on rabbit auricles in relation to acetylcholine synthesis. J. Physiol. 108, 508—524 (1949).

— S. R. KOTTEGODA and A. SHELLEY: Cholinesterase activity in the auricles of the rabbit's heart and their sensitivity to eserine. J. Physiol. 123, 204—213 (1954).

— E. M. LOURIE and U. PARDOE: The presence of acetylcholine in Trypanosoma rhodesiense and its absence from Plasmodium gallinaceum. Brit. J. Pharmacol. 4, 290—294 (1949).

BULLOCK, T. H., and D. NACHMANSOHN: Cholinesterase in primitive nervous systems. J. cell. comp. Physiol. 20, 239—242 (1942).

BURN, J. H., and J. M. WALKER: Anticholinesterases in the heart-lung preparation. J. Physiol. 124, 489—501 (1954).

BUTLER, E. G., and O. E. SCHOTTÉ: Histological alterations in denervated non-regenerating limbs of urodele larvae. J. exp. Zool. 84, 223—239 (1941).

CARMICHAEL, L.: An experimental study in the prenatal guinea pig of the origin and development of reflexes and patterns of behavior in relation to the stimulation of specific receptor areas during the period of active fetal life. Genet. Psychol. Monogr. 16, 337—491 (1934).

CASIDA, J. E.: Comparative enzymology of certain insect acetylesterases in relation to poisoning by organophosphate insecticides. J. Physiol. 127, 20P—21P (1954).

— Comparative enzymology of certain insect acetylesterases in relation to poisoning by organsphosphorus insecticides. Biochem. J. 60, 487—496 (1956).

CHANG, H. C., and J. H. GADDUM: Cholinesters in tissue extracts. J. Physiol. 79, 255—285 (1933).

CHERFURKA, W., and B. N. SMALLMAN: The occurrence of acetylcholine in the housefly, Musca domestica L. Canad. J. Biochem. 34, 731—742 (1956).

CHINO, H.: Enzymatic synthesis and hydrolysis of acetylcholine in the egg of the silkworm, Bombyx mori. Annot. Zool. Japon. **30**, 106—113 (1957).
—, and T. YUSHIMA: On the occurrence of an acetylcholine-like substance in some insect eggs. 2. The change in acetylcholine-like substance content during embryonic development in some insect eggs. Annot. Zool. Japon. **26**, 233—237 (1953).
— — Studies on the appearance and the change of cholinesterase activity in the eggs of some lepidopterous insects. Zool. Mag. Tokyo **63**, 185—188 (1954).
CHOW, K. L., and E. ROY JOHN: Effects of intracerebral injection of anti-cholinesterase drugs on behavior in rats. Science **128**, 781—782 (1958).
COGHILL, G. E.: Anatomy and the problem of behavior. New York: The Macmillan Co. 1929.
— Somatic myogenic action in embryos of Fundulus heteroclitus. Proc. Soc. exp. Biol. (N. Y.) **31**, 62—64 (1933).
COHN, M., J. MONOD, M. R. POLLACK, S. SPIEGELMAN and R. Y. STANIER: Terminology of enzyme formation. Nature (Lond.) **172**, 1096 (1953).
COPENHAVER, W. M.: Initiation of beat and intrinsic contraction rates in the different parts of the Amblystoma heart. J. exp. Zool. **80**, 193—224 (1939a).
— Some observations on the growth and function of heteroplastic heart grafts. J. exp. Zool. **82**, 23—271 (1939b).
COPP, F. C.: Diacid basis. Part I. Compounds related to 1:5-Diphenyl-pentane-pp'-bis (trialkyl-ammonium) salts as anticholinesterases. J. Chem. Soc. **1953**, 3116—3118.
COUTEAUX, R.: Sur l'origine de la sole des plaques motrices. C. R. Soc. Biol. (Paris) **127**, 218—221 (1938).
— Contribution à l'étude de la synapse myoneurale. Thesis presented to the Faculty of Sciences of the U. of Paris. Montreal: Therien Frères Limitée 1947.
DALE, H. H.: Transmission of nervous effects by acetylcholine. Harvey Lect. **32**, 229—245 (1937).
DETWILER, S. R.: Experiments upon midbrain of Amblystoma embryos. Amer. J. Anat. **78**, 115—137 (1946).
— Quantitative studies on locomotor responses in Amblystoma larvae following surgical alterations in the nervous system. Ann. N. Y. Acad. Sci. **49**, 834—855 (1948).
DICKSON, L. U.: The development of nerve endings in the respiratory muscles of the sheep. J. Anat. (London) **74**, 255—267 (1940).
DOMINI, G.: Acetylcholine-esterase activity of some tissues during embryonal development and in the first days after birth. Boll. Soc. ital. Biol. sper. **13**, 1180—1182 (1938).
DURANTE, M.: Cholinesterase in the development of the ascidian, Ciona intestinalis. Experientia (Basel) **12**, 307—308 (1956).
— Cholinesterase in the anterior and posterior hemiembryos of Ciona intestinalis. Acta Embryol. Morph. Exp. **1** (2), 131—133 (1957).
DU SHANE, G. P., and C. HUTCHINSON: The effect of temperature on the development of form and behavior in Amphibian embryos. J. exp. Zool. **87**, 245—258 (1941).
EARL, C. J., and R. H. S. THOMPSON: The inhibitory action of tri-o-cresol phosphate on cholinesterases. Brit. J. Pharmacol. **17**, 261—269 (1952).
ECCLES, J. C., R. M. ECCLES, and P. FATT: Pharmacological investigations on a central synapse operated by acetylcholine. J. Physiol. **131**, 154—169 (1956).
ELKES, J., J. T. EAYRS, and A. TODRICK: In: H. WAELSH, Ed., Biochemistry of the Developing Nervous System, 499—509. New York: Academic Press, Inc. 1955.
—, and A. TODRICK: In: H. WAELSH, Ed., Biochemistry of the Developing Nervous System, 309—314. New York: Academic Press, Inc. 1955.
FELDBERG, W.: Acetylcholine. In: D. RICHTER, Ed., Metabolism of the nervous system, 493—510. New York: Pergamon Press 1957.
—, and M. VOGT: Acetylcholine systhesis in different regions of the central nervous system. J. Physiol. **107**, 373—381 (1948).
FLEXNER, L. B.: The development of the cerebral cortex: a cytological, functional and biochemical approach. The Harvey Lect. Ser. **47**, 156—179 (1952).
— Enzymatic and functional patterns of the developing mammalian brain. In: H. WAELSH, Ed., Biochemistry of the Developing Nervous System, 281—300. New York: Academic Press 1955a.
— Events associated with the development of nerve and hepatic cells. Ann. N. Y. Acad. Sci. **60**, 986—1002 (1955b).
FREEDMAN, A. M., and H. C. HIMWICH: Effect of age on lethality of diisopropyl fluophosphate. Amer. J. Physiol. **153**, 211—126 (1948).
FUKUDA, T., and G. B. KOELLE: The cytological localization of intracellular neuronal acetyl-cholinesterase. J. biophys. biochem. Cytol. **5**, 433—440 (1959).
GEREBTZOFF, M. A.: Histochemical investigations on acetylcholine and cholinesterases. I. Introduction and technique. Acta Anat. **19**, 366—379 (1953).

GEREBTZOFF, M. A.: Appareil cholinestérasique à l'insertion tendineuse des fibres musculaires striées. C. R. Soc. Biol. (Paris) 148, 632—634 (1954).
— Development of cholinesterase activity in the nervous system (observed by a histochemical method). In: H. WAELSH, Ed., Biochemistry of the Developing Nervous System, 315—326. New York: Academic Press, Inc. 1955.
— Nouvelles recherches histochimiques sur l'acétylcholinestérase dans la placenta de cobaye. Ann. Histochim. 2, 3—10 (1957).
— Cholinesterases. New York: Pergamon Press 1959.
— E. PHILIPPOT and M. J. DALLEMAGNE: Recherches histochimiques sur les acétylcholine-et choline-estérases. 2. Activité enzymatique dans les muscles lents et rapides des mammifères et des oiseaux. Acta Anat. 20, 234—257 (1954).
GIACOBINI, E.: The distribution and localization of cholinesterases in nerve cells. Acta physiol. scand. 45, suppl. 151, p. 1 (1959).
GOMORI, D.: Microscopic histochemistry. Chicago: The Chicago U. Press (1952).
GOSS, C. M.: The first contractions of the heart in rat embryos. Anat. Rec. 70, 505—524 (1938).
— First contractions of the heart without cytological differentiation. Anat. Rec. 75, 19—27 (1940).
GUSTAFSON, T.: Enzymatic aspects of embryonic differentiation. In: G. H. BOURNE and J. F. DANIELLI, Eds.: Int. Rev. Cytol. 3, 277—328 (1954).
—, and I. HASSELBERG: Studies on enzymes in the developing sea urchin egg. Exp. Cell Res. 2, 642—672 (1951).
HALL, E. K.: Intrinsic contractility in the embryonic rat heart. Anat. Rec. 3, 381—399 (1951).
HAMBURGER, V.: The mitotic patterns in the spinal cord of the chick embryo and their relation to histogenetic processes. J. comp. Neurol. 88, 221—283 (1948).
—, and H. L. HAMILTON: A series of normal stages in the development of the chick embryo. J. Morph. 88, 49—92 (1951).
HARRIS, J. E., and H. P. WHITING: Structure and function in the locomotory system of the dogfish embryo. The myogenic stage of movement. J. exp. Biol. 31, 501—524 (1954).
HERRICK, C. J.: The brain of the Tiger salamander. Chicago: The U. of Chicago Press 1948.
HESTRIN, S.: The reaction of acetylcholine and other carboxylic derivatives with hydroxylamine and its analytical application. J. biol. Chem. 180, 249—261 (1949).
HIMWICH, H. E., and M. H. APRISON: The effect of age on cholinesterase activity of rabbit brain. In: H. WAELSH, Ed., Biochemistry of Developing Nervous Systems, 301—307. New York: Academic Press, Inc. 1955.
HOEFKE, W., and H. LULLMANN: Der histochemische Nachweis von Cholinesterase im Hühneramnion. Naunyn-Schmiedeberg's Arch. exp. Path. Pharmak. 227, 519—521 (1956).
HOLMSTEDT, B.: Pharmacology of organophosphorus cholinesterase inhibitors. Pharmacol. Rev. 11, 567—688 (1959).
HOOKER, D.: The Origin of Overt Behavior. Ann. Arbor: The U. of Michigan Press 1944.
— The Prenatal Origin of Behavior. Lawrence, Kansas: U. of Kansas Press 1952.
HORNE CRAIGIE, E.: Vascular patterns of developing nervous system. In: H. WAELSH, ED., Biochemistry of the Developing Nervous System, 28—49. New York: Academic Press, Inc. 1955.
HÖRSTADIUS, S.: Experimental researches on the developmental physiology of the sea-urchin. Pubbl. Staz. Zool. Napoli 21, 131—172 (1949).
JASPER, H. H., C. S. BRIDGMAN and L. CARMICHAEL: An ontogenetic study of cerebral electrical potentials in the guinea pig. J. exp. Psychol. 21, 63—71 (1937).
JONES, M., R. M. FEATHERSTONE and S. L. BONTING: The effect of acetylcholine on cholinesterases of chick embryo intestine cultured in vitro. J. Pharmacol. exp. Ther. 116, 114—118 (1956).
JONES, P. E. H., and R. A. MCCANCE: Enzyme activities in the blood of infants and adults. Biochem. J. 45, 464—467 (1949).
JORDAN, W. K., and R. MARCH: The dephosphorylation of nucleotides by developing rat cerebral cortex and cerebellum. In: H. WAELSH, Ed., Biochemistry of the Developing Nervous System, 327—333. New York: Academic Press, Inc. 1955.
KAKUSHKINA, E. A., and A. D. ARKHIPOVA: Changes in activity of cholinesterase in the ontogenesis of mammals. Bull. exp. Biol. Med. 11, 533—535 (1941).
KALOW, W.: Personal communication (1960).
KARCZMAR, A. G.: The role of amputation and nerve resection in the regressing limbs of urodele larvae. J. exp. Zool. 103, 401—427 (1946).
— Limb regeneration and differentiation of "overt behavior" in urodeles as studied by means of their response to chemical agents. Ann. N. Y. Acad. Sci. 60, 1108—1135 (1955).
—, and G. G. BERG: Alkaline phosphatase during limb development and regeneration of Amblystoma opacum and Amblystoma punctatum. J. exp. Zool. 117, 139—164 (1951).

KARCZMAR, A. G., T. KOPPANYI and G. C. SHEATZ: Studies on intravenously injected true cholinesterase. J. Pharmacol. exp. Ther. **102**, 103—111 (1951).

KAVALER, F., and V. M. KIMEL: Biochemical and physiological differentiation during morphogenesis. XV. Acetylcholinesterase activity of the motor cortex of the fetal guinea pig. J. comp. Neurol **96**, 113—119 (1952).

KLÜVER, H.: Discussion. In: G. E. W. WOLSTENHOLME and C. M. O'CONNOR Eds., Neurological basis of behavior, 356—357. Boston: Little, Brown and Co. 1958.

KOELLE, G. B.: The histochemical differentiation of types of cholinesterase and their localizations in tissues of the cat. J. Pharmacol. exp. Ther. **103**, 153—171 (1950).

— The elimination of enzymatic diffusion artifacts in the histochemical localization of cholinesterases and their localizations in the tissues of the cat. J. Pharmacol. exp. Ther. **103**, 153—171 (1951).

— The histochemical localization of cholinesterases in the central nervous system of the rat. J. comp. Neurol. **100**, 211—228 (1954).

— The histochemical identification of cholinesterase in cholinergic, adrenergic and sensory neurons. J. Pharmacol. exp. Ther. **114**, 167—184 (1955).

— E. S. KOELLE and J. S. FRIEDENWALD: The effect of inhibition of specific and nonspecific cholinesterase on the motility of the isolated ileum. J. Pharmacol. exp. Ther. **100**, 180—191 (1950).

KOELLE, W. A., and G. B. KOELLE: The localization of external or functional acetylcholinesterase at the synapses of autonomic ganglia. J. Pharmacol. exp. Ther. **126**, 1—8 (1959).

KOLLROS, J. J.: The development of the optic lobes in the frog. I. The effects of unilateral enucleation in embryonic stages. J. exp. Zool. **123**, 153—187 (1953).

KOPPANYI, T., and A. G. KARCZMAR: Contribution to the study of the mechanism of action of cholinesterase inhibitors. J. Pharmacol. exp. Ther. **101**, 327—344 (1951).

KRAMER, T.: Preliminary report on the innervation of the embryonic chick heart. Anat. Rec. **106**, 210 (only) (1950).

KUHLENBECK, H.: The ontogenetic development of diencephalic centers in the bird's brain (chick) and a comparison with the reptilian and mammalian diencephalon. J. comp. Neurol. **66**, 23—77 (1937).

KUO, Z. Y.: Ontogeny of embryonic behavior in aves. I. The chronology and general nature of the behavior of chick embryo. J. exp. Zool. **61**, 395—430 (1932a).

— Ontogeny of embryonic behavior in aves. III. The structural and environmental factors in embryonic behavior. J. comp. Psych. **13**, 245—171 (1932b).

— Ontogeny of embryonic behavior in aves. XII. Stages in the development of physiological activities in the chick embryo. Amer. J. Psychol. **51**, 361—379 (1938).

— Studies on the physiology of the embryonic nervous system. IV. Development of acetylcholine on the chick embryo. J. Neurophysiol. **2**, 488—493 (1939).

KUPFER, C., and G. B. KOELLE: A histochemical study of cholinesterase during formation of the motor and plate of the albino rat. J. exp. Zool. **116**, 397—415 (1951).

KUSCHINSKY, G., H. LULLMANN and E. MUSCHOLL: Untersuchungen über die Einwirkung von verschiedenen Pharmaka auf die Spontanrhythmik des isolierten Hühnerammion. Naunyn-Schmiedeberg's Arch. exp. Path. Pharmak. **223**, 369—374 (1954).

LARSELL, O.: The nucleus isthmi of the frog. J. Comp. Neurol. **36**, 309—322 (1924).

LEIBSON, R.: Ontogenetic changes in cholinesterase activity in the skeletal muscles of rabbits. Bull. biol. Med. exp. URSS. **7**, 514—517 (1939).

LEWIS, S. E.: Acetylcholine in blowflies. Nature (Lond.) **172**, 1004—1005 (1953).

LEWIS, P. R., and A. F. W. HUGHES: The cholinesterase of developing neurones in Xenopus laevis. In: D. RICHTER, Ed., Metabolism of the Nervous System, 511—513. New York: Pergamon Press 1957.

LINDAHL, P. E.: Contributions to the physiology of form generation in the development of the sea urchin. Quart. Rev. Biol. **17**, 213—227 (1942).

LINDEMAN, V. F.: The cholinesterase and acetylcholine content of the chick retina, with special reference to functional activity as indicated by the pupillary constrictor reflex. Amer. J. Physiol. **148**, 40—44 (1947).

LINDERSTRØM-LANG, K.: The theory of the Cartesian-diver microrespirometer. C. R. Carlsberg, Ser. Chim. **24**, 334—398 (1943).

LISSAK, M., I. TORO, and J. PASZTOR: Untersuchungen über den Zusammenhang des Acetylcholingehaltes und der Innervation des Herzmuskels in Gewebe-Kulturen. Pflügers Arch. ges. Physiol. **245**, 794—801 (1942).

LOEWI, O., and E. NAVRATIL: Über homorale Übertragbarkeit der Herzenwirkung. X. Über das Schicksal des Vagusstoffes. Pflügers Arch. ges. Physiol. **214**, 678—688 (1926).

LORD, K. A., and C. POTTER: Studies on the mechanism of insecticidal action of organophosphorus compounds with particular reference to their antiesterase activity. Ann. appl. Biol. **38**, 495—507 (1951).

LORD, K. A., and C. POTTER: Hydrolysis of esters by extracts of insects. Nature (Lond.) **172**, 679—681 (1953).

MACBRIDE, E. W.: On the development of Echinus esculentus, together with some points in the development of E. miliaris and E. acutus. Phil. Trans. B. **195**, 285—327 (1903).

MARNAY, A., and D. NACHMANSOHN: Sur la repartition de la cholinestérase dans le muscle couturier de la grenouille. C. R. Soc. Biol. (Paris) **125**, 41—43 (1937).

McCANCE, R. A., A. O. HUTCHINSON, R. F. A. DEAN and P. E. H. JONES: Cholinesterase activity of the serum of newborn animals and of colostrum. Biochem. J. **45**, 493—496 (1949).

MCILWAIN, H.: Biochemistry and the Central Nervous System. Boston: Little, Brown and Co. 1955.

MEHES, I., and L. DECSI: Diminution de l'activité acétylcholinestérasique dans la vieillesse. C. R. Soc. Biol. (Paris) **152**, 688—689 (1958).

MEHROTRA, K. N., and B. N. SMALLMAN: Ovicidal action of organo-phosphorus insecticides. Nature (Lond.) **180**, 97—98 (1957).

METCALF, R. L., M. B. MARCH and M. G. MAXON: Substrate preferences of insect cholinesterases. Ann. Ent. Soc. Amer. **48**, 222—228 (1955).

METZLER, C. J., and D. G. HUMM: The determination of cholinesterase activity in whole brains of developing rats. Science **113**, 382—383 (1951).

MITROPOLITANSKAYA, R. L.: On the presence of acetylcholine and cholinesterase in Protozoa, Spongia and Coelenterata. C. R. Acad. Sci. URSS. **31**, 717—718 (1941).

MOOG, F.: The physiological significance of phosphonate esterases. Biol. Rev. **21**, 41—59 (1946).

— The differentiation of enzymes in relation to the functional activities of developing embryo. Ann. N. Y. Acad. Sci. **55**, 57—66 (1952).

NACHMANSOHN, D.: La transmission de l'influx nerveux central. Presse méd. **48**, 942—943 (1938a).

— Cholinestérase dans les tissus embryonnaires. C. R. Soc. Biol. (Paris) **127**, 670—673 (1938b).

— Changements de la cholinestérase dans le muscle strié. C. R. Soc. Biol. (Paris) **128**, 599—673 (1938c).

— Transmission of nerve impulses in the central nervous system. J. Physiol. (Lond.) **93**, 2—3 (1938d).

— Cholinesterase in muscle of developing chick. J. Physiol. (Lond.) **95**, 29—35 (1939a).

— Cholinestérase dans le système nerveux central. Bull. Soc. Chim. biol. (Paris) **21**, 761—796 (1939b).

— On the physiological significance of cholinesterase. Yale J. Biol. Med. **12**, 565—589 (1940a).

— Cholinesterase in brain and spinal cord of sheep embryos. J. Neurophysiol. **3**, 396—589 (1940b).

— Chemical and molecular basis of nerve activity. New York: Academic Press 1959.

NEEDHAM, J.: Chemical embryology. Cambridge: Cambridge U. Press 1931.

— Biochemistry and morphogenesis. Cambridge: Cambridge U. Press 1942.

O'BRIEN, R. D.: Occurrence of cholinesterase in Tenebrio and Tribolium. Nature (Lond.) **172**, 162—163 (1953).

OPPENHEIMER, J. M.: The normal stages of Fundulus heteroclitus. Anat. Rec. **68**, 1—16 (1937).

ORD, M. G., and R. H. S. THOMPSON: Nature of placental cholinesterase. Nature (Lond.) **165**, 927—928 (1950).

ORR, D. W., and W. F. WINDLE: The development of behavior in chick embryos: the appearance of somatic movements. J. comp. Neurol. **60**, 271—285 (1934).

PETERS, J. B., and L. B. FLEXNER: Biochemical and physiological differentiation during morphogenesis. VIII. Quantitative morphologic studies on the developing cerebral cortex of the fetal guinea pig. Amer. J. Anat. **86**, 133—157 (1950).

PETERS, J. B., A. R. VONDERAHE and R. H. POWERS: The functional chronology in developing chick nervous system. J. exp. Zool. **133**, 505—518 (1956).

PIERCE, M. E.: The amnion of the chick as an independent effector. J. exp. Zool. **65**, 443—468 (1933).

POTTER, C., K. A. LORD, J. KENTEN, E. H. SALKELD and D. V. HOLBROOK: Embryonic development and esterase activity of eggs of Pieris brassicae in relation to TEPP poisoning. Ann. appl. Biol. **45**, 361—375 (1957).

POULSON, D. E., and E. J. BOELL: The development of cholinesterase activity in embryos of normal genetically deficient strains of Drosophila Melanogaster. Anat. Rec. **96**, 508 (only) (1946).

RAIHA, C. E.: Tissue metabolism in the human fetus. Cold Spr. Harb. Symp. quant. Biol. **19**, 143—151 (1954).

RAVIN, H. A., S. I. ZACKS and A. M. SELIGMAN: The histochemical localization of acetylcholinesterase in nervous tissue. J. Pharmacol. exp. Ther. **107**, 37—53 (1953).

RICHARDS, A. G., and L. K. CUTCOMP: The cholinesterase of insect nerves. J. comp. Physiol. **26**, 57—61 (1945).

RISLEY, J. E., and D. R. DAVIES: The variation with age of the hydrolysis of choline esters by rat tissues. Biochem. J. **54**, 30 (only) (1953).

ROBERTSON, J. D.: The ultrastructure of adult vertebrate peripheral myelinated nerve fibers in relation to myelinogenesis. J. biophys. biochem. Cytol. **1**, 271—278 (1955).

ROCKSTEIN, M.: The relation of cholinesterase activity to change in cell number with age in the brain of adult worker honeybee. J. cell. comp. Physiol. **35**, 11—24 (1950).

— Physiological aging in the adult worker honeybee. Biol. Bull. **105**, 154—159 (1953).

ROSENZWEIG, M. R., D. KRECH, and E. L. BENNET: Brain chemistry and adaptive behavior. In: H. F. HARLOW, and C. N. WOOLSEY, EDS., Biological and Biochemical Bases of Behavior, 367—400. Madison: U. of Wisconsin Press 1958a.

— — — Brain enzymes and adaptive behavior. In: G. E. W. WOLSTENHOLME and C. M. O'CONNOR, Eds., Neurological Basis of Behavior, 337—358. Boston: Little, Brown & Co. 1958b.

ROTHENBERG, M. A., and D. NACHMANSOHN: Studies on cholinesterase. II. Purification of the enzyme from electric tissue by fractional ammonium sulfate precipitation. J. biol. Chem. **168**, 223—231 (1947).

ROWATT, E.: Relation of pantothenic acid to acetylcholine formation by a strain of Lactobacillus planatarum. J. gen. Microbiol. **2**, 25—39 (1948).

RUBIN, R.: Versuche über die Beziehung des Nervensystems zur Regeneration bei Amphibien. Wilhelm Roux' Arch. Entwickl.-mech. Org. **16**, 21—75 (1903).

RUGH, ROBERTS: Experimental Embryology. Minneapolis: Burgess Publishing Co. 1948.

RUNNSTRÖM, J.: Analytische Studien über Seeigelentwicklung. III. Wilhelm Roux' Arch. Entwickl. mech. Org. **43**, 223—328 (1917).

— Zur experimentellen Analyse der Wirkung des Lithiums auf den Seeigelkeim. Acta Zool. **9**, 365—424 (1928).

RYABINOWSKAYA, A. M.: Cholinesterases in the ontogenesis of mammals. C. R. Acad. Sci. URSS. **26**, 826—828 (1940).

SACKTOR, B.: A comparison of the cytochrome oxidase activity of two strain of houseflies. J. Econ. Entomol. **43**, 837—838 (1950).

SAWYER, C. H.: Choline esterase and behavior in Amblystoma punctatum. Anat. Rec. **28**, 57 (only) (1940).

— Cholinesterase in developing Amblystoma. Proc. Soc. exp. Biol. (N. Y.) **49**, 37—40 (1942).

— Cholinesterase and the behavior problem in Amblystoma. I. The relationship between the development of the enzyme and early motility. II. The effects of inhibiting cholinesterase. J. exp. Zool. **92**, 1—27 (1943a).

— Cholinesterase and the behavior problem in Amblystoma. III. The distribution of cholinesterase in nerve and muscle throughout development. IV. Cholinesterase in nerveless muscle. J. exp. Zoll. **94**, 1—31 (1943b).

— Nature of the early somatic movements in Fundulus heteroclitus. J. cell. comp. Physiol. **24**, 71—84 (1944).

— Further experiments on cholinesterase and reflex activity in Amblystoma larvae. J. exp. Zool. **129**, 561—578 (1955).

—, and W. H. HOLLINSHEAD: Cholinesterase in sympathetic fibers and ganglia. J. Neurophysiol. **8**, 137—154 (1945).

SCHOTTÉ, O. E.: Influences des nerfs sur la régénération des pattes antérieures de Tritons adultes. C. R. Soc. Phys. Hist. nat. (Genève) **39**, 67—70 (1922).

— Nouvelles preuves physiologiques de l'action du système nerveux sympathique dans la régénération. C. R. Soc. Phys. Hist. nat. (Genève) **43**, 140 (1926).

SEAMAN, G. R., and H. K. HOULIHAN: Enzyme system of Tetrahymena gelii (S). II. Acetylcholinesterase activity. Its relation to motility of the organism and to coordinated ciliary action in general. J. cell. comp. Physiol. **37**, 309—322 (1951).

SHAMARINA, N. M.: The cholinesterase content of embryonic muscle. Bull. Biol. med. exp. URSS. **8**, 67—69 (1939).

— The cholinesterase content of the embryonic auricle. Fisiol. Zhur. **28**, 650—656 (1940).

SHAVER, J. R.: Some observations on cytoplasmic particles in early Echinoderm development. In: A. TYLER, R. C. VON BORSTEL and C. B. METZ, Eds., The Beginnings of Embryonic Development. Washington, D. C.: Amer. Assoc. Adv. of Sci. (1957).

SHEN, S. C.: Enzyme development as ontogeny of specific proteins. In: E. G. BUTLER, Ed., Biological Specificity and Growth, 73—92. Princeton: Princeton U. Press 1955.

— Changes in enzymatic patterns during development. In: The Chemical Basis of Development, 416—432. Baltimore: The Johns Hopkins Press 1958.

— P. GREENFIELD and E. J. BOELL: The distribution of cholinesterase in the frog brain. J. comp. Neurol. **102**, 717—744 (1955).

SHEN, S. C., P. GREENFIELD and E. J. BOELL: Localization of acetylcholinesterase in chick retina during histogenesis. J. comp. Neurol. 106, 433—462 (1956).
— — and I. SIPPEL: Application of histochemical technique for cholinesterase to paraffin sections. Proc. Sec. exp. Biol. (N. Y.) 81, 452—455 (1952).
SHUMWAY, W.: Normal stages in the development of Rana pipiens. I. External form. Anat. Rec. 78, 139—147 (1940).
SINGER, M., M. H. DAVIS and E. S. ARKOVITZ: Acetylcholinesterase activity in the regenerating forelimb of the adult newt, Triturus. J. Embryol. exp. Morph. 8, 98—111 (1960a).
— — and M. R. SCHEUING: The influence of atropine and other neuropharmacological substances on regeneration of the forelimb in the adult Urodele, Triturus. J. exp. Zool. 143, 33—46 (1960b).
— Nervous mechanisms in the regeneration of body parts in vertebrates. In: Developing cell systems and their control, 115—133. The Ronald Press Co. 1960.
SIPPEL, T. O.: The growth of succinoxidase activity in the hearts of rat and chick embryos. J. exp. Zool. 126, 205—221 (1954).
— Properties and development of cholinesterase in the hearts of certain vertebrates. J. exp. Zool. 128, 165—184 (1955).
SMITH, C. C., B. JACKSON and C. L. PROSSER: Responses to acetylcholine and cholinesterase content of Cerebratulus. Biol. Bull. 79, 377 (only) (1940).
SMITH, E. H., and A. C. WAGENKNECHT: The occurrence of cholinesterase in the eggs of the peach tree borer and large milk weed bug and its relation to the ovicidal action of parathion. J. Econ. Ent. 49, 777—783 (1956).
— — The ovicidal action of organophosphate insecticides. Canad. J. Biochem. 37, 1135—1144 (1959).
SPEMANN, H.: Embryonic development and induction. New Haven: Yale U. Press 1938.
SPIEGELMAN, S., and A. M. CAMPBELL: The significance of induced enzyme adaptation. In: D. E. GREEN, Ed., Currents in Biochemical Research, 115—116. New York: Interscience Publishers, Inc. 1956.
SPRATT, N., JR.: Nutritional requirements of the early chick embryo. I. The utilization of carbohydrate substrates. J. exp. Zool. 110, 273—298 (1949).
STAUDENMAYER, T.: Die Cholinesterase während der Eientwicklung von Bombyx mori und die ovizide Wirkung von Phosphorsäureester (E 600 und E 605). Z. vergl. Physiol. 37, 416—423 (1955).
— Die Wirkung verschiedener Kontaktinsektizide auf die Atmung von Seidenspinnern. Z. vergl. Physiol. 39, 262—273 (1957).
STEPHENSON, M., and E. ROWATT: The production of acetylcholine by a strain of Lactobacillus planatarum. J. gen. Microbiol. 1, 279—298 (1947).
STRAUS, W. L., JR., and G. WEDDELL: Nature of the first visible contractions of the forelimb musculature in rat fetuses. J. Neurophysiol. 3, 358—369 (1940).
SZEPSENWOL, J., and J. A. CARETTI: Acetylcholine in the chick embryo. I. Its variations in striated muscle and encephalon during development. Rev. Soc. argent. Biol. 18, 300—307 (1942a).
— — Acetilcolina en embryones de pollo. II. Sus variaciones en los differentes centros nerviosos durante el desarrollo. Rev. Soc. argent. Biol. 18, 532—538 (1942b).
TAHMISIAN, T. N.: Enzymes in ontogenesis: cholinesterase in developing Melanoplus differentialis eggs. J. exp. Zool. 92, 199—213 (1943).
TAYLOR, A. C., and J. J. KOLLROS: Stages in the normal development of Rana pipiens larvae. Anat. Rec. 94, 7—23 (1946).
TAYLOR, C. V.: Fibrillar systems in ciliates. In: Protozoa in Biological Research, 191—270. G. N. CALKINS and F. M. SUMMERS, Eds., New York: Columbia U. Press 1941.
TELLO, J. F.: Les differenciations neuronales dans l'embryon du poulet, pendant les premiers jours de l'incubation. Trav. Lab. Rech. Biol., Univ. Madrid 21, 1—93 (1923).
THOMAS, J. A., and D. NACHMANSOHN: La cholinestérase dans les cultures du coeur de l'embryon, chez la poule. C. R. Soc. Biol. (Paris) 128, 577—580 (1938).
TORDA, C.: Cholinesterase activity of embryonic tissues. Biochim. Terap. sper. 25, 532—539 (1938).
VAN DER KLOOT, W. G.: The control of neurosecretion and diapause by physiological changes in the brain of the Cecropia silkworm. Biol. Bull., Wood's Hole 109, 276—294 (1955).
VERZAR, F.: Über glatte Muskelzellen mit myogenem Rhythmus. Pflügers Arch. ges. Physiol. 158, 419—420 (1914).
WATANATE, M. I., and C. M. WILLIAMS: Mitochondria in the flight muscles of insects. I. Chemical composition and enzymatic content. J. gen. Physiol. 34, 675—689 (1951).
WELSH, J. H.: Marine invertebrate preparations useful in the bioassay of acetylcholine and 5-hydroxytryptamine. Nature (Lond.) 173, 955—956 (1954).

WELSH, J. H., and J. E. HYDE: The distribution of acetylcholine in brains of rats of different ages. J. Neurophysiol. **7**, 41—49 (1944).
—, and R. TAUB: The action of acetylcholine antagonists on the heart of Venus mercenaria. Brit. J. Pharmacol. **8**, 327—333 (1953).
—, and S. I. ZACKS: Concerning the significance of the affinity of motor end-plate for Janus green B. Anat. Rec. **105**, 526 (only) (1949).
—, and R. TAUB: The action of choline and related compounds on the heart of Venus mercenaria. Biol. Bull. **95**, 346—353 (1948).
WENGER, B. S.: Cholinesterase activity in different spinal levels of the chick embryo. Fed. Proc. **10**, 268—269 (1951).
WHITING, H. P.: Functional development in the nervous system. In: H. WAELSH, Ed., Biochemistry of the Developing Nervous System, 85—103. New York: Academic Press Inc. 1955.
WILLIAMS, C. U.: Physiology of insect diapause. IV. The brain and prothoracic glands as an endocrine system in the Cecropia silkworm. Biol. Bull., Wood's Hole **103**, 120—138 (1952).
WILLIAMS, C. M.: Isolation and identification of the prothoracic gland hormone of insects. Anat. Rec. **120**, 743—744 (1954).
WINDLE, W. F., and M. F. AUSTIN: Neurofibrillar development in the central nervous system of chick embryos up to 5 days' incubation. J. comp. Neurol. **103**, 431—463 (1936).
WINDLE, W. E., and D. W. ORR: The development of behavior in chick embryos: Spinal cord structure correlated with early somatic motility. J. comp. Neurol. **60**, 287—307 (1934).
YOUNGSTROM, K. A.: On the relationship between cholinesterase and the development of behavior in amphibia. J. Neurophysiol. **1**, 357—363 (1938a).
— Studies on the developing behavior of anura. J. comp. Neurol. **68**, 357—379 (1938b).
— Acetylcholinesterase concentration during the development of the human fetus. J. Neurophysiol. **4**, 473—477 (1941).
YUSHIMA, T.: Distribution of the acetylcholine-like substance in eggs of some lepidopterous insects. Japan. J. Appl. Zool. **21** (2), 20—72 (1956a).
— Two kinds of fluctuation of the acetylcholine-like substance in the paddy borer, Schoenobius incertulas, during the embryonic development. Japan. J. Appl. Zool. **21** (3), 129—131 (1956b).
— Changes in rate of synthesis of acetylcholine in vitro in eggs of the Asiatic rice borer, Chilo suppresalis (WLK.) and the cabbage armyworm, Mamestra brassicae (L.) during embryonic development. J. Econ. Ent. **50**, 440—443 (1957).
—, and H. CHINO: Acetylcholine and cholinesterase in rice stem barer, Chilo simplex. Bull. Oyo-kontyu. **9**, 52—58 (1953a).
— — On the occurrence of an acetylcholine-like substance in some insect eggs. (1) On the muscle stimulating substance in eggs of the rice stem borer, Chilo simplex, and cabbage army-worm, Barathra Brassicae. Annot. Zool. Japan. **26**, 228—232 (1953b).
ZACKS, S. I.: Esterases in the early chick embryo. Anat. Rec. **118**, 509—537 (1954).
—, and J. H. WELSH: Cholinesterase in rat liver mitochondria. Amer. J. Physiol. **165**, 620—623 (1951).
ZAMBOTTI, V., and O. PINOTTI: L'attività colinesterasica, specifica e aspecifica, delle varie parti del cuore di mammifero. Atti Soc. med.-chir. Padova **27**, 43—51 (1949).

Chapter 6

Cytological Distributions and Physiological Functions of Cholinesterases[1]

By

GEORGE B. KOELLE

With 41 Figures

Contents

[1] The work done in the reviewer's laboratory which is described in this chapter was supported largely by research grants (B-282, through C 8) from the National Institute of Neurological Diseases and Blindness, National Institutes of Health, U.S. Public Health Service.

Introduction

With the technical advances of the past few decades, there has been increasing emphasis in neurophysiology and neuropharmacology on studies at the cellular and subcellular levels, as illustrated by most of the chapters in the present volume. The magnitudes and sequences of the electrical signs associated with neuronal activity could be defined accurately only after the development of reliable single unit and intracellular recording techniques. At the same time, the electron microscope has yielded knowledge of the morphological details of nervous tissue well beyond its known physiological correlates. However, the chemistry of the structures and specific reactions involved in nervous function can for the most part be described only at the tissue or relatively gross cellular level, and the cytological details as to where the various reactions occur are largely conjectural.

Of the three known chemical moieties specifically involved in cholinergic transmission, acetylcholine (ACh), choline acetylase (ChAc), and acetylcholinesterase (AChE), these limitations apply fully to the first two (see Chapters 1, 2, and 3), although a recently published bioassay permits the detection of less than 5×10^{-15} mol of ACh in 0.15 μl (NASTUK and LEVINE 1961). The receptor substances with which ACh is assumed to react in producing its characteristic effects are still largely hypothetical (WASER 1960), although this problem is now under direct attack in at least two laboratories (CHAGAS et al. 1957, EHRENPREIS 1960) (see Chapter 15). On the other hand, there is probably no other enzyme, the cytological localization of which has been so extensively described to date as AChE. There are several reasons for this. Acetylcholinesterase (AChE) and the non-specific cholinesterases (non-specific ChE's, pseudo-ChE, butyro-ChE, BuChE) are extremely stable in contrast to most enzymes, and can be subjected to a variety of preparative procedures with little loss of activity. The standard assay methods for cholinesterases (ChE's) are relatively simple and can be made reasonably specific; many have been adapted to micro- and ultramicro-techniques (see Chapter 4). Esterases as a general class are amenable to demonstration by histochemical procedures, and several, of varying degrees of accuracy, have been developed for the ChE's. The fact that the anticholinesterase (anti-ChE) agents are one of the very few classes of drugs for which the mechanism of action can be described at least partially in specific biochemical terms has spurred the efforts of a great many investigators to take advantage of the foregoing factors. The results of such studies to date have probably raised more questions than they have answered. Nevertheless, considered in conjunction with physiological and ultrastructural data, they have allowed certain tentative conclusions to be drawn with reasonable assurance concerning the functions of AChE and ACh, and the basis for the actions of the anti-ChE agents at various sites.

In the present Chapter, consideration will be given first to the methods available for the cytological localization of AChE and the non-specific ChE's, with emphasis on their individual accuracies and limitations. This will be followed by a systematic description of the distributions of the enzymes in the nervous system and elsewhere as derived by the various methods. Finally, the bearing of these findings, along with those from various physiological approaches, on the possible functions of ACh and AChE will be discussed.

Methods

The two types of methods of greatest general value for the cytological localization of ChE's at present are microscopic histochemistry and ultramicro-analysis.

The former has the advantage of allowing much more detailed definition of sites of enzymatic activity in terms of cellular structures. The latter permits a far superior degree of quantitation. A third type of method, fractional centrifugation of homogenates of relatively large samples followed by analysis of the individual fractions, has several limitations, and its applications are more restricted.

A. Microscopic histochemistry

The history, general principles, methods, advantages, and limitations of microscopic histochemistry, particularly as applied to enzymes, have been discussed in several excellent reviews (FRIEDENWALD 1955, GOMORI 1952a, NOVIKOFF 1951, 1955) and monographs (GLICK 1949, GOMORI 1952b, LISON 1953, PEARSE 1960, DEANE et al. 1960). As most of these authors have pointed out, the requirements of a satisfactory histochemical procedure include not only specificity and sensitivity, as do all analytical procedures, but in addition preservation of structure, accuracy of localization, and avoidance of artifacts that may arise from several sources.

Attempts to fulfill maximally any one of the foregoing requirements generally compromise others. For example, preliminary fixation is necessary to maintain optimal structural integrity, but this invariably results in a decrease in enzyme activity; at sites of low initial activity, the enzyme may be inhibited completely. The same relationship is true of fresh-frozen sectioning versus embedding; with the former, enzymatic activity is preserved at the cost of loss of structural detail, whereas with embedding in paraffin or celloidin the reverse is true. These factors will be considered as they apply to the individual methods. They emphasize the value of employing more than one modification of a given technique, and utilizing the information gained from as many techniques as possible, including the other types of methods to be discussed, in arriving at conclusions regarding the relative concentrations of a given enzyme at various sites.

It must be stressed that microscopic histochemical methods, while permitting detection of extremely low concentrations of enzymatic activity, allow by inspection only very general approximations of relative activities. Even with certain techniques that have been developed for recording the optical density of specific areas of stained sections, results can be highly misleading, as has been illustrated graphically by GOMORI (1952b). Such techniques are discussed with the individual methods to which they have been applied.

Finally, with the great improvements that are currently being developed in preparative techniques for electron microscopy, it can be expected that at some future date the most significant histochemical work will be done at this level. At present, relatively few histochemical studies of AChE employing electron microscopy have been published. This in general reflects a laudable conservatism. Only under the best conditions can enzymatic localization be considered reliable at the limits of resolution of light microscopy. Until there is reasonable assurance that such factors as diffusion artifacts and penetration of reagents have been adequately controlled at the level of magnification provided by the electron microscope, results so obtained can offer no particular advantage and may be misleading. However, some of the published results noted below are most encouraging, and every effort should be made to develop suitable methods for electron microscopy.

The individual methods which follow are identified by abbreviations in the subsequent section on cytological localization of the ChE's.

I. Long-chain fatty acid ester methods (LC-Ch)

The first histochemical method published for the localization of cholinesterases was that of GOMORI (1948), in which the choline esters of lauric, myristic, palmitic, and stearic acids were employed as substrates. These esters (GLICK 1941), as well as acetylthiocholine (GLICK 1939), the substrate used in the method which follows, had been shown previously by GLICK to be hydrolyzed by the ChE's of horse serum. The method is based on the following reaction:

$$(CH_3)_3N^+CH_2CH_2OCO(CH_2)_{12}CH_3 \xrightarrow[+ \ H_2O]{(AChE \ or \ BuChE)} \underset{+ \ Choline}{Myristic \ Acid} \xrightarrow{Co^{++}}$$

Myristoylcholine

$$Cobalt \ Myristate \xrightarrow{(H_2S)} CoS$$
(precipitate)

In the original procedure, tissues are fixed in chilled acetone, transferred through alcohol-ether, 4% collodion in alcohol-ether, chloroform, embedded in paraffin, and sectioned. Following hydration, sections are incubated on slides for 2 to 16 hr at 37° in a medium containing 0.004 M substrate, 0.017 to 0.033 M maleate-tris(hydroxymethyl)-aminomethane buffer at pH 7.5 to 7.7, 0.010 to 0.017 M cobaltous chloride, and small amounts of $CaCl_2$, $MgCl_2$, and $MnCl_2$. As the substrate is hydrolyzed, the fatty acid is precipitated as the highly insoluble cobaltous salt. Following a brief rinse in tap water, slides are immersed in yellow ammonium sulfide solution, which converts the cobalt salt to a black precipitate of CoS. Sections are then dehydrated, cleared, and mounted. Subsequently (GOMORI 1952b) it was recommended that the ammonium sulfide solution be made up in 70% alcohol to hasten the reaction.

The method has been modified by other investigators and analyzed critically by PEARSE (1960). Data contained in the original paper indicate that none of the foregoing esters is hydrolyzed by purified preparations of AChE, which led KOELLE and FRIEDENWALD (1949) to conclude that hydrolysis was produced only by non-specific ChE's, and to develop the acetylthiocholine method. However, DENZ (1953) showed that myristoylcholine is hydrolyzed at a significant rate by the AChE of sheep erythrocytes. With his modification of the method (unfixed fresh frozen sections, incubated for 30 min freely floating in a medium containing myristoylcholine, in which the original buffer is replaced by bicarbonate buffer) he obtained excellent localization of AChE at the motor endplates of rat diaphragm. The identity of the enzyme was confirmed by the use of graded concentrations of selective inhibitor. Likewise, with myristoylcholine as substrate and incubating for 24 hr, DE ALMEIDA and COUCEIRO (1955) obtained satisfactory staining of fresh and formalin-fixed frozen sections of rat intercostal muscle and the electric organ of *Electrophorus*.

II. Thiocholine ester methods (ThCh-I-IX)

1. Original method and direct modifications

In extension of GLICK's (1939) earlier report, KOELLE and FRIEDENWALD (1949) found that acetylthiocholine (AThCh) is hydrolyzed by both AChE's and BuChE's at greater velocities than is ACh itself. It therefore appeared to be a promising substrate for histochemical application.

In the original method *(ThCh-I)*, fresh frozen sections or teased preparations were incubated for 10 to 60 min in a medium containing 0.004 M AThCh, 0.002 M CuSO$_4$, 0.008 M glycine, adjusted to pH 8.0, and saturated with copper thiocholine (CuThCh) in order to effect its precipitation as rapidly as formed from the enzymatic liberation of thiocholine. Controls consisted of similar sections pre-incubated for 30 min in 10^{-3} M diisopropyl phosphorofluoridate (diisopropylfluorophosphate, DFP) in saline solution to inactivate all ChE's. Following incubation, sections were rinsed briefly in saline solution and immersed in yellow ammonium sulfide solution to convert the precipitated copper to CuS; presumptive sites of enzymatic activity were visualized as dark brown deposits.

$$AThCh \xrightarrow[+ \ H_2O]{(AChE \ or \ BuChE)} \underset{+ \ HAc}{ThCh} \xrightarrow{Cu^{++}} CuThCh \xrightarrow{H_2S} CuS$$

Acetylthiocholine   Thiocholine   Copper Thio-   Copper
+ Acetic Acid   choline   Sulfide

Additional thiocholine esters and selective inhibitors were investigated to permit the selective localization of AChE and BuChE (KOELLE 1950) *(ThCh-II)*.

It was found that sites of AChE activity could be stained selectively by incubating sections with a low concentration of DFP, which inhibits selectively BuChE, prior to incubation with AThCh. For the localization of BuChE only, butyrylthiocholine (BuThCh) was used as substrate. In the course of the same study, it was found that in the originally employed unbuffered medium, precipitation of CuThCh did not occur until the acid liberated during incubation had reduced the pH considerably. Accordingly, media were then adjusted to pH 6.4 with phosphate buffer.

A further major and some minor modifications were introduced the following year (KOELLE 1951) to bring the method to the stage at which it is used routinely in the author's laboratory at present *(ThCh-III)*. In spite of the fact that most of the AChE is fixed firmly to cellular structures, evidence was obtained that artifacts of localization, particularly false nuclear staining, occurred as the result of diffusion and subsequent adsorption elsewhere of the enzymes, reaction product, or both. The occurrence of partial enzymatic diffusion was demonstrated by assays of the resuspended solid fractions and of the supernatant solutions following centrifugation of cat brain homogenates, which indicated that significant amounts of both AChE and BuChE were present in the latter. In the presence of increasing concentrations of Na_2SO_4, the proportion of enzyme recovered from the solid fraction gradually increased, and recovery was practically complete for AChE in 24%, and for BuChE in 28% Na_2SO_4. When the same concentrations of Na_2SO_4 were incorporated into the incubation media, nuclear staining was virtually eliminated. It is quite possible that the high concentration of the salt served also to minimize diffusion of the reaction product, which has been shown subsequently to be copper thiocholine sulfate $(Cu^+ - SCH_2CH_2N^+(CH_3)_3)SO_4^-$ (MALMGREN and SYLVÉN 1955). The buffer was changed to sodium hydrogen maleate, adjusted to a final pH of 6.0 for the incubation media, and magnesium chloride was added as an activator. Manometric assays showed that at the pH, and at the concentrations of Na_2SO_4, $CuSO_4$, and glycine employed in the histochemical media, the activities of cat AChE and BuChE were reduced approximately to 25% and 50%, respectively, of their activities at pH 7.4 under nearly optimal conditions. Since many of the findings reported in the subsequent sections have been obtained by this method or its modifications, the details of the procedure are given below.

Selective Localization of AChE and BuChE in Cat Tissues (ThCh-III) (KOELLE 1951).

Reagents:

Cu-Gl: 3.75 g glycine, 2.50 g $CuSO_4 \cdot 5 H_2O$, *q.s.* 100.0 ml.
Mal: 9.60 g NaH maleate (TEMPLE 1929), 52.2 ml *N* NaOH, *q.s.* 100.0 ml.
Na_2SO_4: 40% (W/V) Na_2SO_4, adjusted to pH 6.00, stored at 38°.
$MgCl_2$: 2.03 g $MgCl_2 \cdot 6 H_2O$, *q.s.* 10.0 ml.
AThCh: 46 mg acetylthiocholine iodide, 2.4 ml H_2O, 0.8 ml 0.1 *M* $CuSO_4$; centrifuged, supernatant decanted off and saved.
BuThCh: Same, using 50 mg butyrylthiocholine iodide.
CuThCh: Copper thiocholine sulfate; obtained by filtering incubation solutions immediately after removal of slides, storing at 38° for two to four days to permit complete spontaneous hydrolysis of substrate, collecting precipitate by centrifugation and washing with water.
$(NH_4)_2S$: Half-strength concentrated NH_4OH solution saturated with H_2S; stored in refrigerator. Immediately before use, dilute 1.0 ml to 25.0 ml with H_2O, add 2 drops 0.1 *M* $CuSO_4$, mix, filter.

Incubation solutions are prepared by adding the above reagents to test tubes in the amounts and orders listed in table 1-A. The solutions are saturated with the reaction product by adding a trace of CuThCh, stirring to obtain its complete dispersal, and storing in the incubator at 38° for at least fiften min prior to the addition of substrates. In order to minimize spontaneous hydrolysis, substrates (AThCh and BuThCh) are added immediately before the solutions are to be employed, and the solutions are stirred and filtered through Whatman No. 2 filter paper into Coplin jars previously warmed in the incubator.

Table 1-A. *Composition of incubation media for localization of specific (AChE) and non-specific ChE (BuChE) activities (ThCh-III)* (KOELLE 1951)

Solution	Enzyme localized	Reagents							
		Cu-Gl ml	H₂O ml	Mal ml	Na₂SO₄ ml	MgCl₂ ml	CuThCh	AThCh ml	BuThCh ml
A	All ChE's	0.6	0.6	1.5	10.5	0.6	Trace	1.2	—
B	AChE	0.6	2.1	1.5	9.0	0.6	Trace	1.2	—
C	BuChE	0.6	0.6	1.5	10.5	0.6	Trace	—	1.2
D	Control	0.6	2.1	1.5	9.0	0.6	Trace	—	1.2

Slides are kept in the following storage solutions prior to incubation:

DFP: 4.5 ml H₂O, 9.0 ml 40% Na₂SO₄, 1.5 ml 10^{-6} *M* DFP. The DFP solution is prepared within thirty minutes of the time used by serial dilution of a 0.1 *M* stock solution in anhydrous propylene glycol.

B and D: 6.0 ml H₂O, 9.0 ml 40% Na₂SO₄.

A and C: 4.5 ml H₂O, 10.5 ml 40% Na₂SO₄.

Storage solutions are prepared in Coplin jars and kept in a water bath at 30 to 35°.

Tissues are removed immediately after sacrifice and are placed in chilled saline solution. Frozen sections are cut as soon after removal as possible by WHITE and ALLEN's (1951) modification of the method of ADAMSTONE and TAYLOR (1948), and placed immediately on slides. As soon as the sections have thawed and excess moisture has evaporated (requiring about one min), the slides are placed in the appropriate storage solutions. Sections to be stained for AChE (incubation solution B) and controls (incubation solution D) are placed in storage solution *DFP* for 30 min, then transferred to storage solution *B* and *D* until placed in the incubation solutions; sections to be stained for all ChE's (incubation solution A) and for BuChE activity (incubation solution C) are stored in storage solution *A* and *C*, respectively. Following a minimal period of storage, slides are transferred to the incubation solutions for periods of 5 to 60 min at 38°; thirty min is satisfactory for most tissues. They are then transferred to rinse solution 1 (20% Na₂SO₄, saturated with CuThCh) for five min or longer, and immersed for approximately one min in rinse solution 2 (10% Na₂SO₄, saturated with CuThCh) and dipped rapidly (1 to 2 sec) in water, following which they are placed for 20 sec in (NH₄)₂S solution, rinsed rapidly in water, fixed in 10% formalin, dehydrated through alcohols and xylol, and mounted in balsam. The intensity of staining is increased by gold-toning, by any standard method, after removal from the formalin solution. Similar preparations may be counterstained with hematoxylin-eosin or stained by the brilliant cresyl violet or Bielschowsky silver method to facilitate localization of enzymatic activity with respect to various structural details. Any staining encountered in the control sections (solution D) must be discounted in the other sections in assessing sites of AChE (solution B) or BuChE (solution C) activity.

The modification of this procedure recommended by GOMORI (1952b) *(ThCh-IV)* is practically identical. It differs only in that (a) all reagents excepting the substrate are prepared and stored as a stock solution, (b) final concentrations of the individual reagents differ slightly, and (c) saturation with CuThCh is omitted. This modification has the advantage of greater convenience, but does not provide the optimal concentrations of Na₂SO₄ for precipitation of AChE and BuChE. The importance of CuThCh-saturation at pH 6.0 has not been fully assessed, but it is considered a useful precaution particularly for identifying sites of extremely low enzymatic activity.

It was shown later (KOELLE 1955) that homogenates of cat, rabbit, and rhesus monkey brains contain enzymes in addition to AChE and BuChE which can hydrolyze AThCh and BuThCh. In order to distinguish possible staining by such thiolesterases, additional controls containing selective inhibitors of both AChE and non-specific ChE's were introduced *(ThCh-V)*. The results of these studies were confirmed and extended by HOLMSTEDT (1957a, b).

For this purpose, a total of 10 incubation solutions is employed, five of which (A-1 to A-5) contain AThCh as substrate and the remainder (C-1 to C-5), BuThCh (Table 1-B) (KOELLE 1955). The five pairs (A's and C's) of solutions are used with (1) no inhibitor, (2) DFP or Nu 683 (the dimethyl carbamate of [2-hydroxy-5 phenylbenzyl]-trimethylammonium bromide) as a selective inhibitor of BuChE, (3) B.W. 284 (B.W. 284 c 51, 1-5-*bis*-[4-allyl dimethylammonium phenyl]-pentan-3-one dibromide) as a selective inhibitor of AChE, (4) DFP or Nu 683 plus B.W. 284 for the inhibition of both enzymes, and (5) eserine (physostigmine) as a highly selective inhibitor of all ChE's. The appropriate concentration of each inhibitor must be determined for any species under conditions approximating those of the histochemical incubation media. For the three species mentioned, the concentrations causing nearly complete inhibition of the enzymes specified are in the range of 10^{-8} to 3×10^{-8} M for DFP, 6×10^{-8} M for Nu 683, and 10^{-5} to 3×10^{-5} M for B.W. 284 and eserine.

Table 1-B. *Substrate and inhibitor contents of incubation solutions for the selective localization and inhibition of AChE and BuChE in tissues of the cat, rabbit, and rhesus monkey (ThCh-V)* (KOELLE 1955)

Solution	Substrate	ChE's Hydrolizing		Inhibitor	ChE's Inhibited		ChE's Stained	
		AChE	BuChE		AChE	BuChE	AChE	BuChE
A-1	AThCh	+	+	—	—	—	+	+
A-2	AThCh	+	—	DFP or Nu 683	—	+	+	—
A-3	AThCh	+	+	B.W. 284	+	—	—	+
A-4	AThCh	+	+	DFP + B.W. 284	+	+	—	—
A-5	AThCh	+	+	Eserine	+	+	—	—
C-1	BuThCh	—	+	—	—	—	—	+
C-2	BuThCh	—	+	DFP or Nu 683	—	+	—	—
C-3	BuThCh	—	+	B.W. 284	+	—	—	+
C-4	BuThCh	—	+	DFP + B.W. 284	+	+	—	—
C-5	BuThCh	—	+	Eserine	+	+	—	—

The results of staining sections of the superior cervical ganglion of the cat with all 10 solutions are illustrated in Figure 1. By reference to Table 1-B, it will be seen that if A-4, A-5, C-2, C-4, and C-5 are essentially blank (as is the case here), it may be assumed with reasonable certainty that staining in A-2 represents AChE activity, and only sites of BuChE activity are stained in A-3, C-1, and C-3. Staining encountered in the first-mentioned sections might be attributable to enzymes other than AChE or BuChE, incorrect concentrations of inhibitors, non-specific adsorption of copper ion, or other factors, and must be discounted in assessing sites of AChE or BuChE activity in the sections specified as such.

With the use of the additional inhibitors as controls, the thiocholine method appears to be the most specific histochemical method available for AChE or BuChE. As several investigators have pointed out, prolonged incubation with this technique, particularly at sites of high enzymatic activity, results in the deposition of acicular crystals of CuThCh, and eventual diffusion of staining to adjacent areas. However, if the time between sectioning and incubation is minimized, and the incubation period is restricted to a few minutes, a high degree of precision of localization can be obtained (FUKUDA and KOELLE 1959). The modifications employed by COUTEAUX and others (see below) probably permit even greater precision of localization, but at the cost of sensitivity for staining sites of low activity. The above method (*ThCh-III* or *V*) permitted accurate localization of AChE in tissues from animals treated with an irreversible anti-ChE agent, and subsequently with a reactivator, in which no activity could be demonstrated by the ordinary manometric method (RAJAPURKAR and KOELLE 1958). The absolute sensitivity has been approximated by HARRIS et al. (1953). Under certain circumstances, as in the staining of smears of blood and bone marrow, the sensitivity can be increased further by omission of conversion of the initial precipitate to

CuS (ZAJICEK et al. 1954) (see below). The use of the present method at low pH (5.3) has been recommended by BERGNER and O'NEILL (1958) for studying the interaction of oxime reactivators and alkylphosphorylated AChE *in vitro*.

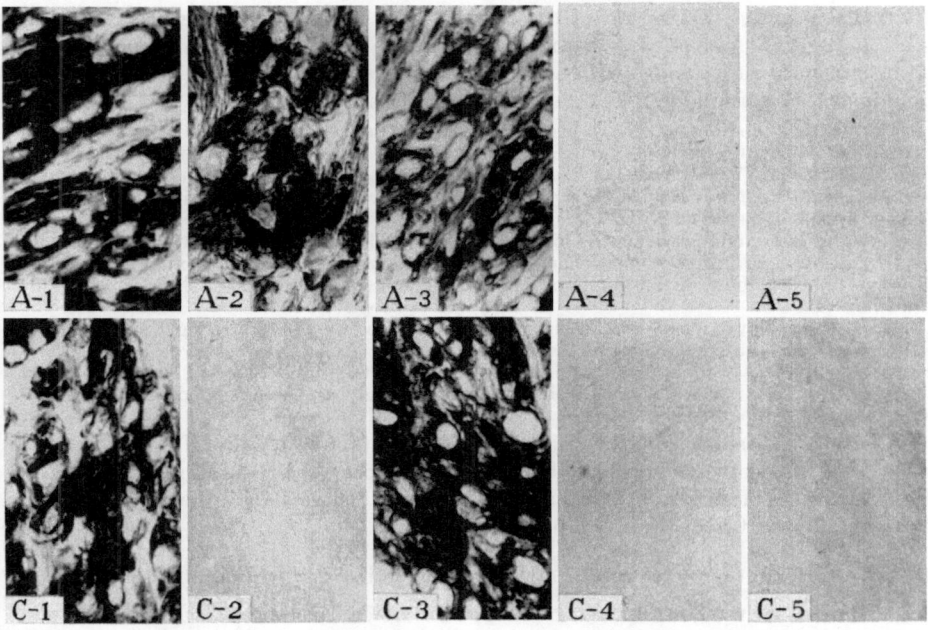

Fig. 1. Superior cervical ganglion, cat. Ten micron sections incubated for two hours in each of the ten solutions described in the text and Table 1-B, developed with $(NH_4)_2S$, and gold-toned. Magnification 250 ×. Substrates: A-AThCh: C-BuThCh. Inhibitors: 1-none; 2-DFP; 3-B.W.284; 4-DFP plus B.W.284; 5-eserine (KOELLE 1955)

2. Modifications employing prior fixation

The most precise localization of AChE published to date with the thiocholine method has been obtained by COUTEAUX (1951) and COUTEAUX and TAXI (1952) at motor endplates of skeletal muscle. This work has been summarized by COUTEAUX (1958).

The chief modifications *(ThCh-VI)* employed consist in fixation in cold neutral 10% formalin for varying periods, incubation of whole muscle or teased preparations in an acetate buffered medium of low pH (in the range of 5.0), from which Na_2SO_4 and CuThCh are omitted, and subsequent paraffin-embedding and sectioning for study at high (× 1,500 to 2,000) magnification. All these steps were introduced as the result of extensive, carefully controlled studies.

COUTEAUX has emphasized the necessity of fixation for preservation of structural detail, but at the same time has recognized the loss of activity entailed; in the case of formalin, TAXI (1952a) showed that the degree of inactivation varies considerably according to the tissue, species, and other factors. Accordingly, COUTEAUX (1958) has recommended that all tissues should be stained both with and without fixation, in order not to overlook sites of low activity, and that the optimal conditions of fixation should be determined for each tissue. The same principle applies to the optimal pH and time of incubation. At levels of pH far below the optimum for the enzyme, diffusion of enzymes, reaction product, or both are apparently minimized in formalin-fixed tissues despite the absence of Na_2SO_4 and CuThCh, but again the exact conditions must be determined indi-

13*

vidually. Prior to incubation with substrate, COUTEAUX incubates tissues in an otherwise identical medium in order to allow the pH of the tissue to attain the level of the medium. Where whole muscle is incubated, the endplates at the surface are presumably sufficiently exposed to the substrates and other reagents for accurate staining. Disruption of the tissue by ice crystals, as occurs with frozen sectioning, is thus avoided. With this modification, the localization of most of the neuromuscular junctional AChE at the level of the subneural apparatus has been demonstrated convincingly, as discussed in a subsequent section.

COUTEAUX's modifications have been employed extensively by several investigators, with certain variations. CÖERS (1953) and GEREBTZOFF (1953) have prepared frozen sections after formalin fixation. The latter author has employed secondary formalin fixation after sectioning, and has incubated at pH levels ranging from 5.0 to 6.8 according to the activity of the enzyme in the tissue being studied *(ThCh-VII)*.

PORTUGALOV and JAKOVLEV (1951) have employed preliminary treatment with cold (—15°) acetone to facilitate penetration of the substrate through lipid-containing membranes. However, their published photo-micrographs of stained motor endplates show considerable diffusion.

The use of polyethylene glycol as an embedding medium for preparing thin (4 to 5 μ) sections of formalin-fixed material prior to staining for AChE has been recommended by RÖHLICH (1956). Alternatively, FREDRICSSON et al. (1960) have reported that if unfixed material is freeze-dried, then embedded in polyethylene glycol, there is good preservation of structure and comparatively little loss of AChE or BuChE activity.

Useful discussions have been given by LEWIS (1961) and by HOLMSTEDT and SJÖQVIST (1961) of the effects produced on both intensity of staining of AChE and BuChE and on structure by various modifications of fixation, embedding, incubation, sulfide-treatment, and mounting.

3. Omission of conversion of metallic thiocholine to corresponding sulfide

As noted above, ZAJICEK et al. (1954) were able to detect AChE in the formed elements of blood and bone marrow by observing directly, under the phase-contrast microscope, the formation of crystals of copper thiocholine sulfate during incubation in the standard medium *(ThCh-III)*. The sensitivity of the method is reflected by their calculation that a single crystal-forming rat platelet ghost, with a surface area of 7×10^{-6} mm², contains only sufficient AChE to hydrolyze 10^{-5} μg AThCh per hour. GIACOBINI (1956) employed the same principle in an elegant study in which single neurons and their constituent parts were isolated by microdissection and observed during incubation in the medium *(ThCh-VIII)*. Relative AChE activities were estimated on the basis of the rate of crystal development. HOLMSTEDT (1957 a, b) modified the standard technique (KOELLE 1951, 1955) by omitting both CuThCh-saturation and final treatment with $(NH_4)_2S$, and by employing N,N'-di*iso*propylphosphorodiamidic fluoride (Mipafox), 4×10^{-6} M, in place of DFP for inhibition of BuChE *(ThCh-IX)*; the former was shown to have greater selectivity than the latter for this purpose, and at the concentration indicated produced complete inactivation of BuChE without affecting AChE.

When silver nitrate or silver sulfate was substituted for the copper salt and glycine omitted, motor endplates developed staining in osmic acid-fixed tissue, without subsequent sulfide treatment, which closely resembled that obtained with CuThCh techniques (BIRKS and BROWN 1960, BROWN 1961). A preliminary account was given of the application of this modification to electron microscopy.

4. Quantitative applications

HELLMANN (1952) utilized $Cu^{64}SO_4$ in place of ordinary $CuSO_4$ in the incubation medium in staining sections of rat diaphragm, and estimated the activity of alcohol-dehydrated sections with a Geiger-Müller counter. He obtained a remarkably constant ratio for the number of endplates to the counts per minute. A histospectrophotometric analysis of the AChE of the motor endplates of rat diaphragms, following treatment with anti-ChE agents, was reported by SOKOLOVSKIY and KOROLEV (1959). The same principle was employed by CREVIER and BÉLANGER (1956) using β-naphthyl acetate and β-carbonaphthoxycholine as substrates (vide infra). While the general criticisms of GOMORI (1952b) mentioned earlier apply to this type of procedure, the motor endplate represents a particularly advantageous structure because of its size, and of the consistency of both its AChE activity and its distribution in the diaphragm.

III. Azo dye coupling methods (Naph-I and -II)

The principle of employing a naphthyl ester as substrate, and incubating sections in the presence of a coupling agent to form a colored precipitate with the liberated naphthol, was introduced by MENTEN et al. (1944) for localizing alkaline phosphatase. It has been applied to the cholinesterases chiefly by SELIGMAN and associates. NACHLAS and SELIGMAN (1949a, b) utilized β-naphthyl acetate and tetrazotized diorthoanisidine for the demonstration of tissue esterases in general. When carbonaphthoxycholine was synthesized and tested, it was found to be a fairly specific substrate for BuChE, and not to be hydrolyzed by AChE (RAVIN, TSOU and SELIGMAN 1951). However, in the same study it was shown that the earlier employed substrate, β-naphthyl acetate, is hydrolyzed at a fairly rapid rate by both BuChE and AChE, as well as by aliesterases.

β-Naphthyl Acetate   β-Naphthol   Tetrazotized Diorthoanisidine

Purple Dye

Several analogs of the ester and various coupling agents were studied by RAVIN, ZACKS and SELIGMAN (1953) to determine the optimal combination for localizing AChE. As a result, they recommended incubating fresh frozen sections on slides for 10 to 20 min at 37° in a filtered medium composed of 10 mg β-naphthyl acetate (initially dissolved in 1 ml actone), 40 mg Fast Blue RR (4-benzoylamino-2,5-dimethoxy aniline), 50 ml 2 M NaCl, 50 ml 0.1 M barbital buffer, pH 7.8, and 5 ml 3% CaCl$_2$. The slides are then rinsed in tap water and mounted in glycerogel *(Naph-I)*.

The limitations of the method as described include low sensitivity, diffusion, and non-specificity. The authors noted that nerve trunks of known AChE activity failed to show localized staining. The published photomicrographs show grossly punctate staining of neurons and considerable diffusion at motor endplates; there is, in addition, considerable background staining of the non-endplate portions of striated muscle fibers. Improved results have been obtained with certain modifications. Although the authors questioned GOMORI's (1950, 1952b) claim that diffusion was reduced by using as substrates esters of α-naphthol, which forms more insoluble dyes on coupling, such was found to be the case by DENZ (1953) in comparing staining of motor endplates with α- and β-naphthyl acetates, and using the same coupling agent as above. The latter author, in the same study, showed also by means of selective inhibitors that staining at the endplates was due to AChE, and that the diffuse staining throughout the myofibrils represented chiefly aliesterase.

Both sensitivity and resolution appear to be improved considerably by a modification introduced recently by DAVIS (1959) *(Naph-II)*.

In this procedure, blood smears are fixed briefly in a cold ($-15°$), 1% solution of osmium tetroxide in dimethylformamide, rinsed in tap water, then incubated for 5 to 120 min in a medium consisting of 15 mg α-naphthyl acetate and 4 drops of pararosaniline ("hexazotized" with $NaNO_2$—HCl immediately prior to addition) in 25 ml $M/15$ Na_2HPO_4, to which is added sufficient $M/15$ KH_2PO_4 to bring the pH to 7.3. The slides are then washed in water, followed by acetone, and dried. Punctate and filamentous staining was noted in erythrocytes, as well as in the various types of leukocytes, but the actual identity of the esterase or esterases involved was not established. Modifications of this method have been employed for studies of the motor endplate (LEHRER and ORNSTEIN 1959) and electric organs (MATHEWSON et al. 1961) by electron microscopy.

Quantitation of staining for AChE and non-specific ChE at the motor endplate by histophotometry has been done by CREVIER and BÉLANGER (1956), using β-naphthyl acetate and β-carbonaphthoxycholine as substrates, and eserine (physostigmine) and excess ACh as selective inhibitors. It was concluded that AChE constituted approximately 90% of the total ChE activity.

IV. Indoxyl ester methods (Ind)

The use of indoxyl acetate and its analogs for the histochemical localization of esterases was introduced independently by BARRNETT and SELIGMAN (1951) and by HOLT (1952). The principle is based upon the autoxidation of the liberated indoxyl to a precipitate of indigo blue.

Indoxyl Acetate   Indoxyl   Indigo Blue

Like the naphthyl acetates, indoxyl acetate and its halogen-substituted analogs are hydrolyzed by many types of esterases, including non-specific esterases, lipases, AChE, non-specific ChE's, and possibly others (PEPLER and PEARSE 1957). The velocity of its hydrolysis by human erythrocyte AChE is approximately half that of ACh, while the velocity with the BuChE of human plasma is somewhat slower (HOLT 1952). Results published by BARRNETT and SELIGMAN with the original procedure indicated extremely diffuse localization of large granular deposits, probably as the result of both delay in oxidation and the nature of the precipitate. With the 5-bromo-analog, HOLT and WITHERS (1952) were somewhat more successful. However, PEPLER and PEARSE (l.c.) considered the procedure less reliable and sensitive for ChE's than ThCh.

In a series of papers, HOLT and associates analyzed and extended this approach with the result that the method has been markedly improved (HOLT 1956). The general requirements of a histochemical procedure for accurate cytological localization were considered first on a theoretical basis (HOLT and O'SULLIVAN 1958). An extensive series of indigogenic compounds was then synthesized (HOLT and SADLER 1958a), and their physical and chemical properties as potential histochemical substrates were studied (HOLT and SADLER 1958b, COTSON and HOLT 1958). For application, 5-bromo-4-chloroindoxyl acetate was chosen as the most satisfactory substrate, and it was found that the addition of potassium ferri- and ferrocya. des in equal concentration (0.005 M) greatly accelerated oxidation of the free i oxyl analogues to the corresponding indigo derivatives, and hence improved the accuracy of localization. The procedure recommended (HOLT 1956) follows (*Ind*).

To a solution consisting of 2 ml 0.1 M tris(hydroxymethyl)-aminomethane buffer, pH 8.5, 1 ml oxidant (potassium ferri- and ferrocyanides, each 0.05 M), 5 ml 2 M NaCl, and 2 ml H_2O, is added 5×10^{-6} mol substrate dissolved in 0.1 ml ethanol or acetone, with rapid mixing and shaking. Fresh frozen sections are incubated freely floating for 5 to 60 min, after which they are transferred to 30% ethanol, containing 0.1% acetic acid; they are then formalin -fixed, counterstained, dehydrated, cleared, and mounted.

With this method, the stain appears as discreet, non-crystalline deposits with diameters ranging as low as 0.5 μ.

V. Thiolacetic acid methods (ThAc)

In accordance with his hypothesis that the final step in the catalytic hydrolysis of substrate by AChE involves acetylation of the esteratic site, with subsequent oxygen-exchange between the carboxylate ion and water, WILSON (1951) showed that the enzyme can combine with undissociated thiolacetic acid, with the elimination of hydrogen sulfide, and subsequent formation of acetic acid:

$$\overset{\text{(AChE)}}{\text{E—H}} + CH_3COSH \longrightarrow \underset{+\ H_2S}{E—COCH_3} \xrightarrow{H_2O} E—H + CH_3COOH$$

This principle was adapted by CREVIER and BÉLANGER (1955) for the histochemical localization of AChE by incubating sections in the presence of thiolacetic acid and lead nitrate *(ThAc)*.

The incubation medium recommended consists of 83 ml 0.1 M Na_2HPO_4 in which are dissolved thiolacetic acid (0.12 M) and lead nitrate (0.001 M), and to which is added 17 ml McIlvaine phosphate-citrate buffer, pH 6.2. Fresh or formalin-fixed frozen sections are dried on slides, incubated for 30 to 60 min at room temperature, washed for 5 min in running water, dehydrated, and mounted.

To date, comparatively little has been published on the use of the thiolacetic acid procedure. Photomicrographs in the original paper showed characteristic staining of motor endplates and neurons. The method was modified by SÁVAY and CSILLIK 1959a), and for use in electron microscopy by BARRNETT and PALADE (1959); the latter authors consistently found staining in the M bands of both cardiac and skeletal muscle, in addition to staining of motor endplates in the latter. As these authors pointed out, specificity can be assured only by the use of selective inhibitors. Another adaptation of the method for electron microscopy was published by ZACKS and BLUMBERG (1961), who noted staining of axoplasmic and sarcoplasmic mitochondria in the vicinity of motor endplates in addition to the sites reported by BARRNETT and PALADE (l.c.).

In the reviewer's laboratory, the following modification of the incubation medium has proven most successful for the staining of sympathetic ganglia and motor endplates of skeletal muscle: 11.3 ml H_2O, 2.0 ml 0.1 M citric acid, 0.60 ml N NaOH, 4.4 ml 2 M sucrose, 0.5 ml M $MgCl_2$, 1.0 ml 0.24 M CH_3COSH (previously neutralized by adding 2.0 ml N NaOH to 0.17 ml CH_3COSH, and H_2O *q.s.* 10.0 ml), 0.2 ml 0.1 M $PbNO_3$, final pH 5.4 (KOELLE, G. B. and GEESEY, C. N., unpublished). For unexplained reasons, staining has not been obtained consistently with all samples of reagent grade thiolacetic acid.

In addition to AChE and BuChE, several other esterases apparently cause staining by this method (WACHSTEIN et al. 1961). Furthermore, the concentrations of reversible inhibitors which inhibit selectively the hydrolysis of ACh and related substrates by AChE and BuChE do not necessarily prevent the hydrolysis of thiolacetic acid by the same enzymes.

It should be noted that motor endplates contain a lead-reactive substance, apparently unrelated to the ChE's, which can produce a pattern of staining resembling superficially that obtained with the foregoing methods (SÁVAY and CSILLIK 1959b). Electron microscopic study has indicated that the staining obtained with concentrated (5%) lead nitrate solutions, in the absence of thiolacetic acid, is confined to the sarcoplasmic columns (ZACKS and BLUMBERG 1961).

B. Micro- and ultramicro-analytical methods

These methods have been treated in Chapter 4, hence only those by means of which the information discussed in the following sections has been obtained, or procedures which are believed to have considerable potential value for similar studies, will be considered here.

For determinations of the AChE or BuChE activity in tissues of moderate activity with samples ranging from a few mg to a few μg, colorimetric methods are most convenient. The hydroxamic acid method of HESTRIN (1949) for determining the residual unhydrolyzed ester following a period of incubation has been adapted by BONTING and FEATHERSTONE (1956) to a micro level. More sensitive, but requiring more exact control of conditions, is the phenol red micro-method of LOWRY et al. (1954) based on the procedure of CROXATTO et al. (1939). When this procedure is utilized with serial sections, and cell counts are performed on alternate sections in accordance with the principle of LINDERSTRØM-LANG (1938—39), it is possible to obtain indirect estimations of the relative enzymatic activities of individual cell-types. A new method which appears promising for micro-determinations is based on the reaction of thiocholine, liberated from AThCh by the enzyme, with 5,5-dithio*bis*-2-nitrobenzoate ion to produce the yellow 5-thio-2-nitrobenzoate ion, which is measured colorimetrically (ELLMAN et al. 1961).

The Cartesian diver microgasometric method, developed originally by LINDERSTRØM-LANG (1937), has been refined further by ZEUTHEN (1953), ZAJICEK and ZEUTHEN (1957), and GIACOBINI (1959a) for determinations of the AChE activities of single neurons and their component parts. With this procedure it has been possible to determine within an accuracy of 5% the AChE activity represented by the liberation of $1 \times 10^{-6} \mu$l CO_2 per hour. The results of these fine studies have been summarized by GIACOBINI (1959b), and will be taken up in the individual sections which follow.

C. Centrifugal fractionation methods

The technique of preparing homogenates of tissues in media of various compositions and densities, separating the cellular components by fractional centrifugation, and subjecting the various fractions to analysis by standard methods was brought into general use by DOUNCE (1943) nearly twenty years ago. The limitations and possible sources of error have been discussed by DUVE and BERTHET (1954), NOVIKOFF (1956), and SCHNEIDER and HOGEBOOM (1956), who have stressed, among other factors, the importance of studying the individual fractions by electron microscopy. The most successful application of the method to the cytological localization of AChE has been reported by TOSCHI and associates (TOSCHI 1959, HANZON and TOSCHI 1959, HOLMSTEDT and TOSCHI 1959). Their findings, and those of others, will be described.

Cytological distribution of cholinesterases

The present section summarizes the findings which have been obtained with the foregoing techniques on the cytological distributions of AChE and non-specific ChE's (e.g., BuChE) in various species. The volume of literature on this subject which has accrued during the past ten years precludes the feasibility of quoting all reports. Consequently, attention has been focused insofar as possible on studies which have included reasonable evidence of specificity, sensitivity, and accuracy of localization, or have contributed new information; observations which are essentially confirmatory, where no controversy exists, generally have been omitted.

It is often impossible to determine the exact priority of observations; for errors of this type the reviewer can offer only his apologies.

The earlier literature reporting the relative concentrations of AChE and non-specific ChE's in homogenates of tissues, and describing the individual properties of such enzymes in various states of purification, has been reviewed thoroughly and critically by AUGUSTINSSON (1948; Chapter 4). In addition, the following reviews and papers may be consulted for further information in the same categories: ORD and THOMPSON (1950), WHITTAKER (1951), DAVIES (1954). The ontogenetic development of ChE's is presented in Chapter 5.

A general summary of the cytological distributions of AChE and BuChE is included in the recent review of HOLMSTEDT (1959). The monograph by GIACOBINI (1959 b) summarizes the studies by himself and associates on ultramicro-quantitative determinations of AChE in individual neurons. GEREBTZOFF's (1959) recent monograph presents in detail the extensive survey conducted over several years in his own laboratory, as well as the work of others, on the histochemical localization of AChE and BuChE in a wide variety of tissues and species. While this represents an extremely valuable contribution, to which reference will be made frequently here, it should be noted that virtually all of its author's work was conducted with the thiocholine method using a low pH, and formalin-fixation before and after sectioning *(ThCh-VII)*. Thus, sensitivity was sacrificed to the advantage of accuracy of localization and preservation of morphological detail. As a consequence, negative findings (e.g., in somatic motor fibers) can in certain instances be attributed to relatively low activity, high sensitivity to formalin, or both.

For a recent survey of the application of several techniques to the histochemical localization of ChE's, the publication of the symposium held in Basel in 1960 should be consulted (SCHWARZACHER 1961).

General considerations; cholinergic and non-cholinergic neurons

The arrangement of material has been dictated by physiological and pharmacological, as well as anatomical, considerations. It is generally conceded that there are four classes of cholinergic nerve fibers: (1) somatic motor fibers to skeletal muscle, (2) preganglionic autonomic fibers to both sympathetic and parasympathetic ganglia, (3) parasympathetic, and a limited number of sympathetic, postganglionic fibers to autonomic effector cells, and (4) some, but by no means all, fibers of the central nervous system. As discussed in detail in the other chapters of the present monograph, the acute pharmacological effects of anti-ChE agents are most evident at the synaptic or neuroeffector sites where the aforementioned groups of fibers terminate. Accordingly, the localization of AChE and BuChE will be discussed first in the first three of these divisions and their effector organs, in the above order. While primary sensory neurons and their specialized terminations are generally assumed to be non-cholinergic, in most cases they contain AChE. These and the special sensory systems will be considered before dealing with the complexities of the central nervous system. Finally, the endocrine glands and miscellaneous sites of AChE activity, for which its functional significance in many cases is still unknown, will be described.

It will be apparent that while some sites, such as the motor endplates of skeletal muscle, have been examined exhaustively by the various techniques mentioned, others, particularly in the central nervous system, have received comparatively little study. It is hoped that calling attention to such hiatuses will stimulate further investigation in these areas.

The general statement can be made at the outset that known cholinergic neurons (e.g., the anterior horn cells) contain high concentrations of AChE throughout their entire lengths, as far as they have been followed, including the dendrites, perikarya, axons, and axonal terminations. Neurons assumed to be non-cholinergic, such as the sensory neurons of the dorsal root ganglia and the adrenergic neurons of the superior cervical ganglia, contain lower concentrations; the absolute values vary from extremely little or none to intermediate, but are distinctly below those of the anterior horn cells of the same species (KOELLE 1951, 1955; GIACOBINI

1959a). Aside from its physiological implications, which will be discussed in the final section, this situation often permits the histochemical identification of cholinergic fibers at peripheral sites provided the proper precautions are observed

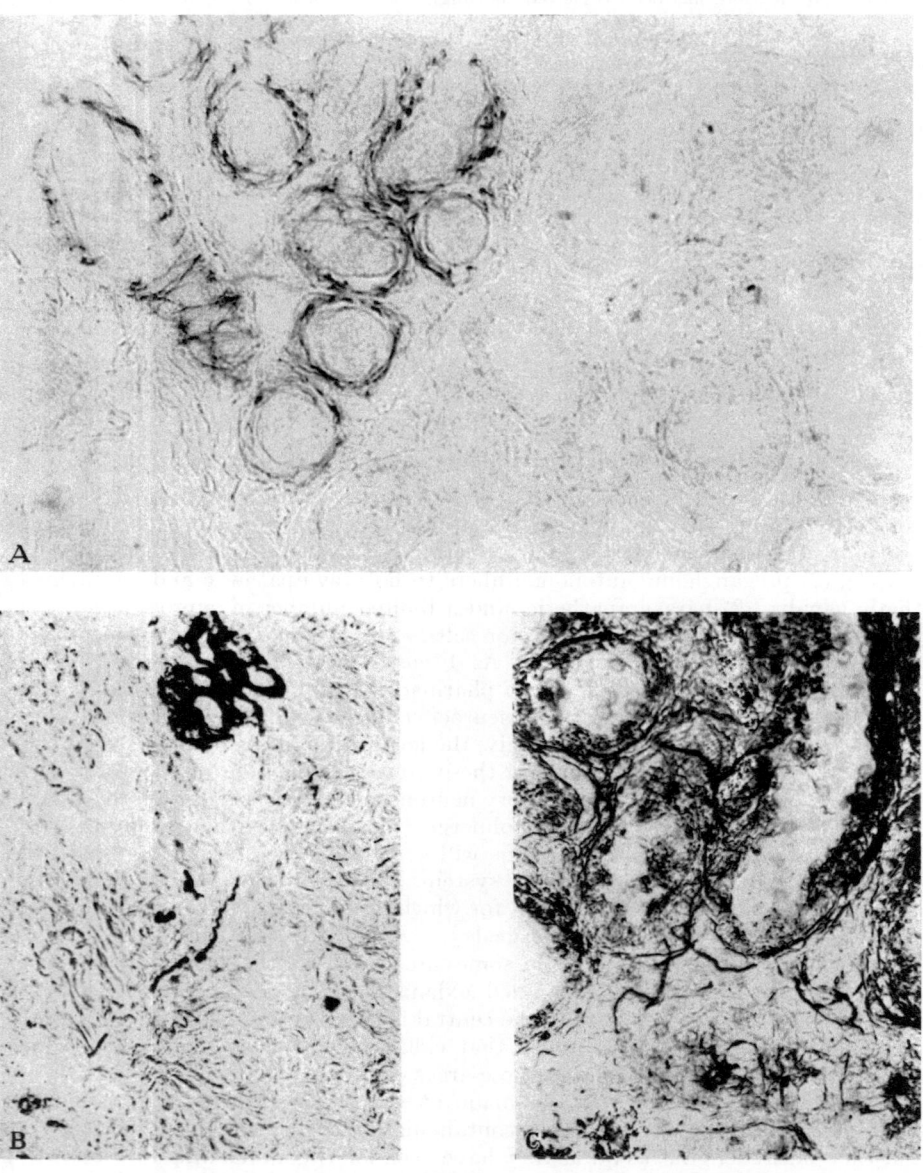

Fig. 2. Dependence upon conditions of staining with *ThCh* method for selective demonstration of cholinergic fibers surrounding human eccrine sweat glands. — A. Demonstration of AChE localized in fibers surrounding the eccrine sweat gland tubules. In the left half of the photograph are seen dark strands encircling each of the eccrine tubules. The dark material is copper sulfide precipitated at sites of AChE activity (*ThCh-III*). In the right half of the photograph are seen the apocrine sweat gland tubules; note the absence of AChE-staining (HURLEY et al. 1953). — B and C. Extremely dense staining for AChE in fibers surrounding human eccrine sweat glands (B, upper part of photograph) and relatively light staining of fibers surrounding apocrine glands (C), with a different modification (*ThCh-IV*) of the method from that used in A (AAVIK 1955)

and the limitations considered (e.g., HURLEY et al. 1953, v.i.). As discussed previously, relative intensities of staining by any of the histochemical procedures provide only a crude approximation of relative concentrations of AChE. In tissue sections, activity will be reduced to a variable extent at different sites if fixatives are employed. Conversely, sites of extremely low AChE activity will stain intensely if thick sections are used, or if the period of incubation is prolonged sufficiently to allow the accumulation of a large amount of reaction product. In some species (e.g., cat), the difference between cholinergic and non-cholinergic neurons with respect to AChE activity is marked, whereas in others (e.g., rabbit) it is considerably less so (KOELLE 1955). Thus, the isolated demonstration of intense staining for AChE of a group of fibers or their terminations by no means implies that they are cholinergic by the usual definition. On the other hand, if it is shown that certain fibers of unknown nature are stained intensely under conditions which result in intense staining of known cholinergic fibers, but in only faint staining of non-cholinergic fibers in the same species, this might be considered presumptive evidence for the identification of the fibers in question as cholinergic.

As an example of this type of distinction, HURLEY et al. (1953) stained sections of human skin for ChE's *(ThCh-III)* and found that the eccrine, but not the apocrine, sweat glands were surrounded by AChE-containing fibers (Fig. 2A). These findings were consistent with pharmacological evidence that the autonomic supply to the former is cholinergic and that to the latter is adrenergic (SHELLEY and HURLEY 1953). With a modified procedure *(ThCh-IV)*, AAVIK (1955) obtained faint staining for AChE in the fibers surrounding the apocrine glands (Fig. 2C), but extreme, diffuse staining in the supply to the eccrine glands (Fig. 2B).

A. Somatic neuro-muscular system

I. Primary motor neurons

High concentrations of AChE have been found throughout the lengths of all primary motor neurons examined. This is demonstrated for the perikarya and initial portions of the processes in a group of anterior horn cells in Fig. 3, and by both the histochemical and ultramicro-analytical data summarized in Table 2. The work of GIACOBINI in the latter category is of particular interest. In the initial series reported (GIACOBINI and HOLMSTEDT 1958), the anterior horn cells of the rat showed a ten-fold variation in AChE concentration, and were separable into two distinct groups with mean values differing by approximately two and one-half-fold. When the series was extended (GIACOBINI 1959a) the mean values fell somewhat, but it was estimated that their ratio remained the same; however, the spread of individual values then reached nearly 100-fold. This raises the question of whether the neurons for which very low values were reported actually contained AChE, or whether the enzyme was associated with presynaptic axonal terminals attached to them. Inasmuch as the cleft between the pre- and postsynaptic membranes has been estimated to be only a few hundred Å, it would seem impossible, with even the most precise microdissection techniques, to assure complete removal of the former. It has been proposed that the Renshaw cells are non-cholinergic neurons in the immediate vicinity of the anterior horn cells, and that the former receive cholinergic innervation from axonal collaterals of the latter (ECCLES et al. 1954). Hence, the cells for which extremely low values were obtained might have been Renshaw cells containing little or no AChE themselves, but perhaps with adherant presynaptic cholinergic *boutons*.

While considerably fewer histochemical studies have been reported on the motor nerve trunks themselves, the presence of high concentrations of AChE in homogenates of the ventral roots of spinal nerves has been documented amply (BURGEN and CHIPMAN 1951, WOLFGRAM 1954, COHEN 1956). SNELL (1957), using

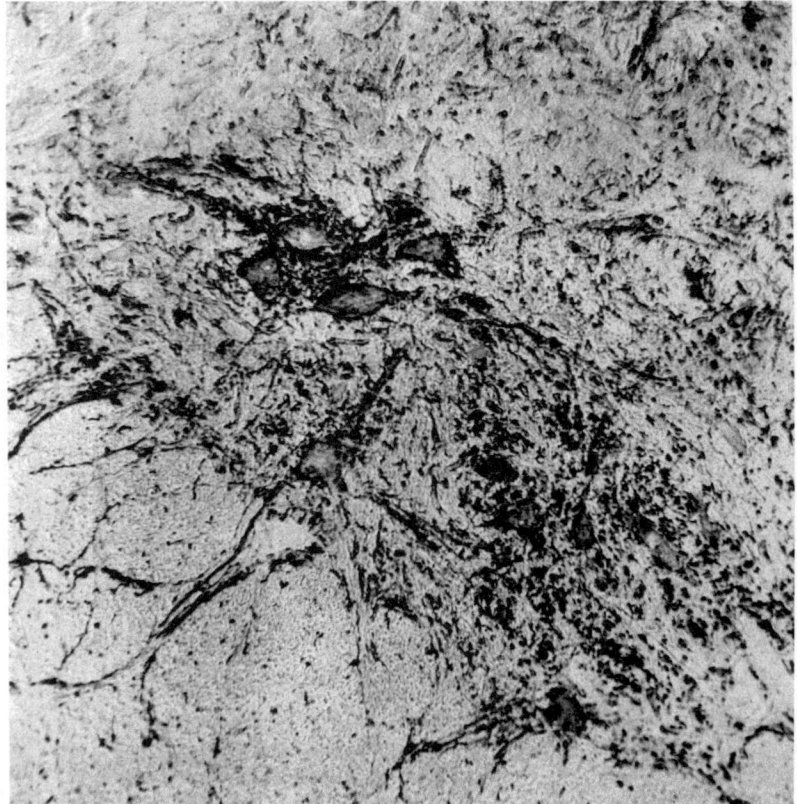

Fig. 3. Anterior horn cells of rat cervical spinal cord. (*ThCh-III*, 10 μ section, incubated 75 minutes with AThCh, uncounterstained, magnification 100 X.) Stained neuronal elements represent AChE; stained glial cells and capillaries represent non-specific ChE (KOELLE 1954)

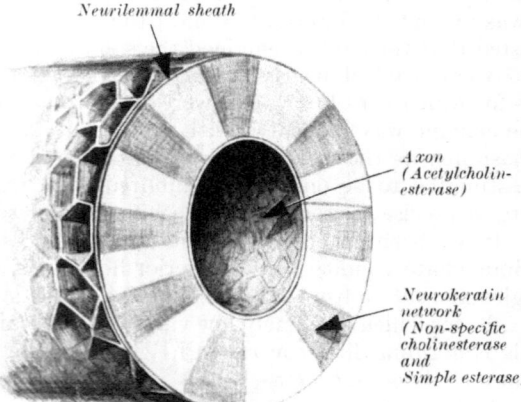

Neurilemmal sheath

*Axon
(Acetylcholin-
esterase)*

*Neurokeratin
network
(Non-specific
cholinesterase
and
Simple esterase)*

Fig. 4. Artist's impression of the nerve. Localization of specific cholinesterase (AChE), non-specific cholinesterase (BuChE), and simple esterase have been labelled; clear areas represent myelin (TEWARI and BOURNE 1960)

a modified thiocholine technique, demonstrated ChE's (types not distinguished) in the axons and neurilemmal sheaths of the sciatic nerve. Following sectioning, enzymatic activity in the distal segment disappeared from the axons but not from the sheaths; high concentrations of ChE were noted in the fibrils growing out of the proximal stump. Strong staining for AChE was noted in the terminal portions of motor axons by BECKETT and BOURNE (1957). While the sciatic is a mixed nerve, the motor component probably constitutes a major portion. In the hypoglossal nerve (C.N. XII), which consists almost exclusively of somatic motor fibers, AChE has been measured quantitatively in homogenates prepared from all levels, including the nucleus of origin, the cranial roots, and several segments along the trunk (KOENIG and KOELLE 1961). Both histochemical (KOELLE 1951) and other (CAVANAGH et al. 1954) evidence indicates that the Schwann sheath cells contain only BuChE, and the axons only AChE. On the basis of the foregoing reports and their additional findings, TEWARI and BOURNE (1960) have proposed that the neurokeratin network, containing the non-specific ChE in addition to simple esterases, oxidative, and other enzymes, forms a series of hexagonal prisms, radiating from the AChE-containing axon and interspersed with the myelin network (Fig. 4).

Table 2. *AChE of primary motor neurons*

Cells	Species	Method[1]	Author	Findings and Comments
Anterior horn cells of spinal cord	Cat	*ThCh-III,V*	KOELLE (1951, 1955)	Moderate to intense staining of all neurons and dendritic and axonal processes as far as can be traced; greatest intensity at neuronal membrane, high in cytoplasm. Identity of AChE confirmed by specific inhibitors.
	Rabbit	*ThCh-V*	KOELLE (1955)	
	Rhesus monkey	*ThCh-V*	KOELLE (1955)	
	Rat	*ThCh-III*	KOELLE (1954)	
Anterior horn cells of spinal cord	Rat	*ThCh-IX*	GIACOBINI and HOLMSTEDT (1958)	Moderate to intense staining of all neurons and dendritic and axonal processes as far as can be traced; greatest intensity at neuronal membrane, high in cytoplasm. Identity of AChE confirmed by specific inhibitors.
Anterior horn cells of spinal cord	Rat	Ultramicro-analysis	GIACOBINI and HOLMSTEDT (1958)	All show high activity but individual cells divisible into two distinct groups with mean values of 3.08 and 7.65×10^{-7} $\mu l CO_2/\mu^3$ per hr, respectively, evolved from AThCh-containing medium.
Anterior horn cells of spinal cord	Rat	Ultramicro-analysis	GIACOBINI (1959)	Individual cells: $0.49-41.0 \times 10^{-7}$ μl CO_2/μ^3 per hr (Means 2.02 and 5.50). Dendrites: 3.41—22.5. Nuclei: 0.46—0.81. Nucleoli: 0.
C.N. III, Nucleus	Rat	*ThCh-III*	KOELLE (1954)	Spindle shaped, moderately heavily stained neurons.
C.N. IV, Nucleus	Rat	*ThCh-III*	KOELLE (1954)	Few small, heavily stained neurons.
C.N. V, Motor Nucleus	Rat	*ThCh-III*	KOELLE (1954)	Large, very heavily stained neurons and fibers.
C.N. VII, Nucleus and Motor Root	Rat	*ThCh-III*	KOELLE (1954)	Large, very heavily stained neurons and fibers.
C.N. X, Dorsal Motor Nucleus	Rat	*ThCh-III*	KOELLE (1954)	Few large neurons and fibers very heavily stained; majority moderately or lightly.
C.N. X, Nucleus ambiguous	Rat	*ThCh-III*	KOELLE (1954)	Large neurons among most heavily stained in brain; smaller cells vary in intensity.
C.N. XI, Nucleus, Root, and Trunk	Rat	*ThCh-III*	KOELLE (1954)	Small neurons exhibiting consistently heavy staining; most axons heavily stained.
C.N. XII, Nucleus, and Root	Rat	*ThCh-III*	KOELLE (1954)	Great variation in size of cells and intensity of staining; larger cells show heaviest staining; some small cells practically unstained.
C.N. XII, Nucleus, Root, and Trunk	Cat	*ThCh-III*	KOENIG and KOELLE (1960)	Intense staining of neurons; detectable staining in roots and throughout lengths of trunk.

[1] Abbreviations for histochemical techniques given in section on methods.

II. Skeletal muscle

1. Motor endplates

The neuromuscular junction has probably been studied more extensively than any other region with respect to both the localization of AChE and the pharmacological action of anti-ChE, cholinomimetic, and cholinergic blocking agents. The latter topic is covered extensively in Chapter 13. The earlier literature on the innervation of skeletal muscle has been reviewed critically by TIEGS (1953). The comparative histology of the motor endplate in various vertebrates was described by COLE (1955). COUTEAUX's (1947) monograph on the detailed morphology of the endplate is a classic in the field.

Prior to the development of histochemical and ultramicro-analytical techniques for AChE, MARNAY and NACHMANSOHN (1938) and FENG and TING (1938) obtained indirect evidence that the AChE of skeletal muscle is concentrated in the areas of termination of the motor nerves. The former authors estimated that the ChE activity of the endplate region is 15,000 to 30,000 times that of the surrounding muscle tissue. This has been extensively confirmed by later, more direct approaches. KOELLE and FRIEDENWALD (1949) showed that in the intercostal muscle of the rat, the distinctive staining *(ThCh-I)* of the motor endplate resembles at least superficially the pictures obtained by COUTEAUX (1947) in selective staining of the subneural apparatus with Janus green. Similar results have been obtained in various species with the subsequent modifications of the thiocholine method *(ThCh-I-IX)* (KOELLE 1950, 1951, COUTEAUX 1951, COUTEAUX and TAXI 1952, PORTUGALOV and JAKOVLEV 1951, CÖERS 1953, GEREBTZOFF 1953, BECKETT and BOURNE 1957, HOLMSTEDT 1957b), the myristoylcholine *(LC-Ch)* and α-naphthyl acetate *(Naph-I)* methods (DENZ 1953), the β-naphthyl acetate method (RAVIN et al. 1953), the indoxyl ester methods *(Ind-I)* (BARRNETT and SELIGMAN 1951, HOLT and WITHERS 1952), and the thiolacetic acid method *(ThAc)* (CREVIER and BÉLANGER 1955). The selective localization of AChE at the endplate region has been demonstrated most unequivocally by the ultramicro-analytical determinations of GIACOBINI and HOLMSTEDT (1960). The activity per unit volume of single endplates, isolated by microdissection, was found to be at least fifty times as high as that of samples taken from other regions of the muscle.

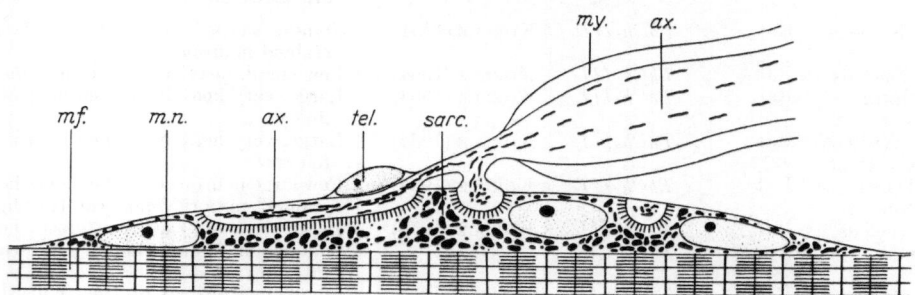

Fig. 5. Schematic drawing of a motor end-plate. *ax.*, axoplasm with its mitochondria; *my.*, myelin sheath; *tel.* teloglia (terminal Schwann cells); *sarc.*, sarcoplasm with its mitochondria; *m.n.*, muscle nuclei; *mf.*, myofibrils. The terminal nerve branches lie in "synaptic gutters" or "troughs." Immediately under the interface axoplasm-sarcoplasm, the ribbon-shaped subneural lamellae, transversely cut, may be seen as rodlets (COUTEAUX 1958)

The most precise histochemical results with light microscopy are unquestionably those of COUTEAUX, who has published a critical summary (COUTEAUX 1958) of his own findings and those of the aforementioned authors as they relate to the detailed structure of the motor endplate revealed by electron microscopy (ROBERTSON 1956, ANDERSSON-CEDERGREN 1959).

As the axon approaches the muscle fiber, it loses its myelin sheath and forms a terminal arborization which lies in a depression of the muscle fiber membrane known as the synaptic gutter (Fig. 5, COUTEAUX 1958). The derivatives of SCHWANN's and HENLE's sheaths remain only on the upper surfaces of the axonal termination and the immediately adjacent portion of the muscle fiber, as the teloglial membrane; contrary to earlier belief, no teloglial sheath is interposed between the lower surface of the axonal termination and the subneural apparatus. The latter represents a modification of the sarcoplasmic surface membrane and the adjacent sarcoplasm. It is composed of a uniform series of infoldings of the sarcoplasmic membrane, which when sectioned at certain angles and stained selectively presents a palisade-like appearance (Fig. 6, COUTEAUX 1958). The axoplasmic surface membrane does not enter the folds; hence, the surface area of the postsynaptic component is considerably greater than that of the presynaptic. By electron microscopy, the axonal and sarcoplasmic membranes appear to form a compound membrane of 5 layers (Figs. 7 and 8, ROBERTSON 1956); the total thickness of the synaptic membrane complex, or the distance between the pre- and postsynaptic sites, ranges from approximately 300 to 500 Å. A three-dimensional reconstruction of an endplate, prepared from a series of electron micrographs, is shown in Figure 9 (ANDERSSON-CEDERGREN 1959).

The highest concentration of AChE appears to be localized postsynaptically at the surface and infoldings of the subneural apparatus; the axonal termination seems to contain relatively a considerably smaller amount. This may be due at least in part to the difference in the surface areas. These distributions are illustrated in Fig. 10 (COUTEAUX and TAXI 1952).

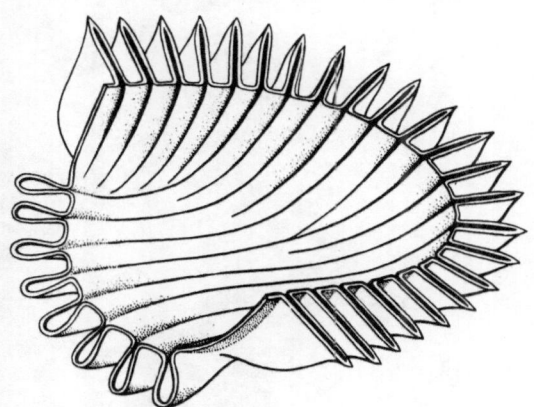

Fig. 6. Schematic three-dimensional presentation of the subneural apparatus at the extremity of a "synaptic gutter". This interpretation is based upon the data hitherto obtained both with the light and the electron microscope (COUTEAUX 1958)

A striking exception to the usual pattern has been noted by COUTEAUX (1961) for the neuromuscular junctions of the dorsal fin muscle of the seahorse, *Hippocampus*. Here, several junctions are distributed along the length of each muscle fiber (as in mammalian extraocular muscles, v.i.), but the enzyme, chiefly AChE *(ThCh-VI, Naph-II)*, is confined entirely to the presynaptic terminals.

While most of the cholinesterase activity of the motor endplate is AChE, DENZ (1953) has shown with a series of selective inhibitors that a small amount of BuChE is also present. It is quite possible that the latter is associated largely with the teloglial surface membrane, as suggested by the findings of SCHWARZACHER (1957), since the Schwann sheath and glial cells elsewhere contain BuChE.

In a recent report, HÄGGQVIST (1960) advanced the proposal that the small diameter motor fibers supplying tonically contracting muscles, which end in *"terminaisons en grappe"* (v.i.), are associated chiefly with BuChE, in contrast with the predominant AChE of the *"terminaisons en plaque"* of phasically contracting muscles supplied by large diameter fibers (v.i.). However, both the technique and the published photomicrographs upon which this conclusion was based are open to question. The author employed concentrations of specific inhibitors (Mipafox and BW 284) which produce selective inhibition of BuChE and AChE, respectively, in the cat *(ThCh-VII)*, without indicating whether the same concentrations apply for this purpose in the rhesus monkey, the species studied. At twice the concentration of BW 284 employed and under very similar conditions otherwise, the AChE of rhesus monkey brain still exhibits definite residual activity and BuChE is partially inhibited (KOELLE 1955). In addition, considerably longer incubation periods were used with BuThCh (3/4 to 2 hr) than with AThCh (5 to 15 min). These results suggest that proportionately more non-specific ChE is present at the endplates of tonic than of phasic muscle, but not necessarily that it exceeds the concentration of AChE at either site. The implications of the author's suggestion are of interest, and warrant more extended investigation.

Most of the conclusions drawn above from histochemical studies at the level of light microscopy have received confirmation from the few electron microscopic

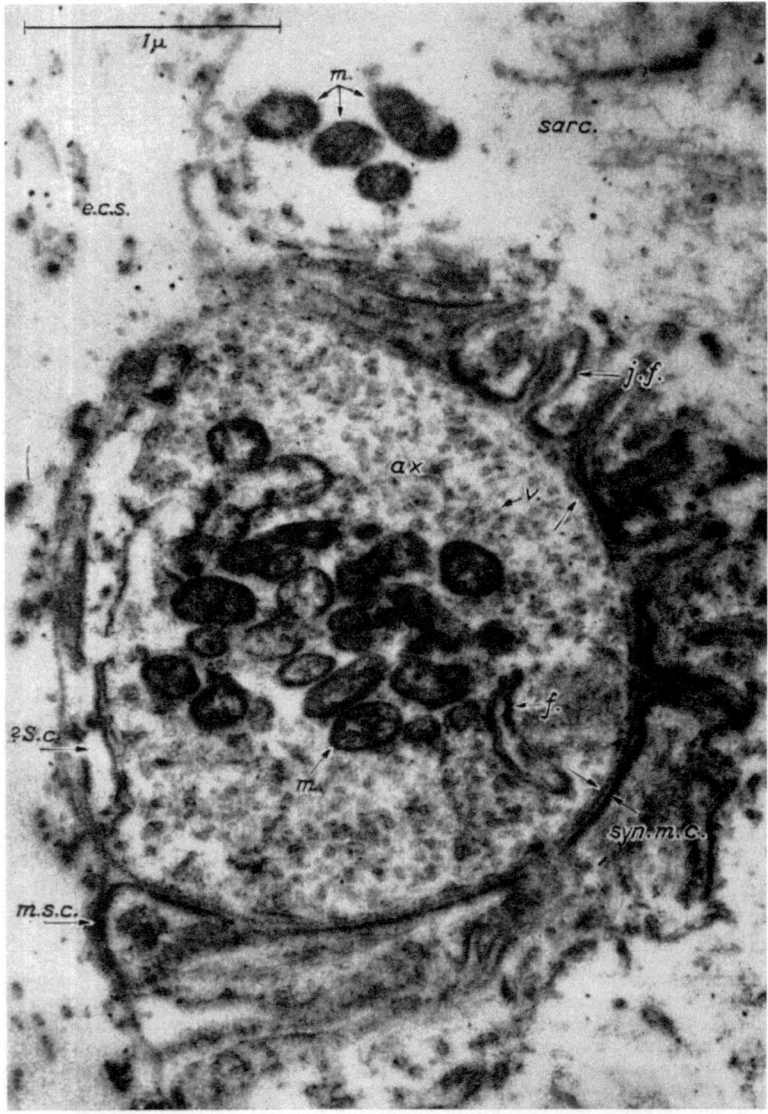

Fig. 7. Electron micrograph of terminal axon embedded in a synaptic gutter. A junctional fold (*j.f.*) in which the light zone of the muscle surface membrane complex is clearly evident is seen to the upper right. The close approximation of the light zones near the origin of the fold is seen here. In this location the dense outer surface material is greatly reduced in amount. The five layers of the synaptic membrane complex (*syn.m.c.*) may be seen at the arrows. The vesicular appearing bodies of the terminal axoplasm and the absence of the axoplasmic filaments are particularly clearly shown here. Note the tubular appearing bodies (*f.*) in terminal axoplasm. At the unlabelled arrow a structure is seen within the synaptic membrane complex which resembles somewhat the axoplasmic vesicular bodies. A layer of cytoplasm(*?S.c.*) which is clearly different from axoplasm is seen between the axoplasm and extracellular space (*e.c.s.*). OsO₄ 4 hours. × 43,000 (ROBERTSON 1956)

investigations published to date. LEHRER and ORNSTEIN (1959) employed the
α-naphthyl acetate-hexazotized pararosaniline technique *(Naph-II)* with OsO₄-
fixed mouse intercostal muscle, which was subsequently embedded and sectioned.
Deposits of the reaction product were noted at two sites of the motor endplate:

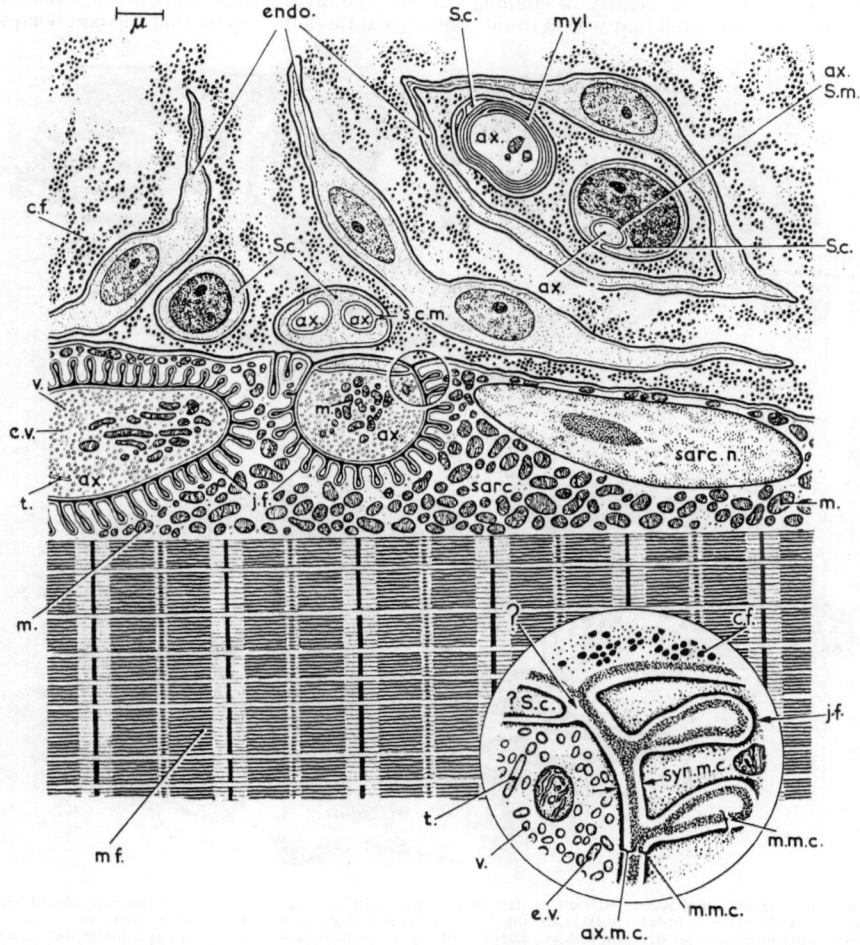

Fig. 8. An interpretative diagram of a myoneural junction in *Anolis*. The double surface membrane complexes
of the Schwann cells *(S.c.)*, muscle fiber, and endoneurial sheath cells *(endo.)* are shown. The manner in which
the muscle surface complex is thrown into the junctional folds of the subneural apparatus is indicated. The five
layers of the compound synaptic membrane complex which separates terminal axoplasm from sarcoplasm may
be seen. The main features of terminal axoplasm and sarcoplasm are included. The continuites of the synaptic,
muscle, and ?Schwann cell surface complexes shown in the diagram represent in part interpretations rather than
direct observations. Furthermore, the inclusion of the surface connecting membranes (mesaxons) in the juxta-
terminal nerve fibers is partly interpretative. The region marked by the circle is enlarged to show more detail.
The continuities between the membrane structures in the region of ?arrow is interpretative. The five layers of
the compound synaptic membrane complex shown between the arrows *syn.m.c.* are discussed in the text.
× ∼ 10,000. Inset × ∼ 60,000 (ROBERTSON 1956)

(1) within the cleft between the axoplasmic and sarcoplasmic membranes, and
between the folds of the latter (Fig. 11), and (2) within the narrower (100 Å) space
between the axoplasmic membrane and that of the superficially situated teloglial
cells.

The authors discussed two possible alternative interpretations of their findings, i.e., that the enzyme is situated extracellularly, within the spaces of the clefts, or within the membranes themselves with the active groups oriented towards the extracellular side. The former viewpoint has also been expressed by ZACKS and BLUMBERG (1961). However, the latter explanation seems more likely to the reviewer on the basis of the comparable apparent disposition of the AChE of the presynaptic terminals of sympathetic ganglia (KOELLE and KOELLE 1959, v.i.). The fact that the density of staining between the sarcoplasmic folds of the subneural apparatus approximated that within the adjacent synaptic cleft suggests that the postsynaptic

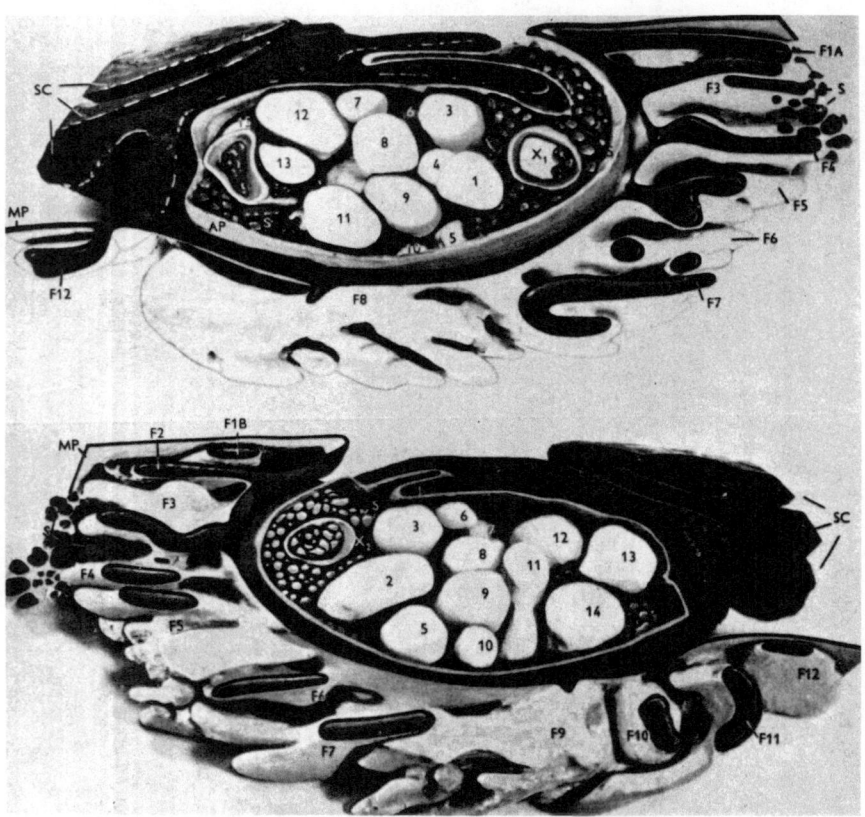

Fig. 9. Three dimensional reconstruction of part of a motor endplate, based on electron micrographs of serial sections. Magnification approximately × 38,000. Labeled items include Schwann cell components (*SC*), a process of which protrudes into an invagination (*I*) of the terminal axon plasma membrane (*AP*); muscle fiber plasma membrane (*MP*) and its folds (*F*, numbered); synaptic vesicles (*S*) in selected regions; mitochondria (nos. 1 to 15); double membrane components (X₁ and X₂). (ANDERSSON-CEDERGREN 1959)

membrane contributed most of the activity, as concluded previously. The lighter staining at the narrower axonal-teloglial cleft might represent externally oriented axonal AChE and, in addition, BuChE of the teloglia, since the procedure does not distinguish between the two enzymes.

BARRNETT (1961), using a further modification of the thiolacetic acid method *(ThAc)* applied earlier to electron microscopy (BARRNETT and PALADE 1959), found the AChE at the motor endplate to be most concentrated at the post-junctional and axonal membranes, with lower concentrations within the primary and secondary synaptic clefts; in addition, bodies within the axonal terminals which resembled the synaptic vesicles were stained (Fig. 12). Staining at the last mentioned site persisted after treatment with 10^{-5} M DFP, which prevented staining at the other sites noted, but not after 10^{-4} M DFP.

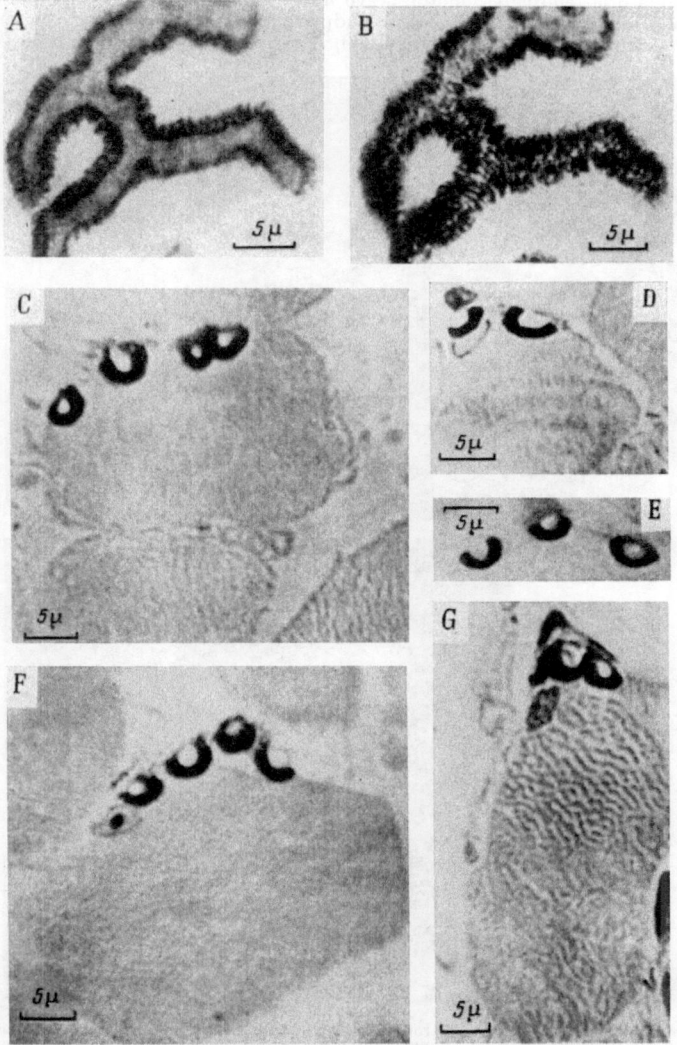

Fig. 10 A– G. Localization of ChE activity at the level of the motor endplate of mouse intercostal muscle. (*ThCh-VI*, formalin fixation; 45 min incubation with AThCh at pH 4.7). A and B. Front view of motor endplate. A, focussed at the border of the synaptic gutters and showing the leveling of the subneural apparatus at the surface; B, focussed at the base. Magnification × 1750. C to G. Cross sections of muscle fibers of different types, showing the endplates at the level of the synaptic junction. In C, the condenser has been adjusted to render the muscle fibers colorless; in the remainder, secondary staining due to carmine is detectable. Magnification × 1500 (COUTEAUX and TAXI 1952)

Several reports have been published describing *differences in individual types of motor endplates*, and the AChE-distribution in various species and at different stages of development (COUTEAUX and TAXI 1952, CÖERS 1953, 1955a, BECKETT and BOURNE 1957, GEREBTZOFF 1959, CSILLIK 1961; see also Chapter 5).

14*

GEREBTZOFF et al. (1954) have suggested that the concentration of AChE is higher in the endplates of rapidly contracting than in slowly contracting muscle; the diameters of the former are in general greater than those of the latter (CÖERS 1955a). The pattern in the extremely rapid extraocular muscles is somewhat similar to that of the intrafusal fibers (v.i.): in addition to multiple equatorial endplates, motor nerve fibers appear to give rise to numerous small branches which innervate series of minute endplate-like structures along the length of the muscle fiber (GEREBTZOFF 1959, KUPFER 1960). Multiple innervation has been reported for

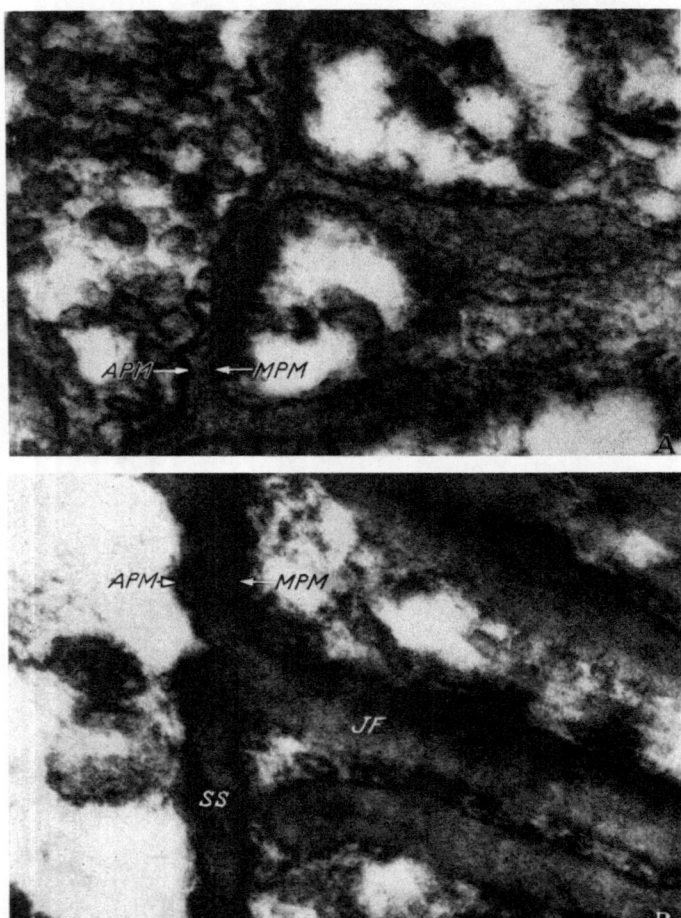

Fig. 11. High magnification (× 200,000) electron micrograph of portion of motor endplate of mouse intercostal muscle stained for ChE activity by the α-naphthyl acetate-hexazotized pararosanilin method (*Naph-II*) (B), and control from which substrate was omitted (A). Axonal terminal with its axonal plasma membrane (*APM*) on the left, muscle plasma membrane (*MPM*) on the right. Azo dye deposited in the synaptic space (*SS*) and junctional folds (*JF*) in B (LEHRER and ORNSTEIN 1959)

other mammalian muscle fibers (FEINDEL et al. 1952, HUNT and KUFFLER 1954), and occurs in many avian muscles (GINSBORG 1960, GINSBORG and MACKAY 1961). The extensive studies of CÖERS and WOLF (1959) on the appearance of AChE in human muscle in various pathological conditions have been assembled as a monograph. It is of interest that in myasthenia gravis marked structural changes have been observed in the endplates, but there is no apparent abnormality in the concentration of AChE (CÖERS and DESMEDT 1959, CÖERS 1961).

In amphibians, the motor endplates are usually extended, straight structures in contrast to the rounded, branching plaques seen in mammals (COUTEAUX 1947, 1958, COUTEAUX and TAXI 1952) (Fig. 13-1, 13-2, 13-3).

The innervation of the segmental muscle fibers of lower vertebrates has been investigated by LEWIS and HUGHES (1960) and MACKAY and PETERS (1961). In *Amphioxus*, ChE activity in the myotomes is represented by diffuse streaks, parallel with the muscle fibers; staining was noted also in nerve bundles in the adjacent septa. Two types of ChE-staining fibers, spaced at regular intervals, have been observed in the myotomes of cyclostomes: fibers stained diffusely throughout their lengths, and those with localized ChE-staining endplates at either end. The same two patterns of staining, but not in the same regular arrangement, were observed in myotomes of the dogfish. In the myotomes of urodeles and larval anurans, ChE-staining endplates are present at both ends of each fiber. Endplates are scattered in the myotomes of the tail of the green lizard and may occur anywhere from the polar to the equatorial regions;

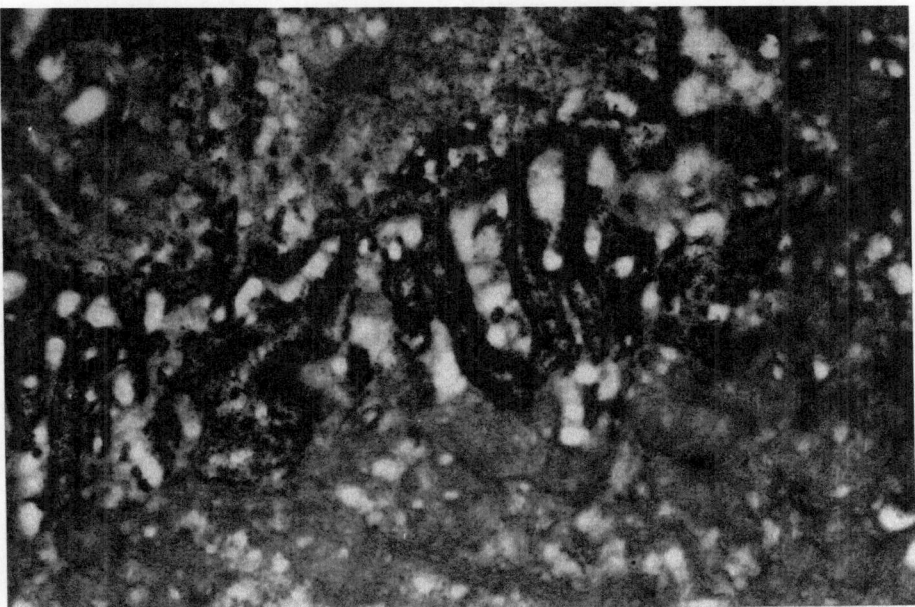

Fig. 12. Electron micrograph of motor endplate stained for ChE activity by modified *ThAc* method. Note heaviest staining at post- and prejunctional membranes, with lighter staining within primary and secondary clefts; additional staining of vesicles within axonal terminal (BARRNETT 1961)

in addition, all fibers show the ChE-staining of the myotendinous junctions which is characteristic of mammalian fibers (v.i.).

HÁMORI (1946), in a report of his own findings, has surveyed the rather limited literature on the localization of ChE in insects. In striated muscle, both the motor nerves and the muscle fibers themselves show staining by various procedures, which is similar to the pattern seen in vertebrates. However, on the basis of both substrate and inhibitor specificity, the enzyme is not a typical AChE (e.g., staining is obtained with BuThCh, but not with AThCh). The extremely rapidly contracting flight muscles of certain insects show multiple endplate-like structures, analogous to those noted in mammalian extraocular muscles (v.s.).

Reports of the effects of sectioning the motor nerve on the AChE of the motor endplates have been extremely variable, according to the species, the particular muscle studied, and the methods employed in determining and calculating relative AChE activities.

In the earlier literature, reviewed by BROOKS and MYERS (1952), the AChE of skeletal muscle (presumably reflecting chiefly that at the motor endplate) was reported to fall, remain unchanged, or rise in various investigations. The instances in which rises were reported probably did not represent actual increases in the absolute amount of AChE, but rather increases in concentration accompanying atrophy and weight loss of the muscle fibers. Whereas most authors found some decrease in the total content of AChE after denervation, BROOKS and MYERS reported no change in the guinea pig serratus anterior as late as five weeks after sectioning of the motor nerve. Quantitative studies with whole muscle homogenate showed that a substantial amount (approximately 30% of control) of AChE persisted in the diaphragm of the rat at 21 days, which remained unchanged up to 42 days following denervation (LÜLL-MANN and MUSCHOLL 1955). BRZIN and ZAJICEK (1958), by means of ultramicro-analysis of

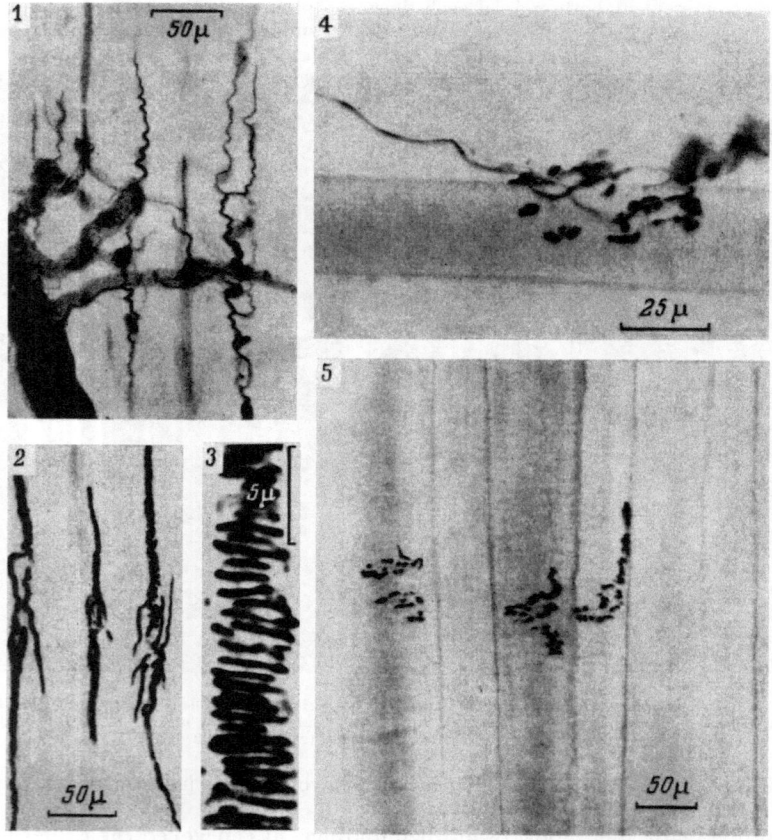

Fig. 13. Frog gastrocnemius end-brushes. *1* — Silver preparation. *2* and *3* — AThCh method *(ThCh-VI)* for AChE; front view of the subneural apparatus without counterstaining (COUTEAUX and TAXI 1952). *4* and *5* — Motor endplates of the "small nerve motor system." 4-Methylene blue method (original photomicrograph from Bavets). 5-AThCh method *(ThCh-VI)* without counterstaining (COUTEAUX 1958)

single endplates of mouse gastrocnemius, found that a high proportion of AChE was present as late as 75 to 85 days after excision of a segment of the sciatic nerve.

In one of the earliest histochemical studies of the effects of denervation *(ThCh-I)*, SAWYER et al. (1950) reported that AChE remained concentrated at the motor endplates of the skeletal muscle of rats, guinea pigs, and rabbits following nerve section and degeneration; no further details were given. KUPFER (1951) found *(ThCh-II)* progressive parallel decreases in the areas of staining of the motor endplates and in the cross-sectional areas of the muscle fibers of the flexors of the forelegs of rats from 9 to 39 days after denervation. In the tongue muscles of the rat, SCHWARZACHER (1957) *(ThCh-III)* noted a decrease in the intensity of staining of the endplates, beginning on the second day after sectioning of the hypoglossal nerve, continuing until the 16th day, and then increasing toward normal coincidentally with regeneration of the nerve fibers. Sávay and Csillik (1956) demonstrated the persistence of AThCh in rat gastrocnemius up to 184 days after denervation, in spite of formalin fixation at two stages *(ThCh-VII)*. Similarly, Cöers (1955b) *(ThCh-VI)* has reported the persistence of some AChE in human motor endplates after disappearance of the axons in patients with complete denervation.

In contrast, Snell and McIntyre (1956) reported the complete disappearance of AChE from the endplates of formalin-fixed guinea pig gastrocnemius 45 days after denervation *(ThCh-VI)*. Bergner (1957) found on repeating this study, but using both formalin-fixed *(ThCh-VI)* and unfixed *(ThCh-IV)* sections, that the latter invariably showed activity at stages when virtually none could be detected in the former; significant staining still occurred in the unfixed sections at the longest post-denervation interval studied (66 days). This exemplifies the importance of Couteaux's (1958) admonition that unfixed tissues should always be included in a series in order not to miss sites of low enzymatic activity; it is possible that denervation renders the residual AChE abnormally sensitive to formalin and other fixatives. It is difficult to assess the significance of the reports of Clodius (1953) and Waser and Hadorn (1961) that AChE disappeared completely from the endplates of mouse hemidiaphragms 120 days following phrenicotomy. In the former instance, formalin fixation was employed, as in the study cited above. This was omitted in the second study, but here staining for AChE was conducted after the tissues had been stored in contact with film at 4° for 5 months, in conjunction with a simultaneous investigation of the fixation of C^{-14}-curarine.

Csillik and Sávay (1958) have suggested that the residual AChE of the denervated subneural apparatus provides the neurotropic factor for the ingrowth of the regenerating axonal terminals. The same phenomenon might operate ontogenetically, since it has been shown that AChE begins to concentrate at the general region of the endplate prior to the entrance of the motor nerve (Kupfer and Koelle 1951). More recently, Csillik (1960) proposed that the motor endplate is formed, both ontogenetically and regeneratively, by the migration of ChE-containing teloblasts (identified as the interstitial cells of Boeke) along the nerve bundles from the neural crest.

Taken together, the foregoing results are in marked contrast with those obtained with the superior cervical ganglion of the cat following preganglionic denervation, in which case nearly all the AChE disappears (v.i.). They provide strong support for the earlier mentioned conclusion that most of the AChE at the neuromuscular junction is postsynaptic. Even under these circumstances, the postsynaptically localized AChE would not necessarily remain fully intact after degeneration of the axons, in view of the marked anatomical and physiological changes which occur. There appears to be no basis for relating to the reduction in AChE activity the changes which occur in the response of striated muscle to the intra-arterial injection or micro-application of ACh following denervation. Such changes as the marked increase in sensitivity and the contractural response to ACh appear to be due largely to the spread of ACh-sensitivity from the endplate region to the eventual involvement of the entire muscle fiber (Axelsson and Thesleff 1959).

2. Musculotendinous junctions

The relatively high concentration of AChE at the *musculotendinous junctions* of the individual fibers of striated muscle was noted first by Couteaux (1953), and has been confirmed and studied in detail in several mammalian species by Gerebtzoff (1953, 1956a, 1957) and by Cöers and Durand (1956), and in the seahorse, *Hippocampus*, by Couteaux (1961). Schwarzacher (1960a, b, 1961) has shown both manometrically and histochemically that the myotendinous enzyme consists entirely of AChE, and that in the rat and cat the activity at each junction

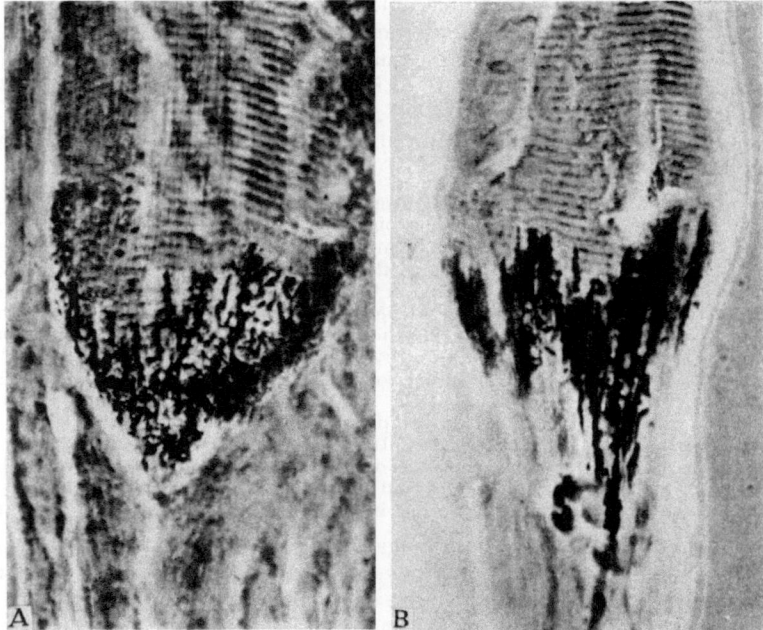

Fig. 14 A and B. A. Whole mount of the myo-tendinous junction of a single muscle fibre, M. opponens digiti minimi, man, stained for AChE by incubation en bloc *(ThCh-III)*, isolation of the single muscle fibre with its myo-tendinous junction under the dissecting microscope. Phase contrast; magnification × 720. B. Isolated muscle fibre end, M. soleus, rat, stained for AChE following fixation in 10% formol for 20 min, and pH = 5.6 of the incubation medium *(ThCh-VI)*. Phase contrast; same magnification (SCHWARZACHER 1960)

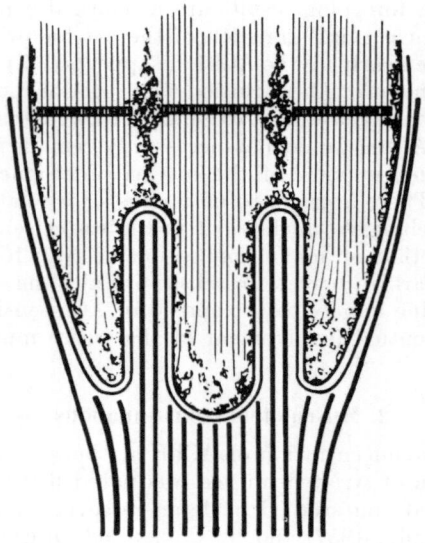

Fig. 15. Diagram of muscletendon junction in frog. Three contracted myofibrils are shown in which the Z band is connected to the fingerlike projections of sarcolemma by way of endoplasmic reticulum. The sarcolemma terminates as a glove around the finger-like muscle fibrils. The tendon fibrils are longitudinally attached to the increased surface of the terminal sarcolemma sheath (EDWARDS et al. 1956)

is approximately 20 to 30% that of the corresponding neuromuscular junction. Its localization is restricted to the surface membrane at the end of the muscle fiber, where no innervation has ever been shown in mammals. GEREBTZOFF (1957) found that the concentration was unaffected by muscular denervation, and was actually increased by tenotomy.

The functional significance of the AChE at this location is unknown. It cannot readily be dismissed as an evolutionary vestige reflecting earlier terminal innervation, as noted in many lower vertebrates, since in species of the latter group both terminal innervation and characteristically distributed myotendinous AChE have been noted concurrently (MACKAY and PETERS 1961). Unlike the neuromuscular junction, the myotendinous junction is not depolarized by ACh, alone or in combination with neostigmine (SCHWARZACHER 1961). The enzyme may be associated with the endoplasmic reticulum, which is highly organized at the musculotendinous junction (EDWARDS et al. 1956) and bears a definite resemblance to the AChE -staining pattern (Fig. 14 and 15).

3. Sarcolemma

In most species, the non-innervated portions of the sarcolemma and adjacent endomysium contain little or no AChE (KOELLE 1955). However, LUNDIN (1958) has shown that these areas in the tail muscle of the guppy *(Lebistes reticulatus)* and goldfish *(Carassius auratus)* produce uniformly intense staining for AChE. Earlier reports (NACHMANSOHN et al. 1941, AUGUSTINSSON 1949) had indicated that in both these species the AChE of the muscles is extremely high, and LUNDIN (1959) has confirmed its identity as a typical AChE. In other fish, such as the bream *(Abramis brama)*, the total AChE and its histochemical distribution do not differ significantly from the usual findings in striated muscle (LUNDIN 1958). The significance of this interesting observation is obscure at present. It may represent phylogenetically a transitional stage, since during embryonic development in rats (KUPFER and KOELLE 1951) and birds (GEREBTZOFF 1955) AChE is distributed diffusely through the muscle fibers, then appears to be more concentrated at the sarcoplasmic membrane before assuming the specific sites of localization described above. Electron microscopic studies have revealed the presence of numerous motor endplates along the muscle fibers of the goldfish (MACKAY and PETERS 1961).

4. Sarcoplasm

BECKETT and BOURNE (1957) noted that in addition to the discreet staining for AChE at the sites discussed above, faint staining was generally present also throughout the sarcoplasm. The possible specific localization of the enzyme at a sarcoplasmic site is suggested by the report of BARRNETT and PALADE (1959), cited previously, of discreet staining *(ThAc)*, presumably due to a ChE, at the swelling of the thick elemental filaments at the M bands in both striated and cardiac muscle of the rat. Additional staining, although of less certain enzymatic specificity, was noted in mitochondria, in round sarcoplasmic bodies, in contraction bands in the area of the Z bands, and in the sarcoplasmic reticulum. The authors suggested the possibility that the ChE associated with the M bands may be identical with the myosincholinesterase found predominantly with L-meromyosin (BEZNÁK 1945, VARGA et al. 1955). When chick embryo skeletal muscle was grown in tissue culture, no endplate-like structures developed, but an AThCh-splitting enzyme accrued in the cytoplasm, particularly in the region of the Z lines (ENGEL 1961). It should be recalled that DENZ (1953) concluded, on the basis of the effects of selective inhibitors, that the diffuse staining *(Naph-I)* of myofibrils was due chiefly to aliesterase. Hence, the exact identities of the ChE's in these various sarcoplasmic locations, as well as their functional significance, remain to be determined.

5. Miscellaneous sites

Additional sites of staining for AChE in skeletal muscle which have been noted by several authors, and were summarized by BECKETT and BOURNE (1957a, b), include (1) structures made up of parallel gutters arranged as a palisade, or "cake frill," around the muscle fiber, (2) parallel gutters, either parallel with or perpendicular to the long axis of the muscle fiber, and (3) spiral gutters wound arround muscle fibers. The functional significance of all these structures is obscure.

6. Muscle spindles

In contrast to the twitch-contracting skeletal muscle fibers which are innervated by large α-fibers, amphibian muscles contain varying proportions of tonically contracting fibers (e.g., the *Tonusbündel* of the frog iliofibular muscle) which are multiply innervated by γ-fibers, or

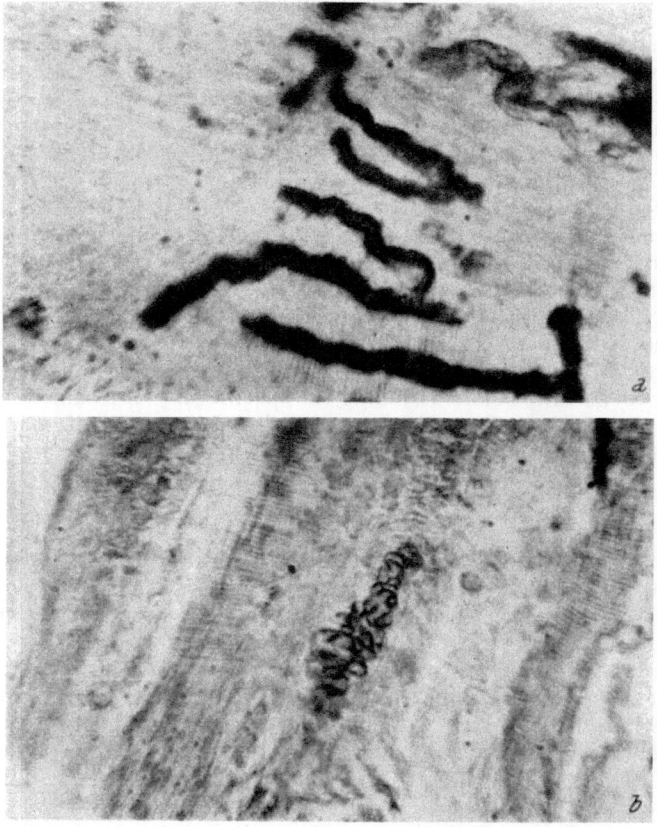

Fig. 16. Cholinesterase staining *(ThCh-VI)* of motor endplates of M. iliofibularis of the frog. Magnification X 900. Upper: Twitch fibers, exhibiting intensive staining. Lower: Tonic fibers of the "tonus bundle" exhibiting light staining (CSILLIK et al. 1961)

the small motor nerve system. The former type responds to nerve impulses by a localized endplate potential, which in turn gives rise to the propagated muscle action potential followed by a rapid, brief contraction; the latter respond only by slow contractures, which are localized to the regions of the multiple endplates (KUFFLER and VAUGHAN WILLIAMS 1953a). These consist of clusters of small, grape-like bodies measuring individually a few micra in diameter, which are located at different levels in each fiber (COUTEAUX 1952) (Fig. 13-4, 13-5). The individual subneural apparatus appears as a small cupule which contains a much lower concentration of AChE than the motor endplates of the twitch-contracting fibers (COUTEAUX 1958, CSILLIK 1961, CSILLIK et al. 1961; Fig. 16). In mammalian muscle, the equivalent system is represented by the intrafusal fibers of the muscle spindles (KUFFLER et al. 1951) in which, however, the total innervation is more complex.

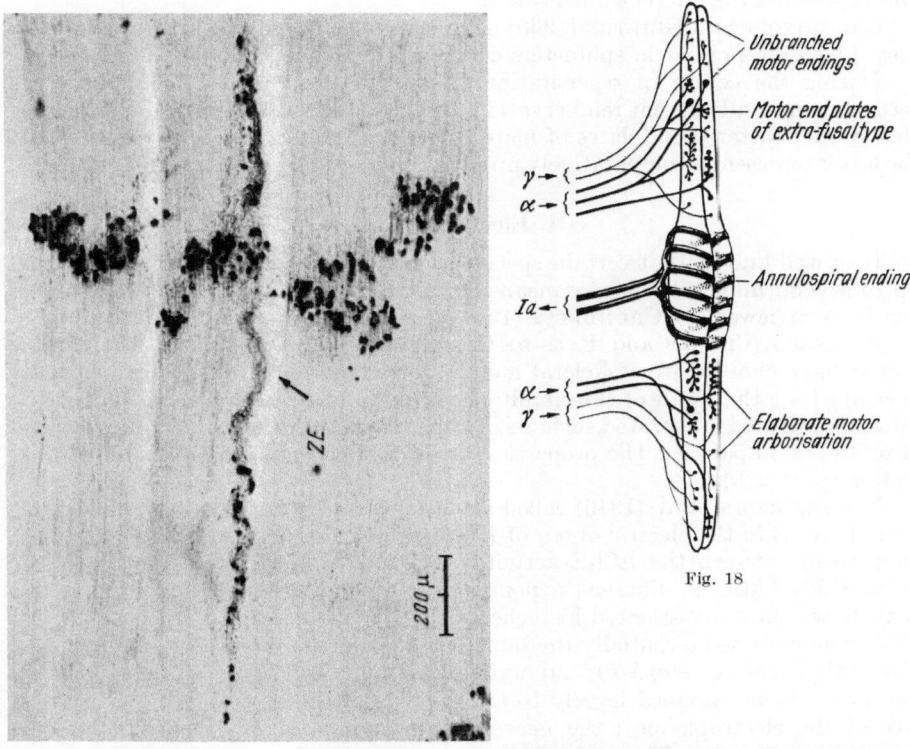

Fig. 17. Low power view of region of terminal innervation in biceps of an infant aged three months, stained for AChE activity *(ThCh-VI)*. The subneural apparatuses of the muscle spindle are spread out along its entire length, except in the equatorial zone (Z.E.) (COËRS and WOOLF 1959)

Fig. 18. Diagram showing nerve fibres and their endings in relation to a muscle spindle. As seen in preparations stained vitally with methylene blue (COËRS and WOOLF 1959)

It was reported first by CÖERS (1954) that human intrafusal muscle fibers, unlike extrafusal fibers, show an extensive distribution of AChE at loci everywhere excepting in the equatorial zone *(ThCh-VI)*. The same general distribution of AChE in the muscle spindles of several mammalian species was noted by GEREB-TZOFF (1955) *(ThCh-VII)*. In addition, non-specific ChE is present throughout the cytoplasm (GOMORI 1948, CSILLIK 1961). The details of the localization of AChE have been investigated by CÖERS and DURAND (1956), and are summarized in the monograph of CÖERS and WOLF (1959), from which Figs. 17 and 18 are taken. Two types of motor endplate have been described, both of which are distributed along most of the length of the fiber in man and the cat, but are most concentrated at the juxta-equatorial region. The ramified endings, which originate presumably from middle-sized α-fibers (COOPER and DANIEL 1956, BOYD 1958), are AChE-rich terminal arborizations similar to those found in extrafusal fibers; their function is not clearly known (GRANIT et al. 1959). The second type of intrafusal motor endplates are scattered, unbranched collaterals, terminating in club-like expansions or verrucose dilatations; these contain a lower concentration of AChE, and resemble the endplates of amphibian tonic fibers; they are probably innervated by the γ-fibers of the small motor nerve system. The equatorial zone of the intrafusal fibers contains the annulo-spiral ending, which is virtually devoid of AChE and represents the afferent innervation.

GEREBTZOFF and GRIETEN (1956) have noted the frequency with which intrafusal fibers are present in sphincters composed of striated muscle.

During the course of regeneration of extrafusal endplates, following nerve sectioning and subsequent reinnervation, they pass through stages which resemble closely the scattered endplates of mature intrafusal fibers; this may suggest that the latter represent a comparatively primitive stage of development (CSILLIK 1961).

III. Electric organs

It is well known that certain species of fish can discharge potentials ranging up to several hundred volts by means of specialized electric organs. The subject has been reviewed by GRUNDFEST (1957 b), and more recently was the topic of a symposium (CHAGAS and PAES-DE-CARVALHO 1961). Apparently, the electric organs have evolved from skeletal muscle fibers; the high voltages and currents developed are the result of the simultaneous discharge, or depolarization, of the similarly oriented innervated surfaces of large numbers of electroplaques, arranged in series and in parallel. The properties of the discharges are discussed in the final section (page 273).

NACHMANSOHN et al. (1946) called attention to the extremely high concentration of AChE in the electric organ of *Electrophorus electricus*, and noted the close parallelism between the AChE activity, the density of electroplaques, and the voltage developed at different regions along its length. The distribution of the enzyme was first investigated histochemically by COUCEIRO and associates (1953, 1955) who obtained essentially the same results with the thiocholine *(ThCh-III)*, β-naphthyl acetate *(Naph-I)*, and myristoylcholine *(LC-Ch)* techniques. Activity was found to be confined largely to the papillae of the innervated, or posterior, face of the electroplaques; the nerve terminals were stained considerably less intensively (Fig. 19). Thus, the pattern is quite similar to that of the motor endplate of skeletal muscle.

MATHEWSON et al. (1961), using the α-naphthyl acetate-hexazotized pararosaniline method *(Naph-II)*, have studied by electron microscopy the fine structure and the AChE-distribution of the electric organs of species representing five different genera. All four marine forms examined (*Narcine, Torpedo, Raia*, and *Astroscopus*) have electroplaques of the electrically inexcitable, or pure endplate, type. In each, AChE was localized in the synaptic cleft and between the folds of the postsynaptic membrane in a pattern analogous to that found at the mouse motor endplate by LEHRER and ORNSTEIN (1959) with the same technique. As in *Electrophorus*, no activity was detected at the non-innervated face of the electroplaques. In the other genus examined, the fresh water electric catfish, *Malapterurus*, no AChE could be detected in the electroplaques.

AUGUSTINSSON and JOHNELS (1958) found that *Malapterurus* was the only genus, of the several studied by them, which is capable of discharging high voltages (up to 400 V) but does not possess proportionately high concentrations of AChE and ACh in the electric organ. Contrary to earlier opinion, the electric organs of this genus also probably are derived from striated muscle (JOHNELS 1956). However, on the basis of their electrical excitability (KEYNES et al. 1961) and limited area of innervation (BALLOWITZ 1899), it is likely that the shock delivered is the result of summated propagated potentials, equivalent to muscle action potentials, where it is unlikely that the ACh-AChE system is involved. COUTEAUX and SZABO (1959) have demonstrated definite AChE activity at the limited synaptic area by means of the thiocholine method *(ThCh-VI)*.

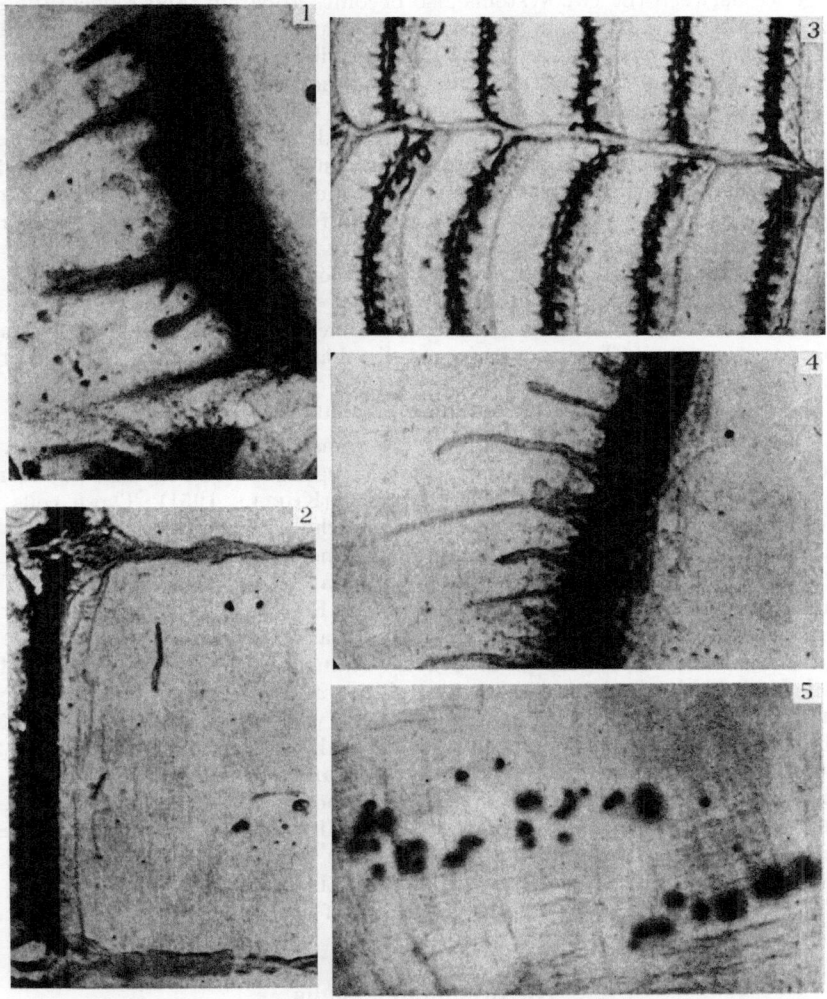

Fig. 19. Localization of AChE in electric organs of *Electrophorus electricus*. 1. Organ of Sachs (*ThCh-III*, × 80). Intense staining at the level of the posterior face, with diffusion toward the papillae of the anterior face; septa colorless. 2. Organ of Sachs (*ThCh-III*, × 80). Stained posterior face of an electroplaque at the left; the adjacent septum and those bounding the electroplaque are completely unstained. 3. Principal organ, mid-region (*Naph-I*, X 30). Posterior papillae stained violet; adjacent longitudinal septa and vertical septa faintly rose colored, as well as the anterior papillae. 4. Organ of Sachs (*Naph-I*, following brief formalin-fixation, × 80). Posterior face stained violet; anterior papillae and septa rose colored. 5. Intercostal muscle of the rat (*ThCh-III*, × 80). Intense staining of subneural apparatus; absence of nuclear staining (COUCEIRO et al. 1953)

B. Autonomic nervous system and effector organs

Anatomically and pharmacologically, the initial portions of the peripheral representations of the somatic motor and autonomic systems show certain similarities. Thus, both take origin from neurons of the antero-lateral columns of the spinal cord and brain stem nuclei, which give rise to myelinated, cholinergic fibers. Their sites of termination, the motor endplates of skeletal muscle and the autonomic ganglia, respectively, are susceptible in common to the actions of a large number of drugs, such as nicotine and d-tubocurarine. However, here the divergence between the two systems also becomes apparent, and reflects the specialized functions which each subserves. There are marked differences, in structural relationships and in the cytological distributions of AChE, between the neuromuscular junctions and the ganglionic synapses; in both respects, certain parasympathetic ganglia (e.g., the ciliary) show what might be considered transitional characteristics, as noted below. Beyond the ganglia, i.e., at the postganglionic fibers, neuroeffector cells and related structures, the autonomic system has no apparent anatomical or physiological counterpart in the somatic neuromuscular system, and analogies with respect to function and the action of drugs are no longer obvious.

The arbitrary inclusion in this section of blood and the placenta, which are obviously not under direct autonomic control, has been done as a matter of convenience. On the other hand the adrenal medulla, which in many respects is the counterpart of the autonomic ganglia, has been included with the other endocrine glands.

I. Preganglionic neurons

In the intermediolateral columns of the spinal cord of the cat, the neurons identified as those giving rise to sympathetic preganglionic fibers show uniformly high to moderate staining for AChE activity (KOELLE 1951). These cells are generally smaller than the anterior horn cells of the same species; as in the latter, staining is most intense in the neuronal membranes, and less so in the cytoplasm *(ThCh-III)*. Analogous neurons of the parasympathetic system have been studied in the brainstem of the rat (KOELLE 1954). The Edinger-Westphal nucleus, from which arise the preganglionic fibers to the ciliary ganglion, consists of small, rounded neurons, all of which are heavily stained by the thiocholine method *(ThCh-III)*. In the dorsal motor nucleus of the vagus, considerable variation was observed; some cells were stained very heavily, whereas others were moderately or lightly stained. Heavily stained neurons in the dorsal motor nucleus of the rabbit have been demonstrated by GEREBTZOFF and VANDERMISSEN (1956).

In an earlier investigation employing the homogenate technique, SAWYER and HOLLINGSHEAD (1945) reported that the cervical sympathetic trunk contains a relatively high concentration of AChE. This has been confirmed both quantitatively and histochemically by KOENIG and KOELLE (1961).

The distribution of AChE at the terminals of the preganglionic fibers is described in the section which follows.

II. Autonomic ganglia

1. General distributions of ganglionic AChE and BuChE

From earlier studies involving analyses of homogenates of the superior cervical and other sympathetic ganglia, it was known that they contain high concentrations of both AChE and BuChE. The marked fall in the former which follows preganglionic denervation led to the conclusion that most of the AChE is localized in the terminals of the preganglionic fibers (SAWYER and HOLLINSHEAD 1945). These findings have been confirmed and considerably amplified by subsequent histochemical investigations.

In the cat, the AChE of all autonomic ganglia examined is confined to the neuronal elements; with the exception of the ganglion cells of the intestinal plexuses (v.i.), the BuChE is restricted to the glial cells (Fig. 1: A-3, C-1, C-3) (KOELLE 1951, 1955). The typical cellular distributions of AChE are illustrated in Fig. 20 (KOELLE and KOELLE 1959) *(ThCh-V)*. In the stellate ganglion (Fig. 20 A), high AChE activity is present in the entering preganglionic axons, their ramifications throughout the protoplasmic tracts of de Castro (the intermingled preganglionic fibers and dendritic fascicles), and their intra- and extra-capsular terminations on the ganglion cells and their dendrites. All the ganglion cells are surrounded by a dense network of AChE-stained fibers which terminate as fine fibrils or expanded bulbs. Numerous partially stained glomerular formations, consisting of intertwined pre- and postsynaptic elements, are also noted. A few

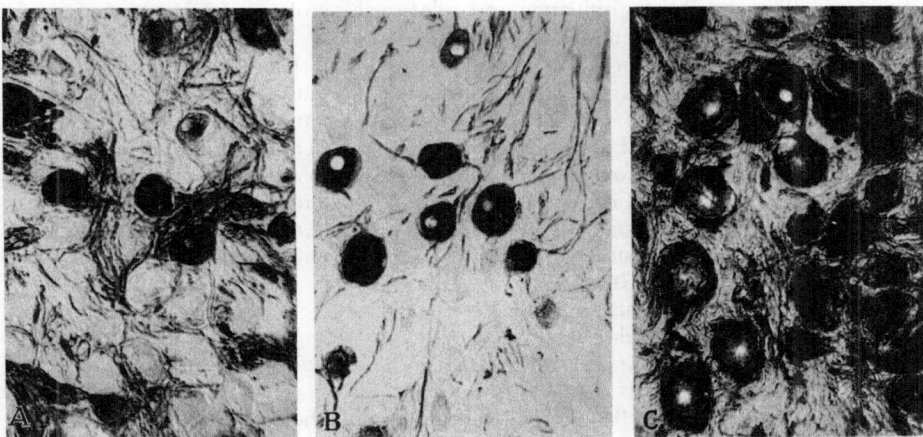

Fig. 20. Autonomic ganglia, cat, stained for acetylcholinesterase activity. Sections (10 μ) incubated 80 min in AThCh medium following selective inhibition of non-specific ChE by DFP *(ThCh-III)*. Magnification× 200. A. Stellate ganglion, normal. B. Stellate ganglion, preganglionically denervated. C. Ciliary ganglion (KOELLE and KOELLE 1959)

stained fibers leave the ganglion with the postganglionic trunks, but the majority of the postganglionic fibers are practically unstained. The identity of most of the stained fibers throughout the ganglion as preganglionic is disclosed by Fig. 20 B, a similarly treated section of the opposite stellate ganglion which had been denervated preganglionically two weeks previously. The small number of residual stained fibers is probably the result of incomplete denervation, or in some cases they may represent the axons of the occasional heavily stained ganglion cells.

The stellate ganglion cells fall into three classes with respect to AChE activity: (1) a small number which are heavily stained, (2) an equivalent number stained moderately or lightly, and (3) the great majority which are stained very faintly (KOELLE 1951, 1955). These observations have received quantitative confirmation by HOLMSTEDT and SJÖQVIST (1959), who employed HOLMSTEDT's (1957b) modified thiocholine method *(ThCh-IX)*. Their approximate percentage figures for the same classes, based on counts of several thousand cells, were for the cat stellate ganglion (1) 7%, (2) 8%, and (3) 85%, and for the superior cervical ganglion (1) 0.5%, (2) 20%, and (3) 80%. The total numbers in classes (1) plus (2) were lower for the superior mesenteric and coeliac ganglia. The only discrepancy between the conclusions of the two investigations is that the former author considered the cells in class (3) to show faint activity, whereas the latter group believed them to be devoid of AChE.

Although the identity of the aforementioned three classes of sympathetic ganglion cells remains to be proven, reasonable conjectures can be proposed for two. In the ciliary ganglion (Fig. 20 C), which gives rise exclusively to cholinergic postganglionic fibers, all the neurons contain high concentrations of AChE. Since the same has been shown also for the neurons of origin of the preganglionic fibers and the somatic motor fibers, all of which are cholinergic, it is likely that the heavily stained sympathetic ganglion cells (class 1) are associated with cholinergic postganglionic sympathetic fibers, such as the vasodilator fibers and those innervating the sweat glands. This assumption was strenghthened by a recent report by SJÖQVIST and FREDRICSSON (1961). The overwhelming majority of faintly stained or unstained neurons (class 3) and their postganglionic fibers are probably adrenergic. The possible significance and relationships of the moderately stained neurons in class (2) are discussed in the final section.

The ganglion cells of Auerbach's plexus throughout the small intestine in the cat likewise show different degrees of staining, but the majority are stained heavily (KOELLE 1955). The same relationship has been assumed here, since there is evidence that the intestinal plexuses give rise to both cholinergic and adrenergic fibers (AMBACHE 1951). However, all the neurons observed in this group are stained heavily for BuChE also, the significance of which is unknown. The only species in which this has been observed at other ganglionic sites is the rat, where occasional neurons of the superior cervical ganglion contain high concentrations of BuChE (KOELLE 1954, GIACOBINI 1957, TAXI 1961).

In the rabbit and rhesus monkey, the patterns of distribution of ganglionic AChE and BuChE are similar to those in the cat, with one general exception: in addition to the small proportion of heavily and moderately stained neurons in the sympathetic ganglia (classes 1 and 2), practically all the remainder show light but definite staining (KOELLE 1955). The same pattern has been reported for man, the mole, and the guinea pig (CAUNA et al. 1961). The proportion of heavily staining sympathetic ganglion cells is considerably higher in the rat (KOELLE 1954, TAXI 1961), whereas in the hedgehog all are stained with relatively high intensity (CAUNA et al. l.c.).

GIACOBINI (1957) has performed quantitative determinations of the AChE of individual autonomic ganglion cells in the rat and frog.

In the rat there was wide variation among individual sympathetic neurons (0.11 to $2.2 \times 10^{-3} \mu l$ CO_2 per hr, from hydrolysis of AThCh), but the majority showed significant activity (mean $= 0.7 \times 10^{-3}$); however, in some cells no activity was detected, even after eight hours' incubation. There was a fairly close correlation between the AChE activities of the neuronal cell bodies and of the immediately adjacent (approximately 200 μ) portions of their axons. These findings may account for the marked reduction in ganglionic AChE (approximately 50%) which has been reported to follow postganglionic axonotomy, in accompaniment with failure of transmission (BROWN and PASCOE 1954), in this species (McLENNAN 1954, BROWN 1958) without necessitating the assumption of an effect on the presynaptic terminals. Activity was uniformly high (1.2 to $4.0 \times 10^{-3} \mu l$) in rat ciliary ganglion cells. In the frog sympathetic ganglion cells, values ranged from 0.13 to $4.4 \times 10^{-3} \mu l$; again, no activity was detected in some.

The distribution of ChE's in the adrenal medulla is described in the section on endocrine glands (E, II).

2. Cytological distinction between external and internal ganglionic AChE; the concept of functional and reserve AChE

The concept that neuronal AChE may be oriented partially externally and partially internally to the cell membrane, and hence exhibit varying degrees of accessibility to different types of inhibitors, was first proposed by SCHWEITZER et al. (1939), and has been extended by NACHMANSOHN (1950), BURGEN and CHIPMAN (1952), and KOELLE and associates (v.i.). This matter has considerable bearing on both the functions of AChE and the actions of anti-ChE agents. Since the most definitive studies have been conducted on autonomic ganglia, these are summarized here.

From measurements of enzymatic inhibition following the administration of 3-di*iso*propylphosphato-N-methyl-pyridinium methylsulfate, BURGEN and CHIPMAN (1952) concluded that most of the AChE of the superior cervical ganglion is oriented towards the exterior of the preganglionic terminations, while that of the neurons of the central nervous system is chiefly intracellular.

KOELLE and STEINER (1956) compared the effects of a tertiary alkylphosphate anticholinesterase agent, 2-diethoxyphosphinylthioethyldimethylamine acid oxalate (217 AO), and its quaternary methiodide analog (217 MI, echothiophate, Phospholine), following their administration to rabbits by various routes. After intravenous injection, the tertiary compound readily reached the brain, but the quaternary compound did not. (This distinction was also found by SCHAUMANN and JOB (1958) from the effects of the two compounds on respiration.) When the quaternary compound was injected in relatively high doses into a lateral ventricle, it became fairly evenly distributed throughout both sides of the brain, and caused marked inhibition of cerebral AChE. Within 24 hours most of the excess compound had disappeared from the cerebrospinal fluid, and presumably from the extracellular fluid, but apparently some persisted in uncombined form at intracellular sites for several days. In spite of this, there was considerable return of AChE activity, at a rate which indicated that both hydrolytic reactivation and synthesis of new enzyme were involved. To explain these results, it was proposed that part of the enzyme is oriented toward the external surface of the neuronal membrane, and part is enclosed within intracellular membranes, possibly of the endoplasmic reticulum, which protected it from the intracellularly located, uncombined inhibitor. The latter fraction was suggested to represent "*reserve AChE*," recently synthesized in the course of the neuron's normal course of protein-turnover, as indicated for neuronal proteins in general by the work of WEISS and HISCOE (1948), PORTER (1953), and PALAY and PALADE (1955). The externally oriented fraction was designated as "*functional AChE*," on the assumption that it is most strategically situated for the rapid hydrolysis of ACh liberated during the course of synaptic transmission. Most of the subsequent studies have been conducted with autonomic ganglia of the cat.

In order to obtain more accurate localization of the cytoplasmic, or *internal neuronal AChE*, cat ciliary ganglia were stained by several modifications of the thiocholine method *(ThCh-III)*, and the results were compared with sections stained by standard histological techniques (FUKUDA and KOELLE 1959). The sharpest patterns were obtained when sections were incubated for very brief periods (3 to 5 min) immediately after cutting, and without fixation. Such slides showed a close superficial resemblance to those stained for Nissl substance with cresyl violet, a method which is considered selective for the ribonucleic acid (RNA) granules adherent to the canaliculi and vesicles of the endoplasmic reticulum (PALAY and PALADE 1955). This tentative localization was strengthened by the recent reports of TOSCHI (1959) and HANZON and TOSCHI (1959) that most of the AChE of cat brain homogenates is associated with remnants of vesicular membranes of the microsome fraction, which is probably composed chiefly of the fragmented endoplasmic reticulum (PALADE and SIEKEVITZ 1956). Further confirmation has been obtained by R. DAVIS (unpublished observations) in the author's laboratory by electron microscopic demonstration of selective staining of the endoplasmic reticulum of chick ciliary ganglion cells with the thiolacetic acid method.

The proposal that only the *external AChE* at the neuronal membrane is immediately functional in the hydrolysis of liberated ACh entails a quantitative pharmacological sequel. Studies in several laboratories with irreversible lipoid-soluble anti-ChE agents, such as di*iso*propyl phosphorofluoridate (DFP), have shown that considerably more than 50 % of the AChE of a given tissue must be inactivated before pharmacological effects dependent upon such inhibition are noted. However, a poorly penetrating compound, which would inhibit the external AChE selectivity, might be expected to produce similar effects after inhibiting a smaller fraction of the total enzyme. This possibility was examined by two approaches.

One approach was provided by the reports of KARCZMAR and HOWARD (1955) and LANDS et al. (1955) on the pharmacology of a *bis*quaternary, reversible, potent anti-ChE agent of high molecular weight, N,N'-*bis*(2-diethylaminoethyl) oxamide *bis*-2-chlorobenzyl chloride (WIN 8077, ambenonium, Mytelase). This compound had been shown to produce typical cholinomimetic effects in various species following the intravenous administration of doses as low as 0.3 μg (0.0005 μmol) per kg. However, it was necessary to give doses of approximately 100 times this amount in order to produce significant inhibition of cholinesterase as detected by standard manometric assays of homogenized tissues from treated animals.

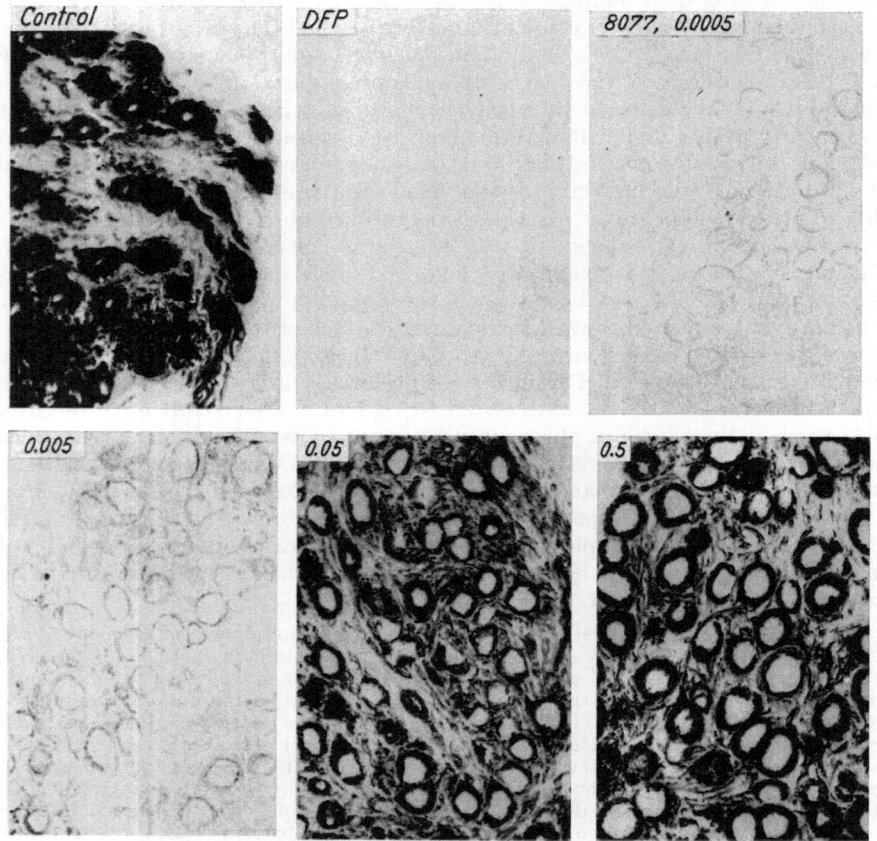

Fig. 21. Sections (10 μ) of ciliary ganglia from cats injected i.v. with doses of ambemonium indicated (micromol/kg), followed five min. later by DFP (20 micromol/kg). Sections washed, stained for AChE by incubation for 80 min in AThCh medium. Magnification × 120 (KOELLE 1957)

To test the possibility that ambenonium might act selectively at sites of external or functional AChE, a series of anesthetized atropinized cats was given single intravenous injections of WIN 8077 in doses ranging from 0.0005 to 0.5 μmol per kg; five min later they received an intravenous dose of DFP (20 μmol per kg) which was sufficient, if given alone, to cause virtually complete inactivation of both the AChE and BuChE of the autonomic ganglia (KOELLE 1957). However, any AChE which was already combined with the reversible inhibitor would be expected to be protected against irreversible inactivation by DFP. Thirty min later, the cats were sacrificed, and the ganglia were removed, sectioned, washed several times, and stained for AChE activity. Examination of the ciliary ganglia revealed that there was definite protection, or reversible inhibition, of a small amount of AChE at the peripheries of the ganglion cells after the pharmacological threshold dose (0.0005 μmol per kg) of ambenonium, and protection of increasing amounts after increasingly larger doses. No AChE was protected within the neuronal cytoplasm, where presumably the *bis*quaternary compound, but not DFP, failed to penetrate (Fig. 21). Comparable results were obtained in the superior cervical and stellate ganglia, and at the motor endplate of intercostal muscle. When 10 μ sections of normal ganglia were exposed *in vitro* to the two inhibitors in the same sequence (i.e., ambenonium, followed by ambenonium plus DFP), the amount of enzyme protected was again proportional to the concentration of the reversible inhibitor, but under these conditions AChE was preserved at all sites, cytoplasmic and peripheral. These results do not, of course, exclude the possibility that the pharmacological actions of ambenonium are due in part to a direct cholinomimetic effect.

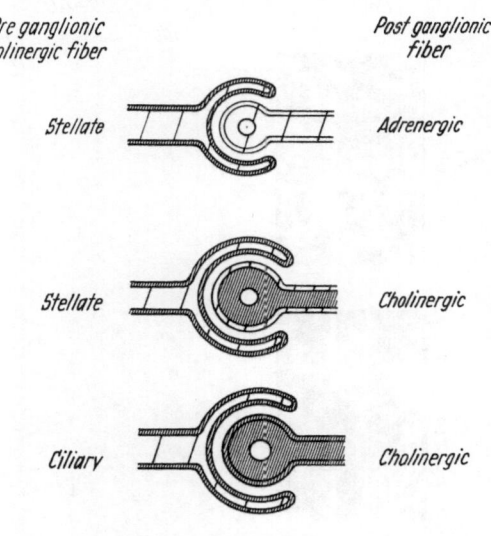

Fig. 22. Diagrammatic representation of distributions of functional (external) and reserve (internal) AChE at synapses of autonomic ganglia. Density of cross-hatching indicates relative concentration of enzymatic activity (KOELLE and KOELLE 1959)

The localization of the external, or ambenonium-inhibited, ganglionic AChE was determined more precisely by conducting similar studies with cats in which various ganglia had been denervated preganglionically one to three weeks previously (KOELLE and KOELLE 1959). The denervated stellate and superior cervical ganglia were found to be practically devoid of external AChE; hence, in their normal counterparts it is essentially entirely presynaptic. In contrast, the concentration of external AChE surrounding the neurons of the denervated ciliary and sphenopalatine ganglia was considerably reduced but by no means abolished; thus, at these locations, external AChE is normally both pre- and postsynaptic. These findings are summarized diagrammatically in Fig. 22; their implications are discussed in the final section. In an earlier study of the ciliary ganglion of the hen, SZENTÁGOTHAI et al. (1954) likewise concluded that AChE is associated with both the pre- and postganglionic membranes. TAXI (1961) has recently made the interesting observation that in this species structures are present in the ciliary ganglion cells which resemble in many respects the neuromuscular junctions of skeletal muscle. In many ganglion cells, the AChE activity is concentrated at one pole, and was still present in this location 10 days following preganglionic denervation.

The second approach to the investigation of the functional significance of the ganglionic external AChE consisted in a quantitative comparison of the pharmacological and AChE-inhibiting effects of the tertiary and quaternary alkylphosphate inhibitors discussed previously, 217 AO and 217 MI, respectively (MCISAAC and KOELLE 1959).

The oil:water partition coefficient of 217 AO is approximately 200 times that of 217 MI, and the latter has approximately three times the anti-ChE potency of the former. It was assumed that 217 AO would penetrate the neuronal membrane readily, but that 217 MI would

act relatively selectively on the external AChE. Cats were prepared for recording ganglionic
action potentials or isotonic contractions of the nictitating membrane during supramaximal
stimulation of the partially resected preganglionic trunk. With this type of preparation,
graded doses of AChE-inhibitors produce first increasing potentiation, then depression, of both
responses (KAMIJO and KOELLE 1952, HOLADAY et al. 1954). After obtaining a series of control
responses, an intravenous injection of one of the drugs was given, and responses were recorded
for the succeeding hour. The superior cervical, stellate, and ciliary ganglia were then removed
for quantitative analysis of AChE activity by the Warburg method and histochemical examination by the ThCh-technique (ThCh-III).

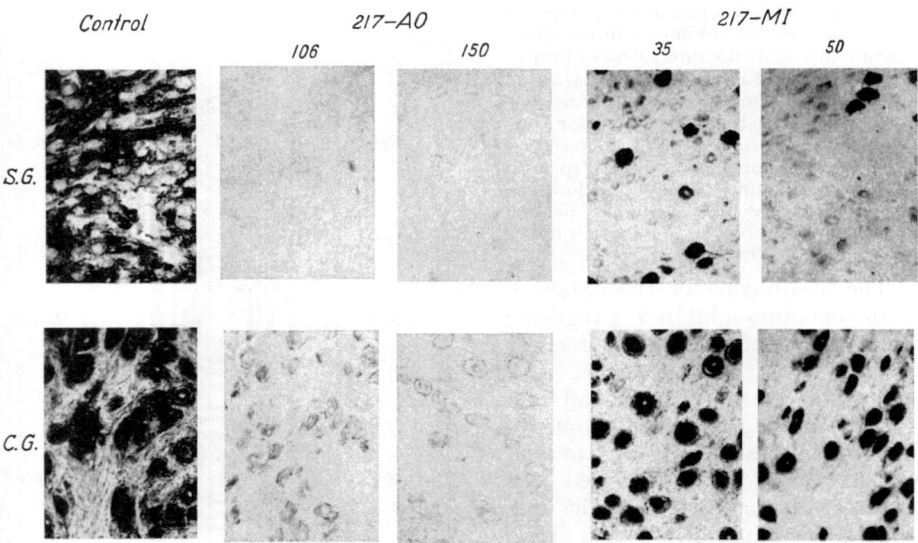

Fig. 23. Sections (10 μ) of the stellate (S.G.) and ciliary (C.G.) ganglia obtained from cats sacrificed 60 min after
receiving 217 AO or 217 MI, and stained for AChE activity (ThCh-III, Magnification × 80). Eighty min. incubation
with substrate. Figures refer to dose administered in μg/kg (MCISAAC and KOELLE 1959)

The doses of the two compounds required to cause equivalent potentiation of responses
were inversely proportional to their anti-ChE potencies. Typical tracings from these experiments are illustrated in Chapter 12, Fig. 5 (p. 548), and results with all cats in the experiments in which contraction of the nictitating membrane was recorded are summarized in
Table 1 of the same chapter (p. 548). From those data, it is apparent that the quaternary
compound, 217 MI, produced far less inactivation of ganglionic AChE than did the tertiary
compound at pharmacologically equivalent doses. The differences were greatest for the ciliary
ganglion, which contains exclusively cholinergic neurons and hence the highest proportion of
internal AChE. The differences in the locations of the residual AChE of the ganglia noted
histochemically are shown in Fig. 23. Whereas 217 AO caused approximately the same degree
of inactivation at all sites, 217 MI acted selectively on the external AChE of the presynaptic
terminals and spared that of the neuronal cytoplasm. The AChE patterns obtained after
administration of the latter agent were thus the reverse of those noted following treatment
with ambenonium and DFP (Fig. 21).

The foregoing findings are consistent with the concept that in the superior
cervical ganglion only the external AChE is directly functional during the process
of ganglionic transmission, and hence inhibition of only this fraction is necessary
for the production of acute pharmacological effects.

The physiological function of the internal or reserve AChE is still uncertain.
In view of the foregoing findings, it was suggested (KOELLE and STEINER 1956,
FUKUDA and KOELLE 1959) that it might represent recently synthesized enzyme
which is subsequently transported from the perikaryon, through the axon, to its
terminations in the course of the neuron's continuous turnover of protein, a pro-

posal made earlier by DALE (1955). However, an investigation of this possibility failed to provide substantiation.

After the systemic administration to cats of doses of DFP sufficient to produce irreversible inactivation of most of the AChE of the hypoglossal nucleus and nerve, no central to peripheral gradient could be detected in the activity of the enzyme during the course of its regeneration (KOENIG and KOELLE 1960, 1961). In fact, the results suggested that AChE is synthesized in the axon at least as rapidly as in the perikaryon. This leaves unanswered the questions of both the function of the cytoplasmic AChE in normal adult neurons, and the mechanism of resynthesis of the AChE of the axons, from which DNA is presumably absent, following the inactivation of AChE by DFP. It is possible that the AChE of the neuronal endoplasmic reticulum functions in the maintenance of the excitable state at that region, in accordance with the suggestion of RUSKA et al. (1958), perhaps by participating in the sodium-pump mechanism (HOKIN et al. 1960). These points have been considered in detail by KOENIG and KOELLE (1961).

III. Autonomic neuroeffector sites

All the postganglionic cholinergic fibers examined exhibit high AChE activity as far as their terminal processes can be traced (KOELLE 1951, SZENTÁGOTHAI 1957, GEREBTZOFF 1959). However, the autonomic effector cells (gland cells, smooth and cardiac muscle fibers) show great variations in their content of AChE and BuChE according to both the individual organ and the species. In many cases it has not been possible to distinguish accurately whether the enzyme is associated with the axonal terminations and plexuses, or with the effector cells. The situation is complicated further by the presence in most organs of a third element, the extensive network of interstitial cells of Cajal. On the basis of its location and histological staining characteristics, and the earlier studies of LEEUWE (1937), MEYLING (1938), and BOEKE (1942), this system has been characterized by several recent authors (JABONERO 1952, TAXI 1952b, MEYLING 1953) as representing a primitive syncytial neuronal network, or "terminal reticulum," interposed between the postganglionic fibers and the effector cells as a means of distributing activating impulses, or functioning to coordinate automatic activity arising from the effector cells themselves. In contrast, HILLARP (1959) has advanced valid arguments for regarding the system merely as a syncytium of supporting glial cells, analogous to the Schwann sheath cells, which encloses the fine, varicose processes of the postganglionic axonal twigs; in this context, the latter would represent the "terminal reticulum," or "fundamental plexus." While it has not been established whether the postganglionic axonal terminations form an actual syncytium or reticulum, or remain as closely associated but independent branches, the latter case seems more likely (HILLARP 1959). SZENTÁGOTHAI (1957) has shown that the axonal terminations represent the major site of AChE activity in the smooth muscle layers of the intestine. In many locations, particularly in the vicinity of Auerbach's plexus in the small intestine of the cat, rabbit, and rhesus monkey, the interstitial cells, or Schwann cells, exhibit high concentrations of BuChE (KOELLE 1951, 1953, 1955). Hence, with respect to the neuronal and glial elements, the distribution of the two enzymes is quite analogous to that in the superior cervical ganglion, described above. Recently it has been suggested that at all sites in the nervous system the glial cells may participate directly in transmission and other active processes (GALAMBOS 1961); this subject is considered in the final section.

Regardless of the question of the function of the interstitial cells, the foregoing points illustrate the difficulty they present with respect to the immediate consideration, the cytological localization of the ChE's. When reliable histochemical procedures become available for electron microscopic studies of autonomic effector organs, it may be necessary to modify present concepts.

The following brief accout may be supplemented by reference to the detailed descriptions and bibliography in GEREBTZOFF's (1959) monograph.

1. Circulatory system

a) Heart

Earlier reports on determinations employing homogenates indicated that cardiac tissue contains significant amounts of both AChE and BuChE, and that the concentrations of both are higher in the atria than in the ventricles (see

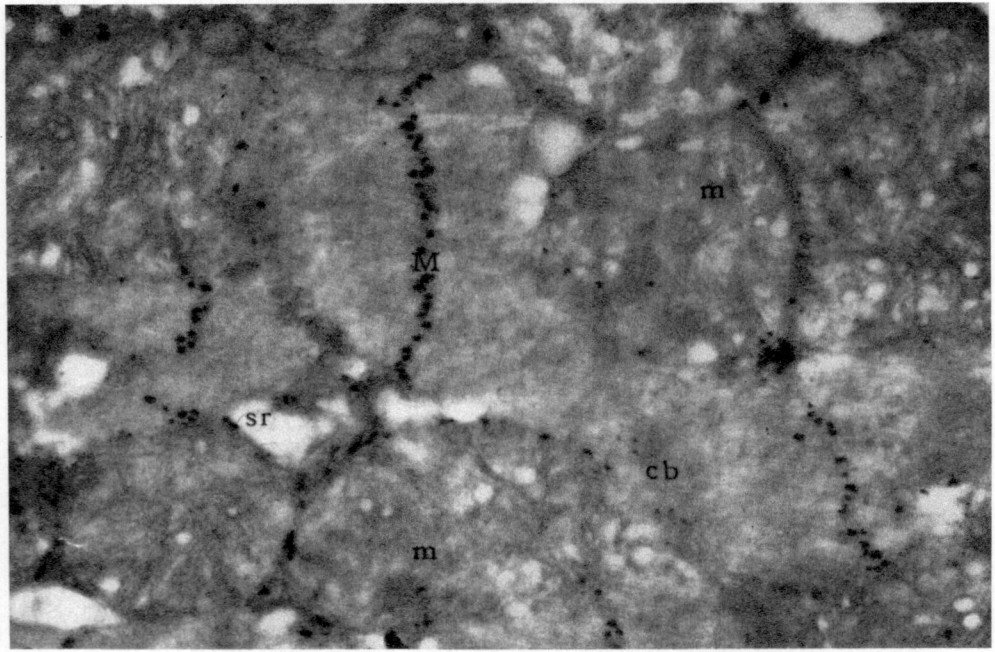

Fig. 24. Section of block of heart muscle incubated for 15 minutes at pH 6.4 in the authors' standard medium (*ThAc*). Alignment of deposits at the M band is not orderly probably because of unequal contraction. Mitochondria (*m*) show many dense deposits, especially on their surfaces; and the sarcoplasmic reticulum (*sr*) and contraction bands (*cb*) contain a few less dense deposits. × 50,000 (BARRNETT and PALADE 1959)

AUGUSTINSSON 1948 for references). These studies have received general confirmation in a recent careful analysis, in which it was noted, hovever, that the frog heart may be devoid of BuChE (GIRARDIER et al. 1960). From the relatively high concentrations recovered from homogenates of beef heart moderator bands, it was concluded by MOMMAERTS et al. (1953) that AChE activity is particularly high in the Purkinje fibers. However, histochemical examination *(ThCh-III)* of several regions of the beef heart revealed that the highest concentrations are present in the neural elements, and that in contrast the AChE and BuChE activities of the myocardial fibers and conducting system are relatively low (KAMIJO and KOELLE 1955). The groups of ganglion cells in the areas of the sino-auricular and atrio-ventricular nodes, which presumably represent the peripheral vagal ganglia, consistently showed intensive staining for AChE, as did their fibers to the adjacent nodal tissue. The Purkinje fibers, while practically unstained, were surrounded by heavily stained nerve trunks and axonal terminations. Nerve fibers elsewhere showed varying degrees of staining. Essentially the same findings have been reported for the heart of the guinea pig, rabbit, dog, sheep, and hog, as well as the ox (Mohr and Gerebtzoff 1954, Dumont and Drouin 1954, Dumont 1957, Il'Ina-Kakueva 1958). Gerebtzoff (1956 b, 1959) has designated the fine, AChE-staining fibers at the surface of the myocardial fibers as a terminal syncytium.

In addition to its efferent autonomic innervation, the hearts of the dog and cat have been shown to contain afferent fibers, forming a plexus in the subendocardium, and complex end organs which contain predominantly BuChE (Holmes 1957).

The faint staining of the myocardial fibers themselves, predominantly for non-specific ChE, has been localized by electron microscopy *(ThAc)* at the M-bands and in mitochondria (Barrnett and Palade 1959, Fig. 24) identically as in skeletal muscle. Butyrocholinesterase is present also in the walls of the cardiac capillaries (Holmes 1957).

b) Blood vessels and lymphatic organs

Because of the small size of the smooth muscle fibers of most blood vessels, such sites represent extremes of the factors discussed above which complicate the histochemical localization of AChE and BuChE in smooth muscle in general, i.e., the difficulty in distinguishing between the association of staining with nerve terminals, interstitial cells, and the muscle fibers themselves. As Gerebtzoff (1959)

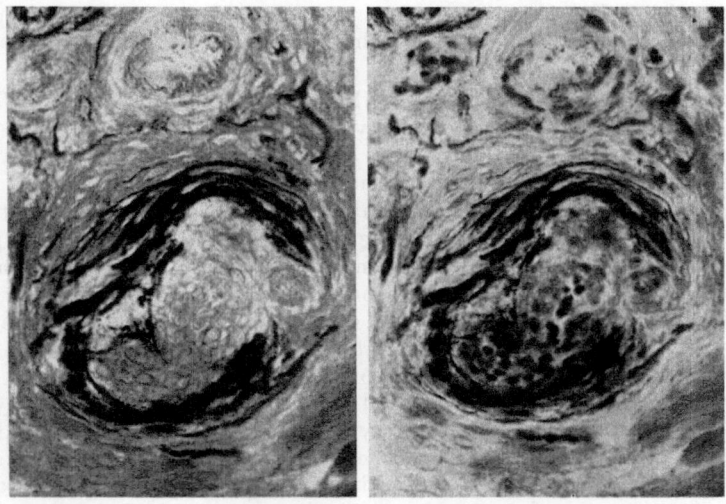

Fig. 25. Acetylcholinesterase around digital arteriovenous anastomoses (A V A's) of human skin. Dark material outlining nerve fibers is copper sulfide precipitated at sites of AChE. *Left:* section counterstained lightly with eosin. *Right:* adjacent serial section counterstained with hematoxylin and eosin. Note large 'epithelioid' cells of media and very narrow lumen of AVA. Absence of fibers about arteriole above AVA is evident also (Hurley and Mescon 1956)

has pointed out, the identification of nerve trunks coursing in association with blood vessels does not implicate the vessels as their sites of termination. Acetylcholinesterase-stained, presumably cholinergic, nerve terminals have been identified among the arteries and veins of various species in varying concentrations in different organs, but in general their distribution is not dense. An outstanding exception to this generalization is the digital arteriovenous anastomosis of human skin, where Hurley and Mescon (1956a) have demonstrated a rich innervation by AChE-containing fibers (Fig. 25), a finding which is consistent with the marked susceptibility of the local circulation to cholinomimetic drugs (MACHT and BADER 1948).

Non-specific ChE has been demonstrated in the walls of capillaries of various organs, particularly in the brain of the rat (KOELLE 1954) and dog (ABRAHAMS et al. 1957). The capillary endothelium of the brain of the toad contains AChE, that of the fish both enzymes, and in several other species neither enzyme is present (BRIGHTMAN and ALBERS 1959). The question has been raised that such staining may be due partially to enzyme adsorbed from the plasma (GEREBTZOFF 1959), but in similar locations it is not prevented by preliminary saline-perfusion.

The spleen, lymph nodes, Peyer's patches, tonsils, and other lymphatic tissues have been shown to stain for AChE in several species (KOELLE et al. 1950, DU-MONT 1955c, D'AGOSTINI and ROSSATTI 1956, ROGISTER and GEREBTZOFF 1958, ELLIS 1959). In most of these tissues, the enzyme has been localized chiefly in the walls of the capillaries which supply the germinal centers of the secondary follicles, with diffuse staining of the immediately adjacent lymphoid elements (D'AGOSTINI and ROSSATTI 1959). The changes which occur during inflammation have been described also by D'AGOSTINI and ROSSATTI (1961).

c) Blood and hematopoietic tissues

In most species, the plasma contains variable concentrations of BuChE or an equivalent ChE, derived chiefly from the liver, and only traces of AChE (AU-GUSTINSSON 1948). Exceptional in this respect are the ruminants, in which the plasma may be practically devoid of both enzymes (GUNTER 1946, ZAJICEK and DATTA 1953).

The wide species variation in the AChE-content of the *erythrocytes*, which are virtually devoid of BuChE, was noted by MENDEL et al. (1943). More recently, ZAJICEK and DATTA (1953) demonstrated a striking inverse relationship between the AChE-content of the erythrocytes and *platelets* of several species. In the sequence: man, cow, guinea pig, horse, rabbit, rat, and cat, the AChE activity of the erythrocytes decreases 100-fold, while that of the platelets increases proportionately. No AChE was detected in human platelets. ZAJICEK (1957) has summarized his subsequent precise histochemical and ultramicro-analytical studies of the AChE contents of individual blood cells and their precursors. The AChE activities of individual megakaryocytes from different species were found to parallel closely the activities of the corresponding platelets (ZAJICEK 1956). In cat marrow preparations, AChE was detected histochemically in promegakaryocytes and "megakaryoblasts," whereas the erythropoietic, granulopoietic, and endothelial cells remained negative. At the other extreme, human preparations showed activity in erythropoietic cells but none in the megakaryocytes (ZAJICEK 1954). From these findings and other considerations, ZAJICEK proposed that the platelets arise from the megakaryocytes, and that their precursors, the megakaryoblasts, and the erythroblasts are derived from a common precursor which contains the factor necessary for AChE-synthesis. It was hypothesized that at the final diferential mitosis of the postulated common precursor, the factor is distributed in different proportions according to the species.

The AChE of both the erythrocytes and platelets is bound tightly to the stroma (PALÉUS 1947, ZAJICEK and DATTA 1953). Various functions have been proposed for erythrocyte AChE, including the regulation of membrane permeability (HOL-LAND and GREIG 1950) and renewal of the phospholipoids of the stroma (DE SANDRE and GHIOTTO 1958). It has also been suggested that the platelets and erythrocytes act jointly as a supply of circulating AChE for functions not related directly to their carrier cells, i.e., as "transport ChE's" for the destruction of ACh which escapes into the circulation from various tissues (KARCZMAR and KOPPANYI 1956).

Granulocytes and lymphocytes probably contain little or no AChE or BuChE (PHILIPPU 1956, literature summarized by ZAJICEK 1957).

2. Respiratory system

Relatively little work has been done on the localization of ChE's in the respiratory system. With an early modification of the ThCh method *(ThCh-II)*, both AChE and BuChE were found in the bronchiolor smooth muscles, scattered groups of pulmonary ganglion cells, nerve trunks, and blood vessels in the cat (KOELLE 1950). MOHR (1955), employing GEREBTZOFF's (1953) modification *(ThCh-VII)*, studied the lungs of several species and obtained fairly consistent results with all. Acetylcholinesterase was noted in the ganglion cells and frequent nerve fibers, particularly in the fine terminals surrounding certain mucous glands. The bronchiolar smooth muscle was stained irregularly for BuChE or non-specific ChE, as were the epithelial goblet cells and mucous gland cells. The ChE of the ciliated respiratory epithelium is discussed in a subsequent section (F, II).

3. Digestive system

a) Salivary glands

In the cat, most of the staining for AChE in the *parotid gland* could be accounted for by the neural elements, including the larger trunks (chiefly postganglionic) and their branches, the occasional ganglion cells, and the pericellular plexuses surrounding the alveoli; staining for BuChE by comparison was extremely faint (KOELLE 1951). These results have received confirmation in measurements of ACh- and BuCh-hydrolysis by homogenates of normal and parasympathetically pre- and postganglionically denervated glands (STROMBLAD 1955). The same general pattern has been reported for the parotid, *submaxillary* and *sublingual glands* in several species by BERTRAND (1955), with the notable exception of intense staining for BuChE in the parotid alveolar cells of the guinea pig. Likewise, SNELL (1958, 1959, 1961b, SNELL and GARRETT 1958) reported the same type of distribution of AChE in all three salivary glands of the rat. By a series of denervation experiments, it was found that most of the intensely stained, presumably cholinergic, fibers in the submaxillary and lingual glands were postganglionic parasympathetic fibers arising from heavily stained ganglion cells within the parenchyma of the glands; the remaining heavily stained trunks represented the preganglionic parasympathetic fibers which enter as small fascicles with the chorda tympani branch to the lingual nerve.

b) Gastrointestinal tract

The ileum reflects the general pattern found throughout the gastrointestinal tract of the cat: AChE is associated with the preganglionic fibers, most of the ganglion cells of Auerbach's plexus, and occasional cells in Meissner's plexus, and the postganglionic fibers distributed among the muscular and glandular elements. Non-specific ChE or BuChE also is present in the ganglion cells, in the interstitial cells, in the membranes of the smooth muscle fibers of all layers, and in the mucosal cells (KOELLE 1951). Similar distributions of the equivalent enzymes have been noted in the duodenum of the rabbit (KOELLE 1953), and in the intestine of the rat and guinea pig (GEREBTZOFF and BERTRAND 1957, DONHOFFER 1959). The latter reference describes in detail the patterns noted throughout the entire gastrointestinal tract of the last two species mentioned. The authors have discussed the possible role of BuChE in digestion and absorption.

c) Liver and pancreas

The *liver* of most species contains predominantly BuChE, and is undoubtedly the source of the same enzyme in the plasma (AUGUSTINSSON 1948). In the cat, it appears to be concentrated in the sinusoidal lining cells, and occurs in decreasing amounts from the central vein to the lobular periphery; the concentration in the parenchymous cells, where it is probably formed, appears to be lower (KOELLE 1951). A similar relationship has been described in the rabbit, whereas in the rat the enzyme is most concentrated in the parenchymatous cells (GEREBTZOFF 1954). The cyclic variation in the distribution of the parenchamytous BuChE of mouse liver with relation to feeding has been described in detail by BERTRAND (1954) and GEREBTZOFF (1961).

The *pancreas* of the dog has long been known to contain high concentrations of predominantly BuChE (MENDEL and RUDNEY 1943). This has been confirmed histochemically by HEBB and HILL (1955a); they found also a marked decrease of BuChE following prolonged stimulation with secretin; unfortunately, localization with the method employed *(ThCh-II)* is compromised by diffusion artifacts, which probably accounts for the intense nuclear staining which was obtained in both acinar and islet cells. The authors failed to find activity in the acinar cells of the pancreas of the other species examined (sheep, goat, horse, rabbit, and cat). In the guinea pig, GEREBTZOFF (1953) noted intense concentrations of BuChE in the cytoplasm of the acinar cells and on the zymogen granules at their apical poles, but no staining of the islet cells. Results similar to the foregoing were obtained by DUMONT (1955a) in the dog and guinea pig; he likewise failed to find significant amounts of BuChE in the rat, rabbit, or sheep pancreas. All investigators have noted the association of AChE with the neural elements of the pancreas.

4. Urogenital system

GRIETEN and GEREBTZOFF (1957) summarized their survey of the ChE's of the urogenital system of the guinea pig, rabbit, mouse, and rat with the statement that AChE is confined chiefly to the postganglionic nerve fibers, and BuChE to the smooth muscle fibers *(ThCh-VII)*. The *kidney* itself was found to be practically devoid of both enzymes excepting for that associated with the vascular and neuronal elements in the hilar region. Additional sites of BuChE activity noted include the epithelium and interstitial cells, as well as the corpora lutea and the atretic follicles of the *ovary*, the gland cells of the *uterine* fundus and horns in the mouse, and the mature *spermatozoa* and *prostate gland* cells in the guinea pig.

The presence in the *placenta* of high concentrations of AChE (ORD and THOMPSON 1950) as well as ChAc (COMLINE 1947, KATO 1960) has been the subject of considerable interest and speculation because of the organ's lack of innervation and relatively brief life-span. GOUTIER-PIROTTE and GEREBTZOFF (1955) have studied the distribution of AChE in the guinea pig placenta at successive stages of development *(ThCh-VII)*.

The enzyme is confined almost entirely to the fetal portion at all stages, and is accompanied in this species by only traces of BuChE. Between the 12th and 14th day, the first appearance of placental AChE was noted in the walls of the mesometrial capillaries in the region destined to become the placental syncytium. A few days later the enzyme was found within the cytoplasm of the interlobular syncytium chiefly at the periphery of its lacunae; since the latter contain maternal blood, this was considered the source of the AChE at that stage. Subsequently, activity was noted throughout the cytoplasm of both the interlobular and marginal syncytia, where it was presumed to be synthesized locally, as well as in the layer of giant cells of Duval, between the marginal syncytium and the ectoplacental entoderm. Towards the end of gestation, activity disappeared from the syncytium and appeared at the periphery of the labyrinthine lacunae, which contain fetal blood. From these observations, and quantitative determinations of the AChE activities of the fetal placenta and blood, the authors suggested that placental AChE beyond the initial stage reflects the organ's hematopoietic activity, which is taken over towards the end of gestation by other tissues. This explanation (see also GEREBT-ZOFF 1961) seems quite reasonable, but it does not, of course, provide any clue to the source or significance of the high placental ChAc activity; the latter enzyme, unlike AChE, is present at most only in traces in erythrocytes (MATHIAS and SHEPPARD 1954) (see also Chapter 5).

C. Sensory systems

I. Ocular

The retina represents a unique situation in which several successive groups of essentially central neurons are distributed in well demarcated layers, with the synaptic regions distinct in most cases from the cell bodies. Nevertheless, the pattern is actually considerably more complicated than this, which probably accounts for the lack of unanimity concerning the cellular localization of the retinal AChE in various species.

It now seems clear that the heavy nuclear staining of the bipolar cells, obtained with techniques in which diffusion was not controlled *(ThCh-II)*, was artifactual (KOELLE and FRIEDENWALD 1950, HEBB et al. 1953, HEBB 1957). With

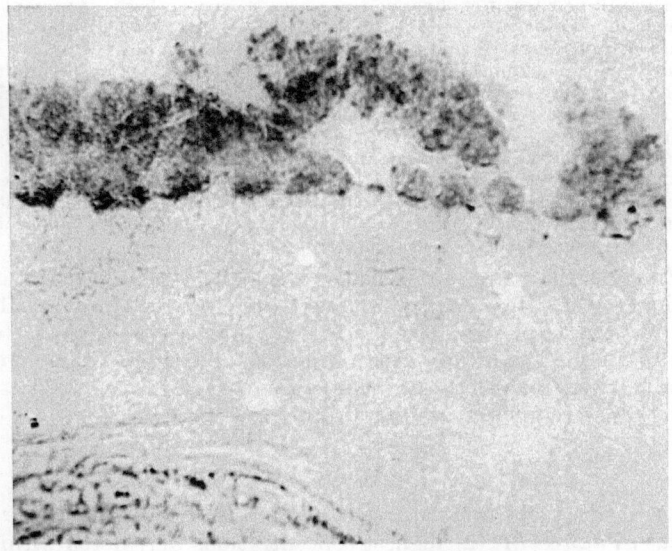

Fig. 26. Acetylcholinesterase of cat retina *(ThCh-III)*. Stained elements identified as perikarya (below) and processes (above) of amacrine cells; bipolar and ganglion cells unstained (KOELLE, FRIEDENWALD et al. 1952)

the modified ThCh method *(ThCh-III)*, the AChE of the cat retina was found to be confined chiefly to two bands, one in the innermost region of the inner nuclear layer, and the other extending from the inner zone of the inner plexiform layer to the outer part of the ganglion cell layer; between the two, within the outer portion of the inner plexiform layer, a paler-staining band was noted (KOELLE et al. 1952, Fig. 26). In the optic nerve, no AChE was found excepting in occasional fibers within the trabeculae separating the main fiber-bundles. From examination of sections of various thicknesses, incubated for different periods, it was concluded that a single type of neural element, the amacrine cell, accounts for most of the retinal AChE, and is therefore probably the only cholinergic type.

The AChE of the outer heavily-staining band was interpreted as representing the amacrine cell bodies, the inner band their axonal terminations on the ganglion cells, and the intermediate lighter-staining zone as their collateral or terminal processes synapsing with the dendrites of the ganglion or bipolar cells. No staining for BuChE was observed. Subsequently, FRANCIS (1953) and LEPLAT and GEREBT-ZOFF (1956) confirmed these general areas of localization in several species, but concluded, from the presence of AChE predominantly in the inner synaptic layer, that the bipolar cells are probably cholinergic. The most extensive and precise study of the retinal AChE to date is the account of SHEN et al. (1956) of the embryological development of AChE in the chick retina (see Chapter 5).

At an early stage, prior to the formation of synaptic connections, AChE was noted in the cytoplasm of all future ganglion cells and amacrine cells; subsequently, lighter staining was seen in the horizontal cells of the outer plexiform layer. At no stage was the enzyme found in the cell bodies of the bipolar cells. At the time of hatching, as in the adult, the distribution of AChE was nearly identical with that noted by KOELLE et al. (l.c.) in the cat. High concentrations were localized in the amacrine and ganglion cells, and in four distinct bands in the inner plexiform layers (see Fig. 7, Chapter 5). The problems of interpretation were defined clearly by SHEN and associates. The four stained synaptic bands represent regions where the axons of both the amacrine and the bipolar cells synapse with the dendrites of the ganglion cells; the same is true of the surfaces of the ganglion cells. At present, there is no direct evidence in the retina, such as exists for the autonomic ganglia, as to whether the enzyme is pre- or postsynaptic at sites of cholinergic transmission, or whether it is present in the cell bodies of cholinergic neurons. As mentioned below (BECKETT et al. 1956), the appearance of AChE in certain neurons during embryological development does not necessarily mean that the enzyme will remain in significant concentrations at the same sites in the adult. Further-more, both the exact synaptic connections and the functions of the amacrine cells are still unknown. Two types have been described in primates: the internal association cells, which may convey impulses laterally between groups of ganglion cells, and the centrifugal bipolar cells, which may transmit impulses peripherally from the ganglion cells to the bipolar or rod and cone cells, and thus take part in an intraretinal reflex mechanism (POLYAK 1941). As SHEN et al. (l.c.) have pointed out ,the contribution of histochemistry to the solution of these questions will require more precise cytological localization of AChE, and a means of localizing ChAc or ACh. (For further discussion, see Chapter 5.)

In fish (FRANCIS 1953) and amphibians (BOELL et al. 1955) AChE is present in both the inner and outer plexiform layers; the enzyme is present also in the fibers of the optic tract and at most of its central synaptic sites in the latter species (SHEN et al. 1955 v.i.). The diffuse distribution of the enzyme at all layers of the human retina reported by EICHNER (1958) cannot readily be interpreted, since insufficient details were given regarding technique.

II. Auditory

CHURCHILL et al. (1956) first reported the detection of AChE in the organ of Corti of the cat *(ThCh-III)*; the highest concentrations were noted within or near the nerve chalices terminating on the inner rows of hair cells, and in nerve fibers oriented toward the organ of Corti. Similar findings and postulated neuronal rela-tionships were published by VINNIKOV and TITOVA (1958). The identification of the stained fibers and their terminals was investigated by the CHURCHILL group (SCHUKNECHT et al. 1959) by a series of denervation experiments.

Destruction of the hair cells themselves, by the injection of streptomycin sulfate into the auditory bulla, caused only minor changes in AChE-staining. Following section and degenera-tion of the acoustic nerve, which presumably contains all the afferent and efferent connections of the organ of Corti, most of the staining disappeared. However, practically the same result was obtained by sectioning selectively the olivocochlear bundle of Rasmussen (Fig. 27), which arises from cell bodies in the medulla, medial to the superior olivary nucleus, decussates, passes through the contralateral saccular ganglion, and divides into fascicles from which fibers are directed toward the organ of Corti (RASMUSSEN 1946, 1953). Stimulation of the bundle causes inhibition of sound-induced action potentials of the acoustic nerve; hence, it apparently represents a feed-back system for suppression of the inflow of activity from the organ of Corti (GALAMBOS 1956).

The above authors therefore concluded that the efferent olivary-cochlear system is cholinergic. The analogy between this and the proposed cholinergic nature of the system represented by the amacrine cells of the retina (v.s.) is striking.

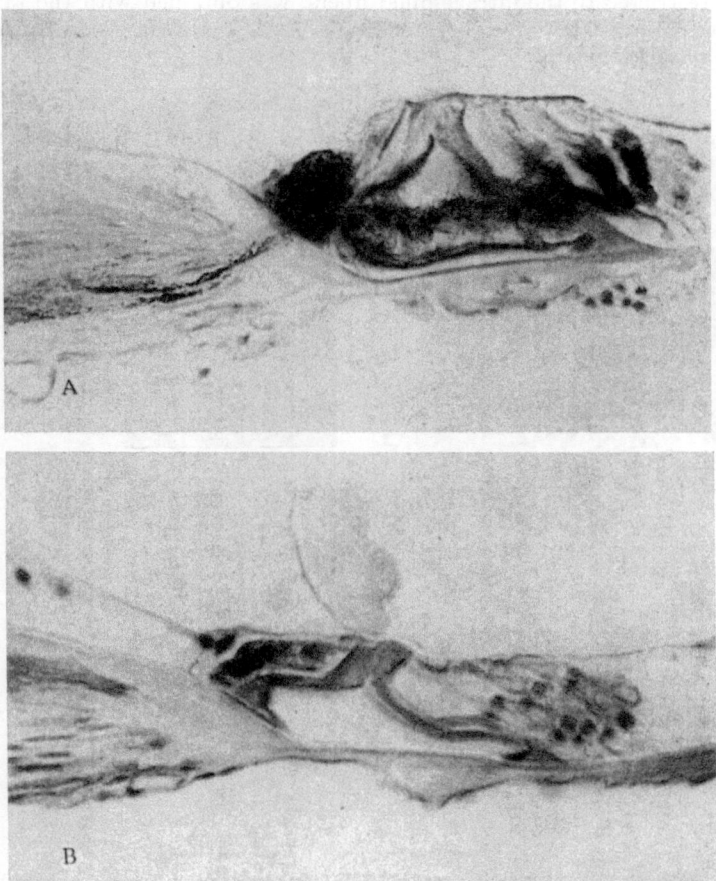

Fig. 27. Acetylcholinesterase of cat organ of Corti (*ThCh-III*). This cat was killed 28 days after the right olivo-cochlear bundle was cut. The stain for AChE is normal in the left (control) organ of Corti (A), and greatly decreased in the right (experimental) organ of Corti (B) (SCHUKNECHT et al. 1959)

III. Gustatory and olfactory

In the foliate papillae of the rabbit, BARADI and BOURNE (1959) reported staining for AChE in the nerve plexuses and individual fibers surrounding the taste buds, and in the intragemmal fibers which penetrate the buds and lie between the taste cells; the latter remained unstained *(ThCh-VI)*. ELLIS (1959) conducted an extensive survey of the ChE's of the tongue in five primate and several additional species. While the thickness of the sections (40 to 100 μ) and prolonged incubation periods (2 to 4 hr) employed limited the precision of localization, from the author's detailed account and illustrations it is clear that both AChE and BuChE are distributed extensively throughout the innervation of the papillae.

In the immediate region of the taste buds, both enzymes were concentrated at the base of each bud in a cup-like socket, which appeared to be continuous with the nerve fibers from the underlying plexus (Fig. 28). The taste buds themselves stained only for AChE; the illustrations suggest that within the taste buds the enzyme is confined to the intragemmal nerve fibers. The same pattern of AChE-staining, restricted to the intragemmal fibers, was obtained with the taste buds of the cat in the reviewer's laboratory *(ThCh-III)* (GEESEY and KOELLE, unpublished observations).

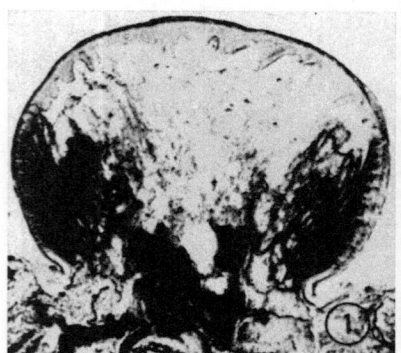 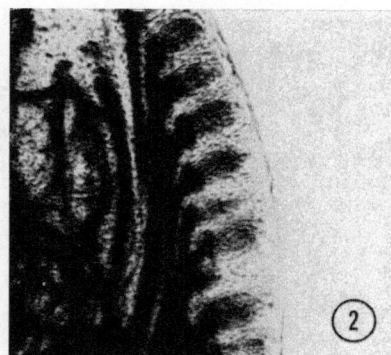

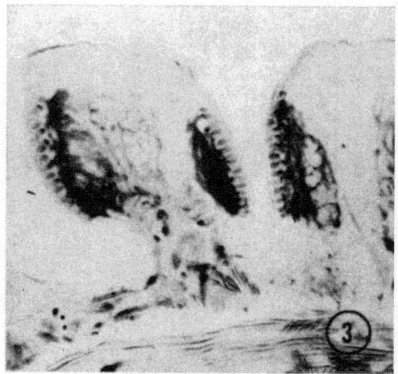

Fig. 28. Acetylcholinesterase of primate tongue *(ThCh-IV,* following formalin fixation). *1.* A median section through a vallate papilla on the tongue of *Macaca nemestrina.* Acetylcholinesterase is present in several nerve cell bodies and in the nerve fibers at the base of the papilla. The rich plexus of reactive nerves beneath the gustatory epithelium and their attachments to the taste buds are clearly shown. AThCh substrate, incubated 2 hours. × 35. *2.* A portion of *1,* at higher magnification. The AChE activity within the taste buds and in the cups at the base of the gemmae can be clearly seen. The nerves beneath the gustatory epithelium are also strongly reactive. AThCh substrate, 2 hour incubation. × 125. *3.* A vertical section through the foliate papillae of *Macaca nemestrina.* The nerves beneath the gustatory epithelium are strongly reactive for AChE; other nerves within the papillae, and the taste buds themselves, have a lower enzymatic response. There is no evidence of basal ganglia. AThCh substrate, incubated 2 hours. × 35 (ELLIS 1959)

A wide variety of nerve fibers in the human tongue were found by EL-RAK-KHAWY and BOURNE (1961) to stain with either AThCh or BuThCh or both. The patterns in the region of the taste buds were for the most part similar to those described above.

BARADI and BOURNE (1959) obtained variable results in attempting to localize the ChE's in the rabbit *olfactory epithelium.* In the majority of sections, staining was noted in the nerve fibers running between the olfactory cells, and in the proximal and distal processes of the olfactory cells themselves. However, the illustrations are difficult to interpret, and in many instances results were negative.

IV. Sensory corpuscles and nerve terminations

It has been pointed out that the concentration of AChE in dorsal roots and their ganglion cells is quite low in comparison with that found in ventral roots and anterior horn cells in most species. In general, the same is true of peripheral sensory terminals when these are contrasted with adjacent parasympathetic and motor nerve endings; it is usually necessary to incubate for prolonged periods to demonstrate AChE at the former sites. This must be considered in assessing the significance of the reports which follow.

The complexities of both classification and anatomical inter-relationships of the various types of sensory corpuscles and terminals have been discussed in detail by CAUNA (1959). The same author (CAUNA 1961) has recently pointed out that practically all possible combinations have been noted with respect to the presence of AChE, BuChE, or both in the preterminal and terminal sensory axons and their associated end organs (Fig. 29). It is thus impossible to generalize on this point; one can only list some of the findings which have been reported, with the hope that their physiological significance will eventually be clarified. The possible participation of ACh in the activation of sensory end organs is discussed in the final section.

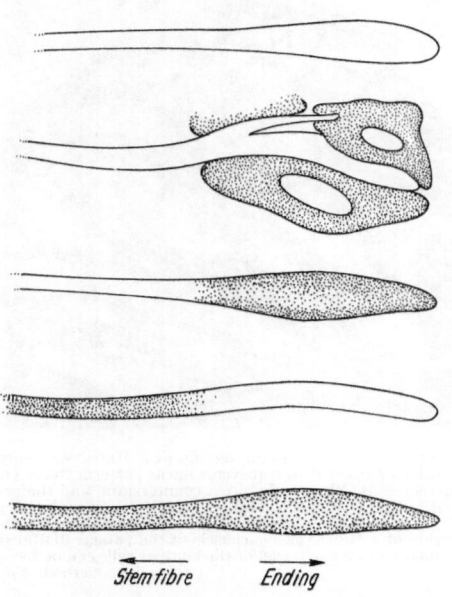

Fig. 29. Diagram showing the range of variation in ChE activity in the sensory nerves and end organs. Presence of a positive ChE reaction with AThCh or BuThCh substrate is indicated by stippling (CAUNA 1961)

1. Sensory corpuscles

Nearly a century ago, KRAUSE (1881) recognized approximately one hundred types of sensory corpuscles. More recently WINKELMANN (1957) concluded from studies employing silver-staining techniques that human skin contains only three basic types: the Meissner corpuscle (including the Merkel-Ranvier tactile disc), the Pacinian (or Vater-Pacini) corpuscle, and the genital or mucocutaneous corpuscle of Krause. From numerous reports, it is apparent that some type of ChE activity is associated with all excepting the Merkel-Ranvier tactile discs.

Several authors have reported the presence of ChE in cutaneous *Meissner's corpuscles* of the rat (CSILLIK and SÁVAY 1954) *(Naph-I)* and man (HURLEY and MESCON 1956 b, BECKETT et al. 1956, THIES and GALENTE 1957) by various modifications of the thiocholine method. This was shown to be BuChE, and to be oriented in a lamellar pattern by HURLEY and MESCON (l.c.) *(ThCh-III)*. CAUNA (1960) and CAUNA and ROSS (1960) established that the enzyme is confined to the plasma membranes of the laminar cells, and that the interdigitating nerve terminals are devoid of detectable ChE's (Fig. 30); by electron microscopy, microvesicles were noted in both the laminar cells and nerve terminals. In the same study, ChE's were shown to be absent from *Merkels's corpuscles* and their associated nerve terminals.

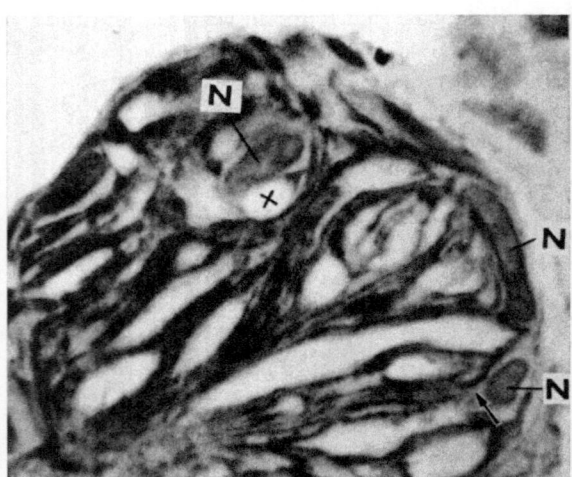 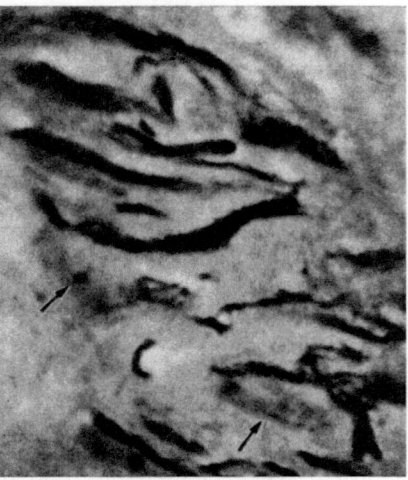

Fig. 30. *Left:* Thin oblique section of a MEISSNER's corpuscle of the palmar digital skin showing positive ChE reaction *(ThCh-VI)* in transverse linear pattern. Nerve endings (unlabelled clear areas) are negative. Nuclei of the laminar cells (N), revealed by a counterstain, and the perinuclear cytoplasm are also negative. The arrow shows continuity of the perinuclear cytoplasm with a ChE-negative zone in the corpuscle. X-shrinkage space. Male, 25 years. (AThCh substrate, 2¹/₄ h incubation, light haematoxylin counterstain, 4 µ, × 2000.) *Right:* Thin oblique section of a MEISSNER's corpuscle of the palmar digital skin showing nerve endings (black) interspersed with the laminar cells. Some nuclei of the laminar cells can be recognized (arrows). Male, 13 years. (Simplified Bielschowsky Gross silver method, 4 µ, × 2000.) (CAUNA 1960)

Pacinian corpuscles of the skin of a variety of species, including man, have been shown to contain ChE (BECKETT et al. 1956, CAUNA and MANNAN 1958, 1959). In this type, staining is most intense in the core; however, these publications did not elucidate whether AChE is present in addition to BuChE (staining was obtained with both AThCh and BuThCh), or any further cytological details of localization. The Pacinian corpuscles of the mesentery of the cat have been shown both histochemically (HEBB and HILL 1955 b) and manometrically (LOEWENSTEIN and MOLINS 1958) to contain chiefly BuChE. With both techniques it was found also that the enzyme is confined largely to the inner core of the corpuscle immediately surrounding the enclosed nerve ending. Synaptic vesicle-like inclusions have been described in the intracorpuscular nerve filament by PEASE and QUILLIAM (1957).

Krause's corpuscles of male and female human genital skin were shown by HURLEY (1958) to contain BuChE *(ThCh-V);* no ChE's were detected in the adjacent nerve fibers.

2. Cutaneous and mucous nerve endings

The sensory fibers which terminate on tactile hairs in various species have been shown to stain with both AThCh and BuThCh, but more consistently with the former substrate (THIES and GALENTE 1957, MONTAGNA and BECKETT 1958, CAUNA 1961); therefore, it seems likely that they contain AChE, and in some cases possibly BuChE as well. The same applies to the simple axial body terminations in various types of skin (CAUNA l.c.) and in the tongue of primates (ELLIS 1959). Unfortunately, most of these studies were conducted with prolonged incubation periods and without the use of selective inhibitors.

With incubation periods of 12 to 20 hr with ThCh-esters, AVERY and RAPP (1958) demonstrated the presence of both AChE and BuChE in human teeth. The former enzyme was detected in the pulpal nerves and along the coronal aspect of the pulp chamber, representing presumably sensory fibers and their terminations. Non-specific ChE was concentrated along the nerves and blood vessels. With shorter incubation periods, no staining was noted, indicating that activity was low, penetration of reagents poor, or both.

3. Chemo- and stretch receptors

The chemoreceptor cells of the carotid body of the cat contain moderate concentrations of BuChE; the distribution of the enzyme is not uniform, but appears to vary considerably between individual cells (KOELLE 1950, 1951; ROSS 1957). In the same reports the concentration of AChE was found to be considerably lower, and was localized in the adjacent nerve fibers. These histochemical findings are consistent with an earlier titrimetric study with respect to the relative concentrations of the two enzymes (HOLLINGSHEAD and SAWYER 1945).

With prolonged incubation, ÁBRÁHÁM (1956) noted staining *(ThCh-VII)* for ChE in the nerve fibers of the pressoreceptors of the carotid sinus and aortic arch of the dog and pig.

Interesting observations on the ChE (probably AChE) activities of the stretch receptor neurons of lobster muscle were reported by MAYNARD and MAYNARD (1960). The slow-adapting type of neuron, which responds to maintained stretch with a continuous discharge and is relatively sensitive to applied ACh, contained a low concentration of ChE in the membrane of the cell body and axon. The fast-adapting type, which develops a phasic, rapidly adapting discharge in response to stretch and requires much higher concentrations of ACh for activation, was stained much more intensively at the same sites. The greatest intensity of staining in both types occurred in the dendritic ramifications and intercalated semitendinous region of the receptor muscle. Cholinesterase was present also in the motor fibers.

D. Central nervous system

The evidence for cholinergic transmission at certain synapses in the central nervous system, while not as direct as for many of the foregeoing peripheral sites, is now reasonably convincing. It has been summarized in several previous reviews (FELDBERG 1945a, 1951, 1954, KOELLE and GILMAN 1949, PERRY 1956, PATON 1958, HOLMSTEDT 1959, MICHELSON 1957, 1961), as well as in Chapter 14 of the present monograph. Early reports on assays of homogenates of samples from various portions of the central nervous system of the dog showed fairly close correlation of the relative concentrations of ACh (MACINTOSH 1941), ChAc (FELDBERG and VOGT 1948), and ChE (NACHMANSOHN 1939) or AChE (BURGEN and CHIPMAN 1951). The limitations of this type of comparison were made apparent by the subsequent histochemical findings on the localization of AChE (v.i.). Many regions in which the total concentration of the enzyme is low contain isolated groups of neurons or their processes which show extremely high activity. This factor, and the likelihood that ACh, ChAc, and AChE are not necessarily concentrated in the same cytological regions of the neuron, may account for the occasional discrepancies in the aforementioned correlations.

Two classes of central neurons have been described in previous sections in conjunction with their corresponding peripheral systems: those giving rise to the motor fibers to skeletal muscle and to the autonomic preganglionic fibers. Both contain extremely high concentrations of AChE, and their fibers are unquestionably cholinergic. As discussed previously, on this basis it seems reasonable to assume that other central neurons which show staining for AChE of equivalent intensity are also cholinergic, whereas those which remain practically unstained are probably non-cholinergic. However, this leaves in question the significance of the comparatively moderate to light AChE activity displayed by a great number of central neurons and fibers. It will be recalled that in the rabbit and monkey practically all the neurons of the sympathetic ganglia, most of which are presumably adrenergic, showed evidence of some degree of AChE activity. It has been suggested that the term "cholinergic" may refer actually to the principal, but not necessarily the exclusive agent participating in transmission by a neuron, and that its relative content of AChE may reflect the extent of participation of ACh (KOELLE 1955, SHEN et al. 1955, BURN and RAND 1960). It should be noted also that in the embryonic human finger, practically all the nerve fibers show high concentrations of AChE, whereas in the adult the activity of many of the corresponding fibers is low (BECKETT et al. 1956). Hence, the persistence of low or intermediate concentrations of AChE may reflect incomplete differentiation of neurons with multiple ontogenetic potentialities. These questions are discussed in the final section.

I. Mammalian

Some of the findings of a histochemical survey of the distribution of AChE in the central nervous system of the rat are presented in Tables 3 to 6 (KOELLE 1954), from which are omitted the heavily-staining somatic motor neurons and the neurons which give rise to preganglionic fibers described previously (see Table 2).

A detailed account of the distribution of AChE in the salivatory centers and other regions of the hindbrain of the rat was published by SHUTE and LEWIS (1960). The same authors (SHUTE and LEWIS 1961) have recently described AChE-staining in several tracts of the rat forebrain, particularly the projections to the hippocampal formation (v.i.). They employed the procedure of sectioning various tracts 4 to 16 days prior to sacrifice, causing the accumulation of AChE on the neuronal side and its loss on the distal side, which facilitated tracing certain pathways. In a survey of the AChE of the rabbit brain, GEREBTZOFF (1959) obtained findings which with few exceptions were similar to those in the rat described below.

The descriptions given in the accompanying tables, from identifications based on CRAIGIE's (1925) atlas, represent 10 μ sections of fresh-frozen rat brain incubated for 75 min in AThCh -medium containing 24% Na_2SO_4, then developed, gold-toned, dehydrated, and mounted *(ThCh-III)*. In the brain and other organs of the rat which have been studied, the non -specific ChE is actually a propionyl-ChE (PrChE) (ORD and THOMPSON 1952). On the basis of the relative rates of hydrolysis of methacholine (MeCh) and benzoylcholine (BzCh), it constitutes approximately 8% of the ChE activity of the whole rat brain (KOELLE 1954). While sites of PrChE activity are revealed also by the above technique, and apparent in the accompanying photomicrographs, simultaneously incubated sections stained selectively showed it to be confined to the capillary walls, vascular smooth muscle fibers, glial cytoplasm (particularly of the fibrous astrocytes of the tracts), and the cytoplasm of some motor neurons which contained also high concentrations of AChE. With essentially the same method *(ThCh-IV)*, PEPLER and PEARSE (1957) were unable to detect PrChE in the fibrous astrocytes, but did find the enzyme in high concentrations in some neurons (e.g., in the medial habenular nucleus) which contained relatively little AChE. Their findings were otherwise in agreement with those presented below.

The assessment of relative AChE activity on the basis of subjective impressions of "intense," "moderate" or "light" staining reactions is admittedly crude. Examples of each type are shown in Fig. 31. Nevertheless, it constitutes the most direct type of evidence available to date on the relative concentrations of the

Table 3. *Regions of the rat central nervous system exhibiting intense staining for AChE* (Neurons giving rise to peripheral motor and preganglionic autonomic fibers omitted; see text for method; from KOELLE 1954)

Region	Stained structures
Reticular formation (medulla)	Scattered neurons and fibers throughout
Nuc. of lateral funiculus (medulla)	Larger neurons most heavily stained
Nuc. of Roller	Scattered neurons and fibers
Ventral nuc. of reticular formation	Neurons and fibers show fairly consistent heavy staining
Nuc. of trapezoid body	Numerous scattered neurons and fibers
Dorsal and median nuc. of the raphe (midbrain)	Small clusters of heavily stained neurons and fibers
Dorsal, caudal ventral and rostral ventral nuc. of lateral lemniscus (midbrain)	Small, scattered, heavily stained neurons and fibers
Cerebellar cortex	Scattered cells in granular layer, mostly of large type; few stellate cells in molecular layer; numerous fibers of medulla
Pontine nuc.	Numerous scattered neurons and fibers very heavily stained
Nuc. interpeduncularis	Thickly clustered very heavily stained neurons and fibers of pars lateralis; occasional neurons of pars medialis
Superior colliculus	Densely-packed, moderately heavily stained neurons of stratum griseum; scattered fibers of non-optic layer of stratum opticum
Fasciculus retroflexus of Meynert	Most fibers heavily stained in cross section
Zona incerta	Few neurons and scattered fibers
Lateral habenular nuc.	Few small neurons and fibers; majority moderately stained
Anterior nuc. of thalamus	Few scattered neurons and numerous fibers of ventro-lateral portion
Lateral nuc. of thalamus	Heavily stained neurons and fibers interspersed with unstained tracts
Caudate nuc.	Very heavily stained, closely-packed neurons and fibers; interspersed bundles of internal capsule largely unstained
Putamen	Densely packed, heavily stained neurons and fibers
Central nuc of amygdala	Scattered, very heavily stained fusiform neurons and fibers
Lateral nuc. of amygdala	Scattered, very heavily stained smaller globular neurons and fibers
Nuc. of lateral olfactory tract	Occasional neurons and fibers (majority unstained)
Tuberculum olfactorium	Densely packed small neurons and fibers
Diagonal band of Broca	Scattered neurons and fibers, many unstained
Nuc. accumbens septi	Numerous neurons and fibers

enzyme in the individual neurons and their constituent parts for most regions of the central nervous system. The exquisite ultramicro-analytical studies discussed below have been confined largely to the spinal cord and cerebral cortex.

The cytological distribution of AChE in the central neurons studied appears to resemble the pattern observed in their peripheral counterparts, in that the intensity of staining is greatest at the membrane, but staining is present also in the cytoplasm, and continues along the length of the processes insofar as they can be traced. However, no quantitative information is available concerning the relative amounts of the enzyme present at these various levels of the central neurons. The presumed function of ACh as a neurohumoral transmitter implies that relatively high concentrations of AChE should be present at synaptic sites. This of course fails to explain the function of the enyzme in the cell bodies of the known cholinergic neurons, since they are at a maximal distance from their

Table 4. *Regions of the rat central nervous system exhibiting moderate staining for AChE* (see text for method; from KOELLE 1954)

Region	Stained structures
Dorsal gray column of cord	Occasional neurons and numerous fibers of dorsal columns and substantia gelatinosa
Nuc. gracilis and cuneatus	Most neurons and fibers, including internal arcuate fibers
Nuc. of lateral funiculus (medulla)	Numerous neurons and fibers
Olivary nuc.	Great variation in intensity; few neurons and fibers moderately stained, majority lightly stained or unstained
Nuc. of fasciculus solitarius	Great variation; some neurons and fibers moderately stained, remainder lightly stained or unstained
Nuc. of Deiters	Numerous large neurons and fibers
Chief vestibular nuc.	Diffuse staining of most neurons and fibers; few unstained
Nuc. emboliformis	Occasional neurons; majority lightly stained or unstained
Dentate nuc.	Diffuse staining of most neurons and fibers; few unstained
Ventral cochlear nuc.	Larger neurons moderately stained
Dorsal and laterodorsal tegmental nuc.	Numerous small, globular neurons stained with varying intensity
Locus coeruleus	Small cluster of small, moderately stained neurons
Pontine nuc.	Occasional neurons, numerous fibers
Inferior colliculus	Few neurons and fibers in nuc. of inf. col.; occasional fibers elsewhere
Posterior nuc. of thalamus	Few small, scattered neurons; majority of fibers
Mammillo-thalamic tract	Most fibers in cross section
Medial lemniscus	Most fibers in cross section
Medial geniculate body	Few scattered small neurons and fibers
Substantia nigra	Variable intensity of staining; few neurons and fibers moderate, remainder light
Lateral geniculate body	Few neurons of dorsal, more of ventral nucleus; scattered fibers
Lateral habenular nuc.	Majority of neurons, scattered fibers
Commissure of Meynert	Few fiber bundles
Medial habenular nuc.	Few neurons and fibers; remainder light
Supraoptic nuc.	Globular neurons and fibers show uniform moderate staining; highly vascular
Anterior nuc. of thalamus	Numerous neurons and fibers of dorso-medial portion
Medial nuc. of thalamus	Occasional neurons and fibers
Nuc. reticularis of thalamus	Occasional small neurons, numerous scattered fibers
Mammillo-thalamic tract	Most fibers in cross section
Medial forebrain bundle	Numerous fibers in cross section of lateral division
Lateral olfactory tract	Most fibers in cross section
Fimbria	Occasional neurons and fibers
Dorsal hippocampal commissure	Occasional neurons and fibers
Neocortex	Rare neurons, majority unstained; scattered fibers

own cholinergic terminals, unless they, too, receive cholinergic presynaptic fibers (see p. 229). Because of the limitations imposed by the blood-brain barrier, it has not yet been possible to localize selectively the external and internal AChE of central neurons in the manner described for the autonomic ganglia. However, evidence for the existence of these two fractions in central neurons has been cited previously (KOELLE and STEINER 1956). In homogenates of both rabbit (NATHAN and APRISON 1955) and rat (TOSCHI 1959) brain, AChE is associated chiefly with membranous structures, represented by the microsomes and mitochondria, whereas the non-specific ChE is present chiefly in the soluble or supernatant fractions (HOLMSTEDT and TOSCHI 1959).

A few generalizations concerning the AChE of the *rat brain* can be drawn from the detailed data listed in the accompanying tables. Activity in the primary

Table 5. *Regions of the rat central nervous system exhibiting light staining for AChE*
(see text for method; from KOELLE 1954)

Region	Stained structures
Dorsal root ganglia of cord	Neurons faintly stained, fibers practically unstained
Dorsal gray column of cord and medulla	Majority of neurons and fibers
Olivary nuc.	Majority of neurons and fibers
Nuc. of fasciculus solitarius	Great variation; most neurons lightly stained or unstained
Chief sensory nuc. of C.N. V	Most neurons and fibers; few more heavily stained neurons near surface
Cerebellar cortex	Scattered fibers in molecular layer
Dorsal longitudinal bundle of Schütz	Scattered small neurons and fibers
Mesencephalic nuc. of C.N. V	Large, globular, very lightly stained neurons
Red nuc.	Large neurons of magnocellular division
Substantia nigra	Majority of neurons and fibers
Posterior commissure (midbrain)	Most fibers lightly stained in cross section
Globus pallidus	Scattered neurons and fibers
Nuc. reuniens	Few lightly stained neurons
Internal capsule	Most fibers lightly stained or unstained, few moderately or heavily

Table 6. *Regions of the rat central nervous system exhibiting slight or no staining for AChE*
(see text for method; from KOELLE 1954)

Region	Stained structures
Cervical cord	Columns of Goll and Burdach, pyramidal tract, ventral funiculus (most fibers), lateral funiculus, tract of Lissauer
Root of C.N. V	Cross section of fibers
Cerebellar cortex	Purkinje cells, numerous small granular cells
Reticular formation of medulla	Numerous small neurons and fibers
Olivary nuc.	Numerous small neurons and fibers
Fasciculus solitarius	Numerous neurons and fibers
Inferior colliculus	Majority of fibers
Posterior nuc. of thalamus	Majority of neurons
Diencephalon	Neurons and fibers of intermediate mass and tuber cinereum
Optic chiasma	Majority of fibers (few lightly stained)
Corpus callosum	Majority of fibers
Lateral olfactory tract	Majority of fibers
Anterior commissure	Most fibers of anterior limb
Medial forebrain bundle	Most fibers of lateral division
Neocortex	Majority of neurons and fibers; few lightly or moderately stained

afferent neurons, as represented by the dorsal roots, their ganglion cells, and their terminations in the spinal cord, is consistently low, whereas that in primary motor neurons, as already stated, is uniformly high. Little or no activity was noted generally in neurons synapsing directly with motor neurons, such as the pyramidal cells and tracts and the neurons of the red nucleus. In the secondary (e.g., gracile and cuneate nuclei) and tertiary (e.g., lateral thalamic nucleus) sensory relay neurons, progressively increasing AChE-activity was observed. Thus, these findings do not support the proposal once offered tentatively by FELDBERG and VOGT (1948) of alteration of central cholinergic and non-cholinergic neurons. In certain correlation centers, particularly of the basal ganglia, activity is extremely high (e.g., caudate and amygdaloid nuclei, putamen), whereas in others it is low (olivary nucleus, globus pallidus). In the cerebellum, considerably more AChE was noted

in scattered, relatively large cells of the granular layer than in the few stained
stellate cells of the molecular layer; stained fibers were present in both layers.
This is consistent with the quantitative findings of ROBINS and SMITH (1953), who
reported that AChE was the only enzyme of eight measured which showed a

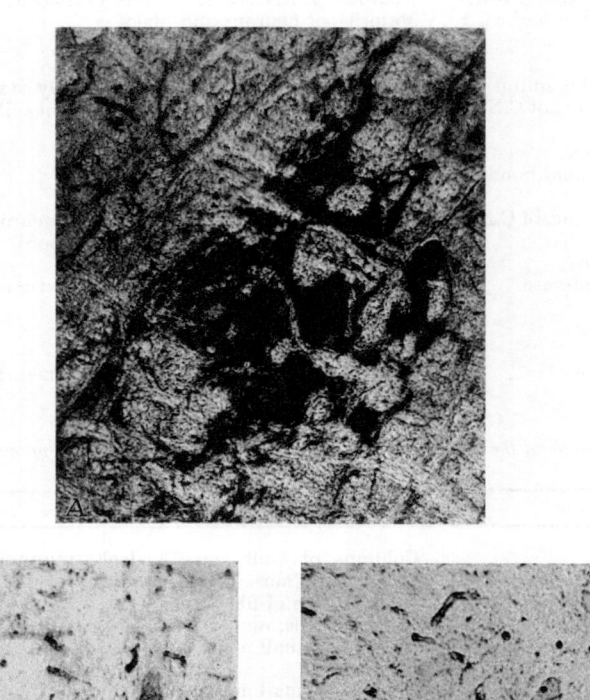

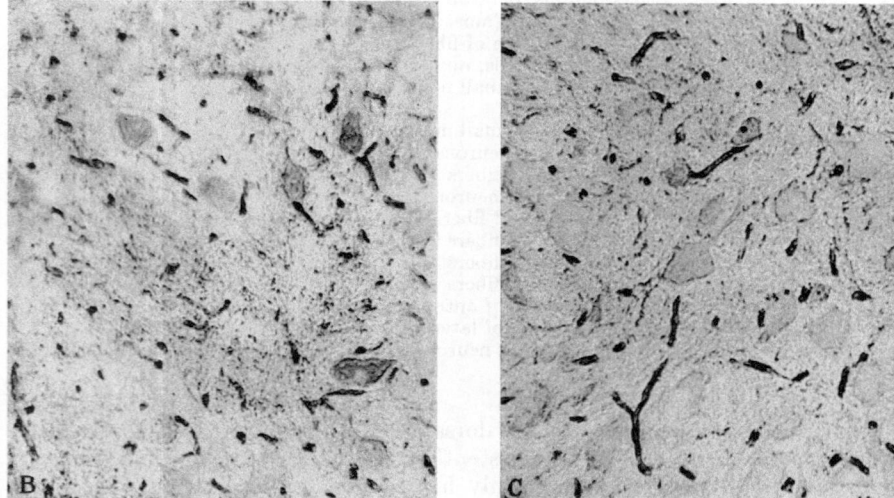

Fig. 31. Cholinesterases of rat central nervous system. Neuronal staining represents AChE, and illustrates neurons
showing intense (I), moderate (M), and light (L) enzymatic activity. Staining of capillaries and glial cells represents
non-specific ChE. (Ten-micron sections, incubated 75 min with AThCh medium [*ThCh-III*], uncounterstained,
magnification × 100.) A. Nucleus ambiguus of medulla (I). B. DEITERS' nucleus (M). C. Red nucleus, magnocellular
division (L) (KOELLE 1954)

higher concentration in the granular than in the molecular layer, and with the
histochemical pattern obtained in the cat by SNELL (1961a). The reticular formation illustrates the frequently observed close interspersion of heavily and lightly
stained neurons.

Areas showing AChE-staining in the study of the rat brain by SHUTE and LEWIS (1961) which were not noted previously included the medial septal nucleus, the interstitial nucleus of the septal part of the median forebrain bundle, the bed nucleus of the stria terminalis, the interstitial nucleus of the ventral hippocampal commissure, and the subfornical organ or intercolumnar tubercle. These authors also found heavy staining in the posterior thalamic or pretectal nucleus, and light staining of the central amygdaloid nucleus, in contrast to the earlier study (KOELLE 1954). Otherwise, their findings were confirmatory. From their examination of previously sectioned pathways, they concluded that cholinergic fibers run caudally from the bed nucleus of the stria to the amygdaloid nucleus, via the lateral portion of the stria terminalis, and from the septal and paraseptal subcortical centers to the hippocampal region, via the cingulum, dorsal fornix, alveus, and fimbria.

There is evidence that the concentration of AChE in central neurons of a given type may be correlated directly with their level of activation by afferent input over varying periods.

PEPLER and PEARSE (1957) reported that procedures which promoted increased secretory activity of the anterior or posterior pituitary (high salt intake, lactation, castration) resulted in increased AChE-staining of certain hypothalamic neurons in the rat. The effect of eye removal at different stages of maturity on the AChE-staining (ThCh, following formalin fixation) of the superior colliculus of mice was investigated by HESS (1960). In this region, the enzyme is concentrated in the stratum zonale and stratum griseum superficiale above, and in the intermediate strata below the stratum opticum; the last mentioned layer remains unstained, and consists of the non-cholinergic fibers of the optic tract, which terminate on presumably cholinergic neurons of the stratum griseum superficiale (HESS 1958, 1960). Removal of an eye at birth resulted consistently in decreased AChE activity of the contralateral stratum griseum superficiale; the difference in intensity of staining from the control side was dependent on the age at sacrifice. It was most marked in animals examined at a relatively early age (e.g., 27 days), and became less so progressively (e.g., 220 days). When the same operation was performed on mature animals, no difference in staining was detected, even after prolonged periods. Similar results were obtained in rabbits and guinea pigs. Two factors were considered as the basis for the marked influence of the age at operation on results: (1) afferent activation might be essential for AChE formation only during early developmental stages, and (2) with advancing development, afferent fibers might converge on the same neurons from other sources (see also Chapter 5).

II. Amphibian

At a considerably lower level in the phylogenetic scale, the brain of the *frog* has been surveyed similarly for AChE by SHEN et al. (1955) who employed essentially the same method *(ThCh-III)*, but with sections from frozen-dried, paraffin-embedded brain. Preliminary assays of homogenates showed that the brain of this species is practically devoid of non-specific ChE, and that the medulla and cerebellum, taken together, and the optic lobe, or mesencephalon, contain high concentrations of AChE, the diencephalon an intermediate, and the hemispheres a low concentration. The absence of non-specific ChE from the spinal cord of the frog, *Rana catesbiana*, and toad, *Bufo boreas halophilus*, was confirmed by CHACKO and CERF (1960) in histochemical studies *(ThCh-V)* employing selective inhibitors.

Histochemically, the neurons of the somatic motor and autonomic nuclei of the frog were very heavily stained, as in the rat. Elsewhere, the heaviest staining was found chiefly in association with the terminations of synaptic processes, or the neuropil, rather than in the neuronal perikarya. The most conspicuously stained single structure was the nucleus isthmi, which is probably homologous with the mammalian medial geniculate body (Fig. 32). Staining was also intense in the medial and lateral habenular nuclei, both in the cell bodies of the cortical zone and in the inner neuropil. This region, along with its intensely stained efferent fibers, the fasciculus retroflexus, is probably an important way-station for impulses from the cerebral hemisphere and preoptic nucleus to the brainstem, particularly the interpeduncular nucleus. In the latter, the cell bodies were unstained, whereas its underlying dense neuropil, containing the spiral terminals of the habenulo-interpeduncular tract, was stained intensely.

Accordingly, this demonstrates a situation within the central nervous system where the neurons were found to exhibit intense AChE activity at all levels, from the cell bodies to their terminations.

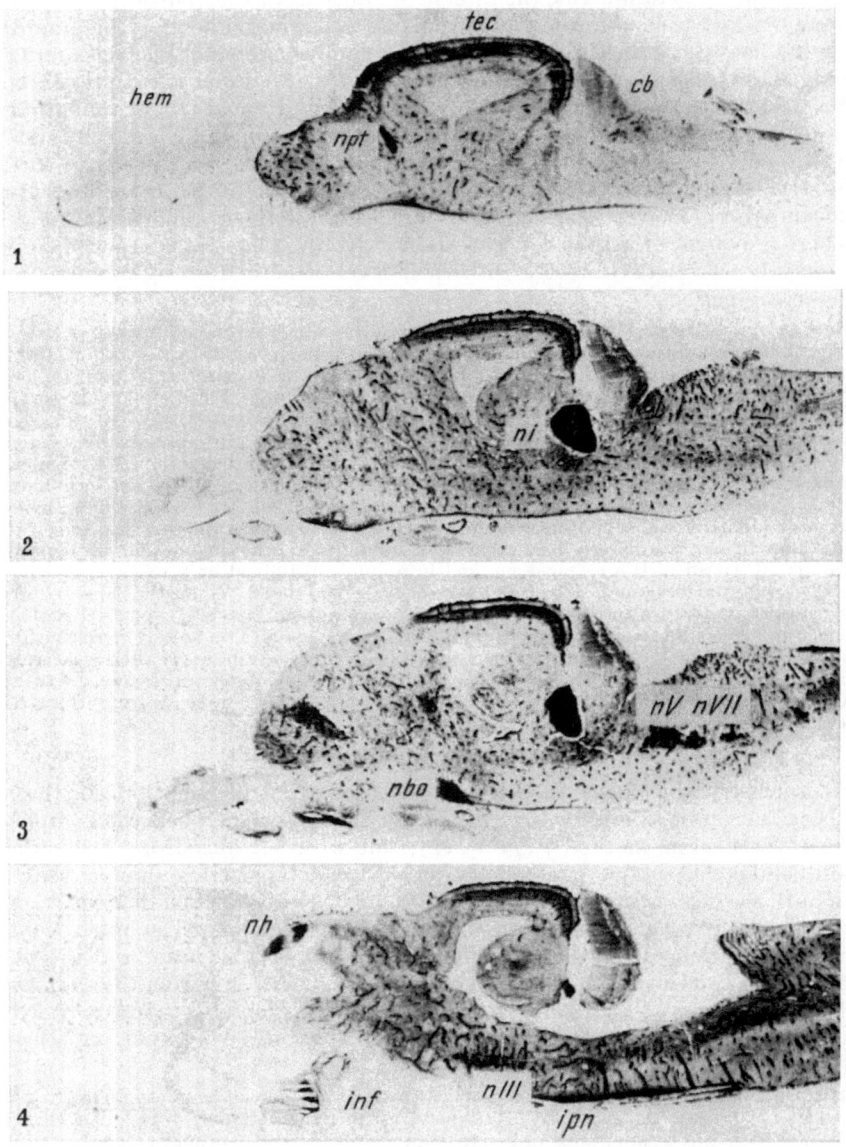

Fig. 32. Histochemical localization of AChE in frog brain. (Sections 15 μ, incubated with AThCh 30 min at 37° C [ThCh-III], uncounterstained, × 14.) Control sections (incubated without substrate or inactivated by alcohol fixation) are completely colorless and photographically nondemonstrable. Note staining of capillaries for AChE. Sagittal sections from a serial section preparation cutting medially. 1. Section through nucleus pretectalis. 2. Section through nucleus isthmi. 3. Section through basal optic nucleus, nucleus isthmi and motor nuclei of the Vth and VIIth nerves. 4. Section through the nucleus habenulae, nucleus of the oculomotor and the interpeduncular neuropil. Abbreviations: cb, cerebellum; hem, cerebral hemisphere; inf, infundibulum; ipn, interpeduncularis neuropil; nbo, nucleus of basal optic nerve; nh, nucleus habenulae; ni, nucleus isthmi; npt, nucleus pretectalis; nIII, nucleus of oculomotor nerve; nV, nucleus of trigeminal nerve; nVII, nucleus of facial nerve; tec, tectum (SHEN et al. 1955)

In contrast to findings in mammals, the optic tract and its various sites of termination (lateral geniculate body, pretectal nucleus, basal optic nucleus, optic tectum) in the frog showed moderately intense staining. Within the well demarcated layers of the optic tectum, staining was associated distinctly with the terminals of the optic tract in layers 15, 11, and 9. It should be noted that in this species a high proportion of the retinal ganglion cells, which give rise to the optic nerve and tract, also showed staining for AChE (BOELL et al. 1955, v.s.). In the optic tectum of the pigeon brain, relatively intense staining for ChE has been noted in both the neuronal and fibrous layers (SCHARRER and SINDEN 1949). In the frog cerebellum, staining was noted in the fibers of both the molecular and granular layers.

The capillary walls, which in the rat contain PrChE, in contrast stained for AChE in all regions of the frog brain excepting the hemispheres. This illustrates the interesting variation among different orders with respect to the staining of the endothelium and neuroglia of the central nervous system for ChE's which has been reported by BRIGHTMAN and ALBERS (1959) and which apparently follows no clear phylogenetic pattern. In the several species examined, the neuroglia were found to contain either non-specific ChE or neither enzyme, whereas the endothelium stained for both enzymes (fish), AChE (toad), non-specific ChE (rat) or neither (turtle, rooster, cat, man).

E. Endocrine system

I. Neurohypophysis and adenohypophysis

In the dog, the neurons of the supraoptic, paraventricular, and suprachiasmatic nuclei, from which are believed to arise the neurosecretory fibers of the neurohypophysis, were shown by ABRAHAMS et al. (1957) to be stained with moderate intensity for AChE *(ThCh-V)*. Similar staining *(ThCh-III)* was noted earlier in the neurons of the supraoptic nucleus of the rat (KOELLE 1954). More recently,

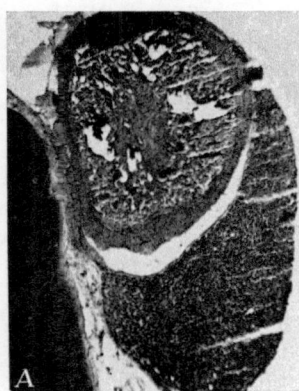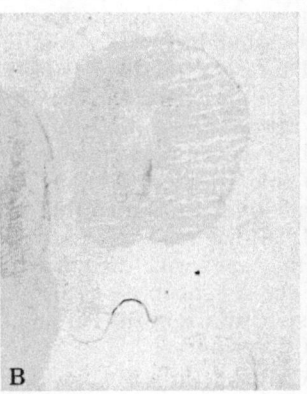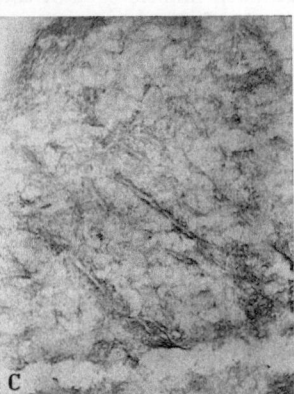

Fig. 33. Section (15 µ) of cat neurohypophysis (above), adenohypophysis (below), and adjacent hypothalamus (left) stained for AChE activity by 120 min incubation in AThCh medium preceded by 30 min incubation with 10⁻⁸ M DFP for selective inhibition of non-specific ChE *(ThCh-V)*. A. Magnification × 13, counterstained with H and E. B. Magnification × 13, no counterstain. C. Portion of neurohypophysis, magnification × 80, no counterstain. All staining in B and C represents AChE activity (KOELLE and GEESEY 1961)

the fibers of the infundibular stalk, and their terminations in the infundibular process of the neurohypophysis in the cat were also shown to stain for AChE *(ThCh-V)* with light to moderate intensity (KOELLE and GEESEY 1961, Fig. 33). Thus, from the collective results in these different species, it appears that AChE is present in significant concentrations along the full length of the hypothalamico-neurohypophyseal tract. The possible functional significance of these observations is considered in the final section. The only evidence of BuChE activity noted in the cat neurohypophysis was in poorly defined structures at its borders, identified tentatively as interstitial cells.

No staining for AChE was noted in the adenohypophysis of the cat, and BuChE-staining was seen only in scattered cells within the gland and at its periphery, similar to those of the neurohypophysis (KOELLE and GEESEY l.c.). DUMONT (1956a, b) reported staining in occasional cells of the adenohypophysis for BuChE in the guinea pig, and for AChE in the rabbit *(ThCh-VII)*, but the identities of these structures were not established.

II. Adrenal medulla and cortex

The *adrenal medulla* is essentially a modified sympathetic ganglion. Embryologically, both the medullary chromaffin cells and the sympathetic ganglion cells originate from the same general region of the neural crest. The predominant secretion of the former, epinephrine in man and most other mammals, is liberated directly into the circulation, whereas the latter release chiefly norepinephrine at their axonal terminations in the immediate vicinity of the effector organs. Like the sympathetic ganglion cells, the chromaffin cells are innervated by preganglionic fibers which regulate their secretory activity.

In the cat, the AChE of the adrenal medulla was shown to be confined to the entering nerve trunks and their intercellular ramifications; originally, no significant concentrations of BuChE were noted (KOELLE 1951). Subsequent studies (COUPLAND and HOLMES 1958) (Fig. 34) employing a modified ThCh procedure have revealed the presence of low concentrations of BuChE in the main nerve bundles, where it apparently is associated with the Schwann cells, and in the smooth muscle cells of the adrenal vein. The presence of only AChE in the meshwork of fine nerve fibers between the chromaffin cells was confirmed. Neither enzyme was detected in the chromaffin cells. Accordingly, the AChE-containing particles of the microsomal fraction obtained from homogenates of ox adrenal medulla by HAGEN (1955) were probably derived chiefly from neural elements. Findings in the rabbit and rat were essentially similar; AChE-positive ganglion cells in the medulla were observed more frequently in the latter species than in the rabbit or cat (COUPLAND and HOLMES 1958). Hence, the distributions of AChE and BuChE in the adrenal medulla are comparable with those found in the sympathetic ganglia. ERÄNKÖ (1958) has reported an interesting selective association of BuChE-containing nerve fiber nets with the noradrenaline-containing cell islets in the rat adrenal medulla; the significance of this observation is unknown. The finding of low concentrations of BuChE in the chromaffin cells by the same author may have been the result of diffusion.

A detailed study of the ChE's of the *adrenal cortex* of the cat, rat, and rabbit was reported also by COUPLAND and HOLMES (1958) (Fig. 34). In all three species, the enzymes are confined to the capsular region and zona glomerulosa, excepting for the nerve trunks which penetrate to the medulla. Diffuse staining for BuChE was noted in the capsular connective tissue of the rat and in the cortical cells of the zona glomerulosa of the cat, but in neither region in the rabbit. However, in each species a capsular or subcapsular nervous plexus showed axonal staining for AChE and coarser staining for BuChE; the latter was associated presumably with the SCHWANN sheaths. The AChE-stained fibers were observed to penetrate only to the level of the zona glomerulosa. Although no physiological implications were drawn by the authors, these results and the earlier histological observations which they cited seem highly suggestive of a nervous control of aldosterone secretion by the zona glomerulosa, in contrast with the control of the secretions of the other layers by the adrenocorticotropic hormone.

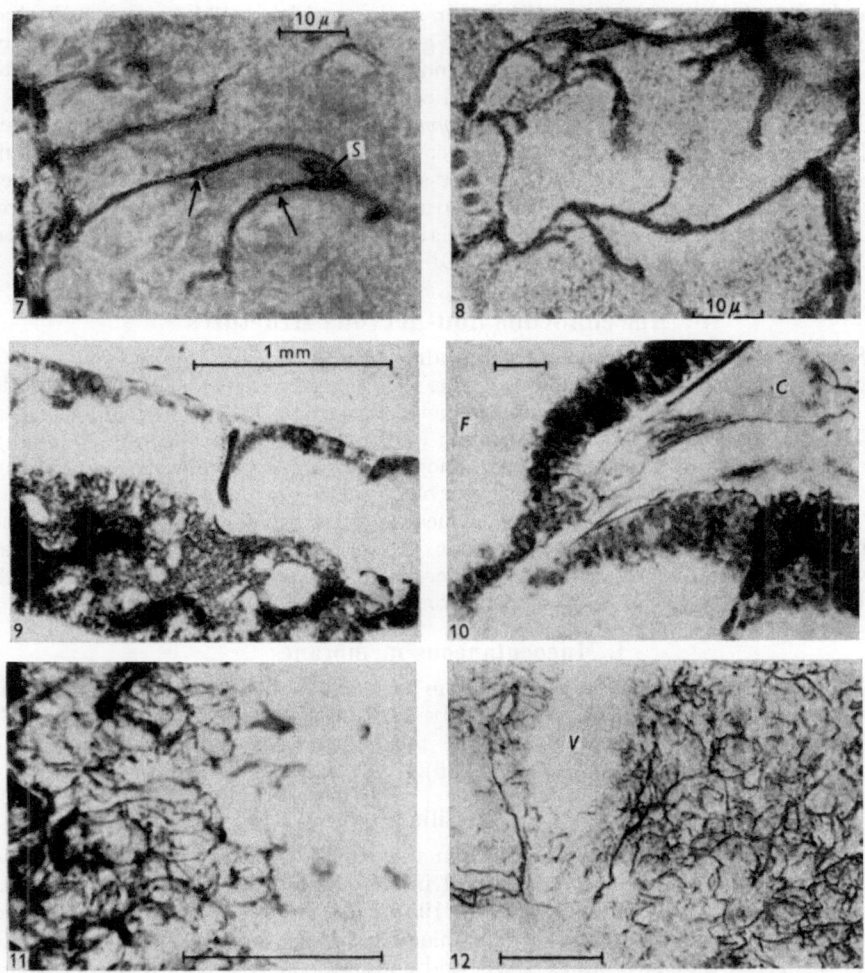

Fig. 34. Cholinesterases of adrenal cortex and medulla (*ThCh-III*, following formalin-fixation). 7. Fine nerve fibers in glomerular zone of rat adrenal. Arrows indicate small ovoid varicosities on ChE-positive strands. A Schwann cell nucleus (S) lies at the point of junction of two fibers. (Incubated 4 hr with AThCh.) 8. Fine strands of the ChE-positive medullary mesh of the rat showing small varicosities and an apparent terminal swelling. (Incubated 4 hr with AThCh.) 9. Cat adrenal. Positive ChE reaction in the zona glomerulosa, medulla, and in nerve fibers; a few fibers may be seen in the capsular region and a large bundle penetrates the gland. (Incubated 20 hr with AThCh.) 10. Cat adrenal showing an indentation of cortex with a positive ChE reaction in the cells of the zona glomerulosa and in nerve fibers. Nerves can be traced from the capsular region (C) into the zona glomerulosa. The cells of the zona fasciculata (F) are negative. (Incubated 20 hr with AThCh.) 11. Nerve mesh in cat adrenal medulla. The clear area on the right of the figure is the zona reticularis. (Incubated 20 hr with AThCh.) 12. Cholinesterase-positive medullary mesh in rabbit. V = venous sinus. (Incubated 5 hr with AThCh.)
(COUPLAND and HOLMES 1958)

III. Thyroid, thymus, parathyroid, and pancreatic islets

Reports on the *thyroid* are somewhat inconsistent and their significance is as yet obscure. DUMONT (1955a) observed in the rabbit, in contrast to several other species, staining for AChE in the perivascular nerve fibers and in the parafollicular cells. The latter localization was reported by SANDRITTER et al. (1956) for the rabbit and for several additional species, in some of which negative results had been obtained by DUMONT. This discrepancy may have resulted from the formalin-fixation employed by the latter author, which could have inactivated the enzyme at sites of low activity. In the guinea pig, DEJARDIN (1955) found only BuChE in the parafollicular cells. It is not known whether these findings relate in any way to nervous control of thyroid secretion.

From a study of the AChE of the *thymus* in several species at various stages of development, ROGISTER et al. (1955) concluded that the enzyme is present in occasional nerve fibers, and in early HASSALL's corpuscles and their forerunner epithelioid and vesicular cells. With maturity, most of the enzyme disappears.

No ChE's have been noted in association with the *parathyroids* (DEJARDIN 1955), or with the *pancreatic islet* cells (DUMONT 1955a).

F. Miscellaneous non-nervous structures

Several tissues have been considered already in which the involvement of the nervous system is either remote or absent, i.e., certain portions of skeletal muscle (A, II, 2—5), the blood and hematopoietic tissue (B, III, 1, c), the placenta (B, III, 4), and certain endocrine glands (E, II and III). In addition, in many autonomic effector organs (e.g., heart, smooth muscle) ACh probably acts both in the transmission of parasympathetic nerve impulses and as a local hormone, as will be discussed. All the foregoing tissues have been classified for convenience with their appropriate functional systems, the major portions of which are under nervous control. The structures considered in the present section are by all evidence completely devoid of nervous control.

I. Mucocutaneous membranes

Frog skin contains a ChE which, on the basis of the relative rates of hydrolysis of various substrates, is probably largely a BuChE or other non-specific ChE; most of the activity is localized in the tela subcutanea (KOBLICK 1958). The placenta has been discussed above (p. 235).

II. Cilia

Both AChE and ChAc are present in the ciliated mucous membrane of the rabbit trachea (KORDIK et al. 1952) and in the ciliated gill filaments of the sea mussel, *Mytilus edulis* (BÜLBRING et al. 1953); in the latter tissue, ACh was also identified chromatographically and by bioassay. These findings, along with the earlier (SEAMAN and HOULIHAN 1951) and simultaneously reported observations of the effects of cholinomimetic, anti-ChE, and anticholinergic agents on ciliary activity in these tissues (v. KORDIK et al. and SEAMAN and HOULIHAN for references) suggest strongly that locally formed ACh is involved intimately in the initiation or control of such activity. Failure to obtain equivalent drug effects on the ciliated epithelium of the frog esophagus (HILL 1957) was apparently due to seasonal variations in sensitivity (BURN and DAY 1958) and the use of phosphate rather than bicarbonate buffer (MILTON 1959). Similar pharmacological actions were reported with explants of human ciliated respiratory epithelium *in vitro*, although extremely high concentrations of drugs were employed (CORSSEN and ALLEN 1959).

III. Unicellular organisms

Acetylcholine has been identified in both a fungus, the rye ergot *Claviceps purpurea* (EWINS 1914), and a bacterium, *Lactobacillus plantarum* (STEPHENSON and ROWATT 1947). The presence of both ACh and an eserine-sensitive enzyme which promotes its hydrolysis in a species of *Paramecium* was reported by BEYER and WENSE (1936). BÜLBRING et al. (1949) found ACh and ChAc in the motile flagellated protozoan, *Trypanosoma rhodesiense*, but not in the non-motile unicellular organism, *Plasmodium gallinaceum*.

SEAMAN and HOULIHAN (1951) reported that homogenates of the ciliated protozoan, *Tetrahymena gelii* S., hydrolyzed ACh, and that the enzymatic activity was blocked by $4 \times 10^{-7} M$ eserine or DFP; ciliary activity in the intact organisms was inhibited reversibly by the same agents at $10^{-3} M$. Subsequently, the ACh-hydrolyzing activity was found to be confined to the fraction composed of pellicular fragments (SEAMAN 1951). From these observations it was concluded that conduction along the pellicular structure connecting the bases of individual cilia is dependent upon AChE. However, TIBBS (1960), employing the same colorimetric assay procedure (HESTRIN 1949), was unable to detect any ACh-hydrolysis by homogenates of a different strain of the same species (*Tetrahymena pyriformis* or *gelii* W.), or in two flagellated protozoans, *Polytoma uvella* and *Polytomella caeca*. The same species of *Tetrahymena* was investigated histochemically by PASTOR and FENNELL (1959); although distinct staining was obtained with the long-chain fatty acid esters of choline *(LC-Ch)* and α- and β-naphthyl acetate *(Naph-I)*, no staining developed following incubation with AThCh or BuThCh *(ThCh-II)* for periods up to 24 hours. With the positively-reacting substrates, inhibition of staining was obtained at an exceedingly high (0.008 M) concentration of eserine, but not at $10^{-4} M$; at the latter concentration, most ChE's are inhibited completely. Accordingly, the presence of a ChE in *Tetrahymena* remains questionable. (See also Chapter 5.)

The presence of an ACh-hydrolyzing enzyme in the sperm of the trout *(Salmo trutta)* and perch *(Perca fluviatilis)*, confined chiefly to the head in the latter species, was reported by TIBBS (l.c.). On the basis of the generally more rapid hydrolysis of MeCh than of BuCh or BzCh, and the inhibition of Ch-hydrolysis by $10^{-5} M$ eserine, it was considered to be an AChE.

In the author's laboratory, little or no AChE or BuChE could be detected manometrically in any of the centrifugation fractions of homogenates of the ameba, *Chaos chaos* (unpublished observations).

Physiological functions of acetylcholine and acetylcholinesterase

In the previous section, the distributions of AChE and non-specific ChE's throughout the body in mammalian and other species were described and illustrated, chiefly on the basis of histochemical observations. In most cases it was possible to indicate only the cells which contain the enzymes, and to assess subjectively their relative concentrations; however, in some instances, the distributions could be described or implied at the subcellular level, and occasionally quantitative ultramicro-analytical data could be given. Isolated descriptions of these types are of little significance in themselves unless they can be correlated, and in some way related to the functional roles of AChE and its physiological substrate, ACh. This has been attempted in the present section. It will be obvious that this involves many controversial issues, concerning several of which diametrically opposed viewpoints are emphasized in the individual chapters throughout the volume. These have been indicated by cross-reference wherever possible. While the opinions and hypotheses to be considered can be modified fairly readily, the observations on which they are based, if carefully controlled, are less ephemeral.

A. Neurohumoral transmission

The role of ACh as a neurohumoral agent, and the primary function of AChE in limiting its transmitter action at synaptic and neuroeffector sites, may seem at first consideration too well established to require either vindication or further explanation. Most of the important pharmacological actions of the anti-ChE agents, which are described in detail in Section III (Chapters 11 to 17), are consistent with this viewpoint; the only fully exceptional interpretation is that of NACHMANSOHN (Chapter 15), which is discussed below. Nevertheless, some important differences in the distributions of AChE at various sites of cholinergic transmission, which have been brought out in the preceding pages, and the demonstration of the presence of the enzyme in varying concentrations in presumably non-cholinergic neurons, as well as in certain non-innervated tissues, have raised several questions which deserve consideration.

I. Cholinergic neurons

Of the four generally acknowledged sites of cholinergic transmission (Fig. 35), the neuromuscular junction (Fig. 35-3) and autonomic ganglia (Fig. 35-2) have been studied in greatest detail with respect to the distributions of AChE and the actions of anti-ChE agents; between these two sites there are several striking differences (see also Chapters 12 and 13). In skeletal muscle, the motor endplates occupy a minute fraction of the total surface of the effector cells, and there is virtually no spatial overlap between the neuroeffector junctions of adjacent fibers. Most of the AChE is postjunctional, a distribution which seems ideal for the rapid termination of the transmitter effect of ACh following its liberation by the nerve terminal and its action at the postjunctional receptor site. This is borne out by the marked prolongation of the endplate potential (EPP), and the repetitive firing

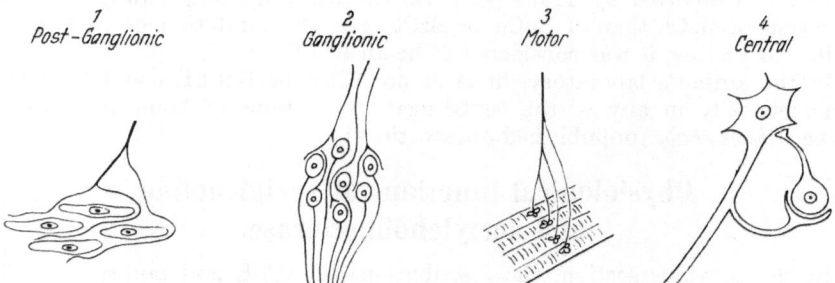

| 1 | 2 | 3 | 4 |
| Post-Ganglionic | Ganglionic | Motor | Central |

Fig. 35. Synaptic and neuroeffector relationships of cholinergic fibers (KOELLE 1961)

of muscle action potentials (MAP's) following a single presynaptic volley which occur after sufficient AChE has been inactivated by an anti-ChE agent (ECCLES et al. 1942, FATT and KATZ 1951). In contrast, the superior cervical ganglion of the cat contains approximately 100,000 ganglion cells, enmeshed within a complicated network of dendrites, presynaptic fibers and their terminals, and capsular glial cells, all of which occupy a volume of a few cubic millimeters. Most of the surface of the individual ganglion cells is covered with terminal boutons (DE CASTRO 1951). As already described, most of the AChE, and virtually all the external or functional AChE, of the superior cervical and stellate ganglia of the cat is presynaptic, whereas in the ciliary and sphenopalatine ganglia it is both pre- and postsynaptic. The ganglionic BuChE in this species is confined to the capsular and intercapsular glial cells. Anticholinesterase agents have been shown to produce some degree of spread and prolongation of the postsynaptic effects of submaximal preganglionic stimulation of the superior cervical ganglion [see references under (1) below], but these actions of the drugs are not nearly so striking as they are at the neuromuscular junction. In fact, it has been calculated that diffusion alone can account for the termination of the transmitter action of ACh in the ganglion (OGSTON 1955, EMMELIN and MACINTOSH 1956). In view of these differences between the neuromuscular junction and the ganglion, and the uncertainty concerning the function of AChE in the latter, VOLLE and KOELLE (1961) investigated several possible physiological roles of AChE in the cat superior cervical ganglion.

Four functions proposed previously for the AChE of sympathetic ganglia and other sites were considered:

(1) Temporal or spatial limitation of the transmitter action of ACh at the postsynaptic site (FELDBERG and VARTIAINEN 1934, ECCLES 1944, HOLADAY et al. 1954).

(2) Rapid hydrolysis of ACh to provide an immediate source of choline for uptake by the presynaptic terminals and resynthesis to ACh (PERRY 1953, 1957).

(3) Protection of the presynaptic terminals against reactivation by self-liberated ACh (KOELLE and KOELLE 1959).

(4) Prevention of accumulation of activating concentrations of ACh liberated during the resting stage (FELDBERG 1945a, b).

With respect to the first proposal, confirmation was obtained of the earlier studies quoted, that inactivation of most of the ganglionic AChE by di*iso*propyl phosphorofluoridate (DFP) resulted in increases in the amplitude and duration of post-tetanic ganglionic after-discharge, and apparent recruitment of additional ganglion cells in response to single supramaximal stimuli delivered to the partially resected preganglionic trunk. However, attempts to obtain more direct evidence of the spread of the area of ganglionic activation following DFP were unsuccessful. No evidence was obtained to support the second proposal; when choline was infused intra-arterially over a wide range of concentrations during preganglionic stimulation at frequencies of 3 to 20 per second, with or without AChE-inactivation by DFP, it only accelerated the rate of failure of postganglionic firing.

Definite support was obtained for the remaining two proposals. Signs of retrograde firing along the preganglionic trunk were obtained only occasionally following the injection of ACh or carbachol (Car) into the ganglion's arterial supply; this probably did not represent antidromic firing from presynaptic terminals, but the activation of centrally displaced ganglion cells and those with recurrent fibers (DOUGLAS et al. 1960). However, the effects of DFP and of denervation on the postganglionic response to injected ACh and Car appeared to implicate

Table 7. *Threshold doses for activation of superior cervical ganglion by intra-arterial injection of ACh and Car* (from VOLLE and KOELLE 1961)

	Mean threshold dose (mμmol ± S.D.)	
	ACh	Car
Normal control	27 ± 13 (21)[1]	2.8 ± 1.1 (8)
Normal post-DFP[2]	0.73 ± 0.50 (13)	2.2 ± 1.1 (7)
Control: post-DFP	38:1	1.3:1
Denervated control	36 ± 15 (19)	71 ± 45 (10)
Denervated post-DFP[2]	3.4 ± 2.8 (14)	6.6 ± 7.2 (8)
Control: post-DFP	11:1	11:1
Control *denervated: normal*.	1.3:1	26:1
Post-DFP *denervated: normal*.	4.6:1	3.0:1
Car: ACh		
Normal control		0.10:1
Normal post-DFP		3.1:1
Denervated control . . .		2.0:1
Denervated post-DFP . .		2.0:1

[1] Number of experiments in parentheses.
[2] 2 μmol, i.a.

the presynaptic axonal terminals as the primary site of action of theses compounds under normal conditions. In this series of experiments, the threshold intra-arterial doses of ACh and of Car were determined for the production of detectable postganglionic firing. Following an intra-arterial injection of DFP (2 μmol), the determinations of the threshold doses were repeated. Similar determinations were conducted on ganglia in which the preganglionic trunks had been resected one to four weeks previously. The mean threshold doses and their standard deviations are summarized in Table 7. In the normal ganglia, the mean threshold doses of ACh and Car for the production of postganglionic firing were 27 and 2.8 mμmol, respectively; these were reduced to corresponding values of 0.73 and 2.2 following DFP. In contrast to the denervation sensitization observed at most sites (CANNON 1939), the mean threshold dose of ACh in the denervated ganglia (36) was slightly higher than in the normal, while that of Car (71) was elevated 26-fold. After DFP, both these values were reduced in the denervated ganglia by 11-fold (3.4 and 6.6, respectively). The interpretation proposed for these results is illustrated in Fig. 36. In the denervated ganglia (lower left), from which both ACh and AChE were presumably absent, the only site of action available to injected ACh and Car was the post-synaptic membrane. Hence, it was suggested that the much lower threshold dose of Car in the normal ganglion (upper left) acted on the presynaptic terminals, causing them in turn to liberate ACh at the synaptic cleft and thus to activate the ganglion cells. However, the normal presynaptic terminals would have been protected against ACh, in contrast to Car, by their sheaths of external AChE; hence the threshold dose of ACh, which was not significantly different in the denervated and normal ganglia, might have acted in the latter at either the pre- or postsynaptic site or both. This effect of the AChE is probably reflected by the marked reduction of the threshold dose of ACh, but not of Car, in the normal ganglia following DFP (upper rigth). The lower threshold doses of both ACh and Car in the DFP-treated normal (upper right) as compared with the DFP-treated denervated (lower right) ganglia suggests that in the former group both drugs acted presynaptically. Two possible explanations were offered for the marked and equal reduction in the threshold doses of both ACh and Car by DFP in the denervated ganglia (lower right). This might represent potentiation of the response of the ganglion cells to ACh and Car as a result of alkylphosphorylation by DFP of non-specific "B-groups" at the receptor site, as sug-

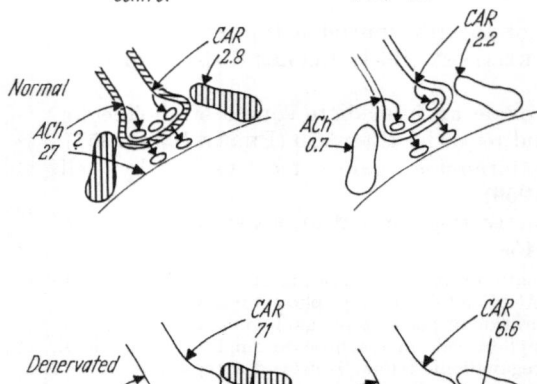

Fig. 36. Diagram depicting threshold intraarterial doses (in mμmol) of ACh and carbachol (CAR) in 4 situations studied. Horizontal cross-hatching represents AChE of presynaptic terminals; vertical cross-hatching, BuChE of capsular glial cells; vesicles, the transmitter (VOLLE and KOELLE 1961)

gested by COHEN and POSTHUMUS (1955, 1957). Alternatively, the BuChE of the capsular glial cells, which is unaffected by denervation (HOLLINGSHEAD and SAWYER 1945, KOELLE 1951), might represent the major barrier to the passage of ACh and Car from the circulation to the postsynaptic site, since both compounds can combine with BuChE (GOLDSTEIN 1951), after which ACh is hydrolyzed relatively slowly, and Car at an insignificant rate (WILSON et al. 1960); their site of binding on the enzyme is probably the same as that which is alkylphosphorylated by DFP (KOELLE 1946).

Following the intra-arterial injection of sufficiently high doses (usually 2 to 3 μmol) of a more potent preparation of DFP than that used in the foregoing experiments, spontaneous postganglionic firing developed consistently within a few minutes after injection, and persisted for several hours. Since this was always seen in acutely, but never in chronically, denervated ganglia it was attributed to the preservation of ACh liberated by the presynaptic terminals during the resting stage. These observations thus provide evidence for the fourth proposed function of the ganglionic AChE.

The explanations given above for the various findings obtained are by no means the only possible ones, and several alternatives were mentioned (VOLLE and KOELLE 1961). However, collectively they suggest that the primary function of the ganglionic AChE, which in the superior cervical ganglion of the cat is localized almost exclusively presynaptically, is the protection of the presynaptic terminals from continuous self re-excitation by the ACh which they liberate during both the resting and active stages. The apparently greater susceptibility of the presynaptic site to excitation by injected ACh, with the consequent excitation of the postsynaptic site by endogenously liberated transmitter, suggests a similar mechanism as the basis for the other recorded pharmacological actions of anti-ChE agents on the ganglion. The spatial spread and prolongation of postsynaptic activation in response to preganglionic stimulation after moderate doses of DFP (proposed function 1), as well as the spontaneous activation of the ganglion cells after high doses (proposed function 4), may be attributed primarily to potentiation of the action of endogenous ACh at the presynaptic terminals, causing them in turn to liberate additonal ACh to produce the resultant effects at the postsynaptic site, i.e., the ganglion cells.

It may be asked why antidromic firing fails to occur along the preganglionic trunk under such circumstances. In the situations described, both endogenous and injected ACh may have produced localized potentials in the fine axonal terminals which, while effective in liberating ACh, were of insufficient magnitude or too distant from the electrogenically excitable portions of the main trunks of the axons to induce conducted impulses. In the pathological state resulting from infection with pseudorabies virus, spontaneous antidromic firing does occur from the superior cervical ganglion, and endogenous ACh is probably directly involved in its production (DEMPSHER and RIKER 1957, DEMPSHER et al. 1959).

At the neuromuscular junction, on the other hand, both the predominantly postjunctional localization of AChE and the more striking direct effects of anti-ChE agents on transmission indicate that the primary role of the enzyme is the limitation of the action of ACh at the postjunctional membrane. However, this proposed difference of the major role of the enzyme from that suggested for the ganglion may be relative. The susceptibility of the motor nerve terminals to excitation by ACh and related compounds has been indicated by the demonstration of antidromic firing along motor fibers after injection of these compounds or of anti-ChE agents (MASLAND and WIGTON 1940, FENG and LI 1941, RIKER et al. 1957, 1959). COUTEAUX's (1961) demonstration of the entirely prejunctional localization of the AChE in the dorsal fin musculature of the seahorse suggests that all degrees of relative distribution, and consequently of functional importance, of the enzyme at the pre- and postjunctional sites may occur in various muscles and species. Likewise, in the ciliary and sphenopalatine ganglia, where the enzyme is oriented externally at both the pre- and postsynaptic sites (SZENTÁGOTHAI et al. 1954, KOELLE and KOELLE 1959), it may serve in equally important capacities at both.

There is hardly sufficient information at the cellular level as yet to permit any reasonable assessment of the major primary functions of AChE at the remaining two sites of cholinergic transmission, the parasympathetically innervated autonomic effector cells and certain regions in the central nervous system (Fig. 35-1 and 35-4). With regard to the former, the most definitive study of the response of effector cells to postganglionic nerve stimulation has been that of BURNSTOCK and HOLMAN (1961); however, this involved adrenergic activation of the guinea pig vas deferens.

In this case, there was at least a superficial resemblance to the events which occur in skeletal muscle following cholinergic activation; each nerve impulse induced partial depolarization of the smooth muscle membrane, and sufficient summation of the individual, localized depolarizations was followed by a spike potential, which was conducted through the adjacent muscle fibers, and contraction. From descriptions of the effects of direct stimulation and of ACh on the smooth muscle membrane of the guinea pig taenia coli, where it causes activation, it is likely that postganglionic cholinergic impulses produce a similar sequence at such sites (BÜLBRING 1957, BÜLBRING et al. 1958, BURNSTOCK 1958). This topic is discussed in the next section (B). Miniature potentials, similar to those recorded at the motor endplate, occur in smooth muscle in the absence of nerve stimulation, but it is uncertain whether these are neurogenic or myogenic in origin (BURNSTOCK and HOLMAN 1961). The nerve terminals contain synaptic vesicles identical with those observed at prejunctional sites elsewhere (CAESAR et al. 1957). There is evidence that in addition to the influence of the extrinsic preganglionic fibers on the intramural ganglion cells of the intestine, they may be activated by 5-hydroxytryptamine liberated from enterochromaffin cells of the mucosa, and that this is the basis of the peristaltic reflex (BÜLBRING 1961).

The striking effects of anti-ChE agents in modifying the activities of smooth muscle and gland cells (see Chapter 11) leave no doubt that the ChE enzymes are essential for terminating the actions of ACh liberated by the corresponding parasympathetic postganglionic fibers, probably during both the resting and active stages; in addition, the enzymes may limit the effects of ACh released by the effector cells themselves (v.i., section B). However, it will be recalled from the previous section that a complicated array of sites of ChE activities is present in such organs; in the gut, these include the AChE and BuChE of the ganglion cells and their processes, and the predominantly BuChE of the muscle fibers, mucosal cells, and interstitial cells. In only a few studies has any attempt been made to determine the effects of selective inhibition of AChE or BuChE. Virtually nothing is known concerning the relative amounts of AChE or BuChE in the individual cell types mentioned, or the orientation of the enzymes with respect to the cell membranes. Hence, one can only postulate by analogy that events occur here which are similar to those suggested for the ganglion.

With regard to cholinergic transmission in the central nervous system, ECCLES and associates (1954, 1956) have shown that anti-ChE agents cause marked prolongation of activation of the RENSHAW cells following stimulation of the corresponding cholinergic motor fibers. As these authors have pointed out, at the central site the transmitter is probably confined within the synaptic cleft until destroyed by enzymatic hydrolysis, since there is less likelihood here than at peripheral sites of its escape by diffusion. The prolongation by anti-ChE agents of the effect recorded at the postsynaptic site might be due primarily to the persistent action of ACh at either the pre- or postsynaptic site, by analogy with the postulated dual action of ACh in sympathetic ganglia and at the motor endplate, just discussed. Only recently has there been any tentative histological identification of the non-cholinergic axonal terminals of the RENSHAW cells on the anterior horn cells (SZENTÁGOTHAI 1958); the cytological distribution and structural characteristics of AChE at the synapses between the cholinergic Golgi II collaterals of the anterior horn cells and the somata of the RENSHAW cells are unknown.

II. Non-cholinergic neurons

1. Adrenergic fibers

It has been pointed out that in the cat the great majority of the sympathetic ganglion cells, presumably those giving rise to adrenergic fibers, contain a scarcely detectable concentration of AChE (KOELLE 1951). A small percentage, which contain concentrations equivalent to that in the cells of the ciliary ganglion, probably constitute cells giving rise to the cholinergic sympathetic fibers, such as the vasodilators and the nerve supply of the sweat glands (SJÖQVIST and FREDRICCSON 1961). Until recently, no functional basis could be offered for the presence of intermediate concentrations of AChE in the remaining sympathetic neurons; in the rabbit and rhesus monkey, and several other species, this type accounts for a considerable percentage of the total (KOELLE 1955). The work of BURN and RAND (1958, 1959, 1960), taken in conjunction with the foregoing discussion, has provided a tentative explanation for these observations. These authors have obtained evidence along several lines that a cholinergic mechanism is involved in the release of norepinephrine by sympathetic fibers.

First, it was shown that in the presence of atropine in doses sufficient to block the muscarinic effects of ACh on peripheral effectors, the intra-arterial injection of ACh or nicotine produced sympathomimetic effects at several sites. These effects were prevented by previous treatment with reserpine, which depletes organs of most of their norepinephrine content, and were restored after a period of infusion with norepinephrine. On the other hand, following reserpine alone, stimulation of sympathetic nerves to many organs produced cholinomimetic effects, which were in turn blocked by atropine (BURN and RAND l.c.). More recently, CHANG and RAND (1960) have found that hemicholinium (α,α'-dimethylethanolamino-4,4'-biaceto-phenone, HC 3) blocks transmission by the sympathetic nerves to several effector organs, and that this effect is reversed by choline. The former compound can prevent transmission at cholinergic terminals, probably by blocking their uptake of choline, and thus limiting the synthesis of ACh (BIRKS and MACINTOSH 1957, GARDINER 1957). From these findings, BURN and RAND have proposed that the so-called adrenergic fibers actually bring about their effects by releasing ACh, and that the latter in turn releases norepinephrine from peripheral stores in the vicinity of the axonal terminals. The exact location of the norepinephrine stores is uncertain; both the nerve terminals themselves and adjacent chromaffin cells have been suggested. However, the former site seems the more likely possibility in view of the observations that sympathetic denervation of various organs (spleen, submaxillary and parotid glands, heart) results in the loss of most of their norepinephrine content (v. EULER and PURKHOLD 1951, COOPER et al. 1961). In contrast to the aforementioned findings, HC 3 over a wide range of concentrations failed to block transmission from the postganglionic sympathetic fibers to the nictitating membrane of the cat, *in situ* (WILSON and LONG 1959) and *in vitro* (GARDINER and THOMPSON 1961).

Accordingly, the terminals of certain postganglionic sympathetic fibers may represent a situation at which the arrival of the nerve impulse liberates first ACh, and it in turn brings about the release from the same site of a different neuro-humoral transmitter, in this case norepinephrine. The concentrations of AChE in the ganglion cell somata, which apparently are paralleled by the relative AChE activities of their fibers insofar as these have been determined quantitatively (GIACOBINI 1957), may reflect the extent of ACh-participation in the liberation of norepinephrine at the terminals. If this is true, the phenomenon may be much more generalized and important in the rabbit and rhesus monkey, for example, where most of the sympathetic ganglion cells contain moderate concentrations of AChE, than in the cat, where the concentration in the great majority is extremely low. The lack of evidence of cholinergic mediation in transmission to the cat's nictitating membrane has been noted (v.s.). Furthermore, the postulated inter-mediate participation of ACh, between the arrival of the nerve impulse and the liberation of norepinephrine, may not be an essential but a facilitatory step. The release of catecholamines by the chromaffin cells of the adrenal medulla is triggered, directly or indirectly, by ACh liberated in their immediate vicinity by cholinergic preganglionic fibers. Although the chromaffin cells appear to be devoid of AChE, the enzyme is readily available in high concentration at the adjacent preganglionic terminals.

2. Hypothalamico-neurohypophyseal tract

It is now generally accepted that the secretions of the neurohypophysis, vasopressin and oxytocin, are synthesized at least in part within the somata of neurons of the hypothalamic supraoptic and paraventricular nuclei, then trans-ported through the corresponding axonal processes, by way of the infundibular stalk, to their terminations in the infundibular process of the neurohypophysis (BARGMANN and SCHARRER 1951, SCHARRER and SCHARRER 1954). On the basis of the effects of anti-ChE agents on the secretion of vasopressin (PICKFORD 1947, DUKE et al. 1950) and of oxytocin (ABRAHAMS and PICKFORD 1956), these processes appear to be under the control of cholinergic fibers. As noted previously, the presence of AChE in light to moderate concentrations along the full length of the hypothalamico-neurohypophyseal tract, but its absence from the fibers terminating on the AChE-stained cells of origin in the supraoptic and paraventricular nuclei, indicates that in these regions only the neurosecretory cells themselves are

17*

cholinergic (ABRAHAMS et al. 1957, KOELLE and GEESEY 1961). It has been shown
by electron microscopy that the neurohypophyses of the rat (PALAY 1957) and
toad (GERSCHENFELD et al. 1960) contain two distinct populations of vesicles:
a larger, highly electron-opaque type, which can be traced back to the nuclei of
origin and presumably represents the endocrine secretions, and smaller, less dense
vesicles which are confined to the terminals and resemble the synaptic vesicles
seen at most presynaptic sites (see Chapter 3). The latter most probably represent
the storage form of ACh and other neurohumoral transmitters (DE ROBERTIS 1958,
WHITTAKER 1959). As proposed previously (ABRAHAMS et al., GERSCHENFELD et al.
l.c.), these findings are strongly suggestive that impulses conducted along the
hypothalamico-neurohypophyseal tract may liberate first ACh, and that it in turn
liberates the endocrine products from the same terminals.

3. Primary afferent fibers

In contrast to the ventral spinal roots and predominantly motor peripheral
nerve trunks, the dorsal roots and predominantly afferent nerves contain extremely low concentrations of ACh (LOEWI and HELLAUER 1938, LISSÁK and
PÁSZTOR 1940, MACINTOSH 1941) and ChAc (HEBB and SILVER 1956, COHEN 1956);
the differential values for AChE activity are not nearly so marked (BURGEN and

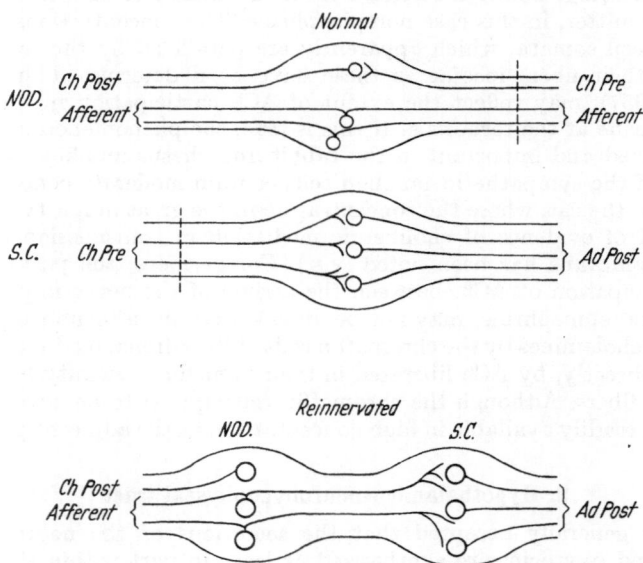

Fig. 37. Diagrammatic representation of synaptic relationships in the normal vagal nodose ganglion (NOD.) and
superior cervical ganglion (S.C.), and in the cross-anastomosed preparations. Transverse dotted lines indicate sites
of sectioning. Fiber types include cholinergic preganglionic and postganglionic (Ch Pre and Ch Post), adrenergic
postganglionic (Ad Post), and afferent (MATSUMURA and KOELLE 1961, modified from DE CASTRO 1951)

CHIPMAN 1951). Both on the basis of these relative values, and the inconclusive
effects of anti-ChE agents on monosynaptic spinal reflexes (e.g., HOLMSTEDT and
SKOGLUND 1953), primary afferent fibers are generally considered to be non-
cholinergic. Yet there have been suggestions that ACh is liberated following their
stimulation (DIKSHIT 1934, BRECHT and CORSTEN 1942). Indirect pharmacological
and histochemical evidence of this has been obtained by MATSUMURA and KOELLE
(1961) in the course of repeating DE CASTRO's (1942, 1951) classical preparation

involving cross-anastomosis between the peripheral afferent vagus and the peripheral cervical sympathetic trunks (Fig. 37). By means of this operation, DE CASTRO (l.c.) was able to establish a functional reflex arc, entirely apart from the central nervous system, consisting of the afferent neurons of the vagal nodose ganglion and the neurons of the superior cervical ganglion, with the central terminals of the former replacing the sympathetic preganglionic fibers.

The original observations were confirmed in 17 cats; then, the effects of several blocking agents [tetraethylammonium (TEA), lysergic acid diethylamide (LSD), carbinoxamine, gamma-aminobutyric acid] and physostigmine were compared with regard to their effects on the response of the nictitating membrane to stimulation of the vagal artificial preganglionic trunk and to the intracarotid injection of various ganglionic stimulants [i.e., ACh, propionylcholine, butyrylcholine, 2-β-imidazol-4'(5')-ylacroloylcholine (murexine), dimethylphenylpiperazinium (DMPP), 5-hydroxytryptamine (5-HT), histamine, adenosine triphosphate (ATP)] (MATSUMURA and KOELLE l.c.). While all the blocking agents produced some degree of reduction in the response to both nerve stimulation and the various stimulant drugs, a fairly high level of specificity was exhibited between pairs of known antagonists (e.g., LSD vs. 5-HT, carbinoxamine vs. histamine). However, only TEA blocked effectively the response to nerve stimulation at the same intraarterial dose level (100 μg) at which it blocked equally the effect of the stimulants which it antagonized (the choline esters and DMPP). There was a remarkable parallelism in the time course of blockade of the response to nerve stimulation and to injected ACh (Fig. 38). Conversely, low doses of physostigmine (2 to 20 μg) potentiated the responses to nerve stimulation and to the choline esters, and produced only reduction in the responses to 5-HT and histamine. Histochemical examination *(ThCh-V)* of the peripheral vagus-reinnervated superior cervical ganglia showed that the regenerated fibers contained AChE in intermediate concentrations, considerably lower than that found in the normal preganglionic fibers at the level of the ganglion (Fig. 39).

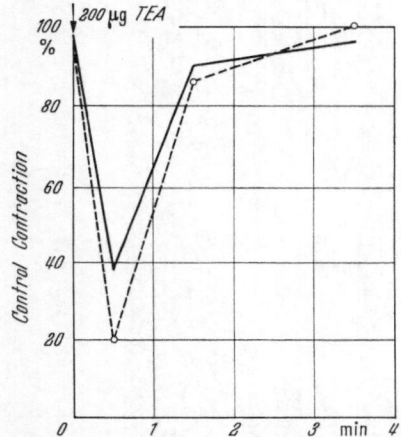

Fig. 38. Effects of TEA on the response of the nictitating membrane to maximal stimulation of the vagal artificial preganglionic trunk (———) and to intra-arterial injection of ACh (x— —x). In addition to original anastomosis, preganglionic sympathetic trunk crushed by cold forceps 42 days prior to experiment (MATSUMURA and KOELLE 1961)

These results suggested that the transmitter of the afferent vagus, under the abnormal condition in which it was studied, was ACh or a similar AChE-hydrolyzable ester. However, in view of the evidence to the contrary mentioned previously, the question may be raised whether an ACh-like compound represents the only, or the chief postsynaptically acting transmitter under normal circumstances. It is possible that ACh may function at the central terminations of the afferent vagus in a manner similar to that proposed above for adrenergic fibers and the neurohypophysis, as a presynaptically acting agent which liberates an unidentified transmitter, to which the sympathetic ganglion cells, however, were relatively insensitive in the experiments described. In this connection, it is of interest that substance P, which has been proposed as the transmitter of primary afferent fibers (ANDREWS and HOLTON 1958), was found to enhance the stimulatory effect of ACh on the superior cervical ganglion but by itself caused no stimulation (BELESIN et al. 1960).

The question of whether ACh or a similar agent functions in the initiation of nerve impulses at the peripheral terminals of primary afferent fibers has long been disputed. Many types of sensory terminals or end organs can be stimulated by the injection of ACh, which effect in turn can be blocked by various anti-ACh drugs, such as hexamethonium, tetraethylammonium, tubocurarine, and nicotine

(GRAY 1959). However, extremely high concentrations of hexamethonium failed to block the responses of the carotid sinus pressoreceptors to their natural stimulus, increased intracarotid pressure (DIAMOND 1955). It is perhaps significant that the tertiary base, nicotine, blocked the response of touch receptors of frog skin to mechanical stimulation as well as to ACh, whereas the *bis*quaternary compound, tubocurarine, blocked only the action of ACh (JARRETT 1956). This suggests that permeability barriers may prevent access of quaternary compounds to possible sites of action of endogenous ACh in normal sensory reception. These and similar

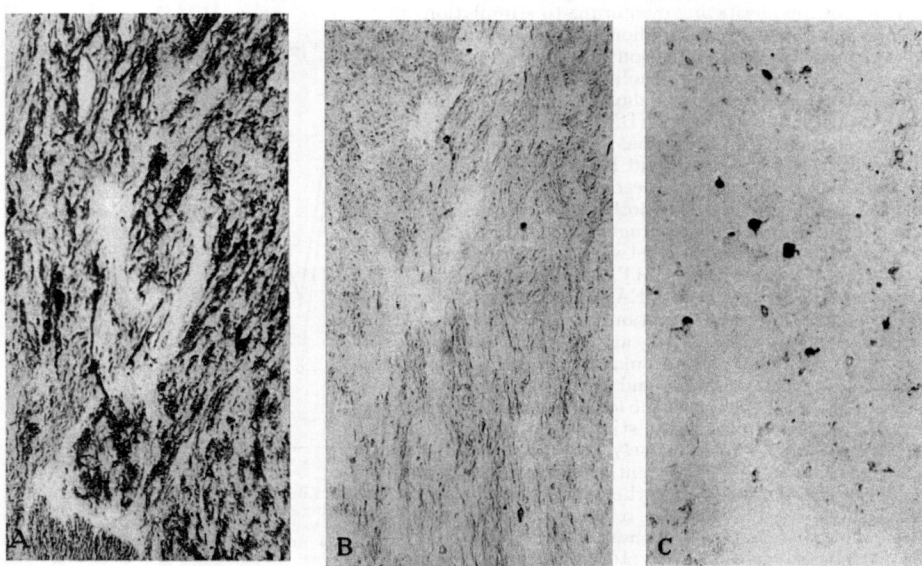

Fig. 39. Sections (10 μ) of normal (A), afferent vagally reinnervated (B), and denervated (C) cat superior cervical ganglia, stained for AChE activity by 60 min incubation in AThCh medium (*AThCh-III*, magnification × 50). The vagally reinnervated ganglion (B) was removed 162 days after the anastomosis, the denervated ganglion (C) 23 days after preganglionic denervation (MATSUMURA and KOELLE 1961)

findings have been held in support of ACh as a peripheral sensory mediator (LILJESTRAND 1954) and, conversely, have been regarded only as artificially induced drug effects (DOUGLAS 1954, GRAY and DIAMOND 1957). The presence of BuChE in several sensory end-organs (e.g., carotid chemoreceptor cells, Pacinian corpuscles, Meissner corpuscles), of low concentrations of AChE in the accompanying nerve fibers, and of synaptic vesicle-like inclusions in the nerve terminals and adjacent cells of Pacinian and Meissner corpuscles has been described in a previous section (pages 239 to 241). On the other hand, in a small series of experiments, cutaneously applied DFP failed to produce detectable modification of crude sensory perception (HURLEY and KOELLE 1958).

The most suggestive evidence of chemically mediated sensory reception lies in the parallelism between the electrical events that have been recorded at certain peripheral afferent terminals, such as the crustacean stretch receptor (EYZAGUIRRE and KUFFLER 1955) and the Pacinian corpuscle (GRAY and SATO 1953, LOEWEN-STEIN 1959), and at sites of cholinergic transmission, including the motor endplate of skeletal muscle (ECCLES and KUFFLER 1941, DEL CASTILLO and KATZ 1955) and the somata of anterior horn cells (COOMBS et al. 1957). The immediate response to pressure in the Pacinian corpuscle is the development of a localized, graded, slowly rising transducer or generator potential, which in all these features resembles the endplate potential (EPP) at the motor endplate, or the postsynaptic potential (PSP) of the anterior horn cell, produced by transmitted nerve impulses or the iontophoretic application of ACh. The non-propagated sensory transducer potential, like the EPP or PSP, initiates a propagated spike, or nerve action potential. This close correspondence of sequential events suggests that the initial response following the application of pressure to the corpuscle may be the liberation of an ACh-like mediator, perhaps from the same nerve terminal at which it acts. At the motor endplate, ACh is without demonstrable effect when it is applied beneath the sarcoplasmic membrane (DEL CASTILLO and KATZ l. c.); hence, its lack of effect during storage prior to its postulated release at the sensory terminal constitutes no objection to the proposal, particularly if the ACh is sequestered within membranous vesicles at the intracellular storage site. CAUNA (1960) has suggested that in MEISSNER's corpuscles ACh may be liberated within the laminar cells which are intercalated between the nerve terminals, and may initiate the impulse by the increase in ion concentration consequent to its local hydrolysis by ChE.

4. Central neurons

The actions of anti-ChE agents surveyed in Chapter 14 provide strong, if indirect, confirmation of the conclusion reached in an earlier review by FELDBERG (1945a) that ACh undoubtedly participates as a neurohumoral transmitter in the central nervous system. Yet, it is equally likely that ACh is not the universal or sole central transmitter. Although there is no other agent for which this role is so well established as that of ACh, the low concentrations of ACh, ChAc, and AChE at many regions of the brain and spinal cord speak against ACh as the primary transmitter at such sites. FELDBERG and VOGT (1948) at one time proposed that there might be an alteration of cholinergic and non-cholinergic neurons within the central nervous system. Although this suggestion is still often quoted, it has since been modified by FELDBERG (1956) to acknowledge the presence of both types, but not in so restricted a pattern.

The principal conclusion derived from the histochemical survey of the AChE of the central nervous system of the rat, described above, was that the concentration of the enzyme in the individual central neurons varies from very high levels, as exhibited by those known to have cholinergic fibers, through moderate, to scarcely detectable levels. In line with the foregoing discussion, it might be suggested that these concentrations reflect the level of ACh-liberation at the corresponding axonal terminals, either as the sole transmitter, or as a presynaptically acting agent which releases other trans-synaptic neurohumoral agents.

III. Summary of the hypothetical roles of ACh and AChE at the pre- and postsynaptic sites

The postulated roles of ACh in synaptic and neuroeffector transmission are summarized in Fig. 40 (KOELLE 1961, 1962). The top diagram represents the steps of the most generally accepted current concept of cholinergic transmission, as depicted by GRUNDFEST (1957a), which consist in (1) the arrival of the conducted nerve action potential (NAP) at the axonal terminal, causing (2) the liberation of ACh (clear vesicles), which diffuses across the synaptic cleft and (3) combiness with a hypothetical receptor substance to bring about a localized depolarization, the postsynaptic potential (PSP); the latter in turn (4) initiates electrogenically the NAP in the second neuron. Largely on the basis of the histochemical and pharmalogical studies described on the superior cervical ganglion, an additional step has been proposed at 2 A in the middle diagram: the immediate action of the liberated ACh on the presynaptic terminal, causing it to release additional quanta of ACh in order to facilitate transmission across the cleft. In effect, this would serve as an amplification mechanism at the terminal. Is hat been suggested that the major function of the presynaptically localized AChE is to prevent perpetuation of this process of self-re-excitation; this was considered the basis of the persistent, spontaneous firing of the postganglionic trunk which followed the intra-arterial injection of a sufficiently high dose of an anti-ChE agent (DFP) into the ganglion (VOLLE and KOELLE l.c.). The relative importance of diffusion and AChE in terminating the action of ACh at the postsynaptic membrane probably varies with the site; at the motor endplates in most skeletal muscle, where the greater part of the AChE is postsynaptic, the enzyme is probably chiefly responsible.

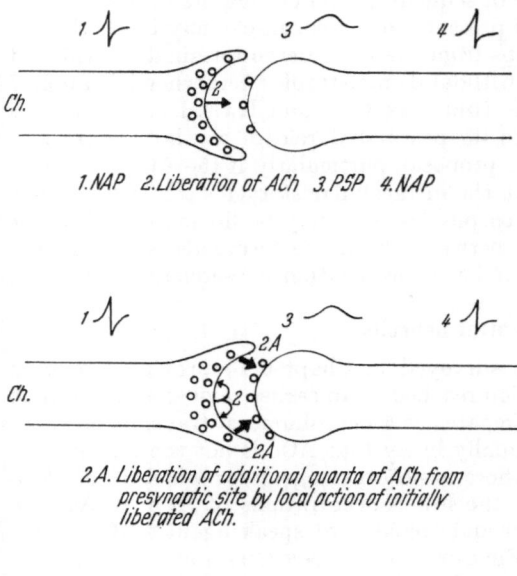

1.NAP   2.Liberation of ACh   3.PSP   4.NAP

2 A. Liberation of additional quanta of ACh from presynaptic site by local action of initially liberated ACh.

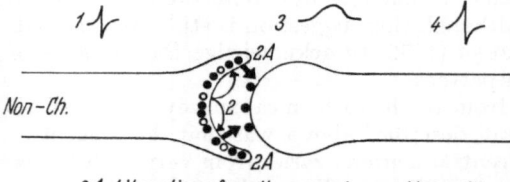

2 A. Liberation of another neurohumoral transmitter from presynaptic site by local action of initially liberated ACh.

Fig. 40. Proposed dual neurohumoral role of ACh. See text for description

The bottom diagram depicts the proposed participation of ACh at the same step, 2 A, in bringing about the release of other neurohumoral transmitters (dark vesicles) in various non-cholinergic neurons, such as adrenergic and sensory fibers, the hypothalamico-neurohypophyseal tract, and perhaps certain central neurons. The varied, and admittedly indirect, evidence for this at the sites mentioned has been presented. With regard to the central topic of the present chapter, the role postulated for ACh provides an explanation of the function of the low to intermediate concentrations of AChE in such neurons and their axonal terminals.

A few ancillary, but equally important items deserve mention in conjunction with the foregoing proposal. First, although the cholinergic transmitter, or "auxiliary transmitter," has been referred to consistently as ACh, this is not meant to exclude the possibility that other choline esters or related compounds may function in such capacities at certain sites. The large number of naturally occurring choline esters which have now been identified (see Chapter 1), and some pharmacological observations (e.g., R. M. ECCLES 1952, KEWITZ 1955) suggest that at some sites the physiological mediator involved may not be ACh alone, but in addition, or instead, a similarly acting compound. The most obvious analogy is the relatively recent identification of norepinephrine, rather than epinephrine, as the transmitter of adrenergic fibers (v. EULER 1948).

Little consideration has been given to the glial cells of the central and peripheral nervous systems aside from reference to the facts that they invest closely all neurons, axons, and junctional sites, and that they contain BuChE or a related non-specific ChE, the function of which has not been established. DE CASTRO (1951), and more recently GALAMBOS (1961), have called attention to the possibility that the glia may participate much more actively in dynamic neural functioning than is generally assumed.

One item cited by the latter author is the report that selective inhibitors of BuChE produce marked effects on the behavior, electroencephalographic pattern, and amplitude of evoked responses in the cat (DESMEDT and LA GRUTTA 1957). Of possible bearing on the same topic is the recent finding that the spontaneous miniature endplate potentials of skeletal muscle, which disappear simultaneously with the loss of vesicles from the axonal terminals shortly after denervation, reappear a few days later and persist at a much lower frequency than normal (BIRKS et al. 1960). Although the entire surface of the muscle becomes responsive to ACh at this stage (AXELSSON and THESLEFF 1959, MILEDI 1959), the miniature endplate potentials are confined to the site of the original neuromuscular junction, and respond in the normal manner to curarine and neostigmine. Since the Schwann cells of the original teloglia continue to invest the endplate, the authors suggested that the slow liberation of ACh from them is the most likely basis of the post-denervation spontaneous potentials. The possibility has also been suggested that the glial cells of the Schwann sheath may participate in the synthesis of axonal AChE (KOENIG and KOELLE 1961). There are no grounds at present for excluding the glial cells from intimate participation in the possible synaptic mechanisms discussed above.

A decade ago it was generally assumed that most drugs which act at peripheral synaptic or neuroeffector sites do so by combining with the postjunctional receptors, and there mimicking or blocking the effects of endogenous neurohumoral transmitters (GOODMAN and GILMAN 1954). While the concept still seems essentially correct in most cases, there has been a number of reports suggesting that many agents act in addition, or even primarily, at the prejunctional terminals, particularly at the neuromuscular junction (e.g., ABDON and BJARKE 1945, RIKER 1960; see Chapter 13 for extensive discussion). The present proposal of a pre- and postjunctional action of ACh in transmission is by no means inconsistent with such suggestions. Moreover, as a working hypothesis it entails the existence of prejunctional ACh-receptors which should have drug affinities which are similar to, but not necessarily identical with, those at the corresponding postjunctional sites, just as drug affinities vary from one postjunctional cholinoceptive site to another. Accordingly, the proposal suggests a physiological function of the presynaptic ACh-receptors implied by the studies indicating excitatory or inhibitory drug effects at the presynaptic site.

Two final points should be mentioned. It is conceivable that in some cases more than one neurohumoral transmitter may be liberated by the same axonal terminal and act at the postjunctional site (KOELLE 1955). On the other hand, at certain synapses transmission probably occurs without the mediation of a neurohumoral transmitter (FURSHPAN and POTTER 1959).

B. Local hormonal role of ACh

In both cardiac and smooth muscle and in many exocrine gland cells, the concentration of BuChE or other non-specific ChE's generally predominates over that of AChE, as described in preceding sections and as ORD and THOMPSON (1950) have shown quantitatively. A notable exception in the cat is the smooth muscle of the iris and ciliary body, which contains almost exclusively AChE, distributed predominantly at the cell membrane in a pattern resembling that of embryonic skeletal muscle (KOELLE et al. 1952, KUPFER and KOELLE 1951). The effects of anti-ChE agents on isolated intestine have been interpreted to indicate both that the BuChE is (KOELLE et al. 1950), and is not (SHELLEY 1955) significantly involved in the hydrolysis of endogenously liberated ACh. In addition to the ChE's, highly active ChAc systems are probably present in the atrial (BURN and KOTTEGODA 1953, DAY 1956) and intestinal (FELDBERG and LIN 1950) muscle fibers. While both these tissues are under the control of postganglionic cholinergic fibers of the parasympathetic system, there is considerable evidence that they themselves continually liberate ACh, as a "local hormone" which is involved in the maintenance of tone, motility, and rhythmicity (see Chapter 11).

As in skeletal muscle, contraction of both cardiac and smooth muscle is directly preceded, and probably triggered, by propagated spikes or action potentials; these are waves of reversed polarization which are conducted over the syncytium of cardiac muscle, and probably directly from cell to cell at intercellular sites of low resistance in smooth muscle (ICHIKAWA and BOZLER 1955, PROSSER and SPERELAKIS 1956), at rates considerably lower than those of the action potentials of skeletal muscle or nerve. The propagated impulses appear to be initiated by rhythmic fluctuations in the resting potential known as pacemaker potentials; in atrial muscle, the latter arise normally from the region of the sinus (ARVANI-TAKI and CARDOT 1937, HUTTER and TRAUTWEIN 1956, MARSHALL and VAUGHAN WILLIAMS 1956), whereas all intestinal muscle fibers appear to generate such localized potentials, with constant shifting of the dominant site (BÜLBRING 1957/58, HOLMAN 1958). These phenomena occur in the absence of nervous control. In response to increased stretch of smooth muscle, the frequency of discharge of conducted potentials, and presumably of pacemaker potentials, is increased (BOZLER 1948, BÜLBRING 1955). In view of the apparent analogy of the pacemaker potentials to the endplate potentials of skeletal muscle (v.s.), it is tempting to attribute the initiation of the former to the action of locally released ACh. However, there is practically no evidence at present to support this concept, although the actions of ACh and related drugs on atrial and smooth muscle have been investigated extensively (see Chapter 11).

The earliest described effects of ACh or vagal stimulation on *atrial muscle* were an increase in the demarcation or resting potential (GASKELL 1887), an increase in potassium output (HOWELL and DUKE 1908), and a shortening of the conducted action potential (SAMOJLOFF 1914). These findings, which were associated originally only with the cardio-inhibitory action of ACh at the sino-atrial node, have been confirmed repeatedly for atrial fibers by modern techniques (BURGEN and TERROUX 1953, HOFFMAN and SUCKLING 1953, TRAUTWEIN et al. 1956). Long after the discovery of the cardio-inhibitory action of ACh, it was found that the addition of ACh to isolated atria can reinstitute spontaneous contractions after these have ceased following their persistence for 30 to 40 hr *in vitro* (BÜLBRING and BURN 1949), or after their abrupt arrest by quinine (BRISCOE and BURN 1954) or cooling below 20° (MARSHALL and VAUGHAN WILLIAMS 1956). Further analysis of the last mentioned effect showed that cooling produces a dissociation between the localized pacemaker potentials at the sinus region and the conducted potentials; although ACh had no apparent effect on the frequency or height of the pacemaker potentials, it re-established coupling between them and the conducted action potentials. It has been suggested that the uncoupling between these two events following cooling may be the result of the failure of formation of endogenous ACh, since atrial ChAc activity falls off steeply below 21° (i.e., the Q_{10} value between 21° and 17° is over 6) (BURN and MILTON 1959).

The best explanation at present for the mechanism by which ACh sustains atrial contraction appears to be the maintenance or increase of the resting membrane potential, through promotion of its permeability to potassium (HARRIS and HUTTER 1956). The critical value of the transmembrane potential for impulse conduction is in the range of 60 mV, below which the rate of sodium entry is too slow to cause depolarization (WEIDMANN 1955). It falls below this level (as estimated from the internal potassium concentration) when contractions cease after prolonged spontaneous contraction *in vitro* (GOODFORD 1959), or (as measured directly by intracellular recording) after cooling (MARSHALL 1957); in the latter case, ACh was shown to raise the potential concomitantly with the reinstitution of contractions. The action of ACh of increasing the conductance of the membrane (TRAUTWEIN et al. 1956), or more specifically its permeabilitiy to potassium, would tend to raise the transmembrane potential from its previous low level toward the maximum to be expected from the relative intra- and extracellular potassium concentrations (TRAUTWEIN and DUDEL 1958). Likewise, the inhibitory effect of ACh on normally contracting atria could result from its hyperpolarizing, or stabilizing, action by the same mechanism (BURGEN and TERROUX 1953, HOFFMAN and SUCKLING 1953). Acetylcholine-induced atrial arrhythmias also appear to result largely from an increase in potassium permeabilitiy; in this case, the crucial effect is the shortening of the spike and of the corresponding refractory period, which converts the orderly progression of the conducted action potential to a disorganized, irregular propagation throughout the affected region of the atrium (BURN 1957, 1961, BRIGGS and HOLLAND 1960). It is of interest that the latter concept can also be traced back to observations recorded over a century ago (HOFFA and LUDWIG 1850, MCWILLIAM 1887).

In contrast to its hyperpolarizing action on atrial muscle, the primary effect of ACh on *intestinal smooth muscle* is a depolarizing one. The evidence that the ACh which is continually liberated from the intestine (FELDBERG and ROSENFELD 1933) arises mainly from non-nervous sources and acts directly on the smooth muscle fibers is based chiefly on the work of FELDBERG and LIN (1949, 1950). These investigators found that neither the spontaneous output of ACh nor the increase in tone or motility produced by eserine was reduced by high concentrations of cocaine which blocked the response to stimulation of the ganglion cells by nicotine. Likewise, the increase in the frequency of spike discharge and in tension which develop in response to stretch, as mentioned above, are independent of nervous intervention; this was demonstrated by EVANS and SCHILD (1953) by means of various blocking drugs and with ganglion cell-free preparations. Is the response to stretch in the absence of neural control the result of increased liberation of ACh? While this seems possible, direct evidence is lacking. The addition of ACh (10^{-7} to 10^{-6} M) to isolated strips of guinea pig taenia coli causes a fall in the resting potential, followed shortly by the initiation or increase in frequency of spikes, along with an increase in tension. These findings have been obtained with both intracellular recording (BÜLBRING 1955, 1957) and the sucrose gap technique (BURNSTOCK and STRAUB 1958). Initially, the conduction velocity of the spikes is increased, and their individual duration is shortened by ACh; both these effects are reversed within a few minutes (BURNSTOCK 1958). The most likely basis of the total primary effects of ACh on the smooth muscle fibers is an increase in the ionic permeability of the cell membranes. This has been demonstrated for potassium (LEMBECK and STROBACK 1955, BORN and BÜLBRING 1956), and probably applies to other ions as well. It is of interest that action potentials in guinea pig taenia coli still occurred when the sodium concentration of the medium was reduced to very low levels (HOLMAN 1958), but did not persist in its total absence, as occurs with crustacean muscle (FATT and KATZ 1953).

Although the conduction of impulses in smooth muscle is dependent upon depolarization of the cell membrane, apparently the contractile process is not. EVANS et al. (1958) showed that after the complete depolarization of a variety of types of smooth muscle by immersion in potassium-Ringer solution, contractions still occurred, at about one-half the original tension, in response to ACh and other drugs. However, ACh-contractions are no longer obtainable after the removal of calcium; furthermore, ACh causes an increase in calcium-uptake by depolarized smooth muscle in potassium-Ringer solution (ROBERTSON 1960), which is reminiscent of the increased calcium-influx associated with contraction of skeletal muscle (BIANCHI and SHANES 1959). From the foregoing and additional evidence (CSAPO 1960, EDMAN and SCHILD 1961) it is possible that ACh promotes the contraction of smooth muscle both by its depolarizing effect on the cell membrane, and more directly by the mobilization of calcium, which in turn acts on the contractile element.

The means by which a given compound, such as ACh, can produce primarily either depolarization (as in intestinal smooth muscle) or hyperpolarization (as in atrial muscle) has been studied extensively by COOMBS et al. (1955), GRUNDFEST (1957a), BOISTEL and FATT (1958), and ECCLES (1959), among others. That this distinction is the basis of the excitatory and inhibitory effects of a single neurohumoral transmitter at various sites was suggested by BACQ and MONNIER (1935). It is now generally agreed that depolarization (i.e., a fall in the membrane potential), which produces excitation, results from a generalized, non-specific increase in the permeability of the membrane to all ions at the postjunctional or effector site. The production of an increase in permeability to small ions only (e.g., potassium, chloride) results in hyperpolarization, or inhibition. To explain situations where the increase is selective for only small cations or small anions, it has been suggested that this is determined by the charge at the "pores" activated by ACh, e.g., that positively charged pores allow selective passage of chloride, and negatively charged, of potassium ions.

The shift from excitation to inhibition produced by high concentrations or the persistent action of ACh, anti-ChE agents, and related drugs at the motor endplate of skeletal muscle and other sites involves additional factors. Initially, the block is associated with prolonged depolarization (BURNS and PATON 1951); however, where measurements have been made, it has been found that repolarization occurs long before recovery from the block takes place (THESLEFF 1955); hence, the persistence of the block may be the result of the loss of potassium from the endplate and its immediate vicinity, a change in the configuration of the receptors, the relative rates of drug-receptor combination and dissociation (PATON 1961), or other factors. This subject is considered extensively for normal and myasthenic muscle in Chapters 13 and 23.

From the findings described previously (pp. 252-253), it seems highly likely that locally formed ACh has also a regulatory effect on the motility of cilia of the vertebrate respiratory and esophageal tracts (KORDIK et al. 1952, BURN and DAY 1958) and of the gill filaments of the mussel (BÜLBRING et al. 1953). While a similar function has been attributed to ACh and AChE in ciliated and flagellated protozoans, the evidence for this is less convincing.

C. Axonal conduction

The case for the direct participation of ACh and AChE in the conduction of propagated impulses in nerve and skeletal muscle has been presented extensively in Chapter 15, and more fully by the same author in a recent monograph (NACH-MANSOHN 1959). According to this hypothesis, stimulation of the neuron or its axon, or of a striated muscle fiber, anywhere along its length leads to the local liberation of ACh, which in turn produces the changes in membrane permeability resulting in the production of the spike (i.e., the nerve or muscle action potential, NAP or MAP). The surrounding eddy current associated with the inflow of Na^+-ions during the rising phase of the spike is considered to trigger the liberation of ACh at the adjacent portion of the membrane, or at the next node of Ranvier, where the process is repeated; the rapid hydrolysis of ACh by AChE is believed to restore membrane permeability to the resting state. Continuation of this sequence along the nerve or muscle fiber is proposed as the explanation for propagation of the impulse. In the terms of the hypothesis, the same process operates at synapses and neuroeffector sites, where transmission is said to be effected by the direct passage of the current across the gap, with the consequent postjunctional liberation of ACh. Accordingly, any essential distinction between the mechanisms underlying axonal conduction and synaptic transmission is precluded.

The hypothesis may be viewed as embracing two concepts: the direct initiation of the propagated NAP by ACh, and the junctional transmission of excitation by the electric current. Regarding the former, it must be admitted that the most widely accepted present hypothesis for the conduction of the nerve impulse (HODGKIN and HUXLEY 1952) provides no explanation for the mechanism underlying the rapid increase in Na^+-, and immediately thereafter in K^+-permeability associated with the spike. However, it appears unlikely to the present reviewer that this role can be attributed to ACh, or certainly not in all mammalian conducting tissues (v.i.). As to the second concept, one can be more explicit. The evidence now appears overwhelming that junctional transmission at most sites is accomplished by neurohumoral mediators, and moreover, that most postjunctional sites are electrically inexcitable (FATT 1954, DEL CASTILLO and KATZ 1956, GRUNDFEST 1957a). There are several distinct differences between propagated action potentials and localized synaptic or transducer potentials (GRUNDFEST 1959) which can hardly be explained away on the basis of geometrical or diffusion-barrier factors (Chapter 15). Accordingly, a unitary hypothesis of axonal conduction and synaptic transmission seems highly unlikely.

The hypothesis has been questioned in several reviews (DALE 1948, KOELLE and GILMAN 1949, FELDBERG 1956) in addition to those quoted above. Nevertheless, because of its ample presentation and defence in the present volume (Chapter 15), it is considered essential to list also some of the major objections to its component concepts. These fall under five headings, the first two of which refer to the postulated mechanism of axonal conduction, and the last three to junctional transmission.

I. Extreme variations in the concentrations of acetylcholine (ACh), choline acetylase (ChAc), and acetylcholinesterase (AChE) in different types of nerves

NACHMANSOHN (1959, Chapter 15) has stressed that the three identifiable components of the cholinergic system (ACh, ChAc, and AChE) are present in all animal nerves and other conducting tissues. Early reports had indicated the near or complete absence of ACh from the optic nerve (LOEWI and HELLAUER 1938, LISSÁK and PÁSZTOR 1940), dorsal roots (LOEWI and HELLAUER l.c., MACINTOSH 1941), and adrenergic nerves (LISSAK 1939), and of ChAc from the optic nerve and dorsal roots (FELDBERG and MANN 1946, HEBB 1954, WOLFGRAM 1954). The significance of these findings was questioned on the grounds of inadequacy of methods (NACHMANSOHN 1959). However, using the most precise methodology and a system which was presumably adequate in all respects, HEBB and SILVER (1956, Chapter 3) obtained values for ChAc in dorsal roots and optic nerve which ranged from 0 to 6 μg ACh per g fresh tissue per hr; the equivalent values for ventral roots ranged from 2,200 to 5,000. Figures obtained in NACHMANSOHN's laboratory (COHEN 1956) show essentially the same spread, although no zero values were reported; thus, the ratio found for the ChAc activities of ventral roots (ox) to dorsal roots (ox) was 240, and the ratio for the ChAc of the ox ventral roots to that of the dorsal roots of the dog or optic nerve of the rabbit was 3,000 (values for ventral roots of the latter two species not given) (Chapter 15, Table 1).

Differences in AChE activities are considerably less marked, but show the same trend. Here it is essential to use selective inhibitors or substrates, since ACh is hydrolyzed by both AChE and non-specific ChE's, and the latter are present in the Schwann sheath cells of all types of fibers (KOELLE 1951). With methacholine (MeCh) as a specific substrate for AChE, BURGEN and CHIPMAN (1951) found the activity of the ventral roots in the dog to be 4.4 times that of the dorsal roots

and 13.5 times that of the optic nerve. These values correspond well with the
rough approximations obtained by histochemical examination (KOELLE 1951,
1955). However, the particular contribution which the latter approach can offer
is best illustrated by findings on the localization of AChE in cross sections of the
optic nerve of the cat (KOELLE et al. 1952). Here, most of the fibers appeared
essentially unstained, whereas a few (presumably postganglionic fibers from the
ciliary ganglion) were stained intensely. Thus, values obtained for homogenates
of whole nerve trunks reflect only the average values of the individual fibers and
by no means imply that the enzyme is present in all. The same principle obviously
applies to ChAc. It is entirely possible that the low values for the latter enzyme
obtained with optic nerves and dorsal roots are attributable to the autonomic
fibers and ganglion cells which may be present at these sites (BOYD 1957), and
not to the afferent fibers which constitute the great majority.

It should be recalled also that GIACOBINI (1957) failed to detect any AChE
activity in some isolated sympathetic ganglion cells following incubation periods
of eight hours in the Cartesian diver apparatus.

On the other hand, findings obtained with the same ultramicro-method (GIACOBINI and
HOLMSTEDT 1960) have provided quantitative confirmation of the localized concentration of
AChE at the subneural apparatus of skeletal muscle observed histochemically in several
laboratories (see p. 206). On the basis of the figures reported for MeCh-hydrolysis, the minimal
value for AChE obtained at the motor endplate was approximately 50 times that at other
regions of the muscle fiber; since the endplates could not be dissected entirely free of adjacent
material, the actual value for the subneural apparatus is probably considerably higher.

II. Effects of ACh, anti-ChE agents, and other drugs on axons

Several years ago it was found that frog sciatic nerve could be bathed for
several hours in a solution containing a high concentration of ACh without producing depolarization or block of conduction (LORENTE DE NÓ 1944), a result which
subsequently was confirmed essentially with single amphibian fibers (JARRETT
1956) and giant axons (HODGKIN 1947). The significance of the original observation
was discounted on the basis that ACh, as a quaternary compound, would not be
expected to penetrate the sheath (NACHMANSOHN 1946). It was then shown that
no observable effect on conduction in the frog sciatic nerve was produced by DFP
or eserine (the former a highly, and the latter a moderately lipoid-soluble compound) excepting at concentrations (ca. 0.01 M) over 100 times those required
to inactivate all detectable AChE; at such high concentrations, only reversible
block ensued with both agents (CRESCITELLI et al. 1946). Under these conditions
it was found that the demarcation potential was increased, suggesting that DFP
was acting non-specifically as a stabilizing agent, rather than producing block by
prolonging the depolarizing action of endogenous ACh (TOMAN et al. 1947). On
the other hand, NACHMANSOHN and associates (BULLOCK et al. 1946a, b, 1947,
FELD et al. 1948, GRUNDFEST et al. 1947) published several studies on the actions
of anti-ChE agents on conduction from which it was concluded that a parallelism
could be demonstrated between conduction block and AChE inhibition; however,
residual AChE concentrations associated with persistence of normal conduction
in different nerves ranged from scarcely detectable amounts (FELD et al. l.c.) to
over 38% (BULLOCK et al. 1946a). These findings and related ones are discussed
from contrasting viewpoints in Chapter 15 and by KOELLE and GILMAN (1949).

It has been pointed out (DAVSON 1951, FATT and KATZ 1952) that if the block
of conduction produced by anti-ChE agents is the result of preservation of
endogenous ACh, rather than due to non-specific stabilization as suggested above,
the hypothesis would require that the block be preceded by a period of prolonga-

tion of the action potential. Failure to demonstrate this was attributed to an additional action of the drugs, i.e., their combination with ACh-receptors in the membrane, thereby blocking the depolarizing action of accumulated ACh (NACH-MANSOHN 1959). Recently results have been published indicating that eserine produced an increase in spike height and prolongation of the action potential when recordings were taken at a node of Ranvier of an isolated frog nerve fiber (DETT-BARN 1960, Chapter 15, Fig. 4). However, this effect seems scarcely significant in contrast to the enormous prolongation of the postjunctional potentials produced by eserine and other anti-ChE agents at sites of cholinergic transmission, such as the motor endplate (ECCLES et al. 1942, ECCLES and MacFARLANE 1949, FATT and KATZ 1951) and in the spinal cord (ECCLES et al. 1954).

Some recent studies of the actions of ACh and related drugs on the non-medullated fibers of the desheathed rabbit vagus by ARMETT and RITCHIE (1960, 1961) have offered some clarification of this matter.

By means of the sucrose gap technique (STÄMPFLI 1954, STRAUB 1957), these investigators found that the addition of ACh (10^{-4} to 10^{-3} M) to the fluid perfusing the isolated nerve produced a fall in the resting potential, a decrease in the spike height, an increase in the positive after-potential, and a slowing of conduction. At the highest concentration tested, complete block sometimes occurred. Similar effects were obtained with "nicotinic" agents, such as carbachol, tetramethylammonium, and nicotine, but little or no effect was seen after "muscarinic" compounds, including arecoline, pilocarpine, methacholine, and bethanechol. Of the anti-ChE agents (0.01 to 1.0 mg/ml), eserine and neostigmine by themselves had no effect on spike height, and DFP caused a slight reduction. When both ACh and the anti-ChE agents were used at near-threshold concentrations, their effects were additive. However, with increase in the concentration of either, the anti-ChE agents consistently reduced the effects of ACh and, similarly, of carbachol. Likewise, the ACh-effects were reduced or blocked by cholinergic blocking agents (tubocurarine, hexamethonium, atropine) which, with the exception of atropine, when used alone had no effect on spike height.

ARMETT and RITCHIE (1961) emphasized that their results gave no reason to infer that ACh plays a role in axonal conduction, particularly in view of the similar effects of anti-ChE agents on the action of ACh and of carbachol. Rather, they suggested the interpretation that ACh receptors, which are present and functional physiologically at synaptic sites, may occur along the axon in an attenuated form. Hence, the effects noted with both anti-ChE agents and cholinergic blocking agents might be due to their competition with added ACh for occupancy of such sites. This proposal is strengthened by the findings of DIAMOND (1959), who compared the effects of intra-arterial injections of ACh on normal and regenerating nerve trunks. When the actions on their terminals were excluded, ACh never caused firing of normal axons, although KCl consistently did so. However, the regenerating terminals regularly responded to ACh, and the effect was potentiated by eserine and blocked by hexamethonium, just as at fully developed terminals. Thus, in their outward growth during embryonic development, the budding axonal terminals may leave along their length sufficient vestige of their ACh-receptors (which may function at the terminals as proposed in Section A) to yield the pharmacological effects described above.

From the evidence in the two foregoing categories, it is extremely difficult to accept the proposed universal role of ACh in the propagation of action potentials. This does not exclude the possibility that it functions in a related, or supporting capacity in those fibers in which ChAc and AChE are present in high concentrations. Analogy might be drawn here to the apparent function of ACh in maintaining the polarization of myocardial fibers, and in promoting depolarization in certain smooth muscle fibers, as discussed in the preceding section (B). Alternatively, ACh might serve to activate the sodium pump mechanism during the resting stage in certain fibers, as discussed below (section D).

The complement of the hypothesis, that junctional transmission is effected by electronic spread of the impulse across the gap just as along the fiber, appears to be inconsistent with the considerations which follow.

III. Irreducible latent period of synaptic and neuroeffector transmission

As GRUNDFEST (1957a) has pointed out, the latency of the response of electric organs to electrical stimulation was noted at the turn of the century by GOTCH (1900) and GARTEN (1910), both of whom suggested that such organs are not directly excitable electrically. This factor has frequently been presented as an argument favoring neurohumoral as opposed to electrotonic transmission, but the possibility could not be overlooked that the delay was due to a decrease in conduction velocity at the fine preterminal axonal twigs (KUFFLER 1948). However, this reservation seems eliminated by measurements of synaptic delay obtained at the giant synapse of the squid by BULLOCK and HAGIWARA (1957). Here it was possible to insert micropipettes into both the pre- and postsynaptic fibers, so that their tips were approximately 2 mm apart, and simultaneous recordings were obtained following preganglionic stimulation. Under these conditions, there was invariably a delay of 1 to 2 msec between the presynaptic spike and the postsynaptic potential. Since both fibers are of large diameter right up to the synapse, the latency could not be explained by geometric factors, but was considered by the authors as demonstration that transmission could not be electrical.

In sharp contrast to these results are the findings of FURSHPAN and POTTER (1959) at one of the exceptional synapses (between the median giant fiber and the motor axon of the crayfish) where electrical transmission apparently does occur; at this site, no latency could be detected between the presynaptic spike and the postsynaptic potential. As noted by the authors, the difference in transmission characteristics between these synapses of the squid and crayfish is striking in view of their gross structural similarities.

IV. Inability of the nerve terminal to provide sufficient current for activation of the postjunctional site

On the basis of intracellular measurements of the endplate potential and of the electrical capacity of the endplate membrane, it has been calculated by FATT and KATZ (1951) that 10^{-7} coulomb flows through a motor endplate following a single impulse when the AChE is inactivated. As they have pointed out, this would require a net flux of approximately 1 $\mu\mu$mol of univalent ions, an amount considerably in excess of the total ionic content estimated for the nerve terminal. Hence, the local current built up at the endplate could not be derived from the action current of the nerve terminal or directly from the flow of ions from it, but must result from the fall in resistance induced at the postsynaptic membrane by a specifically acting chemical transmitter.

Evidence of the same type was also obtained by BULLOCK and HAGIWARA (l.c.) in the study just quoted. The highest deflection recorded postsynaptically, prior to the postsynaptic potential, which could be attributed to the presynaptic spike was 300 μV; allowing for the decrement due to the distance between the recording electrode and the synapse, this would still represent a maximal directly induced potential of less than 1 mV.

V. Electrical inexcitability of most postjunctional membranes, in contrast to the electrical excitability of conducting membranes

The considerable body of evidence on this point has been reviewed by GRUND-FEST (1957) and associates (BENNETT et al. 1961); an extensive list of references can be found in these publications. While the evidence is essentially indirect, it appears to favor overwhelmingly the interpretation indicated.

The unresponsiveness to electrical stimulation of most postjunctional membranes (and probably of many sensory end-organs) is considered one of the major features which distinguishes them from the conductile membranes of axons and muscle fibers (GRUNDFEST 1959, ECCLES 1959). At postjunctional membranes, appropriate neurohumoral transmitters and other chemicals produce localized, graded potentials (PSP) which may be either depolarizing or hyperpolarizing; if the former type is of sufficient magnitude, it induces electrogenically a propagated spike (NAP or MAP) in the adjacent conductile membrane. So distinctive are the PSP and the NAP that it is reasonable to assume that the chemically and electrically excitable regions have distinguishing morphological and chemical properties; however, none has been described to date from either electron microscopic or histochemical examinations. At various regions there is probably an intermingling or mosaic pattern of the two types of excitable membrane, with varying proportions of each (DEL CASTILLO and KATZ 1956).

An important indication of the electrical inexcitability of most postsynaptic membranes is the irreducible latency discussed in the preceding section; in addition, there are other lines of evidence, such as the failure of antidromic impulses to produce characteristic PSP's in the somata of motoneurons (BROCK et al. 1952) or in the apical dendrites of curarized cortical neurons (PURPURA and GRUNDFEST 1956), and the absence of inward current flow at the endplate region of skeletal muscle, in contrast to that recorded elsewhere in the fiber, during the passage of a conducted spike (WERMAN 1960). That certain slow muscle fibers of the frog are totally inexcitable electrically is indicated by their lack of impulse conduction (KUFFLER and VAUGHAN WILLIAMS 1953b, BURKE and GINSBORG 1956).

Probably the oldest observations contributing to this concept are those of duBOIS-REYMOND (1874, 1881) and GARTEN (1910), who noted that the electric organ of *Torpedo* is unresponsive to electrical stimulation following curarization, fatigue, or denervation. Modern approaches have amply confirmed the apparent electrical inexcitability of the electroplaques of this genus, as well as their responsiveness to ACh (FELDBERG and FESSARD 1942, BENNETT et al. 1961). In this connection it is important to recall that these structures represent a highly specialized evolution of muscle fibers. In some genera (e.g., *Electrophorus*) both the postsynaptic membrane (equivalent to the motor endplate) and the conducting membrane are represented, hence they respond with both a characteristic PSP and a spike (ALTAMIRANO et al. 1955). In others, such as *Torpedo* and *Raia*, only the former is present, and hence only a non-propagated PSP occurs (BROCK et al. 1953, BENNETT et al. l.c.). NACHMANSOHN and his associates (1959, Chapter 5), have published a great volume of extremely valuable work on the properties of the AChE and ChAc systems of electric organs, the interactions of ACh and drugs on isolated electroplaques (SCHOFFENIELS 1959), and more recently on the possible separation and partial isolation of the ACh-receptor substance (EHRENPREIS 1960). However, virtually none of these data can be construed as supporting directly the purported role of ACh in the initiation or propagation of conducted impulses, since all these tissues are composed partially or exclusively of typical locally responding postjunctional membranes. An exceptional case is the electric organ of *Sternarchus albifrons*, which apparently is composed entirely of modified axons; in this organ, no AChE activity could be detected (COUCEIRO and DE ALMEIDA 1959).

D. Membrane permeability and active transport

In the foregoing discussion of the postulated roles of ACh at excitable tissues, including nerve, muscle, and gland cells, its primary action has been assumed consistently to be the modification of the ionic permeability of cellular membranes at critical sites. In extension of this concept, a similar function has been proposed for ACh and AChE at other membranes where excitation does not necessarily occur in the same sense, such as erythrocytes, capillaries, and the placenta. Despite the reasonableness of this assumption, and the considerable amount of work that has been done to demonstrate such a role, relatively little concrete evidence to substantiate it has been obtained to date.

Acetylcholine and AChE have been implicated in the control of both passive permeability and active transport. Evidence has been based largely on the demonstration of the presence of one or both of these moieties in membranous structures, and on the effects of anti-ChE agents on the partitioning of various ions. One of the major reservations against acceptance of the proposed causal relationship from most observations of the latter type has been the excessive concentrations of anti-ChE agents required to produce demonstrable changes in the permeability of erythrocytes and other structures.

I. Erythrocytes

On the basis of (1) the decrease in the permeability of erythrocytes to K^+, Na^+, and hemoglobin obtained after treatment with ACh, (2) the increase in permeability produced by eserine, and (3) the mutually antagonistic effects of the two compounds, GREIG and HOLLAND and their associates proposed that the permeability is regulated by the active hydrolysis of ACh by the AChE of the erythrocyte membrane (GREIG and HOLLAND 1949, HOLLAND and GREIG 1950a, b, LINDVIG et al. 1951). Other groups (TAYLOR et al. 1952, GOODMAN et al. 1955, GALE et al. 1958) have indicated that the concentrations of anti-ChE agents required to modify permeability to K^+ are several magnitudes higher than those which produce complete inhibition of AChE.

On the other hand, THOMPSON and WHITTAKER (1952) found that $10^{-4} M$ Paraoxon or di*iso*propyl phosphorofluoridate (DFP) reduced the passive penetration of Na^+ into erythrocytes, while having no effect on its active transport. The reduction in Na^+ permeability produced by DFP was attributed by DAVSON and MATCHETT (1951) to the same type of non-specific effect which is characteristic of most narcotics; under certain circumstances, the latter agents can cause either an increase or a decrease in the permeability of membranes to various ions (DAVSON 1940, 1943). An alternative explanation of the effects of ACh and eserine was offered by PARPART and HOFFMAN (1952), who found that acetic acid reduced the K^+-permeability of erythrocytes to the same extent as did equivalent concentrations of ACh, and that only the action of the latter was blocked by eserine; they therefore attributed the ACh-effect to the acid produced by its enzymatic breakdown.

That AChE can hardly be a universal factor in the control of permeability of erythrocyte membranes is indicated by its absence from the erythrocytes of certain species, notably those in which it is present in relatively high concentrations in the thrombocytes (ZAJICEK 1957). Similarly, AUDITORE et al. (1959) showed that both the efflux and influx of K^+, along concentration gradients, were within normal limits in human erythrocytes from two cases of paroxysmal nocturnal hemoglobinuria, in one of which erythrocyte AChE was undetectable and in the other extremely low.

Perhaps an even greater obstacle to the acceptance of the proposed role of ACh is the extremely low level of ACh (CHANG and GADDUM 1933) and of ACh-synthesis (QUASTEL et al. 1936, BÜLBRING et al. 1949, MATHIAS and SHEPPARD 1954) which could be detected in the erythrocytes of several species, excepting in one study (HOLLAND and GREIG 1952). On the basis of the maximal rate of ACh-synthesis obtained with human erythrocytes (6.3 μg/g/hr), MATHIAS and SHEPPARD (l.c.) calculated that this amount would be less than 1/50th that required to provide the free energy necessary for the accumulation of potassium against a concentration gradient.

II. Brain

The dependence on ChE of the permeability of cerebral tissue to barbital and chloralose was suggested by GREIG and MAYBERRY (1951) on the basis of the findings that physostigmine increased the rates of onset narcosis and uptake of barbital by the brain following intravenous injection. Physostigmine, neostigmine, and DFP have also been reported to enhance the actions of various central stimulants and depressants in mice (GREEN and DAVIS 1956). On the other hand, STRICKLAND and THOMPSON (1955) found no relationship between the concentrations of several anti-ChE agents required to inactivate completely AChE and pseudo-ChE, and those needed to increase the rate of K^+-leakage from chicken brain slices; in all cases, it took considerably higher amounts to produce the latter effect.

While anti-ChE agents have been found to potentiate both the peripheral and central actions of morphine (SLAUGHTER and GROSS 1940, FLODMARK and WRAMNER 1945), neostigmine did not modify the distribution of free morphine in the blood and cerebral tissues (SZERB and McCURDY 1956). Consequently, the suggestion that morphine possesses a cholinomimetic component among its own actions (SLAUGHTER 1950) seems a more likely basis for the potentiating effect of anti-ChE agents than alteration by the latter of the permeability to morphine of the blood-brain barrier or central neurons.

III. Amphibian skin and skeletal muscle; crab gills

Acetylcholinesterase, or non-specific ChE, has been implicated in the active transport of ions by frog skin (KIRSCHNER 1953), frog skeletal muscle (VAN DER KLOOT 1958), and the gills of the fresh water crab, *Eriocheir sinensis* (KOCH 1954), largely on the basis of the ACh-splitting activity of these tissues, and the modification of ion-transport produced by anti-ChE agents and cholinergic blocking drugs. However, in general the same limitation applies to these cases as to most of those discussed above, namely, the high concentrations of drugs required. Accordingly, there remains the question of whether the drug actions, and hence the mechanism of ion-transport, are related to cholinergic systems, or whether the former are non-specific effects of the type discussed by DAVSON (l.c.).

Tetraethylpyrophosphate, when applied to the inside of *frog skin* at a concentration of $6 \times 10^{-3} M$, was found to cause a transient rise, followed by a complete block of the net influx of Na^+, concomitantly with a marked increase in diffusion resistance (defined as electrical D.C. resistance). Application of atropine to the outside, in concentrations of 3×10^{-3} to $1.5 \times 10^{-2} M$, caused an increase in the Na^+-influx (KIRSCHNER l.c.).

Following the observation that several quaternary ammonium-containing basic dyes, at $10^{-3} M$, interfered reversibly with the uptake of NaCl from the medium by the isolated *gills* of *Eriochier*, KOCH (1954, l.c.) and associates found that the same effect was produced, also reversibly, by either physostigmine ($10^{-3} M$) or DFP ($1.9 \times 10^{-3} M$, but not at $10^{-3} M$); the effect of TEPP ($1.9 \times 10^{-3} M$) was not reversed by washing, but was by choline chloride, $10^{-3} M$. Inasmuch as DFP and TEPP are irreversible anti-ChE agents of several magnitudes' higher potency than the dyes employed (AUGUSTINSSON 1948), these data do not present a convincing case that the effects noted were due to ChE-inhibition.

VAN DER KLOOT (l.c.) found that exposure of *frog sartorius muscles* to $5 \times 10^{-4} M$ hexaethyltetraphosphate (HETP, a mixture of organophosphorous compounds in which TEPP is the chief active ingredient) produced a fall in resting potential, concomitantly with a loss of potassium and a rise in sodium. When the muscles were incubated in low-sodium Ringer solution, sodium extrusion was reduced by prior exposure to HETP, and was reduced reversibly by physostigmine (10^{-4} to $10^{-3} M$). The effects of inhibitors of ChAc were inconsistent. Physostigmine, $10^{-3} M$, also prevented the decrease in the ratio of creatine phosphate to total phosphate which otherwise occurred after soaking the muscles in sodium-deficient

18*

Ringer's solution; from this observation it was inferred that physostigmine acted by blocking the expenditure of energy reserves which normally operate in the extrusion of sodium following reduction in its external concentration. The possibility remains that at the concentrations of drugs employed, both the active extrusion of sodium and the passive efflux of creatine phosphate were interfered with by a mechanism, or mechanisms, other than ChE-inhibition. Nevertheless, these studies appear deserving of further pursuit.

IV. Phosphatidic acid cycle

The most concrete proposal regarding a role of ACh in active transport, which has been supported by a considerable amount of data along several lines, is that of L. E. HOKIN and M. R. HOKIN (1960a, b, M. R. HOKIN et al. 1960).

Earlier studies by these investigators indicated that ACh and related drugs which stimulate pancreatic exocrine secretion caused also an increased incorporation of phosphate-P^{32} into the phospholipids of slices of pancreas, and that the latter effect, like secretion, was blocked by atropine (see Chapter 11). The same phenomenon was then demonstrated with several secretory and neural tissues, in most of which the components chiefly involved were phosphoinositide and phosphatidic acid. The increase produced by ACh (10^{-4} or 10^{-5} M, plus 10^{-4} M eserine) was particularly striking (13-fold) in the case of phosphate incorporation into phosphatidic acid in slices of the avian salt gland (HOKIN and HOKIN 1960b), the NaCl secretion of which is probably activated normally by cholinergic fibers (FÄNGE et al. 1958). In the peripheral nervous system of the cat, the highest values for ACh-activated increases in phosphate incorporation into both phosphatidic acid and phosphoinositide (ranging from 31 to 133% greater than controls) were obtained with sympathetic ganglia and the adrenal medulla (HOKIN et al. 1960). Phosphatidic acid (PA) was shown to be formed through the transfer of a phosphate group from adenosine triphosphate (ATP) to a diglyceride by an enzyme termed diglyceride (DG) kinase; the reverse of this reaction, the splitting off of the phosphate to regenerate DG, was accomplished by phosphatidic acid phosphatase (PAP-ase). Both enzymes were obtained from deoxycholate extracts of microsomes from brain (M.R. HOKIN and L. E. HOKIN 1959) and avian salt glands (HOKIN and HOKIN 1960b) in higher concentrations than from similar extracts of other cellular fractions; as discussed earlier, the microsomal fraction is composed to a large extent of fragments of the endoplasmic reticulum, which in the avian salt gland appears to communicate directly with the exterior of the cell (DOYLE 1960).

On the basis of these findings, HOKIN and HOKIN (1960b) have proposed that a PA cycle functions as the sodium pump in the salt gland and in certain neurons, as diagrammed in Fig. 41. According to this schema, each molecule of PA, synthesized at the cytoplasmic side of the membrane, combines with two sodium ions, which are released at the external surface when the PA is split there by PAP-ase; the phosphate released simultaneously is assumed to be returned to the cytoplasm because of a barrier to its external release. A similar mechanism is considered to be involved in the secretion of positively charged organic molecules by various glandular tissues.

The activating effect of ACh on PA-phosphate incorporation is dependent on the integrity of the subcellular membranes, since it could be obtained with cell-free microsomal preparations, but not after freezing, or in hypertonic solutions, or in deoxycholate extracts, although the activities of DG-kinase and PAP-ase were retained in all cases (L. E. HOKIN and M. R. HOKIN 1959). The authors suggested, therefore, that ACh produces a structural modification in the membrane, perhaps to render DG more accessible to its kinase. This is in keeping with a present general concept as to how most hormones probably affect enzymatic reactions (TEPPERMAN and TEPPERMAN 1960). In view of the limited thickness of the microsomal membranes (ca. 100 Å) and the protein-bound state of most of the phosphatidic acid, it was pointed out that the proposed transport mechanism probably involves folding or rotation of the phospholipid carrier rather than diffusion through the membrane. With regard to the functional significance of the increased turnover of PA and phosphoinositide produced by ACh in nervous tissue, the authors suggested that this is probably a specific effect for activation of the neuronal sodium pump during the resting stage, in addition to and independent of its transmitter function at the same sites.

It has been pointed out that the foregoing evidence, while impressive, is incomplete in certain aspects, such as the mechanism for coupling potassium with sodium transport, and the means for the return of phosphate ion to the cytoplasm (WILBRANDT and ROSENBERG 1961). YOSHIDA et al. (1961) found that ouabain, 10^{-5} M, which blocks ion transport at various cell membranes, caused an approximate tripling of the incorporation of phosphate into the PA of mitochondria,

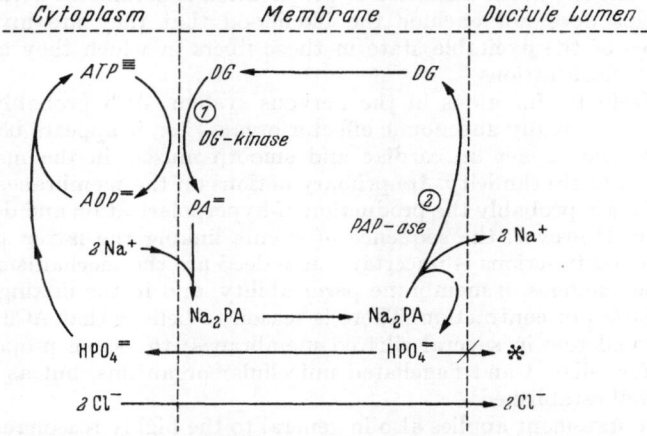

Fig. 41. A schema for the participation of phosphatidic acid as a carrier for the active transport of Na+ ions across the apical membrane of the salt-secreting cell. The scheme is based on a phosphatidic acid-diglyceride cycle catalyzed by enzymes shown to be present in the membrane fraction. The activity of this cycle was found to be greatly increased on stimulation of the tissue with ACh. ATP, adenosine triphosphate; DG, diglyceride; DG-kinase, diglyceride kinase; PA, phosphatidic acid; PAP-ase, phosphatidic acid phosphatase. HPO₄= does not leave the external surface of the membrane (L. E. HOKIN and M. R. HOKIN 1960)

microsomes, and whole slices of guinea pig brain; at the same time it markedly reduced potassium uptake and sodium extrusion, and caused an increase in oxygen uptake. From these findings, and the similar effects on PA turnover produced by potassium, protoveratrine, and ACh, the authors questioned that the phospholipid serves as an ion carrier. On the other hand, TITUS et al. (1961) reported that the same concentration of ouabain caused a transitory increase, followed by a distinct decrease in PA turnover in slices of rabbit brain and several other organs, and that it antagonized the increased PA-phosphate uptake produced by ACh. However, only an increase (18%) in PA turnover was detected with ouabain in slices of sea gull *(L. argentatus)* salt gland. It was suggested that ouabain might act by modifying permeability to phosphate or synthesis of ATP. In spite of these inconsistencies, the concept of the PA cycle presented by the HOKIN's appears to represent both a highly provocative proposal regarding the specific identity of a transport system, and perhaps a true approach to an explanation of a mechanism of action of ACh at the molecular level.

E. Summary and conclusions

In the foregoing discussion, the possible physiological functions of the ACh-AChE system have been considered on the basis of the preceding descriptions of cytological localizations of the latter component, and in the light of information obtained from other methodological approaches. The reviewer has attempted to cite the various proposals as exhaustively as possible and to indicate his own interpretations from consideration of the data which seem most pertinent.

It was concluded that the role of ACh as a neurohumoral transmitter at several synaptic and neuroeffector sites is firmly established. Furthermore, it was proposed that at many junctional regions ACh may act in addition at the presynaptic terminal to effect the liberation of additional quanta of ACh or of other neurohumoral transmitters, in the cases of cholinergic and non-cholinergic neurons, respectively.

From several lines of evidence cited, it appears unlikely that ACh and AChE participate directly in the initiation or propagation of conducted action potentials; however, this does not exclude the likelihood that they are involved in the maintenance of the excitable state in those fibers in which they are present in significant concentrations.

Apart from its functions in the nervous system, ACh probably serves as a local hormone in many autonomic effector organs, i.e., it appears both to be synthesized by and to act on cardiac and smooth muscle in the maintenance of excitability and rhythmicity. Its primary actions on the membranes of these two types of cells are probably the production of hyperpolarization and depolarization, respectively. However, the sequence of events linking the latter actions to the aforementioned functions is uncertain, as indeed are the mechanisms involved in effecting the changes in membrane permeability, and in the linking of the latter to the initiation of contraction. There is reason to believe that ACh has a similar local hormonal role in several ciliated membranes; the same proposal has been advanced for ciliated and flagellated unicellular organisms, but as yet this does not seem well established.

The last statement applies also in general to the highly reasonable suggestions that ACh and AChE may control passive permeability or active transport in several other types of membranes, such as those of erythrocytes and the placenta. The most concrete proposal is that of HOKIN and HOKIN, who have presented evidence that ACh regulates active transport of sodium ions and positively charged organic molecules by a phosphatidic acid system in several glandular and nervous tissues.

It might be noted that from an evolutionary viewpoint, the sequence of presentation which has been used is probably *hysteron-proteron*. With full cognizance of the relative paucity of supporting evidence, it can be surmised that the earliest function of ACh and its associated enzymes in primitive organisms was probably the modification of the passage of various substances across cell membranes. With the development of different types of structural complexity of cellular membranes in accordance with their specialized functions, this role of ACh was retained by many membranes with varying degrees of specificity for particular ions, as for example in cardiac as compared with smooth muscle. In other tissues, this function of ACh may have been lost or replaced by other systems. The highest degree of specialization of the ACh-AChE system itself has been achieved in nervous tissue, where its components and function are concentrated predominantly at junctional sites. At such regions, where the influence of ACh has been extended from a localized to an intercellular one, it may serve both as the trans-junctional mediator of excitation and as the agent for the liberation of other chemical mediators.

At several sites where AChE activity has been demonstrated (e.g., the musculotendinous junctions of skeletal muscle), it was not possible to assign even a tentative function to the enzyme or its substrate. The same may be said of the non-specific ChE's for nearly all their localizations. Further studies may uncover roles at such sites which hitherto have been unsuspected (see Chapters 16, 17, 19). On the other hand, as suggested by the preceding remarks, some sites may represent regions where a function of AChE existed previously but has been lost in the course of phylogenetic development. This suggestion was advanced by MENDEL and associates (1953) with regard to the aliesterases, since their prolonged, nearly complete inhibition had no demonstrable effect on rats of various ages, but interfered with the growth of bacteria, seedlings, and cultures of malignant cells. Furthermore, in the course of ontogenesis AChE may be synthesized at certain sites where its function is evanescent or only potential; the latter suggestion has been mentioned with respect to the possible occurrence of attenuated ACh-receptors along axons in contrast with those at the outgrowing or mature terminals (DIAMOND 1955, ARMETT and RITCHE 1961).

In the chapters (11 to 17) devoted to the pharmacology of the anti-ChE agents, the aforementioned established, speculative, and unknown functions of AChE should be considered in assessing which actions of the individual drugs are dependent on inhibition of AChE activity and which are produced by other mechanisms.

References

AAVIK, O. R.: Cholinesterases in human skin. J. invest. Derm. **24**, 103—106 (1955).
ABDON, N.-O., and T. BJARKE: The mechanism of acetylcholine liberation in striped muscles. Acta pharmacol. (Kbh.) **1**, 1—17 (1945).
ÁBRAHÁM, A.: Über die Struktur und die Endigungen der Aorticusfasern im Aortenbogen des Menschen mit Berücksichtigung der Cholinesterase-Aktivität der Pressorezeptoren. Z. Mikr.-ant. Forsch. **62**, 194—228 (1956).
ABRAHAMS, V. C., G. B. KOELLE and P. SMART: Histochemical demonstration of cholinesterases in the hypothalamus of the dog. J. Physiol. (Lond.) **139**, 137—144 (1957).
—, and M. PICKFORD: The effect of anticholinesterases injected into the supraoptic nuclei of chloralosed dogs on the release of the oxytocic factor of the posterior pituitary. J. Physiol. (Lond.) **133**, 330—333 (1956).
ADAMSTONE, F. B., and A. B. TAYLOR: Rapid preparation of frozen tissue sections. Stain Technol. **23**, 109—116 (1948).
DE ALMEIDA, D. F., and A. COUCEIRO: Resistance to formaldehyde fixation of acetylcholinesterase from the electric tissues and the motor end plate. Ann. Acad. bras. Sci. **27**, 41—47 (1955).
ALTAMIRANO, M., C. W. COATES and H. GRUNDFEST: Mechanism of direct and neural excitability in electroplaques of electric eel. J. gen. Physiol. **38**, 319—360 (1955).
AMBACHE, N.: Unmasking, after cholinergic paralysis by botulinum toxin, of a reversed action of nicotine on the mammalian intestine, revealing the probable presence of local inhibitory ganglion cells in the enteric plexus. Brit. J. Pharmacol. **6**, 51—67 (1951).
ANDERSSON-CEDERGREN, E.: Ultrastructure of motor end plate and sarcoplasmic components of mouse skeletal muscle fiber. J. Ultrastruct. Res., Suppl. **1**, 1—191 (1959).
ANDREWS, T. M., and P. HOLTON: The substance P and adenosinetriphosphate (ATP) contents of sensory nerve on degeneration. J. Physiol. (Lond.) **143**, 45 P—46 P (1958).
ARMETT, C. J., and J. M. RITCHIE: The action of acetylcholine on conduction in mammalian non-myelinated fibres and its prevention by an anticholinesterase. J. Physiol. (Lond.) **152**, 141—158 (1960).
— — The action of acetylcholine and some related substances on conduction in mammalian non-myelinated nerve fibres. J. Physiol. (Lond.) **155**, 372—384 (1961).
ARVANITAKI, A., et H. CARDOT: Tonus automatisme et polarisation du tissu myocardique. Expériences sur l'escargot. Arch. int. Physiol. **45**, 205—240 (1937).
AUDITORE, J. V., R. C. HARTMANN and E. F. COLE: Potassium transport in the acetylcholinesterase-deficient erythrocytes of paroxysmal nocturnal hemoglobinuria (PNH). J. clin. Invest. **38**, 702—706 (1959).
AUGUSTINSSON, K.-B.: Cholinesterases; a study in comparative enzymology. Acta physiol. scand. **15** (Suppl. 52), 1—182 (1948).
— Substrate concentration and specificity of choline ester-splitting enzymes. Arch. Biochem. Biophys. **23**, 111—126 (1949).
—, and A. G. JOHNELS: The acetylcholine system of the electric organ of *Malapterurus electricus*. J. Physiol. (Lond.) **140**, 498—500 (1958).

AVERY, J. K., and R. RAPP: Demonstration of cholinesterase in teeth. Stain Technol. **33**, 31—37 (1958).

AXELSSON, J., and S. THESLEFF: A study of supersensitivity in denervated mammalian skeletal muscle. J. Physiol. (Lond.) **149**, 178—193 (1959).

BACQ, Z. M., et A. M. MONNIER: Recherches sur la physiologie et la pharmacologie du système nerveux autonome. XV. Variations de la polarisation des muscles lisses sous l'influence du système nerveux autonome et de ses mimétiques. Arch. int. Physiol. **40**, 467—484 (1935).

BALLOWITZ, E.: Das elektrische Organ des Afrikanischen Zitterwelses (*Malapterurus electricus* Lacepede). Jena: Fischer 1899.

BARADI, A. F., and G. H. BOURNE: Histochemical localization of cholinesterase in gustatory and olfactory epithelia. J. Histochem. Cytochem. **7**, 2—7 (1959).

BARGMANN, W., and E. SCHARRER: The site of origin of the hormones of the posterior pituitary. Amer. Sci. **39**, 255—259 (1951).

BARRNETT, R. J.: J. biophys. biochem. Cytol. (in press).

—, and G. E. PALADE: Enzymatic activity in the M band. J. biophys. biochem. Cytol. **6**, 163—165 (1959).

—, and A. M. SELIGMAN: Histochemical demonstration of esterases by production of indigo. Science **114**, 579—582 (1951).

BECKETT, E. B., and G. H. BOURNE: Cholinesterase in normal and abnormal human skeletal muscle. J. Neurol. Psychiat. **20**, 191—197 (1957a).

— — The histochemistry of normal and abnormal human muscle. Proc. roy. Soc. Med. **50**, 308—312 (1957b).

— — and W. MONTAGNA: Histology and cytochemistry of human skin. The distribution of cholinesterase in the finger of the embryo and the adult. J. Physiol. (Lond.) **134**, 202—206 (1956).

BELESIN, D., B. RADMANOVIC and V. VARAGIĆ: The effect of substance P on the superior cervical ganglion of the cat. Brit. J. Pharmacol. **15**, 10—13 (1960).

BENNETT, M. V. L., M. WURZEL and H. GRUNDFEST: The electrophysiology of electric organs of marine electric fishes. I. Properties of electroplaques of *Torpedo nobiliana*. J. gen. Physiol. **44**, 757—804 (1961).

BERGNER, A. D.: Histochemical demonstration of the effect of nerve section on cholinesterase activity at motor end plates in the gastrocnemius muscle of the guinea-pig. Brit. J. exp. Path. **38**, 160—163 (1957).

—, and J. J. O'NEILL: A modification of the Koelle technique for use with oximes. J. Histochem. Cytochem. **6**, 72—74 (1958).

BERTRAND, J.: Influence de l'alimentation et du jeune sur la localisation intralobulaire des cholinestérases hépatiques. C. R. Soc. Biol. (Paris) **148**, 1912—1914 (1954).

— Cholinesterases in the salivary glands. C. R. Soc. Biol. (Paris) **149**, 2267—2269 (1955).

BEYER, G., u. T. WENSE: Über den Nachweis von Hormonen in einzelligen Tieren. I. Cholin und Acetylcholin im Paramecium. Pflügers Arch. ges. Physiol. **237**, 417—422 (1936).

BEZNÁK, M.: Mag. Orvosi Arch. **45** (1945).

BIANCHI, C. P., and A. M. SHANES: Calcium influx in skeletal muscle at rest, during activity, and during potassium contracture. J. gen. Physiol. **42**, 803—815 (1959).

BIRKS, R. I., and L. M. BROWN: A method for locating the cholinesterase of a mammalian myoneural junction by electron miscroscopy. J. Physiol. (Lond.) **152**, 5P—7P (1960).

— B. KATZ and R. MILEDI: Physiological and structural changes at the amphibian myoneural junction, in the course of nerve degeneration. J. Physiol. (Lond.) **150**, 145—168 (1960).

—, and F. C. MACINTOSH: Acetylcholine metabolism at nerve-endings. Brit. med. Bull. **13**, 157—161 (1957).

BOEKE, J.: The problem of the interstitial cells in the nervous endformation. Proc. Acad. Sci. Amst. **45**, 208—214 (1942).

BOELL, E. J., P. GREENFIELD and S. C. SHEN: Development of cholinesterase in the optic lobes of the frog *(Rana pipiens)*. J. exp. Zool. **129**, 415—452 (1955).

DU BOIS-REYMOND, E.: Gesammelte Abhandlungen zur allgemeinen Muskel- und Nervenphysik. Leipzig: Veit 1874.

— Dr. CARL SACHS, Untersuchungen am Zitteraal *Gymnotus electricus*. Leipzig: Veit 1881.

BOISTEL, J., and P. FATT: Membrane permeability change during transmitter action in crustacean muscle. J. Physiol. (Lond.) **144**, 176—191 (1958).

BONTING, S. I., and R. M. FEATHERSTONE: Ultramicro assay of the cholinesterases. Arch. Biochem. Biophys. **61**, 89—98 (1956).

BORN, G. V. R., and E. BÜLBRING: The movement of potassium between smooth muscle and the surrounding fluid. J. Physiol. (Lond.) **131**, 690—703 (1956).

BOYD, I. A.: The innervation of mammalian neuromuscular spindles. J. Physiol. (Lond.) **140**, 14P (1958).

BOYD, J. D.: Intermediate sympathetic ganglia. Brit. med. Bull. **13**, 207—212 (1957).

BOZLER, E.: Conduction, automaticity and tonus of visceral muscle. Experientia (Basel) 4, 213—218 (1948).

BRECHT, K., u. M. CORSTEN: Acetylcholin in sensiblen Nerven. Pflügers Arch. ges. Physiol. 245, 160—169 (1942).

BRIGGS, A. H., and W. C. HOLLAND: K^{42} and Cl^{36} fluxes during ACh- and Ca-induced atrial fibrillation. Amer. J. Physiol. 198, 837—840 (1960).

BRIGHTMAN, M. W., and R. W. ALBERS: Species differences in the distribution of extra-neuronal cholinesterases within the vertebrate central nervous system. J. Neurochem. 4, 244—250 (1959).

BRISCOE, S., and J. H. BURN: Quinidine and anticholinesterases on rabbit auricles. Brit. J. Pharmacol. 9, 42—48 (1954).

BROCK, L. G., J. S. COOMBS and J. C. ECCLES: The recording of potentials from motoneurons with an intracellular electrode. J. Physiol. (Lond.) 117, 431—460 (1952).

BROCK, L. G., R. M. ECCLES and R. D. KEYNES: The discharge of individual electroplates in Raia clavata. J. Physiol. (Lond.) 122, 4P (1953).

BROOKS, V. B., and D. K. MYERS: Cholinesterase content of normal and denervated skeletal muscle in the guinea-pig. J. Physiol. (Lond.) 116, 158—167 (1952).

BROWN, G. L., and J. E. PASCOE: The effect of degenerative section of ganglionic axons on transmission through the ganglion. J. Physiol. (Lond.) 123, 565—573 (1954).

BROWN, L. M.: Cholinesterase in the superior cervical ganglion of the rat after preganglionic denervation and axotomy. J. Physiol. (Lond.) 142, 7P—8P (1958).

— A thiocholine method for locating cholinesterase activity by electron microscopy. Histochemistry of Cholinesterase, Symposium, Basel, 1960. Bibl. anat. 2, 21—33 (1961).

BRZIN, M., and J. ZAJICEK: Quantitative determination of cholinesterase activity in individual end-plates of normal and denervated gastrocnemius muscle. Nature (Lond.) 181, 626 (1958).

BÜLBRING, E.: Correlation between membrane potential, spike discharge and tension in smooth muscle. J. Physiol. (Lond.) 128, 200—221 (1955).

— Changes in configuration of spontaneously discharged spike potentials from smooth muscle of the guinea-pig's taenia coli. The effect of electrotonic currents and of adrenaline, acetylcholine and histamine. J. Physiol. (Lond.) 135, 412—425 (1957).

— Physiology and pharmacology of intestinal smooth muscle. Lectures on the Scientific Basis of Medicine 7, 374—397 (1957/58).

— The intrinsic nervous system of the intestine and local effects of 5-hydroxytryptamine. Proc. Fourth Internat. Neurochem. Symp., Varenna, Italy. Regional Neurochemistry, pp. 437—441. Pergamon Press, 1961.

—, and J. H. BURN: Action of acetylcholine on rabbit auricles in relation to acetylcholine synthesis. J. Physiol. (Lond.) 108, 508—524 (1949).

— — and H. SHELLEY: Acetylcholine and ciliary movement in the gill plates of Mytilus edulis. Proc. roy. Soc., Ser. B 141, 445—466 (1953).

— G. BURNSTOCK and M. E. HOLMAN: Excitation and conduction in the smooth muscle of the isolated taenia coli of the guinea-pig. J. Physiol. (Lond.) 142, 420—437 (1958).

— E. M. LOURIE and U. PARDOE: Presence of acetylcholine in Trypanosoma rhodesiense and its absence from Plasmodium gallinaceum. Brit. J. Pharmacol. 4, 290—294 (1949).

BULLOCK, T. H., H. GRUNDFEST, D. NACHMANSOHN, M. A. ROTHENBERG and K. STERLING: Effect of di-isopropyl fluorphosphate (DFP) on action potential and choline esterase of nerve. J. Neurophysiol. 9, 253—260 (1946a).

— — — — Effect of di-isopropyl fluorphosphate (DFP) on action potential and cholinesterase of nerve, II. J. Neurophysiol. 10, 63—78 (1947).

—, and S. HAGIWARA: Intracellular recording from the giant synapse of the squid. J. gen. Physiol. 40, 565—577 (1957).

— D. NACHMANSOHN and M. A. ROTHENBERG: Effects of inhibitors of choline esterase on the nerve action potential. J. Neurophysiol. 9, 9—22 (1946b).

BURGEN, A. S. V., and L. M. CHIPMAN: Cholinesterase and succinic dehydrogenase in the central nervous system of the dog. J. Physiol. (Lond.) 114, 296—305 (1951).

— — The location of cholinesterase in the central nervous system. Quart. J. exp. Physiol. 37, 61—74 (1952).

—, and K. G. TERROUX: On the negative inotropic effect in cat's auricle. J. Physiol. (Lond.) 120, 449—464 (1953).

BURKE, W., and B. L. GINSBORG: The electrical properties of the slow muscle fibre membrane. J. Physiol. (Lond.) 132, 586—598 (1956).

BURN, J. H.: Acetylcholine and cardiac fibrillation. Brit. med. Bull. 13, 181—184 (1957).

— The cause of fibrillation. Canad. med. Ass. J. 84, 625—627 (1961).

—, and M. DAY: The action of tubocurarine and acetylcholine on ciliary movement. J. Physiol. (Lond.) 141, 520—526 (1958).

BURN, J. H., and S. R. KOTTEGODA: Action of eserine on the auricles of the rabbit heart. J. Physiol. (Lond.) **121**, 360—373 (1953).
—, and A. S. MILTON: Choline acetylase activity in the atria and its possible relation to the maintenance of the membrane potential. Brit. J. Pharmacol. **14**, 493—496 (1959).
—, and M. J. RAND: Noradrenaline in artery walls and its dispersal by reserpine. Brit. med. J. **1958** I, 903—908.
— — The cause of the supersensitivity of smooth muscle to noradrenaline after sympathetic degeneration. J. Physiol. (Lond.) **147**, 135—143 (1959).
— — Sympathetic postganglionic cholinergic fibers. Brit. J. Pharmacol. **15**, 56—66 (1960).
BURNS, B. D., and W. D. M. PATON: Depolarization of the motor end-plate by decamethonium and acetylcholine. J. Physiol. (Lond.) **115**, 41—73 (1951).
BURNSTOCK, G.: The effects of acetylcholine on membrane potential, spike frequency, conduction velocity and excitability in the taenia coli of the guinea-pig. J. Physiol. (Lond.) **143**, 165—182 (1958).
—, and M. E. HOLMAN: The transmission of excitation from autonomic nerve to smooth muscle. J. Physiol. (Lond.) **155**, 115—133 (1961).
—, and R. W. STRAUB: A method for studying the effects of ions and drugs on the resting and action potentials in smooth muscle with external electrodes. J. Physiol. (Lond.) **140**, 156—167 (1958).
CAESAR, R., A. EDWARDS and H. RUSKA: Architecture and nerve supply of mammalian smooth muscle tissue. J. biophys. biochem. Cytol. **3**, 867—878 (1957).
CANNON, W. B.: Law of denervation (Hughlings Jackson memorial lecture). Amer. J. med. Sci. **198**, 737—750 (1939).
CAUNA, N.: The mode of termination of the sensory nerves and its significance. J. comp. Neurol. **113**, 169—210 (1959).
— The distribution of cholinesterase in the cutaneous receptor organs, expecially touch corpuscles of the human finger. J. Histochem. Cytochem. **8**, 367—375 (1960).
— Cholinesterase activity in cutaneous receptors of man and of some quadrupeds. Histochemistry of Cholinesterase, Symposium, Basel, 1960. Bibl. anat. **2**, 128—138 (1961).
—, and G. MANNAN: The structure of human digital Pacinian corpuscles (corpuscula lamellosa) and its functional significance. J. Anat. (Lond.) **92**, 1—20 (1958).
— — Development of postnatal changes of digital Pacinian corpuscles (corpuscula lamellosa) in the human hand. J. Anat. (Lond.) **93**, 271—286 (1959).
— N. T. NAIK, D. B. LEAMING and P. ALBERTI: The distribution of cholinesterases in the autonomic ganglia of man and of some mammals. Histochemistry of Cholinesterase, Symposium, Basel, 1960. Bibl. anat. **2**, 90—96 (1961).
—, and L. L. ROSS: The fine structure of Meissner's touch corpuscles of human fingers. J. biophys. biochem. Cytol. **8**, 467—482 (1960).
CAVANAGH, J. B., R. H. THOMPSON and G. R. WEBSTER: The localization of pseudo-cholinesterase activity in nervous tissue. Quart. J. exp. Physiol. **39**, 185—197 (1954).
CHACKO, L. W., and J. A. CERF: Histochemical localization of cholinesterase in the amphibian spinal cord and alterations following ventral root section. J. Anat. (Lond.) **94**, 74—81 (1960).
CHAGAS, C., and A. PAES-DE-CARVALHO (Eds.): Bioelectrogenesis. A comparative survey of its mechanisms, which particular emphasis on electric fishes. Amsterdam: Elsevier Publ. Co. 1961.
— E. PENNA-FRANCA, A. HASSÓN, C. CROCKER, K. NISHIE and E. J. GARCIA: Studies of the mechanisms of curarisation. Ann. Acad. bras. Sci. **29**, 53—62 (1957).
CHANG, H. C., and J. H. GADDUM: Choline esters in tissue extracts. J. Physiol. (Lond.) **79**, 255—285 (1933).
CHANG, V., and M. J. RAND: Transmission failure in sympathetic nerves produced by hemicholinium. Brit. J. Pharmacol. **15**, 588—600 (1960).
CHURCHILL, J. A., H. F. SCHUKNECHT and R. DORAN: Acetylcholinesterase activity in the cochlea. Laryngoscope (St. Louis) **66**, 1—15 (1956).
CLODIUS, L.: Über das Verhalten der Azetylcholinesterase der Endplatte nach Durchtrennung des motorischen Nerven. Schweiz. Arch. Neurol. Psychiat. **81**, 1—10 (1958).
COERS, C.: La détetion histochimique de la cholinestérase au niveau de la jonction neuromusculaire. Rev. belge Path. **22**, 306—315 (1953).
— La localisation histochimique de la cholinestérase dans les fuseaux neuro-musculaires. Bull. Acad. Cl. Sci. Belg. 1000—1002, Nov. 6 (1954).
— Les variations structurelles normales et pathologiques de la jonction neuromusculaire. Acta neurol. belg. **55**, 741—866 (1955a).
— Aspects histologiques de la régénération neuromusculaire au cours de diverses affections du neurone moteur périphérique (régénération collaterale chez l'homme). Acta neurol. belg. **55**, 23—30 (1955b).

Coërs, C.: Application de la méthode de Koelle à l'étude histologique de la jonction neuro-musculaire normale et pathologique. Histochemistry of Cholinesterase, Symposium, Basel, 1960. Bibl. anat. **2**, 139—152 (1961).

—, and J. E. Desmedt: Mise en évidence d'une malformation caractéristique de la jonction neuro-musculaire dans la myasthénie. Acta neurol. belg. **59**, 539—561 (1959).

—, and J. Durand: Données morphologiques nouvelles sur l'innervation des fuseaux neuro-musculaires. Arch. Biol. (Paris) **67**, 685—715 (1956).

—, and A. Z. Woolf: The Innervation of Muscle: A Biopsy Study. Springfield, Illinois: Charles C. Thomas 1959.

Cohen, J. A., and C. H. Posthumus: Mechanism of action of anti-cholinesterases. Acta physiol. pharm. néerl. **4**, 17—36 (1955).

— — The mechanism of action of anti-cholinesterases. III. The action of anti-cholinesterases on the phrenic nerve-diaphragm preparation of the rat. Acta physiol. pharm. néerl. **5**, 385—397 (1957).

Cohen, M.: Concentration of choline acetylase in conducting tissue. Arch. Biochem. **60**, 284—296 (1956).

Cole, W. V.: Motor endings in the striated muscle of vertebrates. J. comp. Neurol. **102**, 671—715 (1955).

Comline, R. S.: Synthesis of acetylcholine by non-nervous tissue. J. Physiol. (Lond.) **105**, 6 P—7 P (1947).

Coombs, J. S., D. R. Curtis and J. C. Eccles: The generation of impulses in motoneurones. J. Physiol. (Lond.) **139**, 232—249 (1957).

— J. C. Eccles and P. Fatt: The specific ionic conductances and the ionic movements across the motoneuronal membrane that produce the inhibitory post-synaptic potential. J. Physiol. (Lond.) **130**, 326—373 (1955).

Cooper, S., and P. M. Daniel: Human muscle spindles. J. Physiol. (Lond.) **133**, 1 P (1956).

Cooper, T., J. W. Gilbert Jr., R. D. Bloodwell and J. R. Crout: Chronic extrinsic cardiac denervation by regional neural ablation. Description of the operation, verification of the denervation, and its effects on myocardial catecholamines. Circ. Res. **9**, 275—281 (1961).

Corssen, G., and C. R. Allen: Acetylcholine: its significance in controlling ciliary activity of human respiratory epithelium in vitro. J. appl. Physiol. **14**, 901—904 (1959).

Cotson, S., and S. J. Holt: Studies in enzyme cytochemistry. IV. Kinetics of aerial oxidation of indoxyl and some of its halogen derivatives. Proc. roy. Soc., Ser. B **148**, 506—519 (1958).

Couceiro, A., and D. F. de Almeida: The electrogenic tissue of some *Gymnotidae*. In C. Chagas and A. Paes-de-Carvelho, Eds., Bioelectrogenesis, 3—13. Amsterdam: Elsevier Publishing Co. 1961.

— — and J. R. C. Freire: Localisation histochimique de l'acetylcholinestérase dans le tissue électrique de l'électrophorus electricus (L). Ann. Acad. bras. Sci. **25**, 205—214 (1953).

— — and M. Miranda: The presence of cholinesterase in the electric tissue of electrophorus electricus by the myristoylcholine method of Gomori. Ann. Acad. bras. Sci. **27**, 49—54 (1955).

Coupland, R. E., and R. L. Holmes: The distribution of cholinesterase in the adrenal glands of the rat, cat and rabbit. J. Physiol. (Lond.) **141**, 97—106 (1958).

Couteaux, R.: Contribution à l'étude de la synapse myoneurale; buisson de Kühne et plaque motrice. Rev. canad. Biol. **6**, 563—711 (1947).

— Remarques sur les méthodes actuelles de détection histochimique des activités cholin-estérasiques. Arch. int. Physiol. **59**, 526—537 (1951).

— Le système moteur à «petites» fibres nerveuses et à contraction «lente»: contribution à son identification histologique sur les muscles de la grenouille. Extrait des Comptes Rendus de l'Association des Anatomistes, XXXIX Réunion, pp. 1—6, 7—9 April. Cler-mont-Ferrand, 1952.

— Particularités histochimiques des zones d'insertion du muscle strié. C. R. Soc. Biol. (Paris) **147**, 1974—1976 (1953).

— Morphological and cytochemical observations on the post-synaptic membrane at motor end-plates and ganglionic synapses. Exp. Cell Res. (Suppl.) **5**, 294—322 (1958).

— Remarques sur la distribution des activités cholinestérasiques dans les muscles striés de l'Hippocampe. Histochemistry of Cholinesterase, Symposium, Basel, 1960. Bibl. anat. **2**, 207—219 (1961).

—, and T. Szabo: Siège de la jonction nerf-électroplaque dans les organs électriques à électroplaques pediculées. C. R. Acad. Sci. (Paris) **248**, 457—460 (1959).

—, et J. Taxi: Recherches histochimiques sur la distribution des activités cholinestérasiques au niveau de la synapse myoneurale. Arch. Anat. micr. Morph. exp. **41**, 352—392 (1952).

Craigie, E. H.: An Introduction to the Finer Anatomy of the Central Nervous System Based Upon that of the Rat. Philadelphia: P. Blakiston's Son and Co. 1925.

Crescitelli, F., G. B. Koelle and A. Gilman: Transmission of impulses in peripheral nerves treated with di-isopropyl fluorophosphate (DFP). J. Neurophysiol. **9**, 241—252 (1946).

CREVIER, M., and L. F. BÉLANGER: Simple method for histochemical detection of esterase activity. Science **122**, 256 (1955).
— — Étude quantitative de l'activité cholinestérasique de la plaque motrice par voie d'histophotometrie. Canad. J. Biochem. **34**, 869—881 (1956).
CROXATTO, H., F. HUIDOBRO, R. CROXATTO et H. SALVESTRINI: Action cholinestérasique du sang veineux pendant l'excitation musculaire directe et indirecte. C. R. Soc. Biol. (Paris) **130**, 236—240 (1939).
CSAPO, A.: Molecular Structure and Function of Smooth Muscle, Vol. I. New York-London: Academic Press 1960.
CSILLIK, B.: Contributions to the development of the myoneural synapses. Ontogenetic aspects of the subneural apparatus. Z. Zellforsch. **52**, 150—162 (1960).
— Cholinesterase active myoneural structures of alpha and gamma efferent fibres. Histochemistry of Cholinesterase, Symposium Basel, 1960. Bibl. anat. **2**, 161—173 (1961).
—, and G. SÁVAY: Cholinesterase activity of sensory nerve endings. A histochemical study. Acta physiol. Acad. Sci. hung. **6**, 379—384 (1954).
— — Die Regeneration der subneuralen Apparate der motorischen Endplatten. Acta neuroveg. (Wien) **19**, 41—52 (1958).
— I. SCHNEIDER u. G. KÁLMÁN: Über die histochemische Struktur tetanischer und tonischer myoneuraler Synapsen. Acta neuroveg. (Wien) **22**, 212—224 (1961).
D'AGOSTINI, N., e B. ROSSATTI: La localizzazione istochimica della colinesterasi specifica nel tessuto linfatico del gatto. Boll. Soc. ital. Biol. sper. **32**, 1534—1536 (1956).
— — The histochemical localization of specific cholinesterase in the lymphatic tissue of mammals. J. Anat (Lond.) **93**, 354—360 (1959).
— — Histochemical features of acetylcholinesterase activity in the lymphatic tissue of man and other mammals. Histochemistry of Cholinesterase, Symposium, Basel, 1960. Bibl. anat. **2**, 236—242 (1961).
DALE, H. H.: Symposium on transmission of effects from the endings of nerve fibres. Nature (Lond.) **162**, 558—560 (1948).
— Junctional transmission of nervous effects by chemical agents. Proc. Mayo Clin. **30**, 5—20 (1955).
DAVIES, D. R.: Cholinesterases and the mode of action of some anticholinesterases. J. Pharm. (Lond.) **6**, 1—26 (1954).
DAVIS, B. J.: Histochemical demonstration of erythrocyte esterases. Proc. Soc. exp. Biol. (N. Y.) **101**, 90—93 (1959).
DAVSON, H.: Ionic permeability. The comparative effects of environmental changes on the permeability of the cat erythrocyte membrane to sodium and potassium. J. cell comp. Physiol. **15**, 317—330 (1940).
— The effects of narcotic substances on permeability. In: The Permeability of Natural Membranes, by H. DAVSON and J. F. DANIELLI, Chapter XVI, 245—257. New York: Macmillan Co. 1943.
— A Textbook of General Physiology. London: Churchill 1951.
—, and P. A. MATCHETT: The non-specific narcotic action of DFP. J. cell. comp. Physiol. **37**, 501—503 (1951).
DAY, M.: The release of substances like acetylcholine and adrenaline by the isolated rabbit heart. J. Physiol. (Lond.) **134**, 558—568 (1956).
DEANE, H. W., R. J. BARRNETT u. A. M. SELIGMAN: Handbuch der Histochemie. Vol. VII, Enzymes. Stuttgart: Gustav Fischer Verlag 1960.
DE CASTRO, F.: Creation of a reflex arc in the sympathetic chain, by anastomosing it with the afferent root of the vagus. New ideas on the synapse. Trab. Inst. Cajal. Invest. biol. **34**, 217—301 (1942).
— Aspects anatomiques de la transmission synaptique ganglionnaire chez les mammifères. Arch. int. Physiol. **59**, 479—525 (1951).
DE DUVE, C., and J. BERTHET: The use of differential centrifugation in the study of tissue enzymes. Int. Rev. Cytol. **3**, 225—275 (1954).
DEJARDIN, M.: Les cholinestérases dans la glande thyroide du cobaye. C. R. Soc. Biol. (Paris) **149**, 621—622 (1955).
DEL CASTILLO, J., and B. KATZ: On the localization of acetylcholine receptors. J. Physiol. (Lond.) **128**, 157—181 (1955).
— — Biophysical aspects of neuro-muscular transmission. In: J. A. V. BUTLER, Ed., Progress in Biophysics and Biophysical Chemistry, vol. VI, 122—170. London: Pergamon Press. 1956.
DEMPSHER, J., and W. K. RIKER: The role of acetylcholine in virus-infected sympathetic ganglia. J. Physiol. (Lond.) **139**, 145—156 (1957).
— T. TOKUMARU and J. ZABARA: A possible role of an inhibitory system in virus-infected sympathetic ganglia of the rat. J. Physiol. (Lond.) **146**, 428—437 (1959).

DENZ, F. A.: On the histochemistry of the myoneural junction. Brit. J. exp. Path. 34, 329—339 (1953).
DE ROBERTIS, E.: Submicroscopic morphology and function of the synapse. Exp. Cell Res. (Suppl.) 5, 347—369 (1958).
DE SANDRE, V. G., u. G. GHIOTTO: Über die Bedeutung der Acetylcholinesterase der Erythrocyten. Helv. med. Acta 25, 235—241 (1958).
DESMEDT, J. E., and G. LA GRUTTA: The effect of selective inhibition of pseudo-cholinesterase on the spontaneous and evoked activity of the cat's cerebral cortex. J. Physiol. (Lond.) 136, 20—40 (1957).
DETTBARN, W. D.: New evidence for the role of acetylcholine in conduction. Biochim. biophys. Acta 41, 377—386 (1960).
DIAMOND, J.: Observations on the excitation by acetylcholine and by pressure of sensory receptors in the cat's carotid sinus. J. Physiol. (Lond.) 130, 513—532 (1955).
— The effects of injecting acetylcholine into normal and regenerating nerves. J. Physiol. (Lond.) 145, 611—629 (1959).
DIKSHIT, B. B.: Action of acetylcholine on the brain and its occurrance therein. J. Physiol. (Lond.) 80, 409—421 (1934).
DONHOFFER, A.: Feinere Lokalisation verschiedener Cholinesterasen der nervösen Darmgeflechte. Acta morph. Acad. Sci. hung. 8, 375—379 (1959).
DOUGLAS, W. W.: Is there chemical transmission at chemoreceptors? Pharmacol. Rev. 6, 81—83 (1954).
— D. W. LYNWOOD and R. W. STRAUB: On the excitant effect of acetylcholine on structures in the preganglionic trunk of the cervical sympathetic: with a note on the anatomical complexities of the region. J. Physiol. (Lond.) 153, 250—264 (1960).
DOUNCE, A. L.: Enzyme studies on isolated cell nuclei of rat liver. J. biol. Chem. 147, 685—698 (1943).
DOYLE, W. L.: The principal cells of the salt-gland of marine birds. Exp. Cell. Res. 21, 386—393 (1960).
DUKE, H. N., M. PICKFORD and J. A. WATT: The immediate and delayed effects of di-isopropylfluorophosphate injected into the supraoptic nuclei of dogs. J. Physiol. (Lond.) 111, 81—88 (1950).
DUMONT, L.: Localisations histochimiques des cholinestérases dans le pancréas. C. R. Soc. Biol. (Paris) 149, 736—737 (1955a).
— Localisation histochimique d'acétylcholinestérase dans la thyroide de lapin. C. R. Acad. Sci. (Paris) 240, 1946—1948 (1955b).
— Localisations histochimiques d'acétylcholinestérase dans la rate et les ganglions lymphatiques. C. R. Soc. Biol. (Paris) 149, 960—964 (1955c).
— Localisation histochimique d'acétylcholinestérase dans l'adénohypophyse du lapin. C. R. Acad. Sci. (Paris) 242, 296—298 (1956a).
— Localisation histochimique de la cholinestérase dans l'adénohypophyse du cobaye. C. R. Soc. Biol. (Paris) 150, 728—732 (1956b).
— Histochemical localization of acetylcholinesterase in the nodal regions of the mammalian heart. Ann. Histochem. 2, 19—26 (1957).
—, et M. DROUIN: Histochemical determination of acetyl-cholinesterase in the myocardium. C. R. Acad. Sci. (Paris) 238, 274—277 (1954).
ECCLES, J. C.: The nature of synaptic transmission in a sympathetic ganglion. J. Physiol. (Lond.) 103, 27—54 (1944).
— Excitatory and inhibitory synaptic action. Ann. N. Y. Acad. Sci. 81/2, 247—264 (1959).
— R. M. ECCLES and P. FATT: Pharmacological investigations of a central synapse operated by acetylcholine. J. Physiol. (Lond.) 131, 154—169 (1956).
— P. FATT and K. KOKETSU: Cholinergic and inhibitory synapses in a pathway from motoraxon collaterals to motoneurones. J. Physiol. (Lond.) 126, 524—562 (1954).
— B. KATZ and S. W. KUFFLER: Effect of eserine on neuromuscular transmission. J. Neurophysiol. 5, 211—230 (1942).
—, and S. W. KUFFLER: The endplate potential during and after the muscle spike potential. J. Neurophysiol. 4, 486—506 (1941).
—, and W. V. MACFARLANE: Actions of anti-cholinesterases on endplate potential of frog muscle. J. Neurophysiol. 12, 59—80 (1949).
ECCLES, R. M.: Responses of isolated curarized sympathetic ganglia. J. Physiol. (Lond.) 117, 196—217 (1952).
EDMAN, K. A. P., and H. O. SCHILD: Interaction of acetylcholine, calcium and depolarization in the contraction of smooth muscle. Nature (Lond.) 190, 350—352 (1961).
EDWARDS, G. A., H. RUSKA, P. DE S. SANTOS and A. VALLEJO-FREIRE: Comparative cytophysiology of striated muscle with special reference to the role of the endoplasmic reticulum. J. biophys. biochem. Cytol. (Suppl.) 2, 143—156 (1956).

EHRENPREIS, S.: Isolation and identification of the acetylcholine receptor protein of electric tissue. Biochim. biophys. Acta **44**, 561—577 (1960).

EICHNER, D.: Zur Histologie und Topochemie der Netzhaut des Menschen. Z. Zellforsch. **48**, 137—186 (1958).

ELLIS, R. A.: Cholinesterases in the mammalian tongue. J. Histochem. Cytochem. **7**, 156—163 (1959).

ELLMAN, G. L., K. D. COURTNEY, V. ANDRES Jr. and R. M. FEATHERSTONE: A new and rapid colorimetric determination of acetylcholinesterase activity. Biochem. Pharmacol. **7**, 88—95 (1961).

EL-RAKHAWY, M. T., and G. H. BOURNE: Cholinesterases in the human tongue. Histochemistry of Cholinesterase, Symposium, Basel, 1960. Bibl. anat. **2**, 243—255 (1961).

EMMELIN, N., and F. C. MACINTOSH: The release of acetylcholine from perfused sympathetic ganglia and skeletal muscles. J. Physiol. (Lond.) **131**, 477—496 (1956).

ENGEL, W. K.: Cytological localization of cholinesterase in cultured skeletal muscle cells. J. Histochem. Cytochem. **9**, 66—72 (1961).

ERÄNKÖ, O.: Differential demonstration of acetylcholinesterase and nonspecific cholinesterase in the adrenal medulla of the rat. Nature (Lond.) **182**, 183—184 (1958).

VON EULER, U. S.: Identification of the sympathomimetic ergone in adrenergic nerves of cattle (sympathin N) with laevo-noradrenaline. Acta physiol. scand. **16**, 63—74 (1948).

—, and A. PURKHOLD: Effect of sympathetic denervation on the noradrenaline and adrenaline content of the spleen, kidney, and salivary glands in the sheep. Acta physiol. scand. **24**, 212—217 (1951).

EVANS, D. H. L., and H. O. SCHILD: The reactions of plexus-free circular muscle of cat jejunum to drugs. J. Physiol. (Lond.) **119**, 376—399 (1953).

— — and S. THESLEFF: Effects of drugs on depolarized plain muscle. J. Physiol. (Lond.) **143**, 474—485 (1958).

EWINS, A. J.: Acetylcholine; a new active principle of ergot. Biochem. J. **8**, 44—49 (1914).

EYZAGUIRRE, C., and S. W. KUFFLER: Processes of excitation in the dendrites and in the soma of single isolated nerve cells of the lobster and crayfish. J. gen. Physiol. **39**, 87—119 (1955).

FÄNGE, R., K. SCHMIDT-NIELSEN and M. ROBINSON: Control of secretion from the avian salt gland. Amer. J. Physiol. **195**, 321—326 (1958).

FATT, P.: Biophysics of junctional transmission. Physiol. Rev. **34**, 674—710 (1954).

—, and B. KATZ: An analysis of the end-plate potential recorded with an intra-cellular electrode. J. Physiol. (Lond.) **115**, 320—370 (1951).

— — Some problems of neuro-muscular transmission. In: Cold Spring Harbor Symposia on Quantitative Biology, vol. XVII (The Neuron). Lancaster, Pennsylvania: The Science Press 1952.

— — The electrical properties of crustacean muscle fibres. J. Physiol. (Lond.) **120**, 171—204 (1953).

FEINDEL, W., J. R. HINSHAW and G. WEDDELL: The pattern of motor innervation in mammalian striated muscle. J. Anat. (Lond.) **86**, 35—48 (1952).

FELD, E. A., H. GRUNDFEST, D. NACHMANSOHN and M. A. ROTHENBERG: Effect of di-isopropyl fluorophosphate (DFP) on action potential and cholinesterase of nerve. IV. J. Neurophysiol. **11**, 125—132 (1948).

FELDBERG, W.: Present views on the mode of action of acetylcholine in the central nervous system. Physiol. Rev. **25**, 596—642 (1945a).

— Synthesis of acetylcholine by tissue of the central nervous system. J. Physiol. (Lond.) **103**, 367—402 (1945b).

— Some aspects in pharmacology of central synaptic transmission. Arch. int. Physiol. **59**, 544—560 (1951).

— Central and sensory transmission. Pharmacol. Rev. **6**, 85—93 (1954).

— Acetylcholine. In: D. RICHTER, Ed., Metabolism of the Nervous System, 493—510. London: Pergamon Press 1956.

—, and A. FESSARD: The cholinergic nature of the nerves to the electric organ of the *Torpedo (Torpedo marmorata)*. J. Physiol. (Lond.) **101**, 200—216 (1942).

—, and R. C. Y. LIN: The effect of cocaine on the acetylcholine output of the intestinal wall. J. Physiol. (Lond.) **109**, 475—487 (1949).

— — Synthesis of acetylcholine in the wall of the digestive tract. J. Physiol. (Lond.) **111**, 96—118 (1950).

—, and T. MANN: Properties and distribution of enzyme system which synthesizes acetylcholine in nervous tissue. J. Physiol. (Lond.) **104**, 411—425 (1946).

—, u. P. ROSENFELD: Der Nachweis eines acetylcholinartigen Stoffes im Pfortader-Blut. Pflügers Arch. ges. Physiol. **232**, 212—235 (1933).

—, and A. VARTIAINEN: Further observations on the physiology and pharmacology of a sympathetic ganglion. J. Physiol. (Lond.) **83**, 103—128 (1934).

FELDBERG, W., and M. VOGT: Acetylcholine synthesis in different regions of the central nervous system. J. Physiol. (Lond.) **107**, 372—381 (1948).

FENG, T. P., and T. H. LI: Studies on the neuromuscular junction. XXIII. A new aspect of the phenomena of eserine potentiation and post-tetanic facilitation in mammalian muscles. Chin. J. Physiol. **16**, 37—54 (1941).

—, and Y. C. TING: Studies on the neuromuscular junction. XI. A note on the local concentration of cholinesterase at motor nerve endings. Chin. J. Physiol. **13**, 141—143 (1938).

FLODMARK, S., and T. WRAMNER: The analgetic action of morphine, eserine and prostigmine studied by a modified Hardy-Wolff-Goodell method. Acta physiol. scand. **9**, 88—96 (1945).

FRANCIS, C. M.: Cholinesterase in the retina. J. Physiol. (Lond.) **120**, 435—439 (1953).

FREDRICSSON, B., K. FUXE, B. HOLMSTEDT and F. SJÖQVIST: Preservation of cholinesterase and its histochemical demonstration after freeze-drying and polyethylene glycol embedding. Acta morph. neerl.-scand. **3**, 107—114 (1960).

FRIEDENWALD, J. S.: Histochemistry: a review. Pharmacol. Rev. **7**, 83—96 (1955).

FUKUDA, T., and G. B. KOELLE: The cytological localization of intracellular neuronal acetylcholinesterase. J. biophys. biochem. Cytol. **5**, 433—440 (1959).

FURSHPAN, E. J., and D. D. POTTER: Transmission at the giant motor synapses of the crayfish. J. Physiol. (Lond.) **145**, 289—325 (1959).

GALAMBOS, R.: Suppression of auditory nerve activity by stimulation of efferent fibers to cochlea. J. Neurophysiol. **19**, 424—437 (1956).

— A glia-neural theory of brain function. Proc. nat. Acad. Sci. (Wash.) **47**, 129—136 (1961).

GALE, G. R., I. W. BROWN Jr. and G. S. EADIE: Cholinesterase activity and potassium permeability in human erythrocytes. Proc. Soc. exp. Biol. (N. Y.) **98**, 297—299 (1958).

GARDINER, J. E.: Experiments on the site of action of a choline acetylase inhibitor. J. Physiol. (Lond.) **138**, 13P—14P (1957).

—, and J. W. THOMPSON: Lack of evidence for a cholinergic mechanism in sympathetic transmission. Nature (Lond.) **191**, 86 (1961).

GARTEN, S.: Die Produktion von Electrizität. Handbuch vergleichender Physiologie **3**, 105 (1910).

GASKELL, W. H.: On the action of muscarin upon the heart, and on the electrical changes in the non-beating cardiac muscle brought about by stimulation of the inhibitory and augmentor nerves. J. Physiol. (Lond.) **8**, 404—415 (1887).

GEREBTZOFF, M. A.: Recherches histochimiques sur les acétylcholine- et choline-estérases. I. Introduction et technique. Acta anat. (Basel) **19**, 366—379 (1953).

— La localisation histochimique des cholinestérases hépatiques. C. R. Soc. Biol. (Paris) **148**, 397—398 (1954).

— Les quatre localisations de l'acétylcholinestérase dans les muscles striés des mammifères et des oiseaux. C. R. Soc. Biol. (Paris) **149**, 823—826 (1955).

— Contribution à la morphologie comparée des appareils cholinestérasiques myo-neurales et musculo-tendineux des vertèbres. Ann. Histochim. **1**, 145—159 (1956a).

— Recherches sur l'innervation cholinergique comparée du coeur de mammifère et de tortue. Ann. Histochim. **1**, 166—175 (1956b).

— L'appareil cholinestérasique musculo-tendineux: Structure, développement, effet de la dénervation et de la ténotomie. Acta physiol. pharm. néerl. **6**, 419—427 (1957).

— Cholinesterases: A Histochemical Contribution to the Solution of Some Functional Problems. New York: Pergamon Press 1959.

— About humoral cholinesterases. Histochemistry of Cholinesterase, Symposium, Basel, 1960. Bibl. anat. **2**, 228—235 (1961).

—, et J. BERTRAND: Gradients d'activité cholinestérasique dans la muqueuse du tube digestif. Ann. Histochim. **2**, 149—162 (1957).

—, et J. GRIETEN: Abondance de fibres intrafusales dans les muscles striés des viscères. C. R. Soc. Biol. (Paris) **150**, 1013 (1956).

— E. PHILIPPOT et M. J. DALLEMAGNE: Recherches histochimiques sur les acétylcholine- et choline-estérases. II. Activité enzymatique dans les muscles lents et rapides des mammifères et des oiseaux. Acta anat. (Basel) **20**, 234—257 (1954).

—, et L. VANDERMISSEN: Étude de la relation spatiale entre acétylcholinestérase et recepteur de l'acétylcholine. Ann. Histochim. **1**, 221—229 (1956).

GERSCHENFELD, H. M., J. H. TRAMEZZANI and E. DE ROBERTIS: Ultrastructure and function in neurohypophysis of the toad. Endocrinology **66**, 741—762 (1960).

GIACOBINI, E.: Histochemical demonstration of AChE activity in isolated nerve cells. Acta physiol. scand. **36**, 276—290 (1956).

— Quantitative determination of cholinesterase in individual sympathetic cells. J. Neurochem. **1**, 234—244 (1957).

— Quantitative determination of cholinesterase in individual spinal ganglion cells. Acta physiol. scand. **45**, 238—254 (1959a).

GIACOBINI, E.: The distribution and localization of cholinesterases in nerve cells. Acta physiol. scand. **45** (Suppl. 156), 1—45 (1959b).
—, and B. HOLMSTEDT: Cholinesterase content of certain regions of the spinal cord as judged by histochemical and Cartesian diver technique. Acta physiol. scand. **42**, 12—27 (1958).
— — Cholinesterase in muscles: A histochemical and microgasometric study. Acta pharmacol. (Kbh.) **17**, 94—105 (1960).
GINSBORG, B. L.: Spontaneous activity in muscle fibres of the chick. J. Physiol. (Lond.) **150**, 707—717 (1960).
—, and B. MACKAY: A histochemical demonstration of two types of motor innervation in avian skeletal muscle. Histochemistry of Cholinesterase, Symposium, Basel, 1960. Bibl. anat. **2**, 174—181 (1961).
GIRARDIER, L., F. BAUMANN et J. M. POSTERNAK: Recherches sur les cholinestérases cardiaques. Helv. physiol. pharmacol. Acta **18**, 467—481 (1960).
GLICK, D.: Further studies on the specificity of choline esterase. J. biol. Chem. **130**, 527—534 (1939).
— Some additional observations on the specificity of cholinesterase. J. biol. Chem. **137**, 357—362 (1941).
— Techniques of Histo- and Cytochemistry. New York: Interscience Publishers 1949.
GOLDSTEIN, A.: Properties and behavior of purified human plasma cholinesterase. III. Competitive inhibition by prostigmine and other alkaloids with special reference to differences in kinetic behavior. Arch. Biochem. **34**, 169—188 (1951).
GOMORI, G.: Histochemical demonstration of sites of choline esterase activity. Proc. Soc. exp. Biol. (N. Y.) **68**, 354—358 (1948).
— Sources of error in enzymatic histochemistry. J. Lab. clin. Med. **35**, 802—809 (1950).
— The histochemistry of esterases. Int. Rev. Cytol. **1**, 323—335 (1952a).
— Microscopic Histochemistry: Principles and Practice. Chicago: Chicago University Press 1952b.
GOODFORD, P. J.: The loss of potassium from isolated rabbit atria. J. Physiol. (Lond.) **145**, 221—224 (1959).
GOODMAN, J. R., L. H. MARRONE and M. C. SQUIRE: Effect of in vivo inhibition of cholinesterase on potassium diffusion from the human red cell. Amer. J. Physiol. **180**, 118—120 (1955).
GOODMAN, L., and A. GILMAN: The Pharmacological Basis of Therapeutics, 2nd ed., Chapter XIX, 389—421. New York: The Macmillan Co. 1954.
GOTCH, F.: The physiology of electrical organs. In: E. SCHAFER, Ed., Textbook of Physiology. New York: Macmillan Co. 1900.
GOUTIER-PIROTTE, M., and M. A. GEREBTZOFF: Acetylcholinesterase in the guinea pig placenta; initial results of histochemical and biochemical research. Arch. int. Physiol. **63**, 445—457 (1955).
GRANIT, R., O POMPEIANO and B. WALTMAN: Fast supraspinal control of mammalian muscle spindles; extra- and intrafusal co-activation. J. Physiol. (Lond.) **147**, 385—398 (1959).
GRAY, J. A. B.: Initiation of impulses at receptors. In: J. FIELD, Ed., Handbook of Physiology, Sect. I: Neurophysiology, Vol. I, Chapter IV, 123—145. Washington, D. C.: American Physiological Society 1959.
—, and J. DIAMOND: Pharmacological properties of sensory receptors and their relation to those of the autonomic nervous system. Brit. med. Bull. **13**, 185—188 (1957).
—, and M. SATO: Properties of the receptor potential in Pacinian corpuscles. J. Physiol. (Lond.) **122**, 610—636 (1953).
GREEN, V. A., and J. E. DAVIS: Modification of CNS drug action by anticholinesterases. Fed. Proc. **15**, 431 (1956).
GREIG, M. E., and W. C. HOLLAND: Studies on the permeability of erythrocytes. I. The relationship between cholinesterase activity and permeability of dog erythrocytes. Arch. Biochem. **23**, 370—384 (1949).
—, and T. C. MAYBERRY: The relationship between cholinesterase activity and brain permeability. J. Pharmacol. **102**, 1—4 (1951).
GRIETEN, J., et M. A. GEREBTZOFF: Les cholinestérases dans l'appareil uro-génital. Ann. Histochim. **2**, 127—140 (1957).
GRUNDFEST, H.: General problems of drug actions on bioelectric phenomena. Ann. N. Y. Acad. Sci. **66**/3, 537—591 (1957a).
— The mechanisms of discharge of the electric organs in relation to general and comparative electrophysiology. Progr. Biophys. **7**, 3—71 (1957b).
— Synaptic and ephaptic transmission. In: J. FIELD, Ed., Handbook of Physiology, Section I: Neurophysiology, Vol. I, 147—197. Washington, D. C.: American Physiological Society. 1959.

GRUNDFEST, H., D. NACHMANSOHN and M. A. ROTHENBERG: Effect of di-isopropyl fluorophosphate (DFP) on action potential and cholinesterase of nerve. III. J. Neurophysiol. 10, 155—164 (1947).

GUNTER, J. M.: Absence of pseudo-cholinesterase from the tissues of ruminants. Nature (Lond.) 157, 369 (1946).

HAGEN, P.: The distribution of cholinesterase in the chromaffin cell. J. Physiol. (Lond.) 129, 50—52 (1955).

HÄGGQVIST, G.: Cholinesterases and innervation of skeletal muscles. Acta physiol. scand. 48, 63—70 (1960).

HÁMORI, J.: Cholinesterases in insect muscle innervation with special reference to insecticide effects of DDT and DFP. Histochemistry of Cholinesterase, Symposium, Basel, 1960. Bibl. anat. 2, 194—206 (1961).

HANZON, V., and G. TOSCHI: Electron microscopy on microsomal fractions from rat brain. Exp. Cell Res. 16, 256—271 (1959).

HARRIS, C., B. S. COHEN and A. D. BERGNER: Correlation of manometric and histochemical techniques in the study of cholinesterase activity. J. Histochem. Cytochem. 1, 405—414 (1953).

HARRIS, E. J., and O. F. HUTTER: The action of acetylcholine on the movements of potassium ions in the sinus venosus of the heart. J. Physiol. (Lond.) 133, 58P—59P (1956).

HEBB, C. O.: Acetylcholine metabolism of nervous tissue. Pharmacol. Rev. 6, 39—43 (1954).
— The problem of identifying cholinergic neurones in the retina. Acta physiol. pharm. neerl. 6, 621—631 (1957).
—, and K. J. HILL: Distribution of cholinesterases in the mammalian pancreas. Quart. J. exp. Physiol. 40, 168—175 (1955a).
— — Pseudocholinesterase in Pacinian corpuscles. Nature (Lond.) 175, 597 (1955b).
—, and A. SILVER: Choline acetylase in the central nervous system of man and some other mammals. J. Physiol. (Lond.) 134, 718—728 (1956).
— — A. A. B. SWAN and E. G. WALSH: A histochemical study of cholinesterases of rabbit retina and optic nerve. Quart. J. exp. Physiol. 38, 185—191 (1953).

HELLMANN, K.: Quantitative histochemical demonstration of cholinesterase by means of radioactive copper. J. Physiol. (Lond.) 117, 77P—78P (1952).

HESS, A.: Optic centers and pathways after eye removal in fetal guinea pigs. J. comp. Neurol. 109, 91—116 (1958).
— The effects of eye removal on the development of cholinesterase in the superior colliculus. J. exp. Zool. 144, 11—23 (1960).

HESTRIN, S.: The reaction of acetylcholine and other carboxylic acid derivatives with hydroxylamine and its analytical application. J. biol. Chem. 180, 249—261 (1949).

HILL, J. R.: The influence of drugs on ciliary activity. J. Physiol. (Lond.) 139, 157—166 (1957).

HILLARP, N.-A.: The construction and functional organization of the autonomic innervation apparatus. Acta physiol. scand. 46 (Suppl. 157), 1—38 (1959).

HODGKIN, A. L.: The effect of potassium on the surface membrane of an isolated axon. J. Physiol. (Lond.) 106, 319—340 (1947).
—, and A. F. HUXLEY: A quantitative description of membrane current and its application to conduction and excitation in nerve. J. Physiol. (Lond.) 117, 500—544 (1952).

HOFFA, M., u. G. LUDWIG: Einige neue Versuche über Herzbewegung. Z. rat. Med. 9, 107—144 (1850).

HOFFMAN, B. F., and E. E. SUCKLING: Cardiac cellular potentials: effect of vagal stimulation and acetylcholine. Amer. J. Physiol. 173, 312—320 (1953).

HOKIN, L. E., and M. R. HOKIN: The mechanism of phosphate exchange in phosphatidic acid in response to acetylcholine. J. biol. Chem. 234, 1387—1390 (1959).
— — The role of phosphatidic acid and phosphoinositide in transmembrane transport elicited by acetylcholine and other humoral agents. Int. Rev. Neurobiol. 2, 99—136 (1960a).
— — Studies on the carrier function of phosphatidic acid in sodium transport. I. The turnover of phosphatidic acid and phosphoinositide in the avian salt gland on stimulation of secretion. J. gen. Physiol. 44, 61—85 (1960b).

HOKIN, M. R., and L. E. HOKIN: The synthesis of phosphatidic acid from diglyceride and adenosine triphosphate in extracts of brain microsomes. J. biol. Chem. 234, 1381—1386 (1959).
— — and W. D. SHELP: The effects of acetylcholine on the turnover of phosphatidic acid and phosphoinositide in sympathetic ganglia, and in various parts of the central nervous system in vitro. J. gen. Physiol. 44, 217—226 (1960).

HOLADAY, D. A., K. KAMIJO and G. B. KOELLE: Facilitation of ganglionic transmission following inhibition of cholinesterase by DFP. J. Pharmacol. exp. Ther. 111, 241—254 (1954).

HOLLAND, W. C., and M. E. GREIG: Studies on permeability. II. The effect of acetylcholine and physostigmine on the permeability to potassium of dog erythrocytes. Arch. Biochem. 26, 151—155 (1950a).
— — Studies on the permeability of erythrocytes. III. The effect of physostigmine and acetylcholine on the permeability of dog, cat and rabbit erythrocytes to sodium and potassium. Amer. J. Physiol. 162, 610—615 (1950b).
— — Synthesis of acetylcholine by human erythrocytes. Arch. Biochem. 39, 77—79 (1952).
HOLLINGSHEAD, W. H., and C. H. SAWYER: Mechanisms of carotid body stimulation. Amer. J. Physiol. 144, 79—86 (1945).
HOLMAN, M. E.: Membrane potentials recorded with high-resistance micro-electrodes; and the effects of changes in ionic environment on the electrical and mechanical activity of the smooth muscle of the taenia coli of the guinea-pig. J. Physiol. (Lond.) 141, 464—488 (1958).
HOLMES, R. L.: Cholinesterase activity in the atrial wall of the dog and cat heart. J. Physiol. (Lond.) 137, 421—426 (1957).
HOLMSTEDT, B.: A modification of the thiocholine method for the determination of cholinesterase. I. Biochemical evaluation of selective inhibitors. Acta physiol. scand. 40, 322—330 (1957a).
— A modification of the thiocholine method for determination of cholinesterase. II. Histochemical application. Acta physiol. scand. 40, 331—337 (1957b).
— Pharmacology of organophosphorus cholinesterase inhibitors. Pharmacol. Rev. 11, 567—688 (1959).
—, and F. SJÖQVIST: Distribution of acetocholinesterase in the ganglion cells of various sympathetic ganglia. Acta physiol. scand. 47, 284—296 (1959).
— — Some principles about histochemistry of cholinesterase with special reference to the thiocholine method. Histochemistry of Cholinesterase, Symposium, Basel, 1960. Bibl. anat. 2, 1—10 (1961).
—, and C. R. SKOGLUND: Action of dimethyl-amido-ethoxy-phosphoryl cyanide (Tabun) a cholinesterase inhibitor on the spinal reflexes in the cat. Acta physiol. scand. 29, 410—427 (1953).
—, and G. TOSCHI: Enzymic properties of cholinesterases in subcellular fractions from rat brain. Acta physiol. scand. 47, 280—283 (1959).
HOLT, S. J.: A new principle for the histochemical localization of hydrolytic enzymes. Nature (Lond.) 169, 271—273 (1952).
— The value of fundamental studies of staining reactions in enzyme histochemistry, with reference to indoxyl methods for esterases. J. Histochem. Cytochem. 4, 541—552 (1956).
—, and D. G. O'SULLIVAN: Studies in enzyme cytochemistry. I. Principles of cytochemical staining methods. Proc. roy. Soc. 148, 465—480 (1958).
—, and P. W. SADLER: Studies in enzyme cytochemistry. II. Synthesis of indigogenic substrates for esterases. Proc. roy. Soc. 148, 481—494 (1958a).
— — Studies in enzyme cytochemistry. III. Relationships between solubility, molecular association and structure in indigoid dyes. Proc. roy. Soc. 148, 495—505 (1958b).
—, and R. F. J. WITHERS: Cytochemical localization of esterases using indoxyl derivatives. Nature (Lond.) 170, 1012—1014 (1952).
HOWELL, W. H., and W. W. DUKE: The effect of vagus inhibition on the output of potassium from the heart. Amer. J. Physiol. 21, 51—63 (1908).
HUNT, C. C., and S. W. KUFFLER: Motor innervation of skeletal muscle: multiple innervation of individual muscle fibres and motor unit function. J. Physiol. (Lond.) 126, 293—303 (1954).
HURLEY, H. J.: Non-specific cholinesterase in specialized sensory nerve-endings of human genital skin. Brit. J. Derm. 70, 284—287 (1958).
—, and G. B. KOELLE: The effect of inhibition of non-specific cholinesterase on perception of tactile sensation in human volar skin. J. invest. Derm. 31, 243—245 (1958).
—, and H. MESCON: Cholinergic innervation of the digital arterio-venous anastomoses of human skin. A histochemical localization of cholinesterase. J. appl. Physiol. 9, 82—84 (1956a).
— — Localization of non-specific cholinesterase in MEISSNER's corpuscles in human skin. Brit. J. Derm. 68, 290—293 (1956b).
— W. B. SHELLEY and G. B. KOELLE: The distribution of cholinesterases in human skin, with special reference to eccrine and apocrine sweat glands. J. invest. Derm. 21, 139—147 (1953).
HUTTER, O. F., and W. TRAUTWEIN: Vagal and sympathetic effects on the pacemaker fibres in the sinus venosus of the heart. J. gen. Physiol. 39, 715—733 (1956).
ICHIKAWA, S., and E. BOZLER: Monophasic and diphasic action potentials of the stomach. Amer. J. Physiol. 182, 92—96 (1955).

IL'INA-KAKUEVA, E. I.: A histochemical study of the cholinesterase activity of the nerve cells and conducting system of the heart. Bull. exp. Biol. Med. **46**, 1270—1273 (1958).

JABONERO, V.: Die interstitiellen Zellen des vegetativen Nervensystems und ihre vermutliche Analogie zu anderen Elementen. Acta neuroveg. (Wien) **5**, 1—24 (1952).

JARRETT, A. S.: The effect of acetylcholine on touch receptors in frog's skin. J. Physiol. (Lond.) **133**, 243—254 (1956).

JOHNELS, A. G.: On the origin of the electric organ in *Malapterurus electricus*. Quart. J. micr. Sci. **97**, 455—464 (1956).

KAMIJO, K., and G. B. KOELLE: The relationship between cholinesterase inhibition and ganglionic transmission. J. Pharmacol. exp. Ther. **105**, 349—357 (1952).

— — The histochemical localization of specific cholinesterase in the conduction system of beef heart. J. Pharmacol. exp. Ther. **113**, 30 (1955).

KARCZMAR, A. G., and J. W. HOWARD: Antagonism of d-tubocurarine and other pharmacologic properties of certain bis-quaternary salts of basically substituted oxamides (WIN 8077 and analogs). J. Pharmacol. exp. Ther. **113**, 30 (1955).

—, and T. KOPPANYI: Changes in transport cholinesterase levels and responses to intravenously administered acetylcholine and benzoylcholine. J. Pharmacol. exp. Ther. **116**, 245—253 (1956).

KATO, J.: Choline acetylase of human placenta. J. Biochem. **48**, 768—772 (1960).

KEWITZ, H.: Über die Aktionssubstanz in sympathischen Ganglien. Naunyn-Schmiedeberg's Arch. exp. Path. Pharmak. **225**, 111—114 (1955).

KEYNES, R. D., M. V. L. BENNETT and H. GRUNDFEST: Studies on morphology and electrophysiology of electric organs. II. *Malapterurus electricus*. In: C. CHAGAS and A. PAES-DE-CARVALHO, Eds., Bioelectrogenesis, 102—112. Amsterdam: Elsevier Publishing Co. 1961.

KIRSCHNER, L. B.: Effect of cholinesterase inhibitors and atropine on active sodium transport across frog skin. Nature (Lond.) **172**, 348—349 (1953).

KOBLICK, D. C.: The characterization and localization of frog skin cholinesterase. J. gen. Physiol. **41**, 1129—1134 (1958).

KOCH, H. J.: Cholinesterase and active transport of sodium chloride through the isolated gills of the crab *Eriochier sinensis* (M. Edw.). In: J. A. KITCHING, Ed., Recent Developments in Cell Physiology, 15—27. London: Butterworths Publ. Ltd. 1954.

KOELLE, G. B.: Protection of cholinesterase against irreversible inactivation by di-isopropyl fluorophosphate (DFP) *in vitro*. J. Pharmacol. exp. Ther. **88**, 232—237 (1946).

— The histochemical differentiation of types of cholinesterases and their localizations in tissues of the cat. J. Pharmacol. exp. Ther. **100**, 158—179 (1950).

— The elimination of enzymatic diffusion artifacts in the histochemical localization of cholinesterases and a survey of their cellular distributions. J. Pharmacol. exp. Ther. **103**, 153—171 (1951).

— Cholinesterases of the tissues and serum of rabbits. Biochem. J. **53**, 217—226 (1953).

— The histochemical localization of cholinesterases in the central nervous system of the rat. J. comp. Neurol. **100**, 211—228 (1954).

— The histochemical identification of acetylcholinesterase in cholinergic, adrenergic and sensory neurons. J. Pharmacol. exp. Ther. **114**, 167—184 (1955).

— Histochemical demonstration of reversible anticholinesterase action at selective cellular sites *in vivo*. J. Pharmacol. exp. Ther. **120**, 488—503 (1957).

— A proposed dual neurohumoral role of acetylcholine: its functions at the pre- and post-synaptic sites. Nature (Lond.) **190**, 208—211 (1961).

— A new general concept of the neurohumoral functions of acetylcholine and acetylcholinesterase. J. Pharm. (Lond.) **14**, 65—90 (1962).

—, and J. S. FRIEDENWALD: A histochemical method for localizing cholinesterase activity. Proc. Soc. exp. Biol. (N. Y.) **70**, 617—622 (1949).

— — The histochemical localization of cholinesterase in ocular tissue. Amer. J. Ophthal. **33**, 253—256 (1950).

—, and C. N. GEESEY: Localization of acetylcholinesterase in the neurohypophysis and its functional implications. Proc. Soc. exp. Biol. (N. Y.) **106**, 625—628 (1961).

—, and A. GILMAN: Anticholinesterase drugs. Pharmacol. Rev. **1**, 166—216 (1949).

— E. S. KOELLE and J. S. FRIEDENWALD: The effect of inhibition of specific and non-specific cholinesterase on the motility of isolated ileum. J. Pharmacol. exp. Ther. **100**, 180—191 (1950).

—, and E. C. STEINER: The cerebral distributions of a tertiary and a quaternary anticholinesterase agent following intravenous and intraventricular injection. J. Pharmacol. exp. Ther. **118**, 420—434 (1956).

— L. WOLFAND, J. S. FRIEDENWALD and R. A. ALLEN: Localization of specific cholinesterase in ocular tissues of the cat. Amer. J. Ophthal. **35**, 1580—1584 (1952).

19*

Koelle, W. A., and G. B. Koelle: The localization of external or functional acetylcholinesterase at the synapses of autonomic ganglia. J. Pharmacol. exp. Ther. **126**, 1—8 (1959).

Koenig, E., and G. B. Koelle: Acetylcholinesterase regeneration in peripheral nerve after irreversible inactivation. Science **132**, 1249—1250 (1960).

— — Mode of regeneration of acetylcholinesterase in cholinergic neurons following irreversible inactivation. J. Neurochem. **8**, 169—188 (1961).

Kordik, P., E. Bülbring and J. H. Burn: Ciliary movement and acetylcholine. Brit. J. Pharmacol. **7**, 67—79 (1952).

Krause, W.: Die Nervenendigung innerhalb der terminalen Körperchen. Arch. mikr. Anat. **19**, 53—136 (1881).

Kuffler, S. W.: Physiology of neuro-muscular junctions: electrical aspects. Fed. Proc. **7**, 437—446 (1948).

—, C. C. Hunt and J. P. Quilliam: Function of medullated small-nerve fibers in mammalian ventral roots: efferent muscle spindle innervation. J. Neurophysiol. **14**, 29—54 (1951).

—, and E. M. Vaughan Williams: Small-nerve junctional potentials. The distribution of small motor nerves to frog skeletal muscle, and the membrane characteristics of the fibres they innervate. J. Physiol. (Lond.) **121**, 289—317 (1953a).

— — Properties of the 'slow' skeletal muscle fibres of the frog. J. Physiol. (Lond.) **121**, 318—340 (1953b).

Kupfer, C.: Histochemistry of muscle cholinesterase after motor nerve section. J. cell. comp. Physiol. **38**, 469—471 (1951).

— Motor innervation of extraocular muscle. J. Physiol. (Lond.) **153**, 522—526 (1960).

—, and G. B. Koelle: A histochemical study of cholinesterase during the formation of the motor end plate of the albino rat. J. exp. Zool. **116**, 399—414 (1951).

Lands, A. M., A. G. Karczmar, J. W. Howard and A. Arnold: An evaluation of the pharmacologic actions of some bis-quaternary salts of basically substituted oxamides (WIN 8077 and analogs). J. Pharmacol. exp. Ther. **115**, 185—198 (1955).

Leeuwe, H.: Over de interstitieele Cel (Cajal). Utrecht: Schotanus & Jens 1937.

Lehrer, G. M., and L. A. Ornstein: A diazo coupling method for the electron microscopic localization of cholinesterase. J. biophys. biochem. Cytol. **6**, 390—406 (1959).

Lembeck, F., and R. Strobach: Kaliumagbabe aus glatter Muskulatur. Naunyn-Schmiedeberg's Arch. exp. Path. Pharmak. **228**, 130—131 (1955).

Leplat, G., and M. A. Gerebtzoff: Localisation de l'acétylcholinestérase et des médiateurs diphénoliques dans la rétine. Ann. Oculist. (Paris) **189**, 121—128 (1956).

Lewis, P. R.: The effect of varying the conditions in the Koelle technique. Histochemistry of Cholinesterase, Symposium, Basel, 1960. Bibl. anat. **2**, 11—20 (1961).

—, and A. F. W. Hughes: Paterns of myo-neural junctions and cholinesterase activity in the muscles of tadpoles of *Xenopus laevis*. Quart. J. micr. Sci. **101**, 55—67 (1960).

Liljestrand, G.: Transmission at chemoreceptors. Pharmacol. Rev. **6**, 73—78 (1954).

Linderstrøm-Lang, K.: Principle of the Cartesian diver applied to gasometric technique. Nature (Lond.) **140**, 108 (1937).

— Distribution of enzymes in tissue and cells. Harvey Lect. **34**, 214—245 (1938/39).

Lindvig, P. E., M. E. Greig and S. W. Peterson: Studies on permeability. V. The effects of acetylcholine and physostigmine on the permeability of human erythrocytes to sodium and potassium. Arch. Biochem. **30**, 241—250 (1951).

Lison, L.: Histochimie et Cytochimie Animales. Principes et Méthodes, Ed. 2. Paris: Gauthier-Villars 1953.

Lissák, K.: Effects of extract of adrenergic fibers on frog heart. Amer. J. Physiol. **125**, 778—785 (1939).

—, and J. Pásztor: Acetylcholingehalt sensibler Nerven. Pflügers. Arch. ges. Physiol. **244**, 120—124 (1940).

Loewenstein, W. R.: The generation of electric activity in a nerve ending. Ann. N. Y. Acad. Sci. **81/2**, 367—387 (1959).

—, and D. Molins: Cholinesterase in a receptor. Science **128**, 1284 (1958).

Loewi, O., and H. Hellauer: Über das Acetylcholin in peripheren Nerven. Pflügers Arch. ges. Physiol. **240**, 769—775 (1938).

Lorente de Nó, R.: Effects of choline and acetylcholine chloride upon peripheral nerve fibers. J. cell. comp. Physiol. **24**, 85—97 (1944).

Lowry, O. H., N. R. Roberts, M.-L. Wu, W. S. Hixon and E. J. Crawford: The quantitative histochemistry of brain. II. Enzyme measurements. J. biol. Chem. **207**, 19—37 (1954).

Lüllmann, H., and E. Muscholl: Über das Verhalten der Cholinesterase und des Gewichtes denervierter Rattenzwerchfelle. Naunyn-Schmiedeberg's Arch. exp. Path. Pharmak. **225**, 486—490 (1955).

Lundin, S. J.: On the location of cholinesterase in fishes. Experientia (Basel) **14**, 131—132 (1958).

LUNDIN, S. J.: Acetylcholinesterase in goldfish muscles. Biochem. J. 72, 210—214 (1959).

MACHT, M. B., and M. E. BADER: Iontophoresis with acetyl-beta-methyl-choline and blood flow through the hand at low environmental temperatures. J. appl. Physiol. 1, 205—214 (1958).

MACINTOSH, F.: The distribution of acetylcholine in the peripheral and central nervous system. J. Physiol. (Lond.) 99, 436—442 (1941).

MACKAY, B., and A. PETERS: Terminal innervation of segmental muscle fibres. Histochemistry of Cholinesterase, Symposium, Basel, 1960. Bibl. anat. 2, 182—193 (1961).

MALMGREN, H., and B. SYLVÉN: On the chemistry of the thiocholine method of Koelle. J. Histochem. Cytochem. 3, 441—445 (1955).

MARNAY, A., and D. NACHMANSOHN: Choline esterase in voluntary muscle. J. Physiol. (Lond.) 92, 37—47 (1938).

MARSHALL, J. M.: Effects of low temperatures on transmembrane potentials of single fibers of the rabbit atrium. Circulation Res. 5, 664—669 (1957).

—, and E. M. VAUGHAN WILLIAMS: Pacemaker potentials. The excitation of isolated rabbit auricles by acetylcholine at low temperatures. J. Physiol. (Lond.) 131, 186—199 (1956).

MASLAND, R. L., and R. S. WIGTON: Nerve activity accompanying fasciculation produced by prostigmin. J. Neurophysiol. 3, 269—275 (1940).

MATHEWSON, R., A. WACHTEL and H. GRUNDFEST: Fine structure of electroplaques. In: C. CHAGAS and A. PAES-DE-CARVALHO, Eds., Bioelectrogenesis, 25—53. Amsterdam: Elsevier Publishing Co. 1961.

MATHIAS, P. J., and C. W. SHEPPARD: An upper limit for acetylcholine content and synthesis in human erythrocytes. Proc. Soc. exp. Biol. (N. Y.) 86, 69—74 (1954).

MATSUMURA, M., and G. B. KOELLE: The nature of synaptic transmission in the superior cervical ganglion following reinnervation by the afferent vagus. J. Pharmacol. exp. Ther. 134, 28—46 (1961).

MAYNARD, E. A., and D. M. MAYNARD: Cholinesterase in the crustacean muscle receptor organ. J. Histochem. Cytochem. 8, 376—379 (1960).

McISAAC, R. J., and G. B. KOELLE: Comparison of the effects of inhibition of external, internal, and total acetylcholinesterase upon ganglionic transmission. J. Pharmacol. exp. Ther. 126, 9—20 (1959).

McLENNAN, H.: Acetylcholine metabolism of normal and axotomized ganglia. J. Physiol. (Lond.) 124, 113—116 (1954).

McWILLIAM, J. A.: Fibrillar contraction of the heart. J. Physiol. (Lond.) 8, 296—310 (1887).

MENDEL, B., D. B. MUNDELL and H. RUDNEY: Studies on cholinesterase. III. Specific tests for true cholinesterase and pseudo-cholinesterase. Biochem. J. 37, 473—476 (1943).

— D. K. MYERS, I. E. UYLDERT, A. C. RUYS and W. M. DE BRUYN: Ali-esterase inhibitors and growth. Brit. J. Pharmacol. 8, 217—224 (1953).

—, and H. RUDNEY: Studies on cholinesterase; cholinesterase and pseudo-cholinesterase. Biochem. J. 37, 59—63 (1943).

MENTEN, M. L., J. JUNGE and M. H. GREEN: A coupling histochemical azo dye test for alkaline phosphatase in the kidney. J. biol. Chem. 153, 471—477 (1944).

MEYLING, H. A.: Bau und Innervation von Glomus caroticum und Sinus caroticus. Acta neerl. morph. 1, 193—288 (1938).

— Structure and significance of the peripheral extension of the autonomic nervous system. J. comp. Neurol. 99, 495—535 (1953).

MICHELSON, M. J.: The Physiological Role of Acetylcholine and the Investigation of New Drug Substances (in Russian). Leningrad: Leningrad Medical Institute 1957.

— Pharmacological evidences of the role of acetylcholine in the higher nervous activity of man and animals. Activitas nervosa superior 3, 140—147 (1961).

MILEDI, R.: Acetylcholine sensitivity of partially denervated frog muscle fibres. J. Physiol. (Lond.) 147, 45P—46P (1959).

MILTON, A. S.: The action of tubocurarine on ciliary movement. Brit. J. Pharmacol. 14, 323—326 (1959).

MOHR, E.: Les cholinestérases dans l'appareil respiratoire. C. R. Soc. Biol. (Paris) 149, 828—830 (1955).

—, et M. A. GEREBTZOFF: Recherches histochimiques sur les acétylcholine- et choline-estérases. III. Localisations dans le coeur de mammifère. Acta anat. (Basel) 22, 143—151 (1954).

MOMMAERTS, W. F. H. M., P. A. KHAIRALLAH and M. F. DICKENS: Acetylcholinesterase in the conductive tissue of the heart. Circulation Res. 1, 460—465 (1953).

MONTAGNA, W., and E. B. BECKETT: Cholinesterases and alpha esterases in the lip of the rat. Acta anat. (Basel) 32, 256—261 (1958).

NACHLAS, M. M., and A. M. SELIGMAN: The histochemical demonstration of esterase. J. nat. Cancer Inst. 9, 415—425 (1949a).

NACHLAS, M. M., and A. M. SELIGMAN: The comparative distribution of esterase in the tissues of five mammals by a histochemical technique. Anat. Rec. 105, 677—687 (1949b).
NACHMANSOHN, D.: Chemical mechanism of nerve activity. Ann. N. Y. Acad Sci. 47/4, 395—428 (1946).
— Chemical and Molecular Basis of Nerve Activity. New York: Academic Press 1959.
— C. W. COATES and R. T. COX: Electric potential and activity of cholinesterase in the electric organ of *Electrophorus electricus* (Linnaeus). J. gen. Physiol. 25, 75—88 (1941).
— — and M. A. ROTHENBERG: Studies on cholinesterase. II. Enzyme activity and voltage of the action potential in electric tissue. J. biol. Chem. 163, 39—48 (1946).
NACHMANSOHN, D.: Cholinestérase dans le système nerveux central. Bull. Soc. Chim. biol. (Paris) 21, 761—796 (1939).
NACHMANSOHN, D.: Studies on permeability in relation to nerve function. I. Axonal conduction and synaptic transmission. Biochim. biophys. Acta 4, 78—95 (1950).
NASTUK, W. L., and L. LEVINE: A microbioassay for acetylcholine. Proc. Soc. exp. Biol. (N. Y.) 106, 502—505 (1961).
NATHAN, P., and M. H. APRISON: Cholinesterase activity in cytoplasmic particles from rabbit brain. Fed. Proc. 14, 106—107 (1955).
NOVIKOFF, A. B.: The validity of histochemical phosphatase methods on the intracellular level. Science 113, 320—324 (1951).
— Histochemical and cytochemical staining methods. In: R. C. MELLORS, Ed., Analytical Cytology, Chapter 2. New York: McGraw-Hill 1955.
— Electron microscope: cytology of cell fractions. Science 124, 969—972 (1956).
OGSTON, A. G.: Removal of acetylcholine from a limited volume by diffusion. J. Physiol. (Lond.) 128, 222—223 (1955).
ORD, M. G., and R. H. S. THOMPSON: The distribution of cholinesterase types in mammalian tissues. Biochem. J. 46, 346—352 (1950).
— — Pseudo-cholinesterase activity in the central nervous system. Biochem. J. 51, 245—251 (1952).
PALADE, G. E., and P. SIEKEVITZ: Liver microsomes. J. biophys. biochem. Cytol. 2, 171—200 (1956).
PALAY, S. L.: The fine structure of the neurohypophysis. In: H. WAELSCH, Ed., Ultrastructure and Cellular Chemistry of Neural Tissue, Chapter II, 31—49. New York: Hoeber-Harper 1957.
—, and G. E. PALADE: The fine structure of neurons. J. biophys. biochem. Cytol. 1, 69—88 (1955).
PALÉUS, S.: On the localization of the specific cholinesterase in human blood. Arch. Biochem. 12, 153—154 (1947).
PARPART, A. K., and J. F. HOFFMAN: Acidity versus acetylcholine and cation permeability of red cells. Fed. Proc. 11, 117 (1952).
PASTOR, E. P., and R. A. FENNELL: Some observations on the esterases of Tetrahymena pyriformis W. II. Some factors affecting alisterase and cholinesterase activity. J. Morph. 104, 143—158 (1959).
PATON, W. D. M.: Central and synaptic transmission in the nervous system (pharmacological aspects). Ann. Rev. Physiol. 20, 431—470 (1958).
— A theory of drug action based on the rate of drug-receptor combination. Proc. roy. Soc. (Lond.), Ser. B, 154, 21—69 (1961).
PEARSE, A. G. E.: Histochemistry, Theoretical and Applied, 2nd edition. Boston: Little Brown and Co. 1960.
PEASE, D. C., and T. A. QUILLIAM: Electron microscopy of the Pacinian corpuscle. J. biophys. biochem. Cytol. 3, 331—342 (1957).
PEPLER, W. J., and A. G. E. PEARSE: The histochemistry of the esterases of rat brain, with special reference to those of the hypothalamic nuclei. J. Neurochem. 1, 193—202 (1957).
PERRY, W. L. M.: Acetylcholine release in the cat's superior cervical ganglion. J. Physiol. (Lond.) 119, 439—454 (1953).
— Central and synaptic transmission (pharmacological aspects). Ann. Rev. Physiol. 18, 279—308 (1956).
— Transmission in autonomic ganglia. Brit. med. Bull. 13, 220—226 (1957).
PHILIPPU, A. J.: Cholinesterase of leucocytes. Amer. J. Physiol. 184, 145—146 (1956).
PICKFORD, M.: The action of acetylcholine on the supraoptic nucleus of the chloralosed dog. J. Physiol. (Lond.) 106, 264—270 (1947).
POLYAK, S. L.: The Retina. Chicago: University of Chicago Press 1941.
PORTER, K. R.: Observations on a submicroscopic basophilic component of cytoplasm. J. exp. Med. 97, 727—750 (1953).
PORTUGALOV, V. V., and V. A. JAKOVLEV: Localization of cholinesterase in striated muscles. Dokl. Akad. Nauk SSSR (in Russian) 78, 1021—1024 (1951).

PROSSER, C. L., and N. SPERELAKIS: Transmission in ganglion-free circular muscle from the cat intestine. Amer. J. Physiol. 187, 536—545 (1956).

PURPURA, D. P., and H. GRUNDFEST: Nature of dendritic potentials and synaptic mechanisms in cerebral cortex of cat. J. Neurophysiol. 19, 573—595 (1956).

QUASTEL, J. H., M. TENNENBAUM and A. H. M. WHEATLEY: Choline ester formation in, and choline esterase activities of, tissues in vitro. Biochem. J. 30, 1668—1681 (1936).

RAJAPURKAR, M. V., and G. B. KOELLE: Reactivation of DFP-inactivated acetylcholinesterase by monoisonitroacetone (MINA) and diacetylmonoxime (DAM) "in vivo." J. Pharmacol. exp. Ther. 123, 247—252 (1958).

RASMUSSEN, G. L.: The olivary peduncle and other fiber projections of the superior olivary complex. J. comp. Neurol. 84, 141—220 (1946).

— Further observations of the efferent cochlear bundle. J. comp. Neurol. 99, 61—74 (1953).

RAVIN, H. A., H. C. TSOU and A. M. SELIGMAN: Colorimetric estimation and histochemical demonstration of serum cholinesterase. J. biol. Chem. 191, 843—857 (1951).

— S. I. ZACKS and A. M. SELIGMAN: The histochemical localization of acetylcholinesterase in nervous tissue. J. Pharmacol. exp. Ther. 107, 37—53 (1953).

RIKER, W. F.: Pharmacologic considerations in a re-evaluation of the neuromuscular synapse. Arch. Neurol. 3, 488—499 (1960).

— J. ROBERTS, F. G. STANDAERT and H. FUJIMORU: The motor nerve terminal as the primary focus for drug-induced facilitation of neuromuscular transmission. J. Pharmacol. exp. Ther. 121, 286—312 (1957).

— G. WERNER, J. ROBERTS and A. S. KUPERMAN: Pharmacologic evidence for the existence of a presynaptic event in neuromuscular transmission. J. Pharmacol. exp. Ther. 125, 150—158 (1959).

ROBERTSON, J. D.: Some features of the ultrastructure of reptilian skeletal muscle. J. biophys. biochem. Cytol. 2, 369—392 (1956).

ROBERTSON, P. A.: Calcium and contractility in depolarized smooth muscle. Nature (Lond.) 186, 316—317 (1960).

ROBINS, E., and D. E. SMITH: A quantitative histochemical study of eight enzymes of the cerebellar cortex and subjacent white matter in the monkey. Metabolic and Toxic Diseases of the Nervous System 32, 305—327 (1953).

ROGISTER, G., E. L. DUMOULIN et M. A. GEREBTZOFF: Recherches histochimiques sur les acétylcholine- et choline-estérases. 4. L' acétylcholinestérase dans le thymus et la mesure biochimipue de son activité. Acta anat. (Basel) 25, 361—371 (1955).

—, et M. A. GEREBTZOFF: Recherches histochimiques sur les acétylcholine- et choline-estérases. V. Localization dans les éléments figures du sang et dans les organes hemopoiétiques. Acta anat. (Basel) 32, 39—50 (1958).

RÖHLICH, P.: Demonstration of acetylcholinesterase on motor endplates after embedding in polyethylene glycol. Nature (Lond.) 178, 1398 (1956).

ROSS. L. L.: A cytological and histochemical study of the carotid body of the cat. Anat. Rec. 129, 433—456 (1957).

RUSKA, H., G. A. EDWARDS and R. CAESAR: A concept of intracellular transmission of excitation by means of the endoplasmic reticulum. Experientia (Basel) 14, 117—120 (1958).

SAMOJLOFF, A.: Die Vagus- und Muskarin-Wirkung auf die Stromkurve des Froschherzens. Arch. ges. Physiol. 155, 471—552 (1914).

SANDRITTER, W., E. KUMMER, G. PILLAT and L. ROWE: Zur Histochemie und Funktion der parafollikulären Zellen in der Schilddrüse. Klin. Wschr. 31/32, 871—872 (1956).

SÁVAY, G., and B. CSILLIK: The effect of denervation on the cholinesterase activity of motor end plates. Acta morph. Acad. Sci. hung. 6, 289—297 (1956).

— — Beiträge zur Methodik der histochemischen Cholinesterase-Reaktion. Acta histochim. (Jena) 6, 307—314 (1959a).

— — Lead reactive substances in peripheral synapses. Experientia (Basel) 15, 396—397 (1959b).

SAWYER, C. H., C. DAVENPORT and L. M. ALEXANDER: Sites of cholinesterase activity in neuromuscular and ganglionic transmission. Anat. Rec. 106, 287—288 (1950).

—, and W. H. HOLLINSHEAD: Cholinesterases in sympathetic fibers and ganglia. J. Neurophysiol. 8, 137—153 (1945).

SCHARRER, E., and B. SCHARRER: Hormones produced by neurosecretory cells. Recent Progr. Hormone Res. 10, 183—240 (1954).

—, and J. SINDEN: A contribution to the "chemoarchitectonics" of the optic tectum of the brain of the pigeon. J. comp. Neurol. 91, 331—336 (1949).

SCHAUMANN, W., and C. JOB: Differential effects of a quaternary cholinesterase inhibitor, phospholine, and its tertiary analogue, compound 217-AO, on central control of respiration and on neuromuscular transmission, the antagonism by 217-AO of the respiratory arrest caused by morphine. J. Pharmacol. exp. Ther. 123, 114—120 (1958).

Schneider, W. C., and G. H. Hogeboom: Biochemistry of cellular particles. Ann. Rev. Biochem. **25**, 201—224 (1956).

Schoffeniels, E.: Ion movements studied with single isolated electroplax. Ann. N. Y. Acad. Sci. **81**/2, 285—306 (1959).

Schuknecht, H. F., J. A. Churchill and R. Doran: The localization of acetylcholinesterase in the cochlea. Arch. Otolaryng. (Chicago) **69**, 549—559 (1959).

Schwarzacher, H. G.: Der histochemisch nachweisbare Cholinesterasegehalt in Muskelplatten nach Durchschneidung des motorischen Nerven. Acta anat. (Basel) **31**, 507—521 (1957).

— Untersuchungen über die Skeletmuskel-Sehnenverbindung. II. Histochemische Lokalisation der Acetylcholinesterase und Untersuchungen über ihre mögliche Funktion an der Muskelfaser-Sehnenverbindung. Acta anat. (Basel) **42**, 318—332 (1960a).

— Untersuchungen über den Cholinesterasegehalt der Skeletmuskel-Sehnenverbindung. Arch. int. Pharmacodyn. **128**, 330—342 (1960b).

— (Ed.): Histochemistry of Cholinesterase (Symposium, Basel, 1960). Bibl. Anat. **2**, 1—255 (1961).

— Acetylcholinesterase in mammalian myo-tendinous junction. Histochemistry of Cholinesterase, Symposium, Basel, 1960, Bibl. anat. **2**, 220—227 (1961).

Schweitzer, A., E. Stedman and S. Wright: Central action of anticholinesterases. J. Physiol. (Lond.) **96**, 302—336 (1939).

Seaman, G. R.: Localization of acetylcholinesterase activity in the protozoan *Tetrahymena geleii* S. Proc. Soc. exp. Biol. (N. Y.) **76**, 169—170 (1951).

—, and R. K. Houlihan: Enzyme systems in *Tetrahymena geleii* S. II. Acetylcholinesterase activity. Its relation to motility of the organism and to coordinated ciliary action in general. J. cell. comp. Physiol. **37**, 309—321 (1951).

Shelley, H.: A correlation between cholinesterase inhibition and an increase in muscle tone in rabbit duodenum. Brit. J. Pharmacol. **10**, 26—35 (1955).

Shelley, W. B., and H. J. Hurley Jr.: The physiology of the human axillary apocrine sweat gland. J. invest. Derm. **20**, 285—297 (1953).

Shen, S. C., P. Greenfield and E. J. Boell: The distribution of cholinesterase in the frog brain. J. comp. Neurol. **102**, 717—743 (1955).

— — — Localization of acetylcholinesterase in chick retina during histogenesis. J. comp. Neurol. **106**, 433—462 (1956).

Shute, C. C. D., and P. R. Lewis: The salivatory centre in the rat. J. Anat. (Lond.) **94**, 59—73 (1960).

— — The use of cholinesterase techniques combined with operative procedures to follow nervous pathways in the brain. Histochemistry of Cholinesterase, Symposium, Basel, 1960. Bibl. anat. **2**, 34—39 (1961).

Sjöqvist, F., and B. Fredricsson: Cholinesterase distribution in the sympathetic nervous system of the cat. Biochem. Pharmacol. **8**, 18 (1961).

Slaughter, D.: Neostigmine and opiate analgesia. Arch. int. Pharmacodyn. **83**, 143—148 (1950).

—, and E. G. Gross: Some new aspects of morphine action. Effect on intestine and blood pressure; toxicity studies. J. Pharmacol. exp. Ther. **68**, 96—103 (1940).

Snell, R. S.: Changes in the histochemical appearances of cholinesterase in a mixed peripheral nerve following nerve section and compression injury. Brit. J. exp. Path. **38**, 479—482 (1957).

— The histochemical appearances of cholinesterases in the parasympathetic nerves supplying the submandibular and sublingual salivary glands of the rat. J. Anat. (Lond.) **92**, 534—543 (1958).

— The histochemical appearances of cholinesterase in the parotid salivary gland of the rat. Z. Zellforsch. **49**, 330—338 (1959).

— The histochemical localisation of cholinesterase in the central nervous system. Histochemistry of Cholinesterase, Symposium, Basel, 1960. Bibl. anat. **2**, 50—58 (1961a).

— The innervation of the salivary glands. A study of cholinesterase in nerves. Histochemistry of Cholinesterase, Symposium Basel, 1960. Bibl. anat. **2**, 97—110 (1961b).

—, and J. R. Garrett: The effect of postganglionic sympathectomy on the histochemical appearances of cholinesterase in the nerves supplying the submandibular and sublingual salivary glands of the rat. Z. Zellforsch. **48**, 201—214 (1958).

—, and N. McIntyre: Changes in the histochemical appearances of cholinesterase at the motor end plate following denervation. Brit. J. exp. Path. **37**, 44—48 (1956).

Sokolovskiy, V. V., and N. V. Korolev: Determination of the degree of inactivation of cholinesterase by a histospectrophotometric method. Tsitologoya **1**, 177—182 (1959).

Stämpfli, R.: A new method for measuring membrane potentials with external electrodes. Experientia (Basel) **10**, 508—509 (1954).

STEPHENSON, M., and E. ROWATT: The production of acetylcholine by a strain of Lactobacillus planatarum. J. gen. Microbiol. 1, 279—298 (1947).

STRAUB, R. W.: Sucrose-gap apparatus for studying the resting and action potential in
mammalian non-medullated fibres. J. Physiol. (Lond.) 135, 2P—4P (1957).

STRICKLAND, K. P., and R. H. S. THOMPSON: On the mechanism of the potassium loss from
brain slices induced by cholinesterase inhibitors. Biochem. J. 60, 468—475 (1955).

STROMBLAD, R.: Acetylcholine inactivation and acetylcholine sensitivity in denervated salivary glands. Acta physiol. scand. 34, 38—58 (1955).

SZENTÁGOTHAI, J.: Einige Bemerkungen zur Struktur der peripheren Endausbreitung vegeta-
tiver Nerven. Acta neuroveg. (Wien) 15, 417—445 (1957).

— The anatomical basis of synaptic transmission of excitation and inhibition in motoneurons.
Acta morph. Acad. Sci. hung. 8, 287—309 (1958).

— A. DONHOFFER and K. RAJKOVITS: Die Lokalisation der Cholinesterase in der interneuralen
Synapse. Acta histochim. 1, 272—281 (1954).

SZERB, J. C., and D. H. McCURDY: Concentration of morphine in blood and brain after intravenous injection of morphine in non-tolerant, tolerant and neostigmine-treated rats. J.
Pharmacol. exp. Ther. 118, 446—450 (1956).

TAXI, J.: Action du formol sur l'activité de diverses préparations de cholinestérases. J. Physiol.
Path. gén. 44, 595—599 (1952a).

— Cellules de Schwann et "cellules interstitielles de Cajal" au niveau des plexus nerveaux
de la musculeuse intestinale du cobaye: retour aux définitions. Arch. Anat. micr. Morph.
exp. 41, 281—304 (1952b).

— La distribution des cholinestérases dans divers ganglions du système nerveux autonome
des vertébrés. Histochemistry of Cholinesterase, Symposium, Basel, 1960. Bibl. anat. 2,
73—89 (1961).

TAYLOR, I. M., J. M. WELLER and A. B. HASTINGS: The effect of cholinesterase and choline
acetylase inhibitors on the potassium concentration gradient and potassium exchange of
human erythrocytes. Amer. J. Physiol. 168, 658—665 (1952).

TEMPLE, J. M.: Sodium maleate: a buffer for the pH region of 5.2 to 6.8. J. Amer. chem.
Soc. 51, 1754—1755 (1929).

TEPPERMAN, J., and H. M. TEPPERMAN: Some effects of hormones on cells and cell constituents.
Pharmacol. Rev. 12, 301—353 (1960).

TEWARI, H. B., and G. H. BOURNE: Histochemical localization of specific and non-specific
cholinesterases and simple esterase in myelinated nerves. Exp. Cell Res. 21, 245—248 (1960).

THESLEFF, S.: The mode of neuromuscular block caused by acetylcholine, nicotine, decamethonium and succinylcholine. Acta physiol. scand. 34, 218—231 (1955).

THIES, W., and L. F. GALENTE: Zur histochemischen Darstellung der Cholinesterasen im
vegetativen Nervensystem der Haut. Hausarzt 8, 69—75 (1957).

THOMPSON, E. H., and V. P. WHITTAKER: Cholinesterase activity and sodium transport in
the human red cell. Biochim. biophys. Acta 9, 700—701 (1952).

TIBBS, J.: Acetylcholinesterase in flagellated systems. Biochim. biophys. Acta 41, 115—122
(1960).

TIEGS, O. W.: Innervation of voluntary muscle. Physiol. Rev. 33, 90—144 (1953).

TITUS, E., D. NICHOLLS and J. KANFER: Effects of ouabain on incorporation of P³² into
phospholipids. Fed. Proc. 20, 279 (1961).

TOMAN, J. E. P., J. W. WOODBURY and L. A. WOODBURY: Mechanism of nerve conduction
block produced by anti-cholinesterases. J. Neurophysiol. 10, 429—441 (1947).

TOSCHI, G.: A biochemical study of brain microsomes. Exp. Cell Res. 16, 232—255 (1959).

TRAUTWEIN, W., and J. DUDEL: Zum Mechanismus der Membranwirkung des Acetylcholin an
der Herzmuskelfaser. Pflügers Arch. ges. Physiol. 266, 324—334 (1958).

— S. W. KUFFLER and C. EDWARDS: Changes in membrane characteristics of heart muscle
during inhibition. J. gen. Physiol. 40, 135—145 (1956).

VAN DER KLOOT, W. G.: The effect of enzyme inhibitors on the resting potential and on the
ion distribution of the sartorius muscle of the frog. J. gen. Physiol. 41, 879—900 (1958).

VARGA, E., T. KONIG, E. KISS, T. KOVACS and L. HEGEDUS: On the cholinesterase activity
of myosin. Acta physiol. Acad. Sci. hung. 7, 171—173 (1955).

VINNIKOV, A., and L. K. TITOVA: Presence and distribution of acetylcholinesterase in the
organ of Corti in animals who are in a state of relative rest, and under the conditions of
acoustic effect. Dokl. Akad. Nauk SSSR (in Russian) 119, 164—168 (1958).

VOLLE, R. L., and G. B. KOELLE: The physiological role of acetylcholinesterase (AChE) in
sympathetic ganglia. J. Pharmacol. exp. Ther. 133, 223—240 (1961).

WACHSTEIN, M., E. MEISEL and C. FALCON: Histochemistry of thiolacetic acid esterase: a
comparison with nonspecific esterase with special regard to the effect of fixatives and
inhibitors on intracellular localization. J. Histochem. Cytochem. 9, 325—339 (1961).

WASER, P. G.: The cholinergic receptor. J. Pharm. (Lond.) 12, 577—594 (1960).
—, and I. HADORN: Relations of cholinergic receptors to acetylcholinesterase of end-plates in denervated muscle. Histochemistry of Cholinesterase, Symposium, Basel, 1960. Bibl. anat. 2, 155—160 (1961).
WEIDMANN, S.: The effect of the cardiac membrane potential on the rapid availability of the sodium-carrying system. J. Physiol. (Lond) 127, 213—224 (1955).
WEISS, P., and H. B. HISCOE: Experiments on the mechanism of nerve growth. J. exp. Zool. 107, 315—395 (1948).
WERMAN, R.: Electrical inexcitability of the synaptic membrane in the frog skeletal muscle fibre. Nature (Lond.) 188, 149—150 (1960).
WHITE, R. T., and R. A. ALLEN: An improved clinical microtome for sectioning frozen tissue. Stain Technol. 26, 137—138 (1951).
WHITTAKER, V. P.: Specificity, mode of action and distribution of cholinesterases. Physiol. Rev. 31, 312—343 (1951).
— The isolation and characterization of acetylcholine-containing particles from brain. Biochem. J. 72, 694—706 (1959).
WILBRANDT, W., and T. ROSENBERG: The concept of carrier transport and its corollaries in pharmacology. Pharmacol. Rev. 13, 109—183 (1961).
WILSON, H., and J. P. LONG: The effect of hemicholinium (HC-3) at various peripheral cholinergic transmitting sites. Arch. int. Pharmacodyn. 120, 343—352 (1959).
WILSON, I. B.: Mechanism of hydrolysis. II. New evidence for an acylated enzyme as intermediate. Biochim. biophys. Acta 7, 520—525 (1951).
— M. A. HATCH and S. GINSBURG: Carbamylation of acetylcholinesterase. J. biol. Chem. 235, 2312—2315 (1960).
WINKELMANN, R. K.: The primary organized sensory ending in human skin. A.M.A. Arch. Derm. 76, 225—235 (1957).
WOLFGRAM, F. J.: Relative amounts of choline acetylase and cholinesterases in dorsal and ventral roots of cattle. Amer. J. Physiol. 176, 505—507 (1954).
YOSHIDA, H., T. NUKADA and H. FUJISAWA: Effect of ouabain on ion transport and metabolic turnover of phospholipid of brain slices. Biochim. biophys. Acta 48, 614—615 (1961).
ZACKS, S. I., and J. M. BLUMBERG: The histochemical localization of acetylcholinesterase in the fine structure of neuromuscular junctions of mouse and human intercostal muscle. J. Histochem. Cytochem. 9, 317—324 (1961).
ZAJICEK, J.: Studies on the histogenesis of blood platelets. Acta haemat. (Basel) 12, 238—244 (1954).
— Studies on the histogenesis of blood platelets. II. Quantitative determination of acetylcholinesterase activity in single megakaryocytes from various mammals. Acta haemat. (Basel) 15, 296—302 (1956).
— Studies on the histogenesis of blood platelets and megakaryocytes. Acta physiol. scand. 138 (Suppl. 40), 1—32 (1957).
—, and N. DATTA: Investigation on the acetylcholinesterase activity of erythrocytes, platelets and plasma in different animal species. Acta haemat. (Basel) 9, 115—121 (1953).
—, and E. ZEUTHEN: Quantitative determination of cholinesterase activity in individual cells. Exp. Cell Res. 11, 568—579 (1957).
— B. SYLVÉN and N. DATTA: Attempts to demonstrate acetylcholinesterase activity in blood and bone-marrow cells by a modified thiocholine technique. J. Histochem. Cytochem. 2, 115—121 (1954).
ZEUTHEN, E.: Growth as related to the cell cycle in single-cell cultures of Tetrahymena piriformis (formerly Colpidium piriformis or Tetrahymena geleii). J. Embryol. exp. Morph. 1, 239—249 (1953).

Chapter 7

The Active Site of Acetylcholinesterase and Related Esterases and its Reactivity towards Substrates and Inhibitors

By

J. A. COHEN and R. A. OOSTERBAAN

With 30 Figures

Contents

Introduction

The purpose of the present chapter is to review the available data on the structure of the active site of acetylcholinesterase (AChE) and on the way this active site reacts with the substrates and inhibitors of the enzyme. In the present review the term "active site" will refer to those regions of the enzyme surface where the substrate is localized and activated during the enzymic action. No attempt is made to include information on the enzyme, its substrates, or inhibitors which does not directly contribute to an understanding of the structure of the active site or its reactivity. For these many alternative aspects outside the scope of the present paper the reader is referred to excellent articles available in the literature including those by AUGUSTINSSON (1948 and 1951 c), HOLMSTEDT (1959), NACHMANSOHN and WILSON (1951), WHITTAKER (1951), ZELLER (1958) and chapters 4, 8, and 9 of the present handbook

The material has been arranged as follows. The first sections deal with those aspects of the interaction of AChE with substrates and inhibitors that provide essential information on its active site. Much attention is devoted to relevant structural properties of these compounds and to the kinetics of their interaction with the enzyme. Thus, in an indirect way an as yet incomplete picture will be drawn of the active site.

In the final section the direct evidence obtained by chemical analysis of the active site itself is reviewed. This direct approach gives the most explicit information on the active site and is therefore extensively treated. Unfortunately, the availability and purity of AChE are at present prohibitive with regard to chemical analysis of its active site. Therefore practically all the analytical data in this section refer to other esterases. It will be shown, however, that it is permissible within limits to interpret chemical data obtained on other esterases in terms of structural properties of the active site of AChE. In the same section the significance of the active sites of AChE and other esterases as possible components of pharmacological receptors will be mentioned.

The interaction of acetylcholinesterase with substrates

Acetylcholinesterase, the predominant acetylcholine (ACh)-decomposing enzyme of nervous tissue and erythrocytes, is distinguished from other esterases by a number of characteristics. The most essential is its substrate specificity. Its natural substrate is ACh, and this ester is split according to reaction (1).

$$CH_3—N^{(+)}—CH_2—CH_2—O—\overset{O}{\overset{\|}{C}}—CH_3 + H_2O \underset{}{\overset{AChE}{\rightleftarrows}}$$

with the CH_3 groups on the nitrogen,

$$H^+ + CH_3—\overset{O}{\overset{\|}{C}}—O^- + CH_3—N^{(+)}—CH_2—CH_2OH$$

$$(1)$$

Propionylcholine is split at a lower rate, and butyrylcholine is hardly split at all but in fact strongly inhibits the enzyme's action on the other two esters (cf. AUGUSTINSSON and NACHMANSOHN 1949 a).

Acetylcholinesterase has been isolated for purposes of biochemical investigation mainly from electric organs of certain marine organisms and from erythrocytes. The methods have been recently described in a review by AUGUSTINSSON (1957), which might be extended by the procedure of CLAIRE LAWLER (1958). In the same review methods for the estimation of the enzymic activity have been summarized. For more information on the subject the reader may also be referred to the chapter by AUGUSTINSSON (4) in the present book.

It is generally agreed that the interaction of AChE with substrate is adequately described by the familiar formulation proposed by MICHAELIS-MENTEN:

$$EH + S \underset{k_1}{\overset{k_2}{\rightleftharpoons}} EHS \xrightarrow{k_3} EH + \text{products} \tag{2}$$

where EH is free enzyme and EHS is the Michaelis enzyme-substrate complex. Generally an equilibrium is established, as demonstrated by HESTRIN (1949, 1950).

During the hydrolysis of ACh an acetylated enzyme is formed from EHS as an intermediate, accompanied by liberation of choline. The acetylated enzyme is subsequently split by water to give acetic acid and free enzyme. The remarkable efficiency of the enzymic catalysis of ACh hydrolysis is expressed in the high turnover number of AChE.

The turnover number (TN) of AChE gives a good index of the speed at which the active site reacts with ACh. It is defined as the number of substrate (ACh) molecules reacting per minute per active site. Obviously the use of TN has sense only when the conditions of the activity test are well defined.

NACHMANSOHN and WILSON (1951) and ROTHENBERG and NACHMANSOHN (1947) found that 1 mg of protein of a highly purified preparation of eel AChE splits 75 g ACh per hour under their experimental conditions (temperature 37°, medium 0.13 M NaCl, 0.04 M MgCl$_2$, 0.025 M NaHCO$_3$, and 0.018 M ACh, equilibrated with 5% CO$_2$ — 95% N$_2$). A similar preparation was subjected to ultracentrifugation. The molecular weight (MW) of the enzymically most active component was estimated at approximately 3×10^6. Combination of these data gives a turnover for AChE of 20×10^6 molecules ACh/min/molecule AChE. Obviously this figure requires division by the number of active sites per molecule enzyme to arrive at a true TN as described above. In order to find a true TN, MICHEL and KROP (1951) estimated the number of active sites per mg of eel AChE by inhibiting it with ^{32}P labelled di*iso*propyl phosphorofluoridate (DF^{32}P). Assuming that every active site reacts irreversibly with one molecule of DFP, the amount of ^{32}P per mg of completely inhibited enzyme preparation will give the number of active sites per mg. They calculated a TN of 4.9×10^5 molecules ACh/min/molecule active site (= molecule DFP) (pH 7.4, temp. 38°, ionic strength 0.14). Identical results were obtained for preparations of varying purity. ROTHENBERG and NACHMANSOHN (1947) concluded that AChE of MW 3×10^6 possessed 48 active sites. Another possible interpretation is that the MW of 3×10^6 represents an aggregation of smaller molecules of MW 63,000. SERLIN and FLUKE (1956) exposed dried films of AChE to electron, proton, or α-particle bombardment, and calculated for the radiosensitive unit of the enzyme a MW of 105,000. Assuming a cylindrical shape, the unit was established to be 360 Å long and to have a diameter of 21 Å.

BERRY (1951), using dicyclohexylphosphorofluoridate (DCFP) instead of DF^{32}P, calculated a TN for human red cell AChE of 1.61×10^5 molecules ACh/min/molecule active site (= molecule DCFP). The number of active sites was calculated from the amount of DCFP bound per mg of completely inhibited enzyme preparation.

COHEN et al. (1955a, 1955b) and COHEN and WARRINGA (1953) developed a method allowing them to use the DF^{32}P method of MICHEL and KROP (1951) on partly purified preparations of ox red cell AChE. They incubated the AChE preparation with unlabelled DFP in the presence of butyrylcholine. This ester protects the active site of AChE against the attack of DFP but all other DFP sensitive groups in the preparation are irreversibly blocked. After removal of the butyrylcholine and the excess DFP by dialysis, the active sites of AChE become free and are then specifically labelled by DF^{32}P. Different preparations gave a TN of 2.55 to 3.51 × 10^5 molecules ACh/min/active site (= molecule DFP). The best estimate is 2.95×10^5 (manometric technique, 37°, Krebs-Ringer NaHCO$_3$, 10^{-2} M ACh).*

It is also generally accepted that two groups at the active site of the enzyme are essential in bringing about the hydrolysis of substrate: the esteratic site where

---

*) See for additional results H. CLAIRE LAWLER: J. biol. Chem. **236**, 2296—2301 (1961) and I. B. WILSON and M. A. HARRISON: J. biol. Chem. **236**, 2292—2295 (1961).

the ester bond is activated, and the anionic site, consisting of one or more negative groups which interact by ionic bonding with the cationic N^+-atom of the choline residue and supporting the enzyme-substrate attraction by van der Waals forces.

In the following sections we propose to represent the data in this field which are relevant to an understanding of the properties of the active site. For this purpose we shall deal consecutively with the main factors which determine the enzyme-substrate interaction. These factors are:

A. The concentration of the substrate;
B. The structure of the substrate;
C. The effect of the pH;
D. The effect of the presence of inorganic ions;
E. The effect of the temperature.

A. The concentration of the substrate

I. Substrate inhibition

When the initial reaction velocity (v) of the hydrolysis of ACh by AChE is plotted against the concentration of the substrate (S) a curve is obtained (Fig. 1) which deviates from the typical rectangular hyperbola of enzyme reactions obeying Michaelis-Menten kinetics (Fig. 2).

It will be seen from Fig. 1 that starting at low substrate concentrations the initial reaction velocity increases until an optimal concentration of substrate is reached. It has been found that this concentration lies at approximately 3×10^{-3} M ACh. At higher concentrations the reaction is inhibited. The type of curve which is found when an enzyme reaction is inhibited at high substrate concentration is usually called a "bell-shaped" curve; it has been described for AChE by AUGUSTINS-SON (1948), BODANSKY (1946), NACHMANSOHN and ROTHENBERG (1944, 1945) and SCHAEFER (1947).

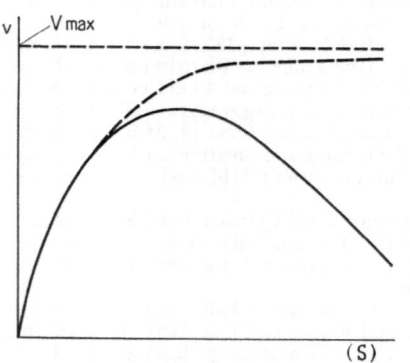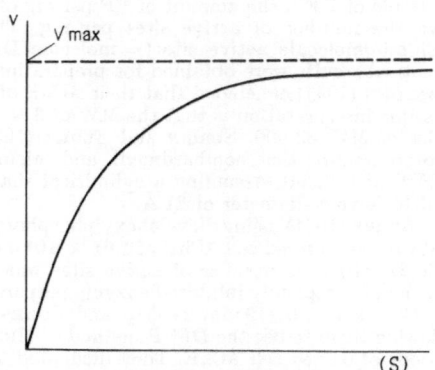

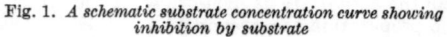

Fig. 1. *A schematic substrate concentration curve showing inhibition by substrate*　　Fig. 2. *Hyperbolic form of typical substrate concentration curve*

The phenomenon was first noticed by ALLES and HAWES (1940) for red cell AChE and explained by the assumption that an inactive complex was formed consisting of one mole of enzyme and two or more moles of substrate. The formation of this complex by ACh at high substrate concentrations is readily explained by the assumption that at high substrate concentration each of two sites of the enzyme surface attracts a substrate molecule. It is understandable that in this complex the substrate would not be in an optimal steric position for activation of the ester bond, resulting in decrease of enzymic activity. Thus, already in 1943 ZELLER and BISSEGGER (1943, cf. ZELLER 1958) postulated on account of the inhibition of AChE by excess ACh the presence of two essential groups at the surface of this enzyme.

Substrate inhibition is responsible for the existence of an optimal concentration of ACh with respect to hydrolysis by AChE. This optimal concentration, (S) opt, has been determined by a number of authors using enzyme preparations of varying purity and was usually found to fall within the range of 2.5 to 3×10^{-3} M ACh (AUGUSTINSSON 1946, 1949, AUGUSTINSSON and NACHMANSOHN 1949b, BERGMANN et al. 1950a, VAN DER MEER 1953, NACHMANSOHN and ROTHENBERG 1944, 1945, SHUKUYA 1951a, ZELLER and BISSEGER 1943).

The consistency of most of the results suggests that the (S) opt is independent of the purity of the enzyme preparation. The occasional divergent values reported are probably due to unusual experimental conditions (ALLES and HAWES 1940, MENDEL and RUDNEY 1945). WILSON and BERGMANN (1950b) argued that the optimal substrate concentration should on theoretical grounds increase at non optimal pH values (see paragraph C); they proved experimentally the validity of their argument for pH values below the optimal pH; the same was done by HEILBRONN (1954) and GRAUERS (1952).

Moreover, various authors have reported that the (S) opt increases with the ionic strength (see paragraph D of this section).

II. Kinetics of enzyme-substrate interaction

The kinetics of the interaction of AChE with its substrates is firmly rooted in the general theory of enzyme kinetics of which excellent surveys are available (ALBERTY 1956b, CHANCE 1953, DIXON and WEBB 1958, HUENNEKENS 1953, The Mechanism of Enzyme Action 1954, eds. W. D. McELROY and B. GLASS, Discussions of the Faraday Society no. 20, 1955).

In this section, in accordance with the general purpose of this review, only those kinetic treatments of the action of AChE will be dealt with which provide essential and specific information with regard to the structure of the active site of this particular enzyme and its interaction with substrate. The same principle will be followed when later attention will be focussed on interaction of AChE with inhibitors. This restriction is responsible for the omission of kinetic analyses which are not specific for or even applicable to AChE, e.g., those performed at enzyme concentrations of the order of that of the reactants by GOLDSTEIN (1944) and STRAUSS and GOLDSTEIN (1943).

It has been mentioned that the simplest form of representing the action of AChE according to the classical Michaelis-Menten theory (Equation 2) is incomplete because it does not account for the formation of the acetyl enzyme intermediate. Equation (3)

$$\text{EHS} \xrightarrow{k_4} \text{E-acyl} + \text{alcohol} \xrightarrow[\text{H}_2\text{O}]{k_5} \text{EH} + \text{acid} + \text{alcohol} \qquad (3)$$

expresses the situation in a more satisfactory manner. This is not in contradiction to the formulation of equation (2), but it means that k_3 is complicated because it is composed of at least two reaction velocity constants (k_4 and k_5).

There is considerable circumstantial evidence for the hypothesis that an acyl enzyme, E-acyl, is formed as an intermediate in the hydrolysis of ACh by AChE. It is derived partly from the demonstration that AChE has a catalytic action with regard to a number of chemical reactions which are easily understandable on the basis of an acyl enzyme intermediate; they include:

1. The synthesis at low pH of ACh and propionylcholine (COLLIER and SOLVONUK 1955, HESTRIN 1949, 1950) from the corresponding fatty acid + choline and of butyrylcholine from tributyrin + choline (WILSON et al. 1950).

2. The synthesis of propionylcholine and butyrylcholine from choline + acid anhydride (BERGMANN et al. 1953a).

3. The formation of hydroxamic acid from ethyl acetate (COLLIER and SOLVONUK 1955, WILSON et al. 1950), ACh (HESTRIN 1950), and the smaller members of the fatty acid series (HESTRIN 1949, 1950, WILSON et al. 1950).

Further arguments may, according to WILSON et al. (1950), be derived from the fact that for the synthesis of choline esters form choline and fatty acids by AChE a low pH is required; this may be interpreted as an indication of the importance of the electrophily of the substrate carboxyl carbon atom which is favourable for acyl enzyme formation. The same author demonstrated also that many acetyl substrates are hydrolyzed at an equal rate in spite of large differences in Km; this would also argue in favour of a common intermediate, the acetyl enzyme. The hydrolysis of thiolacetic acid yielding hydrogen sulphide (see page 309) may be explained along the same line (WILSON 1951b). Also the transfer of ^{18}O from $H_2{}^{18}O$ into one of the two oxygen atoms of acetic acid during enzymic hydrolysis of ACh, as demonstrated by STEIN and KOSHLAND (1953), is in agreement with the formation of an acyl enzyme intermediate.

Finally, it is virtually certain that certain esterases related to AChE form acyl intermediates during their enzymic action. In the case of chymotrypsin such intermediates have actually been isolated (BALLS and ALDRICH 1955, BALLS and WOOD 1956). Since, as will be shown in the last section, there is strong reason to believe that the esteratic site of AChE is very similar to that of these related esterases, its action too may be expected to involve acyl intermediates.

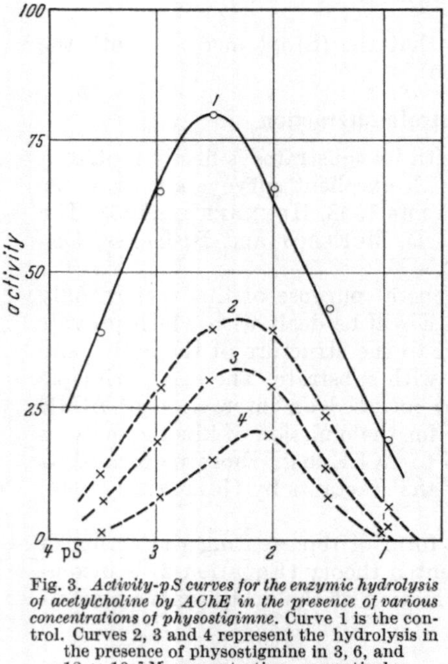

According to (2), the reaction is first order with regard to enzyme concentration and the velocity $v = k_3$ (EHS). It is also first order with regard to substrate at low substrate concentration as follows from (2) and the left hand part of the curve of Fig. 2. At higher substrate concentrations it should become zero order, as it does in Fig. 2, but in fact it follows the pattern of Fig. 3 due to inhibition by high concentrations of substrate. The substrate concentration curve has a bell shape but the curve has a flat maximum that corresponds to a wide range of substrate concentrations. Therefore, also in this case zero order kinetics prevail within a considerable zone (AUGUSTINSSON 1948). However the maximum activity is no longer represented as it is in classical Michaelis-Menten kinetics by

$$V_{max} = k_3 \, (\text{EH}_t)$$

where (EH_t) represents the concentration of the initial enzyme present and V_{max} the maximal velocity.

Fig. 3. *Activity-pS curves for the enzymic hydrolysis of acetylcholine by AChE in the presence of various concentrations of physostigmine.* Curve 1 is the control. Curves 2, 3 and 4 represent the hydrolysis in the presence of physostigmine in 3, 6, and 18×10^{-7} M concentration, respectively. From AUGUSTINSSON (1949b)

The substrate inhibition of AChE can be represented by HALDANE's theory (HALDANE 1930, cf. MURRAY 1930), assuming the possibility of the formation, in addition to the normal Michaelis complex EHS, of an inactive complex EHS_2 (supercomplex) consisting of one enzyme and two substrate molecules as follows,

$$\text{EHS} + \text{S} \rightleftarrows \text{EHS}_2 \text{ (diss. constant } K_2) \tag{4}$$

$$(\text{EHS}_2) = \frac{(\text{EHS})(\text{S})}{K_2} \, .$$

The reaction velocity under conditions of substrate inhibition is given by equation (5).

$$v = \frac{V_{max}(S)}{Km + (S) + \frac{(S)^2}{K_2}} \tag{5}$$

For the steady state $\frac{d(EHS)}{dt} = 0$ of equation (2) where the rate of formation and removal of EHS are equal,

$$(EH)(S) k_1 = k_2(EHS) + k_3(EHS). \tag{6}$$

For the concentration of free enzyme (EH)

$$(EH) = (EH_t) - (EHS) - \frac{(EHS)(S)}{K_2}$$

Assuming that $(EH_t) \ll (S)$, the expression (S) in the formula is not corrected for enzyme-bound substrate and equalizes the total substrate concentration. Substitution of (EH) in (6) and rearrangement gives

$$\frac{(EHS)}{(EH_t)} = \frac{(S)}{\frac{k_2 + k_3}{k_1} + (S) + \frac{(S)^2}{K_2}} \; ;$$

substitution of $\frac{(EHS)}{(EH_t)} = \frac{v}{V_{max}}$ and $\frac{k_2 + k_3}{k_1} = Km$ (Michaelis-Menten constant) yields

$$v = \frac{V_{max}(S)}{Km + (S) + \frac{(S)^2}{K_2}}. \tag{7}$$

Formula (7) describes the bell-shaped curve as represented in Fig. 1. It is obtained when (S) or log(S) is plotted against v. In the latter case the "bell" is symmetrical around an axis corresponding to the optimal substrate concentration. Formula (7) simplifies into (8) when K_2 is very large or (S) very small,

$$v = \frac{V_{max}(S)}{Km + (S)}. \tag{8}$$

This is the familiar Michaelis expression of a rectangular hyperbola: $Km = (S)$ at half maximal velocity. Using this expression, Km and V_{max} may be easily computed, e.g., from a Lineweaver-Burk plot of $1/v$ against $1/(S)$ (Fig. 4); for this purpose, the linear segment of the curve of Fig. 4 corresponding to low values of (S), or the linear extrapolated extension of this segment should be used. Because of substrate inhibition, the maximal velocity observed experimentally never actually reaches V_{max} as may be seen from the same figure. The experimental maxi-

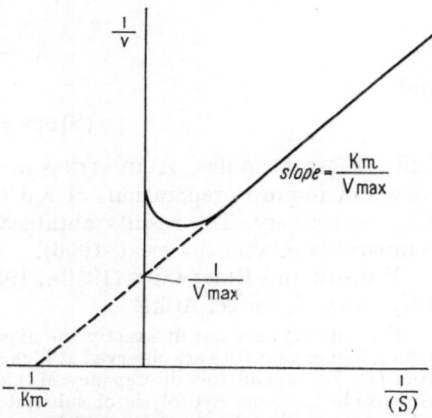

Fig. 4. *Determination of Km and V$_{max}$ in the case of substrate inhibition.* The reciprocals of Km and V_{max} are found at the intercepts of the curve with the $\frac{1}{(S)}$ — and $\frac{1}{v}$ axis, respectively

mal velocity is reached at the (S)opt which may be obtained by differentiation of expression (7). It is found that

$$(S)opt = \sqrt{Km \cdot K_2} \tag{9}$$

The Km read from the graph is equal to $\frac{k_2 + k_3}{k_1}$ from equation (2). It is not equal to k_2/k_1, i.e., the dissociation constant of the Michaelis complex. It would be of considerable interest to known this dissociation constant because it could provide valuable information on the nature of the ACh-AChE Michaelis complex. Fortunately, the Km computed may serve the same purpose since it has been shown that for many enzyme-substrate systems $Km = \dfrac{k_2 + k_3}{k_1}$ simplifies into $Km = k_2/k_1$, because $k_2 \gg k_3$ (BERNHARD 1955b, BOTTS and MORALES 1953, LAIDLER 1955a, MORALES 1955). WILSON (1952b) has demonstrated with regard to AChE that variation of substrate may cause considerable variation of Km, but only limited change of k_3 (Table 1). This suggests that also for AChE the above

Table 1. *Values of Km, k_3, and concentration range for several substrates*

Substrate	Concentration range	Km	Relative k_3 [1]
Ethyl acetate	$5 \times 10^{-2} - 3 \times 10^{-1}$	5×10^{-1}	12
Ethyl chloroacetate	$5 \times 10^{-3} - 2 \times 10^{-2}$	3×10^{-2}	13
*Iso*amyl acetate	$6 \times 10^{-4} - 5 \times 10^{-3}$	8×10^{-3}	11
Dimethylaminoethyl acetate	$1 \times 10^{-3} - 1 \times 10^{-1}$	1×10^{-3}	38
Acetylcholine	$4 \times 10^{-4} - 1 \times 10^{-1}$	4.5×10^{-4}	100
Acetic anhydride	$5 \times 10^{-4} - 6 \times 10^{-3}$	4×10^{-4}	13
Dithiolacetic acid	$3 \times 10^{-4} - 3 \times 10^{-3}$	2×10^{-4}	18
Acetylthiocholine	$2 \times 10^{-4} - 1 \times 10^{-2}$	1.2×10^{-4}	100

[1] For ACh = 100. From WILSON and BERGMANN (1950b).

approximation for Km, viz. k_2/k_1, seems justified. Therefore substitution of $K_S(k_2/k_1)$ for Km in formulas (7) and (9) is permissible. These formulas now convert into

$$v = \frac{V_{max}\,(S)}{K_S + (S) + \dfrac{(S)^2}{K_2}}, \tag{10}$$

and

$$(S)\text{opt} = \sqrt{K_S \cdot K_2}. \tag{11}$$

Using these formulas, AUGUSTINSSON (1948) calculated form substrate-activity curves of impure preparations of red cell AChE a pK_S* and a pK_2* of 3.2 and 1.8, respectively. The results obtained with purified preparations of AChE are comparable (GREGOIRE et al. 1956).

WILSON and BERGMANN (1950a, 1950b) arrived at values of 3.58 and 1.53 for pK_S and pK_2 for eel AChE.

Formula (7) does not fit exactly the experimentally obtained values of the "bell" curve; in fact, higher velocities are observed at high substrate concentrations than would be predicted from (7). To explain this discrepancy MYERS (1952c) postulated that the EHS_2 complex is responsible for some hydrolysis of substrate. To provide a better fit for the experimental points he introduced a factor y, which expresses the ratio of substrate hydrolysis by EHS and EHS_2, respectively. Thus, equation (12) is developed:

$$v = V_{max}\, \frac{(S) + y(S)}{K_S + (S) + \dfrac{(S)^2}{K_2}}. \tag{12}$$

When $y = 0.1$, a remarkably good fit is achieved, as may be seen from Fig. 5 where activity is plotted against pS. MYERS (1952c) showed also that (S)opt as well as K_S and K_2 are functions of the ionic strength.

---

* Instead of the actual values of the dissociation-constants and the (S)opt, their negative logarithms are often used and expressed as pK_S, pK_2, and p(S)opt, respectively.

Another objection to the Haldane equation (7) is that in the integrated form fits it inadequately the experimental points of plots of substrate concentration against time for experiments where substrate hydrolysis is allowed to evolve to near-completion. Corrections for this deviation have been proposed by SCHAEFER (1947) (cf. HARDEGG et al. 1956, HARDEGG and SCHAEFER 1952, SCHAEFER and MAIER 1949).

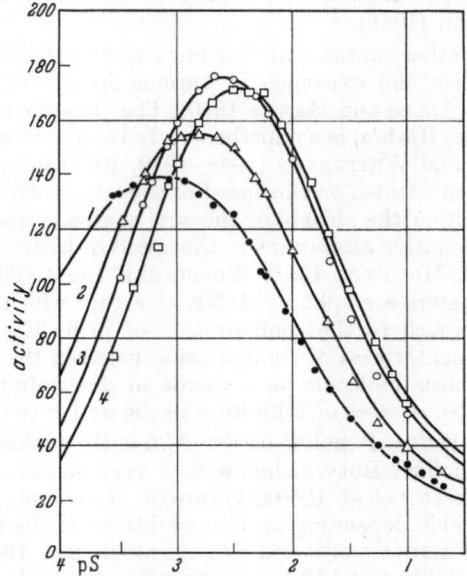

Fig. 5. *Substrate concentration activity curves for AChE*. Experimental results obtained for the hydrolysis of ACh by red cell AChE in the presence of various concentrations of NaCl increasing in order from (1) to (4). The ordinate gives the enzyme activity as $\mu l\, CO_2/0.1$ ml erythrocyte hemolysate/20 min; the abscissa gives the negative logarithm of the molar concentration of ACh. The theoretical curves were calculated from equation (7) assuming $y = 0.1$ (see text). The best theoretical curves were obtained using the following values:

M concn. of NaCl added to the 0.025 M NaHCO$_3$ medium	K_2 $\times 10^4$ M	K_3 $\times 10^2$ M	K_3/K_2	$(S)_{opt}$ $\times 10^3$ M	V_{opt}	V_{max}
—	0.55	1.10	200	0.78	140	157
0.02[1]	1.10	1.21	110	1.15	146	169
0.05	1.9	1.35	70	1.60	156	190
0.10[1]	2.6	1.55	60	2.05	168	208
0.20	3.7	1.8	50	2.70	175	221
0.50	5.5	2.2	40	3.65	171	221

[1] To avoid unnecessary confusion on the graph, these two curves were not included in Fig. 5. From MYERS (1952c)

A final correction which may be mentioned has been proposed by WILSON (1952b). It concerns the Km which is usually calculated from enzyme reactions at maximal velocity assuming that all enzyme molecules, (EH_t), interact with substrate. In fact, due to the pH dependence of the active group of the enzyme, the amount of enzyme available for the interaction with substrate is a function of pH. WILSON proposed the following equation for the effective Km at pH 7.3:

$$\text{Effective } Km = 1.5\,\frac{k_2 + k_3}{k_1}$$

B. The structure of the substrate

In the first part of this section data on substrate specificity of AChE will be summarized succintly. In the next part these will be used to explore the properties of the active site of this enzyme.

20*

I. Substrate specificity of AChE

It is generally perhaps somewhat too readily agreed that ACh is the physiological substrate of AChE. However, many more esters are hydrolyzed by this enzyme; they represent changes with respect to ACh which may concern either the acyl- or the alcohol residue or both. Many esters that have been tested are listed by AUGUSTINSSON (1948).

The situation was rather confused at first but cleared considerably with regard to aliphatic esters when the existence of various species of ACh-hydrolyzing enzymes was realised (ALLES and HAWES 1940). The enzymic hydrolysis of these esters by cholinesterases (ChE's) is comprehensively treated in a survey by WHITTAKER (1951). ADAMS and WHITTAKER (1948, 1949, 1950) investigated the effect of chain-branching of substrates on the speed of their hydrolysis; they concluded that such changes in either the alcohol or the acyl chains in homologous series of esters effected similar relative alterations in the speed of hydrolysis (cf. MOUNTER and WHITTAKER 1950, MOUNTER 1951, WHITTAKER 1953). These authors have shown that aliphatic esters are split by AChE at a rate which is determined by their closeness of approach to the configuration of ACh. They emphasized the importance of complimentariness of configuration between the active center and the substrate or inhibitor molecule as a factor in determining specificity and strength of binding of substrates or inhibitors to the active center.

In the homologous series of choline esters, ACh is the best substrate, followed closely by propionylcholine. Butyrylcholine is a very slugish substrate and its hydrolysis may (BERGMANN et al. 1950a, HARDEGG et al. 1956, UNDERHAY 1957) or may not be measurable depending on the conditions of the test (ADAMS 1949, AUGUSTINSSON 1949, NACHMANSOHN and ROTHENBERG 1944, 1945). It is certainly a strong competitive inhibitor of AChE with regard to the hydrolysis of good substrates; this, coupled with the excellent substrate properties of butyrylcholine towards butyrocholinesterase (BuChE), makes it a useful agent for the analysis of mixtures of ChE's (COHEN et al. 1949).

AUGUSTINSSON (1949) reported on the pS-activity relationship for the choline esters, including acetyl-β-methylcholine, and WHITTAKER (1951) on the relation between the length of the acyl chain and the speed of hydrolysis.

It is curious that no inhibition by high substrate concentrations was observed for dimethylaminoethyl acetate (WILSON 1952b, WILSON and BERGMANN 1950a); this phenomenon was reported also for esters carrying no positive charges, such as triacetin (ADAMS 1949, AUGUSTINSSON 1948, 1949, 1950b, BODANSKY 1946, WHITTAKER 1949); the pS-activity curve of these substrates does not show the "bell shape". BERGMANN and SHIMONI (1953) reported that the same applies to noncharged aliphatic esters (ADAMS 1949, BALDRIDGE et al. 1955, WILSON 1952b) amongst which is the carbon analogue of ACh, β,β-dimethylbutyl acetate (ADAMS 1949). This ester is notable for its rapid hydrolysis by AChE, showing that the cationic site is no absolute condition for proper binding of the substrate at the active site. In the case of these compounds the absence of substrate inhibition is readily explained on account of the lacking of a cationic site; the latter is necessary to cause the addition of a substrate molecule to the active EHS complex to give the inactive EHS_2 complex (see A. 1).

Conversely, uncharged alkyl halogenoacetates (ADAMS and WHITTAKER 1950, BERGMANN 1955, BERGMANN et al. 1956, McNAUGHTON and ZELLER 1949, ZELLER and BISSEGER 1943) do show the phenomenon of substrate inhibition (BERGMANN et al. 1950b, BERGMANN and SHIMONI 1953).

Carboxyl acid anhydrides (BERGMANN et al. 1953a, 1953b, WILSON 1952b) are hydrolyzed by AChE and thus have borne upon the concept of an acyl enzyme complex in normal substrate hydrolysis (see A. 2).

It has been known for a long time that substituted phenyl esters are hydrolyzed (WHITTAKER 1951, ZELLER et al. 1949); more recently this was confirmed by MOUNTER and WHITTAKER (1953) and UNDERHAY (1957) using purified preparations. Other compounds that are split are indoxyl- and α-naphthyl esters (UNDERHAY 1957) and salicylyl- and acetyl salicylyl choline (AUGUSTINSSON 1948, 1950a, ZELLER et al. 1949). BERGMANN et al. (1958), KOELLE (1950), KOELLE and FRIEDENWALD (1949), and WILSON (1952b) showed the hydrolysis of acetyl thiocholine by AChE, as had been shown earlier with BuChE by GLICK (1939).

The interesting hydrolysis by AChE of dithiolacetic acid ($CH_3 \cdot CO \cdot SS \cdot CO \cdot CH_3$) into acetic acid, thiolacetic acid, and sulphur (WILSON 1952b), and that of thiolacetic acid into hydrogen sulphide and acetic acid should be mentioned (WILSON 1951b).

II. Stereochemical specificity

AUGUSTINSSON and ISACSHEN (1957) and HOSKIN and TRICK (1955) have shwon that only the D-form of acetyl-β-methylcholine (methacholine, Mecholyl) is attacked by AChE. According to AMMAN and MEYER (1959), AChE from various brain tissues hydrolyzes preferably the L-configuration of the choline ester of mandelic acid (possessing an asymmetrical C-atom in the acid residue). BERGMANN et al. (1950a) found that for the inhibition of AChE by amino acids the L-configuration was required.

FRIESS et al. (1958) studied inhibition by trimethyl (2-piperidinopropyl)-ammonium. They reported that the (*d*) isomer was more effective than the (*l*) isomer. AARON et al. (1958) showed that (l)-0-ethyl S-(2-ethylthioethyl) ethylphosphonothioate attacked AChE much more rapidly than the *d*-form.

III. Interpretation of substrate specificity of AChE with respect to properties of the active site

The study of the kinetics of the hydrolysis by AChE of a variety of substrates from many different classes has greatly contributed to our understanding of the active site and its mode of action. We have already had many opportunities to show how the use of different substrates can elucidate certain properties of AChE, such as the *Km* and various kinetic constants.

In the previous section it was mentioned that the absence of substrate inhibition when uncharged substrates are used agrees with and confirms Haldane's theory elaborated in A. 1. Moreover, the hydrolysis of carboxylic acid anhydrides was shown to be relevant in the present context insofar as it confirmed the theory of the acyl enzyme intermediate in the course of AChE action. The formation of H_2S from thiolacetic acid corroborates this theory; it is explained by the reaction sequence:

$$CH_3COSH + EH \rightleftharpoons EH \cdot CH_3COSH$$
$$\downarrow$$
$$\dot{E}\!-\!COCH_3 + H_2S$$
$$H_2O \downarrow$$
$$EH + CH_3COOH$$

Table 1, which was given earlier, presented the *Km* and the k_3 values for a number of substrates which varied greatly in *Km* and relatively little in k_3. WILSON (1952b) used these data to corroborate his hypothesis that *Km* is determined essentially by k_2/k_1, the dissociation constant of the EHS complex. Moreover, he calculated the contribution of the cationic group of substrates to their overall binding force from the hydrolysis data of dimethylaminoethyl acetate between pH 6 and 10. In this range the substrate converts from the ionized into the un-ionized form which is reflected by an accompanying increase of the Km. Assuming that Km is equivalent to k_2/k_1, and using the BRØNSTED equation, he calculated a distance of 6.3 to 6.5 Å (NACHMANSOHN and WILSON 1951, WILSON and BERGMANN 1950a) for the nearest approach between the cationic site of the substrate and the singly charged anionic site of the enzyme (see Table 2). Earlier, ADAMS and WHITTAKER (1950) established this distance at 5 to 6 Å, using slightly different experimental conditions.

Table 2. *The effect of positive electrical charge on the binding forces of substrates and inhibitors*

Reactants	$\dfrac{K^{\cdot}}{K}$	Distance (Å)			References
		(14)	(15)	(16)	
Physostigmine$^+$	20		6.5		WILSON and BERGMANN (1950a)
Physostigmine$^\circ$	16		5.4	6.7	WILSON (1954)
N-Methylnicotinamide$^+$ Nicotinamide$^\circ$	8		5.8	7.7	WILSON (1954)
Dimethylaminoethanol$^+$ Isoamyl alcohol$^\circ$	30 30		5.0 5.7	6.3	WILSON (1954) WILSON (1952b)
Dimethylaminoethyl acetate$^+$ Isoamyl acetate$^\circ$	8	6.6			BERNHARD (1955a)
Dimethylaminoethyl acetate$^+$ Dimethylaminoethyl acetate$^\circ$	20		6.5		WILSON and BERGMANN (1950a)
Choline$^+$ — AChE	29			5.3	ADAMS and WHITTAKER (1950)
Choline$^+$ — BuChE	29		5.6		BERNHARD (1955a)
Butyrocholinesterase (BuChE): Acetylcholine$^+$ 3,3-dimethylbutyl acetate$^\circ$	1.3				ADAMS and WHITTAKER (1950)

The figures in column 3 were calculated from $\dfrac{K^{\cdot}}{K}$ using equation (14), (15), or (16) given at page 311. $^+$ charged species of reactant; $^\circ$ uncharged species of reactant. For further explanation see text.

The contribution of electrostatic interaction of the anionic site of AChE with charged sub-strates and inhibitors to the total binding force, expressed as the free energy change (ΔF), may be computed from the thermodynamic equation (13):

$$\Delta F = - \mathrm{RT} \ln \frac{K}{K^{\cdot}} . \tag{13}$$

In this formula $K^{\cdot}$ is the dissociation constant of the enzyme complex of AChE with an ionized substrate or inhibitor, and K that with the same compound in unionized form. Alternatively, K may represent interaction of AChE with another uncharged molecule provided that it would not differ from the corresponding $K^{\cdot}$ for reasons other than the difference in electric charge between the compounds compared (*viz.*, ACh and the geometrically related 3,3-di-methylbutyl acetate). A third approach is the comparison of the dissociation constant of the EHS- or EHI-complex of AChE and that of BuChE with respect to the same charged substrate or inhibitor. Butyrocholinesterase is thought to be intimately related to AChE but to lack an anionic site. The relevant equation is:

$$\Delta F = - \mathrm{RT} \ln \frac{K^{\cdot} \mathrm{BuChE}}{K^{\cdot} \mathrm{AChE}} .$$

The ΔF calculated as suggested should be equal to the Coulomb interaction between the anionic site of AChE, which is supposed to possess a single charge, and the charged atom as computed from the Brønsted-Christiansen-Scatchard equation (cf. HAMMETT 1940, BERNHARD 1955a):

$$\Delta F = \frac{\varepsilon^2 \, N Z_A Z_B}{Dr} \cdot \frac{e^{-\varkappa(a_i - r)}}{1 + \varkappa a_i} \tag{14}$$

where ε is unit charge, N the Avogrado number, Z_A and Z_B the valency of the ions, D the effective dielectric constant, and r the distance between the centres of charge A and B. The second term of the equation represents a correction for the shielding action of the ions in the solution with respect to the electric field between A and B. It is the Debye-Hückel correction for the ionic composition of the medium applicable at low ionic strength for small, symmetrical ions. a_i is the distance of nearest approach of the ions of the medium to the central ion, A; in $\varkappa = \sqrt{(8 \, \varepsilon^2 / D \, k \, T)} \, \mu$, k is the Boltzmann constant and μ the ionic strength. The Debye-Hückel factor must be applied whenever, e.g., by steric action, the distance between the ionogenic group of the reactant and the anionic site of the enzyme becomes larger than the distance a_i of the salt ions to the anionic site. Low values for $K/K^{\cdot}$ and consequently for ΔF are an indication that this situation may prevail. Conversely, high values of $K/K^{\cdot}$ argue against steric hindrance, $a_i \sim r$, and formula (14) converts into

$$\Delta F = \frac{\varepsilon^2 N Z_A Z_B}{Dr} \cdot \frac{1}{1 + \varkappa r} \, . \tag{15}$$

It is equivalent with the alternative form

$$\log \frac{K}{K^{\cdot}} = \frac{\varepsilon^2 Z_A Z_B}{2.3 \, D r k T} \cdot \frac{1}{1 + \varkappa r} \text{ with } k = \mathrm{R/N} \, .$$

At ionic strength zero, (15) converts into equation (16),

$$\Delta F = \frac{\varepsilon^2 N Z_A Z_B}{Dr} \, , \tag{16}$$

the classical Coulomb equation. It follows form Table 2 that the effect of the ionic strength implies a considerable correction.

WILSON (1952b) found very good agreement between the difference in dissociation constants of AChE with ethyl acetate, isoamyl acetate, and ACh and the expected differences in ΔF of the respective EHS complexes as calculated from the Van der Waals forces of the methyl groups and the Coulomb forces of the positive N-atom of quaternary ammonium inhibitors. The same study showed that the substrates acetic acid anhydride and dithiolacetic acid which lack a cationic structure have a Km which is of the order of that of ACh. This result underscores the importance of the electrophilic carbon in the interaction of substrate with the esteratic site. Moreover, WILSON (1952b) demonstrated that the introduction of a 4th methyl group into the trimethylammonium ion did not influence its binding by AChE. On the other hand, the difference in Km between dimethylaminoethyl acetate and ACh suggests that the situation is complicated. This, coupled with the fact that dimethylaminoethyl acetate is not subject to substrate inhibition, prompted Wilson to the hypothesis that during substrate inhibition deformation of the AChE molecule takes place. BALDRIDGE et al. (1955) and FRIESS and BALDRIDGE (1956c) studied the cis-isomers of the acetates of 2-trimethyl-amino-cyclopentanol and the corresponding cyclohexanol. They found that these esters are better substrates than ACh, and concluded that the distance between the anionic and the esteratic site on the AChE surface amounts to approximately 2.5Å, where as the mean separation distance between the N and the O-atom in the $N-CH_2-CH_2O$-chain of ACh was calculated at 2.3 Å (FRIESS and McCARVILLE 1954a). In this connection it is interesting to recall the conclusion of BERNHARD (1955a) that ACh appears to be 1.0 Å too short; this conclusion was based on electrostatic energy calculations on the assumption that the excellent inhibitor physostigmine provides a veracious reflection of the enzyme surface. WHITTAKER (1954) pointed out that if an inhibitor like neostigmine with a longer carbonyl-nitrogen distance and a 10^4 times greater affinity for AChE than ACh was taken as having the unstrained configuration, the calculated difference in binding energy would correspond to an appreciable degree of deformation in the substrate.

BERGMANN et al. (1958) observed that the hydrolysis of acetylthiocholine and of phenyl acetate and its derivatives by AChE is pH independent in the pH range 7.5 to 9.5. In contrast, the hydrolysis of ACh is very much pH dependent in this range (see Fig. 6). These authors explained this pH-dependence by assuming that the acidic group of the esteratic site is capable of forming a hydrogen bridge to the ethereal oxygen of ACh. They suggested that the formation of this bond is not possible at high pH, or when the character of the ester linkage of the substrate is changed, such as happens in acetylthiocholine and the phenyl acetates.

C. The effect of the pH

In agreement with the policy followed in the arrangement of this review, general pH kinetics will be dealt with only insofar as it is of direct impact on the present subject. For more extensive background of pH-enzyme kinetics, the reader is referred to ALBERTY (1956b), M. DIXON (1953), HALDANE (1930), LAIDLER (1955b) and WALEY (1953).

It should be realized that during the enzymic action the pH may affect the enzyme, the substrate, or both. As far as the substrate is concerned, the main influence of the pH is connected with the degree of dissociation of ionizing groups, in particular the status of the N-atom of the amino-alcohol. When choline is involved, the N is present in the quaternary form in the usual p_H range and therefore essentially pH-independent. Thus, when ACh is the substrate, the pH variations formed must be ascribed to changes of the enzyme.

Figure 6 represents a pH-activity curve as described by BERGMANN et al. (1958) for the hydrolysis of ACh by eel AChE. The curve shows a maximum at a pH between 8 and 9. Many authors have confirmed the existence of a definite pH optimum for the hydrolysis of ACh by AChE. The most likely value for this optimum lies at pH 8.25 (BERGMANN et al. 1956, 1958, GRAUERS 1952, HEILBRONN 1954, HESTRIN 1950, SHUKUYA and SHINODA 1956, WILSON and BERGMANN 1950b).

WILSON and BERGMANN (1950a, 1950b) and WILSON (1954) considered the decreasing enzyme activity on either side of the pH optimum to be due to the influence of the ionization state of a basic and an acidic group on AChE, with ionization constants of pK_b and pK_a, respectively. Their kinetic analysis is based on this dualism of the active esteratic site. Form the pH-activity curve of the hydrolysis of ACh they calculated the values given in Table 3. Some evidence for the existence of an acidic group on the esteratic site has already been reported above; it is implied in the work of BERGMANN et al. (1958), who explained the pH dependence of ACh hydrolysis, as opposed to the pH independence of that of

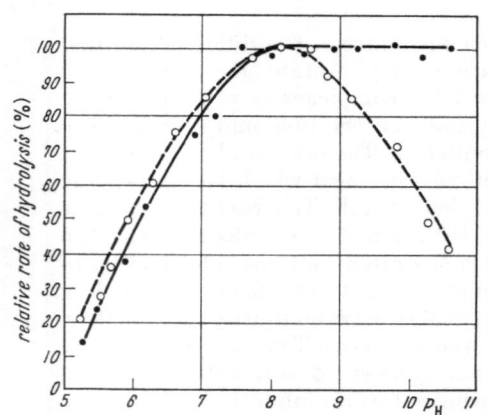

Fig. 6. *Hydrolysis of choline esters by eel AChE as a function of* pH. Substrates: ACh, 5×10^{-3} M (○) and acetylthiocholine, 6×10^{-3} M (●). Temperature 27°. From BERGMANN et al. (1958)

acetylthiocholine and phenyl acetates, as due to the existence of an acidic group capable of hydrogen bonding with ACh but not with the other esters. WILSON (1954) on the other hand suspected that the acidic group was not involved in substrate binding. He re-examined his experimental data on the assumption that a mechanism prevailed where the dissociation of the acidic group is essentially that of an acidic group in the EHS complex, dissociating into $ES^- + H^+$. LAIDLER (1955c) extended this approach with the hypothesis that the supercomplex EHS_2 is also liable to dissociate; the pK_a value which he derived on the basis of this assumption was considerably higher than that of WILSON.

Table 3. *Dissociation constants of active groups in acetylcholinesterase*

Source	Substrate or inhibitor	pK$_a$	pK$_b$	pK$_{anion}$	References
Electrophorus electricus	acetylcholine	9.3	7.2	—	[1]
Electrophorus electricus	acetylcholine	10.4	6.3	—	[2]
Electrophorus electricus	acetylcholine	10.3	7.2	—	[3]
Human red cells	acetylcholine	—	6.1	—	[4]
Torpedo marmorata	propyl fluoroacetate	9.0	6.2	—	[5]
Torpedo marmorata	propyl chloroacetate	9.0	6.2	—	[5]
Torpedo marmorata	tetraethylammonium Br	—	—	6.3	[5]
Electrophorus electricus	ethyl chloroacetate	9.6	6.7	—	[5]
Electrophorus electricus	ethyl bromoacetate	9.0	6.5	—	[5]
Electrophorus electricus	tetraethylammonium Br	—	—	6.2	[5]
Bovine red cells	acetylcholine	—	6.6	—	[6]

References: [1] WILSON and BERGMANN (1950b); [2] WILSON (1954); [3] LAIDLER (1955c); [4] SHUKUYA and SHINODA (1956); [5] BERGMANN et al. (1956); [6] MOUNTER et al. (1957a).

A difficulty that is met in the calculation of the pK values of the esteratic site is the possible contribution by the anionic site. To eliminate this influence, BERGMANN et al. (1956) calculated pK values of the esteratic site from the pH-activity curve of the enzymic hydrolysis of uncharged halogenoacetyl esters (cf. BERGMANN 1955).

From the values presented in Table 3 it follows that the pK refering to the basic group of the esteratic site is approximately 6.5. This is generally taken as evidence for the hypothesis that an imidazole residue of histidine operates at the active site (BERGMANN 1955, BERGMANN et al. 1956, MOUNTER et al. 1957a, WILSON 1954, WILSON and BERGMANN 1950b). The hypothesis is based primarily on kinetic evidence; it will be dealt with further in the last section in relation to other esterases. The imidazole hypothesis is further supported by pK studies on the inhibition of AChE by organophosphorus compounds which will be mentioned in the next section.

As a possible chemical group for the anionic site, the β-carboxylic group of aspartic acid or the γ-carboxylic group of glutamic acid may qualify. It should be noted, however, that the pK's of these groups (3.65 and 4.25, respectively) differ considerably with the values presented in Table 3. In this connection BERGMANN et al. (1956) have ventured the opinion that protonized imidazole at the esteratic site may influence the dissociation of the carboxylic group at the anionic site. In connection with their hypothesis that two negative groups may be concerned, BERGMANN et al. (1956, cf. BERNHARD 1955a) have suggested that the anionic site may contain an α-glutamyl-α-glutamyl peptide situated near the esteratic site. The problem of the chemical nature of the anionic site can not be considered to be solved as yet, nor would it be prudent to express at this stage a preference for one of the two possibilities mentioned.

For the mathematical analysis of the pH effect, obviously a chemical model of the enzyme action should be selected. For this purpose WILSON and BERGMANN (1950b) used the hypothesis that the esteratic site of the active center of AChE, EH, may convert into inactive forms by either donating or receiving a proton as follows:

$$\mathrm{EH_2^+} \xrightleftharpoons{+\mathrm{H^+}} \mathrm{EH} \xrightleftharpoons{-\mathrm{H^+}} \mathrm{E^-}\,.$$

Depending on pH, three forms of AChE may now occur, viz., EH, $\mathrm{EH_2^+}$ and $\mathrm{E^-}$. When it is further postulated that only EH reacts with substrate, the following reactions will prevail:

$$\mathrm{EH} \rightleftarrows \mathrm{E^-} + \mathrm{H^+}, \text{ with } K_{EH}$$

$$\mathrm{EH_2^+} \rightleftarrows \mathrm{EH} + \mathrm{H^+}, \text{ with } K_{EH_2^+}$$

$$\mathrm{EHS} + \mathrm{S} \rightleftarrows \mathrm{EHS_2}, \text{ with } K_2$$

$$\text{and } \mathrm{EH} + \mathrm{S} \underset{k_2}{\overset{k_1}{\rightleftarrows}} \mathrm{EHS} \xrightarrow{k_3} \mathrm{EH} + \text{ products, with}$$

$$Km = \frac{k_2 + k_3}{k_1}\,,$$

In the steady state $v = k_3(\mathrm{EHS})$. After calculation of EHS from the equilibria above, and from $(\mathrm{EHS}) = (\mathrm{EH}_t) - (\mathrm{E^-}) - (\mathrm{EH_2^+}) - (\mathrm{EHS_2})$ assuming that (EH) is negligible, substitution gives

$$v = \frac{k(\mathrm{EH}_t)\,(\mathrm{S})}{Km\left[\dfrac{(\mathrm{H^+})}{K_{EH_2^+}} + 1 + \dfrac{K_{EH}}{(\mathrm{H^+})}\right] + (\mathrm{S}) + \dfrac{(\mathrm{S})^2}{K_2}}\,. \qquad (17)$$

(S)opt is derived from (17) by differentiation with respect to (S):

$$(\mathrm{S})\mathrm{opt} = \sqrt{Km \cdot K_2 \left[\frac{(\mathrm{H^+})}{K_{EH_2^+}} + 1 + \frac{K_{EH}}{(\mathrm{H^+})}\right]}\,. \qquad (18)$$

(S)opt proves to be a function of pH. The $(\mathrm{H^+})$opt is found by differentiation of (17) with respect to $(\mathrm{H^+})$

$$(\mathrm{H^+})\mathrm{opt} = \sqrt{K_{EH_2^+} \cdot K_{EH}}\,. \qquad (19)$$

Formula (17) may be converted by relating v to v°, the velocity at optimal pH. With $K_{EH_2^+} \gg K_{EH}$ (as is actually the case),

$$\frac{v^\circ}{v} = 1 + \frac{Km\,(\mathrm{H^+})}{K_{EH_2^+}\left[Km + (\mathrm{S}) + \dfrac{(\mathrm{S})^2}{K_2}\right]} + \frac{Km \cdot K_{EH}}{\left[Km + (\mathrm{S}) + \dfrac{(\mathrm{S})^2}{K_2}\right]} \cdot \frac{1}{(\mathrm{H^+})}\,. \qquad (20)$$

For $(\mathrm{H^+}) > (\mathrm{H^+})$opt, the second $(\mathrm{H^+})$ term is negligible; therefore, v°/v will be linear with respect to $(\mathrm{H^+})$. For $(\mathrm{H^+}) < (\mathrm{H^+})$opt, the first $(\mathrm{H^+})$ term is negligible; therefore, v°/v will be linear with respect to $1/(\mathrm{H^+})$. The relationship between v and (S) may be represented graphically using the following equation derived from (17):

$$\frac{(\mathrm{S})}{v} = \frac{1}{k(\mathrm{EH}_t)}\left[Km\left(\frac{(\mathrm{H^+})}{K_{EH_2^+}} + 1 + \frac{K_{EH}}{(\mathrm{H^+})}\right) + (\mathrm{S}) + \frac{(\mathrm{S})^2}{K_2}\right]\,. \qquad (21)$$

If substrate inhibition is negligible, $\left[(S) \gg \dfrac{(S)^2}{K_2} \right]$, the plot of $(S)/v$ versus (S) will be linear.

WILSON and BERGMANN (1950a) have shown that the experimental data with regard to the influence of p_H on the hydrolysis of ACh by AChE fits excellently into the equations developed, the $(S)/v$ against (S) plot is linear, and (S)opt depends on pH (confirmed by GRAUERS 1952 and HEILBRONN 1954). LAIDLER (1955c) has given the mathematical treatment for the assumption that both EH and EHS can release a proton.

D. The effect of the presence of inorganic ions

For the older literature on the effect of inorganic ions on AChE the reader is referred to the review by AUGUSTINSSON (1948).

Most studies have been concerned with the activation of AChE by divalent cations. Unfortunately, only very few have been performed on purified preparations although, particularly for this type of work, this is necessary to obtain unequivocal results. NACHMANSOHN (1940) showed activation of eel AChE by Ba^{++}, Ca^{++}, Mg^{++} and Mn^{++}, increasing in this order; 2×10^{-5} M Mn^{++} gave an activation of 14 times. VAN DER MEER (1953) reported 100% activation by Ca^{++} (5×10^{-3} M) of crude and purified red cell AChE (ACh conc. 10^{-2} M). MYERS (1952c) reported 50% activation under these circumstances for crude hemolysates.

With regard to $MgCl_2$, rather conflicting conclusions have been reached. FRIESS and McCARVILLE (1954a) found that complexing agents inhibit the enzyme activity down to 4% of the original value at Mg^{++} concentrations of 0.01 M; they concluded that Mg is essential for enzymic activity. Under similar conditions WILSON and CABIB (1954) observed an inhibition of only 20% and concluded that AChE should not be classified as a metallo-enzyme.

Table 4. *The effect of storage on the Mg^{++} activation of acetylcholinesterase*

pH	Added Mg^{++}, M	Versene M	Activity after dilution		
			0 hr	21 hr	62 hr
7.4	0.016		100	100	100[1]
7.4	0		15	50	76
8.2	0	0.014	18	79	91

Dilution stored at 3—4°. Tests run at $25.12 \pm 0.02°$ in substrate (3.34×10^{-3} M) and phosphate (1.2×10^{-2} M).
[1] The absolute activity in this standard run with Mg^{++} present was found to have dropped only 1% from that observed at 0 hours. From FRIESS et al. (1954).

Table 4 summarizes the results of FRIESS et al. (1954). It shows a curious effect on the activity of AChE after dilution. The rise of activity in the absence of added metal, coupled with the activating effect of versene suggests that the original preparation contained an inhibiting metal, which gradually dissociated after dilution. According to DIXON and WEBB (1958) this probably means that the effect of Mg^{++} in raising the activity to a constant value is due to a displacement of the inhibitor and not to direct activation.

The activation by univalent inorganic cations (Na^+, K^+, and Li^+) is probably non-specific and due only to increase in ionic strength. Compared with divalent ions, higher concentrations (NACHMANSOHN 1940) are usually required to obtain equivalent activation. Moreover the effect of divalent ions is additive with respect to that of the monovalent.

According to some authors monovalent ions may, in addition to increasing the ionic strength, possess a more specific action (MENDEL and RUDNEY 1945, MYERS, 1950, 1951, 1952c). These authors reported a shift of the optimal substrate concentration to lower values when monovalent ions are added. This shift was not observed by AUGUSTINSSON (1948) or VAN DER MEER (1953). From the curves of MYERS (1952c) (Fig. 5) it follows that at the usual concentration of substrate (10^{-3} M ACh) and NaCl the effect of monovalent cations on substrate hydrolysis is negligible. FRIESS and McCARVILLE (1954a) found that in a medium of 3.33×10^{-3} M ACh + 0.01 M $MgCl_2$ no activation could be achieved on purified eel AChE by increasing the ionic strength from 0.176 to 0.563.

Summarizing the available evidence, it appears that AChE is no metallo-enzyme and that the activation by Na^+, K^+, Li^+, Mg^{++} and Ca^{++} ions occurring at the usual substrate concentration is highly dependent on the experimental conditions. As an optimal ionic medium, 0.15 M NaCl + 0.01 to 0.04 M $MgCl_2$ is recommended.

E. The effect of the temperature

Studies of the effect of temperature on the hydrolysis of substrates by AChE has provided useful information on its mechanism of action (cf. CHADWICK 1957).

WILSON and CABIB (1956) using equation (8) determined the Km of eel AChE for various substrates and found that it varied little over a temperature range between 15 and 30°. This temperature independence of Km was reported also for red cell AChE towards ACh (SHUKUYA 1953).

Investigation of the dependence of k_3 on temperature was also very instructive. It has been shown earlier [equation (3)] on page 303 that the complete enzymic action for AChE, neglecting for a moment the inhibition at high substrate concentration, may be written as follows:

$$ EH + S \underset{k_2}{\overset{k_1}{\rightleftharpoons}} EHS \xrightarrow{k_4} E\text{-acyl} + alcohol \xrightarrow[k_5]{H_2O} EH + acid \qquad (22) $$

$$ \xrightarrow{k_3} $$

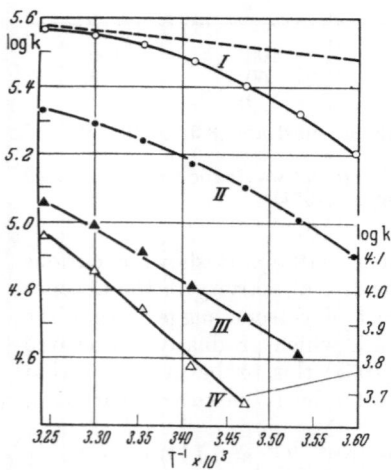

Fig. 7. *Arrhenius plot of log k versus T^{-1}*. Dotted line is drawn as an estimated asymptote to curve for substrate I and represents log k_5. Substrates used: acetylcholine (I), dimethylaminoethyl acetate (II), methylaminoethyl acetate (III), amino-ethyl acetate (IV). From WILSON and CABIB (1956)

According to this equation k_3, which was defined earlier (page 301) by the equation $v = k_3(\text{EHS})$, represents at least two reactions with velocity constants k_4 and k_5. WILSON and CABIB (1956) have tried to establish which part of the overall velocity constant k_3 could at various temperatures be allocated to k_4 and to k_5, respectively. Using the data of v versus (S) plots for various temperatures, they plotted $\log k_3$ versus $1/T$ according to Arrhenius. The slope of this type of graph, that should give straight lines, expresses the activation energy E in units of energy ($^e\log k = {}^e\log A - \dfrac{E}{RT}$, where A is a probability term and R the gas constant). They thus obtained a curve with a downward slope for ACh, whereas for other acetyl substrates of lower affinity (large Km) straight lines were observed (Fig. 7). Therefore, in the latter case it is likely that the energy of activation is determined by one velocity constant which may be either k_4 or k_5 at all temperatures. All acetyl substrates used must give an identical acetyl enzyme complex, and correspondingly must have an identical k_5. The difference in slope observed for different acetyl substrates must therefore be due to variations in k_4, the formation of the acetyl enzyme complex.

The non-linear curve for ACh is likely to be due to varying contributions of k_4 and k_5, depending on temperature. The authors concluded that for sluggish substrates (high Km), k_4 is rate limiting; whereas for good substrates (small numerical values of Km) like ACh, k_5 (hydrolysis of acyl enzyme) is rate limiting at high temperatures, and k_4 (formation of acyl enzyme) at low temperatures. For ACh, k_4 and k_5 are equal at 3°. The constant k_5 may be found by extrapolation to high values of T. It should be equal for all acetyl substrates; its logarithm ($\log k_5$) varies between 5.65 and 5.56 at 35°. The activation energy for purified eel AChE is 1.7 ± 0.4 kcal/mole (WILSON and CABIB 1956), and 3.7 kcal/mole for red cell AChE (SHUKUYA 1953) under normal conditions.

The Interaction of AChE with Inhibitors

The inhibitors of AChE, the anticholinesterase (anti-ChE) agents, may be divided into reversible and irreversible inhibitors. We shall use the term reversible to indicate that the enzyme-inhibitor complex dissociates freely on removal of the free inhibitor by dialysis or otherwise, showing that there is an equilibrium between free inhibitor and enzyme. With irreversible inhibitors, no such equilibrium is established and the enzyme activity does not, or at least not readily, return on mere dialysis. The distinction between substrates and inhibitors and between reversible and irreversible inhibitors is by no means absolute. There is a continuous transition from substrates, through reversible inhibitors, to irreversible inhibitors. Under certain circumstances, a distinct hydrolysis of butyrylcholine by AChE may be registered; the hydrolysis of ACh is, however, markedly impeded by butyrylcholine. The strong inhibitor (3-acetoxyphenyl)trimethylammonium is slowly split by AChE (WESCOE et al. 1950) to give another inhibitor, (3-hydroxyphenyl)trimethylammonium. The essentially reversible character of a reversible inhibitor may be obscured by very strong bonding to the enzyme, as in the case of polymethylene bis [(m-hydroxyphenyl)ammonium chloride, methylcarbamate] (HERZFELD and STUMPF 1956, KRAUPP et al. 1955).

In agreement with the purpose of this chapter the reversible and irreversible inhibitors (see Tables 5 and 6) will be treated in as far as they provide information on the active site of AChE. More complete listings at the same classes of compounds, with ancillary data, can be found in chapters 8 and 9, respectively.

A. Reversible inhibitors

I. Kinetics of the interaction of AChE with reversible inhibitors

The reversible inhibitors may be divided into competitive and non-competitive inhibitors. In the case of competitive inhibitors, substrate and inhibitor influence each other's affinity for the enzyme molecule. This may mean that substrate and inhibitor compete for one and the same site at the AChE molecule, or merely that they hinder each other's attachment to separate sites. The formation of the enzyme-substrate complex will be hampered, but its hydrolysis will be unaltered. Thus, in either case the maximal velocity (at excess substrate) will be equal to V_{max}, i.e., the maximal velocity for the uninhibited enzyme, but the $K\acute{m}$ will increase with regard to Km; the $K\acute{m}$ is the apparent Michaelis constant. It is the concentration of substrate at half-maximal velocity in the presence of inhibitor.

Table 5. *List of selected reversible inhibitors of acetylcholinesterase*

Formula	Name		$K_i \times 10^4$	References
$(CH_3)_4\overset{+}{N}$	tetramethylammonium		162"	Wilson (1952b)
$(CH_3)_3\overset{+}{N}H$	trimethylammonium		135" 189^	Wilson (1952b)
$(CH_3)_2\overset{+}{N}H_2$	dimethylammonium		1080^	Wilson (1952b)
CH_3NH_3	methylammonium		6300^	Wilson (1952b)
$(C_2H_5)_4\overset{+}{N}$	tetraethylammonium		45"	Wilson (1952b)
$(CH_3)_3\overset{+}{N}-CH_2-CH_2OH$	trimethylethanolammonium (choline)		45"	Wilson (1952b)
$(CH_3)_2\overset{+}{N}H-CH_2-CH_2OH$	dimethylethanolammonium		45"	Wilson (1952b)
$(CH_3)_2CH-CH_2-CH_2OH$	isoamylalcohol		1350"	Wilson (1952b)
$(CH_3)_2\overset{+}{N}H-CH_2-CH_2-CH_3$	dimethylpropylammonium		36"	Wilson (1952b)
$CH_3NH_2-CH_2-CH_2OH$	methylethanolammonium		630"	Wilson (1952b)
$\overset{+}{N}H_3-CH_2-CH_2OH$	ethanolammonium		2520^	Wilson (1952b)
$(CH_3)_3\overset{+}{N}-(CH_2)_n-CH_3$	tetramethylammonium	n = 0	135^	Bergmann and Segal (1954)
	trimethylethylammonium	n = 1	61.2	Bergmann and Segal (1954)
	trimethylpropylammonium	n = 2	27	Bergmann and Segal (1954)
	trimethylbutylammonium	n = 3	18	Bergmann and Segal (1954)
	trimethylpentylammonium	n = 4	13.5	Bergmann and Segal (1954)
	trimethylhexylammonium	n = 5	6.21	Bergmann and Segal (1954)
	trimethylheptylammonium	n = 6	5.4	Bergmann and Segal (1954)
$(CH_3)_3\overset{+}{N}-(CH_2)_n-\overset{+}{N}(CH_3)_3$	tetramethylenebis(trimethylammonium)	n = 4	774	Bergmann and Segal (1954)
	pentamethylenebis(trimethylammonium)	n = 5	432	Bergmann and Segal (1954)
	hexamethylenebis(trimethylammonium) (hexamethonium)	n = 6	171	Bergmann and Segal (1954)
	heptamethylenebis(trimethylammonium)	n = 7	108	Bergmann and Segal (1954)
	octamethylenebis(trimethylammonium)	n = 8	21.6	Bergmann and Segal (1954)

Structure	Name	Value	Reference
$n = 9$	nonamethylenebis(trimethylammonium)	2.7	BERGMANN and SEGAL (1954)
$n = 10$	decamethylenebis(trimethylammonium) (decamethonium)	0.18	BERGMANN and SEGAL (1954)
$n = 12$	dodecamethylenebis(trimethylammonium)	0.073	BERGMANN and SEGAL (1954)
$(CH_3)_2N$— cyclohexyl —OH	2-dimethylaminocyclohexanol (cis)	0.4″	FRIESS (1957)
$(CH_3)_3\overset{+}{N}$— cyclohexyl —OH	trimethyl[(2-hydroxycyclohexyl)ammonium] (cis) (trans)	0.11= 0.21=	BALDRIDGE et al. (1955) cf FRIESS and BALDRIDGE (1956c)
$(CH_3)_3\overset{+}{N}$— cyclopentyl (HO)	trimethyl[(2-hydroxycyclopentyl)ammonium] (cis) (trans)	7.5= 8.9=	FRIESS and BALDRIDGE (1956c)
$(CH_3)_3\overset{+}{N}$— cyclohexyl —$N(CH_3)_2$	2-dimethylaminocyclohexyltrimethyl ammonium (cis) (trans)	2.35= 2.9=	MASTERSON and FRIESS (1958)
$(CH_3)_3\overset{+}{N}$—CH_2—CH_2Cl	trimethyl[(2-chloroethyl)ammonium]	0.012″	FRIESS and McCARVILLE (1954b)
$(CH_3)_3\overset{+}{N}$—CH_2—$CHCl$—CH_3	trimethyl[(2-chloropropyl)ammonium]	1.68=	FRIESS and BALDRIDGE (1956b)
$(CH_3)_3\overset{+}{N}$—CH_2—CH_2—$N(CH_3)_2$	trimethyl[(2-dimethylaminoethyl)ammonium]	0.0083″	FRIESS and McCARVILLE (1954b)
$(CH_3)_2N$—CH_2—CH_2—N (piperidine)	1-(2-dimethylaminoethyl)piperidine	0.0064″	FRIESS (1957)
$(CH_3)_2N$—CH_2—CH(CH_3)—CH_2—N (piperidine)	1-(2-dimethylaminopropyl)piperidine	1.0=	FRIESS and BALDRIDGE (1956b)
$(CH_3)_2N$—CH_2—CH(CH_3)—N (piperidine)	1-(2-dimethylamino-1-methylethyl)piperidine	1.04=	FRIESS and BALDRIDGE (1956b)

Table 5 (continued)

Formula	Name	$K_f \times 10^5$	References
$(CH_3)_3\overset{+}{N}$—CH_2—CH_2—N (piperidino)	trimethyl(2-piperidinoethyl)ammonium	0.0016"	FRIESS (1957) cf. FRIESS and BALDRIDGE (1956b)
$(CH_3)_3\overset{+}{N}$—CH—CH_2—N, CH_3	trimethyl(2-piperidinopropyl)ammonium dl d l	0.91= 1.6= 2.8= 0.67=	FRIESS and BALDRIDGE (1956c); FRIESS et al. (1958)
$(CH_3)_3\overset{+}{N}$—CH_2—N, CH_3	trimethyl(1-methyl-2-piperidino ethyl)-ammonium	1.45=	FRIESS and BALDRIDGE (1956c)
$(CH_3)_2N$—CH_2—CH_2—N (pyrrolidine)	1-(2-dimethylaminoethyl)pyrrolidine	0.0049"	FRIESS (1957)
$(CH_3)_3\overset{+}{N}$—CH_2—CH_2—N (pyrrolidine)	trimethyl 2-(1-pyrrolidinyl)-ethyl ammonium	0.0023"	FRIESS (1957)
$(CH_3)_3\overset{+}{N}$-phenyl	phenyltrimethylammonium	3.8=	WILSON and QUAN (1958)
$(CH_3)_3\overset{+}{N}$-phenyl-OH	(3-hydroxyphenyl)trimethylammonium	0.031=	WILSON and QUAN (1958)
$(CH_3)_3\overset{+}{N}$-phenyl-OH	(4-hydroxyphenyl)trimethylammonium	2.3=	WILSON and QUAN (1958)
$(CH_3)_3\overset{+}{N}$-phenyl-OH	(2-hydroxyphenyl)trimethylammonium	0.52=	WILSON and QUAN (1958)
$(CH_3)_3\overset{+}{N}$-phenyl-OCH_3	(3-methoxyphenyl)trimethylammonium	0.75=	WILSON and QUAN (1958)

Structure	Name	Value	Reference
	(4-methyl-3-hydroxyphenyl)trimethyl-ammonium	0.0099=	Wilson and Quan (1958)
	(3-hydroxyphenyl)ethyldimethylammonium (Tensilon, edrophonium)	0.033"	Wilson (1955b)
	(2-hydroxyphenyl)trimethylammonium dimethylcarbamate RO1-4987	0.0072"	Foldes et al. (1958)
	(2-hydroxybenzyl)trimethylammonium dimethylcarbamate RO2-9147	0.001"	Foldes et al. (1958)
	(3-hydroxybenzyl)trimethylammonium dimethylcarbamate RO2-0907	0.05"	Foldes et al. (1958)
	(3-hydroxyphenyl)trimethylammonium dimethylcarbamate (neostigmine)	0.0028" 0.016"	Foldes et al. (1958) Augustinsson and Nachmansohn (1949b), cf. Wilson and Bergmann (1950a); Nachmansohn and Wilson (1951)

Table 5 (continued)

Formula	Name	$K_I \times 10^6$	References
	physostigmine (eserine)	0.0061''	AUGUSTINSSON and NACHMANSOHN (1949b), cf. WILSON and BERGMANN (1950a); NACHMANSOHN and WILSON (1951)
NH_2—CH_2—COOH	glycine ethyl glycinate	2700 270	BERGMANN et al. (1950b)
$(CH_3)_2N$—CH_2—CH_2—$\overset{\text{O}}{\underset{\parallel}{C}}$—$CH_3$	1-dimethylamino-3-butanone	45	BERGMANN et al. (1950b)
$(C_2H_5)_2N$—CH_2—CH_2—$C\equiv N$	β-diethylaminopropionitrile	20	BERGMANN et al. (1950b)
$(CH_3)_2N$—CH_2—CH_2—$C\equiv N$	β-dimethylaminopropionitrile	67	BERGMANN et al. (1950b)
	N-methylnicotinamide methyl sulphate	67	BERGMANN et al. (1950b)
	nicotinic acid (R=OH) nicotinamide (R=NH₂) N,N-diethylnicotinamide (R=N(C₂H₅)₂) β — acetylpyridine (R=CH₃) ethyl nicotinate (R=OC₂H₅)	2700 450 15 18 6.3	BERGMANN et al. (1950b)
	neostigmine(reference) [trimethylenebis (oxy-m-phenylene)] bis(trimethylammonium iodide) CT 2842	pI₅₀ = 8 pI₅₀ = 7.3	FUNKE et al. (1954) FUNKE et al. (1954)

Structure	Compound	pI_{50}	Reference
HO–⟨C₆H₃(OH)⟩–O–(CH₂)₃–O–⟨C₆H₃⟩–N(CH₃)₃⁺ ; 2 I⁻ ; N(CH₃)₃⁺	{trimethylene*bis*[oxy(5-hydroxy-*m*-phenylene)]}*bis*(trimethylammonium iodide) CT 3116	$pI_{50} = 9.7$	FUNKE et al. (1954)
R–C(=O)–O–⟨C₆H₃⟩–O–(CH₂)₃–O–⟨C₆H₃⟩–N(CH₃)₃⁺ ; 2 I⁻ ; O–C(=O)–R ; N(CH₃)₃⁺ ; R = N(CH₃)₂	{3-[3-(*m*-dimethylaminophenoxy)propoxy]-5-hydroxyphenyl}-trimethyl ammonium iodide methiodide, dimethyl carbamate CT 3152	$pI_{50} = 9.2$	FUNKE et al. (1954)
R–C(=O)–O–⟨C₆H₃⟩–O–(CH₂)₃–O–⟨C₆H₃⟩–O–C(=O)–R ; 2 I⁻ ; N(CH₃)₃⁺ ; N(CH₃)₃⁺ ; R = N(CH₃)₂	{trimethylene *bis* [oxy(5-hydroxy-*m*-phenylene)]}*bis*(trimethylammonium iodide), *bis*(dimethylcarbamate) CT 3113	$pI_{50} = 9.0$	FUNKE et al. (1954)
[(CH₃)₃N⁺ ; I⁻ ; O–C(=O)–N(CH₃)–(CH₂)₄–]₂	octamethylene bis (*m*-hydroxyphenyl) ammonium chloride, methylcarbamate BC 47	$pI_{50} = 9.4$	KRAUPP et al. (1955)

For a number of compounds the values of K_i were calculated from the known C_{50} values using the relation $K_i = 0.09 \times C_{50}$ computed from equation

$$\frac{v}{v'} = 1 + \frac{(I)}{K_i\left[1 + \dfrac{(S)}{K_m} + \dfrac{(S)^2}{K_m K_2}\right]}$$

assuming an ionic strength $= 0.25$ and concentration of ACh $= 4 \times 10^{-3}$ M and substituting K_m and K_2 values as given by WILSON (1952b) for the system AChE—ACh at pH 7.3 and 37°. The indices of the K_i values refer to the ionic strength in the ranges 0.1—0.15 (=), 0.15—0.25 ("), 0.25—0.30 ('), 0.30—0.45 (^).

Table 6. *Organophosphorus anticholinesterase agents*

Formula	Name	Remarks[1]
C_2H_5O P—O—P OC_2H_5 / C_2H_5O, OC_2H_5 / O O	tetraethyl pyrophosphate (TEPP)	$k_2 = 2.1 \times 10^6$, eel AChE, pH 7.4, 25°, MICHEL (1955) $k_2 = 3.3 \times 10^6$, sheep red cell AChE, pH 7.6, 37°, ALDRIDGE and DAVISON (1952a)
$(CH_3)_2CHO$ P O / $(CH_3)_2CHO$ F	diisopropyl phosphorofluoridate (DFP)	$k_2 = 1.9 \times 10^4$, eel AChE, pH 7.4, 25°, MICHEL (1955) $k_2 = 9.5 \times 10^4$, human cell AChE, pH 7.4, 25°, JANDORF et al. (1955b)
n-C_3H_7O P O / n-C_3H_7O $OCH=CCl_2$	di-n-propyl 2,2-dichlorovinyl phosphate (DDP)	$k_2 = 2.8 \times 10^5$, eel AChE $k_2 = 1.3 \times 10^6$, human cell AChE, pH 7.4, 25°, JANDORF (1956b)
C_2H_5O P O / C_2H_5O O—⟨⟩—NO_2	diethyl-4-nitrophenylphosphate (Paraoxon, E 600, Mintacol)	$k_2 = 1.1 \times 10^6$, sheep red cell AChE, pH 7.6, 37°, ALDRIDGE and DAVISON (1952a, 1952b)
C_2H_5O P O / C_2H_5O S—⟨⟩—NO_2	0,0-diethyl-S-(4-nitrophenyl) phosphorothioate	$k_2 = 9.7 \times 10^5$, sheep red cell AChE, pH 7.6, 37°, ALDRIDGE and DAVISON (1952b)
C_2H_5O P O $CH_3SO_4^-$ / C_2H_5O O ⟨⟩—$\overset{+}{N}(CH_3)_3$	3-(diethylphosphato)-N-trimethyl anilinium methyl sulphate (diethylphosphostigmine)	$pI_{50} = 7.4$, human red cell AChE, pH 7.4 (approx.), 20 min, 37°, HOBBIGER (1954b)
C_2H_5O P O $CH_3SO_4^-$ / C_2H_5O O [quinolinium ring] N CH_3	3-(diethylphosphato)-N-methylquinolinium methyl sulphate	$pI_{50} = 9.8$ human red cell AChE, pH 7.4 (approx.), 37°, 20 min, HOBBIGER (1954b)
C_2H_5O P O / C_2H_5O S—CH_2—CH_2—$\overset{+}{N}(CH_3)_3$ I^-	0,0-diethyl-S-2-trimethylammonium-methyl phosphonothiolate iodide	$pI_{50} = 8.4$[2] human red cell AChE, pH 7.5, 25°, 120 min $k_2 = 1.2 \times 10^5$, electric ray AChE, pH 7.5, 25°, TAMMELIN (1957b and 1958b)
$(CH_3)_2N$ P O / C_2H_5O $C\equiv N$	ethyl-N-dimethyl phosphoramidocyanidate (Tabun)	$pI_{50} = 7.95$[3] human red cell AChE, pH 7.4, 25°, 60 min, AUGUSTINSSON (1953a)
CH_3 P O / $(CH_3)_2CHO$ F	isopropyl methylphosphonofluoridate (Sarin)	$k_2 = 6.3 \times 10^7$, eel AChE, pH 7.4, 25°, MICHEL (1955) $k_2 = 1.5 \times 10^7$, human red cell AChE, pH 7.4, 25°, JANDORF (1956b)

Table 6 (continued)

Formula	Name	Remarks[1]
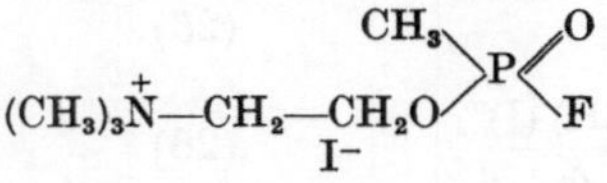 $(CH_3)_3\overset{+}{N}-CH_2-CH_2O$ ... $\underset{I^-}{}$ ... P with CH_3, O, F	2-trimethylammonium-ethyl methyl phos-phonofluoridate iodide	$pI_{50} = 10.0$[2]) human red cell AChE, pH 7.5, 25°, 30 min, TAMMELIN (1958a, 1958b)
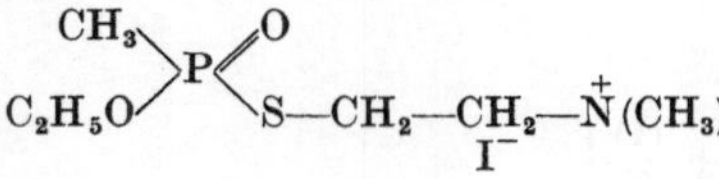 C_2H_5O ... P with CH_3, O, $S-CH_2-CH_2-\overset{+}{N}(CH_3)_3$ ... $\underset{I^-}{}$	0-ethyl-S-trimethyl-ammoniumethyl methylphosphono-thioate iodide	$pI_{50} = 9.1$[2]) human red cell AChE, pH 7.5, 25°, 120 min, TAMMELIN (1957b, 1958a) $k_2 = 4.2 \times 10^6$, electric ray AChE, pH 7.5, 25°, TAMMELIN (1958b)

[1]) In this column k_2 is the second order rate constant (1/mole. min); [2]) TEPP gives $pI_{50} = 7.5$; [3]) TEPP gives $pI_{50} = 6.79$.

In the case of non-competitive inhibition there will be separate sites on the AChE molecule to accomodate substrate and inhibitor. Substrate and inhibitor will not influence each other's interaction with the enzyme molecule, but the rate of hydrolysis will be decreased, because the enzyme molecules which have combined with inhibitor are not available for substrate hydrolysis, although they may be combined with substrate as well. In other words, the maximal velocity in the presence of inhibitor, V'_{max}, will be less than V_{max} of the uninhibited enzyme, but Km' (i.e., the substrate concentration at half V_{max}) will be equal to Km.

It is evident that for our present purpose, i.e., the study of the active site of AChE, non-competitive inhibitors and those competitive inhibitors which do not directly interact with the active site are far less interesting than the fully competitive inhibitors which actually compete with the substrate for one and the same site.

FRIEDENWALD and MAENGWYN-DAVIES (1954) have given general equations for competitive and non-competitive inhibition, and also for the mixture of competitive and non-competitive effects where Km as well as V_{max} of the uninhibited enzyme are altered in the presence of the inhibitor (cf. MASTERSON and FRIESS 1958). Since the analysis of the mixed type is too complicated to allow straightforward interpretation in the frame of the present problem, it will not be further elaborated.

a) Competitive inhibition

It was stated above that fully competitive inhibition is the most interesting interaction in the present context; in this case substrate and inhibitor compete for one and the same active site on the AChE molecule. The following reactions take place:

$$EH + S \underset{k_2}{\overset{k_1}{\rightleftarrows}} EHS \overset{k_3}{\underset{H_2O}{\longrightarrow}} EH + products \qquad (23)$$

$$\text{with } Km = \frac{k_2 + k_3}{k_1},$$

$EHS + S \rightleftarrows EHS_2$ with dissociation constant K_2, and $EH + I \rightleftarrows EHI$ with dissociation constant Ki and inhibitor I. The most convenient equations are obtained when v, the velocity for uninhibited enzyme is related to v', the velocity in the presence of inhibitor. We find for v (see p. 305):

$$v = \frac{V_{max}(S)}{Km + (S) + \dfrac{(S)^2}{K_2}}. \qquad (24)$$

In the presence of inhibitor the rate of hydrolysis will depend entirely on the fraction EHS of the total available enzyme (EH_t) that is formed:

$$\frac{v'}{V_{max}} = \frac{(EHS)}{(EH_t)} \, . \tag{25}$$

$$\text{Now } (EH_t) = (EH) + \frac{(EH)\,(S)}{Km} + \frac{(EH)\,(S)^2}{Km\,K_2} + \frac{(EH)\,(I)}{K_i} \, . \tag{26}$$

After substitution of (26) in (25) yielding

$$\frac{v'}{V_{max}} = \frac{(EHS)}{(EH)\left[1 + \dfrac{(S)}{Km} + \dfrac{(S)^2}{Km\,K_2} + \dfrac{(I)}{K_i}\right]} \, ,$$

and substitution of $\dfrac{(EHS)}{(EH)}$ by $\dfrac{(S)}{Km}$ [reaction (23)] we arrive at

$$v' = \frac{V_{max}\,(S)}{Km\left[1 + \dfrac{(S)}{Km} + \dfrac{(S)^2}{Km\,K_2} + \dfrac{(I)}{K_i}\right]} \, , \tag{27}$$

and

$$\frac{v}{v'} = 1 + \frac{(I)}{K_i\left[1 + \dfrac{(S)}{Km} + \dfrac{(S)^2}{Km\,K_2}\right]} \, . \tag{28}$$

When substrate inhibition is neglected,

$$\frac{v}{v'} = 1 + \frac{(I)}{K_i\left[1 + \dfrac{(S)}{Km}\right]} \, . \tag{29}$$

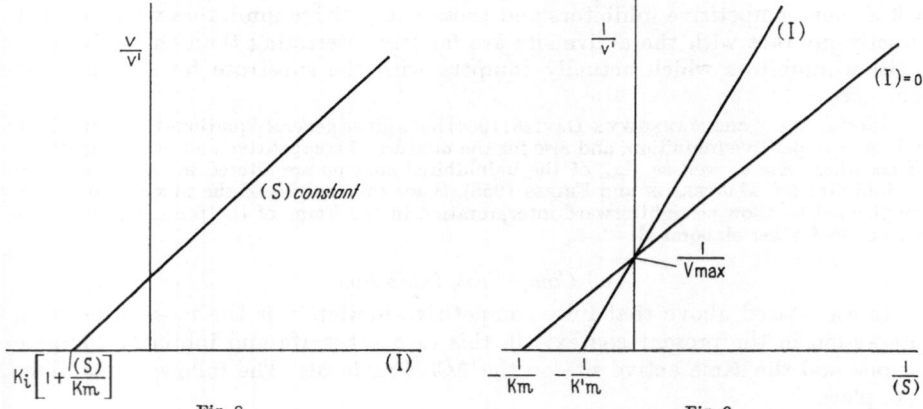

Fig. 8

Fig. 8. *Schematic plot of $\dfrac{v}{v'}$ against (I) for competitive inhibition with (S) constant*

Fig. 9. *Schematic plot of $\dfrac{1}{v'}$ against $\dfrac{1}{(S)}$ for competitive inhibition.* The reciprocal of the apparent Michaelis constant $K'm = Km\left[1 + \dfrac{(I)}{K_i}\right]$ is found at the intercept of the curve with the $\dfrac{1}{(S)}$ axis and is dependent on (I). The reciprocal of V_{max} is found at the intercept of the curve with the $\dfrac{1}{v'}$ axis and is independent of (I)

When (S) is kept constant, equations (28) and (29) may be graphically represented (Fig. 8) as plots of v/v' versus (I). A straight line is obtained; the intercept with the (I)-axis gives

$$K_i\left[1 + \frac{(S)}{Km} + \frac{(S)^2}{Km\,K_2}\right] \text{ and}$$

$$K_i\left[1 + \frac{(S)}{Km}\right], \text{ respectively.}$$

With known values for Km, K_2, and (S), K_i may be calculated. The graph may also be used to read the value for (I) at $v/v' = 2$, i.e., the $(I)_{50}$, the concentration of inhibitor for 50% inhibition. $(I)_{50}$ is sometimes called C_{50}; $pI_{50} = -\log C_{50}$. Rearrangement of equations (27) and (29) gives

$$\frac{1}{v'} = \frac{1}{V_{max}} + \frac{1}{V_{max}} \cdot \frac{1}{(S)} \left[Km + \frac{(S)^2}{K_2} + \frac{Km(I)}{K_i} \right] \tag{30}$$

and

$$\frac{1}{v'} = \frac{1}{V_{max}} + \frac{1}{V_{max}} \cdot \frac{Km}{(S)} \left[1 + \frac{(I)}{K_i} \right] . \tag{31}$$

It follows from (31) that a plot of $\dfrac{1}{v'}$ against $\dfrac{1}{(S)}$ for (I) constant gives a straight line; $\dfrac{1}{V_{max}}$ is given by the intercept with the $\dfrac{1}{v'}$ axis and the reciprocal value of $Km \left[1 + \dfrac{(I)}{K_i} \right]$ is given by the intercept with the $\dfrac{1}{(S)}$ axis (Fig. 9). $\dfrac{1}{V_{max}}$ does not depend on $Km \left[1 + \dfrac{(I)}{K_i} \right]$, implying that it is also independent from the concentration of inhibitor, which is typical for competitive inhibition. This simply means that at high substrate concentration all available enzyme is present in the form of the active EHS complex. For $(I) = 0$ the intercept with the $\dfrac{1}{(S)}$ axis corresponds to Km. $Km \left[1 + \dfrac{(I)}{K_i} \right]$ is known as the apparent Michaelis constant Km'. From $Km' = Km \left[1 + \dfrac{(I)}{K_i} \right]$ follows $K_i = \dfrac{(I)}{\dfrac{Km'}{Km} - 1}$. When substrate inhibition prevails [equation (30)], the $\dfrac{1}{v'}$ against $\dfrac{1}{(S)}$ plot is not linear.

Differentiating (27) with regard to (S) gives

$$\frac{dv'}{d(S)} = Km \left[1 + \frac{(I)}{K_i} \right] - \frac{(S)^2}{K_2} .$$

For (S) opt $\dfrac{dv'}{d(S)} = 0$ and

$$(S) \text{opt} = \sqrt{K_2 Km \left[1 + \frac{(I)}{K_i} \right]} = \sqrt{K_2 Km'} . \tag{32}$$

It follows that the optimal substrate concentration, (S)opt, is increased by the presence of a competitive inhibitor [cf. equations (9) and (32)] and increases with (I); this has been experimentally confirmed (see Fig. 3) (AUGUSTINSSON 1948, 1951a, AUGUSTINSSON and NACHMANSOHN 1949b, BERGMANN et al. 1950a, BRZIN and ŽUPANČIČ 1956).

b) Non-competitive inhibition

We shall deal here only with the practically important simple situation of fully non-competitive inhibition where the interactions of the substrate and of the inhibitor with AChE do not mutually influence each other's affinity for the enzyme. In this situation it seems reasonable to assume that the dissociation constants with regard to I of the inhibitor-enzyme complexes, EHI, EHIS, and $EHIS_2$, will be equal and that the inhibitor is in equilibrium with (EH_i), i.e., all initially present enzyme (including EH, EHS, and EHS_2). Moreover, it is assumed that only the EHS complex is active and subject to substrate hydrolysis; the enzyme-substrate-inhibitor-complex EHIS and the enzyme-double substrate-inhibitor complex $EHIS_2$ are supposed to be as inactive as EHI.

From $EH + I \rightleftarrows EHI$, with dissociation constant K_i, follows

$$\frac{(EH_i) - (EHI)}{(EHI)} = \frac{K_i}{(I)} \quad \text{and}$$

$$(EHI) = \frac{(I)}{K_i + (I)} \cdot (EH_i) .$$

Since we are dealing with non-competitive inhibition, all initially present enzyme (EH_t) (including EH and EHI) is also in equilibrium with substrate. However, only $(EH_t)-(EHI) = \dfrac{K_i}{K_i+(I)}$. (EH_t) will be available for the formation of active hydrolysable EHS complex. For the reaction velocity in the absence of inhibitor was calculated [equation (24)]

$$v = \frac{V_{max}\,(S)}{Km + (S) + \dfrac{(S)^2}{K_2}} \;.$$

When V'_{max} is the maximal velocity in the presence of inhibitor, it will be related to the V_{max} (in the absence of inhibitor) as the available enzyme (EH_t-EHI) is related to (EH_t). Thence,

$$V'_{max} = V_{max} \cdot \frac{K_i}{K_i + (I)} \quad \text{and}$$

$$v' = \frac{V_{max}\cdot(S)}{Km + (S) + \dfrac{(S)^2}{K_2}} \cdot \frac{K_i}{K_i + (I)} \;. \tag{33}$$

The ratio of the reaction velocities is

$$\frac{v}{v'} = \frac{K_i + (I)}{K_i} = 1 + \frac{(I)}{K_i} \;. \tag{34}$$

It follows from the above equations that for every concentration of inhibitor, v/v' is independent of the substrate concentration. V'_{max} is smaller than V_{max} for

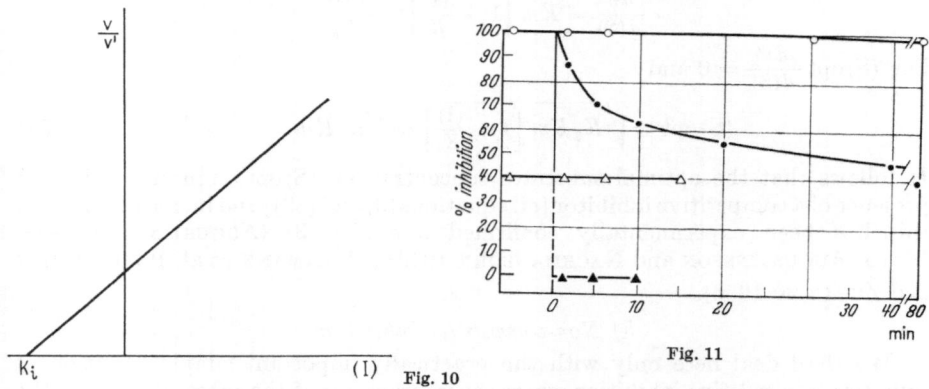

Fig. 10. *Schematic plot of* $\dfrac{v}{v'}$ *against (I) for non-competitive inhibition.* K_i *is found at the intercept of the curve with the (I) axis. The slope of the curve is independent of (S)*

Fig. 11. *Rate of dissociation of AChE complexes of edrophonium and neostigmine.* At zero time two portions of a solution of the enzyme in 2×10^{-6} M neostigmine (o) and in 2×10^{-6} M edrophonium ($\triangle$) were diluted 40 times, one with 2×10^{-6} M drug (same symbols) and one without drug (● and ▲ respectively). Assays requiring one minute were made at various times after dilution. From WILSON (1955b)

the uninhibited enzyme, but Km is unchanged. The K_i may be read from a plot of v/v' versus (I) as the reciprocal value of the slope. For non-competitive inhibition this slope is independent of the concentration of substrate (Fig. 10). Competitive can be distinguished experimentally from non-competitive inhibitors only when the equilibrium of substrate-inhibitor-enzyme is established with sufficient speed (compare the behaviour of edrophonium and neostigmine as demonstrated in Fig. 11).

Usually, the kinetics of inhibition are satisfactorily described by the simple equations quoted. The use of very powerful anti-ChE agents may, however, lead to situations where the concentrations of enzyme and inhibitor are of the same order, and prompt a somewhat more complicated treatment. In particular, the equations which are expressed in terms of free inhibitor then require correction. GOLDSTEIN (1944) and STRAUSS and GOLDSTEIN (1943), in their exhaustive treatment of the significance of relative concentrations of enzyme, substrate, and inhibitor for kinetic analysis, have dealt with this situation by the development of equations expressed in terms of total inhibitor concentrations. For the reaction $EH + I \rightleftarrows EHI$ with dissociation constant K_i,

$$K_i = \frac{(EH_t - EHI)(I - EHI)}{(EHI)},$$

where EH_t and I represent the total concentrations of enzyme and inhibitor, respectively. Introducing $i = \frac{(EHI)}{(EH_t)}$ as the fraction of total enzyme that is combined with inhibitor leads to

$$(I) = \frac{K_i \, i}{1-i} + i \, (EH_t). \qquad (35)$$

This equation demonstrates the partition of the total molar concentration of inhibitor between an enzyme-bound and a free component. Using the specific concentrations $(I)' = \frac{(I)}{K_i}$ and $(EH_t)' = \frac{(EH_t)}{K_i}$ simplifies (35) to

$$(I)' = \frac{i}{1-i} + i \, (EH_t)'. \qquad (36)$$

When the specific enzyme concentration $(EH_t)'$ is small, equation (36) simplifies into

$$(I)' = \frac{i}{1-i}. \qquad (37)$$

In this case the enzyme-bound fraction of inhibitor is negligible with regard to its total concentration, and the system is in zone A according to the terminology of STRAUSS and GOLDSTEIN. When $\frac{i}{1-i}$ is negligible with regard to $i(EH_t)'$, (36) converts into

$$(I)' = i(EH_t)'. \qquad (38)$$

The system is now in zone C of SRAUSS and GOLDSTEIN, when practically all inhibitor molecules are bound to the enzyme. In all other cases the system is in zone B which is described by the complete formula (36).

It is obvious that for the approximations which underlie equations (37) and (38), the ratio between the concentrations of enzyme and inhibitor and also the K_i are relevant. The zones are determined as follows:

$(EH_t)' < 0.1$ zone A
$(EH_t)' \; 0.1 - 100$ zone B
$(EH_t)' > 100$ zone C .

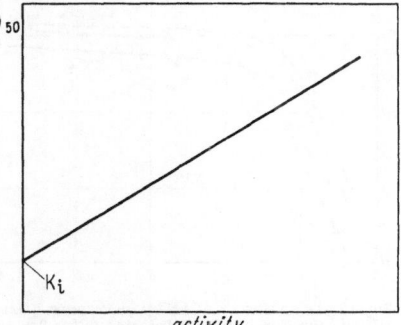

Fig. 12. *Determination of K_i for highly effective inhibitors of AChE. K_i appears as the intercept with the $(I)_{50}$ axis of the curve of the enzymic activity against $(I)_{50}$*

From equation (35) it follows, as was pointed out by MYERS (1952a), that at an inhibitor concentration $(I)_{50}$ resulting in 50% inhibition where $(EHI) = \frac{1}{2}(EH_t)$,

$$(I)_{50} = K_i + \frac{1}{2}(EH_t). \qquad (39)$$

When $(I)_{50}$ is determined at different enzyme concentrations, a linear curve is obtained from which K_i may be read as the intercept on the $(I)_{50}$ axis (see Fig. 12). Its value does not depend on the absolute but on the relative enzyme concentration, and the latter may be plotted as the enzyme's activity. Using equation (39) the enzyme concentration may now be calculated from known values of $(I)_{50}$ and K_i. For a proper estimation of $(I)_{50}$, the equilibrium between (EH) and (I) should not be disturbed by the substrate. In other words, non-competitive conditions should prevail. This is possible even for competitive inhibitors provided that the activity is measured within a few minutes of adding the substrate to the inhibited enzyme; the system behaves then as a non-competitive one. In practice the concentration of AChE employed will usually amount at most to 10^{-9} M (active group), as may be derived from the figures given for the turnover number of AChE (p. 301); 10 ml of such a solution hydrolyses approximately 4 μmole ACh/min. Since (EH_i) is calculated from the difference between $(I)_{50}$ and K_i, the values of (EH_i) and K_i should be compatible. Only very strong inhibitors of $K_i < 10^{-10}$ M can be used. On the other hand, the determination of the K_i of this type of inhibitor is highly inaccurate because extrapolation to enzyme activity zero is required (Fig. 12). At the usual enzyme concentrations (approx. 10^{-9} M), all inhibitors with $K_i < 10^{-10}$ M will show only very small variation in $(I)_{50}$. It will amount to half of the enzyme concentration. For the characterization of this type of inhibitor the estimation of the bimolecular rate constant of the enzyme-inhibitor reactions seems more adequate. To obtain absolute values, (EH) should now be known and be of the order of (I). Another complication, that is sometimes met, is destruction of the inhibitor in the course of its reaction with the enzyme, followed by liberation of the latter. Kinetics for this situation are given by MYERS (1952a, 1952b).

II. The structure of reversible inhibitors in relation to the active site of AChE

Very many compounds with anti-ChE action are available as a result of large synthetic programs induced by the pharmacological importance of anti-ChE agents (cf. AUGUSTINSSON 1948, HEYMANS 1951, KOELLE and GILMAN 1949), and of the search for inhibitors which might be used as tools to distinguish between various esterases such as AChE, BuChE, aliesterase, etc. (ADAMS and THOMPSON 1948, AUSTIN and BERRY 1953, BAYLISS and TODRICK 1956, FULTON and MOGEY 1954, HAWKINS and MENDEL 1949, HOLMSTEDT 1957, JACOB and FUNKE 1953, MYERS 1951, 1953, MYERS and MENDEL 1949, PULVER and DOMENJOZ 1951; for reviews, cf. AUGUSTINSSON 1957, HOLMSTEDT 1959).

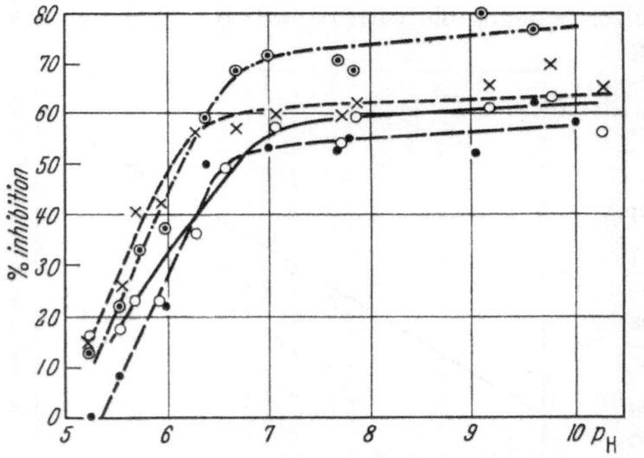

Reversible, fully competitive inhibitors may react with the anionic site, the esteratic site, or both. Representative for the first class of inhibitors of AChE are the alkylated ammonium ions. From the K_i values of mono-, di- and trimethylammonium derivatives, WILSON (1952b) concluded that the Coulomb interaction is augmented by dispersion forces at a rate of a change in ΔF of 1.2 k cal per methyl group; addition of the third methyl group did not increase the binding force of the N^+ with AChE. The Coulomb interaction was computed by comparison of the K_i for the dimethylethanolammonium ion and its carbon analogue isoamylalcohol. The nearest approach between the N^+ and the anionic site was calculated at 5.7 Å. Earlier, work of NACHMANSOHN and WILSON (1951) and WILSON and BERGMANN (1950a) was quoted; using the Brønsted equation, they arrived at a value of 6.3 to 6.5 Å (the reader is referred to Table 2).

Fig. 13. *Inhibition of AChE by quaternary ammonium salts as function of* pH. Substrate: ACh 3.3×10^{-3} M. Inhibitors used: neostigmine 8×10^{-5} M (●), acetophenone *m*-trimethylammonium iodide 8×10^{-5} M (○), choline 1.10^{-2} M (⊙) and tetraethylammonium bromide 5×10^{-3} M (×). From BERGMANN and SHIMONI (1952c)

BERGMANN et al. (1956) and BERGMANN and SHIMONI (1952a, 1952c) attempted to compute the dissociation constant of the anionic site from the pH dependence of the inhibition of AChE by aliphatic quaternary ammonium ions (Fig. 13). By rapid estimation of the activity of the inhibited AChE, non-competitive conditions could be simulated and the dissociation constant (pK_{anion}) of the inhibitor-enzyme complex could be estimated; pK_{anion} values thus obtained are summarized in Table 3. BERGMANN (1955), BERGMANN et al. (1950b), BERGMANN and SEGAL (1954) and BERGMANN and SHIMONI (1951) showed a linear relationship to exist between the pI_{50} and the number (n) of carbon atoms of a homologous series of monoquaternary ammonium salts of the general formula:

$$(CH_3)_3\overset{+}{-}N{-}(CH_2)_n{-}CH_3 \ .$$

A change in $\varDelta F$ per methylene group of 300 cal/mole was calculated at 20° for AChE, and of 500 cal/mole at 37° for BuChE (Fig. 14). Some of the bis-quaternary

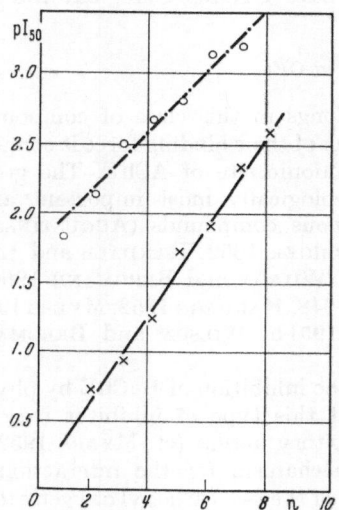

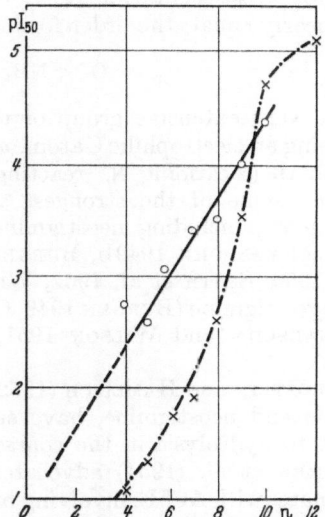

Fig. 14. pI_{50} values of N-alkyl trimethylammonium ions as function of the number of carbon atoms n. AChE (O) (temp. 23°, ACh 4 × 10⁻³ M), BuChE (x) (temp. 37°, ACh 6 × 10⁻³ M). From BERGMANN (1955)

Fig. 15. pI_{50} values of bis-quaternary ammonium ions of the structure $(CH_3)_3\overset{+}{N}{-}(CH_2)_n{-}\overset{+}{N}(CH_3)_3$, as function of n. AChE (x), BuChE (O). Temperature 37°, ACh 4 × 10⁻³ M. From BERGMANN (1955)

nitrogen compounds of the general formula: $(CH_3)_3\overset{+}{N}{-}(CH_2)_n{-}\overset{+}{N}(CH_3)_3$ are strong inhibitors of AChE (BARLOW and ING 1948, KIMURA et al. 1949, TODRICK 1954). The high affinity of these compounds towards AChE has been interpreted by BERGMANN (1955) and BERGMANN and SEGAL (1954, 1955) as confirmation of the operation of 2 anionic sites on the enzyme surface. In the bis-quaternary series, pI_{50} increases with chain length and is practically maximal at $n = 10$ (Fig. 15). The strong binding of this compound is not merely ascribed to the increase of the dispersion forces with chain length, but also to the favorable distance between the nitrogen functions in relation to the distance of the hypothetical two anionic sites on the enzyme surface. BERGMANN (1955) and BERGMANN et al. (1956) suggested that the two anionic sites may consist of the γ-carboxylic groups of an α-glutamyl-α-glutamyl peptide in the vicinity of the esteratic site. BERNHARD (1955a) criticized BERGMANN's results. He argued that these may be adequately explained on the basis of an AChE model possessing only one anionic site. At present, BERGMANN's interpretation assuming 2 anionic sites seems preferable, being less factitious. The question whether both anionic sites are involved in substrate hydrolysis remains open (cf. NACHMANSOHN and WILSON 1951).

BERGMANN et al. (1950a), comparing the inhibitive properties of amides, dipeptides, esters, ketones, and nitriles, found that compounds possessing an electrophilic C atom interact with the basic group of the esteratic site and thus cause competitive inhibition. A fair correlation exists between electrophily and inhibitory power in the nicotinic acid series where R in formula

is substituted (see Table 5). The order of increasing electrophily of the carbon atom for substituents for R is: $O^- < NH_2 < OEt < NMe_2 < Me$, but the last 3 are nearly equal; the order for inhibition is:

$$O^- < NH_2 < NEt_2 < Me < OEt \, .$$

The very extensive group of urethanes belongs in this class of compounds possessing an electrophilic C atom, although much of their binding force is connected with their cationic N^+ reacting with the anionic site of AChE. The group harbours some of the strongest and pharmacologically most important anti-ChE agents, including neostigmine and analogous compounds (AUGUSTINSSON and NACHMANSOHN 1949b, BURGEN 1949, HOBBIGER 1952, RANDALL and LEHMANN 1950, SMITH et al. 1952, WILSON 1955b, WILSON and BERGMANN 1950a) and physostigmine (BURGEN 1949, COHEN et al. 1948, HARDEGG 1952, MYERS 1950, NACHMANSOHN and WILSON 1951, SHUKUYA 1951b, WILSON and BERGMANN (1950a).

GOLDSTEIN and HAMLISCH (1952), studying the inhibition of BuChE by physostigmine and neostigmine, have suggested that this type of inhibitor may be subject to hydrolysis in the course of its inhibitory action (cf. MYERS 1952b). KOLBEZEN et al. (1954) advocated a third mechanism for the interaction of carbamates with AChE, involving binding of one of the two carboxyl oxygen atoms with a positive locus of the esteratic site related to the three point attachement of ACh on AChE proposed by PFEIFFER (1948).

neostigmine (Prostigmine)   physostigmine

Neostigmine is positively charged in the whole pH range of AChE activity, but physostigmine is a tertiary amine which dissociates in this range. WILSON and BERGMANN (1950a) demonstrated that, accordingly, the inhibitory action of neostigmine is inherantly pH-independent, whereas that of physostigmine decreases when the pH increases from 6 to 10. The electrophilic carbon atom of the carbonyl group of the urethanes, reacting with the basic group of the esteratic site, may account for the residual activity of the uncharged physostigmine molecule. The same applies to those phenylcarbamates which, although devoid of a positive locus, were shown by KOLBEZEN et al. (1954) to inhibit AChE. Comparative studies of a number of substituted ammonium phenylcarbamates have been carried out by FOLDES et al. (1958) and WILSON and QUAN (1958), who showed that phenylcarbamates with a distance of 4.7 to 5.3 Å between the N and the C=O function are the strongest inhibitors (Fig. 16). The conclusion seems justified that the urethanes react by means of their electrophilic carbon atom with the basic group of the esteratic, and with their cationic $\overset{+}{N}$ group with the anionic site of AChE. Interaction by means of oxygen with an acidic group of the esteratic site, as suggested by KOLBEZEN et al. (1954), is not excluded. However, the fact that inhibition by quaternary ammonium ions hardly changes at alkaline pH (BERGMANN and SHIMONI 1952c) has been inter-preted in the case of neostigmine as an indication that the acidic group of the esteratic site does not interact with the carbamate group of the inhibitor (WILSON 1951a). The authors concluded that since the acidic group apparently does not react with neostigmine it probably does not operate in the binding of ACh by AChE, but may be involved in the hydrolysis of the enzyme-substrate complex. It was mentioned earlier that BERGMANN et al. (1958), from the pH independence of the hydrolysis of acetylthiocholine and of phenyl acetates at high pH in contrast with the pH dependence of the hy-drolysis of ACh, arrived at the opposite conclu-sion. The authors ascribed the failure of the acidic group to react to the absence of a typical etheral oxygen in acetylthiocholine and the phenyl ace-tates; this is in contrast to the presence of a typ-ical etheral oxygen in ACh. It might be argued that the ethereal oxygen in neostigmine is not typical either, and that therefore its failure to react with the acidic group may not be typical for the situation which prevails in substrate hy-drolysis.

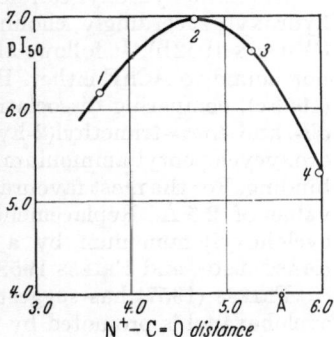

Fig. 16. *Relation between* pI_{50} *and* $\overset{+}{N} - C = O$ *distance.* The pI_{50} of ure-thane inhibitors versus red cell AChE is plotted against their $\overset{+}{N} - C = O$ distance. 1 = (2-hydroxyphenyl) tri-methylammonium dimethylcarbama-te, 2 = (2-hydroxybenzyl)trimethyl-ammonium dimethylcarbamate, 3 = (3-hydroxyphenyl)trimethylammoni-um dimethylcarbamate (neostigmine), 4 = (3-hydroxybenzyl)trimethylam-monium dimethylcarbamate. From FOLDES et al. (1958)

Powerful inhibitors of AChE are found also amongst the phenolic quaternary ammonium ions (RANDALL 1950), such as (3-hydroxyphenyl)ethyldimethylammo-nium chloride (edrophonium, Tensilon) (RANDALL 1951, WESCOE et al. 1950).

$$(CH_3)_2C_2H_5\overset{+}{N}-\underset{OH}{\underset{\displaystyle\bigcirc}{}}$$

edrophonium (Tensilon)

The contribution by the phenolic hydroxyl to the binding forces has been investi-gated by WILSON and QUAN (1958). Introduction of a hydroxyl group in the 3-position of the phenyltrimethylammonium strengthened the binding forces by a factor of 120 ($\Delta F = -2$ k cal/mole), but introduction of a methoxy group only by a factor of 5. This indicates that a hydrogen bond favours the interaction be-tween AChE and the 3-hydroxy derivative. A methyl group introduced in the 4-position of the (3-hydroxyphenyl)trimethylammonium ion gives additional gain in binding forces, presumably by directing the hydroxyl group to a favourable steric position. The weakening of the action of edrophonium in alkaline medium may be explained by dissociation of the phenolic OH, resulting in breakdown of the hydrogen bond. Strong binding occurs with the dimethylcarbamates of the (2-hydroxyphenyl)-, (3-hydroxybenzyl)-, and particularly the (3-hydroxyphenyl)- trimethylammonium ion, indicating, according to WILSON and QUAN (1958), that in these cases not only the quaternary nitrogen is bound but that also a bond will be formed with the esteratic site. These investigators moreover suggest, on account of atom models, that the hydroxyl hydrogen of (3 hydroxyphenyl)-trimethylammonium ion too is directed towards the esteratic site, which itself is situated at a distance of approximately 5 Å from the anionic site.

Aliphatic hydroxyl can not be expected to form hydrogen bonds like phenolic hydroxyl; accordingly, choline is no more active than trimethylpropylammonium (WILSON 1952 b). It follows also that the oxygen of the choline hydroxyl group is not bound to AChE either. BALDRIDGE et al. (1955) and FRIESS and BALDRIDGE (1956 c), comparing dissociation constants of the AChE complexes with choline, *cis*- and *trans*-trimethyl(2-hydroxycyclohexyl)ammonium, and trimethyl (2-hydroxycyclopentyl)ammonium, concluded that a hydroxyl function can contribute to binding. For the most favourable distance between N and O they found a minimum value of 2.5 Å. Replacement of the hydroxyl group of trimethyl(2-hydroxycyclohexyl)ammonium by a dimethylamino group seems to be unfavourable (MASTERSON and FRIESS 1958).

FRIESS (1957) has suggested that the inhibitory action of 2-dimethylaminocyclohexanol is promoted by the capability of this compound to form the zwitterion:

$$\text{(CH}_3)_2\overset{+}{\text{NH}} \quad \overset{-}{\text{O}} \quad .$$

The compound would thus posses a combination of a polymethylsubstituted N atom and an atom of high electron density. It is exactly this combination that, according to the theory developed by these authors, leads to highly active compounds. The basis of this theory is formed by experiments involving the substitution of the OH group of choline by Cl, dimethylamino-, or cyclic, N-containing 5- or 6-ringed compounds which are very strong inhibitors (FRIESS and McCARVILLE 1954a, 1954b, cf. FRIESS 1957). This was explained by the authors on account of interaction between the esteratic site of AChE with an atom or "region" of high electron density, such as Cl or $-\ddot{\text{N}} <$. Accordingly, protonisation of the heterocyclic $-\ddot{\text{N}} <$ leads to considerable reduction of the affinity of the inhibitor towards AChE (FRIESS and BALDRIDGE 1956a). Branching of the N—C—C—N chain greatly diminishes the inhibitory power of compounds of this type (FRIESS and BALDRIDGE 1956b). On the other hand, the third methyl group of the trimethylammonium group scarcely contributes to the binding forces (FRIESS and BALDRIDGE 1956b, FRIESS and McCARVILLE 1954a). In addition to these compounds, FRIESS et al. (1957) studied some other compounds with a heterocyclic quaternized nitrogen function.

The CT compounds of the general formula

$$R_1\text{—}\underset{\underset{\overset{+}{\text{N}}(\text{CH}_3)_3}{|}}{\bigcirc}\text{—O—(CH}_2)_3\text{—O—}\underset{\underset{\overset{+}{\text{N}}(\text{CH}_3)_3}{|}}{\bigcirc}\text{—}R_2 \quad ,$$

with R_1 and R_2 representing H, OH, OCH_3, or a carbamyl group, form another group of very strong inhibitors (DEPIERRE and FUNKE 1954, FUNKE et al. 1952, 1954, TREFOUEL 1952).

Very effective inhibitors are the compounds where one or both R functions represent N-dimethylcarbamyl groups (see Table 5). FUNKE et al. (1952) initially reported extremely low C_{50} values for these compounds (10^{-16} M and 10^{-14} M for CT 3152 and CT 3113, respectively) but later corrected these to approximately 10^{-9} M, which is in agreement with the findings of LEVIN and JANDORF (1955).

B. Irreversible inhibitors

Many reversible inhibitors have an irreversible character as a result of very slow dissociation of the enzyme-inhibitor complex. In the case of irreversible inhibitors, however, there is no true dissociable enzyme-inhibitor complex at all, but a chemical reaction takes place to form a compound from which the inhibitor is never recovered in unaltered, active form, although active enzyme may be set free (reactivation, not reversion). Thus MYERS (1952b) suggested that after inhibition of AChE by 2-(N-N-dimethylcarbamyl-oxy)-5-phenylbenzyl trimethylammonium bromide, N-N-dimethylcarbamyl-AChE is formed, and AChE is regenerated by release of the N-N-dimethylcarbamyl group. MYERS (1956) obtained stable inactive N-N-diethylcarbamyl-AChE after inhibition by N-N-diethylcarbamylfluoride; he reported similar results with other organic fluorides (MYERS and KEMP 1954).

I. Kinetics of the interaction of AChE with irreversible inhibitors

The inhibition of AChE by an irreversible inhibitor may be described as a bimolecular reaction as follows

$$AChE + PX \rightarrow AChE \cdot P + X' .$$

Theoretically the maximal inhibition is determined by the concentration of the reactants only, but actually such factors as stability of the inhibitor against hydrolysis, purity of the AChE preparation, absorption phenomena, etc. may have considerable influence. It is therefore desirable to express the effectivity of an irreversible inhibitor by giving the bimolecular rate constant of its reaction with AChE. Often, however, only C_{50} (or pI_{50}) is mentioned, a value which depends heavily on the experimental conditions.

The bimolecular or second order rate constant, k_2, which characterizes bimolecular reaction kinetics is determined experimentally from the equation

$$\frac{dX}{dt} = k_2 (EH_i - X) (I - X) ,$$

which on integration yields

$$k_2 \cdot t = \frac{2.303}{(EH_i - I)} \log \frac{(I) \cdot (EH_i - X)}{(EH_i) (I - X)} , \tag{40}$$

where (EH_i) and (I) are the initial molar concentrations of AChE and inhibitor, and X the number of moles per liter of each reacting in an interval of t minutes. From (40) follows:

$$t = \frac{2.303}{k_2 (EH_i - I)} \log \frac{(EH_i - X)}{(I - X)} + \frac{2.303}{k_2 (EH_i - I)} \log \frac{(I)}{(EH_i)} . \tag{41}$$

Plotting $\log \frac{(EH_i - X)}{(I - X)}$ *versus* t yields a straight line with slope

$$\frac{2.303}{k_2 (EH_i - I)} . \tag{Fig. 17}$$

In order to use formula (40), not only the concentration of the inhibitor but also that of the enzyme should be known; however, it is of importance only in those circumstances where these concentrations are comparable. When excess inhibitor is present, the reaction follows

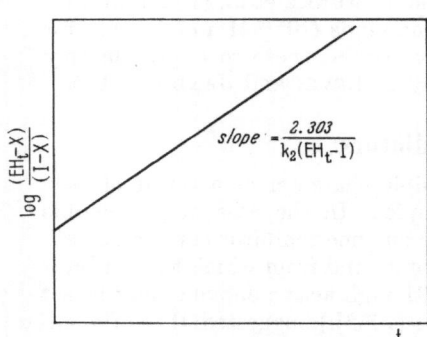

Fig. 17. *Determination of the second order rate constant, k_2, from a plot of log $\dfrac{(EH_t - X)}{(I - X)}$ against time (t)*

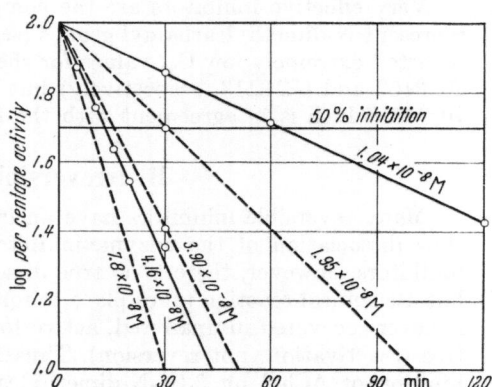

Fig. 18. *Time course of inhibition of AChE by diethyl-4-nitrophenylphosphate as function of concentration.* The straight lines demonstrate the pseudo first order kinetics for the reactions involved. From ALDRIDGE (1950)

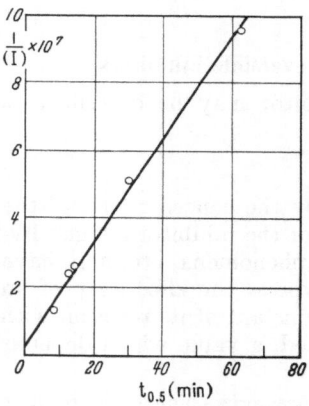

Fig. 19. *Relation between inhibitor concentration and time required to reach 50% inhibition.* Time for 50% inhibition ($t_{0.5}$) is inversely proportional to the concentration of inhibitor $(I)_{50}$. Inhibitor used: diethyl-4-nitrophenylphosphate (E 600). From ALDRIDGE (1950)

pseudo first order kinetics:

$$k_2 \cdot t = \frac{2.303}{(I)} \log \frac{(EH_t)}{(EH_t - X)} .\qquad(42)$$

Knowledge of the absolute concentration of enzyme is then not required to find k_2. The ratio $(EH_t)/(EH_t - X)$ may be found experimentally by measuring the enzyme activity, Ao, before $(t = o)$ and t minutes after incubation with the inhibitor (At). Substitution of Ao and At in (42) gives:

$$k_2 t = \frac{2.303}{(I)} \cdot \log \frac{Ao}{At} ,\qquad(43)$$

and from (43)

$$t = \frac{2.303}{k_2(I)} \log \frac{Ao}{At} .\qquad(44)$$

k_2 may be calculated from the slope of a plot of log $\dfrac{Ao}{At}$ versus t (Fig. 18). From (44), equation (45) may be derived which relates inhibitor concentration to the period required to obtain 50% inhibition ($t_{0.5}$).

$$t_{0.5} = \frac{2.303}{k_2(I)} \log 2 \qquad(45)$$

A plot of $t_{0.5}$ against $1/(I)$ will be linear (Fig. 19).

II. The structure of irreversible inhibitors in relation to the active site of AChE

The most important group of irreversible anti-ChE agents is formed by the organophosphorus compounds. They have been excellently reviewed by HOLMSTEDT (1959) in an article which extends and completes previous reviews (cf. BALLS and JANSEN 1952, FUKUTO 1957, HOLMSTEDT 1951, SAUNDERS 1957, SCHRADER 1952), and are covered in fuller detail by the same authors in Chapter 9 of the present volume.

A number of this type of inhibitors is presented in Table 6. For our purpose—elucidation of the interaction with the active site of AChE—reference to only a few representative members of this group will suffice.

It was soon realized that these compounds act by phosphorylation of enzymes, giving rise to irreversible inhibition not only of AChE (AUGUSTINSSON 1953b, AUGUSTINSSON and NACHMANSOHN 1949b, BOURSNELL and WEBB 1949, BURGEN 1949, GOLDSTEIN and HAMLISCH 1952, McNAUGHTON and ZELLER 1949, NACHMANSOHN et al. 1948) but also of many other enzymes (cf. ALDRIDGE 1957, MOUNTER et al. 1957b). A number of these will be mentioned in the last section of this chapter. For several enzymes the reaction is stoichiometric and may be described as follows:

$$\text{EH} + \boxed{\text{P}}\text{—X} \rightarrow \text{E—}\boxed{\text{P}} + \text{H}^+ + \text{X}^-. \tag{46}$$

The reaction is accompanied by proton release (BALLS and JANSEN 1952, HARTLEY and KILBY 1950, JANDORF et al. 1955b, JANSEN and BALLS 1952, JANSEN et al. 1949, 1950, 1951). MICHEL (1952) and MICHEL and KROP (1951), using ^{32}P labelled diisopropyl phosphorofluoridate (DF^{32}P), showed that in the case of AChE the phosphorus atom is tightly bound to the enzyme, as had been shown previously with regard to BuChE (BOURSNELL and WEBB 1949) and chymotrypsin (JANSEN et al. 1952). The chemical nature of the interaction of enzymes with organophosphorus inhibitors is borne out by the high values (approx. 10 to 15 k cal/mole) found for the activation energy.

The organophosphorus compounds react with AChE according to bimolecular kinetics, as described in the previous paragraph (ALDRIDGE 1950, AUGUSTINSSON and NACHMANSOHN 1949b, JANDORF 1956b, JANDORF et al. 1955b, TAMMELIN 1958b). JANDORF et al. (1955b) have listed the rate constants of the interaction of various enzymes with organophosphorus inhibitors including those of AChE with DFP, isopropyl methylphosphonofluoridate (Sarin), and tetraethyl pyrophosphate (TEPP). The difference in rate constants between the reactions of AChE with DFP and with Sarin, respectively, is particularly striking (Table 7). Other authors have also reported the high specificity of certain phosphorus compounds (ALDRIDGE 1953a, AUSTIN and BERRY 1953, McNAUGHTON and ZELLER 1949, MYERS 1952b, TAMMELIN 1958a, cf. AUGUSTINSSON 1957). These differences between members of the same group will at least partly reflect the adaptation of the inhibitor to the AChE surface. This led ALDRIDGE (1954) to compare the affinity of a series of inhibitors of AChE with the hydrolysis by this enzyme of substrates of corresponding structure; this study clearly revealed the importance of steric factors in substrates and inhibitors.

Table 7. *Bimolecular rate constants for the reaction between esterases and organophosphorus compounds*

	DFP	TEPP	Sarin
Eel AChE	1.9×10^6	2.1×10^6	6.3×10^7
Human red cell AChE	9.5×10^4	2.1×10^6	1.5×10^7
BuChE	1.5×10^7	5.0×10^7	4.4×10^6
Chymotrypsin	2.0×10^4	1.1×10^3	1.7×10^4
Trypsin	8.3×10^2	9.7×10^1	1.2×10^3

The figures are given in 1/mole min. From JANDORF et al. (1955b).

However, the contribution of the binding energy of the P—X bond to the effectiveness of inhibitors is also of great importance, as was clearly established by ALDRIDGE (1954) and ALDRIDGE and DAVISON (1952a), who demonstrated a correlation between the lability of the P—X bond in diethyl phosphoryl compounds of phenol- and thiophenol derivatives, and their inhibitory power (Fig. 20).

A similar relationship was found by FUKUTO and METCALF (1956) to exist with respect to the inhibitory action on fly brain AChE of a number of organophosphorus compounds. A striking exception is formed by di-*n*-propyl 2,2-dichlorovinyl phosphate and its fluoro analogue; both compounds have a similar inhibitory power but the former is much more stable against hydrolysis than the latter (JANDORF 1956b).

FUKUTO (1957) in a review article, considered the relationship between chemical structure and reactivity of these compounds. The correlation found between the reaction velocity of these compounds with AChE and the speed of hydrolysis in alkaline medium indicated that chemically both reactions evolve similarly.

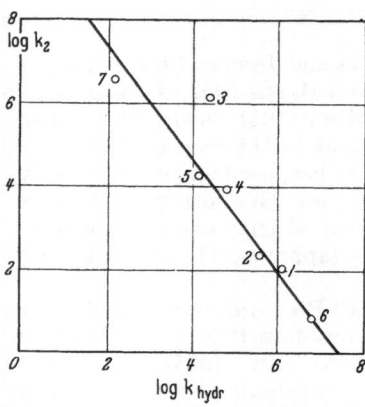

Fig. 20. *The relation between stability to hydrolysis (37° at pH 7.6) and inhibitory power.* The negative logarithm of the hydrolysis constant ($-\log k_{hydr.}$) of a number of diethylphosphoryl-derivatives is plotted against the logarithm of the bimolecular rate constant for the reaction of red cell AChE and inhibitor ($\log k_2$). Inhibitors used: 1 = diethyl-4-chlorophenyl phosphate, 2 = diethyl-2-chlorophenyl phosphate, 3 = diethyl-4-nitrophenyl phosphate, 4 = diethyl-3-nitrophenyl phosphate, 5 = diethyl-2-nitrophenyl phosphate, 6 = diethyl-phenyl phosphate, 7 = tetraethyl pyrophosphate. From ALDRIDGE (1954)

BLUMENTHAL and HERBERT (1945) using ^{18}O-rich water demonstrated that alkaline hydrolysis of phosphotriesters rapidly brings about the break of one P—O bond, presumably by nucleophilic attack on the P-atom. Accordingly, enzymic hydrolysis of, e.g., diethyl-4-nitrophenyl phosphate (Paraoxon, Mintacol, E 600):

$$C_2H_5O\diagdown\!\!\!\underset{C_2H_5O\diagup}{\overset{\overset{\displaystyle O}{\|}}{P}}\!\!-O-\!\!\!\bigcirc\!\!\!-NO_2$$

is likely to involve nucleophilic attack by the enzyme on the phosphorus atom. This analogy between enzymic and alkaline hydrolysis is also borne out by the observation by AUGUSTINSSON and HEIMBURGER (1954) that when horse plasma reacts with ethyl-N-dimethyl phosphoramidocyanidate (Tabun) the cyanide ion is set free. The same occurs at alkaline hydrolysis, but acid hydrolysis results in release of the dimethylamido group (LARSSON 1952).

In the group of compounds under consideration of the general formula

$$R_1O\diagdown\!\!\!\underset{R_2}{\overset{\overset{\displaystyle O}{\|}}{P}}\!\!-X$$

the electrophilic character of the phosphorus atom is determined by the substituents for R_1, R_2, and X, where R_1 is alkyl, R_2 alkyl, alkoxy or amido, and X halogen (e.g., F), aryloxy, cyano, or otherwise.

When the series of phosphorofluoridates,

$$R_1O\diagdown\!\!\!\underset{R_1O\diagup}{\overset{\overset{\displaystyle O}{\|}}{P}}\!\!-F,$$

is considered, substitution of R_1 by methyl-, ethyl- or *iso*propyl will lead to decrease of the electrophily of the phosphorus atom and consequently of the rate of hydrolysis in the order given, because this is the order of increasing electron donating power of the substituent groups. Replacement of F in the molecule of DFP by Cl, a halogen of lesser electro-negativity, will decrease the electrophily of the P atom and its anti-ChE action (MACKWORTH and WEBB 1948, MAZUR and BODANSKY 1946; cf. FUKUTO 1957). The correlation between anti-AChE action of inhibitors and the electrophilic character of the central phosphorus atom is simulated by the relationship between the binding force at the esteratic site of AChE with substrates and the electrophilic character of the carbon atom of the latter. This parallelism has been pointed out by WILSON (1952c, WILSON and BERGMANN (1950a), and ALDRIDGE (1953b). They postulated that phosphorylation of AChE by inhibitors would be the counterpart of acylation of the enzyme by substrates, the difference being that in the latter case substrate hydrolysis would follow whereas the phosphorylated enzyme would be stable. Both phosphorylation and acylation would be localized at the esteratic site. That one and the same active site is involved is very plausible in view of the strong protection afforded by substrate against the attack by organophosphorus agents on AChE (ALDRIDGE 1950, 1954, BAIN 1949, COHEN et al. 1951, HOBBIGER 1954a, MICHEL and KROP 1951, TAMMELIN 1958b) (Fig. 21). Reversible inhibitors (AUGUSTINSSON 1950b, 1953a, AUGUSTINSSON and GRAHN 1952, BERGMANN and SHIMONI 1952b, KOELLE 1946, TAKAGI 1953, TAMMELIN 1958b) may also protect aginst organophosphorus compounds. The similarity of the reaction of AChE with substrates, on the one hand, and inhibitors on the other is further demonstrated by the pH activity curves of TEPP (WILSON and BERGMAN 1950a) and Tabun (AUGUSTINSSON 1953a), which correspond well with a pH activity curve for substrate hydrolysis, i.e., inhibition is strongest when the status of the active site is most favourable for substrate hydrolysis.

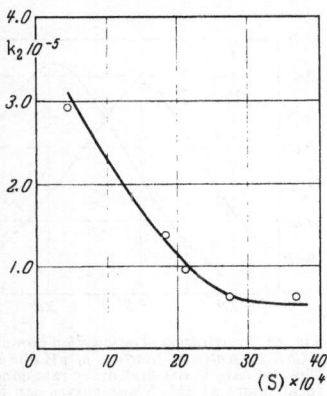

Fig. 21. *Reaction velocity of 2-trimethylammoniumethyl methylphosphonofluoridate (iodide).* Second order velocity constant k_2 for the inhibition of red cell AChE is shown as function of the concentration of ACh. Inhibitor is added after the substrate. From TAMMELIN (1958b)

Compounds differing only with regard to the X-group yield identical phosphorylated AChE compounds, as has been shown by ALDRIDGE and DAVISON (1952b) for the structures

$$\begin{matrix} MeO \\ MeO \end{matrix} \!\!\!\!\! \diagdown\!\!\!\! P-X, \text{ where}$$

$$X = F, \quad O-\!\!\!\langle\bigcirc\rangle\!\!\!-NO_2, \quad S-\!\!\!\langle\bigcirc\rangle\!\!\!-NO_2, \text{ or}$$

$$-O-P \diagup\!\!\!\!\overset{OMe}{\underset{OMe}{\diagdown}}$$

ALDRIDGE (1950) postulated originally that 0,0-diethyl 0-(4-nitrophenyl) phosphorothioate (E 605, Parathion), the sulphur analogue of E 600, would be of the same order of effectiveness as the latter and attack AChE in an analogous way. He modified his opinion later (ALDRIDGE and DAVISON 1952a, 1952b), and so did other authors (DIGGLE and GAGE 1951, GAGE 1953). Although the situation is not yet entirely clear, it is obvious that the phosphorothionates and -dithionates are considerably weaker inhibitors *in vitro* than the corresponding oxygen compounds (BORKE and KIRCH 1956, HOLMSTEDT 1951); it is likely that this weaker action is due to a reduction of the electrophilic properties of the phosphorus atom (cf. FUKUTO 1957).

☞ As has been remarked earlier, steric requirements of the enzyme surface also exert considerable influence on the affinity of phosphorus compounds for AChE. Such factors are at the basis of the strong inhibitory power of agents like *iso*-propyl methylphosphonofluoridate (Sarin) (cf. HOLMSTEDT 1951).

Many attempts have been made to synthesize phosphorus compounds of high specificity for AChE by the introduction of groups of high affinity for the AChE surface. Thus the "phosphostigmines", where the carbamyl groups of neostigmine-like compounds is replaced by a substituted phosphoryl residue (ANDREWS et al. 1952, BURGEN and HOBBIGER 1951, HOBBIGER 1954b, MYERS 1952b, 1954), have been prepared. The importance of the quaternary ammonium group in these and other compounds follows from the observation that the corresponding tertiary N compounds are weaker inhibitors (ANDREWS et al. 1952, 1954, HOBBIGER 1954a, 1954b).

3 - (Diethylphosphato) - N - methyl-quinolinium methylsulphate may be considered to belong to the same group. The contribution of the quaternary ammonium group of these compounds is certainly determined by its affinity for the anionic site of AChE.

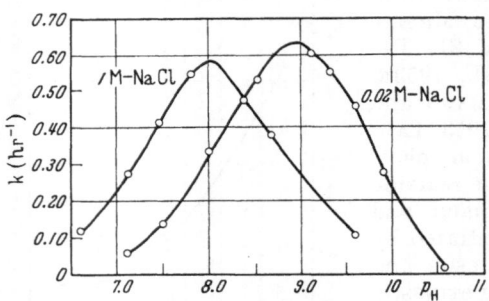

Fig. 22. *Reactivation of tetramethyl pyrophosphate inhibited AChE by water as function of* pH *and salt concentration.* The ordinate is the first order rate constant (k) in reciprocal hours at 25°. These curves can be reproduced by assuming that both an acidic and a basic group are essential for reactivation. Suitable pK's are about 7.4 and 8.7 for 1 M NaCl and about 8.2 and 9.6 for 0.02 M NaCl. From WILSON et al. (1958)

Another interesting group of related compounds was developed by GHOSH and NEWMAN (1955) and TAMMELIN (1957a, 1957b, 1957c, 1958a, 1958b) who introduced the dimethylamino-ethanol and choline esters of organophosphorus acids and their thio-analogues. The dialkoxy- and the methyl-alkoxy phosphorylcholines are poor inhibitors (TAMMELIN 1957b, 1958b). The methyl-fluorophosphoryl-cholines (TAMMELIN 1957a) and the organophosphoryl thiocholines, however, are very potent inhibitors (TAMMELIN 1957b). Reactivation experiments taught that during the reaction of AChE with 0,0-diethyl-S-2-trimethylammonium-ethyl-phosphonothioate iodide and 0-*iso*propyl-S-trimethylammonium-methyl-methyl phosphonothioate iodide, the thiocholine residue is released (TAMMELIN 1958a) After reaction of AChE with 2-trimethylammonium-ethyl-methylphosphonofluoridate iodide the choline residue probably remains associated with the phosphorus atom, since the thus inhibited AChE is refractory against reactivation by pyridine-2-aldoxime methiodide (P-2-AM), presumably because the choline residue prevents the binding of the quaternary ammonium of the reactivator at the anionic site (ENANDER 1958).

The stability of the phosphorylated AChE is evidently conditioned by the chemical structure of the phosphoryl group. WILSON (1951c) showed that diethyl phosphoryl AChE slowly dephosphorylates spontaneously to give the active free enzyme; diethyl phosphoryl eel AChE requires about 4 weeks at pH 7 and 7° to reach 50% hydrolysis (cf. ALDRIDGE 1953b, 1954, AUGUSTINSSON 1953a, DAVISON 1953, 1955). This spontaneous reactivation has a pH optimum which depends on the ionic strength (WILSON et al. 1958). The curves of Fig. 22 can be explained on account of the operation of an acidic and a basic group which are both essential for reactivation. In 0.02 M NaCl, the pK's for these groups are 8.2 and 9.6, and in 1 M NaCl, 7.4 and 8.7, respectively. Dimethyl phosphoryl AChE decomposes faster (ALDRIDGE 1953 b, 1954); after $1\frac{1}{2}$ hour (37°, pH 7.8) 50% of this compound is hydrolyzed following first order kinetics (ALDRIDGE and DAVISON 1953, DAVISON 1955); this process also has a pH optimum (DAVISON 1955). Di-n-propyl phosphoryl enzyme is also subject to spontaneous hydrolysis (DAVISON 1955), but after inhibition of AChE by diisopropyl phosphorofluoridate no spontaneous reactivation is observed (DAVISON 1955, HOBBIGER 1951, WILSON 1951 c, WILSON and GINSBURG 1955 b, WILSON and MEISLICH 1953); the same applies to Sarin (CHILDS et al. 1955) and Tabun (AUGUSTINSSON 1953 a). Spontaneous reactivation underlines the analogy between AChE interaction with substrates and phosphorus inhibitors. This follows from the reaction sequence which, by extending equation (46), may be written as follows:

$$EH + \boxed{P}\,X \rightleftarrows [EH \cdot P—X] \rightarrow E—\boxed{P} + H^+ + X^-$$

$$\downarrow H_2O$$

$$EH + \boxed{P}—OH\,.$$

However, the occurrence of a reversible AChE-inhibitor intermediate, comparable with the enzyme-substrate Michaelis complex, has not been experimentally demonstrated yet. The claim that such a AChE-inhibitor complex, analogous to the reversible AChE-substrate complex occurs (NACHMANSOHN et al. 1947) was later shown to be wrong, being based on faulty technique (ALDRIDGE 1950, WILSON and COHEN 1953). The analogy with substrate hydrolysis is also borne out by the pH dependence of the inhibition reaction. Thus, AUGUSTINSSON (1953 a) and

Table 8. *The effect of the phosphoryl group on the ageing of phosphorylated AChE*

Phosphoryl group	"Ageing" (%)	Conditions	References
$\begin{array}{l}CH_3 \\ \diagdown \\ (CH_3)_2 \cdot CHO \diagup \end{array}$ P=O	60% in 4 hours	37°, pH 7.2[2]	[1]
$\begin{array}{l}(CH_3)_2CHO \\ \diagdown \\ (CH_3)_2CHO \diagup \end{array}$ P=O	40% in 3 hours 45% in 3 hours 70% in 8 hours	25°, pH 7.4[1] 25°, pH 7[1] 37°, pH 7.45[2]	[2] [3] [4] cf [1]) and [5]
$\begin{array}{l}C_2H_5O \\ \diagdown \\ C_2H_5O \diagup \end{array}$ P=O	0% in 3 hours 31% in 24 hours	25°, pH 7[1] 25°, pH 7[1]	[3] [3] cf [1]) and [5]
$\begin{array}{l}CH_3O \\ \diagdown \\ CH_3O \diagup \end{array}$ P=O	10% in 3 hours 100% in 24 hours	25°, pH 7[1] 25°, pH 7[1]	[3] [3]

[1] Eel AChE.
[2]) Red cell AChE.
References: [1]) DAVIES and GREEN (1956); [2]) JANDORF et al. (1955 b); [3]) WILSON (1955a); [4]) HOBBIGER (1956); [5]) HOBBIGER (1955).

WILSON and BERGMANN (1950a) have stressed the importance of a basic group of a pK of approx. 6.5 for the inhibition reaction. The interference by diazonium compounds in the binding by AChE of ACh and organophosphorus compounds has been referred to in evidence of the assumption that a tyrosine and particularly a histidine residue may be operating at the active site (HOLLAND and KLEIN 1956,

MOUNTER et al. 1957a). The significance of the inhibition of AChE by the non-specific agent dinitrofluorobenzene (MOUNTER et al. 1957a) will be dealt with in section 3 in relation to other enzymes. At any rate, the pH-dependence of the inhibition reaction provides more circumstantial evidence that an imidazole group of histidine is involved in the function of the esteratic site of AChE.

Spontaneous hydrolysis is counteracted by another spontaneous reaction termed ageing, which leads to a very stable AChE-phosphoryl compound which is refractory to spontaneous or induced reactivation. The chemical basis of this reaction will be elaborated in the next section. Table 8 summarizes some data on the ageing process. It follows first order kinetics (DAVIES and GREEN 1956) and can be accelerated by lowering the pH (DAVIES and GREEN 1956, HOBBIGER 1956, MICHEL 1958) or by increasing the temperature (HOBBIGER 1956, JANDORF et al. 1955b). Both spontaneous reactivation and ageing depend strongly on the structures of the phosphoryl substituents.

III. Induced reactivation of phosphorylated AChE

It has been mentioned that a number of phosphoryl-AChE complexes are subject to spontaneous hydrolysis in aqueous medium. This reaction is accelerated in the presence of nucleophilic agents, called reactivators, such as choline, imidazole, pyridine, and particularly hydroxylamine (WILSON 1951c, 1952c). The reaction is accompanied by recuperation of the enzymic activity (JANDORF et al. 1955a).

Systematic investigations have stimulated the development of various very powerful reactivators related to hydroxylamine, in particular a number of oximes and hydroxamic acids. In Table 9 some representative specimens are listed.

The subject of reactivators is dealt with separately in the present volume by HOBBIGER (Chapter 21), and has also been reviewed elsewhere (DAVIES and GREEN 1958, HOLMSTEDT 1959, WILSON 1955a). Here we shall confine ourselves to those data that are relevant to the structure of the active site.

Kinetic analysis of the reactivation of phosphorylated AChE by choline, pyridine-2-aldoxime methiodide (P-2-AM) (GREEN and SMITH 1958b), and hydroxamic acids (WILSON 1952c) showed that at high concentrations of reactivator, pseudo first order reactions occurred, and at lower concentrations, second order reactions prevailed. It may be inferred that an intermediary complex of reactivator and phosphorylated enzyme is formed during the reactivation.

Like the spontaneous reactivation of phosphorylated AChE, the reactivator catalyzed process shows a pH optimum; this was shown for the hydroxamic acids, hydroxylamine, pyridine, P-2-AM and others by WILSON (1955a) and WILSON et al. (1958), and for mono-isonitrosoacetone (MINA) by DAVIES and GREEN (1956). The =NOH group of the hydroxamic acids and the oximes owes its nucleophilic character to its oxygen atom. It is particularly evident at alkaline pH, when it dissociates into =NO$^-$; this follows from the reaction kinetics of these agents with the organophosphorus compounds (GREEN and SAVILLE 1956, SWIDLER and STEINBERG 1956). Hydroxylamine and pyridine (JANDORF 1956a), on the other hand, react as free bases. The nucleophilic properties of the =NOH compounds increase with the dissociation constant. According to DAVIES and GREEN (1956), the observed pH dependence of the reactivation by means of MINA agrees with a reaction of the oxime anion with a protonized form of phosphorylated AChE. For the pK of this protonized group, a value of approximately 7.5 was calculated. The decrease of reactivation at increasing pH is due to dissociation of this protonized group. From pH-reactivation curves of the hydroxamic acids, WILSON (1955a) and WILSON et al. (1955) estimated the pK of the protonized group of AChE to be 8.2. The protonized group may be identical with the acidic group of the esteratic site. It may be objected that the pK of 8.2 is considerably lower than that found by WILSON for the acidic group of AChE. It should, however, be recognised that a lowering of the pK of this group by phosphorylation of AChE may be involved. The reactivators with the strongest nucleophilic properties may not be very effective because they have high $pK's$, and may in fact only dissociate into the active =NO$^-$ form at pH values where the necessary protonized group is dissociated. However, it is certain that the effect of these reactivators is not exclusively due to the nucleophily of a particular atom, but that other interactions with the enzyme cooperate. Thus, DAVIES and GREEN (1958) and GREEN and SMITH (1958a) have

Table 9. *List of selected reactivators*

Formula	Name	Concn.	A	Remarks
$(CH_3)_3\overset{+}{N}$—CH_2—CH_2OH	choline	3×10^{-1}	0.004	TEPP inhibited eel AChE. pH 7.0, 25°, 0.1 M NaCl, 1.5×10^{-3} M EDTA, 3×10^{-2} M phosphate. The figures in column A are taken from WILSON et al. (1955), (Fig. 2 and Fig. 3), and represent the first order rate constants (min⁻¹)
[pyridine structure]	pyridine	5×10^{-2}	0.006	
H_2NOH	hydroxylamine	5×10^{-2}	0.025	
[nicotinhydroxamic acid structure] C—NHOH	nicotinhydroxamic acid	5×10^{-2}	0.003	
[nicotinhydroxamic acid methiodide structure] C—NHOH, I⁻, CH₃	nicotinhydroxamic acid methiodide	5×10^{-2}	0.04	
[pyridine-aldoxime structure] CH=NOH	pyridine-2-aldoxime	2.5×10^{-2}	0.0045	TEPP inhibited eel AChE. pH 7.0, 25°, 0.1 M NaCl, 10^{-4} M EDTA, 10^{-3} M phosphate. The figures in column A represent the first order rate constants (min⁻¹)
	pyridine-3-aldoxime	1.0×10^{-2}	0.0016	
	pyridine-4-aldoxime	1.0×10^{-2}	0.0048	
[pyridinium methiodide structure] CH=NOH, I⁻, CH₃	pyridine-2-aldoxime methiodide	10^{-5}	0.14	
	pyridine-2-aldoxime methiodide	10^{-5}	0.23[1]	
	pyridine-2-aldoxime methiodide-*syn*	10^{-3}	0.057[1]	
	3-hydroxypyridine-2-aldoxime methiodide	10^{-4}	0.02	
[1-pyridinium-3-(pyridinium-4-aldoxime)-propane dibromide structure] CH=NOH, 2 Br⁻, CH₂—CH₂—CH₂	1-pyridinium-3-(pyridinium-4-aldoxime)-propane dibromide	—	800	TEPP inhibited human red cell AChE. 37°, 0.025 M NaHCO₃—N₂—5% CO₂, 10^{-2} M ACh. The figures in column A represent the potency as reactivator with P-2-AM taken as 100. HOBBIGER et al. (1958)
[1-3-bis-(pyridinium-4-aldoxime)-propane dibromide structure] CH=NOH CH=NOH, 2 Br⁻, CH₂—CH₂—CH₂	1-3-*bis*-(pyridinium-4-aldoxime)-propane dibromide	—	2200	
[isonitrosoacetone structure] CH₃—C—CH, O, NOH	*iso*nitrosoacetone	—	6.8	TEPP inhibited human red cell AChE. pH 7.4, 25°, 0.07 M NaCl, 0.15 M KCl, 10^{-3} M KH₂PO₄, 5×10^{-3} M Na-diethylbarbiturate. The figures in column A represent the second order rate constants (1/mole min). DAVIES and GREEN (1956)
[diisonitrosoacetone structure] CH—C—CH, O, NOH NOH	di*iso*nitrosoacetone	—	8.4	
[picolinohydroxamic acid hydrochloride structure] C—NHOH, Cl⁻, H, O	picolinohydroxamic acid hydrochloride	—	2.9	
	reference compound: nicotinhydroxamic acid methiodide	—	0.3	

[1] Experiments at pH 8.0. WILSON et al. (1958).

suggested that the superior action of substances like 2-oxo-aldoximes, pyridine-hydroxamic acids, picolinohydroxamic acid, and pyrimidine-2-hydroxamic acid is partly due to the formation of a hydrogen bond between the phorphorylated AChE and the carbonyl oxygen atom of the first, or a heterocyclic nitrogen atom of the following compounds.

Reactivators possessing a cationic quaternary nitrogen group show a steeper decrease of activity with pH than compounds lacking this group; for the latter compounds, this decrease corresponds merely with protonisation of the $=NO^-$ group. In the former an additional contribution to the decrease is afforded by protonization of the anionic site of AChE, leading to weakening of its interaction with the cationic group of the reactivator.

All available evidence indicates that reactivation is best with agents which fit snugly at the AChE suface. Choline loses its properties as a reactivator when a methyl group is removed from the N-atom to give dimethylaminoethanol. Reactivation by stilbamidine and hydroxy-stilbamidine is also related to the affinity of these compounds for the enzyme surface, which is indicated by their strong inhibiting action on AChE (WILSON 1952c).

Strong reactivators have been developed on the basis of knowledge of the active surface of AChE. Thus, introduction of a quaternary ammonium function into reactivators to fit the free anionic site of phosphorylated AChE greatly improved their efficacy, as appears form the highly effective action of, e. g. nicotin-hydroxamic acid methiodide and picolinohydroxamic acid (WILSON and MEISLICH 1953, WILSON and GINSBURG 1955b, WILSON et al. 1955; cf. WILSON 1955a). Table 9 accentuates the special assets of P-2-AM. This agent was developed by WILSON and GINSBURG (1955b) and CHILDS et al. (1955). It may be noted that methylation of the N-atom of pyridine-2-aldoxime increases its activity by a factor of 70,000, in spite of the accompanying decrease of its nucleophilic properties (lower pK). There is little doubt that the spectacular potency of this compound is based on its steric adaptation to the AChE surface.

WILSON (1959) and WILSON et al. (1958) accomplished a comparative study on the effectiveness of a number of P-2-AM isomers. Departing from the conception of molecular complementariness, they were able to interpret their results in terms of steric properties of the AChE surface. Thus, it is significant for the structure of the active site of AChE that the *anti*-configuration of P-2-AM is far more effective than the *syn*-configuration.* Excellent fit of P-2-AM into the phosphorylated AChE is concordant with the model of the enzyme surface derived from the structure of the very effective reversible inhibitor, neostigmine. From earlier studies (WILSON and QUAN 1958), it was likely that in combining with the enzyme the carbamate group occupies the position as indicated with regard to the ring (planar model), and that the position of the carboxyl carbon atom will correspond with the position of the P atom in phosphorylated AChE.

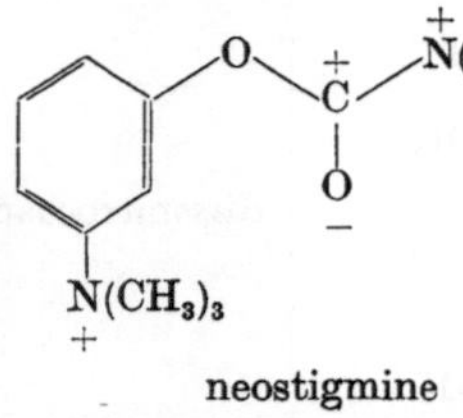

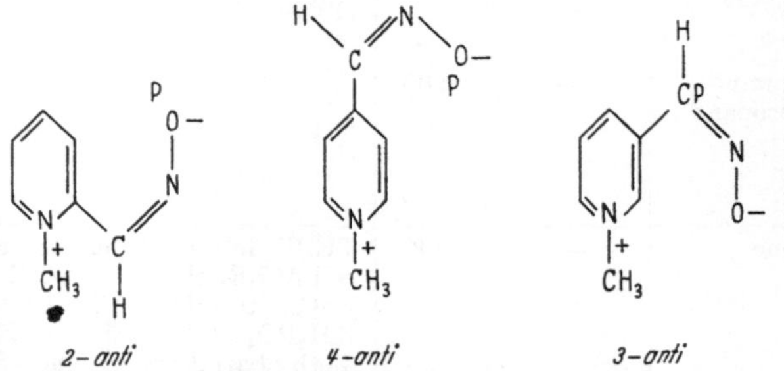

Fig. 23. *Position of the nucleophilic oxygen atom of PAM compounds on the surface of phosphorylated AChE.* The spacial relationship of the phosphorus atom with regard to the quaternary nitrogen agrees with that of the carbamate carbon atom with respect to the quaternary nitrogen of neostigmine. The picture shows the favourable structures of the 2- and 4-isomers. From WILSON (1959)

neostigmine

Taking the quaternary N atom of the ring as origin, and the ring axis as ordinate, coordinates of 3.42 and 3.32 Å are calculated for the position of the P atom. Fig. 23 gives the *anti*-configurations of PAM compounds, indicating how these would be bound to the phosphorylated enzyme with the quaternary N of PAM and the P atom of phosphorylated AChE in the required position. The figure shows that the position of the nucleophilic oxygen atom with

* See additional information E. J. POZIOMEK and D. N. KRAMER: Org. Chem. **26**, 423—427 (1961).

regard to the P atom is favourable in P-2-AM and P-4-AM, but very unfavourable in P-3-AM. This explains why of 2 compounds of nearly equal nucleophilic properties, like P-2-AM and P-3-AM, the former is a highly effective reactivator and the latter a very poor one. The model explains also why substitution into the P-2-AM ring decreases the effectivity.

The effect of quaternary N-possessing reactivators is antagonized by compounds which may compete for the anionic site of AChE, e.g., alkylammonium ions (WILSON 1952c). Also, the decreased effectivity of P-2-AM in the presence of salt is readily explained along the same line by reduction of the Coulomb interaction with the anionic site (WILSON et al. 1958).

Earlier, the strong inhibiting action of bis-quaternary ammonium compounds in comparison with those possessing only one quaternary N function was mentioned. Similarly, *bis*-quaternary oximes have been developed, and some are remarkably potent reactivators (even 20 times as strong as P-2-AM towards DFP- or TEPP-inactivated AChE) (HOBBIGER et al. 1958, HOBBIGER and SADLER 1958). This may be interpreted as further evidence of 2 anionic sites at the AChE surface.

The stability of the enzyme-phosphorus bond depends strongly on the other substituents at the P atom. The resistance of attack by water and reactivators increases in the following order: dimethyl-, diethyl-, di*iso*propyl phosphoryl AChE. The ratio of the rate constants for reactivation of diethyl- and di*iso*propyl phosphoryl AChE is given in Table 10. This ratio is far smaller for reactivators lacking a cationic group than for those which possess such a group (with the exception of hydroxylamine). This has been interpreted as further indication of the importance of the anionic site in the sense that the directed action of the reactivator is disturbed as a result of steric hindrance by the *iso*propyl groups.

Table 10. *The ratio of the rate constant for the reactivation of diethylphosphoryl enzyme (k_a) to that of diisopropyl phosphoryl enzyme (k_b)*

Reactivators	k_a/k_b
Without cationic centre	
Nicotinhydroxamic acid	3.5
*Iso*nicotinhydroxamic acid	2
Picolinohydroxamic acid	6
Chloroacethydroxamic acid	9
Pyridine[1]	8
Imidazole[1]	5
Hydroxylamine	40
With a cationic centre	
Nicotinhydroxamic acid methiodide	30
*Iso*nicotinhydroxamic acid methiodide	90
Picolinohydroxamic acid methochloride	120
Betaine hydroxamic acid	60
Glycinehydroxamic acid	20
Choline[1]	100
Pyridinoacethydroxamic acid[1]	200
Trimethylamine oxide	100

[1] The reactivation of di*iso*propyl enzyme was in these cases poor; therefore, there may be an error in the ratio of as large as 50%. From WILSON (1955a).

The chemical analysis of the active site of esterases related to acetylcholinesterase

A. Introduction

In the previous sections information was given on the structure and properties of the active site of AChE which had been obtained in reference to the properties of substrates and inhibitors and to the interaction of these with the enzyme.

Various properties and interactions of the active site of AChE are summarized graphically in the diagrams of Fig. 24.

In this section the emphasis will be laid on evidence emanating from chemical analysis of the enzyme molecule itself and particularly of its active site. As before, the term "active site" will refer to those regions of the enzyme surface where the substrate is localized and activated during the enzymic action. It is not necessarily a part of the molecule which when isolated would be capable of simulating the properties of the complete enzyme; its configuration as occurring within the intact native protein molecule depends, apart from its amino acid composition and sequence, on the secondary and tertiary structures of the latter. It is this subtle configuration that is probably required for complete enzymic activity. This is lost when isolation withdraws the active site from the influence of those forces that prevail in the intact native molecule.

We have seen in the preceding chapters that the active site of AChE comprises at least two distinct structures, an anionic and an esteratic site. The anionic site is likely to consist of one or more free carboxylic groups. In the previous section was mentioned the work of BERGMANN et al. (1956) who provided some kinetic data which might indicate that not one but two anionic sites, each consisting of a glutamic acid residue, may be involved. No direct chemical analysis of the anionic site (s) has so far been possible. The most formidable obstacle against this direct attack has been the impossibility of obtaining sufficient quantities of pure AChE.

Although lack of adequate material is equally prohibitive with regard to direct chemical attack on the esteratic site of AChE itself, considerable progress has been made towards the elucidation of its chemical structure. This was made possible by inferring that the esteratic site of AChE is probably very similar to that of other related esterases which can be obtained in sufficient quantity and quality to allow chemical analysis. This conclusion is based on the following facts.

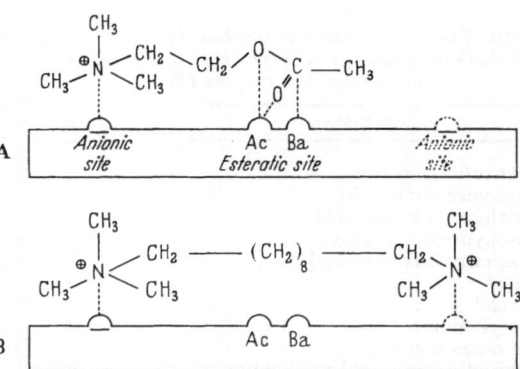

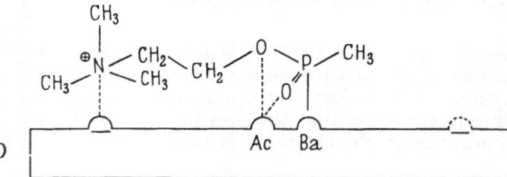

Fig. 24. *Schematic representation of the interaction of ACh and inhibitors with the active site of AChE.* The active site is composed of one or two anionic sites and the esteratic site containing an acidic group (Ac) and a basic group (Ba). In the figure are demonstrated the interactions of AChE with ACh (A) and with decamethonium (B). The structure of AChE after its reaction with dipropyl phosphorofluoridate and 2-trimethylammonium ethyl methylphosphonofluoridate iodide are represented in C and D, respectively

Chemical analysis by many workers of esterases of greatly varying substrate specificity, such as trypsin, chymotrypsin (ChTr), liver ali esterase, BuChE, and thrombin, showed all these enzymes to have a very similar structure on their esteratic site, arranged around a serine residue (COHEN et al. 1959). These data substantiated the hypothesis (COHEN et al. 1955b) that a number of DFP-sensitive enzymes carry a very similar structure reacting with DFP. It was suggested that this common structure (the B group) is closely associated with the general properties of enzymic hydrolysis. The substrate specificity, however, would be determined by additional chemical groups on or near the active site, and also by the secondary and tertiary structures of the native protein molecule. It is now almost generally agreed that all the enzymes involved have a comparable mechanism of action consisting in acylation of the esteratic site at a serine hydroxyl followed by hydrolysis of the acyl enzyme complex. They are all inhibited by organophosphorus anti-ChE agents which act, as will be shown presently, by phosphorylating rather than acylating the serine hydroxyl group of the active site. The interactions with both substrates and organophosphorus inhibitors are pH dependent in a range which suggests the catalytic involvement of a histidine residue. Acetylcholinesterase has been shown to belong to this group as far as mechanism of action is concerned (i.e., acylation of the enzyme by substrate followed by hydrolysis of the complex); moreover it is strongly inhibited by organophosphorus compounds, and in the course of this inhibition it is phosphorylated at the serine hydroxyl group. Finally, an imidazole group of histidine has been suspected to operate catalytically at the AChE surface. Therefore, the conclusion seems warranted that the esteratic site of AChE will carry the B group structure and that analytical data on the active site of the whole group of related esterases may be expected to be relevant to the esteratic site of AChE. Accordingly, in the present section, the chemical data available on the active site of this group of esterases will be dealt with in detail.

B. The imidazole group

In agreement with the data reported with regard to the pH dependence of AChE, analysis of the influence of pH on the rate of substrate hydrolysis by related enzymes has shown that again an ionizable group of pK 6 to 8 is involved in the enzymic action (DIXON and NEURATH 1957a, 1957b, DIXON et al. 1958c, GUT-FREUND and STURTEVANT 1956a, MARTIN et al. 1959, MOUNTER et al. 1957a, SCHONBAUM et al. 1959). The merits of this method of determination of the pK of enzymic groups have been explored by ALBERTY (1956a, 1956b).

Similarly, the inhibition of a number of esterases by organophosphorus agents depends on pH. MOUNTER et al. (1957a) showed that for this reaction also, a group with a pK within the range of 6 to 8 is essential. Most authors believe that this group is the imidazole ring of a histidine residue at the active site. However, much caution should be observed with respect to such interpretations (FRAENKEL-CONRAT 1956). When amino acid side-chain groups occur in different environments, their properties may greatly vary from those of the free amino acids. Thus BARNARD and STEIN (1958) have shown that the pK of the imidazole group may be strongly influenced by its environment, and this type of effect is also to be expected in proteins. Moreover, other side-chains in protein will be susceptible to similar variations of pK, depending on the overall protein structure in which they are embedded. These variations may very well bring some of them into the pK range of the free imidazole group (EDSALL 1943).

More support for the significance of imidazole has issued from experiments with model compounds. It could actually be shown that imidazole and its derivatives under certain circumstances are capable of accelerating the hydrolysis of esters. The relevant work has been recently summarized by DIXON et al. (1958c) in a review to which the reader is referred. Thus, catalysis of p-nitrophenyl acetate by imidazole has led BENDER and TURNQUEST (1957a, 1957b) to a general theory of a base-catalyzed ester hydrolysis (Fig. 25). Similar experiments and theories have been proposed by BENDER and TURNQUEST (1957b) and BRUICE and SCHMIR (1956, 1957), but the latter authors suggested the reaction sequence shown in Fig. 26 to explain the effectiveness of N-methyl imidazole, which could not possibly replace imidazole in the reaction sequence of Fig. 25 involving the loss of a proton. However, there are considerable qualitative and quantitative differences between the catalytic action on hydrolysis of esters such as p-nitrophenyl acetate by imidazole, and that by enzymes like ChTr. Therefore, if it is true that an imidazole group operates in the esteratic site of enzymes it must have been greatly modified by its environment.

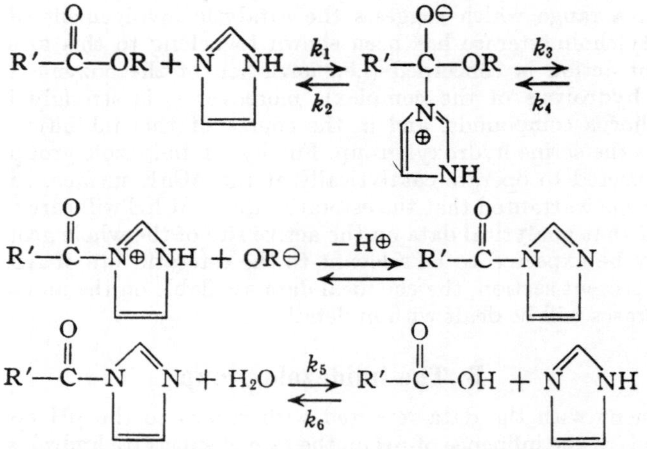

$$R'-\overset{O}{\overset{\|}{C}}-OR + N\diagup NH \underset{k_2}{\overset{k_1}{\rightleftarrows}} R'-\overset{O^{\ominus}}{\underset{\overset{\oplus}{N}-\diagdown NH}{\overset{|}{C}}}-OR \underset{k_4}{\overset{k_3}{\rightleftarrows}}$$

$$R'-\overset{O}{\overset{\|}{C}}-N^{\oplus}\diagup NH + OR^{\ominus} \xrightarrow{-H^{\oplus}} R'-\overset{O}{\overset{\|}{C}}-N\diagup N$$

$$R'-\overset{O}{\overset{\|}{C}}-N\diagup N + H_2O \underset{k_6}{\overset{k_5}{\rightleftarrows}} R'-\overset{O}{\overset{\|}{C}}-OH + N\diagup NH$$

Fig. 25. *Proposed mechanism for the catalysis of the hydrolysis of p-nitrophenyl acetate by imidazole.* The hydrolysis involves the catalytic attack on the ester by imidazole *via* an intermediary imidazole-ester complex to give N-acetylimidazole. It is subsequently hydrolyzed by water into acetate ions and imidazole. According to BENDER and TURNQUEST (1957a)

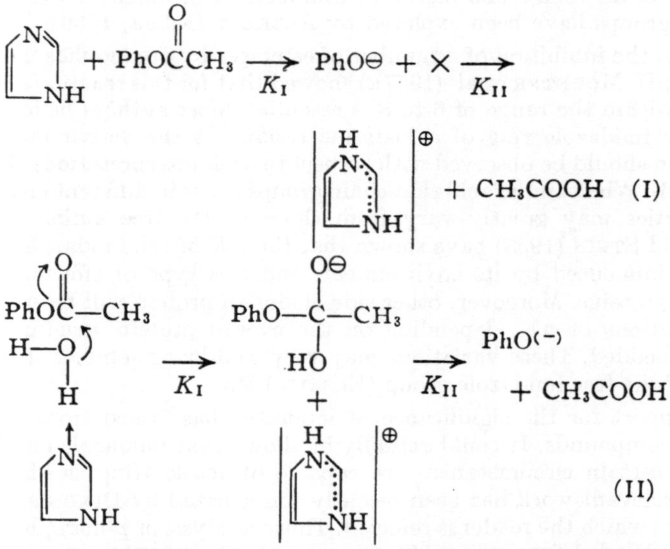

$$N\diagup NH + PhO\overset{O}{\overset{\|}{C}}CH_3 \xrightarrow{K_I} PhO^{\ominus} + X \xrightarrow{K_{II}}$$

$$\left[N\diagup NH \right]^{\oplus} + CH_3COOH \quad (I)$$

$$\begin{array}{c} PhO\overset{O}{\overset{\|}{C}}-CH_3 \\ H-O \\ H \\ \uparrow \\ N\diagup NH \end{array} \xrightarrow{K_I} \begin{array}{c} PhO-\overset{O^{\ominus}}{\underset{HO}{\overset{|}{C}}}-CH_3 \\ + \\ \left[N\diagup NH \right]^{\oplus} \end{array} \xrightarrow{K_{II}} \begin{array}{c} PhO^{(-)} \\ + CH_3COOH \\ \\ (II) \end{array}$$

Fig. 26. *Two reaction schemes for the hydrolysis of phenyl acetates by imidazole as a basic catalyst.* In (I) imidazole reacts directly with phenyl acetate to form an intermediate, X, of unknown character and phenoxide ion. Subsequently X reacts with water to form acetic acid and imidazole. In (II) imidazole-bound water reacts with phenyl acetate to form an unstable intermediate. This intermediate decomposes into acetic acid and phenoxide ion. Reaction scheme (I) is favored by the authors. According to BRUICE and SCHMIR (1957)

Direct chemical evidence for the presence of an imidazole group in the active site is also available. The subject has been recently reviewed by BARNARD and STEIN (1958) and DAVIES and GREEN (1958). This type of evidence emanates from attempts to establish a parallelism between the presumed capability of certain agents to block histidine residues of an enzyme and the degree of interference they may offer with respect to the reaction of the enzyme with substrates and inhibitors. Thus, evidence for the presence of imidazole has been obtained by MOUNTER et al. (1957a) using non-specific blocking agents like 2,4-dinitrofluoro-benzene (DNFB), photo-oxydation, and diazonium coupling for AChE, trypsin, and other hydrolases, including fluorophosphatases and thrombin. Similar observations have been reported by other authors with regard to ChTr. Thus, WEIL et al. (1953) and JANDORF et al. (1955b) have shown that destruction by selective photo-oxydation of one of the two histidines of ChTr destroys the enzyme's activity and its power of combining with organophosphorus agents. Other investigators (HARTLEY 1956, MASSEY and HARTLEY 1956, WHITAKER and JANDORF 1956) have shown that the reaction of DNFB with ChTr reduces the activity of the enzyme in proportion to the extent of the reaction of DNFB with one of its two histidine residues. The same type of evidence with regard to ChTr, using DNFB, was offered by FRAENKEL-CONRAT (1956) and SORM and RYCHLIK (1952); whereas MASSEY et al. (1955) and HARTLEY and MASSEY (1956), using fluorescent aryl sulfonyl chlorides, arrived at similar conclusions. WOOD and BALLS (1955), however, found that peroxidase oxidation of ChTr resulted in al loss of 50% of the activity with oxidation of one tryptophan and no histidine or other residues. The authors did not exclude the presence of imidazole at the active site, but suggested an auxiliary role for a tryptophan group.

The value of these results is naturally qualified by the fact that the methods and reagents involved are of limited specificity; secondary effects are therefore not excluded.

As has been mentioned earlier, very good evidence is available to demonstrate that organophosphorus compounds, like DFP, react specifically at the esteratic site of ChE's and other esterases (ALDRIDGE 1957, BALLS and JANSEN 1952, BARNARD and STEIN 1958, HOLMSTEDT 1959, JANSEN et al. 1950, KOELLE and GILMAN 1949, RIKER 1953, SCHRADER 1952).

It could be demonstrated that the enzymes concerned were inhibited by low concentrations of DFP. Where the molecular weight of the enzyme was known (in the case of trypsin and ChTr), it was found that one mole of enzyme reacted with one mole of DFP to give complete inhibition; correspondingly, when inhibition was only partial, its degree was always linearly related to the amount of DP (diisopropyl phosphoryl) bound (ASHBOLT and RYDON 1957, BALLS and JANSEN 1952, JANDORF et al. 1955b). Other evidence is provided by the well-known ability of substrates to prevent inhibition by DFP, indicating competition for a common active site (ALDRIDGE 1950, COHEN et al. 1955b, N. GREEN 1953). Finally, it is now generally accepted that the inhibition by DFP involves a permanent phosphorylation of the active site analogous to the transient acylation of this site in the course of normal substrate hydrolysis (WILSON et al. 1950).

Kinetic, pH, and chemical evidence of the same type that was used to demonstrate the significance of imidazole in substrate hydrolysis points also to its significance with regard to the coupling of the active site with organophosphorus inhibitors. MOUNTER et al. (1957a) showed that for the inhibition of a number of esterases by organophosphorus agents a group of pK 6 to 8 is essential. In experiments referred to earlier, WHITTAKER and JANDORF (1956) showed that the inhibition by DNFB of ChTr closely parallels the reaction of DNFB with one of the histidine residues, and that the capacity subsequently to bind DFP corresponds with the free portion of the enzyme. Conversely, DFP protects one histidine from DNFB (FRAENKEL-CONRAT 1956). The destruction by photo-oxydation of one of the two histidines (and two tryptophans) of chymotrypsin destroys the enzyme's power of combining with organophosphorus compounds (JANDORF et al. 1955b,

WEIL et al. 1953). Conversely, the DP group, when introduced in ChTr, will protect histidine (and tryptophan groups) from photo-oxydation.

Necessarily the same caution should be observed with regard to evaluation of this evidence, based on the reaction with inhibitors, as was recommended with regard to the reaction of enzymes with substrates.

Altogether an impressive body of circumstantial evidence has been accumulated to support the conclusion that an imidazole group operates at the active site of esterases. However, this evidence is based on pH and kinetic data which are intrinsically inconclusive for reasons mentioned before, and on chemical reactivity with agents which by their lack of specificity can no more be expected to produce unequivocal results.

C. The B group in the hydrolysates of phosphorylated esterases

It is obvious that straightforward interpretation with regard to the chemical structure of the active site could be expected from studies involving a specific reaction of the active site of an enzyme, followed by the analysis of the groups involved. Therefore, we shall deal in detail with work based on such a specific reaction, *viz.*, the property of many esterases to react with DFP to form an enzymically inactive compound. The value of the method is stressed by the fact that removal of the DP group from inhibited enzymes by nucleophilic agents leads to restoration of the enzyme's activity (see Chapter 21).

The results obtained from such investigations of the DFP reactive group of a number of esterases have been recently discussed by COHEN et al. (1959) and by NEURATH et al. (1958). The technical approach is generally as follows.

The enzyme is first completely inhibited by ^{32}P (or ^{14}C)-labelled DFP; sometimes *iso*propyl methylphosphonofluoridate (Sarin) is used. Consequently, the isolated ^{32}P-labelled protein is hydrolyzed, using hydrochloric acid or proteolytic enzymes or a combination of both. The radioactive break-down products must be isolated from unlabelled material. This is effected by familiar methods of isolation, like chromatography and electrophoresis on columns and on filter paper. The purified radioactive fragments may then be analyzed. The first study of this kind was undertaken by SCHAFFER et al. (1953) with ChTr inhibited by DF^{32}P. After degradation of the inhibited enzyme with hydrochloric acid, about 30% of the ^{32}P was recovered as serine phosphate. These results have been confirmed and extended by these and other authors. Thus, 0-serine phosphate has been isolated from the following DFP inhibited enzymes: ChTr (SCHAFFER et al. 1953), ali esterase and AChE from red cell stroma, and BuChE (COHEN et al. 1955b), eel AChE (SCHAFFER et al. 1954), trypsin, and horse liver ali esterase (COHEN et al. 1955b, JANSZ et al. 1959b, 1959c). Similarly larger fragments, *viz.*, ^{32}P-bearing peptides (P peptides) were isolated from enzymes inhibited by radioactive DFP or Sarin using hydrochloric acid or enzymic hydrolysis. All pertinent results are presented in Table 11.

It will be seen that as far as ChTr is concerned all authors agree on an amino acid sequence

$$\overset{\overset{\textstyle ^{32}P}{\textstyle |}}{\text{Gly—Asp—Ser—Gly}}$$

of the active site around the ^{32}P-label; the latter is invariably found attached to the serine residue. The data of OOSTERBAAN et al. (1958a, 1958b) are not in agreement with those of SCHAFFER et al. (1957) and TURBA and GUNDLACH (1955) as far as the further sequence of larger peptides is concerned. The former authors found

$$^{32}\text{P}$$
$$|$$
Gly—Asp—Ser—Gly—Gly—Pro—Leu ;

the latter,

$$^{32}\text{P}$$
$$|$$
Gly—Asp—Ser—Gly—Glu—Ala .

As far as trypsin is concerned, the most complete sequence reported by DIXON et al. (1958 a, 1958 b),

NH₂　　　　　　　　　　　　　　　　　　　　　　³²P
|　　　　　　　　　　　　　　　　　　　　　　　　|
(Asp—Ser—Cys—Glu—Gly—Gly—Asp—Ser—Gly—Pro—Val—Cys—Ser—Gly—Lys),
　　　　　　|　　　　　　　　　　　　　　　　　　　　　　　　　　|
　　　　　SO₃⁻　　　　　　　　　　　　　　　　　　　　　　　　SO₃⁻

agrees with earlier reports on the composition and structure of smaller peptides as presented in Table 11.

Table 11 includes also structures of phosphorylated peptides of DFP-inhibited thrombin, liver ali esterase and BuChE. Phosphoglucomutase represents a special case since it is a non-hydrolytic enzyme (transferase). Furthermore, the relevant peptides were not obtained by inhibition of the enzyme with DF³²P, but by phosphorylating it during normal enzyme action (KOSHLAND and ERWIN 1957, KOSHLAND et al. 1958).

Apart from the isolation of serine phosphate from enzymes inhibited by organophosphorus compounds, there is now very good evidence that the di*iso*-propyl phosphoryl group (DP) is attached at the hydroxyl oxygen of the serine residue of the peptides examined. For detailed information on this evidence, the reader is referred to the paper by COHEN et al. (1959). The evidence is based on analysis of the DP-peptides from horse liver aliesterase and ChTr (JANSZ et al. 1959 b, 1959 c, OOSTERBAAN et al. 1958 a, 1958 b), and on the identical behaviour after alkaline hydrolysis of DP peptides and that of synthetic 0-phosphorylated serine derivatives as reported by RILEY et al. (1953). In either case, alkaline hydrolysis splits off the phosphoryl group with simultaneous dehydratation of the serine. A reasonable inference, therefore, is that all phosphorylated enzymes which on mild enzymic hydrolysis yield these peptides have the DP-group attached at the serine oxygen.

Earlier we stressed the strong evidence available to indicate that DFP reacts with the active site of esterases to produce a stable, phosphorylated, inhibited enzyme, whereas the substrates react analogously with the same group to produce a labile acylated enzyme. Using the techniques now under discussion, it was possible to provide substantial evidence to this effect after the work of HARTLEY and KILBY (1954), BALLS and ALDRICH (1955) and BALLS and WOOD (1956) had shown the way to isolate the labile intermediate acetyl ChTr formed during the hydrolysis of *p*-nitrophenyl acetate (NPA) by ChTr. OOSTERBAAN and VAN ADRICHEM (1958) prepared ¹⁴C acetyl ChTr by allowing ChTr to react on ¹⁴C-labelled NPA. The ¹⁴C enzyme was first hydrolyzed with pepsin and then with pancreatin. The ¹⁴C peptides were isolated and analyzed. One of these peptides possessed an amino acid sequence which was completely identical to that of the DP-peptide as shown in Table 11. The acetyl group is almost certainly attached to the serine oxygen (BENOITON et al. 1960, COHEN et al. 1959).

Closer examination of the phosphorylated peptides of ChTr, trypsin, *BuChE*, thrombin, and horse liver ali esterase reveals that the phosphorylated serine

Table 11. *Amino acid compositions and sequences in the active sites of enzymes*

Labelled enzyme	Hydrolysis method	Amino acid composition or sequence	References
Chymotrypsin-DFP	HCl	$\overset{\text{P}}{\mid}$ GLY—ASP—SER—GLY	Schaffer et al. (1957)
	HCl	$\overset{\text{P}}{\mid}$ ASP—SER—GLY (Glu, Ala, Gly)	Turba and Gundlach (1955)
	"Cotazym"	$\overset{\text{P}}{\mid}$ GLY—ASP—SER—GLY—GLY—PRO—LEU	Oosterbaan et al. (1958a, 1958b)
Chymotrypsin-Sarin	HCl	$\overset{\text{P}}{\mid}$ GLY—ASP—SER—GLY—GLU—ALA (Val)	Schaffer et al. (1956, 1957)
	Papain	$\overset{\text{P}}{\mid}$ GLY—ASP—SER—GLY—GLU—ALA (Val, His, Pro, Leu, Cys, Thr)	Schaffer et al. (1956, 1957)
Trypsin-Sarin	HCl	$\overset{\text{P}}{\mid}$ ASP—SER—GLY	Schaffer et al. (1958)
Trypsin-DFP	Trypsin	NH_2—ASP—SER—CYS—GLU—GLY—GLY—ASP—SER—GLY—PRO—VAL—CYS—SER—GLY—LYS (with SO_3H under CYS residues and P above SER)	Dixon et al. (1958a, 1958b)
	Chymotrypsin	Gly, Asp, Ser, Gly, Pro, Val, Cys, Ala, Glu, Lys	Dixon et al. (1956b)

	Peptide structure	Hydrolysis	Reference
"Cotazym"	P | Gly, Asp, Ser, Gly, Pro, Val		OOSTERBAAN et al. (1956)
Liver aliesterase-DFP	P | GLY–GLU–SER–ALA–GLY–GLY–(GLU,SER)	Pepsin	JANSZ et al. (1959b, 1959c)
Butyrocholinesterase-DFP	P | PHE–GLY–GLU–SER–ALA–GLY–(ALA,ALA,SER)	Pepsin	JANSZ et al. (1959a)
Thrombin-DFP	P | ASP–SER–GLY and P | Asp, Ser, Gly, Glu, Ala	HCl	GLADNER and LAKI (1958)
Phosphoglucomutase	PO_3H_2 | ASP–SER–(Gly, Glu,) and PO_3H_2 | ASP–SER–(Gly, Glu, Ala, Val, Thr, Leu)	HCl or Proteolysis	KOSHLAND and ERWIN (1957); KOSHLAND et al. (1958) *)
Chymotrypsin-NPA	$O=C–CH_3$ | GLY–ASP–SER–GLY–GLY–PRO–LEU	Pepsin and "Cotazym"	COHEN et al. (1959)

Remarks: P in the peptide structures denotes the phosphorylgroup originating from DFP or Sarin. GLY-etc = amino acid residue in established sequence. GLY, = amino acid residue in unknown sequence.
Gly, etc = sequence and exact number of residues unknown. NPA = p-nitrophenyl acetate.

*) Recently C. MILSTEIN and F. SANGER [Biochem. J 79, 456—469 (1961)] found the sequence THR. ALA. P-SER. HIS-ASP (or ASP-NH2).

residue is always preceded by a dibasic amino acid (Asp or Glu). It is followed by a glycine or a closely related alanine residue. Moreover, it was found that the dibasic acid is preceded by a glycine residue. Particularly the sequence, dibasic amino acid-serine, appears significant and not fortuitous.

The data reported in this section provide evidence that in addition to the amino acid histidine, the following sequence occurs in the active site of esterases:

$$\text{Gly}-\frac{\text{Asp}}{\text{Glu}}-\text{Ser}-\frac{\text{Gly}}{\text{Ala}}.$$

This sequence represents the best description of the B group available at present*.

D. The mode of action of esterases

We shall now try to develop a picture to visualize the way in which the imidazole and the B group sequence

$$\text{Gly}-\frac{\text{Asp}}{\text{Glu}}-\text{Ser}-\frac{\text{Gly}}{\text{Ala}}$$

(in particular the serine hydroxyl and the free carboxylic group of the dibasic amino acid residue) might operate in the active site of esterases. This picture should be consistent with generally accepted concepts about the mode of action of the enzymes under consideration.

WILSON et al. (1950) introduced the hypothesis that enzymic ester hydrolysis might follow the same course as alkaline hydrolysis, in the sense that a nucleophilic group on the active site of the enzyme would play the role of the OH⁻ ion; it would be acylated during the reaction.

As far as AChE is concerned, the considerations whereupon this hypothesis is based have been given in a previous section (BENDER and KEMP 1957, HARTLEY and KILBEY 1954, SPRINSON and RITTENBERG 1951, WILSON 1951b). Most convincing in this respect has been the work of BALLS and ALDRICH (1955) and BALLS and WOOD (1956), who succeeded in isolating acetyl ChTr from the reaction of ChTr on NPA, and of DIXON and NEURATH (1957a) who demonstrated likewise the formation of acyl enzyme in the course of trypsin-catalyzed ester hydrolysis. Consequently, the following discussion will be based on a mechanism involving the formation of acyl enzyme accompanied by release of the alcohol residue, and followed by hydrolysis of the intermediate to yield acid and free enzyme. Moreover, the assumption seems justified that DFP reacts with the enzyme in an analogous way to form a stable phosphoryl enzyme. The significance of each of the groups of the active site will be examined against the background of this mechanism.

I. The imidazole group of histidine

Many authors believe that the imidazole group is the primary acceptor for the acyl and the phosphoryl residue, respectively. This concept is strongly favoured by the results of model experiments (see above). However, DIXON et al. (1956a), following the reaction between ChTr and NPA spectrophotometrically, were unable to register an increase of the absorption at 245 mμ (the absorption maximum for acetyl imidazole) during the formation of the acetyl ChTr. Likewise GUTFREUND and STURTEVANT (1956b), in studying the same reaction, showed that the acylation does not involve a basic group.

The process of "ageing" observed in DFP inhibited cholinesterases has often been interpreted as evidence for imidazole as the initial site of phosphorylation. The activity of freshly phosphorylated ChE may be restored by the action of

---

*) Recently F. SANGER and D. C. SHAW demonstrated the sequence Thr. P-Ser. Met. Ala for a DFP-Sensitive proteïnase from *B. Subtilis*. [Nature (Lond.) **187**, 872 (1960)].

nucleophilic agents. On storage, however, "ageing" occurs, a process by which the inhibited enzyme gradually loses its ability to be reactivated. The process is usually explained as an intramolecular migration of the phosphoryl group from histidine to an adjacent serine residue (HOBBIGER 1955, JANDORF et al. 1955b). This explanation is consistent with the lability of phosphoryl imidazole and the stability of 0-phosphoryl serine derivatives. However, this ageing process has been observed only in ChE's. Moreover it has been shown recently that another mechanism is responsible for the ageing process.

JANSZ et al. (1959a) found that the peptide isolated from *BuChE* which had been inhibited by DFP carried a mono*iso*propylphosphoryl (MP) instead of the usual DP-group. Further studies (BERENDS et al. 1959; cf. COHEN et al. 1959) showed that this MP-group was present also in older preparations of DFP-inhibited BuChE; freshly inhibited enzymes carried a DP-group. There was always a close quantitative parallelism between the amount of ageing, i.e., that part of the inhibition that could not be overcome by reactivation, and the fraction of the enzyme that was MP-bound. Conversely, the fraction of DP-bound enzyme corresponded closely with that part of the inhibition that could still be reversed by incubation with reactivators like pyridine 2-aldoxime methiodide.

The results of a representative experiment are summarized in Fig. 27. They show clearly that ageing of DFP-inhibited BuChE consists in conversion of a reactivatable DP-enzyme into a non-reactivatable MP-enzyme. COHEN et al. (1959) have been able to show the existence of a similar mechanism for AChE; aged DFP inhibited AChE carries a MP-group. Studies on BuChE with ^{14}C and ^{32}P labelled DFP (BERENDS et al. 1959, COHEN et al. 1959) showed that during ageing the *iso*propyl group came free in the solvent as *iso*propanol; it was apparently not attached to another site of the enzyme protein.

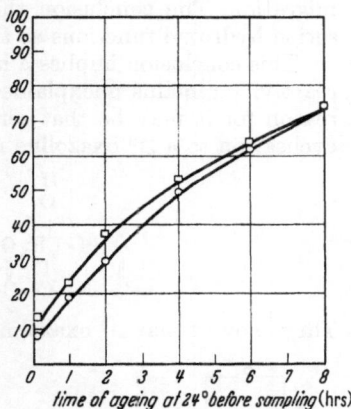

Fig. 27. *Relation between conversion of DP- into MP-Butyrocholinesterase and the ageing process.* □ = percentage of ageing; ○ = percentage of conversion of DP-enzyme into MP-enzyme. From COHEN et al. (1959)

The data so far presented do not argue in favour of a concept of assigning to imidazole the role of carrier for the acyl or phosphoryl group in isolated acyl and phosphoryl enzymes, respectively. On the other hand, the imidazole group may well be involved in reactions leading to acylation or de-acylation of enzymes. Kinetic analysis of both processes on the system ChTr-NPA demonstrated the importance of a group with a pK of 6 to 8 (DIXON and NEURATH 1957a). Little or nothing is known about how imidazole may influence the acylation. The role of imidazole in de-acylation seemed fairly well established when DIXON and NEURATH (1957c) showed spectrophotometrically that de-acylation of acetyl ChTr was accompanied by the formation of an acetyl imidazole intermediate. Recently, however, doubt has been thrown on the significance of these spectrophotometric data as evidence for the role of imidazole in de-acylation, since SPENCER and STURTEVANT (1959) demonstrated that the acetylated enzyme studied by DIXON and NEURATH was not on the pathway of the enzyme reaction.

T. VISWANATHA and LIENER (1960) reported that they succeeded in isolating enzymatically active peptides from peptic hydrolysates of acetyl trypsinogen. These peptides were devoid of histidine (not more than 0.1 mole of histidine per mole of peptide in good preparations). These results may be of great interest for the final evaluation of the significance of histidine.

23*

II. The serine hydroxyl

The attachment of phosphoryl groups at a serine hydroxyl of inhibited enzymes has long been considered an artifact. It was thought that in the course of degradation or isolation procedures, or during ageing the phosphoryl group migrated from the active site to a serine residue. Consequently, the significance of serine phosphate and phosphoryl peptides isolated from inhibited enzymes seemed doubtful. However, it soon became apparent that from many different esterases very similar phosphoryl seryl peptides could be isolated by a variety of methods (hydrochloric acid, various proteolytic enzymes); moreover, a confirming acetyl seryl peptide was obtained from acetyl ChTr. These results have established the significance of the serine residue at the active site, and of the concept of the B group; moreover, as discussed above, the ageing process can no longer be taken as evidence for migration. The conclusion therefore seems justified that in these esterases the serine hydroxyl functions as the acyl and phosphoryl acceptor.

This conclusion implies a high reactivity of the serine hydroxyl, and this high reactivity remains unexplained by the present knowledge of the active site. The reason for it may be that serine is incorporated in a special structure, e.g., by cyclisation to a Δ^2 oxazoline ring as suggested by PORTER et al. (1958).

They showed that Δ^2 oxazolines may react with DFP to give products that yield

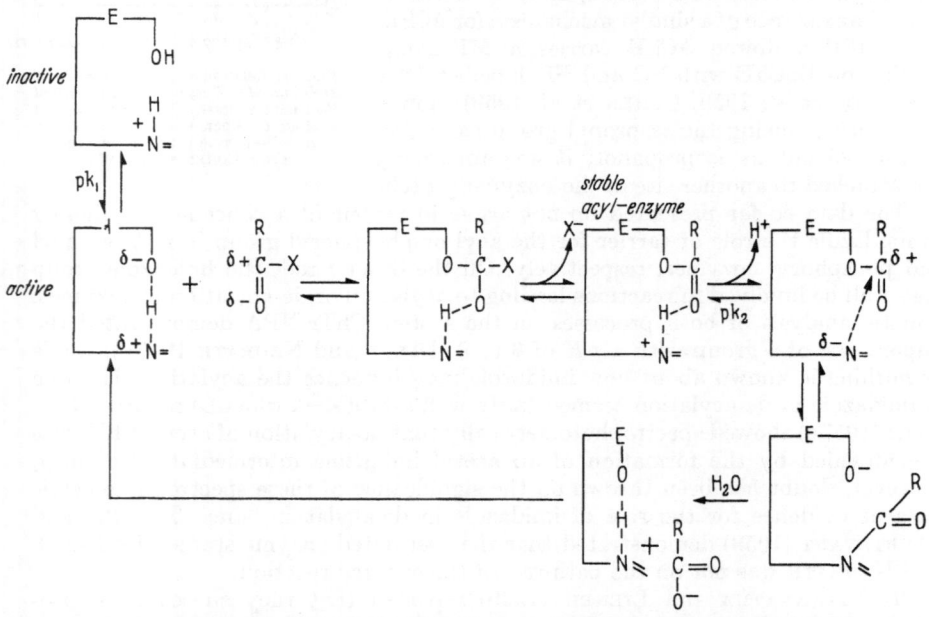

Fig. 28. *Proposed mechanism of enzymic hydrolysis.* The active center is postulated to involve hydrogen bonding between a serine hydroxyl and an uncharged imidazole nucleus. The nucleophilic oxygen of the hydroxyl attacks the carbonyl function of the substrate. Expulsion of the alcoholic part of the ester is accompanied by the formation of acylated enzyme. The next step involves the nucleophilic attack of the imidazole nitrogen on the newly formed ester linkage in the acylated enzyme leading to formation of acyl imidazole. The latter is rapidly hydrolyzed by water into acid and active enzyme. According to CUNNINGHAM (1957)

0-phosphoryl ethanolamines on acid hydrolysis. Another possibility would be that other groups, on the strength of their steric position, could induce high reactivity in the serine hydroxyl. BROUWER (1957), CUNNINGHAM (1957) and WESTHEIMER (1957) have suggested that imidazole might be in such a position. CUNNINGHAM (1957) proposed a detailed mechanism for the enzymic action of ChTr consistent with data available at the time (pK for acylation and de-acylation, pH- and denaturation stabilization of acyl enzyme, and occurrence of acyl imidazole during de-acylation) (Fig. 28). Various other mechanisms involving the imidazole group, the serine hydroxyl, or both have been proposed (DAVIS and GREEN 1958).

III. The carboxyl group

As discussed before, the available evidence on the chemical structure of the active site favours the concept that the amino-N of the essential serine is linked to the α-carboxyl of a dibasic amino acid residue. It seems likely that this sequence (Asp—Ser or Glu—Ser) is an obligatory property of the active site. It will, therefore, be necessary that models explaining the enzymic action of the esterases under consideration should take account of this residue and its function by including a functional free carboxyl group in the right position. Reaction schemes and models that fail to account for this group seem less satisfactory.

The significance of this residue with regard to the functional characteristics of the active site, *viz.*, substrate hydrolysis and reactivity towards organophosphorus compounds, has been discussed by COHEN et al. (1959). For instance, the free carboxyl group of the dibasic amino acid could serve as acceptor for the substrate alcohol just as serine serves as acceptor for its acyl residue. It is conceivable that in the active enzymes the serine hydroxyl and this carboxyl group are linked to give an internal ester. Substrate hydrolysis would then involve transesterification; in this process the imidazole group could take part, e.g., by promoting acylation or de-acylation.

A second possibility accounts for recently reported properties of the carboxyl group with regard to ester hydrolysis. Several authors (BENDER et al. 1958a, 1958b, EDWARDS 1950, 1952, GARRETT 1957, MORAWETZ and ORESKES 1958, ZIMMERING et al. 1957) have demonstrated that an internal carboxylate ion in the right position relative to the ester bond may participate catalytically in the hydrolysis. The hydrolysis of acetylsalicylic acid may be regarded as a classical example. The acceleration of the hydrolysis is almost certainly attributable to an intramolecular attack of the carboxylate ion on the carboxyl carbon atom of the ester to produce an intermediate (mixed) anhydride, which is subsequently rapidly hydrolyzed. The hypothesis that a free carboxyl group is involved in the last stages of substrate hydrolysis has also been used in the reaction scheme of RYDON (1958) (Fig. 29).

It has been proposed by BERNHARD and GUTFREUND (1956) that catalysis by the enzyme ficin is dominated by a group with a pK of approximately 4.3, presumedly an ionized carboxyl group, which is rate-determining for the breakdown of an acyl thiol enzyme compound; similarly, SMITH and PARKER (1958) have demonstrated that in papain a carboxylate ion participates in the hydrolysis of the thiol ester intermediate. It was suggested by BENDER et al. (1958b) that the mixed anhydride mechanism for intramolecular catalysis operates during the action of such SH enzymes. COHEN et al. (1959) extended the hypothesis to include the intermediate 0-acyl seryl enzymes formed during esteratic action. The significance of the dicarboxylic acid residue was supposed to be the furnishing of a carboxylate ion in a steric position suitable to enable it to catalyze the hydrolysis

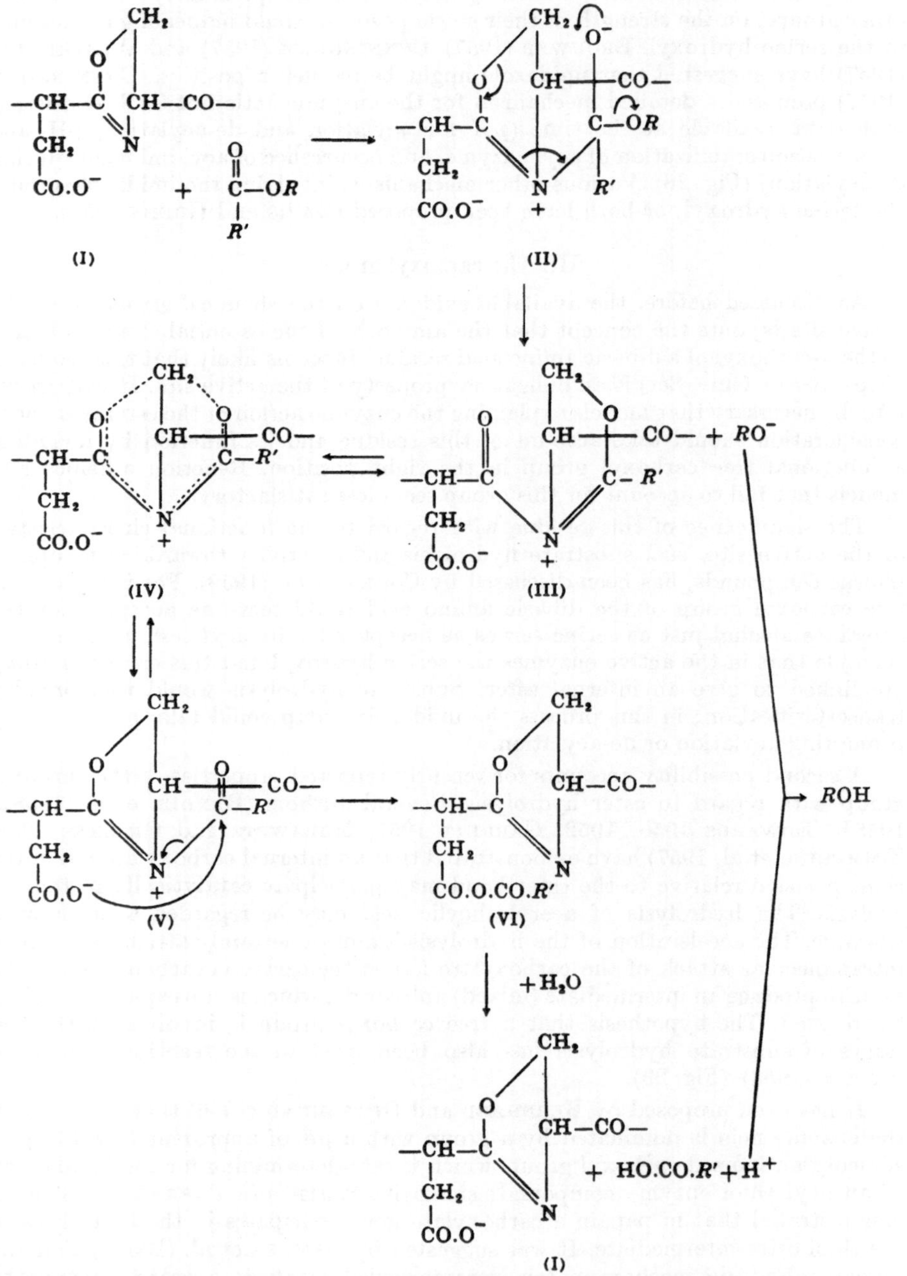

Fig. 29. *Proposed mechanism for the oxazoline function for ester hydrolysis.* The intermediate II results from a nucleophilic attack of the oxazoline nitrogen on the ester. After expulsion of the alkoxide ion (RO⁻), III is formed, which is in equilibrium with IV and V. In the next stage the ionized carboxyl group of the aspartic acid residue attacks the carbonyl group with the formation of an acid anhydride, VI. Finally VI undergoes hydrolysis, possibly assisted by a suitably placed histidine residue. According to RYDON (1958)

of either S-acyl cysteyl (in the case of SH enzymes) or 0-acyl seryl formed during esteratic or proteolytic action; the catalytic action would consist in a nucleophilic attack on the ester carboxyl carbon atom, leading to a labile acid anhydride. If this hypothesis is true, it would involve the presence of a dicarboxylic amino acid residue preceding not only the serine residue in the active site of esterases, but

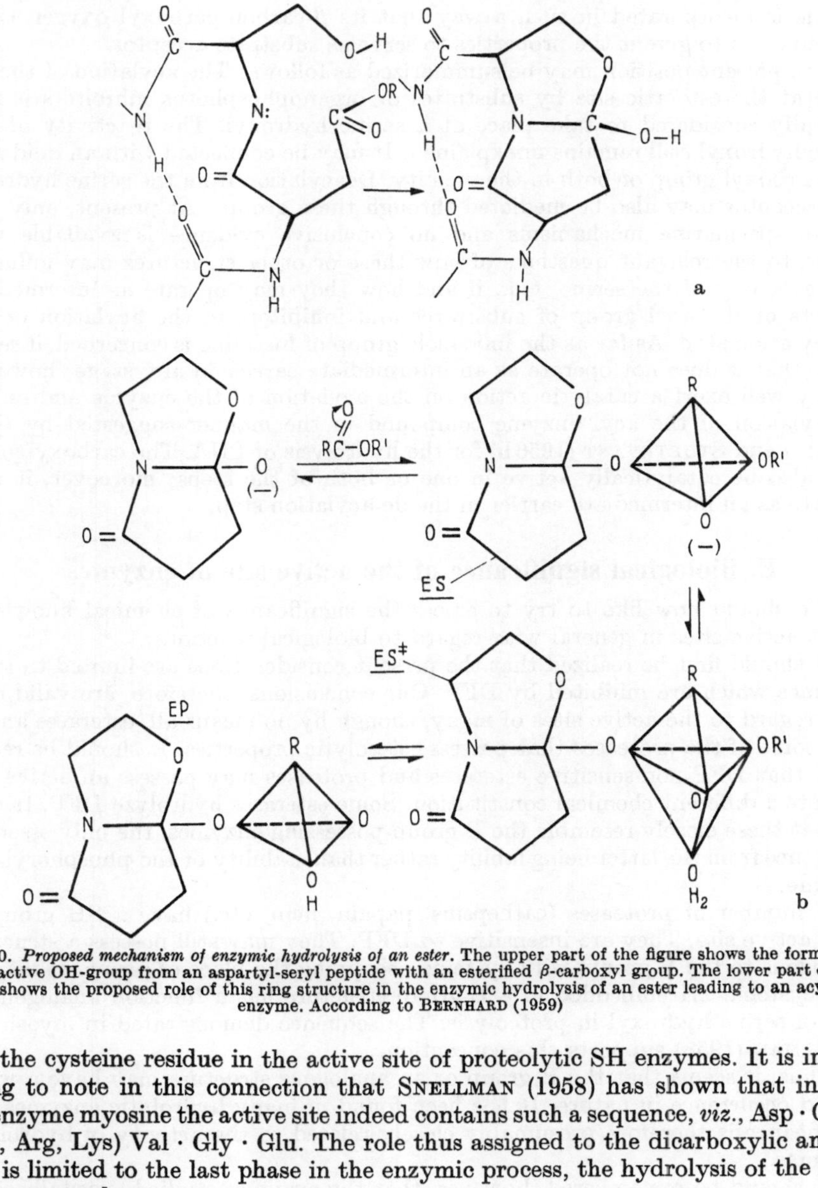

Fig. 30. *Proposed mechanism of enzymic hydrolysis of an ester.* The upper part of the figure shows the formation of an active OH-group from an aspartyl-seryl peptide with an esterified β-carboxyl group. The lower part of the figure shows the proposed role of this ring structure in the enzymic hydrolysis of an ester leading to an acylated enzyme. According to BERNHARD (1959)

also the cysteine residue in the active site of proteolytic SH enzymes. It is interesting to note in this connection that SNELLMAN (1958) has shown that in the SH enzyme myosine the active site indeed contains such a sequence, *viz.*, Asp · Cys · (Tyr, Arg, Lys) Val · Gly · Glu. The role thus assigned to the dicarboxylic amino acid is limited to the last phase in the enzymic process, the hydrolysis of the acyl enzyme complex.

Attempts to relate the reactivity of serine hydroxyl groups with the free carboxyl group of the active site are still very speculative. SMITH (1958) has suggested that the reactive group at the active site of papain involves an internal thiol ester in which the free carboxyl group participates. Another mechanism (Fig. 30) to account for the reactivity of the aspartyl-seryl sequence in ChTr has recently been proposed by BERNHARD (1959), in the form of a double ring model involving the seryl and the preceding aspartyl group, that seems to account satisfactorily for some properties of the active site; in this model the aspartyl residue is incorporated in such a way that its β-carbon carboxyl oxygen is activated so as to give it the properties to serve as substrate acceptor.

The present position may be summarized as follows: The acylation of the enzyme at the esteratic site by substrates or organophosphorus inhibitors is now generally considered to take place at a serine hydroxyl. The reactivity of this serine hydroxyl still remains unexplained. It may be connected with an imidazole or a carboxyl group or both in the vicinity. Deacylation from the serine hydroxyl to a receptor may also be mediated through these groups. At present, only tentative, speculative mechanisms and no conclusive evidence is available with regard to the relevant questions of how these or other structures may influence the reactivity of the serine, c.q., if and how they may operate as intermediate carriers of the acyl group of substrates and inhibitors in the acylation or the de-acylation step. As far as the imidazole group of histidine is concerned, it seems likely that it does not operate as an intermediate carrier in any stage; however, it may well exert a catalytic action on the acylation of the enzyme and on the de-acylation of the acyl enzyme compound in the manner suggested by GUT-FREUND and STURTEVANT (1956 b) for the hydrolysis of PNA. The carboxyl group may also be catalytically active in one or both of the steps; moreover, it may operate as an intermediate carrier in the de-acylation step.

E. Biological significance of the active site of enzymes

We should now like to try to assess the significance of chemical knowledge about active sites in general with regard to biological reactions.

It should first be realized that the present considerations are limited to those enzymes which are inhibited by DFP. Our conclusions, therefore, are valid only with regard to the active sites of many, though by no means all, esterases and of only some of the proteases that possess esterolytic properties. It should be recognized that DFP-non-sensitive esterases and proteases may possess an active site of quite a different chemical constitution. Some esterases hydrolyze DFP. It may be that these closely resemble the B group-possessing enzymes, the only essential difference from the latter being lability rather than stability of the phosphorylated enzyme.

A number of proteases (cathepsins, papain, ficin, etc.) have a SH group in their active site. They are insensitive to DFP. They may still possess a structure analogous to the B group, with cysteine occupying the place of serine. It may be that cysteine-SH embedded in a B group structure has a function analogous to that of serine hydroxyl in proteolysis. The sequence demonstrated in myosin by SNELLMAN (1958) supports this conception.

Thus, it seems that the B group or an analogous structure may have a widespread occurrence in nature. It has been found in many hydrolytic enzymes. Its significance is therefore presumably closely related to the activity of hydrolytic enzymes.

It should be remembered, however, that the enzymes studied, crystallized or otherwise purified, are often the sorry results of a series of maltreatments to which a protein has been subjected on its way from its natural biological position, in harmony with the total of the organism, into the test tube. Therefore, the obvious conclusion that *in vitro* hydrolytic ability represents the only *in vivo* function of isolated proteins is not always tenable, and has often proved wrong. It is certainly warranted for proteins like ChTr and trypsin that occur in the intestinal tract of animals, where they break proteins down into metabolites that are readily absorbed into the general circulation. Correspondingly, with regard to the *in vivo* function of these enzymes the significance of the B group will be that of a structure, arranged in such a way within the enzyme macromolecule, that it favours the hydrolysis of substrates. In this process the macrostructure is acylated at the serine hydroxyl site followed by de-acylation, i.e., transfer of the acyl group to the acceptor, water.

It is certain that a number of enzymes that *in vitro* hydrolyze substrates act *in vivo* as transferring enzymes owing to the presence of acceptors other than water. In this connection, it is of great interest that KOSHLAND and ERWIN (1957) and KOSHLAND et al. (1958) have suggested that a non-hydrolytic enzyme, phosphoglucomutase, possesses the B group structure at its active site. These results provide chemical support for the concept that hydrolases may be considered as a special class of transferases. The general mechanism of all these enzymes is acylation or phosphorylation of the serine hydroxyl at the active site, followed by transfer of the acyl or phosphoryl group to an acceptor which may be water, an alcohol, or something else.

In other cases, isolated proteins with hydrolytic action *in vitro* may *in vivo* have enzymic activities other than hydrolysis or transfer; they may *in vivo* even be endowed with other than enzymic properties of high biological significance. The muscle protein myosin is a good illustration of this. ŽUPANČIČ (1953) has forwarded the hypothesis that cell receptors of many, if not most, biologically active substrates may be identical with enzymes which inactivate the substances concerned.

Likewise, it may very well be that the main function *in vivo* of AChE, an enzyme which is found in cholinergic receptors and in the membrane of erythrocytes, is not the breakdown of ACh. HOLLAND and KLEIN (1956) and HOLLAND et al. (1952) have suggested that the function of AChE is associated with permeability processes. Interaction of ACh with AChE protein embedded in receptor structures may lead to the triggering of changes of permeability in those structures. Acetylcholinesterase may thus be involved in sodium transport (KOBLICK 1959) and in mechano-electric conversion in Pacinian bodies (LOEWENSTEIN and MOLINS 1958). It is also conceivable that some esterases may *in vivo* be involved in permeability processes in the sense that they may be able to transfer the acyl group of esters through membranes, passing it first toward receptors and from there onward; similarly, they may promote the passage of the alkoxy group of esters. The concept of enzyme catalyzed group-transfer through membranes has been elaborated by MITCHELL and MOYLE (1958). STEIN (1958) showed that a polypeptide of the red cell membrane may be essential for the permeation of glycerol; the terminal histidine amino-group of this peptide was essential. A relation with the imidazole of the active site of esterases might be considered in this connection. Clearly, studies of the active site of these esterases may thus provide information on permeability of membranes. Accordingly, in the present context many of the results presented concerning the active site of esterases may in future prove to be of the utmost relevance with regard to the understanding of the chemical composition and biological function of acetylcholine receptors.

References

AARON, H. S., H. O. MICHEL, B. WITTEN and J. I. MILLER: The stereochemistry of asymmetric phosphorus compounds. II. Stereospecificity in the irreversible inactivation of cholinesterases by enantiomorphs of an organophosphorus inhibitor. J. Amer. chem. Soc. **80**, 456—458 (1958).

ADAMS, D. H.: The specificity of the human erythrocyte cholinesterase. Biochim. biophys. Acta **3**, 1—14 (1949).

— and R. H. S. THOMPSON: The selective inhibition of cholinesterases. Biochem. J. **42**, 170 to 175 (1948).

— and V. P. WHITTAKER: The specificity of the human erythrocyte cholinesterase. Biochem. J. **43**, XIV (1948).

— — The cholinesterases of human blood. I. The specificity of the plasma enzyme and its relation to the erythrocyte cholinesterase. Biochim. biophys. Acta **3**, 358—366 (1949).

— — The cholinesterases of human blood. II. The forces acting between enzyme and substrate. Biochim. biophys. Acta **4**, 543—558 (1950).

ALBERTY, R. A.: Kinetic effects of the ionization of groups in the enzyme molecule. In: Symposium on structure of enzymes and proteins 1955, Gatlinburg, Tenn. The Wistar Institute of Anatomy and Biology, Philadelphia, 1956. Suppl. 1 to J. cell. comp. Physiol. **47** (1956a).

— Enzyme kinetics. In: F. F. NORD, Ed. Advanc. Enzymol. **17**, 1—64 (1956b).

ALDRIDGE, W. N.: Some properties of specific cholinesterase with particular reference to the mechanism of inhibition by diethyl p-nitrophenyl thiophosphate (E 605) and analogues. Biochem. J. **46**, 451—460 (1950).

— Differentiation of true and pseudo cholinesterase by organophosphorus compounds. Biochem. J. **53**, 62—67 (1953a).

— The inhibition of erythrocyte cholinesterase by tri-esters of phosphoric acid. 3. The nature of the inhibitory process. Biochem. J. **54**, 422—448 (1953b).

— Anticholinesterases. Inhibition of cholinesterase by organophosphorus compounds and reversal of this reaction. Mechanism involved. Chem. and Ind., 473—476 (1954).

— Organophosphorus compounds and esterases. Ann. Repts. Progr. Chem. **53**, 294—305 (1957).

— and A. N. DAVISON: The inhibition of erythrocyte cholinesterase by tri-esters of phosphoric acid. I. Diethyl p-nitrophenyl phosphate (E 600) and analogues. Biochem. J. **51**, 62—70 (1952a).

— — Inhibition of erythrocyte cholinesterase by tri-esters of phosphoric acid. II. Diethyl p-nitrophenyl thionphosphate (E 605) and analogues. Biochem. J. **52**, 663—671 (1952b).

— — Mechanism of inhibition of cholinesterases by organophosphorus compounds. Biochem. J. **55**, 763—765 (1953).

ALLES, G. A., and R. C. HAWES: Cholinesterases in the blood of man. J. biol. Chem. **133**, 375—390 (1940).

AMMAN, R., and H. MEYER: Zur stereochemischen Spezifität der Cholin- bzw. Acetylcholinesterase. Hoppe-Seylers Z. physiol. Chem. **314**, 198—204 (1759).

ANDREWS, K. J. M., F. R. ATHERTON, F. BERGEL and A. L. MORRISON: The synthesis of neurotropic and musculotropic stimulators and inhibitors. Part V. Derivatives of aminophenyl phosphates as anticholinesterases. J. chem. Soc. 780—784 (1952).

— — — — Anticholinesterases, hydroxypyridine and hydroxyquinoline. J. chem. Soc. 1638 (1954).

ASHBOLT, R. F., and H. N. RYDON: The action of diisopropyl phosphorofluoridate and other anticholinesterases on amino acids. Biochem. J. **66**, 237—242 (1957).

AUGUSTINSSON, K. B.: Specificity of cholin esterase in *Helix pomatia*. Biochem. J. **40**, 343—349 (1946).

— Cholinesterases. A study in comparative enzymology. Acta physiol. scand. **15**, suppl. 52 (1948).

— Substrate concentration and specificity of choline ester-splitting enzymes. Arch. Biochem. **23**, 111—126 (1949).

— Hydrolysis of noncholine esters by acetylcholinesterase from human erythrocytes. Acta chem. scand. **4**, 948—956 (1950a).

— Enzymic hydrolysis of triacetin by acetylcholinesterase and its inhibition by various compounds. Acta chem. scand. **4**, 1149—1150 (1950b).

— Comparison between acetylcholinesterase activity of helix blood and cobra venom. I. Hydrolysis of acetylcholine and its inhibition by various compounds. Acta chem. scand. **5**, 699—711 (1951a).

— Comparison between acetylcholinesterase activity of helix blood and cobra venom. II. Hydrolysis of certain choline and noncholine esters. Acta chem. scand. **5**, 712—723 (1951b).

— Acetylcholine esterase and cholinesterase. In: J. B. SUMNER and K. MYRBÄCK, Eds., The Enzymes, vol. I, part 1, 443—472. New York: Academic Press Inc. publishers, 1951c.

Augustinsson, K. B.: Biochemical studies with tabun and allied compounds. Ark. Kemi 6, 331—350 (1953a).
— Mintacol (diethyl p-nitrophenylphosphate). Svensk.farm. T. 57, 261—267 (1953b).
— Assay methods for cholinesterases. In: D. Glick, Ed., Meth. biochem. Anal. 5, 1—63 (1957).
— and M. Grahn: Protection of cholinesterases by procaine against inactivation by tabun in vitro. Acta physiol. scand. 27, 10 (1952).
— and G. Heimbürger: Enzymatic hydrolysis of organophosphorus compounds. II. Analysis of reaction products in experiments with Tabun and some properties of blood plasma tabunase. Acta chem. scand. 8, 762—767 (1954).
— and T. Isacshen: The enzymatic hydrolysis of the β-methyl derivatives of acetylcholine and acetylthiocholine. Acta chem. scand. 11, 750—751 (1957).
— and D. Nachmansohn: Distinction between acetylcholine-esterase and other choline-ester-splitting enzymes. Science 110, 98—99 (1949a).
— — Studies on cholinesterase. VI. Kinetics of the inhibition of acetylcholine esterase. J. biol. Chem. 179, 543—559 (1949b).
Austin, L., and W. K. Berry: Two selective inhibitors of cholinesterase. Biochem. J. 54, 695—701 (1953).
Bain, J. A.: Mechanism of the inhibition of rat brain cholinesterase by diisopropylfluorophosphate, tetraethyl pyrophosphate and eserine. Proc. Soc. exp. Biol. (N. Y.) 72, 9—13 (1949).
Baldridge, D., W. J. McCarville and S. L. Friess: Nature of the acetyl cholinesterase surface. III. Enzymatic response to cis-trans isomers in the cyclohexane series as mapping agents. J. Amer. chem. Soc. 77, 739—741 (1955).
Balls, A. K., and F. L. Aldrich: Acetylchymotrypsin. Proc. nat. Acad. Sci. (Wash.) 41, 190—196 (1955).
— and E. F. Jansen: Stoichiometric inhibition of chymotrypsin. In: F. F. Nord, ed. Advanc. Enzymol. 13, 321—343 (1952).
— and H. N. Wood: Acetylchymotrypsin and its reaction with ethanol. J. biol. Chem. 219, 245—256 (1956).
Barlow, R. B., and H. R. Ing: Curarelike action of polymethylene bis-quaternary ammonium salts. Nature (Lond.) 161, 718 (1948).
Barnard, E. A., and W. D. Stein: The roles of imidazole in biological systems. In: F. E. Nord, ed. Advanc. Enzymol. 20, 51—111 (1958).
Bayliss, B. J., and A. Todrick: The use of a selective acetylcholinesterase inhibitor in the estimation of pseudocholinesterase activity in rat brain. Biochem. J. 62, 62 (1956).
Bender, M. L., and K. C. Kemp: Oxygen-18 studies of the mechanism of the α-chymotrypsin catalyzed hydrolysis of esters. J. Amer. chem. Soc. 79, 111—116 (1957).
— and B. W. Turnquest: The imidazole-catalyzed hydrolysis of p-nitrophenyl acetate. J. Amer. chem. Soc. 79, 1652—1655 (1957a).
— — General basic catalysis of ester hydrolysis and its relationship to enzymatic hydrolysis. J. Amer. chem. Soc. 79, 1656—1662 (1957b).
— F. Chloupek and C. Neveu: Intramolecular catalysis of hydrolytic reactions. III. Intramolecular catalysis of carboxylate ion in the hydrolysis of methyl hydrogen phthalate. J. Amer. chem. Soc. 80, 5384—5387 (1958a).
— Y. L. Chow and F. Chloupek: Intramolecular catalysis of hydrolytic reactions. J. Amer. chem. Soc. 80, 5380—5384 (1958b).
Benoiton, L., H. N. Rydon, R. A. Oosterbaan, M. E. van Adrichem and J. A. Cohen: The structures of some acetyl-serine peptides from acetylchymotrypsin. Nature (Lond.) 187, 596—597 (1960).
Berends, F., C. H. Posthumus, I. van der Sluys and F. A. Deierkauf: The chemical basis of the "Ageing Process" of DFP-inhibited pseudocholinesterase. Biochim. biophys. Acta 34, 576—578 (1959).
Bergmann, F.: Fine structure of the active surface of cholinesterases and the mechanism of enzymic ester hydrolysis. Disc. Faraday Soc. 20, 126—134 (1955).
— S. Rimon and R. Segal: Effect of pH on the activity of eel esterase towards different substrates. Biochem. J. 68, 493—499 (1958).
— and R. Segal: The relationship of quaternary ammonium salts to the anionic sites of true and pseudo cholinesterase. Biochem. J. 58, 692—698 (1954).
— — The characterization of tissue cholinesterase. Biochem. biophys. Acta 16, 513—519 (1955).
— — A. Shimoni and M. Wurzel: The pH-dependence of enzymic ester hydrolysis. Biochem. J. 63, 684—690 (1956).
— and A. Shimoni: Quaternary ammonium salts as inhibitors of acetylcholinesterase. Biochim. biophys. Acta 7, 483—484 (1951).

BERGMANN, F., and A. SHIMONI: Quaternary ammonium salts as inhibitors of acetylcholine esterase. II. The pH dependence of the inhibitory effects of quaternary ammonium salts, and the dissociation constant of the anionic site. Biochim. biophys. Acta 8, 347—348 (1952a).
— — Quaternary ammonium salts as inhibitors of acetylcholinesterase. Biochim. biophys. Acta 8, 520—525 (1952b).
— — Quaternary ammonium salts as inhibitors of acetylcholinesterase. II. pH Dependence of the inhibitory effects, and the dissociation constant of the anionic site. Biochim. biophys. Acta 9, 473—477 (1952c).
— — The enzymic hydrolysis of alkyl fluoroacetates and related compounds. Biochem. J. 55, 50—57 (1953).
— I. B. WILSON and D. NACHMANSOHN: Acetylcholinesterase. IX. Structural features determining the inhibition by amino acids and related compounds. J. biol. Chem. 186, 693 to 703 (1950a).
— — — The inhibitory effect of stilbamidine, curare and related compounds and its relationship to the active groups of acetylcholine esterase action of stilbamidine upon nerve impulse conduction. Biochim. biophys. Acta 6, 217—224 (1950b).
— M. WURZEL and E. SHIMONI: The enzymic hydrolysis of acid anhydrides. Biochem. J. 55, 888—891 (1953a).
— — — Hydrolysis of anhydrides by esterases. Nature (Lond.) 171, 744—745 (1953b).
BERNHARD, S. A.: A simple model of molecular specificity in enzyme-substrate systems. I. Theory and applications to the system acetylcholinesterase-substrate. J. Amer. chem. Soc. 77, 1966—1972 (1955a).
— A simple model of molecular specificity in enzyme-substrate systems. II. The correlation of the Michaelis constant with the inhibition constant. J. Amer. chem. Soc. 77, 1973—1974 (1955b).
— Symposium on enzyme reaction mechanisms, Gatlinburg, Tenn., 1—4 April 1959. J. cell. comp. Physiol. 54, 188—199 (1959).
— and H. GUTFREUND: Ficin-catalyzed reaction: The affinity of ficin for some arginine derivatives. Biochem. J. 63, 61—64 (1956).
BERRY, W. K.: The turnover number of cholinesterase. Biochem. J. 49, 615—620 (1951).
BLUMENTHAL, E., and J. B. M. HERBERT: The mechanism of the hydrolysis of trimethyl orthophosphate. Trans. Faraday Soc. 41, 611—617 (1945).
BODANSKY, O.: Cholinesterase. Ann. N. Y. Acad. Sci. 47, art. 4, 521—547 (1946).
BORKE, M. L., and E. R. KIRCH: A note on chemical constitution and biological activity of some derivatives of thiophosphoric acid. J. Amer. pharm. Ass. 45, 817—818 (1956).
BOTTS, J., and M. MORALES: Analytical description of the effects of modifiers and of enzyme multivalency upon the steady state catalyzed reaction rate. Trans. Faraday Soc. 49, 696—707 (1953).
BOURSNELL, J. C., and E. C. WEBB: Reaction of esterases with radioactive diisopropylfluorophosphate. Nature (Lond.) 164, 875 (1949).
BROUWER, D. M.: The role of the imidazole group in the hydrolytic action of chymotrypsin. Thesis 1957, University of Leyden, The Netherlands.
BRUICE, T. C., and G. L. SCHMIR: The catalysis of the hydrolysis of p-nitrophenyl acetate by imidazole and its derivatives. Arch. Biochem. 63, 484—486 (1956).
— — Imidazole catalysis. I. The catalysis of the hydrolysis of phenyl acetate by imidazole. J. Amer. chem. Soc. 79, 1663—1667 (1957).
BRZIN, M., and A. O. ŽUPANČIČ: The mode of action of tubocurarine. Brit. J. Pharmacol. 11, 428—430 (1956).
BURGEN, A. S. V.: The mechanism of action of anticholinesterase drugs. Brit. J. Pharmacol. 4, 219—228 (1949).
— and F. HOBBIGER: The inhibition of cholinesterases by alkylphosphates and alkyl phenol phosphates. Brit. J. Pharmacol. 6, 592—605 (1951).
CHADWICK, L. E.: Temperature dependence of cholinesterase activity. Influence Temp. Biol. Systems, Paper Symposium, Storrs, Conn. 1956, 45—59 (Pub. 1957).
CHANCE, B.: Biological reactions. Part 1: Reaction kinetics of enzyme-substrate compounds. In: S. L. FRIESS and A. WEISSBERGER, Eds., Techn. Org. Chem. 8, 627—667 (1953).
CHILDS, A. F., D. R. DAVIES, A. L. GREEN and J. P. RUTLAND: The reactivation by oximes and hydroxamic acids of cholinesterase inhibited by organo-phosphorus compounds. Brit. J. Pharmacol. 10, 462—465 (1955).
CLAIRE LAWLER, H.: A simplified procedure for the partial purification of acetylcholinesterase from electric tissue. J. biol. Chem. 234, 799—801 (1958).
COHEN, J. A., F. KALSBEEK and M. G. P. J. WARRINGA: Reversibility of the inhibition of true cholinesterase by physostigmine. Biochim. biophys. Acta 2, 549 (1948).

COHEN, J. A., F. KALSBEEK and M. G. E. J. WARRINGA: The significance of butyrylcholine in the testing of cholinesterase-containing preparations. Acta brev. neerl. Physiol. 17, no 1—4, 32—36 (1949).
— R. A. OOSTERBAAN, H. S. JANSZ and F. BERENDS: The active site of esterases. J. cell. comp. Physiol. 54, 231—244 (1959).
— — and M. G. P. J. WARRINGA: The turnover number of ali-esterase, pseudo- and true cholinesterase and the combination of these enzymes with diisopropylfluorophosphate. Biochim. biophys. Acta 18, 228—235 (1955a).
— — and H. S. JANSZ: The chemical structure of the reactive group of esterases. Disc. Faraday Soc. 20, 114—119 (1955b).
— and M. G. P. J. WARRINGA: Methods to estimate the turnover number of preparations of ox red cell cholinesterase. Biochim. biophys. Acta 11, 52—58 (1953).
— — and B. R. BOVENS: Protection of true cholinesterase against diisopropyl fluorophosphonate by butyrylcholine. Biochim. biophys. Acta 6, 469—476 (1951).
COLLIER, H. B., and P. F. SOLVONUK: Acylation reactions in the presence of acetylcholinesterase of human erythrocytes. Biochim. biophys. Acta 16, 583—588 (1955).
CUNNINGHAM, L. W.: Proposed mechanism of action of hydrolysis enzymes. Science 125, 1145—1146 (1957).
DAVIES, D. R., and A. L. GREEN: The kinetics of reactivation by oximes of cholinesterase inhibited by organophosphorus compounds. Biochem. J. 63, 529—535 (1956).
— — The mechanism of hydrolysis by cholinesterase and related enzymes. In: F. F. NORD, Ed., Advanc. Enzymol. 20, 283—319 (1958).
DAVISON, A. N.: Return of cholinesterase activity in the rat after inhibition by organo phosphorus compounds. 1 diethyl p-nitrophenyl phosphate (E 600, Paraoxon). Biochem. J. 54, 583—590 (1953).
— Return of cholinesterase activity in the rat after inhibition by organophosphorus compounds. Biochem. J. 60, 339—346 (1955).
DEPIERRE, F., et M. A. FUNKE: Anticholinestérasiques. II. Dérivés analogues à la prostigmine. Influence de la structure chimique sur l'intensité et la sélectivité de l'action antiacétylcholinestérasique. C. R. Acad. Sci. (Paris) 239, 370—372 (1954).
DIGGLE, W. M., and J. C. GAGE: Cholinesterase inhibition in vitro by 0-0-diethyl 0-p-nitrophenyl thiophosphate (Parathion, E 605). Biochem. J. 49, 491—494 (1951).
DIXON, G. H., W. J. DREYER and H. NEURATH: The reaction of p-nitrophenyl acetate with chymotrypsin. J. Amer. chem. Soc. 78, 4810 (1956a).
— S. GO and H. NEURATH: Peptides with ¹⁴C-diisopropylphosphoryl following degradation of ¹⁴C-DIP-trypsin with α-chymotrypsin. Biochim. biophys. Acta 19, 193—195 (1956b).
— D. L. KAUFMANN and H. NEURATH: Amino acid sequence in the region of diisopropylphosphoryl binding in DIP-trypsin. J. Amer. chem. Soc. 80, 1260—1261 (1958a).
— — Amino acid sequence in the region of diisopropylphosphoryl binding in diisopropylphosphoryl-trypsin. J. biol. Chem. 233, 1373—1381 (1958b).
— and H. NEURATH: Acylation of the enzymatic sites of chymotrypsin and trypsin. Fed. Proc. 16, 173 (1957a).
— — Acylation of the enzymatic site of Δ-chymotrypsin by esters, acid anhydrides and acid chlorides. J. biol. Chem. 225, 1049—1059 (1957b).
— — An intermediate in the deacylation of mono-acetyl-chymotrypsin having the properties of acetyl imidazolyl. J. Amer. chem. Soc. 79, 4558—4559 (1957c).
— — and J. F. PECHERE: Proteolytic Enzymes. In: J. M. LUCK, Ed. Ann. Rev. Biochem. 27, 489—532 (1958c).
DIXON, M.: The effect of pH on the affinities of enzymes for substrates and inhibitors. Biochem. J. 55, 161—171 (1953).
— and E. C. WEBB: "Enzymes", Longmans, Green and Co., London, New York, Toronto. London and Colchester: Printed by Spottiswoode, Ballantyne and Co. Ltd. 1958.
EDSALL, J. T.: Dipolar ions and acid-base equilibria (chapter 4); Some relations between acidity and chemical structure (chapter 5). In: E. J. COHN and J. T. EDSALL, Eds., Proteins, Amino Acids and Peptides. New York: Reinhold Publ. corp. 1943.
EDWARDS, L. J.: The hydrolysis of aspirin. A determination of the thermodynamic kinetics by ultra-violet spectrophotometry. Trans. Faraday Soc. 46, 723—735 (1950).
— The hydrolysis of aspirin. Part 2. Trans. Faraday Soc. 48, 696—699 (1952).
ENANDER, I.: Experiments with methyl-fluorophosphorylcholine inhibited cholinesterases. Acta chem. scand. 12, 780—781 (1958).
FOLDES, F., G. VAN HEES, D. L. DAVIS and S. P. SHANOR: The structure-action relationship of urethane type cholinesterase inhibitors. J. Pharmacol. 122, 457—464 (1958).
FRAENKEL-CONRAT, H.: The chemistry of proteins and peptides. In: J. M. LUCK, Ed., Ann. Rev. Biochem. 25, 291—330 (1956).

FRIEDENWALD, J. S., and G. D. MAENGWYN-DAVIES: Elementary kinetic theory of enzymatic activity. In: W. D. McELROY and B. GLASS, Eds., The Mechanism of Enzyme Action, 154—191. Baltimore: The John Hopkins Press 1954.

FRIESS, S. L.: The acetylcholinesterase surface. VIII. Further observations on bifunctional inhibition of the enzyme. J. Amer. chem. Soc. 79, 3269—3273 (1957).

— and H. D. BALDRIDGE: Nature of the acetylcholinesterase surface. IV. The control of enzymatic inhibition by basicity in the substitued ethylenediamines. J. Amer. chem. Soc. 78, 199—202 (1956a).

— — The acetylcholinesterase surface. V. Some new competitive inhibitors of moderate strength. J. Amer. chem. Soc. 78, 966—968 (1956b).

— — The acetylcholinesterase surface. VI. Further studies with cyclic isomers as inhibitors and substrates. J. Amer. chem. Soc. 78, 2482—2485 (1956c).

— and W. M. McCARVILLE: Nature of the acetyl cholinesterase surface. I. Some potent competitive inhibitors of the enzyme. J. Amer. chem. Soc. 76, 1363—1367 (1954a).

— — Nature of the acetyl cholinesterase surface. II. The ring effect in enzymatic inhibitors of the substituted ethylenediamine type. J. Amer. chem. Soc. 76, 2260—2261 (1954b).

— A. A. PATCHETT and B. WITKOP: The acethyl cholinesterase surface. VII. Interference with surface binding as reflected by enzymatic response to turicine, betonicine and related heterocycles. J. Amer. chem. Soc. 79, 459—462 (1957).

— E. R. WHITCOMB, B. T. HOGAN and P. A. FRENCH: The action of some diamine optical antipodes on acetylcholinesterase inhibition and on conduction in desheathed bullfrog sciatic nerve. Arch. Biochem. 74, 451—457 (1958).

— I. B. WILSON and E. CABIB: The Mg (II) activation of acetylcholinesterase. J. Amer. chem. Soc. 76, 5156—5157 (1954).

FUKUTO, T. R.: The chemistry and action of organic phosphorus insecticides. In: R. L. METCALF, Ed., Advances in Pest Control Research, vol. I, 147—192. New York: Interscience Publishers, inc. 1957.

— and R. METCALF: Structure and insecticidal activity of some diethyl substituted phenyl phosphates. J. Agr. Food Chem. 4, 930—935 (1956).

FULTON, M. P., and G. A. MOGEY: Some selective inhibitors of true cholinesterase. Brit. J. Pharmacol. 9, 138—144 (1954).

FUNKE, A., J. BAGOT et F. DEPIERRE: Anticholinestérasiques. I. Synthèse de diphénoxyalcanes porteurs d'une ou deux fonctions phénoliques libres. C. R. Acad. Sci. (Paris) 239, 329—331 (1954).

— F. DEPIERRE and M. W. KRUCKER: Exaltation de l'activité anticholinestérasiques des sels d'ammonium quaternaires des phénoxyalcanes par l'introduction de groupements uréthanes. C. R. Acad. Sci. (Paris) 234, 762—764 (1952).

GAGE, J. C.: A cholinesterase inhibitor derived from 0,0-diethyl 0-p-nitrophenyl thiophosphate in vivo. Biochem. J. 54, 426—430 (1953).

GARRETT, E. R.: The kinetics of solvolysis of acyl esters of salicylic acid. J. Amer. chem. Soc. 79, 3401—3408 (1957).

GHOSH, R., and J. F. NEWMAN: A new group of organophosphorus pesticides. Chem. and Ind., 118 (1955).

GLADNER, J. A., and K. LAKI: The activity site of thrombin. J. Amer. chem. Soc. 80, 1263 (1958).

GLICK, D.: The specificity of choline esterase. J. biol. Chem. 130, 527 (1939).

GOLDSTEIN, A.: Mechanism of enzyme-inhibitor-substrate reactions. Cholinesterase-eserine-acetylcholine system. J. gen. Physiol. 27, 529 —580 (1944).

— and R. E. HAMLISCH: Properties and behavior of purified human plasma cholinesterase. IV. Enzymatic destruction of the inhibitor prostigmine and physostigmine. Arch. Biochem. 35, 12—22 (1952).

GRAUERS, S.: The influence pf pH on the enzymic hydrolysis of acethylcholine. Acta chem. scand. 6, 1223—1231 (1952).

GREEN, A. L., and B. SAVILLE: The reaction of oximes with isopropyl methylphosphonofluoridate (sarin). J. chem. Soc. 1956, 3887—3892.

— and H. J. SMITH: The reactivation of cholinesterase inhibited with organophosphorus compounds. 1. Reactivation by 2-oxo-aldoximes. Biochem. J. 68, 28—31 (1958a).

— — The reactivation of cholinesterase inhibited with organophosphorus compounds. 2. Reactivation by pyridinealdoxime methiodides. Biochem. J. 68, 32—35 (1958b).

GREEN, N.: Competition among trypsin inhibitors. J. biol. Chem. 205, 535—551 (1953).

GRÉGOIRE, J., N. LIMOZIN and J. GRÉGOIRE: Activity of cholinesterase. III. Application of the spectrographometric method to the study of the influence of salt concentrations on the affinity of purified cholinesterases for acetylcholine. Bull. Soc. Chim. biol. (Paris) 38, 147—163 (1956).

GUTFREUND, H., and J. M. STURTEVANT: Mechanism of chymotrypsin-catalyzed reactions. Proc. nat. Acad. Sci. (Wash.) **42**, 719—728 (1956a).
— — The mechanism of the reaction of chymotrypsin with p-nitrophenyl acetate. Biochem. J. **63**, 656—661 (1956b).
HALDANE, J. B. S.: The Enzymes. London: Longmans Green 1930.
HAMMETT, L. P.: Physical Organic Chemistry. New York: Mc. Graw-Hill Book Company Inc. 1940.
HAMMOND, B. R., and H. GUTFREUND: The mechanism of ficin-catalysed reactions. Biochem. J. **72**, 349—357 (1959).
HARDEGG, W.: Zur Kinetik der Cholinesterasen-Hemmung durch Prostigmin. Naunyn-Schmiedeberg's Arch. exp. Path. Pharmak. **214**, 540—555 (1952).
— D. BECHINGER and R. DOHRMANN: Importance of Schaefer's equation for our interpretation of the kinetics of cholinesterase. Pflügers Arch. ges. Physiol. **263**, 33—47 (1956).
— and H. SCHAEFER: The kinetics of cholinesterase, with an improvement of the Warburg apparatus. Pflügers Arch. ges. Physiol. **255**, 136—153 (1952).
HARTLEY, B. S.: The site of action of inhibitors of α-chymotrypsin. Biochem. J. **64**, 27 p (1956).
— and B. A. KILBY: Inhibition of chymotrypsin by diethyl p-nitrophenyl phosphate. Nature (Lond.) **166**, 784—785 (1950).
— — The reaction of p-nitrophenyl esters with chymotrypsin and insulin. Biochem. J. **56**, 288—297 (1954).
— and V. MASSEY: The active centre of chymotrypsin. I. Labelling with a fluorescent dye. Biochim. biophys. Acta **21**, 58—70 (1956).
HAWKINS, R. D., and B. MENDEL: Studies on cholinesterase. 6. The selective inhibition of true cholinesterase in vivo. Biochem. J. **44**, 260—264 (1949).
HEILBRONN, E.: pH Dependence of choline esterase activity at various substrate and inhibitor concentrations. Acta chem. scand. 8, 1368—1372 (1954).
HERZFELD, E., and CH. STUMPF: Untersuchungen über die Cholinesterasehemmwirkung der Polymethylen-bis-(n-methyl-carbaminoyl-m-trimethyl-ammoniumphenole). Arch. int. Pharmacodyn. **107**, 33—44 (1956).
HESTRIN, S.: Acylation reactions mediated by purified acetylcholinesterase. J. biol. Chem. **180**, 879—881 (1949).
— Acylation reactions mediated by purified acetylcholinesterase II. Biochim. biophys. Acta **4**, 310—321 (1950).
HEYMANS, C.: Les substances anticholinestérasiques exposés annuels de Biochimie médicale. 12me série 1951. Paris: Masson et Cie.
HOBBIGER, F. W.: Inhibition of cholinesterases by irreversible inhibitors in vitro and in vivo. Brit. J. Pharmacol. **6**, 21—30 (1951).
— The mechanism of anticurare action of certain neostigmine analogues. Brit. J. Pharmacol. **7**, 223—236 (1952).
— The inhibition of cholinesterase by 3-(diethoxyphosphinyloxy)-N-methylquinolinium methylsulphate and its tertiary base. Brit. J. Pharmacol. **9**, 159—165 (1954a).
— Anticholinesterases. A comparison between the in vitro activity and the in vivo action of certain organic phosphates. Chem. and Ind. **1954b**, 1574.
— Effect of nicotinhydroxamic acid methiodide on human plasma cholinesterase inhibited by organophosphates containing a dialkylphosphate group. Brit. J. Pharmacol. **10**, 356—362 (1955).
— Chemical reactivation of phosphorylated human and bovine true cholinesterase. Brit. J. Pharmacol. **11**, 295—303 (1956).
— D. G. O'SULLIVAN and P. W. SADLER: New potent reactivators of acetocholinesterase inhibited by tetraethyl pyrophosphate. Nature (Lond.) **182**, 1498—1499 (1958).
— and P. W. SADLER: Protection by oximes of bispyridinium ions against lethal diisopropyl phosphonofluoridate poisoning. Nature (Lond.) **182**, 1672—1673 (1958).
HOLLAND, W. C., C. E. DUNN and M. E. GREIG: Studies on permeability. VII. Effect of several substrates and inhibitors of acetyl cholinesterase on permeability of isolated auricles to Na and K. Amer. J. Physiol. **168**, 546—556 (1952).
— and R. L. KLEIN: Effects of diazonium salts on erythrocyte fragility and cholinesterase activity. Amer. J. Physiol. **187**, 501—504 (1956).
HOLMSTEDT, B.: Synthesis and pharmacology of dimethylamido-ethoxyphosphoryl cyanide (tabun) together with a description of some allied anticholinesterase compounds containing the N-P bond. Acta physiol. scand. suppl. 90. **25**, 11—120 (1951).
— A modification of the thiocholine method for the determination of cholinesterase. I. Biochemical evaluation of selective inhibitors. Acta physiol. scand. **40**, 322—330 (1957).
— Pharmacology of organophosphorus cholinesterase inhibitors. Pharmacol. Rev. **11**, 567—688 (1959).

HOSKIN, F. C. G., and G. S. TRICK: Stereospecificity in the enzymic hydrolysis of tabun and acetyl-β-methylcholine chloride. Canad. J. Biochem. Physiol. **33**, 940—947 (1955).

HUENNEKENS, F. M.: Biological reactions. Part 1. Measurement and General theory. In: S. L. FRIESS and A. WEISSBERGER, Eds., Techn. Org. Chem. 8, 535—627 (1953).

JACOB, J., and A. FUNKE: Relation between chemical structure and anticholinesterase properties of a group of selective inhibitors of cell acetylcholinesterase of the dog. C. R. Acad. Sci. (Paris) **237**, 1809—1811 (1953).

JANDORF, B. J.: Chemical reactions of nerve gases in neutral solution. I. Reactions with hydroxylamine. J. Amer. chem. Soc. 78, 3686—3691 (1956a).

— Mode of action of pesticides. Mechanism of reaction of di-n-propyl-2, 2-dichlorovinyl phosphate (DDP) with esterases. J. Agr. Food. Chem. 4, 853—858 (1956b).

— E. A. CROWELL and A. P. LEVIN: Role of hydroxamic acids in prevention and reversal of cholinesterase inactivation by DFP and sarin. Fed. Proc. **14**, 231 (1955a).

— H. O. MICHEL, N. K. SCHAFFER, R. EGAN and W. H. SUMMERSON: The mechanism of reaction between esterases and phosphorus-containing anti-esterases. Disc. Faraday Soc. 20, 134—142 (1955b).

JANSEN, E. F., and A. K. BALLS: The inhibition of β and γ chymotrypsin and trypsin by diisopropyl fluorophosphate. J. biol. Chem. **194**, 721—727 (1952).

— A. L. CURL and A. K. BALLS: Reaction of α-chymotrypsin with analogues of diisopropyl fluorophosphate. J. biol. Chem. 190, 557—562 (1951).

— M. D. FELLOWS NUTTING and A. K. BALLS: Mode of inhibition of chymotrypsin by diisopropylfluorophosphate. I. Introduction of phosphorus. J. biol. Chem. **179**, 201—204 (1949).

— — R. JANG and A. K. BALLS: Mode of inhibition of chymotrypsin by diisopropylfluorophosphate. II. Introduction of isopropyl and elimination of fluorine as hydrogen fluoride. J. biol. Chem. 185, 209—220 (1950).

— R. JANG and A. K. BALLS: The inhibition of purified, human plasma cholinesterase with diisopropyl fluorophosphate. J. biol. Chem. **196**, 247—253 (1952).

JANSZ, H. S., D. BRONS and M. G. P. J. WARRINGA: Chemical nature of the DFP-binding site of pseudocholinesterase. Biochim. biophys. Acta 34, 573—575 (1959a).

— C. H. POSTHUMUS and J. A. COHEN: On the active site of horse liver ali esterase. I. The reaction of the enzyme with diisopropylphosphorofluoridate. Biochim. biophys. Acta **33**, 387—395 (1959b).

— — — On the active site of horse liver ali esterase. II. Amino acid sequence in the DFP binding site of enzyme. Biochim. biophys. Acta 33, 396—403 (1959c).

KIMURA, K. K., C. UMRA and C. C. PFEIFFER: Diatropine derivatives as proof that d-tubocurarine is a blocking moiety containing twin atropine-acetylcholine prosthetic groups. J. Pharmacol. **95**, 149—154 (1949).

KOBLICK, D. C.: An enzymatic ion exchange model for active sodium transport. J. gen. physiol. **42**, 635—645 (1959).

KOELLE, G. B.: Protection of cholinesterase against irreversible inactivation by diisopropyl fluorophosphate in vitro. J. Pharmacol. 88, 232—237 (1946).

— The histochemical differentiation of types of cholinesterases and their localizations in tissues of the cat. J. Pharmacol. 100, 158—179 (1950).

— and J. S. FRIEDENWALD: A histochemical method for localizing cholinesterase activity. Proc. Soc. exp. Biol. (N. Y.) 70, 617—622 (1949).

— and A. GILMAN: Anticholinesterase drugs. Pharmacol. Rev. 1, 166—216 (1949).

KOLBEZEN, M. J., R. L. METCALF and T. R. FUKUTO: Insecticidal activity of carbamate cholinesterase inhibitors. J. Agr. Food Chem. 2, 864—870 (1954).

KOSHLAND, D. E., and M. J. ERWIN: Enzyme catalysis and enzyme specificity-combination of amino acids at the active site of phosphoglucomutase. J. Amer. chem. Soc. 79, 2657 to 2658 (1957).

— W. J. RAY and M. J. ERWIN: Protein structure and enzyme action. Fed. Proc. 17, 1145 to 1150 (1958).

KRAUPP, O., CH. STUMPF, E. HERZFELD and B. PILLAT: Pharmakologische Eigenschaften einiger langwirksamer Cholinesterase-Hemmkörper aus der Reihe der Polymethylen-bis-(carbaminoyl-m-trimethylammoniumphenole). Arch. int. Pharmacodyn. 102, 281—303 (1955).

LAIDLER, K.: Some kinetic and mechanistic aspects of hydrolytic enzyme action. Disc. Faraday Soc. 20, 83—96 (1955a).

LAIDLER, K. I.: The influence of pH on the rate of enzyme reactions. Trans. Faraday Soc. 51, part 1: 528—539, part 2: 540—550, part 3: 550—561 (1955b).

— The influence of pH on the rates of enzyme reactions. Part 3: Analysis of experimental results for various enzyme systems. Trans. Faraday Soc. 51, 550—561 (1955c).

LARSSON, L.: A spectrophotometric study in the infra-red of the hydrolysis of dimethyl amidoethoxyphosphoryl cyanide (tabun). Acta chem. scand. 6, 1470—1476 (1952).

LEVIN, A. P., and B. J. JANDORF: Inactivation of cholinesterase by compounds related to neostigmine. J. Pharmacol. **113**, 206—211 (1955).

LOEWENSTEIN, R. W., and D. MOLINS: Cholinesterase in a receptor. Science **128**, 1284 (1958).

MACKWORTH, J. F., and E. C. WEBB: Inhibition of serum cholinesterase by alkyl fluophosphates. Biochem. J. **42**, 91—95 (1948).

MARINI, M. A., and G. P. HESS: Reactivity and interrelationship of intermediates in the hydrolysis of p-nitrophenyl acetate catalysed by chymotrypsin. Nature (Lond.) **184**, 113 to 114 (1959).

MARTIN, C. J., J. GOLUBOW and A. E. AXELROD: A rapid and sensitive spectrophotometric method for the assay of chymotrypsin. J. biol. Chem. **234**, 204—298 (1959).

MASSEY, V., W. F. HARRINGTON and B. S. HARTLEY: Certain physical properties of chymotrypsin and chymotrypsinogen using the depolarization of fluorescence technique. Disc. Faraday Soc. **20**, 24—32 (1955).

— and B. S. HARTLEY: The active centre of chymotrypsin; Reaction with dinitrofluorobenzene. Biochim. biophys. Acta **21**, 361—367 (1956).

MASTERSON, D. S., and S. L. FRIESS: The acetylcholinesterase surface. IX. Dependence of competitive inhibition by diaminocyclohexane derivatives on substrate level. J. Amer. chem. Soc. **80**, 5687—5689 (1958).

MAZUR, A., and O. BODANSKY: The mechanism of in vitro and in vivo inhibition of cholinesterase activity by diisopropylfluorophosphate. J. biol. Chem. **163**, 261—276 (1946).

McNAUGHTON, R. A., and E. A. ZELLER: On the specificity and differentiation of cholinesterases. Proc. Soc. exp. Biol. (N. Y.) **70**, 165—167 (1949).

MEER, C. VAN DER: Effect of calcium chloride on choline esterase. Nature (Lond.) **171**, 78—79 (1953).

MENDEL, B., and H. RUDNEY: Effect of salts on true cholinesterase. Science **102**, 616—617 (1945).

MICHEL, H. O.: Reaction of diisopropylfluorophosphate (DFP) with red blood cell cholinesterase. Fed. Proc. **11**, 259 (1952).

— Kinetics of the reactions of cholinesterase chymotrypsin and trypsin with organophosphorus inactivators. Fed. Proc. **14**, 255 (1955).

— Development of resistance of alkyl-phosphorylated cholinesterase to reactivation by oximes. Fed. Proc. **17**, 275 (1958).

— and S. KROP: The reaction of cholinesterase with diisopropylfluorophosphate. J. biol. Chem. **190**, 119—125 (1951).

MITCHELL, P., and J. MOYLE: Group-translocation: A consequence of enzyme-catalyzed group-transfer. Nature (Lond.) **182**, 372—373 (1958).

MORALES, F.: If an enzyme-substrate modifier system exhibits non-competitive interaction, then, in general, its Michaelis constant is an equilibrium constant. J. Amer. chem. Soc. **77**, 4169—4170 (1955).

MORAWETZ, H., and I. ORESKES: Intramolecular bifunctional catalysis of ester hydrolysis. J. Amer. chem. Soc. **80**, 2591—2592 (1958).

MOUNTER, L. A.: The specificity of cobra venom cholinesterase. Biochem. J. **50**, 122—128 **54**, 551—559 (1953).

— H. C. ALEXANDER, K. D. TUCK and L. T. H. DIEN: The pH dependence and dissociation constants of esterases and proteases treated with diisopropylfluorophosphate. J. biol. Chem. **226**, 867—872 (1957a).

— — — — The reactivity of esterases and proteases in the presence of organo-phosphorus compounds. J. biol. Chem. **226**, 873—879 (1957b).

— and V. P. WHITTAKER: The esterases of horse blood. 2. The specificity of horse erythrocyte cholinesterase. Biochem. J. **47**, 525—530 (1950).

— — The hydrolysis of esters of phenol by cholinesterases and other esterases. Biochem. J. (1951).

MURRAY, D. R. P.: Inhibition of esterases by excess substrate. Biochem. J. **24**, 1890—1898 (1930).

MYERS, D. K.: Effect of electrolytes on cholinesterase inhibition. Arch. Biochem. **27**, 341—347 (1950).

— Differentiation of three types of competitive cholinesterase inhibitors. Arch. Biochem. **31**, 29—40 (1951).

— Studies on cholinesterase. 7. Determination of the molar concentration of pseudo-cholinesterase in serum. Biochem. J. **51**, 303—311 (1952a).

— Studies on cholinesterase. 8. Determination of reaction velocity constants with a reversible inhibitor of pseudo-cholinesterase. Biochem. J. **52**, 46—53 (1952b).

— Effect of salt on the hydrolysis of acetylcholine by cholinesterases. Arch. Biochem. **37**, 469—487 (1952c).

MYERS, D. K.: Cholinesterase. IX. Species variation in the specificity pattern of the pseudocholinesterases. Biochem. J. 55, 67—79 (1953).
— Studies on selective esterase inhibitors. Thesis, Amsterdam 1954.
— Cholinesterase. X. Return of cholinesterase activity in the rat after inhibition by carbamoyl fluorides. Biochem. J. 62, 556—563 (1956).
— and A. KEMP: Inhibition of esterases by the fluorides of organic acids. Nature (Lond.) 173, 33—34 (1954).
— and B. MENDEL: Investigation on the use of eserine for the differentiation of mammalian esterases. Proc. Soc. exp. Biol. (N. Y.) 71, 357—360 (1949).
NACHMANSOHN, D.: Action of ions on choline esterase. Nature (Lond.) 145, 513—514 (1940).
— and M. A. ROTHENBERG: Specificity of cholinesterase in nervous tissue. Science 100, 454 to 455 (1944).
— — Cholinesterase. I. The specificity of the enzyme in nerve tissue. J. biol. Chem. 158, 653—666 (1945).
— — and E. A. FELD: The in vitro reversibility of cholinesterase inhibition by diisopropyl-fluophosphate (DFP). Arch. Biochem. 14, 197—211 (1947).
— — — Studies on cholinesterase. V. Kinetics of the enzyme inhibition. J. biol. Chem. 174, 247—256 (1948).
— and I. B. WILSON: The enzymic hydrolysis and synthesis of acetylcholine. In: F. F. NORD, Ed., Advanc. Enzymol. 12, 259—339 (1951).
NEURATH, H., G. H. DIXON and J. F. PECHÈRE: Certain aspects of the structure and active sites of α-chymotrypsin and trypsin. In: Symposium on Proteins, IVth Intern. Congress of Biochemistry, Vienna. London: Pergamon Press Ltd. 1958.
OOSTERBAAN, R. A., and M. E. VAN ADRICHEM: Isolation of acetyl peptides from acetyl-chymotrypsin. Biochim. biophys. Acta 27, 423—425 (1958).
— H. S. JANSZ and J. A. COHEN: The chemical structure of the reactive group of esterases. Biochim. biophys. Acta 20, 402—403 (1956).
— P. KUNST, J. VAN ROTTERDAM and J. A. COHEN: The reaction of chymotrypsin and diisopropylphosphorofluoridate. Isolation and analysis of diisopropylphosphorylpeptides. Biochim. biophys. Acta 27, 549—555 (1958a).
— — — — The reaction of chymotrypsin and diisopropylphosphorofluoridate. The structure of two DP-substitutes peptides from chymotrypsin-DP. Biochim. biophys. Acta 27, 556 to 563 (1958b).
PFEIFFER, C. C.: Nature and spatial relationship of the prosthetic chemical groups required for maximal muscarinic action. Science 107, 94—96 (1948).
PORTER, G. R., H. N. RYDON and J. A. SCHOFIELD: Nature of the reactive serine residue in enzymes inhibited by organophosphorus compounds. Nature (Lond.) 182, 927 (1958).
PULVER, R., and R. DOMENJOZ: The specificity of esterase inhibitors. Experientia (Basel) 7, 306—307 (1951).
RANDALL, L. O.: Anticurare action of phenolic quaternary ammonium salts. J. Pharmacol. 100, 83—93 (1950).
— Synthetic curarelike agents on their antagonists. Ann. N. Y. Acad. Sci. 54, 460—479 (1951).
— and G. LEHMANN: Pharmacological properties of some neostigmine analogs. J. Pharmacol. 99, 16—32 (1950).
RIKER, W. F., jr.: Excitatory and anti-curare properties of acetylcholine and related quaternary ammonium compounds at the neuromuscular junction. In: L. S. GOODMAN, Ed., Pharmacol. Rev. 5, no. 1, 1—86 (1953).
RILEY, G., J. H. TURNBULL and W. WILSON: O. phosphoryl serine derivatives. Chem. and Ind. 1953, 1181.
ROTHENBERG, M. A., and D. NACHMANSOHN: Cholinesterase. III. Purification of the enzyme from electric tissue by fractional ammonium sulfate precipitation. J. biol. Chem. 168, 223—231 (1947).
RYDON, H. N.: A possible mechanism of action of esterases inhibitable by organo-phosphorus compounds. Nature (Lond.) 182, 928—929 (1958).
SAUNDERS, B. C.: Phosphorus and fluorine. The chemistry and toxic action of their organic compounds. Cambridge: University Press 1957.
SCHAEFER, H.: The properties of cholinesterase in normal blood. Pflügers Arch. ges. Physiol. 249, 405—430 (1947).
—, and E. MAIER: Critique and procedure for cholinesterase determinations in blood. Biochem. Z. 319, 420—438 (1949).
SCHAFFER, N. K., R. R. ENGLE, L. SIMET and R. W. DRISKO: Phosphopeptides from chymotrypsin and trypsin after inactivation by ^{32}P labeled DFP and sarin. Fed. Proc. 15, 347 (1956).

SCHAFFER, N. K., R. P. LANG, L. SIMET and R. W. DRISKO: Phosphopeptides from acid-hydrolyzed ^{32}P labeled isopropyl methylphosphonofluoridate-inactivated trypsin. J. biol. Chem. 230, 185—192 (1958).
— C. S. MAY and W. H. SUMMERSON: Serine phosphoric acid from diisopropylphosphoryl chymotrypsin. J. biol. Chem. 202, 67—76 (1953).
— — — Serine phosphoric acid from diisopropylphosphoryl derivative of eel cholinesterase. J. biol. Chem. 206, 201—207 (1954).
— L. SIMET, S. HARSHMAN, R. R. ENGLE and R. W. DRISKO: Phosphopeptides from acid-hydrolyzed ^{32}P labelled diisopropylphosphoryl chymotrypsin. J. biol. Chem. 225, 197—206 (1957).
SCHONBAUM, G. R., K. NAKAMURA and M. L. BENDER: Direct spectrophotometric evidence for an acyl-enzyme intermediate in the chymotrypsin-catalyzed hydrolysis of 0-nitrophenyl cinnamate. J. Amer. chem. Soc. 81, 4746—4747 (1959).
SCHRADER, G.: Die Entwicklung neuer Insektizide auf Grundlage von organischen Fluor- und Phosphorverbindungen. Monographie no. 2, 2. Aufl. Weinheim: Verlag Chemie 1952.
SERLIN, I., and D. J. FLUKE: The size and shape of the radiosensitive acetylcholinesterase unit. J. biol. Chem. 223, 727—736 (1956).
SHUKUYA, R.: Mechanism of action of cholinesterase. I. Differences in pS-activity curves of cholinesterases of human erythrocytes and serum. J. Japan. biochem. Soc. 23, 129—133 (1951a).
— Kinetics of human blood cholinesterase. J. Biochem. (Tokyo) 38, 225—236 (1951b).
— Kinetics of human blood cholinesterase. II. The temperature effect upon cholinesterase activity. J. Biochem. (Tokyo) 40, 135—140 (1953).
—, and M. SHINODA: Kinetics of the human blood cholinesterase. V. The inhibition of acetylcholinesterase and cholinesterase by hydrogen ion and tetraethylammonium bromide. J. Biochem. (Tokyo) 43, 315—326 (1956).
SMITH, C. M., H. L. COHEN, E. W. PELIKAN and K. R. UNNA: Mode of action of antagonists to curare. J. Pharmacol. 105, 391—399 (1952).
SMITH, E. L.: Active site of papain and covalent "high-energy" bonds of proteins. J. biol. Chem. 233, 1392—1397 (1958).
—, and M. J. PARKER: Kinetics of papain action. III. Hydrolysis of benzoyl-1-arginine ethyl ester. J. biol. Chem. 233, 1387—1391 (1958).
SNELLMAN, O.: A peptide material from myosin containing sulfhydryl groups. Acta chem. scand. 12, 503—510 (1958).
SÖRM, F., and I. RYCHLIK: Enzyme activity of dinitro derivatives of α-chymotrypsin. Chem. listy 46, 465—468 (1952).
SPENCER, T., and J. M. STURTEVANT: The mechanism of chymotrypsin-catalyzed reactions. III. J. Amer. chem. Soc. 81, 1874—1882 (1959).
SPRINSON, D. B., and D. RITTENBERG: Nature of the activation process in enzymatic reactions. Nature (Lond.) 167, 484 (1951).
STEIN, S. S., and D. E. KOSHLAND: Mechanism of hydrolysis of acetylcholine catalyzed by acetylcholinesterase and by hydroxide ion. Arch. Biochem. 45, 467—468 (1953).
STEIN, W. D.: N terminal histidine at the active centre of a permeability mechanism. Nature (Lond.) 181, 1662—1663 (1958).
STRAUS, O. H., and A. GOLDSTEIN: Zone behavior of enzymes. Illustrated by the effect of dissociation constant and dilution on the system cholinesterase-physostigmine. J. gen. Physiol. 26, 559—585 (1943).
SWIDLER, R., and G. M. STEINBERG: The kinetics of isopropyl methylphosphonofluoridate (Sarin) with benzohydroxamic acid. J. Amer. chem. Soc. 78, 3594—3598 (1956).
TAKAGI, H.: The relation between the action of various drugs and the activity of specific cholinesterase in the brain. II. Protection of the cholinesterase activity from cholinesterase inhibitors by anticholinergic drugs. Folia pharmacol. jap. 49, 89—95 (1953).
TAMMELIN, L. E.: Methyl-fluoro-phosphorylcholines. Acta chem. scand. 11, 859—865 (1957a).
— Dialkoxy-phosphorylthiocholines. Alkoxymethyl-phosphoryl-thiocholines and analogous choline esters. Acta chem. scand. 11, 1340—1349 (1957b).
— Isomerisation of ω-dimethylamino-ethyldiethyl thionophosphate. Acta chem. scand. 11, 1738—1744 (1957c).
— Choline esters. Substrates and inhibitors of cholinesterases. Svenska Kemi. Tidskr. 70, 157—181 (1958a).
— Organophosphorylcholines and cholinesterases. Ark. Kemi 12, 287—298 (1958b).
TODRICK, A.: The inhibition of cholinesterases by antagonists of acetylcholine and histamine. Brit. J. Pharmacol. 9, 76—83 (1954).
TRÉFOUËL, J.: Exaltation de l'activité anticholinestérasique des sels d'ammonium quaternaires des phénoxyalcanes par l'introduction de groupements uréthanes. C. R. Acad. Sci. (Paris) 234, 762—764 (1952).

Turba, F., and G. Gundlach: Aminosäure-sequenz in der Umgebung des reaktiven Serin-restes im Chymotrypsin-Molekül. Biochem. Z. **327**, 186—188 (1955).

Underhay, E. E.: The hydrolysis of indoxyl esters by esterases of human blood. Biochem. J. **66**, 383—390 (1957).

Viswanatha, T., and I. E. Liener: The peptic activation of acetyltrypsinogen. Physico-chemical properties of the active derivative. Biochim. biophys. Acta **37**, 389 (1960).

Waley, S. G.: Some aspects of the kinetics of enzymic reactions. Biochim. biophys. Acta **10**, 27—34 (1953).

Weil, L., S. James and A. R. Buchert: Photo-oxidation of crystalline chymotrypsin in the presence of methylene blue. Arch. Biochem. **46**, 266—278 (1953).

Wescoe, W. C., W. F. Riker and W. L. Beach: Studies on the interrelationships of certain cholinergic compounds. III. The reactions between 3-acetoxy phenyl-trimethylammonium methylsulfate, 3-hydroxy phenyltrimethylammonium bromide and cholinesterases. J. Pharmacol. **99**, 265—276 (1950).

Westheimer, F. H.: Hypothesis for the mechanism of action of chymotrypsin. Proc. nat. Acad. Sci. (Wash.) **43**, 969—975 (1957).

Whitaker, J. R., and B. J. Jandorf: Specific reactions of dinitrofluorobenzene with active groups of chymotrypsin. J. biol. Chem. **223**, 751—764 (1956).

Whittaker, V. P.: The specificity of pigeon-brain cholinesterase. Biochem. J. **44**, proc. 46 (1949).

— Specificity, mode of action and distribution of cholinesterases. Physiol. Rev. **31**, 312—343 (1951).

— The specificity of pigeon-brain cholinesterase. Biochem. J. **54**, 660—664 (1953).

— In Progress in Stereochemistry, p. 317—318. Ed. Klyne. London: Butterworths.

Wilson, I. B.: Mechanism of enzymic hydrolysis. I. Role of the acidic group in the esteratic site of acetylcholinesterase. Biochim. biophys. Acta **7**, 466—470 (1951a).

— Mechanism of hydrolysis. II. New evidence for an acylated enzyme as intermediate. Biochim. biophys. Acta **7**, 520—525 (1951b).

— Acetylcholinesterase. XI. Reversibility of tetraethyl pyrophosphate inhibition. J. biol. Chem. **190**, 111—117 (1951c).

— Acetylcholinesterase. The mechanism of enzymic activity. Baskerville chem. J. City Coll. N. Y. **3**, no. 1, 7—12 (1952a).

— Acetylcholinesterase. XII. Further studies of binding forces. J. biol. Chem. **197**, 215—225 (1952b).

— Acetylcholinesterase. XIII. Reactivation of alkyl phosphate-inhibited enzyme. J. biol. Chem. **199**, 113—120 (1952c).

— The mechanism of enzyme hydrolysis studied with acetylcholinesterase. In: W. D. McElroy and B. Glass, Eds., The Mechanism of Enzyme Action, 642—657. Baltimore: The John Hopkins Press 1954.

— Promotion of acetylcholinesterase activity by the anionic site. Disc. Faraday Soc. **20**, 119—125 (1955a).

— The interaction of tensilon and neostigmine with acetylcholinesterase. Arch. int. Pharmacodyn. **104**, 204—213 (1955b).

— Molecular complementarity and antidotes for alkylphosphate poisoning. Fed. Proc. **18**, 752—758 (1959).

—, and F. Bergmann: Studies on cholinesterase. VII. The active surface of acetylcholine esterase derived from effects of pH on inhibitors. J. biol. Chem. **185**, 479—489 (1950a).

— — Acetylcholinesterase. VIII. Dissociation constants of the active groups. J. biol. Chem. **186**, 683—692 (1950b).

— — and D. Nachmansohn: Acetylcholinesterase. X. Mechanism of the catalysis of acylation reactions. J. biol. Chem. **186**, 781—790 (1950).

—, and E. Cabib: Is acetylcholinesterase a metallo enzyme? J. Amer. chem. Soc. **76**, 5154 to 5156 (1954).

— — Acetylcholinesterase: Enthalpies and entropies of activation. J. Amer. chem. Soc. **78**, 202—207 (1956).

—, and M. Cohen: The essentiality of acetylcholinesterase in conduction. Biochim. biophys. Acta **11**, 147—156 (1953).

—, and S. Ginsburg: A powerful reactivator of alkylphosphate-inhibited acetylcholinesterase. Biochim. biophys. Acta **18**, 168—170 (1955a).

— — Reactivation of acetylcholinesterase inhibited by alkylphosphates. Arch. Biochem. **54**, 569—571 (1955b).

— — and E. K. Meislich: The reactivation of acetylcholinesterase inhibited by tetraethyl pyrophosphate and diisopropylfluorophosphate. J. Amer. chem. Soc. **77**, 4286—4291 (1955).

— — and C. Quan: Molecular complementariness as basis for reactivation of alkyl phosphate-inhibited enzyme. Arch. Biochem. **77**, 286—296 (1958).

WILSON, I. B., and E. K. MEISLICH: Reactivation of acetylcholinesterase inhibited by alkyl-phosphates. J. Amer. chem. Soc. 75, 4628—4629 (1953).
—, and C. QUAN: Acetylcholinesterase studies on molecular complementariness. Arch. Biochem. 73, 131—143 (1958).
WOOD, H. N., and A. K. BALLS: Enzymatic oxidation of α-chymotrypsin. J. biol. Chem. 213, 297—304 (1955).
ZELLER, E. A.: Enzymes of snake venoms and their biological significance. In: F. F. NORD, Ed., Advanc. Enzymol. 20, 283—318 (1958).
——, and A. BISSEGER: Influence of drugs and chemotherapy on enzyme reactions. III. Cholinesterases of brain and erythrocytes. Helv. chim. acta 26, 1619—1630 (1943).
— F. A. FLEISHER, R. A. McNAUGHTON and J. S. SCHWEPPE: New substrates for cholinesterase. Proc. Soc. exp. Biol. (N. Y.) 71, 526—529 (1949).
ZIMMERING, P. E., E. W. WESTHEAD jr., and H. MORAWETZ: Hydrolytic enzyme models. I. Effect of neighboring carboxyl on the reactivity of ester and anilide groups. Biochim. biophys. Acta 25, 376—381 (1957).
ŽUPANČIČ, A. O.: The mode of action of acetylcholine. A theory extended to a hypothesis on the mode of action of other biologically active substances. Acta physiol. scand. 29, 63—71 (1953).

Chapter 8

Structure-Activity Relationships of the Reversible Anticholinesterase Agents*

By

J. P. LONG

Contents

Introduction

Since the classical work of CRUM-BROWN and FRAZIER nearly one hundred years ago, which demonstrated that relatively simple alterations in chemical structure could modify substantially the pharmacological properties of alkaloids, interest in Structure-Activity Relationships (SAR) has been ever increasing. Never before has the chemically oriented biologist had such a formidable list of com-

---

* This work was aided by a grant from the United States Public Health Service (RG B-1396).

pounds to consider. In association with any given pharmacological action, there are many compounds which obviously have similar structures, but there are also many where chemical similarities are not so apparent. On the basis of what have appeared to be "similar" chemical compounds, many of the SAR advances have occurred in autonomic pharmacology. The approach that has been used with cholinesterase inhibitors has certainly yielded many active compounds, with the net result of advancement in both therapeutic application and our understanding of drug-enzyme interaction. If workers concerned had not used the principles of SAR in their design of drugs, progress which resulted would probably have been considerably less.

However there are certain limitations always present in any discussion of SAR—whether it be with respect to cholinesterase inhibitors or any other class of agents. The following limitations may be present and are often ignored in biological testing, especially when general conclusions are drawn from the work: (1) The problem of whether two compounds are acting by the same mechanism. Unless there is evidence that this is so, little constructive information can be drawn from any SAR comparison. (2) Altered physiological response following administration of a compound is usually interpreted as a measurement of drug-receptor interaction. However, one compound may readily reach the site of action, whereas another compound may reach the site of action in lower concentrations (i.e., it may be bound to plasma proteins, have difficulty in penetration of membranes, etc.). The interpretation from an SAR viewpoint in such cases could be erroneous. (3) Very few of the experiments have incorporated statistical design. Any discussions of SAR based on apparent differences in activity can also be very misleading. (4) Discussion of SAR on the basis of data collected by various investigators in separate laboratories is subject to considerable error. Consideration of the I_{50} values presented by various workers for physostigmine or neostigmine will illustrate this point.

Since no one has ever characterized a receptor chemically or defined a drug-receptor interaction in such terms, one or more of the above limitations of SAR can be raised for each study. At best, every SAR worker can offer only evidence that these objections may or may not be valid. The following principles are offered as lines of evidence only and should not be regarded as criteria of proof.

If the compounds are obviously chemical analogs (as in a homologous series), they probably possess similar pharmacological actions. Of course, one notable exception is the huge field of biological antagonists, but even here the evidence is that at least some of the points on the receptor are the same as for the normal substrate. As far as autonomic agents are concerned, homologous series usually represent agents that vary quantitatively and not qualitatively. Another check that should be included in biological evaluation is the activities of the compounds *in vivo* as compared with those *in vitro*. If the same relative activity holds in these two types of tests, this is suggestive of similar mechanisms, and also serves as a check of the possibility of variations in their ability to reach the site of action. Another very useful check when using reversible agents is to compare the activities against a reversible antagonist. With proper experimental design and incorporation of various test objects one can obtain suggestive evidence that the SAR comparisons are valid.

The text of this chapter discusses the "reversible inhibitors of cholinesterase." Unfortunately, only a few workers have made any attempt to elucidate the type of inhibition involved. Various tests for competitive inhibition (LINEWEAVER and BURK 1934; GOLDSTEIN 1944) have been described and should be applied to at least key members of a given series. This can provide good evidence that at least some of the points for substrate interaction of the enzyme surface are the same for inhibitor and substrate.

For competitive inhibition of an enzyme, fulfillment of at least two requirements would be expected. First, the geometry of the inhibiting molecule would be expected to be complementary with that of the surface of the enzyme. This probably would not necessarily apply to the entire drug molecule, but the geometry of the molecule must be such that there will be no interference with the approach of the functional groups in the molecule to the reactive sites on the receptor surface. This is probably the reason for quantitative differences often seen with geometrical isomers, and even more with stereoisomers. In this case we have paired compounds that have the same physical and chemical properties (other than the rotation of polarized light), hence the most likely explanation for differences in biological activity is due to spatial aspects. This is probably as good evidence as there is for drug-receptor interactions, as well as evidence for at least three-point attachment on the receptor surface (BECKETT 1956; LONG et al. 1956). The second requirement expected to be fulfilled for competitive inhibition is that the inhibiting molecule possesses opposite (but not necessarily equal) charges to that of the receptor. The spacing of the charges on the inhibiting molecule would be expected to be a close approximation to the interatomic spacings of the points for attachment on the receptor surface. However this does not mean that one can necessarily measure interatomic distances on the inhibitor and have a space model of the receptor. If the substrate attaches at two or more points on the receptor, and simultaneous association at both points is essential for activity, the inhibitor could produce inhibition by combining with only one point on the receptor that is essential for substrate attachment, and some site where the substrate does not attach. At any rate both geometrical and charge requirements must be met before a compound can act as a competitive inhibitor.

Another nebulous area that can be considered in an SAR approach is what type(s) of bonding takes place when there is a drug-receptor interaction. Several types of bonding between two chemical compounds are well known. As far as the reversible inhibitors are concerned the types of polar (electrostatic) bonds in order of decreasing strength are as follows: ion-ion > ion-dipole > dipole-dipole > Van der Waal's forces = induced dipole-induced dipole. These are the basic types of bonding that are undoubtedly involved in certain drug-receptor interaction. Also there is the problem of orienting a molecule (lining up the opposite charges on molecule and receptor) so that an interaction can occur. This probably involves the stronger and more "long range" forces. If the geometries of the inhibitor and receptor are highly complementary, then short range forces such as Van der Waal's and induced dipole-induced dipole probably contribute much to the total association energy of the complex.

Little attention has been given to the resulting complex following drug-receptor interaction. Does a molecule (such as neostigmine) produce inhibition by "removing" or altering charges on the enzyme surface, and thus directly or indirectly prevent normal substrate activity? Another possible mechanism for competitive inhibition may involve the close association (but not neutralization of charges) of the drug and enzyme. This would tend to shield the receptor surface from the normal substrate. Whatever the mechanism by which the competitive inhibitors act, there are certainly many chemical similarities within a homologous series. At least from an SAR point of view, a molecule can react only with another molecule, or ion, and it is certain that parts of each molecule combine or associate with other molecules.

A. Terminology and abbreviations

The terminology in this area is often confusing and the meaning of terms used by some authors is not clear. Following is the list of abbreviations that will be used in this chapter.

Abbreviation	Definition
SAR	Structure-Activity Relationship
ACh	Acetylcholine
ChE	Cholinesterase
AChE	Acetylcholinesterase (aceto-, true-, specific, or e-type cholinesterase)
BuChE	Butyrocholinesterase, used synonymously with pseudo, non-specific, or S-type cholinesterase
anti-ChE	Anticholinesterase
pI_{50}	Negative logarithm of the molar concentration needed to produce 50% inhibition of cholinesterase
I_{50}	Molar concentration for 50% inhibition

The material in this chapter is presented primarily in tabular form. In general, the structures, activities on various cholinesterases, and references to authors will be shown. The classification of compounds will be based on either similarity of chemical structures or similarity of pharmacological properties.

B. Physostigmine and related alkaloids

JOBST and HESSE nearly one hundred years ago unknowingly began the study of the field of reversible cholinesterase inhibitors with the isolation of physostigmine (eserine) (HENRY 1949). The suggestion was not made for many years that the action of physostigmine on the heart was due to inhibition of acetylcholine (ACh)-destruction by an esterase normally present in the tissues. ENGELHART and LOEWI (1930) and MATTHES (1930) demonstrated that the inactivation of acetylcholine was largely enzymic in character, and that physostigmine was highly specific in its ability to inhibit the enzyme. Following the original observations cited above, that physostigmine was highly active in inhibiting cholinesterase, this compound was used by many investigators as a reference standard when evaluating new cholinesterase inhibitors. Most workers have found that physostigmine is almost equally effective for acetylcholinesterase (AChE) and nonspecific cholinesterase or butyrocholinesterase (BuChE) (for example see BODANSKY 1946 and AUGUSTINSSON and NACHMANSOHN 1949). The molar concentration required for 50% inhibition of either type of cholinesterase usually has been reported to vary between 10^{-6} and 10^{-8} M. Apparently most, if not nearly all, of the peripheral pharmacological properties reported for this compound are due to the inhibition of cholinesterase. The action of physostigmine on the central nervous system appears to be very complex.

Although many alkaloids (HENRY 1949) other than physostigmine have been isolated from the Calabar bean, apparently they have not been investigated for anticholinesterase (anti-ChE) activity. The decomposition products of physostigmine are shown below.

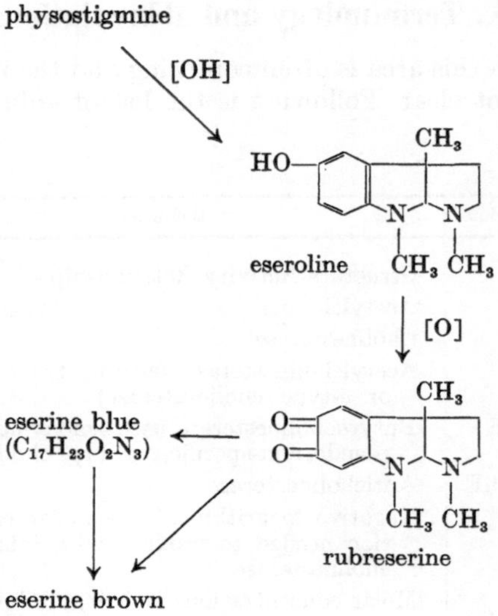

physostigmine

[OH]

HO—<chemical structure: eseroline>CH₃ ... N ... N ... CH₃ CH₃

eseroline   CH₃ CH₃

[O]

eserine blue   O=<chemical structure: rubreserine>CH₃
(C₁₇H₂₃O₂N₃)   O=   N   N
                        CH₃ CH₃
                      rubreserine

eserine brown

ELLIS (1943) and ELLIS et al. (1943 a, b) reported the following values for inhibition of horse serum BuChE.

	I_{50}
physostigmine salicylate	4×10^{-8}
rubreserine	9.9×10^{-6}
eserine blue	5.7×10^{-6}
eseroline and eserine brown	inactive

The above decomposition products are interesting in that the stepwise oxidation of eseroline produces compounds that alternate in their ability to inhibit serum BuChE. Even though rubreserine and eserine blue are only about 1/100 as active as physostigmine, these compounds demonstrate that the methyl carbamate group found in physostigmine is not essential for anti-ChE activity.

The activity of the methyl quaternary analog of physostigmine has been evaluated against various test objects and reported to be quantitatively similar to physostigmine; however it possesses less anti-ChE activity (AESCHLIMANN and REINERT 1931; SCHWEITZER et al. 1939).

C. From physostigmine to neostigmine

Following the structural elucidation of physostigmine (STEDMAN and BARGER 1925), there was rapid progress in the development of synthetic anti-ChE compounds. The work of STEDMAN and co-workers stands as one of the high points in the structure-activity area and places them among the pioneers of this method of experimental approach which has yielded many active therapeutic agents in most branches of medicine.

Very early they reasoned that the two linked pyrollidine rings in physostigmine may not be essential for activity. The approach used was the assumption that methyl carbamates of simple phenols might yield active compounds. The experimental reasoning used by STEDMAN and co-workers in dissecting the physostigmine molecule into its active components is outlined as follows:

essential moiety   non-essential moiety

The simplest analogs studied were the methyl carbamates of basically substituted phenols. They evaluated whether the carbamate and amino N should be *o*, *m*, or *p* to each other for maximal activity. This series was prepared and tested originally only for miotic activity; these first synthetic cholinesterase inhibitors are shown in Table 1 (STEDMAN 1926). This early work demonstrated that the basic grouping outlined would produce active compounds, and phenyl carbamate substitution was not found to be favorable for activity, at least in this series. They noted that conversion of the *m*-tertiary substituted compounds to quaternary compounds intensified the activity, while the quaternary analogs of the *o* and *p* substituted compounds were devoid of miotic activity. The observation that the more acidic phenols (*o* and *p* substituted) tended to possess less activity led to the preparation and evaluation of benzylsubstituted compounds, especially since the investigators had already observed activity with the methyl carbamate derivative of hordenine (Table 1).

Table 1. *The effect of position isomerism on miotic activity in a series of substituted hydroxyaniline derivatives*

Position	R	R₁	Miotic activity
para	HCl	CH₃	+
para	CH₃I	CH₃	—
para	HCl	C₂H₅	—
para	CH₃I	C₂H₅	—
meta	HCl	H	+
meta	HCl	CH₃	+
meta	CH₃I	CH₃	+
meta	HCl	C₂H₅	—
meta	CH₃I	C₂H₅	+·
meta	CH₃I	C₆H₅	—
ortho	HCl	CH₃	+
ortho	CH₃I	C₂H₅	—
ortho	HCl	C₂H₅	+
ortho	CH₃I	C₂H₅	—
H *p*-CH₃NCOOC₆H₄CH₂CH₂N(CH₃)₂			+
H *p*-C₆H₅NCOOC₆H₄CH₂CH₂N(CH₃)₂			—

STEDMAN (1926).

The same general pattern of activity for the benzyl derivatives as outlined for the phenol derivatives was observed. The structures and miotic properties are shown in Table 2 (STEDMAN 1929). These compounds were prepared to obtain more stable derivatives (apparently many of the compounds outlined in Table 1 readily decomposed in a warm solution), to evaluate more fully their "acidic" hypothesis, and to reduce any inductive interaction between the ring nitrogen and the carbamate grouping.

This series of compounds demonstrated that the methyl urethanes of the isomeric hydroxybenzyldimethylamines have the following order of activity — $o > p > m$. In this series, conversion of the tertiary amines to the quaternary analogs increased the activity of the *ortho*, diminished that of the *meta*, and abolished that of the *para* compounds. The observations that the quaternary derivatives of "*meta* phenol" (Table 1) and "*ortho* benzyl" (Table 2) are the more active compounds indicate that the increase in activity may be related to a formal charge, and not to inductive effects of the quaternary nitrogen atom. Also, the interatomic distance in the *meta* phenols between the quaternary nitrogen atom and the carbonyl group is approximately the same as that found in the *ortho*-benzyl structure. The observation that simple urethanes are inactive indicated to them that the urethane grouping by itself was not sufficient for activity, but that phenyl substituted urethanes are essential. This suggested that it was the entire molecule that was active as a miotic and not a urethane decomposition product.

Table 2. *The effect of position isomerism on miotic activity in a series of substituted hydroxybenzylamine derivatives*

Position	R	R$_1$	Miotic activity
meta	HCl	CH$_3$	+ +
meta	CH$_3$I	CH$_3$	+
meta	HCl	C$_2$H$_5$	—
meta	CH$_3$I	C$_2$H$_5$	—
meta	HCl	C$_6$H$_5$	—
para	HCl	CH$_3$	+ + +
para	CH$_3$I	CH$_3$	—
para	HCl	C$_2$H$_5$	—
ortho	HCl	CH$_3$	+ + + +
ortho	CH$_3$I	CH$_3$	+ + + + +
ortho	CH$_3$I	C$_2$H$_5$	—
urethane of choline			—
urethane of tropine			—

STEDMAN (1929).

The next advance came with the synthesis of further benzyl substituted compounds. This series led to the development of the first useful synthetic miotic agent, appropriately named "miotine" (STEDMAN 1929). The structures of miotine and related analogs are listed in Table 3 (EASSON and STEDMAN 1933).

Miotine contains an asymmetric carbon atom, so that it exists in the form of two stereoisomers. Because the earlier attempts to separate the stereoisomers were unsuccessful (STEDMAN 1929; WHITE and STEDMAN 1931), the compound was used clinically first as the racemic mixture. Early studies demonstrated that the pharmacological properties of miotine resembled those of physostigmine both qualitatively and quantitatively (STEDMAN and STEDMAN 1929; WHITE and STEDMAN 1931; BACQ and BROWN

Table 3. *Miotic activity of various analogs of miotine*

R	Miotic activity
CH$_2$	+
CH-(CH$_3$)-d,l-(miotine)	+ +
CH(C$_2$H$_5$)	+
CH(C$_3$H$_7$)	+
CH(C$_6$H$_5$)	0
C(CH$_3$)$_2$	+ + +

EASSON and STEDMAN (1933).

1937; SCHWEITZER et al. 1939). MATTHES (1930) included miotine along with physostigmine in his experiments when demonstrating that these compounds inhibited approximately to the same extent the esterase for ACh found in the blood. EASSON and STEDMAN (1933) reported that miotine was more active than physostigmine as a cholinesterase inhibitor. The isomers were separated (MACDONALD and STEDMAN 1932), and studies indicated that the l-isomer is the active component, at least when evaluated on isolated rabbit intestinal strips (EASSON and STEDMAN 1933). Removal of the assymetric carbon by dimethyl substitution increased the miotic activity considerably over that observed for miotine. It is interesting to speculate that this dimethyl substitution product may have approximately the same activity as l-miotine. Substitution with a group larger than methyl on the carbon appeared unfavorable for activity, and phenyl substitution resulted in inactivation. Apparently the methyl quaternary analog of miotine was less active (SCHWEITZER et al. 1939). The introduction of a methoxy group *para* to the alkyl side chain of miotine also reduced the activity (AESCHLIMANN and REINERT 1931).

The compounds were evaluated biochemically first for their ability to inhibit liver esterase (STEDMAN and STEDMAN 1931), and later for various other esterases including guinea pig serum esterase (STEDMAN and STEDMAN 1932). In both of these studies the authors used either methylbutyrate or tributyrin as substrate. The relative activities of the position isomers, using liver and serum esterase, are outlined in Table 4 (STEDMAN and STEDMAN 1931, 1932). The compounds were

Table 4. *Antiesterase activity of various mono-substituted carbamate derivitives*

Series	Salt	Substrate	Activity of isomers	Esterase
phenyl (table 1)	HCl	methylbutyrate	$m > p > o$	liver esterase
benzyl (table 2)	HCl	methylbutyrate	$m > p > o$	liver esterase
miotine (table 3)	HCl	methylbutyrate	$m = p > o$	liver esterase
phenyl	CH_3I	methylbutyrate	$m \gtrless p > o$	liver esterase
benzyl	CH_3I	methylbutyrate	$p > o > m$	liver esterase
miotine	CH_3I	methylbutyrate	$o > p \gtrless m$	liver esterase
phenyl	HCl	tributyrin	$m > p > o$	liver esterase
benzyl	HCl	tributyrin	$o > m > p$	liver esterase
miotine	HCl	tributyrin	$m > o > p$	liver esterase
phenyl	CH_3I	tributyrin	$o > p = m$	liver esterase
benzyl	CH_3I	tributyrin	$p > o > m$	liver esterase
miotine	CH_3I	tributyrin	$o > p = m$	liver esterase
phenyl	HCl	tributyrin	$m > p = o$	guinea pig serum
benzyl	HCl	tributyrin	$m = p > o$	guinea pig serum
miotine	HCl	tributyrin	$o = m = p$	guinea pig serum
phenyl	CH_3I	tributyrin	$o = p > m$	guinea pig serum
benzyl	CH_3I	tributyrin	$m = p > o$	guiena pig serum
miotine	CH_3I	tributyrin	$o = m = p$	guinea pig serum

STEDMAN and STEDMAN (1931, 1932).

much more active when tributyrin was used as a substrate. With tributyrin the most active compound was the hydrochloride of the m-dimethylaminophenyl ester of methylcarbamic acid. The relative activities of the compounds tested depended on both the substrate and the esterase. In most cases the anti-esterase activity of the quaternary was lower than that of the corresponding tertiary analog. The miotic activity did not always correspond with the esterase inhibiting activity. This discrepancy may be related in part to limited penetration in experiments, *in vivo*, but more likely the difficulty they had in explaining their results is related to their selection of esterases other than acetylcholinesterase.

D. Neostigmine and analogs

AESCHLIMANN and REINERT (1931) reported on various pharmacological properties of analogs of miotine and neostigmine (Prostigmine) (Tables 5 and 6). They
did not do any esterase studies, so the question remains as to whether the activity
reported was due to direct muscarinic action, cholinesterase inhibition, or in the
case of the rabbit intestine, which was stimulated, "nicotinic" effects. Since
arecoline and analogs (HUNT and RENSHAW 1929) and derivatives of 3-hydroxy-
piperidine (SCHUELER 1956) are known muscarinic agents, the compounds in their
series may have this component of action. However, in all probability most of the
analogs of miotine and neostigmine produce their pharmacological action entirely
or in part by the inhibition of cholinesterase. The simple structural analogs, compounds 1 to 7 (Table 5), appear to be relatively inactive. Substitution of a
2-methoxy group in miotine appears to reduce activity slightly. Physostigmine-
like activity was strongest in methyl-, dimethyl-, allyl-, benzyl-, and methyl-
phenyl-carbamic esters of phenol bases. The activity appeared weak in ethyl- and
phenyl-, and was absent in diethyl- and diallyl-carbamic esters. The quaternary
salts of the aromatic bases were more active than the corresponding tertiary
derivatives. When the basic radical was in the side-chain, the difference was less
marked or reversed.

One of the major problems with miotine and physostigmine is that both compounds are quite unstable in solution. This appears to be true, in general, for
mono-methyl carbamates (STEDMAN 1926). With this series it was observed that
the dialkylphenylcarbamates are relatively stable and highly active — especially
those in which the carbamate group is *meta* to an alkylated quaternary nitrogen
substituent.

Following the demonstration by AESCHLIMANN and REINERT (1931) that neostigmine is a very active cholinesterase inhibitor and that it is stable in solution,
many workers have and are still synthesizing and evaluating analogs of this
compound. BLOCH (1939) first reported the activity of compounds in which the
carbamate grouping of neostigmine was replaced by a hydroxyl group and
esterified. For esterification he used either acetic or *iso*butyric acid. Both of these
compounds are less active than neostigmine when evaluated for inhibition of
human or dog serum BuChE (Table 7). This was the first suggestion that the
carbamate grouping is not essential for activity. Apparently these compounds have
not been evaluated using AChE. It was later demonstrated that at least the
acetyl derivative undergoes rather rapid hydrolysis *in vivo*, and that the *meta*
hydroxy-phenyl-trimethylammonium derivative may be the active compound.

The possible structural modifications of neostigmine, as with almost any
chemical compound, are nearly without limit. The two most common points of
structural alteration are the carbamate and the ammoniacal groups. A number of
compounds has also been prepared in which various groups have replaced hydrogen atoms in the phenyl ring. Tables 5 to 22 illustrate the structural variations
that have been reported by various workers.

BLASCHKO et al. (1949) studied the influence of structural variation of the
quaternary head as well as various other modifications of the neostigmine structure
(Table 8). Stepwise replacement of methyl groups by ethyl groups on the quaternary nitrogen atom led first to an increase in anti-ChE activity, reaching a maximum with the diethyl-methyl derivative, and then decreasing sharply in activity
with the triethyl derivative. The dimethyl tertiary analog is much less active
than the parent compound. BLASCHKO et al. (1949) also compared the effects of
various other structural modifications. They demonstrated that the quaternary

Table 5. *Molar concentrations of various carbamate derivatives required for miotic action and isolated intestine stimulation*

N-$(CH_3)_2 \cdot$ HCl benzene ring —O—R

Compound No.	R	Miotic action — cat (concentration for activity)	Isolated rabbit intestine (molar conc. for excitation)
1	$COOC_2H_5$	1% (inactive)	2×10^{-5}
2	CO-(bis)	insoluble	
3	$CONHCH_3$	5%	1×10^{-4}
4	$CONHCH_2CH=CH_2$	2% (inactive)	0.5×10^{-6}
5	$CONHCH_2C_6H_5$	insoluble	
6	$CONHC_6H_5$	—	—
7	$CON(CH_3)_2$	1% (slight)	1×10^{-5} (inactive)

R, R_1 benzene ring —O—C(=O)—N(H)—CH_3

	R	R_1		
8	$N(C_2H_5)_2$	H	—	1×10^{-6}
9	p-$N(CH_3)CH_2CH_2N(C_2H_5)_2$	H	2% (inactive)	2×10^{-5} (inactive)
10	$CH(CH_3)N(CH_3)_2$	H	0.1—0.5%	0.2×10^{-6}
11	$CH(CH_3)N(CH_3)_2$	2-OCH_3	0.5%	1×10^{-5}
12	$\overset{+}{N}(CH_3)_2(C_2H_5)$ Br^-	H	—	—
13	$\overset{+}{N}(C_2H_5)_2(CH_3)$ I^-	H	0.5%	0.5×10^{-7}
14	p-$\overset{+}{N}(CH_3)_3$ I^-	H	—	1×10^{-5}
15	$CH(CH_3)N(CH_3)_2$	6-OCH_3	0.5%	1×10^{-5}
16	o-$CH_2N(C_2H_5)_2$	H	1%	2×10^{-5}
17	p-$CH_2CH_2N(CH_3)_2$	H	2%	0.254×10^{-6}
18	$CH(CH_3)\overset{+}{N}(CH_3)_3$ I^-	6-OCH_3	0.5%	2×10^{-6}
19	o-$CH_2\overset{+}{N}(CH_3)(C_2H_5)_2$ I^-	H	1% (inactive)	1×10^{-5}
20	p-$CH_2CH_2\overset{+}{N}(CH_3)_3I$	H	0.1%	0.2×10^{-6}
21			0.5%	1×10^{-5} (inactive)
22			1% (inactive)	2×10^{-5}
23			0.25%	0.2×10^{-6}
	physostigmine		0.1%	0.2×10^{-6}

AESCHLIMANN and REINERT (1931).

Table 6. *Molar concentrations of various analogs of neostigmine required for miotic action and intestine stimulation*

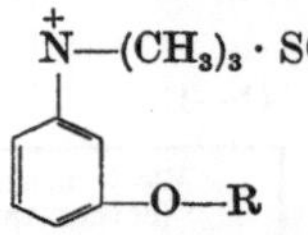

$$\overset{+}{N}-(CH_3)_3 \cdot SO_4CH_3^-$$

—O—R

Compound No.	R	Miotic action — cat (concentration for activity)	Isolated rabbit intestine (molar conc. for excitation)
1	H	2% (inactive)	1×10^{-6}
2	$COCH_3$	1%	5×10^{-6}
3	$COOC_2H_5$	5% (inactive)	1×10^{-5}
4	$CH_3CONHCH_3$	2% (inactive)	1×10^{-5} (inactive)
5	CO-(bis)	1% (inactive)	1×10^{-5}
6	$CONH_2$	1% (inactive)	5×10^{-6}
7	$CONHCH_3$	1%	0.5×10^{-6}
8	$CONHCH_2CH{=}CH_2$	1%	0.5×10^{-6}
9	$CONHC_2H_5$	1%	—
10	$CONHCH_2C_6H_5$	1% (inactive)	0.5×10^{-6}
11	$CONHC_6H_5$	1% (inactive)	2×10^{-6}
12	$CONHNHC_6H_5$	1% (inactive)	0.3×10^{-6}
neostigmine	$CON(CH_3)_2$	0.5%	0.4×10^{-6}
13	$CON(C_2H_5)_2$	4% (inactive)	2×10^{-5} (inactive)
14	$CON(CH_2CH{=}CH_2)_2$	4%	2×10^{-5}
15	$CON\langle\rangle$ 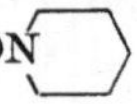	2% (inactive)	1×10^{-5}
16	$CON{<}^{CH_3}_{C_6H_5}$	2% (slight)	0.4×10^{-6}
physostigmine		0.1%	0.2×10^{-6}

AESCHLIMANN and REINERT (1931).

nitrogen atom could be incorporated into the ring, as in pyridinium (e.g., pyrido-stigmin, Mestinon), as a substituted pyridine, or as a substituted quinoline (No. 38), or could be removed by one carbon, as in miotine, and still maintain fairly high anti-ChE activity.

Two papers, one by LEHMANN (1946) and the other by AESCHLIMANN and STEMPEL (1946) published in the Emil Barell Jubilee Volume, summarize much of the work these authors have done with analogs of neostigmine. AESCHLIMANN and STEMPEL (1946) reported the activities of a comprehensive series of disubstituted carbamate analogs of neostigmine (Table 9). The phenyl-methylcarbamate analog of neostigmine demonstrated a sharp reduction in activity when compared with neostigmine. However, halogen (bromine or chlorine) in the *para* position of the phenyl ring greatly increased the activity when compared with that of the unsubstituted analog. This increase in activity probably is not due

Table 7. *Isosteres of neostigmine*

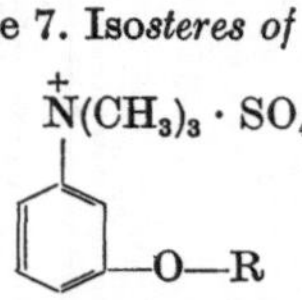

$$\overset{+}{N}(CH_3)_3 \cdot SO_4CH_3^-$$

—O—R

Compound	R	% Inhibition (25 mg/l) human serum BuChE	dog serum BuChE
1. neostigmine	$OCON(CH_3)_2$	94	89
2	$OCOCH_3$	30	60
3	$OCOCH(CH_3)_2$	40	73

BLOCH (1939).

to an inductive effect of halogens, since an electron-donor group (*p*-methyl) also demonstrated activity greater than neostigmine. This is supported further by the lack of activity observed for the *ortho* halogen derivatives. These results may

Table 8. *The effect of various substitutions on the cationic head and related compounds of neostigmine*

Compound	R	R'	R''	X	pI$_{50}$	
					dog caudate nucleus AChE	horse serum BuChE
neostigmine	CH_3	CH_3	CH_3	CH_3SO_4	7.4	7.2
Ro 1-3392	CH_3	CH_3	C_2H_5	I	8.0	7.3
Ro 1-3393	CH_3	C_2H_5	C_2H_5	I	8.2	8.0
Ro 1-5208	C_2H_5	C_2H_5	C_2H_5	I	7.2	7.4
RO 1-5220/5	CH_3	CH_3	OH	Cl	4.5	4.8
NU 683					6.2	8.5
Ro 1-5130 (pyrido-ostigmin)					6.4	5.8
miotine					7.2	6.4
38					7.1	7.6
Nu 1250	R = Cl				7.4	7.9
NU 1197	R = CH_3				6.9	7.1

BLASCHKO et al. (1949).

indicate a position of additional attachment of these compounds on the receptor surface. Substitution of both carbamate methyl groups by larger aliphatic or aromatic groups does not appear to be favorable for activity.

LEHMANN (1946) reported a series in which the substitutions in the quaternary head, carbamate group, and phenyl ring were varied. In this series the quaternary head was one carbon removed from the phenyl ring. The structures and anti-ChE activities are shown in Tables 10 and 11. These studies indicate that trimethyl-ammonium compounds with either phenyl or benzyl groups substituted on the phenyl ring *para* to the carbamate group may retain activity equal to that of neostigmine. Cyclohexyl in place of phenyl does not appear to be as active. Further structural alterations of the quaternary head and carbamate group lead to reduction in activity. Ring substitution in the position *ortho* to carbamate greatly reduces the activity of these compounds.

Table 9. *Variations in substitutions on the carbamate group of neostigmine*

$$\underset{}{\overset{+\;\;Br^-}{N}(CH_3)_3}$$

phenyl ring with $-O-\overset{O}{\overset{\|}{C}}-N\overset{R_1}{\underset{R_2}{\diagup}}$

Compound	R_1	R_2	Relative anti-ChE activity
Ro 2-			(neo-stigmine = 1)
neostigmine	CH_3	CH_3	1
0613	CH_3	C_6H_5	1/20
1250	CH_3	$C_6H_4Cl\ (p)$	5
1489	CH_3	$C_6H_4Br\ (p)$	2
1526	CH_3	$C_6H_3Br_2\ (o, p)$	1—2
1197	CH_3	$C_6H_4CH_3\ (p)$	> 1
1208	CH_3	$C_6H_4CH_3\ (m)$	1/5
1243	CH_3	$C_6H_4Cl\ (m)$	> 1/5
1249	CH_3	$C_6H_4Cl\ (o)$	> 1/5
1214	CH_3	$C_6H_4CH_3\ (o)$	> 1/100
1173	CH_3	$C_6H_3(CH_3)_2\ (m, p)$	1/5
0658	CH_3	$C_6H_3(CH_3)_2\ (o, m)$	> 1/100
1331	$CH(CH_3)_2$	$CH(CH_3)_2$	1/100
2058	$CH_2\overset{CH_3}{\underset{\|}{C}}=CH_2$	$CH_2\overset{CH_3}{\underset{\|}{C}}=CH_2$	< 1/100
2697	C_6H_5	C_6H_5	> 1/10

AESCHLIMANN and STEMPEL (1946).

HAWKINS and GUNTER (1946) reported that Nu-683 (Table 12) is a highly selective inhibitor of BuChE when compared with the compound's ability to inhibit AChE. HAWKINS and MENDEL (1949) demonstrated that the *p*-chloro-phenyl methyl carbamate analog of neostigmine (Nu-1250) is a highly selective inhibitor of AChE.

RANDALL and LEHMANN (1950) studied a series of neostigmine analogs in which the carbamate group was replaced by various other groups (Table 13). Similar anti-ChE activity was found for the 3-OH derivative (Ro 2-2561) and for the acetyl ester (Ro 2-2017). The acetyl derivative appears to be unstable at a slightly alkaline pH and is readily hydrolyzed to yield the parent hydroxy compound. In this series of compounds the absence of the carbamate group of neo-stigmine leads to compounds that are no more than 1/100th as active. The low anti-ChE activity found for these compounds is believed to be responsible for the relatively weak intestinal stimulating and miotic properties observed. The above authors did not believe that the anticurare and direct stimulating effects on striated muscle could be explained entirely by the cholinesterase-inhibiting properties.

Wescoe et al. (1950) also reported on the acetyl derivative of the "Tensilon" (edrophonium) series. Their work agrees with the conclusions of Randall and Lehmann (1950). Wescoe et al. (1950) demonstrated further that the acetyl and hydroxy derivatives are of the same order of activity. These results are shown

Table 10. *Effects of amine, carbamate, and ring substitutions on anti-ChE activity*

Compound	R	R₁	R₂	R₃	Relative anti-ChE activity
Ro 2-					(neostigmine = 1)
0683 (NU 683)	CH_3	CH_3	CH_3	C_6H_5	1
0683/1	CH_3	CH_3	H	C_6H_5	1/10
0772	CH_3	N O (morpholine)		C_6H_5	1/100
0800	CH_3	CH_3 ...... CH_3 (tetrahydroisoquinoline)		OC_6H_5	1/10
0803	CH_3			C_6H_5	1/10
0809	CH_3	CH_3	CH_3	C_6H_{11}	1/10
0812	CH_3	N (piperidine)		C_6H_5	1/10
0834	CH_3	CH_3	CH_3	COC_6H_5	1
0855	$CH(CH_3)_2$	CH_3	CH_3	C_6H_5	1/1,000
0918	CH_3	CH_3	CH_3	SC_6H_5	1/5
1071	CH_3	C_2H_5	C_2H_5	C_6H_5	1/10
1113	CH_3	CH_3	CH_3	$\overset{CH_3}{\underset{CH_3}{C}}{-}C_6H_5$	1/10
1128	CH_3	N (pyrrolidine)		C_6H_5	> 1/10
1405	CH_3	N (piperidine)		C_6H_5	—
1560	$\overset{CH_3}{\underset{C_6H_4CH_3(p)}{}}$	CH_3	CH_3	C_6H_5	—

Lehmann (1946).

in Table 14. They suggested that on the basis of their low AChE-inhibiting activity, the compounds' physiological properties are due to some other mechanism of action. They also demonstrated by the Lineweaver-Burk plot that the compounds compete with one another for access to ChE's.

Macfarlane et al. (1950), Cohen and Unna (1951), and Smith et al. (1952) carried out extensive investigations of *m*-hydroxyphenyl-trialkylammonium compounds; the activities of these compounds against various AChE's are tabulated in Table 15. These workers found that the most active compound as a cholinesterase inhibitor is the diethylmethyl derivative (Ro 2-980), which is approximately equal to neostigmine in activity. Increasing or decreasing the size of the

25*

Table 11. *Additional analogs with various amine, carbamate, and ring substitutions*

Compound	R	R_1	R_2	R_3	Relative anti-ChE activity
Ro 2-					(neostigmine = 1)
0734	CH_3	CH_3	CH_3	C_6H_5	1
0906	CH_3	CH_3	CH_3	C_6H_{11}	1/1,000
0911	CH_3	(ring N)		C_6H_{11}	< 1/1,000
1122*	CH_3	(ring N)		C_6H_{11}	1/1,000
1151	CH_3	(ring N—O)		C_6H_{11}	1/10,000
1210	CH_3	(ring N—O with CH_3, CH_3)		C_6H_5	inactive

* Tertiary of Ro 2-0911.
LEHMANN (1946).

Table 12. *Specificity of NU 683 and NU 1250*

Enzyme-Substrate	M Conc. of NU 683	% Inhibition
human plasma-benzoyl choline.	5×10^{-9}	66
human erythrocyte-acetyl-β-methyl choline	5×10^{-9}	4
human plasma-benzoyl choline.	1×10^{-8}	92
human erythrocyte-acetyl-β-methyl choline	1×10^{-8}	15
dog plasma-benzoyl choline	2.5×10^{-8}	55
dog plasma-benzoyl choline	5×10^{-8}	91

HAWKINS and GUNTER (1946).

Enzyme	M Conc. of ACh substrate	I_{50}
human erythrocyte	0.0012	approx. 5×10^{-9}
human plasma	0.06	approx. 10^{-4}
horse erythrocyte	0.0012	approx. 10^{-8}
horse serum	0.06	approx. 5×10^{-8}

HAWKINS and MENDEL (1949).

Table 13. *Substituted amine and carbamate analogs of neostigmine*

$$\overset{+}{N}(R)_3 \quad Br^-$$

Compound	R	R_1	Potency against electric eel AChE
Ro-			(neostigmine = 1)
neostigmine	CH_3	$OCN(CH_3)_2$ (C=O)	1
2-2979	CH_3	H	$< 1/100$
2-3218	$CH_3(C_2H_5)_2$	H	$< 1/100$
2-2561	CH_3	OH	$< 1/100$
2-2017 (iodide)	CH_3	$OC-CH_3$ (C=O)	1/100
2-2651 (iodide)	$CH_3(C_2H_5)_2$	$OC-CH_3$ (C=O)	1/100
2-2650	CH_3	$OC-C_6H_5$ (C=O)	$< 1/100$
2-2794	CH_3	$OC-C_6H_4Cl(m)$ (C=O)	$< 1/100$
2-2856	CH_3	$OC-C_6H_{11}$ (C=O)	$< 1/100$
2-2732	CH_3	$OC-CH_2C_6H_5$ (C=O)	$< 1/100$
2-2951	CH_3	$OC-CH=CHC_6H_5$ (C=O)	$< 1/100$
2-2906	CH_3	$OC-C_6H_4NH_2(p)$ (C=O)	1/100
2-2789	CH_3	$OC-C_6H_4CH_3(p)$ (C=O)	$< 1/100$
2-2783	CH_3	$OC-C_6H_4CH_3(m)$ (C=O)	$< 1/100$
2-2798	CH_3	$OC-C_6H_4Cl(p)$ (C=O)	1/100
2-2788	$CH_3(C_2H_5)_2$	$OC-C_6H_5$ (C=O)	$< 1/100$
2-2765	$C_6H_5\overset{O}{C}-O-\langle\text{ring}\rangle-\overset{+}{N}(CH_3)_3$		$< 1/100$

Table 13. (contd.)

Compound	R	R_1	Potency against electric eel AChE
2-2952	ortho isomer of above		$< 1/100$
2-2748	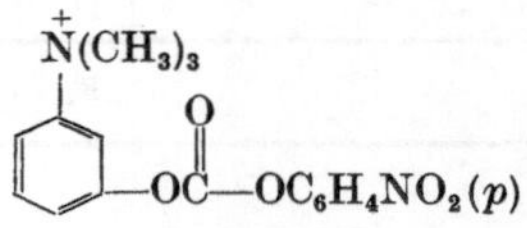		$< 1/100$
2-2649	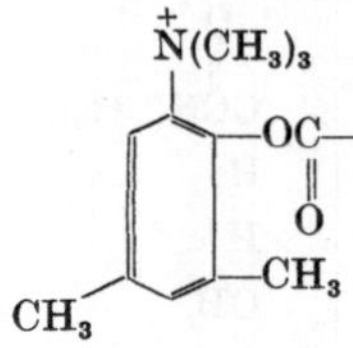		$< 1/100$
2-2819	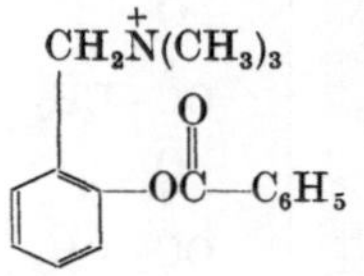		$< 1/100$

RANDALL and LEHMANN (1950).

quaternary head resulted in a decrease of the anti-ChE activity. Similar results have been reported for analogs of neostigmine (see Table 8).

HOBBIGER (1952) also evaluated the activity of various esterified hydroxy-alkylphenylamine derivatives. The anti-ChE activities are tabulated in Table 16. He concluded that the ester linkage is rapidly hydrolyzed by human serum BuChE (especially with Ro 2-2651), and that the pharmacological action is probably due in part to the corresponding phenolic analog.

Table 14. *Activity of edrophonium analog and acetylated form*

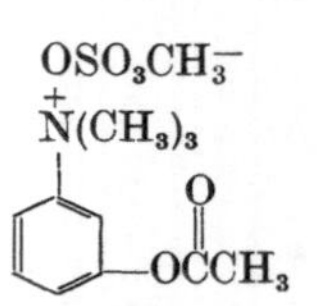

NU 2017
(Ro 2-2017)
I_{50}

human erythrocyte 2.5×10^{-5} M

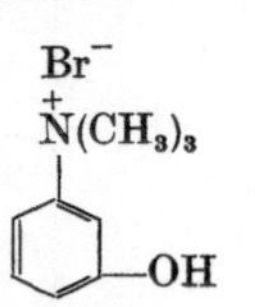

NU 2561
(Ro 2-2561)
I_{50}

human erythrocyte 2.5×10^{-5} M
human serum 8×10^{-4} M

WESCOE et al. (1950).

BURGEN and HOBBIGER (1951) reported a series of alkylphenolphosphates in which the carbamate grouping of neostigmine was replaced by the various phosphates. The anti-ChE activities of these compounds are listed in Table 17. The dimethyl phosphate (Ro 3-0412) is completely reversible. The diethyl derivative is similar to tetraethylpyrophosphate (TEPP) in that it is partially reversible. Substitutions larger than diethyl produced completely irreversible compounds. All of the compounds are more active inhibitors of human plasma BuChE than

Table 15. *Alkyl amino substituted analogs of edrophonium*

$$\begin{array}{c} R_1 \\ \overset{+}{N}\!-\!R_2 \\ R_3 \\ \text{(phenyl)} \\ -OH \end{array}$$

Compound	R_1	R_2	R_3	I_{50} Values for		
				electric eel AChE[1, 2]	bovine erythrocyte[1] AChE	rat brain[3] AChE
Ro 2-						
2561	CH_3	CH_3	CH_3	4.0×10^{-5}	4.8×10^{-5}	1×10^{-4}
3198 (edrophonium, Tensilon)	CH_3	CH_3	C_2H_5	1.3×10^{-5}	3.4×10^{-5}	5×10^{-5}
980	CH_3	C_2H_5	C_2H_5	5×10^{-6}	3.1×10^{-5}	
3709	C_2H_5	C_2H_5	C_2H_5	2.5×10^{-5}	2×10^{-4}	
neostigmine				3×10^{-6}	4×10^{-7}	

[1] SMITH et al. (1952).
[2] COHEN and UNNA (1951).
[3] MACFARLANE et al. (1950).

human red cell AChE. Even the completely reversible analog is about 10 times more active in inhibiting BuChE than in affecting AChE.

FOLDES et al. (1958) evaluated a series of neostigmine analogs in which the interatomic $\overset{+}{N}$ to $C=O$ distances were varied (Table 18). In this series the less complex structures (Ro 1-4987, Ro 2-9147, neostigmine, Ro 2-0907) were more

Table 16. *Alkyl amino and acylated analogs of edrophonium*

$$CH_3\!-\!\overset{+}{N}\!\!<\!\!\begin{array}{c} R \\ R_1 \end{array}$$
$$\text{(phenyl)}-R_2$$

Compound	R	R_1	R_2	I_{50} for human red cell AChE
Ro 2-				
2650	CH_3	CH_3	$OC\overset{O}{\overset{\|}{C}}C_6H_5$	1.4×10^{-5}
2651	C_2H_5	C_2H_5	$OC\overset{O}{\overset{\|}{C}}CH_3$	6×10^{-6}
2783	CH_3	CH_3	$OC\overset{O}{\overset{\|}{C}}C_6H_4CH_3\,(m)$	1.1×10^{-5}
3198 (edrophonium, Tensilon)	CH_3	C_2H_5	OH	4×10^{-6}
neostigmine				3.5×10^{-8}

HOBBIGER (1952).

active inhibitors of plasma BuChE than of red cell AChE. The maximum activity for both types of cholinesterase was exhibited by Ro 2-9147, where the $\overset{+}{N}$ to $C=O$ distance is 4.7 Å. Increasing or decreasing this critical interatomic distance led to a reduction in activity; the distance is more critical for AChE. This is further evidence that AChE contains two sites of attachment, and BuChE has only one (see also BERGMAN and SEGAL 1954, and BERGMAN 1956). Substitution in the R_5 position results in sharp reduction in activity. This is probably due to steric

Table 17. *Inhibition of cholinesterases by dialkylphosphostigmines*

$$CH_3SO_4^-$$
$$\overset{+}{N}(CH_3)_3$$

Compound	R	I_{50} Values for	
		human red cell AChE	human plasma BuChE
Ro 3-			
0412	CH_3	7.5×10^{-8}	6.3×10^{-9}
0340	C_2H_5	8×10^{-8}	1.2×10^{-9}
0411	$CH\overset{CH_3}{\underset{CH_3}{<}}$	2.1×10^{-7}	3×10^{-9}
0397	$C\overset{H\ \ CH_3}{\underset{CH_2CH_3}{<}}$	1.6×10^{-7}	9×10^{-9}
neostigmine		1.1×10^{-7}	6.9×10^{-7}

BURGEN and HOBBIGER (1951).

hindrance of the carbonyl group, since the cyclohexyl substitution would not be expected to exert much inductive effect. Substitutions in the R_4 position (analogs of NU-683) do not seem to alter the activity of the parent compound.

WILSON and QUAN (1958) reported on the SAR of a series of phenyltrimethyl-ammonium analogs in relation to their "binding" strengths (Table 19). The introduction of the 3-OH group increased the binding strength by a factor of 120. This marked increase in binding strength is very suggestive of strong hydrogen bonding (having a $\overset{+}{N}$ to OH distance of about 5 Å). A sharp decrease in activity was noted when the hydroxyl group was moved to the 4-position. In all probability this was due to an increase in the $\overset{+}{N}$ to OH interatomic distance. The 2-OH compound (No. 4) was intermediate in activity, and probably represented a compound that had too short an $\overset{+}{N}$ to OH interatomic distance. Also, the hydrogen may be partly associated with the cationic site on the nitrogen. Compound No. 5 further illustrates the importance of the presence of a free hydrogen for hydrogen bond formation. The difference in activity of the methyl isomers, (compounds Nos. 6, 7 and 8) may be due to some factor other than the influence on hydrogen bonding, since the 4- and 6-methyl derivatives would be expected to have a trend in activity different from that observed for the 5-methyl derivative. Replacement of the hydroxyl groups in compounds 2, 3, and 4 with methyl groups (11, 12, and 13) resulted in a reduction in activity. Even though the hydrogens in a methyl group can undergo bonding, the bond energy is much less than that observed for a hydroxy hydrogen.

Table 18. *The effect of ring position isomerisom on anti-ChE activity*

$$O=C-N-CH_3$$

R_5 —ring— R_2, R_3, R_4, O, R_1, Br^-

Compound	R_1	R_2	R_3	R_4	R_5	I_{50} values for human plasma BuChE	human red cell AChE
Ro 1-4987	CH_3	$\overset{+}{N}(CH_3)_3$	H	H	H	1.8×10^{-7}	7.3×10^{-7}
Ro 2-7920	⬡—Cl	$\overset{+}{N}(CH_3)_3$	H	H	H	1.5×10^{-5}	1.5×10^{-6}
Ro 2-7921	⬡—CH_3	$\overset{+}{N}(CH_3)_3$	H	H	H	3.9×10^{-5}	2.9×10^{-6}
Ro 2-9147	CH_3	$CH_2\overset{+}{N}(CH_3)_3$	H	H	H	4.5×10^{-8}	9.0×10^{-7}
Ro 2-0683 (NU-683)	CH_3	$CH_2\overset{+}{N}(CH_3)_3$	H	⬡	H	3.2×10^{-9}	9.0×10^{-7}
Ro 2-0809	CH_3	$CH_2\overset{+}{N}(CH_3)_3$	H	⬡	H	4.3×10^{-9}	4.9×10^{-7}
Ro 2-0800	CH_3	$CH_2\overset{+}{N}(CH_3)_3$	H	⬡—O—	H	2.9×10^{-8}	6.2×10^{-7}
Ro 2-0918	CH_3	$CH_2\overset{+}{N}(CH_3)_3$	H	⬡—S—	H	2.1×10^{-8}	1.3×10^{-7}
Ro 2-0906	CH_3	$CH_2\overset{+}{N}(CH_3)_3$	H	H	⬡	1.1×10^{-6}	2.5×10^{-4}
Ro 2-0911	CH_3	$CH_2-\overset{+}{N}-CH_3$ (piperidine)	H	H	⬡	10^{-4}	3.3×10^{-3}
Ro 2-0812	CH_3	$CH_2-\overset{+}{N}-CH_3$ (piperidine)	H	⬡	H	7.1×10^{-8}	1.4×10^{-6}
neostigmine	CH_3	H	$\overset{+}{N}(CH_3)_3$	H	H	5.6×10^{-8}	2.3×10^{-7}
Ro 2-1250	⬡—Cl	H	$\overset{+}{N}(CH_3)_3$	H	H	1.1×10^{-5}	1.3×10^{-8}
Ro 2-1197	⬡—CH_3	H	$\overset{+}{N}(CH_3)_3$	H	H	7.0×10^{-6}	7.5×10^{-8}
Ro 2-0907	CH_3	H	$CH_2\overset{+}{N}(CH_3)_3$	H	H	1.3×10^{-7}	5.2×10^{-6}

FOLDES et al. (1958).

Table 19. *Ring position isomers of edrophonium analog and derivatives*

$$\overset{+}{N}(CH_3)_3$$

Compound	R₁	R₂	R₃	R₄	R₅	I 50 for electric eel AChE
1	H	H	H	H	H	4.4×10^{-4}
2	H	OH	H	H	H	3.2×10^{-6}
3	H	H	OH	H	H	2.7×10^{-4}
4	OH	H	H	H	H	6.3×10^{-5}
5	H	OCH₃	H	H	H	9×10^{-5}
6	H	OH	CH₃	H	H	1.2×10^{-6}
7	H	OH	H	CH₃	H	2.5×10^{-6}
8	H	OH	H	H	CH₃	1.1×10^{-5}
9	H	OH	H	H	OCH₃	6.2×10^{-6}
0	H	OH	OCH₃	H	H	1.4×10^{-5}
11	H	H	CH₃	H	H	3.5×10^{-4}
12	H	CH₃	H	H	H	1.4×10^{-4}
13	CH₃	H	H	H	H	4.9×10^{-4}

WILSON and QUAN (1958).

E. Heterocyclic analogs of neostigmine

The incorporation of the nitrogen atom into a heterocyclic ring has long been considered a possible structural alteration for the production of active anti-ChE agents. STEDMAN (1926) prepared two derivatives of 8-hydroxyquinoline but did not report their pharmacological activities. AESCHLIMANN and REINERT (Table 5) reported that certain carbamate derivatives of 8-hydroxyquinoline were active intestinal stimulating agents. The anti-ChE properties of the dimethylcarbamate of quaternized 8-hydroxytetrahydroquinoline (Tetramethoquine) have been reported by BROWN et al. (1950).

WUEST and SAKAL (Table 20) reported on a large series of quaternized carbamic esters of 3-pyridol, which exhibited anti-ChE and parasympathomimetic activity. Dimethylurethane substitution produced more active compounds, as indicated by the reduction in activity when this group was replaced by diethyl- or diphenyl-urethane. The activity observed was intermediate when methyl plus some other group was placed on the carbamate nitrogen. The monomethylcarbamates were relatively inactive. The "oxygens" of the carbamate portion could be replaced by the sulfur isostere and retain moderate activity. One of the more interesting features was that the introduction of an iodine atom in the 2-position resulted in a sharp increase in activity (compound 40). Substitutions of up to three methyl groups for hydrogen atoms on the benzene ring did not appear to alter the activity greatly.

Another large series of 3-pyridol derivatives was reported by STEMPEL and AESCHLIMANN (1952); their results are shown in Tables 21 and 22. Table 21 lists the activity of the various tertiary derivatives. The most potent members are Ro 2-2126 and Ro 2-2219. These compounds are approximately equal to neo-stigmine in activity, and apparently are much better absorbed following oral administration. The quaternary derivatives (Table 22) are about as active as the

Table 20. *Pyridyl substituted analogs of neostigmine*

$$\underset{R_3}{}\overset{\overset{+}{N}-R_2 \quad Br^-}{\underset{R_1}{\bigcirc}}$$

No.	R_1	R_2	R_3	Inhibition of bovine erythrocyte AChE at 3×10^{-9} mol/cc (Compound No. 10 = 1)
1	OC—N(CH$_3$)$_2$ (O)	methyl	H	> 1/7
2	OC—N(CH$_3$)$_2$ (O)	ethyl	H	1/6
3	OC—N(CH$_3$)$_2$ (O)	n-propyl	H	1/7
4	OC—N(CH$_3$)$_2$ (O)	isopropyl	H	1/15
5	OC—N(CH$_3$)$_2$ (O)	n-butyl	H	> 1/6
6	OC—N(CH$_3$)$_2$ (O)	n-amyl	H	< 1/7
7	OC—N(CH$_3$)$_2$ (O)	n-hexyl	H	> 1/15
8	OC—N(CH$_3$)$_2$ (O)	n-heptyl	H	> 1/15
9	OC—N(CH$_3$)$_2$ (O)	2-hydroxyethyl	H	> 1/7
10	OC—N(CH$_3$)$_2$ (O)	benzyl	H	1
11	OC—N(CH$_3$)$_2$ (O)	4-NO$_2$-benzyl	H	1
12	OC—N(CH$_3$)$_2$ (O)	4-OCH$_3$-benzyl	H	> 1/7
13	OC—N(CH$_3$)$_2$ (O)	2-napthylmethyl	H	1
14	OC—N(CH$_3$)$_2$ (O)	2-phenylethyl	H	1
15	OC—N(CH$_3$)$_2$ (O)	2-thienylmethyl	H	1
16	OC—N(CH$_3$)$_2$ (O)	benzhydryl	H	< 1/75

Table 20. (contd.)

No.	R_1	R_2	R_3	Inhibition of bovine erythrocyte AChE at 3×10^{-9} mol/cc (Compound No- 10 = 1)
17	$\overset{\text{O}}{\overset{\|}{\text{OC}}}$—$N(CH_3)_2$	allyl	H	1/4
18	$\overset{\text{O}}{\overset{\|}{\text{OC}}}$—$N(CH_3)_2$	methallyl	H	$< 1/7$
19	$\overset{\text{O}}{\overset{\|}{\text{OC}}}$—$N(CH_3)_2$	methylene	H	$< 1/33$
20	$\overset{\text{O}}{\overset{\|}{\text{OC}}}$—$N(CH_3)_2$	1,2-ethylene	H	$> 1/4$
21	OH	benzyl	H	$< 1/75$
22	$OCOCH_3$	methyl	H	$< 1/75$
23	$OCONHCH_3$	benzyl	H	$< 1/75$
24	$OCON(C_2H_5)_2$	benzyl	H	$< 1/75$
25	$OCON(CH_3)CH_2(C_6H_5)$	benzyl	H	> 1
26	$OCON(CH_2C_6H_5)_2$	benzyl	H	—
27	$OCON(CH_3)C_6H_4Cl\,(p)$	benzyl	H	> 1
28	$OCON(C_6H_5)_2$	methyl	H	—
29	$OCON(CH_2)_4$ [1]	benzyl	H	$< 1/30$
30	$OCON$⟨ ⟩O	benzyl	H	$< 1/75$
31	$OCO_2N(CH_3)_2$	benzyl	H	$< 1/75$
32	$SCON(CH_3)_2$	benzyl	H	1/15
33	$OCON(CH_3)_2$	benzyl	6-methyl	$> 1/7$
34	$OCON(CH_3)_2$	benzyl	6-styryl	$< 1/75$
35	H	benzyl	2,6-dimethyl	—
36	$OCON(CH_3)_2$	methyl	2,6-dimethyl	$> 1/4$
37	$OCON(CH_3)_2$	methyl	2,4,6-trimethyl	1/30
38	$OCON(CH_3)_2$	methyl	2,4,5-trimethyl	—
39	$OCON(CH_3)_2$	benzyl	2,4,5-trimethyl-6-benzyl	$< 1/75$
40	$OCON(CH_3)_2$	methyl	2-iodo	> 1
41	$OCONHCH_3$	methyl	2-iodo	—

[1] N, N-tetramethylenecarbamyloxy

WUEST and SAKAL (1951).

above compounds when given by the parenteral route, but are much less effective when given by the oral route. The dimethylcarbamates in this series are the most active derivatives.

Table 21. *Pyridyl substituted analogs of miotine*

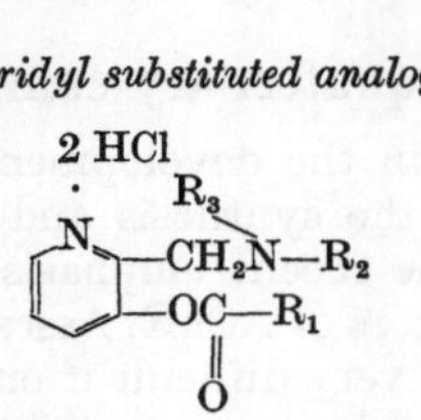

2 HCl

Compound	R₁	R₂	R₃	Anti-ChE activity (neostigmine = 1)
Ro 2-				
2126	$N(CH_3)_2$	CH_3	CH_3	1
2235	$N(CH_3)_2$	CH_3	H	—
2219	$N(CH_3)_2$	C_2H_5	C_2H_5	1
2255	$N(CH_3)_2$	CH_3	$CH_2C_6H_5$	< 0.1
2256	$N(CH_3)_2$	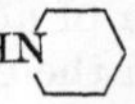 HN ⬡		0.1
2288	$N(CH_3)C_6H_5$	C_2H_5	C_2H_5	< 0.1
2421	$N[CH(CH_3)_2]_2$	CH_3	CH_3	⩽ 0.1

STEMPEL and AESCHLIMANN (1952).

Table 22. *Alterations in the amine and carbamate groups of pyridyl analogs*

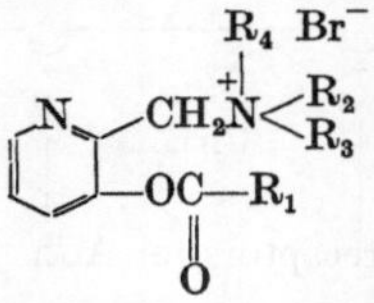

R_4 Br^-

Compound	R₁	R₂R₃	R₄	Anti-ChE activity (neostigmine = 1)
Ro 2-				
1658	$N(CH_3)_2$	CH_3	CH_3	1
1976	$N(CH_3)C_6H_4Br(p)$	CH_3	CH_3	0.1
2007	$N(CH_3)C_6H_4CH_3(p)$	CH_3	CH_3	0
2043	$N[CH(CH_3)_2]_2$	CH_3	CH_3	0
2550	CH_3	CH_3	CH_3	0
2817	C_6H_5	CH_3	CH_3	0
3128	$CH(C_6H_5)_2$	CH_3	CH_3	0
2016	$N(CH_3)_2$	C_2H_5	CH_3	1
2400	$N(CH_3)_2$	C_2H_5	C_2H_5	1/4
2750	$N(CH_3)_2$	$n\text{-}C_3H_7$	CH_3	1/2—1
3124	$N(CH_3)_2$	$i\text{-}C_3H_7$	CH_3	1/2
2279	$N(CH_3)_2$	$n\text{-}C_4H_9$	CH_3	1/4
2227	$N(CH_3)_2$	$CH_2C_6H_5$	CH_3	0
2253	$N(CH_3)_2$	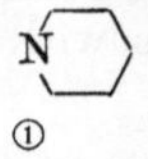 N ⬡	CH_3	1/4
2267	$N(CH_3)_2$	①		0

① $R_2 = C_6H_5$, $R_3 = CH_2CH_2\overset{+}{N}(CH_3)(C_2H_5)_2Br^-$.

STEMPEL and AESCHLIMANN (1952).

F. Bis-quaternary compounds

The most recent advances in the development of competitive cholinesterase inhibitors have resulted from the synthesis and pharmacological evaluation of *bis*-quaternary compounds. The recent emphasis has been directed toward the development of selective inhibitors of AChE. Assessment of the structural requirements of these various series is very difficult if one attempts to go from series to series. However, within the various series there are many examples of high structural specificity. A more challenging question is, why are two quaternary heads required for high activity in these various series? In most of these series, the monoquaternary analogs are either inactive or at least there is a sharp reduction in activity when compared with their *bis* analogs. On a single cholinesterase molecule there may be as many as 48 different "receptors" for ACh (MICHEL and KROP 1951). The basic ChE molecule has a molecular weight of about 105×10^3, but the molecular weight of the total molecule may be as high as 3×10^6 (SERLIN and FLUKE 1956). There are several theoretical possibilities that should be considered to explain the mechanism of action of these agents. At least some of the possible points for attachment on the enzyme surface are outlined below.

a) There is a possibility that these compounds may be bracketing the receptor on the cholinesterase molecule and shielding this site from ACh. A schematic outline of this may be represented as follows:

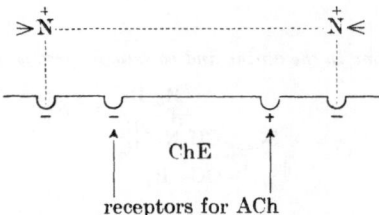

b) Another possibility is that these agents may combine with the same site as the cationic head of acetylcholine and some other negatively charged site on the cholinesterase molecule. This suggestion may be outlined as follows:

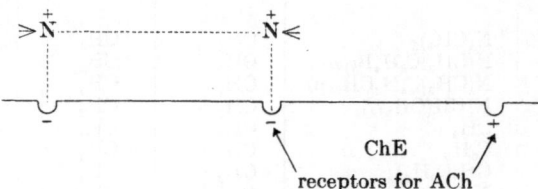

With this type of binding one of the sites for acetylcholine attachment would be blocked, and perhaps the second site of inhibitor-cholinesterase interaction would serve to stabilize or increase the total bond energy of the association. With this type of interaction, a competitive relationship would be expected. Likewise an inhibiting molecule may combine with both the anionic and cationic sites for ACh (KOELLE 1957).

c) Perhaps there is a repetition of the cationic site for acetylcholine on the cholinesterase molecule. This may allow attachment of the inhibiting compound at two cationic sites and "shielding" of the esteratic site. This possibility could be outlined as follows:

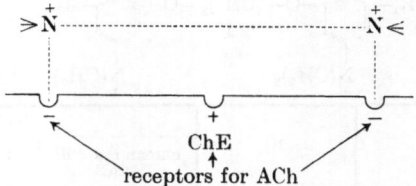

With this theoretical explanation an acetylcholine molecule would have the choice of two "cationic sites" and a common "esteratic" site. Most of the *bis*-quaternary compounds have an interatomic distance between the nitrogens of about 14 Å, which is approximately the same interatomic distance as that between the nitrogens of two molecules of acetylcholine linked through the acyl carbons.

d) The above considerations involve only one cholinesterase molecule. The possibility of an inhibitor binding from one molecule to another molecule may be yet an alternative suggestion (Long and Schueler 1954). If this were the mechanism, one would need to postulate that the cholinesterase molecules are relatively rigid in their relationship to each other. An outline of this possibility is as follows:

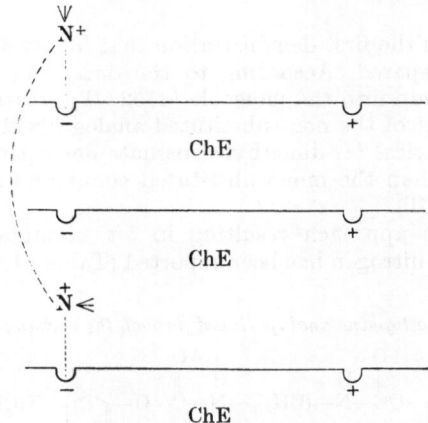

Whether the speculations outlined above are correct or not cannot be stated at this time. To study these and other theoretical possibilities is challenging and may offer leads to drug-receptor interactions at sites other than on the cholinesterase molecule. The possibility of intramolecular attachment could be more fully evaluated by studying *tris* and higher homologs. As yet, compounds of this type have not been reported.

Funke et al. (1952) reported originally that some *bis* neostigmine analogs linked together with 1, 3-dihydroxy propane possessed extremely high activity when evaluated against dog red cell AChE. Later studies indicated activity not as high as originally reported, but still probably as active a series of compounds as had yet been synthesized (Funke et al. 1954; Depierre and Funke 1954). Levin and Jandorf (1955) re-evaluated selected members of this series, using human red cell AChE, and found activity comparable to that reported by Depierre and Funke (1954). The data of both workers are shown in Table 23. However, there can be little doubt that this series contains highly active AChE

Table 23. bis *Neostigmine analogs linked with 1,3-propylene diol*

$$R_1-\overset{\underset{\displaystyle N(CH_3)_3}{|}}{\bigcirc}-O-(CH_2)_3-O-\overset{\underset{\displaystyle N(CH_3)_3}{|}}{\bigcirc}-R_2 \qquad 2\,I^-$$

Compound	R_1	R_2	I_{50} Values for		
			human red cell[1] AChE	dog plasma[2] BuChE	dog red cell[2] AChE
2842 CT	H	H	9.9×10^{-7}	1×10^{-3}	5×10^{-8}
3443 CT	OH	H	—	5×10^{-5}	1×10^{-9}
3116 CT	OH	OH	—	5×10^{-5}	2×10^{-10}
3152 CT	$O\overset{\displaystyle O}{\overset{\|}{C}}N(CH_3)_2$	H	1.4×10^{-9}	5×10^{-9}	6×10^{-10}
3113 CT	$O\overset{\displaystyle O}{\overset{\|}{C}}N(CH_3)_2$	$O\overset{\displaystyle O}{\overset{\|}{C}}N(CH_3)_2$	3.5×10^{-9}	5×10^{-8}	1×10^{-9}
neostigmine			6.9×10^{-8}	1×10^{-8}	1×10^{-8}

[1] LEVIN and JANDORF (1955).
[2] FUNKE et al. (1954), DEPIERRE and FUNKE (1954).

inhibitors; it represents the first demonstration that highly active *bis* quaternary compounds can be prepared. According to the data, the introduction of one dimethylcarbamate group into the molecule (3152 CT) greatly increased activity in comparison with that of the non-substituted analog (2842 CT). It is also to be noted that the symmetrical *bis*-dimethylcarbamate derivative (3113 CT) did not have greater activity than the monosubstituted compound (3152 CT) or the dihydroxy analog (3116 CT).

Another interesting approach resulting in *bis* neostigmine analogs linked through the carbamate nitrogen has been reported (Table 24, KRAUPP et al. 1955;

Table 24. bis *Neostigmine analogs linked through the carbamate substitution*

$$\left[(CH_3)_3N-\bigcirc-O\overset{\underset{\displaystyle}{\overset{\displaystyle O}{\|}}}{C}-\overset{\displaystyle H}{N}-(CH_2)_n-\overset{\displaystyle H}{N}-\overset{\overset{\displaystyle O}{\|}}{C}-O-\bigcirc-N(CH_3)_3\right]^{2+}\;2\,X^-$$

Compound	n	pI$_{50}$	
		dog erythrocyte AChE	dog serum BuChE
BC-30	4	5.7	5.2
BC-37	6	8.5	7.1
BC-18	8	9.0	7.4

$$\left[(CH_3)_3N-\bigcirc-O\overset{\overset{\displaystyle O}{\|}}{C}-\underset{\underset{\displaystyle CH_3}{|}}{N}-(CH_2)_n\underset{\underset{\displaystyle CH_3}{|}}{N}-\overset{\overset{\displaystyle O}{\|}}{C}-O-\bigcirc-N(CH_3)_3\right]^{2+}\;2\,X^-$$

BC-40	6	8.4	7.6
BC-47	8	9.4	7.9
BC-48	10	10.0	8.2

KRAUPP et al. (1955).

KLUPP et al. 1955). The tests *in vitro* indicated that the methyl carbamate derivatives have approximately the same activity as the non-methylated derivatives (compare BC-40 and BC-47 with BC-38 and BC-8). However, methylation of the carbamate nitrogen decreases the action *in vivo* somewhat, but these compounds show less spontaneous hydrolysis than the non-methylated analogs. It is obvious from the data reported that increasing the chain length between the two neostigmine molecules results in marked increase in activity. It would be interesting to know whether or not the distance found in BC-48 is optimal. The activity of BC-48 indicates that this compound is among the most active reversible inhibitors of AChE yet reported. HERZFELD et al. (1957) reported that the pyridine analog of BC-40 had pI_{50} values of 5.7 and 6.95 for serum BuChE and red cell AChE, respectively.

Table 25. *Anti-ChE activity of polymethylene bis quinolinium bromides*

n	pI_{50} dog caudate nucleus AChE
6	5.3
7	6.2
8	6.5
9	6.7
10	7.2

BARLOW and HIMMS (1955).

BARLOW and HIMMS (1955) reported the AChE-inhibiting properties of *bis* quinolines (Table 25). With these compounds there was a progressive increase in activity as the number or methylene groups was increased from six to ten. This gradual increase in activity was cited by the authors as support for their suggestion that only those *bis*-onium compounds which are able to become attached to the esteratic sites of the enzyme will show a maximum or a large increase in activity with the octamethylene member of the series. SMITH et al. (1953) reported the activity of a large series of *bis*-tetrahydroisoquinolines (Table 26). In this series activity tended to increase to the apparent maximum with the twelve methylene analog. It is interesting to note that the secondary amine analog of the C-8 derivative is as active as the quaternary derivative.

Table 26. *Anti-ChE activity of polymethylene bis isoquinolinium derivatives*

Compound	Y	R	I_{50} (M $\times$ 10^5) bovine erythrocyte AChE
4 A	$(CH_2)_4$	CH_3	100.0
6 A	$(CH_2)_6$	CH_3	10.0
7 A	$(CH_2)_7$	CH_3	1.0
8 A	$(CH_2)_8$	CH_3	0.96
8 Sec amine[1]	$(CH_2)_8$	H	0.90
9 A	$(CH_2)_9$	CH_3	0.70
10 A	$(CH_2)_{10}$	CH_3	0.80
10	$(CH_2)_{10}$	(CH_3) (C_2H_5)	1.0
10- 6,7,8-trimethoxy	$(CH_2)_{10}$	CH_3	1.0
12 A	$(CH_2)_{12}$	CH_3	0.94
12 B	$(CH_2)_{12}$	CH_3	0.60

6,7-dimethoxy-2-methyl 1,2,3,4-tetrahydro-isoquinoline methiodide	> 100.0
Tubocuarine chloride	> 100.0
Decamethonium bromide	30.0
Neostigmine bromide	0.09

[1] Chloride.

SMITH et al. (1953).

HAZARD et al. (1953) compared the activity of *bis* pyridines and *bis* 3-pyridyl carbamates (Table 27). In both series of compounds, increasing the distance between the quaternary nitrogens from 5 to 10 methylene groups led to sharp

Table 27. *Activity of* bis *pyridines and* bis *pyridyl-3-carbamates*

Compound	n	mg/1.6 ml for 25% inhibition	
		human serum BuChE	rabbit brain AChE
1	5	5	> 10
2	6	0.05	10
3	10	0.005	0.001

4	5	5	> 10
5	6	1.5	> 10
6	10	0.15	0.5
eserine		5×10^{-6}	1×10^{-5}

HAZARD et al. (1953).

increases in activity against both AChE and BuChE. This is another example suggesting that the *bis* quaternary compounds bind at two anionic sites, at least for optimal activity, and indicating that BuChE, as well as AChE, may possess a second anionic site.

Table 28. *Anti-ChE activity of derivatives of biphenyl and of* bis
(piperidinomethyl-5-coumaranyl) ketone

Compound	Positions	R	A	I 50 Values	
				dog plasma BuChE	dog red cell AChE
1446 F	o-o'	HCl	—	1×10^{-4}	1×10^{-4}
1466 F	m-m'	HCl	—	6×10^{-4}	6×10^{-6}
1389 F	p-p'	HCl	—	3×10^{-4}	3×10^{-7}
3220 CT	p-p'	HCl	C=O	1×10^{-4}	2×10^{-7}
3326 CT	p-p'	CH$_3$I	C=O	1×10^{-4}	2×10^{-7}

3157 CT		HCl	—	3×10^{-4}	3×10^{-6}
3297 CT		CH$_3$I	—	3×10^{-4}	3×10^{-6}
3191 CT		HCl	O	3×10^{-4}	3×10^{-6}
3235 CT		HCl	CH$_2$	3×10^{-4}	3×10^{-6}
3204 CT		HCl	C=O	3×10^{-4}	1×10^{-7}
3318 CT		CH$_3$I	C=O	1×10^{-4}	1×10^{-8}
neostigmine				1×10^{-7}	1.3×10^{-7}

FUNKE et al. (1953), JACOB and FUNKE (1953), JACOB (1955).

A series of selective acetylcholinesterase inhibitors that are derivatives of *bis* coumaranyl ketone was reported by FUNKE et al. (1953), JACOB and FUNKE (1953), and JACOB (1955) (Table 28). The maximal activity was reached when the two coumarin moieties were separated by an acyl group, and the piperidine nitrogens were quaternized with methyl groups (3318 CT). This particular compound is among the most active selective inhibitors yet reported for AChE. The author reported that the "one-half" molecule of 3318 CT was virtually inactive as an inhibitor of dog red blood cell AChE. This highly selective activity has been used as a tool to evaluate different types of cholinesterase (PAULESU et al. 1955). The high selectivity against AChE has been confirmed in two additional studies (JACOB 1956; PAULESU 1956).

Table 29. *Disubstituted benzyl derivatives of methylene, ketone, and carbinol*

$$R_1\!\!-\!\!\bigcirc\!\!-\!\!CH_2\!\!-\!\!A\!\!-\!\!CH_2\!\!-\!\!\bigcirc\!\!-\!\!R_2$$

Compound	R_1	R_2	A	pI$_{50}$ rat brain AChE	pI$_{50}$ horse serum BuChE
71C48	+NMe$_3$I	+NMe$_3$I	CH$_2$	6.1	3.6
61C47	+NMe$_3$I	+NMe$_3$I	CO	6.7	3.2
25C48	+NMe$_2$EtI	+NMe$_2$EtI	CO	7.7	< 3.0
297C50	+NMe$_2$AllI	+NMe$_2$AllI	CO	7.8	< 3.0
298C50	+NMe$_2n$PrI	+NMe$_2n$PrI	CO	7.8	< 3.0
312C50	+NMe$_2n$BuBr	+NMe$_2n$BuBr	CO	5.9	3.5
19C51	+NMe$_2$CH$_2$PhCl	+NMeCH$_2$PhCl	CO	5.3	4.8
455C50	+NMeEt$_2$I	+NMeEt$_2$I	CO	7.5	< 3.0
153C47	+NMe$_3$I	H	CO	4.0	3.0
26C48	+NMe$_3$I	OMe	CO	4.6	3.2
143C48	+NMe$_3$I	+NMe$_3$I	CHOH	5.7	< 3.0
101C48	+NMe$_3$I	OMe	CHOH	3.9	< 3.0
316C50	+NMe$_2$EtI	+NMe$_2$EtI	CHOH	5.9	< 3.0
495C50	+NMeEt$_2$I	+NMeEt$_2$I	CHOH	6.3	< 3.0
	eserine			6.5	8.0
	neostigmine			6.6	7.6

COPP (1953), FULTON and MOGEY (1954).

The activity of a large series of substituted *bis* phenyl ketones was reported by FULTON and MOGEY (1954, Table 29). These compounds are also quite selective as inhibitors of AChE. Maximal activity was reached when the quaternary groups were substituted with a total of 4 or 5 carbon atoms each (25C48, 297C50 and 298C50). Increasing the size of the quaternary head with the dimethyl-butyl grouping resulted in a sharp decrease in activity. The activity was further reduced in the dimethyl-benzyl analog. In this series, too, it should be noted that the monoquaternary analogs are relatively inactive (153C47, 26C48, and 101C48). All of the derivatives are relatively inactive as inhibitors of BuChE.

An interesting example of the marked influence of geometrical isomerism on the type and degree of inhibition was reported by BOVET-NITTI and BOVET (1953, Table 30). The *ortho* phthalyl substituted esters are relatively selective inhibitors of BuChE, while the *para* derivatives are selective inhibitors of AChE. The *ortho* substituted analogs were further evaluated by BARSTAD et al. (1959), and these results are shown in Table 31. With this isomer, they too found relatively high selectivity for BuChE. Apparently, it makes little difference in the pattern of anti-ChE activity whether or not the choline moiety has a *B*-methyl group. Triethyl substitution is as favorable for activity as the trimethyl.

A series of P, P' disubstituted biphenyl derivatives was reported by LONG and SCHUELER (1954). The compounds are shown in Table 32. In this series marked differences in activity were produced by altering the structures of the quaternary nitrogen groups. The alkyl derivatives were relatively inactive, but maximal

Table 30. *Substituted phthalic acid and isomers*

$$R = -CH_2CH_2\overset{+}{N}(C_2H_5)_3$$
$$I^-$$

$$R' = -CH_2CH_2\overset{+}{N}(C_2H_5)_2C_3H_7$$
$$I^-$$

Compound		electric eel AChE	horse serum BuChE
306 IS		no inhib.	$pI_{50} = 5$
449 IS		no inhib.	$pI_{50} = 6$
302 IS		$pI_{50} = 5$	no inhib.
452 IS		$pI_{50} = 6$	weak inhib. $pI_{50} = 2.2$

BOVET-NITTI and BOVET (1953).

activity was found where pyridinium, and especially 2- and 3-methylpyridinium groups, were substituted at both ends of the molecule. The 4-methyl pyridine analog demonstrated a sharp reduction in activity. Compound No. 11, Table 32, was found to be virtually devoid of cholinesterase inhibiting activity, but it was observed that the compound was very toxic. Later studies suggest that this compound has pharmacological properties different from those of its close analogs which are due possibly to interferance with the synthesis and/or release of ACh from sites of cholinergic transmission.

FLEMING et al. (1957) evaluated further various methyl pyridine analogs of substituted benzidine (Table 33). Here, too, the optimal activity tended to be found in the 3-methyl derivative; at least there was a sharp reduction in the activity of the 4-methyl isomer. If the methyl groups merely influenced the charge on the nitrogen atoms of these compounds, one would expect similar activities with the 2- and 4-position isomers and dissimilar activities from the 2- and 3-isomers. The comparatively high activity of the 3-methylpyridinium compound suggests that the methyl group on the pyridine ring is involved in attachment at some additional site. An alternate explanation could be that groups about the cationic site on the cholinesterase molecule may hinder the attachment of the 4-position

Table 31. *Additional analogs of phthalic acid derivatives*

Compound	R_1	R_2	R_3	R_4	I_{50} Values		
					human plasma BuChE	horse serum BuChE	rat brain AChE
330IS	H	CH_3	CH_3	CH_3	1.0×10^{-4}	1.0×10^{-4}	3.4×10^{-2}
Tx1	H	C_2H_5	CH_3	CH_3	7.0×10^{-5}	1.8×10^{-5}	7.0×10^{-2}
Tx2	CH_3	CH_3	CH_3	CH_3	3.5×10^{-5}	5.0×10^{-4}	1.0×10^{-1}
Tx3	CH_3	CH_3	CH_3	C_2H_5	7.8×10^{-6}	7.5×10^{-5}	3.2×10^{-2}
Tx4	CH_3	CH_3	C_2H_5	C_2H_5	6.6×10^{-6}	4.7×10^{-5}	2.1×10^{-2}
Tx5	CH_3	C_2H_5	C_2H_5	C_2H_5	2.0×10^{-5}	5.5×10^{-5}	3.1×10^{-2}

BARSTAD et al. (1959).

isomer and offer no interference with 2- or 3-substituted derivatives. Steric hindrance, however, would not account for the increased activity noted for the 2- or 3-substituted compounds.

The activity of a diphenyl ether analog was first reported by HERMANN and TUST (1956), and additional compounds were studied by MARSHALL and LONG (1959). These data are shown in Table 34. The same general pattern of action can be noted as has been discussed for the biphenyl and benzidine series. One obvious difference is that separation of the phenyl rings by an oxygen or methylene group results in a sharp reduction in activity. This may suggest that resonance between the two phenyl rings contributes to activity in the biphenyl series.

The first "open chain" *bis*-carbamate analogs were reported by KLUPP et al. (1953). Their results are shown in Table 35. In addition to this reference, maximal activity has also been reported for BC-9 (n = 8) by KRAUPP et al. (1953). Also STUMPF (1955) reported that BC-9 was more active as an inhibitor of AChE than of BuChE. The data shown in Table 35 indicate that in this series the degree of selectivity is related to the chain length. The closer the carbamate nitrogens are together, the greater is the tendency for selective inhibition of BuChE.

One of the most complete series of *bis*-quaternary cholinesterase inhibitors has been reported from the group at Sterling-Winthrop Research Institute. Their observations were an outgrowth of the report by HOPPE et al. (1955) that the neuromuscular blocking agent, benzoquinonium (Mytolon), possessed considerable

Table 32. bis *Phenacyl derivatives*

$$R-CH_2-C(=O)-\text{(biphenyl)}-C(=O)-CH_2-R$$

No.	R	I_{50} bovine erythrocyte AChE
1	(2-CH$_3$, N-CH$_3$ pyridinium)	8×10^{-10}
2	(3-CH$_3$ pyridinium, N—)	10^{-9}
3	(pyridinium, N—)	10^{-9}
4	HOCH$_2$CH$_2$CH$_2$—(pyridinium N—)	2×10^{-7}
5	(piperidinium, N$^+$–CH$_2$CH$_3$)	3×10^{-7}
6	(phenyl)—CH$_2$N$^+$(CH$_3$)(CH$_3$)—	5×10^{-6}
7	CH$_3$—(4-pyridinium N—)	5×10^{-6}
8	(CH$_3$CH$_2$)$_3$N$^+$—	4×10^{-6}
9	O(morpholinium N$^+$–CH$_3$)—	3×10^{-6}
10	(CH$_3$)$_3$N$^+$—	6×10^{-5}
11	HOCH$_2$CH$_2$N$^+$(CH$_3$)(CH$_3$)—	$\ll 10^{-5}$
12	neostigmine	8.5×10^{-8}

LONG and SCHUELER (1954).

Table 33. *Various* bis *substituted derivatives of benzidine*

$$R\text{(pyridinium)}N^+CH_2-C(=O)-N(H)-\text{(biphenyl)}-N(H)-C(=O)-CH_2-N^+\text{(pyridinium)}R \quad 2\,Br^-$$

Compound	R	I_{50} bovine erythrocyte AChE	I_{50} dog serum BuChE
1	H	3.8×10^{-7}	4.5×10^{-3}
2	2-CH$_3$	3.6×10^{-7}	7.1×10^{-5}
3	3-CH$_3$	8.9×10^{-8}	4.0×10^{-2}
4	4-CH$_3$	4.5×10^{-6}	4.5×10^{-4}
neostigmine	—	7.9×10^{-8}	1.3×10^{-6}

FLEMING et al. (1957).

cholinesterase-inhibiting activity (Table 36). These analogs demonstrated that the benzyl (especially 2-chlorobenzyl) substituted quaternary were much more active than the trialkyl quaternary compounds. One of the obvious dissection moieties

Table 34. *Anti-ChE activity of* bis *substituted biphenyl, biphenyl ether, and biphenyl methane derivatives*

$$R-CH_2C(O)-\langle\text{ring}\rangle-A-\langle\text{ring}\rangle-C(O)-CH_2R$$

Compound	R	A	I_{50} bovine erythro-cyte AChE
HC-3	HOCH$_2$CH$_2$N$^+$(CH$_3$)(CH$_3$)—	—	$> 2.9 \times 10^{-3}$
1	HOCH$_2$-pyridinium—	—	2.0×10^{-6}
2	HOCH$_2$-pyridinium—	—	1.9×10^{-7}
3	HOCH$_2$CH$_2$—N$^+$(CH$_3$)(CH$_3$)—	O	7.9×10^{-4}
4	HOCH$_2$-pyridinium—	O	2.9×10^{-6}
5	HOCH$_2$-pyridinium—	O	1.2×10^{-5}
6	HOCH$_2$-pyridinium—	O	8.6×10^{-5}
7[1]	pyridinium—	O	3.2×10^{-6}
8	HOCH$_2$CH$_2$N$^+$(CH$_3$)(CH$_3$)—	CH$_2$	1.5×10^{-5}

[1] HERMANN and TUST (1956), rat brain AChE.
MARSHALL and LONG (1959).

of the "benzoquinolinium" nucleus would be substituted oxamides, and the original report on the cholinesterase inhibiting action of a number of these was published by ARNOLD et al. (1954). Various pharmacological properties in relation to their cholinesterase inhibiting action have been reported (LANDS and KARCZMAR 1957;

LANDS et al. 1958; LEMME et al. 1959). The above workers have studied many of the possible structural alterations in the oxamide series. The cholinesterase

Table 35. bis *Polymethylene carbamate derivatives*

$$(CH_3)_3\overset{+}{N}-CH_2CH_2O\overset{O}{\overset{\|}{C}}-\overset{H}{N}-(CH_2)_n-\overset{H}{N}-\overset{O}{\overset{\|}{C}}-OCH_2CH_2\overset{+}{N}(CH_3)_3$$
$$I^- \qquad\qquad\qquad\qquad\qquad\qquad\qquad\qquad\qquad I^-$$

Compound	n	pI_{50}	
		dog caudate nucleus AChE	horse serum BuChE
BC-4	0	1.0	3.5
BC-12	4	4.0	3.7
BC-16	6	4.9	5.0
BC-9	8	6.8	5.9
BC-14	10	5.8	5.8
physostigmine		7.0	7.0

KLUPP et al. (1953).

inhibiting activity was discussed by LANDS et al. (1958), and the major points from an SAR consideration are summarized in Tables 37 to 40. The cholinesterase

Table 36. *Anti-ChE activity of a series of N, N′ bis (diethylaminopropyl) quinone derivatives*

Compound	R_1	R_2	R_3	X	Potency against bovine erythrocyte AChE (neostigmine = 100)
benzoquinonium Cl	C_2H_5	C_2H_5	⬡—CH_2	Cl	25.0
Win 7846	C_2H_5	C_2H_5	C_2H_5	Br	1.8
Win 3317	C_2H_5	C_2H_5	CH_3	Br	1.1
Win 7558	CH_3	CH_3	C_2H_5	Br	0.4
Win 5424	CH_3	CH_3	CH_3	Br	0.03
Win 7665	C_2H_5	C_2H_5	NO_2—⬡—CH_2	Cl	0.6
Win 7775	C_2H_5	C_2H_5	⬡(NO_2)—CH_2	Cl	11.0
Win 7758	C_2H_5	C_2H_5	Cl—⬡—CH_2	Cl	11.0
Win 7789	C_2H_5	C_2H_5	⬡(Cl)—CH_2	Cl	210.0

HOPPE et al. (1955).

inhibiting properties were greatly enhanced by benzyl substitution in the quaternary group. Also one of the most interesting features of this series is that selected

Table 37. *N, N' bis (Diethylaminoethyl) — oxamide —* bis *benzylhalide quaternary salts*

$$
\left[\begin{array}{c} \text{O} \\ \parallel \\ \text{—C—N—CH}_2\text{CH}_2\overset{+}{\underset{|}{\text{N}}}\overset{\text{X}^-}{\overset{|}{\text{—C}_2\text{H}_5}}\underset{\text{C}_2\text{H}_5}{} \\ \underset{\begin{array}{c}\text{CH}_2 \\ | \end{array}}{\text{H}} \end{array} \right]_2
$$

Compound	R	X	Potency against bovine erythrocyte AChE (neostigmine = 100)
1	H	Cl	3.6
2	2-F	I	5.1
ambenonium	2-Cl	Cl	580.0
3	2-Br	Br	4100.0
4	2-I	Br	770.0
5	2-OCH$_3$	Cl	14.0
6	2-*mono*-Cl	Cl	430.0
7	2—CH$_3$	Br	80.0
8	3-Cl	Cl	55.0
9	4-Cl	Cl	14.0
10	3,4-*di*-Cl	Cl	2.4
11	4-OCH$_3$	Cl	< 0.1

LANDS et al. (1958).

substitution in the *ortho* position of the phenyl group greatly enhanced the anti-ChE activity (Table 37). The order of activity (Br > Cl > I > F) does not follow either the size of the halogen or the expected inductive effects of these substitutions. This series suggests that on the AChE enzyme at about 5 to 6 Å from the

Table 38. *Anti-ChE activity of higher homolog derivatives of oxalic acid*

$$
(\text{C}_2\text{H}_5)_2\overset{\text{X}^-}{\overset{+}{\underset{\text{CH}_2}{\text{N}}}}\text{(CH}_2)_n\text{—N—C—(CH}_2)_r\text{—C—N—(CH}_2)_n\overset{\text{X}^-}{\underset{\text{CH}_2}{\overset{+}{\text{N(C}_2\text{H}_5)_2}}}
$$

Compound	n	r	x	Approx. N—N distance (Å)	Potency against bovine erythrocyte AChE (neostigmine = 100)
ambenonium	2	0	Cl	11.5—12.0	580.0
12	2	2	Cl	14.1—14.6	23.0
13	2	4	Cl	16.7—17.2	9.0
14	2	6	Cl	19.3—19.8	53.0
15	3	0	Cl	14.1—14.6	20.0
16	4	0	I	16.7—17.2	340.0
17	5	0	I	19.3—19.8	650.0

LANDS et al. (1958).

site for attachment of the cationic head there may be a positive center for halogen attachment. If this is the reason for increased activity, one would have to postulate further that this center must be specific with respect to size. That is, the chlorine atom may be too small, and iodine too large. This may account also for the decreased activity observed for the 2-OCH$_3$ compound (No. 5). Substitutions in other than the 2 position are not favorable for anti-ChE activity (compounds 8 to 11).

Table 38 demonstrates the influence of varying the interatomic distances between the nitrogen centers in this series of compounds (11.5 Å to 20 Å). Increasing

Table 39. *The effect of alterations in substitution in the nitrogen center of ambenonium*

Compound	R	Potency against bovine erythrocyte AChE (neostigmine = 100)	Compound	R	Potency against bovine erythrocyte AChE (neostigmine = 100)
ambenonium	C$_2$H$_5$	580	15	C$_2$H$_5$	20
18	CH$_3$	3	22	CH$_3$	1
19	CH$_2$CH$_2$CH$_3$	17	23	N	8
20	N	8	24	N	1.5
21	N	4	25	O N	7.6

LANDS et al. (1958).

the interatomic distances by adding methylene groups between the two carbonyl groups led to a decrease in activity (see ambenonium, compounds 12 to 14). This is good evidence that one or both of the carbonyl groups may be involved in attachment on the receptor surface. This possibility is strengthened further by the observation that increasing the N to N cationic distances by adding methylene groups between the amide and cationic N leads to a progressive increase in anti-ChE activity (compounds 15 to 17). The compounds in Table 39 demonstrate the high structural requirements for the substituents on the cationic head. Increasing or decreasing the size from diethyl results in a sharp decrease in activity. Even with rigid substituents (pyrrol and piperidine), which would have approximately the same volume factor, the anti-ChE activity is still relatively weak. This is also true where the amide N and cationic N are separated by three methylene groups.

That the *bis*-quaternary groups are apparently essential in this series of compounds is illustrated by the series of monoquaternary analogs outlined in Table 40. Compound 31, the monochlorobenzyl analog of ambenonium, is the only compound showing significant AChE inhibiting properties. This compound, of course, lacks the second quaternary group as well as the benzyl substitution. At any rate, the one-half molecule (No. 26) is relatively inactive. Using these compounds as models

Table 40. *The inhibition of AChE by monoquaternary compounds related to ambenonium*

$$(C_2H_5)_2\overset{+}{\underset{\underset{\overset{\displaystyle CH_2}{|}}{|}}{N}}-CH_2-CH_2-\overset{H}{\underset{|}{N}}-\overset{O}{\overset{||}{C}}-R \quad Cl^-$$

Compound	Structure	Approx. N—N distance (Å)	Potency against bovine erythrocyte AChE (neostigmine = 100)
26	H	5.5	0.2
27	CH_3	7.0	< 0.1
28	$\overset{O}{\overset{||}{C}}OC_2H_5$	9.5—10	6.4
29	$\overset{O}{\overset{||}{C}}NHC_3H_7$	10.5—11.0	6.6
30	$(CH_2)_4\overset{O}{\overset{||}{C}}OC_2H_5$	16.0—16.5	0.2
31	$\overset{O\ H}{\overset{||\ |}{C}}N(CH_2)_2N(C_2H_5)_2$	11.5—12.0	31.0
32	$\overset{O}{\overset{||}{C}}NH(CH_2)_3N(C_2H_5)_2$	12.8—13.3	6.2

LANDS et al. (1958).

Table 41. *Polymethylene* bis *trimethylammonium analogs*

$$(CH_3)_3\overset{+}{N}-(CH_2)_n-\overset{+}{N}(CH_3)_3$$

n	I_{50}			
	human plasma[1] BuChE	electric eel[1] AChE	rabbit erythrocyte[2] AChE	% inhibition at conc. of 1.25×10^{-3} rabbit serum benzyol-ChE[2]
4	4.7×10^{-2}	8.6×10^{-2}		
5	2.1×10^{-2}	4.8×10^{-2}		
6	1.1×10^{-2}	1.9×10^{-2}		
7	3.4×10^{-3}	1.2×10^{-2}	3.5×10^{-3}	
8	1.9×10^{-3}	2.4×10^{-3}	1.0×10^{-3}	
9	6.2×10^{-4}	3.0×10^{-4}	1.2×10^{-4}	
10	1.2×10^{-4}	2.0×10^{-5}	4.5×10^{-5}	8
11			1.8×10^{-5}	
12		8.2×10^{-6}	5.6×10^{-6}	35
18			1.4×10^{-5}	97
eserine			7.1×10^{-8}	

[1] BERGMANN and SEGAL (1954).
[2] PATON and ZAIMIS (1949).

for the receptor (see introduction), LANDS et al. (1958) concluded that the esteratic site on the cholinesterase molecule is not narrower than 3 Å or wider than 6 Å.

PATON and ZAIMIS (1949) and BERGMANN and SEGAL (1954) evaluated the cholinesterase inhibiting activities of various polymethylene bis-trimethylammonium salts; the results are shown in Table 41. PATON and ZAIMIS moted an increase in AChE inhibitory activity up to twelve methylene groups. The C-18 analog demonstrated a reduction in activity. They found the compounds considerably less active when evaluated on rabbit plasma cholinesterase. BERGMANN and SEGAL (1954) studied part of the same series and noted an increase in activity as the chain length was increased. A plot of the log I_{50} versus the number of linking methylene groups yielded a straight line for plasma BuChE and a sigmoid curve for electric eel AChE. The explanation offered by these workers is that electric eel AChE has two anionic sites, while human plasma BuChE contains only one. BARLOW (1955) observed that members of his *bis*-choline series demonstrated some inhibition of the two types of cholinesterase (Table 42). The acetoxy analogs were less active.

Table 42.
Polymethylene analogs of bis *choline derivatives*

$$HOCH_2CH_2\overset{\overset{\displaystyle CH_3}{|+}}{\underset{\underset{\displaystyle CH_3}{|}}{N}}{-}(CH_2)_n{-}\overset{\overset{\displaystyle CH_3}{|+}}{\underset{\underset{\displaystyle CH_3}{|}}{N}}{-}CH_2CH_2OH$$

n	% Inhibition with concentration of 10^{-3} M	
	dog caudate nucleus AChE	horse serum BuChE
5	0	33
8	78	62
9	80	82
10	89	93
11	100	94
12	100	98

BARLOW (1955).

G. Miscellaneous compounds

The following compounds embrace many of the classes of agents known to pharmacologists. One may raise the question as to whether most of the agents described below have cholinesterase inhibiting properties strong enough to have any bearing on their primary actions. However, sometimes it is just as important to know the relatively inactive compounds as those showing greater activity. It will be noted in reading the following series that most of the compounds listed inhibit cholinesterase in concentrations of 10^{-2} M to 10^{-4} M. LEVY (1947) and AUGUSTINSSON (1948) have reported detailed surveys of the earlier literature, and most of the following references pertain to work published during the past eleven years. Some earlier references are included for comparative purposes. This section will present many of the types of compounds studied, and a general range of their activities.

I. Amino acids, amines and derivatives

BERGMANN et al. (1950) reported the following values for inhibition of *Electrophorus electricus* acetylcholinesterase:

Amino acid	M conc.	% Inhibition	Amino acid	M conc.	% Inhibition
glycine	0.3	50	l-glutamic	0.04	20
l-alanine	0.12	30	d-glutamic	0.06	0
β-alanine	0.06	0	l-histidine	0.06	0
d,l-serine	0.12	13	l-proline	0.06	12
l-leucine	0.1	50	l-lysine	0.12	14
d,l-leucine	0.06	8	l-arginine	0.03	50
d,l-phenylalanine	0.06	30	d-arginine	0.24	25
l-tryptophan	0.06	18	creatine	0.03	50
p-aminobenzoic acid	0.06	23	creatinine	0.14	50
l-aspartic acid	0.08	50	nicotinic acid	0.3	50
l-glutamic acid	0.18	50	d-picolinic acid	0.1	50
trigonelline	0.18	50	betaine	0.12	50

Amides, dipeptides and esters

Amino acid	M conc.	% Inhibition		M conc.	% Inhibition
acetamide	2.0	39			
acetylglycine	0.3	20			
glycylglycine	0.12	18			
hippuric acid	0.06	24			
l-asparagine	0.06	50			
l-glutamine	0.2	50			
nicotinamide	0.05	50			
N′-methylnicotinamide methyl sulfate				0.0075	50
Coramine (nikethamide)				0.005	50
ethyl glycinate				0.03	50
ethyl picolinate				0.007	50
ethyl nicotinate				0.0007	50
β-acetylpyridine				0.002	50
β-dimethylaminobutanone				0.005	50
β-trimethylammonium butanone methyl sulfate				0.0064	50
β-dimethylaminopropionitrile				0.0075	50
β-trimethylammonium propionitrile methyl sulfate				0.0075	50
β-diethylaminopropionitrile				0.0022	50

The above study demonstrates that amino acids are weak inhibitors of AChE. However, some have been reported to be activators of serum BuChE. They inhibit the enzyme in concentrations from 0.03 to 0.3 M. The l-form of the stereoisomers is more active, therefore suggesting that the receptor is stereospecific. Esterification of the carbonyl group of amino acids tends to increase the inhibiting activity.

The I_{50} for indole is 10^{-2} M for human serum BuChE, and the methyl quaternary derivative is twice as active (WAELSCH and RACKOW 1942). Serotonin has an I_{50} of 5×10^{-3} for human serum BuChE, and is somewhat less active when evaluated on red cell AChE (LANGEMANN 1954). Histamine exhibits only weak activity against dog serum BuChE (FROMMEL et al. 1944). No inhibition by guanidine of serum BuChE was observed, but very large doses may produce activation (MINOT 1939). Iodoacetamide has been reported to be virtually inactive when evaluated on cat serum BuChE (WELS and PEPKE 1947). BENSON (1948) reported that epinephrine (adrenaline) in concentrations of 6×10^{-3} M inhibited 50% of the cholinesterase activity of swine caudate nucleus and parotid gland. He demonstrated that the potentiation of acetylcholine by adrenaline correlates with the inhibiting effects of the latter on cholinesterase. Adrenaline also inhibits cholinesterase of the frog rectus abdominus muscle (BELENKOV 1949). Adrenaline oxidized with bromine has an I_{50} value of 10^{-4} when evaluated on human serum BuChE, but adrenaline shows no inhibition when oxidized with either catechol or iodate (WAELSCH and RACKOW 1942). KASWIN (1939) reported that a concentration of 1/7,000 of quaternary N-methyladrenaline inhibited by 50% horse serum

BuChE. This is approximately twice as active as adrenaline. Using human red blood cell AChE and serum BuChE, NAESS and SKRAMSTAD (1954) reported that hydralazine (hydrazinophthalazine) was equally effective for both types of cholinesterase and that the I_{50}'s are approximately 10^{-3} M.

II. Analgesics

BERNHEIM and BERNHEIM (1936) reported that morphine and apomorphine were quite active as inhibitors of rat brain cholinesterase. These authors reported the 100% inhibitory dose, which makes comparisons with other data difficult. They did suggest that much of the pharmacological properties of these agents might be explained by their cholinesterase inhibiting properties. SLAUGHTER and Lackey (1940) were unable to confirm the above observations. They reported no inhibition of serum BuChE activity *in vitro* with concentrations of morphine up to 1 mg/0.5 ml. They did observe some depression of dog serum BuChE when the experiment was carried out *in vivo*. WRIGHT and SABINE (1943) demonstrated that inhibition depended on the source of the enzyme, and suggested that this might be related to differences in action on an organ level observed with the analgesics. EADIE et al. (1948) suggested that cholinesterase inhibition has nothing to do with analgesia, but may be related to the peripheral side-effects, e.g., cholinomimetic stimulation, as well as the emetic action (KUHN and SURLES 1938). FROMMEL (1951) evaluated a series of compounds and was unable to find any correlation between analgesic activity and cholinesterase inhibition. YOUNG et al. (1955) studied a series of morphinan derivatives and concluded that analgesia and intestinal effects are probably not dependent on anti-ChE activity. A similar conclusion was recently drawn by FOLDES et al. (1959) who evaluated a large series of analgesic agents. The data presented suggested that analgesia and the intestinal stimulating action of analgesic agents are not related to their cholinesterase inhibiting activity. The cholinesterase inhibiting potency of various analgesics is as follows:

Compound	Cholinesterase	Molar I_{50} or conc. used	Reference
morphine	dog serum	0.5 mg/ml	WRIGHT (1941)
morphine	rabbit brain	0.7 mg/ml	WRIGHT (1941)
morphine	human serum	7×10^{-3}	GOLDSTEIN (1951)
morphine	bovine erythrocyte	1.4×10^{-3}	BLOHM and GONZALES (1951)
morphine	horse serum	7.5×10^{-4}	BLOHM and GONZALES (1951)
morphine	bovine erythrocyte	27% 10^{-3}	YOUNG et al. (1955)
morphine	human plasma	4.0×10^{-3}	FOLDES et al. (1959)
morphine	human erythrocyte	9.8×10^{-4}	FOLDES et al. (1959)
Levorphan	bovine erythrocyte	95% 10^{-3}	YOUNG et al. (1955)
Levorphan	human plasma	7.1×10^{-4}	FOLDES et al. (1959)
Levorphan	human erythrocyte	5.6×10^{-5}	FOLDES et al. (1959)
d-isoamidone	dog serum	0.6 mM	GREIG and HOWELL (1948)
d-isoamidone	rat brain	>4.8 mM	GREIG and HOWELL (1948)
l-isoamidone	dog serum	0.08 mM	GREIG and HOWELL (1948)
l-isoamidone	rat brain	0.6 mM	GREIG and HOWELL (1948)
d-amidone	dog serum	0.8 mM	GREIG and HOWELL (1948)
d-amidone	rat brain	4.8 mM	GREIG and HOWELL (1948)
l-amidone	dog serum	0.2 mM	GREIG and HOWELL (1948)
l-amidone	rat brain	2.4 mM	GREIG and HOWELL (1948)
codeine	bovine erythrocyte	0% 10^{-3} M	YOUNG et al. (1955)
dihydrocodeine	human plasma	3.9×10^{-3}	FOLDES et al. (1959)
dihydrocodeine	human erythrocyte	>10^{-2}	FOLDES et al. (1959)
dihydrohydroxycodeine	human plasma	>10^{-2}	FOLDES et al. (1959)
dihydrohydroxycodeine	human erythrocyte	3.3×10^{-3}	FOLDES et al. (1959)

Compound	Cholinesterase	Molor I_{50} or conc. used	Reference
14-hydroxydihydro-morphinone	human plasma	4.6×10^{-3}	FOLDES et al. (1959)
14-hydroxydihydro-morphinone	human erythrocyte	4.6×10^{-3}	FOLDES et al. (1959)
meperidine	human plasma	2.2×10^{-3}	FOLDES et al. (1959)
meperidine	human erythrocyte	$>10^{-2}$	FOLDES et al. (1959)
alphaprodine	huamn plasma	5×10^{-4}	FOLDES et al. (1959)
alphaprodine	human erythrocyte	3.4×10^{-3}	FOLDES et al. (1959)
dextromorphan	bovine erythrocyte	$41\% \quad 10^{-3}$	YOUNG et al. (1955)
racemorphan	bovine erythrocyte	$65\% \quad 10^{-3}$	YOUNG et al. (1955)
dextrallorphan	bovine erythrocyte	$25\% \quad 10^{-3}$	YOUNG et al. (1955)
levomethorphan	bovine erythrocyte	$0\% \quad 10^{-3}$	YOUNG et al. (1955)
dextromethorphan	bovine erythrocyte	$0\% \quad 10^{-3}$	YOUNG et al. (1955)
levallorphan	bovine erythrocyte	$76\% \quad 10^{-3}$	YOUNG et al. (1955)
levallorphan	human plasma	8.5×10^{-5}	FOLDES et al. (1955)
levallorphan	human erythrocyte	4.0×10^{-5}	FOLDES et al. (1955)
N-allylnormorphine	bovine erythrocyte	1.5×10^{-3}	BLOHM and GONSALES (1951)
N-allylnormorphine	bovine erythrocyte	$36\% \quad 10^{-3}$	YOUNG et al. (1955)
N-allylnormorphine	horse serum	3.8×10^{-4}	BLOHM and GONSALES (1951)
N-allynormorphine	human plasma	2.0×10^{-4}	FOLDES et al. (1959)
N-allylnormorphine	human erythrocyte	9.8×10^{-4}	FOLDES et al. (1959)

Conclusions similar to the above results were drawn by CANNARA and ATZORI (1953), who used various analgesics to compare inhibition of enzyme obtained from various sources. It appears that from the above series of analgesics there is no relationship between cholinesterase inhibiting properties and analgesic activity.

III. Antibiotics

VINCENT et al. (1949) reported that streptomycin is a more active inhibitor of serum BuChE than of AChE, but in both cases the concentrations employed were very high. Chloramphenicol demonstrates no inhibitory action unless a concentration of 10^{-2} M is used (VINCENT and PARANT 1950). Penicillin in large doses depresses for a short time guinea pig serum cholinesterase by 15 to 20%, and also produces some inhibition of frog rectus abdominis cholinesterase (FROMMEL et al. 1946).

IV. Anticholinergic drugs

Atropine has been evaluated by several workers, and the I_{50} values for serum BuChE range from about 10^{-3} to 10^{-4}M (KASWIN 1939; GOLDSTEIN 1951; LULLMANN et al. 1952; HARDEGG et al. 1955; VINCENT and PARANT 1956).

Atropine appears to be less active against AChE than on serum BuChE (LULLMANN et al. 1952; VINCENT and PARANT 1956), and has been reported to activate cholinesterase in some concentrations (PARTENI and CORNEANU 1954). Apoatropine is about one hundred and fifty times more active than atropine against dog serum BuChE and ten times as active against nerve cholinesterase (VINCENT and PARANT 1956). TODRICK (1954) evaluated the inhibition of rat brain and intestinal mucosa cholinesterase by a large series of anticholinergic and antihistaminic agents. Comparing in vitro the inhibiting activities on brain and muscle AChE, the ratio of the first activity to the second was found to be between 5 and 60. GYERMEK (1955) studied a series of derivatives of atropine, homatropine, benzoyl-tropine, and tropine, and found the ratio of activities on AChE/BuChE to be high for the anticholinergic agents and low for the curariform ones. In general, the anticholinergic activity was proportionate to the inhibitory effect upon BuChE. The ganglionic blocking or the curariform effect varied in proportion to the AChE blocking potency. All compounds in both series had I_{50}'s between 10^{-2} and 10^{-5} M.

V. Anticoagulants

GROSSMAN et al. (1950) studied a series of ethyl biscoumacetate analogs at 2.2×10^{-4} M, using human serum BuChE. The compound with the unsubstituted 4 position (dicoumarol) exhibited 27% inhibition. Increasing the size of the ester component led to a gradual increase in activity.

VI. Anticonvulsants

Compound	M conc.	Inhibition	Cholinesterase	Reference
barbiturates—see central nervous system depressants				
trimethadione	10^{-3}	inactive	rat brain	BAIN (1950)
trimethadione	10^{-2}	99%	human serum	TORDA and WOLFF (1947)
trimethadione	10^{-2}	100%	frog brain	TORDA and WOLFF (1947)
phenacetylurea	10^{-3}	inactive	rat brain	BAIN (1950)
diphenylhydantoin	10^{-3}	inactive	rat brain	BAIN (1950)
diphenylhydantoin	10^{-2}	99%	human serum	TORDA and WOLFF (1947)
diphenylhydantoin	10^{-2}	94%	frog brain	TORDA and WOLFF (1947)
hydantoin	10^{-2}	100%	human serum	TORDA and WOLFF (1947)
hydantoin	10^{-2}	100%	frog brain	TORDA and WOLFF (1947)
diallylmalonylurea	10^{-2}	100%	human serum	TORDA and WOLFF (1947)
diallylmalonylurea	10^{-2}	93%	frog brain	TORDA and WOLFF (1947)

VII. Antihistaminics

VINCENT (1950) reported that Antergan and Neoantergan (pyrilamine) inhibit serum cholinesterase in concentrations of 20 μg/ml. TODRICK (1954) reported that promethazine has an I_{50} for rat brain cholinesterase of 1.6×10^{-3} M, and for rat intestinal mucosa cholinesterase of 2.8×10^{-5} M.

VIII. Antimalarial drugs

WRIGHT and SABINE (1948) studied the inhibition of human plasma cholinesterase by chloroquine, quinacrine, plasmochin, quinidine, quinine and paludrine. The first four drugs exhibited typical competitive inhibition; paludrine showed a combination of competitive and non-competitive types and quinine failed to fit the theoretical curves. The drugs were much more effective inhibitors of plasma BuChE than of red blood cell AChE; quinidine is an excellent selective inhibitor of the former. WAELSCH and NACHMANSOHN (1943) reported that quinacrine at 1×10^{-5} M was an equally effective inhibitor of electric eel, human serum, and human red cell cholinesterase. Quinine is effective at 10^{-3} to 10^{-4} M (NACHMANSOHN 1939, 1943; HASE et al. 1949; GOLDSTEIN 1951).

IX. Antipyretic analgesics

PULVER (1954) reported that phenylbutazone inhibits markedly the hydrolysis of acetylsalicyclic acid by rabbit serum in concentrations of 1 to 20 mg per hundred ml. Inhibition of the hydrolysis of procaine and caramiphen (Panparnit) was also observed. MIKHEL'SON (1946) reported that the following compounds in the molar concentrations listed produced 30 to 70% inhibition of "blood" cholinesterase: antipyrine (5.3×10^{-2}); aminopyrine (1.3×10^{-2}); acetanilide (7.4×10^{-3}); acetophenetidin (2.8×10^{-3}).

X. Bile acids

SCHACTER and DVORKIN (1942) reported that bile salts do not enhance the actions of acetylcholine, and the characteristic depressor response seen following intravenous administration must be due to a mechanism other than the inhibition of cholinesterase. However, ERDMANN and HENNE (1954) demonstrated that certain bile acids do have anti-ChE effects on the intestine both *in vitro* and *in vivo*. They reported that desoxycholic acid was most active. To demonstrate the above property requires larges amounts of acids, and with the normal therapeutic dosage range it is questionable whether there is inhibition of cholinesterase.

XI. Central nervous system depressants

The following outline lists the compounds, concentrations, inhibition, and cholinesterases that have been evaluated.

Compound	M conc.	Inhibition	Cholinesterase	Reference
sodium bromide	10^{-2}	activation	human serum	TORDA and WOLFF (1947)
sodium bromide	10^{-2}	activation	frog brain	TORDA and WOLFF (1947)
phenobarbital	10^{-2}	96%	human serum	TORDA and WOLFF (1947)
phenobarbital	10^{-2}	95%	frog brain	TORDA and WOLFF (1947)
phenobarbital	10^{-3}	inactive	rat brain	BAIN (1950)
phenobarbital	10^{-1}	25%	dog erythrocyte	HEIM and RHODE (1943)
barbital	10^{-3}	96%	human serum	TORDA and WOLFF (1947)
barbital	10^{-3}	94%	frog brain	TORDA and WOLFF (1947)
barbital	5×10^{-2}	25%	dog erythrocyte	HEIM and ROHDE (1943)
pentobarbital	10^{-3}	95%	human serum	TORDA and WOLFF (1947)
pentobarbital	10^{-3}	95%	frog brain	TORDA and WOLFF (1947)
hexobarbital	5×10^{-2}	25%	dog erythrocyte	HEIM and ROHDE (1943)
chloral hydrate	5×10^{-3}	I_{50}	rat brain	DYBING and DYBING (1955)
chloral hydrate	5×10^{-3}	40%	dog erythrocyte	HEIM and ROHDE (1943)
trichloroethanol	1×10^{-2}	approx. I_{50}	rat brain	DYBING and DYBING (1955)
tribromoethanol (Avertin)	10^{-2}	3%	rat brain	DYBING and DYBING (1955)
ethyl alcohol	10^{-2}	3%	rat brain	DYBING and DYBING (1955)

XII. Central nervous system stimulants

The activity of various central nervous system stimulants is shown below.

Compound	M conc.	Inhibition	Cholinesterase	Reference
strychnine	1.1×10^{-4}	43%	electric eel	NACHMANSOHN (1938,1939)
strychnine	1.6×10^{-4}	I_{50}	rat brain	BAIN (1950)
strychnine	10^{-3}	58%	human serum	TORDA and WOLFF (1947)
strychnine	10^{-3}	65%	frog brain	TORDA and WOLFF (1947)
strychnine	4×10^{-3}	I_{50}	human serum	GOLDSTEIN (1951)
strychnine	4×10^{-3}	I_{50}	horse serum	HASE et al. (1949)
nicotine	5×10^{-3}	I_{50}	rat brain	BAIN (1950)
nicotine	5×10^{-4}	32%	electric eel	NACHMANSOHN (1939)
pentylenetetrazol	10^{-3}	inactive	rat brain	BAIN (1950)
pentylenetetrazol	10^{-3}	92%	human serum	TORDA and WOLFF (1947)
picrotoxin	10^{-3}	92%	human serum	BAIN (1950)
picrotoxin	10^{-3}	76%	human serum	TORDA and WOLFF (1947)
picrotoxin	10^{-3}	78%	frog brain	TORDA and WOLFF (1947)
camphor	10^{-2}	100%	human serum	TORDA and WOLFF (1947)
amphetamine	5×10^{-2}	I_{50}	human serum	GOLDSTEIN (1951)

XIII. Dyes

The molar I_{50} concentration with human red cell AChE for methylene blue is 2.7×10^{-5} and for 2-methyl-1,4-naphthoquinone is $> 3.1 \times 10^{-3}$ (TAYLOR et al. 1952). CHOUTEAU and MORAND (1956) demonstrated that injection of trypan blue in the dog was able to lower markedly serum cholinesterase levels. Similar observations were made for brilliant cresyl blue using human serum BuChE; concentrations of approximately 20 mg/ml produced 50% inhibition (MORAND and GAY 1953). The pI_{50} values of the following compounds for horse serum were reported by HASE et al. (1949): 1,1'-diethyl 4,4'-monomethinequinocyamine iodide (5.4); p-dimethylamino benzylidinal epidine ethylbromide (5.6); 4-(d-pyridyl-amino) ethenylquinoline ethiodide (5.4).

XIV. General anesthetics

TORDA (1943) reported that both chloroform and ether inhibit cat muscle cholinesterase *in vitro*, and that chloroform is about forty times as active as ether. ADRIANI and ROVENSTINE (1941) reported that no inhibition of human serum BuChE was observed with nitrous oxide, ethylene, cyclopropane, ethyl ether, divinyl ether, chloroform or paradehyde when saturated solutions were used. Ether and chloroform during deep general anesthesia did not inhibit cat serum BuChE. (MIQUEL 1946).

XV. Hormones

TORDA (1943a) reported the following depression of steer brain cholinesterase by the hormones listed; the amount in 2 ml used is shown in brackets: follutein [5 IU] — 24%; estrone suspension [100 IU] — 22%; progestin [1 IU] — 18%; testosterone propionate [25 mg] — 19%; pitressin [2 IU] — 13%; pitocin [5 IU] 0%. Due to the low water solubility of some of these hormones, the above author could not evaluate accurately the amounts dissolved.

XVI. Inorganic ions and substituted inorganic compounds

MOUNTER and WHITTAKER (1953) studied a very large series of various heavy metal salts, and also included a summary of values obtained by earlier workers. A large number of metallic ions was evaluated as activators or inhibitors of serum BuChE by FROMMEL et al. (1944). Fluoride poisoning was demonstrated not to be related to inhibition of cholinesterase (DYBING and LOE 1956). A large series of arylarsonic and diarlyarsinic acids was evaluated by FREEDMAN and DOAK (1955) for cholinesterase inhibition. The activity of complex ions was studied by DWYER et al. (1952).

XVII. Local anesthetics

Compound	M conc.	Inhibition	Cholinesterase	Reference
procaine	2.4×10^{-3}	I_{50}	electric eel	SKOU (1956a)
procaine	3.2×10^{-4}	I_{50}	human erythrocyte	SKOU (1956b)
procaine	1.6×10^{-3}	inactive	dog erythrocyte	GREIG et al. (1950)
procaine	2×10^{-4}	I_{50}	human serum	GOLDSTEIN (1951)
cocaine	2.6×10^{-3}	I_{50}	electric eel	SKOU (1956a)
cocaine	2.2×10^{-3}	I_{50}	human erythrocyte	SKOU (1956b)
cocaine	6.0×10^{-3}	I_{50}	dog caudate	BLASCHKO et al. (1947)

Compound	M conc.	Inhibition	Cholinesterase	Reference
tropacocaine	3.5×10^{-4}	I_{50}	electric eel	Skou (1956a)
tropacocaine	1.8×10^{-4}	I_{50}	human erythrocyte	Skou (1956b)
dibucaine	6.7×10^{-4}	I_{50}	electic eel	Skou (1956a)
dibucaine	3.2×10^{-4}	I_{50}	human erythrocyte	Skou (1956b)
dibucaine	1.6×10^{-3}	25%	dog erythrocyte	Greig et al. (1950)
methoxyphenamine	1.6×10^{-3}	18%	dog erythrocyte	Greig et al. (1950)
mesidicaine	1.6×10^{-3}	14%	dog erythrocyte	Greig et al. (1950)
pyrrolocaine	1.6×10^{-3}	44%	dog erythrocyte	Greig et al. (1950)
butacaine	1.6×10^{-3}	68%	dog erythrocyte	Greig et al. (1950)
tetracaine	4×10^{-4}	I_{50}	electric eel	Skou (1956a)

XVIII. Quaternary compounds, miscellaneous

Compound	M conc.	Inhibition	Cholinesterase	Reference
choline	2×10^{-3}	10.6%	rat diaphragm	Stovner (1956)
choline	5×10^{-3}	21%	rat diaphragm	Stovner (1956)
choline	5.5×10^{-2}	I_{50}	human plasma	Bergmann and Wurzel (1953)
choline	4.0×10^{-3}	I_{50}	electric eel	Bergmann and Wurzel (1953)
tetramethyl-ammonium	2.5×10^{-2}	I_{50}	electric eel	Bergmann and Wurzel (1953)
tetramethyl-ammonium	6.0×10^{-2}	I_{50}	human plasma	Bergmann and Wurzel (1953)
tetraethylammonium	4.0×10^{-2}	I_{50}	human plasma	Bergmann and Wurzel (1953)
tetraethylammonium	3×10^{-3}	I_{50}	electric eel	Bergmann and Wurzel (1953)
tetraethylammonium	6×10^{-3}	I_{50}	human serum	Kensler and Elsner (1951)
tetra-n-propyl-ammonium	5.5×10^{-3}	I_{50}	human plasma	Bergmann and Wurzel (1953)
tetra-n-propyl-ammonium	1.5×10^{-4}	I_{50}	electric eel	Bergmann and Wurzel (1953)
tetra-n-butyl-ammonium	2×10^{-3}	I_{50}	human plasma	Bergmann and Wurzel (1953)
$(CH_3)_3\overset{+}{N}-CH_2CH_2\overset{\overset{\displaystyle O}{\|}}{C}-OCH_3$	1.6×10^{-2}	I_{50}	bovine erythrocyte	Bass et al. (1950)
hexamethonium	1.6×10^{-3}	I_{50}	human plasma	Bergmann and Wurzel (1953)
hexamethonium	$< 10^{-1}$	I_{50}	electric eel	Bergmann and Wurzel (1953)
decamethonium	6×10^{-5}	I_{50}	human plasma	Bergmann and Wurzel (1953)
decamethonium	2.5×10^{-5}	I_{50}	electric eel	Bergmann and Wurzel (1953)
decamethonium	0.1 as active as neostigmine		bovine erythrocyte	Hoppe et al. (1955)
decamethonium	2.5×10^{-5}	I_{50}	electric eel	Bergmann et al. (1950)
decamethonium	4.5×10^{-5}	I_{50}	rabbit erythrocyte	Paton and Zaimis (1949)
decamethonium	1.5×10^{-5}	I_{50}	rabbit serum cholinesterase	Cogni (1950—1951)
d-tubocurarine chloride	1.5×10^{-4}	I_{50}	serum	Cogni (1950—1951)
d-tubocurarine chloride	1.2×10^{-3}	I_{50}	nerve	Cogni (1950—1951)

The acetylenic quaternary analogs of acetylcholine are active at about 10^{-3} M (Jacob and Olomucki 1952).

XIX. Vesicants

The inhibition of rat brain cholinesterase by a large series of β-chlorinated amines was reported by Bain (1950).

Compound	I_{50} M
methyl *bis* (β-chloroethyl) amine	1.2×10^{-4}
ethyl *bis* (β-chloroethyl) amine	1.8×10^{-4}
propyl *bis* (β-chloroethyl) amine	2.0×10^{-4}
butyl *bis* (β-chloroethyl) amine	4.5×10^{-4}
metho *bis* (β-chloroethyl) amine	4.0×10^{-4}
benzyl *bis* (β-chloroethyl) amine	0.3×10^{-4}
diethyl (β-dichloro*iso*propyl) amine	3.0×10^{-4}
diethyl (β-dichloro*iso*butyl) amine	2.6×10^{-4}
N-(2-(2-biphenyloxy) ethyl)-N-(2-chloroethyl butylamine)	2.5×10^{-5}
N-(2-bromoethyl)N-ethyl)N-ethyl-1-naphthylenemethylamine	3.0×10^{-5}
N-(2-chloroethyl) dibenzylamine	3×10^{-4}

N-methylamine HCl (DDM) 8.7×10^{-5}, human brain   ADAMS and THOMPSON (1948)
N-methylamine HCl (DDM) 8.7×10^{-5}, human erythrocyte   ADAMS and THOMPSON (1948)

Using brain cholinesterase, β, β'-dichlorodiethyl-N-methyl amine hydrochloride (DDM) has been demonstrated to be somewhat reversible (THOMPSON 1942) and to be a selective inhibitor of AChE (ADAMS and THOMPSON 1948). THOMPSON (1947) also demonstrated that DDM was considerably more active than either carbomethoxy-β-chloroethylnitrosamine or mustard gas.

XX. Vitamins

Compound	M conc.	Inhibition	Cholinesterase	Reference
thiamine*	6×10^{-3}	I_{50}	rat plasma	GJONE and SKRAMSTAD (1955)
thiamine*	2×10^{-3}	I_{50}	horse or rat serum	GLICK (1939)

     * Probably non-competitive. Thiamine does not reactivate cholinesterase that has been inhibited by eserine (DE BETTENCOURT and CARDOSO 1948). *d,l*-Tocopheryl phosphate is a weak inhibitor of cholinesterase, being believed to act as an anionic detergent; its effect *in vitro* bears no relation to the physiological action of vitamin E (VAN DER MEER and NIEUWERKERK 1951).

XXI. Xanthine derivatives

     A number of studies has been directed toward demonstrating that some of the pharmacological properties of xanthine derivatives are related to their cholinesterase inhibiting activity. However, as the following data indicate, these compounds are at best only very weak inhibitors.

Compound	M conc.	Inhibition	Cholinesterase	Reference
caffeine	5×10^{-2}	approx. I_{50}	dog serum	VINCENT and PARANT (1954)
caffeine	5×10^{-2}	0	human serum	VINCENT and PARANT (1954)
caffeine	4×10^{-3}	approx. I_{50}	sheep brain	VINCENT (1950)
caffeine	$> 2 \times 10^{-2}$	I_{50}	dog serum	VINCENT (1950)
theobromine	2×10^{-3}	approx. I_{50}	sheep brain	VINCENT (1950)
theobromine	$\gg 2 \times 10^{-3}$	I_{50}	dog serum	VINCENT (1950)
theophylline	2×10^{-2}	approx. I_{50}	sheep brain	VINCENT (1950)
theophylline	$> 2 \times 10^{-2}$	I_{50}	dog serum	VINCENT (1950)
theophylline ethylene- diamine				
(aminophylline)	1×10^{-2}	approx. I_{50}	sheep brain	VINCENT (1950)
(aminophylline)	2×10^{-2}	approx. I_{50}	dog serum	VINCENT (1950)

     BOUNAMEAUX and GOFFART (1948, 1949) demonstrated that caffeine in pharmacological doses does not inhibit either BuChE or AChE.

Literature

ADAMS, D. H., and R. H. S. THOMPSON: Selective inhibition of cholinesterases. Biochem. J. **42**, 170—175 (1948).

ADRIANI, J., and E. A. ROVENSTINE: The effect of anesthetic drugs on activity of cholinesterase. Anesthesia and Analgesia **20**, 109—111 (1941).

AESCHLIMANN, J. A., and M. REINERT: Pharmacological action of some analogues of physostigmine. J. Pharmacol. **43**, 413—444 (1931).

—, and A. STEMPEL: Festschr. EMIL BARELL, Basel, p. 306 (1946).

ARNOLD, A., A. E. SORIA and F. K. KIRCHNER: A new anticholinesterase oxamide. Proc. Soc. exp. Biol. (N. Y.) **87**, 393—394 (1954).

ARON, E., A. D. HERSCHBERG and E. FROMMEL: Influence des acides amines sur la cholinestérase. Helv. physiol. pharmacol. Acta **2**, 495—505 (1944).

AUGUSTINSSON, K.-B.: Cholinesterases — A study in comparative enzymology. Acta physiol. scand. **15**, 1—179, Suppl. 52 (1948).

—, and D. NACHMANSOHN: Comments and Communications — Distinction between acetylcholine-esterase and other choline estersplitting enzymes. Science **110**, 98 (1949).

BACQ, Z. M., and G. L. BROWN: Pharmacological experiments on mammalian voluntary muscle in relation to the theory of chemical transmission. J. Physiol. (Lond.) **89**, 45—60 (1937).

BAIN, J. A.: Inhibition of rat brain cholinesterase by B-chlorinated amines. Amer. J. Physiol. **160**, 187—194 (1950).

BARLOW, R. B.: A series of polymethylene bis acetoxyethyl-dimethylammonium salts. Brit. J. Pharmacol. **10**, 168—172 (1955).

—, and J. M. HIMMS: The anticholinesterase activity of polymethylene bisquinolinium salts. Brit. J. Pharmacol. **10**, 173—174 (1955).

BARSTAD, J. A. B., K. H. S. KRAMSTAD and S. OKSNE: Some bisquaternary phthalyl esters as pseudocholinesterase inhibitors and neuro-muscular blocking agents. Arch. int. Pharmacodyn. **121**, 395—403 (1959).

BASS, W. B., F. W. SCHUELER, R. M. FEATHERSTONE and E. G. GROSS: Preliminary studies on the "reversed carboxyl" analogue of acetylcholine. J. Pharmacol. **100**, 465—481 (1950).

BECKETT, A. H.: Analgesics and their antagonists: some steric and chemical considerations. J. Pharm. (Lond.) **8**, 848—859 (1956).

BELENKOV, N. Yu.: Action of adrenaline on cholinesterase activity. Fiziol. Zhur. U.S.S.R. (Russian) (J. Physiol.) **34**, 223—227 (1948), C. A. **42**, 8338a.

BENSON, W. M.: Inhibition of cholinesterase by adrenaline. Proc. Soc. exp. Biol. (N. Y.) **68**, 598—601 (1948).

BERGMANN, F.: The Physical Chemistry of Enzymes, p. 126 (No. 20, Discussions of the Faraday Society) Aberdeen University Press 1956.

—, and R. SEGAL: Relations of quaternary ammonium salts to the anionic sites of true and pseudo cholinesterase. Biochem. J. **58**, 692—698 (1954).

—, I. B. WILSON and D. NACHMANSOHN: Acetylcholinesterase IX. Structural features determining the inhibition by amino acids and related compounds. J. biol. Chem. **186**, 693 to 703 (1950).

— — — The inhibitory effect of stilbamidine, curare and related compounds and its relationship to the active groups of acetylcholine esterase. Biochim. biophys. Acta **6**, 217—224 (1950a).

—, and M. WURZEL: The active surface of pseudo-cholinesterase and the possible role of this enzyme in conduction. Biochim. biophys. Acta **11**, 440—441 (1953).

BERNHEIM, F., and M. L. C. BERNHEIM: Action of drugs on the cholinesterase of the brain. J. Pharmacol. **57**, 427—436 (1936).

DE BETTENCOURT, J. M., and M. R. CARDOSO: Aneurine et inhibition de là cholinestérase par l'ésérine. C. R. Soc. Biol. (Paris) **142**, 1149 (1948).

BLASCHKO, H., E. BULBRING and T. C. CHOU: Tubocurarine antagonism and inhibition of cholinesterases. Brit. J. Pharmacol. **4**, 29—32 (1949).

—, T. C. CHOU and I. WAJDA: Inhibition of esterases by paludrine. Brit. J. Pharmacol. **2**, 116—120 (1947).

BLOCH, H.: Darstellung und Pharmakologie des Isobutyryl — 3-oxyphenyltrimethylammonium-methylsulfats und einiger Verwandter Verbindungen. Naunyn-Schmiedeberg's Arch. exp. Path. Pharmak. **193**, 292—304 (1939).

BLOHM, T. R., and W. G. WILLMORE: Effects of N-allylmorphine on cholinesterases. Proc. Soc. exp. Biol. (N. Y.) **77**, 718—721 (1951).

BODANSKY, O.: Cholinesterase. Ann. N. Y. Acad. Sci. **47**, 521—547 (1946).

BOUNAMEAUX, Y., and M. GOFFART: Activité anticholinestérasique de la caféine. C. R. Soc. Biol. (Paris) **142**, 1193—1194 (1948).
— — Pouvoir anticholinesterasique de la caféine, de la theophylline et de la theobromine. Arch. int. Pharmacodyn. **80**, 361—377 (1949).
BOVET-NITTI, F., and D. BOVET: Bis (2-diaethylaminoethyl)-benzol-dicarbonsäureester-dialkyljodide als spezifische Hemmstoffe der Truecholinesterase und der Pseudo-cholinesterase. Naunyn-Schmiedeberg's Arch. exp. Path. Pharmak. **220**, 52—61 (1953).
BOVET, D., S. COUVOISIER, R. DUCROT and R. HORCLOIS: Propriétés curarisantes du di-iodo-éthylate de bis (quinoéyl-oxy-8) 1.5 pentane. C. R. Acad. Sci. (Paris) **223**, 597—600 (1946).
BROWN, B. B., E. TAYLOR and H. H. WERNER: A comparative study of tetramethoquin, a new parasympathetic stimulant, neostigmine and physostigmine. Arch. int. Pharmacodyn. **81**, 276—283 (1950).
BÜLBRING, E., and F. DEPIERRE: The action of synthetic curarizing compounds on skeletal muscle and sympathetic ganglia both normal and denervated. Brit. J. Pharmacol. **4**, 22—28 (1949).
BURGEN, A. S., and F. HOBBIGER: The inhibition of cholinesterases by alkylphosphates and alkylphenolphosphates. Brit. J. Pharmacol. **6**, 593—601 (1951).
CANNARA, A., and A. M. ATZORI: Comparative research on the action of some phenantherene alkaloids of opium and their derivatives on serum cholinesterase of different species. (Italian) Med. sper. **24**, 318—330 (1953). C. A. **50**, 8067 C.
CASIER, H.: Action de diverses substances sur les cholinestérase sanguines. Arch. int. Pharmacodyn. **82**, 155—180 (1950).
CHOUTEAU, J., and P. MORAND: Inhibition partielle de l'activité cholinestérasique sérique chez le chien.par injection de bleu trypan. C. R. Soc. Biol. (Paris) **150**, 209—212 (1956).
COGNI, G.: Inhibiting action of some new curare like compounds on cholinesterase. (Italian) Atti. Soc. lombarda sci. med. biol. **6**, 162—166 (1950—1951). C. A. **47**, 2376 b.
COHEN, H. L., and K. R. UNNA: Correlation between cholinesterase inhibition and acetylcholine potentiation of some phenolic quaternary ammonium compounds. J. Pharmacol. **103**, 340—341 (1951).
COPP, F. C.: Diacid bases. I. Compounds related to 1,5-diphenylpentane-P,P'- *bis* (trialkylammonium) salts as anticholinesterases. J. chem. Soc. 3116—3118 (1953).
DEPIERRE, F., and A. FUNKE: Anticholinestérasiques. II. Dériviés analogues à la prostigmine. Influence sur la structure chimique sur l'intensité et la séelivité de l'action antiacétyl-cholinestérasique. C. R. Acad. Sci. (Paris) **239**, 370—372 (1954).
DWYER, F. P., E. C. GYARFAS, W. P. ROGERS and J. H. KOCH: Biological activity of complex ions. Nature (Lond.) **170**, 190—191 (1952).
DYBING, F., and O. DYBING: Anticholinesterase and anticurare effects of chloral hydrate and trichloroethanol. Acta pharmacol. (Kbh.) **11**, 398—404 (1955).
EADIE, G. S., F. BERNHEIM and D. B. FITZGERALD: The inhibition of the cholinesterase of rat brain by methadon. J. Pharmacol. **94**, 19—21 (1948).
EASSON, L. H., and E. STEDMAN: Studies on the relationship between chemical constitution and physiological action. Biochem. J. **27**, 1257—1266 (1933).
ELLIS, S.: Studies on physostigmine and related substances. IV. Chemical studies on physostigmine break down products and related epinephrine derivatives. J. Pharmacol. **79**, 364 to 372 (1943).
—, O. KRAYER and F. L. PLACHTE: Studies on physostigmine and related substances. II. The destruction of physostigmine in buffered solutions and in serum. J. Pharmacol. **79**, 295 to 308 (1943 a).
— — — Studies on physostigmine and related substances. III. Breakdown products of physostigmine; their inhibitory effect on cholinesterase and their pharmacological action. J. Pharmacol. **79**, 309—319 (1943 b).
ENGELHART, E., u. O. LOEWI: Fermentative Azetylcholinspaltung im Blut und ihre Hemmung durch Physostigmine. Naunyn-Schmiedeberg's Arch. exp. Path. Pharmak. **150**, 1—13 (1930).
ERDMANN, W. D., and H. F. HENNE: Spasmolytische Wirkungen von Gallensäuren auf Glattmuskelige Organe. Arch. int. Pharmacodyn. **98**, 45—65 (1954).
EVANS, F. T., P. W. S. GRAY, H. LEHMANN and E. SILK: Sensitivity to succinylcholine in relation to serum cholinesterase. Lancet **262**, 1229—1230 (1952).
FLEMING, W. J., J. P. LONG, R. J. WULF and R. M. FEATHERSTONE: Some pharmacologic properties of a new series of cholinesterase inhibitors. J. Pharmacol. **121**, 113—118 (1957).
FOLDES, F. F., and M. H. AVEN: The inhibition of the hydrolysis of procaine and 2-chloro-procaine in plasma by neostigmine and dimethylcarbamate of (2-hydroxy-5-phenylbenzyl) trimethylammonium bromide (Ro 2-683). J. Pharmacol. **105**, 253—258 (1952).

FOLDES, F. F., E. G. ERDOS, N. BAART, J. ZWART, and E. K. ZSIGMOND: Inhibition of human cholinesterases by narcotic analgesics and their antagonists. Arch. int. Pharmacodyn. 120, 286—291 (1959).
—, G. VAN HEES, D. L. DAVIS and S. P. SHANER: The structure-action relationships of urethane type cholinesterase inhibitors. J. Pharmacol. 122, 457—464 (1958).
FREEDMAN, D., and G. O. DOAK: The anticholinesterase activity of arylarsonic and diarylarsinic acids. J. Amer. chem. Soc. 77, 6374—7376 (1955).
FROMMEL, E., E. ARON, A. D. HERSCHBERG, J. PIQUET and A. GOLDFEDER: Influence de l'histamine sur l'action de l'acétylcholine et de la cholinestérase. Helv. physiol. pharmacol. Acta 2, 111—120 (1944).
—, M. BECK, BECK, I. T. D. MELKONIAN, R. WYSS, F. VALLETTE and M. DUCOMMUN: The relation of opium alkaloids to cholinergy. Actualités pharmacol. 3, 157—181 (1951). C. A. 49, 5685i.
—, A. GOLDFEDER and J. PIQUET: Some secondary effects of penicillin on experimental animals; influence on cholinesterase and ascorbic acid. Acta pharmacol. (Kbh.) 2, 207—211 (1946).
—, A. D. HERSCHBERG and J. PIQUET: Effects des ions inorganiques sur l'activité de la cholinestérase sérique. Helv. physiol. pharmacol. Acta 2, 169—191 (1944).
FULTON, M. P., and C. A. MOGEY: Some selective inhibitors of true cholinesterase. Brit. J. Pharmacol. 9, 138—144 (1954).
FUNKE, A., J. BAGOT and F. DEPIERRE: Anticholinestérasiques. I. Synthèse de diphénoxyalcanes porteurs d'une ou deux fonctions phenoliques librés. C. R. Acad. Sci. (Paris) 239, 329—331 (1954).
—, F. DEPIERRE and M. W. KRUCKER: Exaltation de l'activité anticholinestérasique des sels d'ammonium quaternaire des phénoxyalcanes par l'introduction de groupements uréthanes. C. R. Acad. Sci. Nr. 7, 762—764 (1952).
—, J. JACOB and K. DANIKEN: Propriétés analgésiques et anticholinestérasiques du dichlorhydrate et du diiodométhylate de la bis (pipéridinométhyl-coumaranyl-5) cetone. C. R. Acad. Sci. (Paris) 236, 149—151 (1953).
GLICK, D., and W. ANTOPOL: The inhibition of choline esterase by thiamine (Vitamin B₁). J. Pharmacol. 65, 389—394 (1939).
GOLDSTEIN, A.: The mechanism of enzyme-inhibitor-substrate reactions illustrated by the cholinesterase-physostigmine-acetylcholine system. J. gen. Physiol. 27, 529—580 (1944).
— Properties and behaviors of purified human plasma cholinesterase. III. Competitive inhibition by prostigmine and other alkaloids with special reference to differences in kinetic behavior. Arch. Biochem. 34, 169—188 (1951).
GREIG, M. E., W. C. HOLLAND and P. E. LINDVIG: The anesthetization of the rabbit cornea by nonsurface anesthetics. Brit. J. Pharmacol. 5, 461—464 (1950).
GREIG, M. R., and R. S. HOWELL: Comparison of effects of d- and l-isomers of amidone and isoamidone on cholinesterase. Proc. Soc. exp. Biol. (N. Y.) 68, 352—354 (1948).
GROSSMANN, V., I. M. HAIS and B. KASALICKY: Inhibition of human serum cholinesterase by some 4 hydroxycoumarin derivatives. Nature (Lond.) 165, 276 (1950).
GYERMEK, L.: Cholinergic blocking substances. VII. Correlations between anticholinergic and cholinesterase blocking effects. Acta physiol. Acad. Sci. hung. 8, 43—48 (1955).
HARDEGG, W., R. DOHRMANN u. D. BECHINGER: Weitere Untersuchungen über die Kinetik der Cholinesterasen und ihre Beeinflussung durch Atropin. Naunyn-Schmiedeberg's Arch. exp. Path. Pharmak. 224, 55—65 (1955).
HASE, I. E., Y. MIZUNO and N. KALAYANAGI: Inhibitory effect of cyanine and styryl dyes upon cholinesterase. (Japanese.) Bull. Chem. Soc. Japan 22, 250—255 (1949). C. A. 45, 7176e.
HAWKINS, R. D., and J. M. GUNTER: Studies on cholinesterase. V. Selective inhibition of pseudocholinesterase in vivo. Biochem. J. 40, 192—197 (1946).
—, and B. MENDEL: Cholinesterase. VI. Selective inhibition of true cholinesterase in vivo. Biochem. J. 44, 260—264 (1949).
HAZARD, R., J. CHEYMOL and E. CORTEGGIANI: Effets anticholinestérasiques et action sensibilisante sur l'acétylcholine de quelques curares de synthèse. Naunyn-Schmiedeberg's Arch. exp. Path. Pharmak. 220, 62—68 (1953).
HEIM, F., and W. ROHDE: Die Wirkung Hehrerer Narkotica auf die Aktivität der Cholinesterase des Blutes. Naunyn-Schmiedeberg's Arch. exp. Path. Pharmak. 202, 215—218 (1943).
HENRY, T. A.: The Plant Alkaloids, Ed. 4. Philadelphia: Blakiston, 1949.
HERMANN, R. G., and R. H. TUST: Studies on a new cholinesterase inhibitor. J. Pharmacol. 117, 75—81 (1956).
HERZFELD, E., O. KRAUPP, K. PATEISKY and CH. STUMPF: Pharmakologische und Klinische Wirkungen des Cholinesterasehemmkörpers Hexamethylen-bis-(N-methyl-carbaminoyl-1-methyl-3-oxy-pyridinium-bromid (BC-51)). Wien. klin. Wschr. 69, 245—271 (1957).

424   Literature

HOBBIGER, F.: The mechanism of anticurare action of certain neostigmine analogues. Brit. J.
    Pharmacol. **7**, 223—236 (1952).
HOLTON, P., and H. R. ING: Specificity of the trimethylammonium group in acetylcholine.
    Brit. J. Pharmacol. **4**, 190—196 (1949).
HOPPE, J. O., and A. ARNOLD: Influence of alkyl substitution in the onium nitrogen centers
    of Mytolon. Fed. Proc. **11**, 358—359 (1952).
—, J. E. FUNNELL and H. LAPE: The effects of structural variation in the quaternary nitrogen
    centers of benzoquinonium chloride upon neuromuscular blocking activity. J. Pharmacol.
    115, 106—119 (1955).
HUNT, R., and R. R. RENSHAW: Action of certain heterocyclic compounds on the autonomic
    nervous system. J. Pharmacol. **35**, 75—84 (1929).
JACOB, J.: Propriétés antiacétylcholinestérasiques spécifiques du diiodométhylate de la
    bis (piperidinométhylcoumaranyl-5) cétone (3318 CT). I. Relations entre la structure
    chimique et le pouvoir antiacétylcholinestérasique-pouvoirs inhibiteurs, in vitro et in vivo.
    Arch. int. Pharmacodyn. **101**, 446—468 (1955).
— Propriétés antiacétylcholinestérasiques spécifiques du diiodomethylate de la *bis* (piperidino-
    méthyl coumaranyl 5) cétone (3318 CT). II. Propriétés pharmacologiques. Arch. int.
    Pharmacodyn. **106**, 395—436 (1956).
—, and A. FUNKE: Relations entre la structure chimique et les propriétés anticholinestérasiques
    d'un groupe d'inhibiteurs sélectifs de l'acétycholinestérase globulaire du chien. C. R. Acad.
    Sci. (Paris) **237**, 1809—1811 (1953).
—, and A. OLOMUCKI: Comportement de divers sels d'ammonium quaternaire acétyléniques
    vis-à-vis des cholinestérases sérique et globulaire. C. R. Acad. Sci. (Paris) **235**, 263—264
    (1952).
JACOBI, H. P., P. A. STOESZ and A. R. MCINTYRE: *d*-Tubocurarine chloride and enzyme
    activity. J. Pharmacol. **99**, 350—357 (1950).
KARCZMAR, A. G.: Antagonism between a *bis*-quaternary oxamide, Win 8078, and depolarizing
    and competitive blocking agents. J. Pharmacol. **119**, 39—47 (1957).
—, and J. W. HOWARD: Antagonism of *d*-tubocurarine and other pharmacologic properties
    of certain *bis* quaternary salts of basically substituted oxamides. J. Pharmacol. **113**, 30—39
    (1955).
KASWIN, A.: Action inhibitrice des ammoniums quaternaires sur l'activité de la cholinestérase
    du sérum sanguin. C. R. Soc. Biol. (Paris) **130**, 859—862 (1939).
KENSLER, C. J., and R. W. ELSNER: Tetraethylammonium and cholinesterase activity. J.
    Pharmacol. **102**, 196—199 (1951).
KOELLE, G.: Histochemical demonstration of reversible anticholinesterase action at selective
    cellular sites *in vivo*. J. Pharmacol. **120**, 488—503 (1957).
KLUPP, H., O. KRAUPP, H. G. SCHWARZACHER u. CH. STUMPF: Cholinesterase-Hemmwirkung
    und pharmakologische Eigenschaften von Octamethylen-*bis*-carbaminoyl-*m*-trimethyl-
    ammoniumphenol. Arch. int. Pharmacodyn. **101**, 205—227 (1955).
— — H. STORMANN u. E. STUMPF: Über die pharmakologischen Eigenschaften einiger Poly-
    methylen-Dicarbaminsäure-bis-cholinester. Arch. int. Pharmacodyn. **96**, 161—182 (1953).
KRAUPP, O., H. KLUPP, H. STORMANN u. E. STUMPF: Cholinesterase-Hemmwirkung und
    neuro-muskuläre Wirksamkeit von bis-choline Polymethylen-dicarbaminsäureestern.
    Naunyn-Schmiedeberg's Arch. exp. Path. Pharmak. **222**, 180—182 (1954).
—, CH. STUMPF, E. HERZFELD u. B. PILLAT: Pharmakologische Eigenschaften einiger lang-
    wirksamer Cholinesterase-Hemmkörper aus der Reihe der Polymethylen-*bis*-(Carbaminoly-
    m-Trimethylammoniumphenole). Arch. int. Pharmacodyn. **102**, 281—303 (1955).
KUHN, H. H., and D. SURLES: The action of various members of the morphine series and
    emetine on the cholinesterase of the brain. Arch. int. Pharmacodyn. **58**, 88—92 (1938).
LANDS, A. M., J. O. HOPPE, A. ARNOLD and F. K. KIRCHNER: An investigation of the structure-
    activity correlations within a series of ambenonium analogs. J. Pharmacol. **123**, 121—127
    (1958).
— — A. G. KARCZMAR and A. ARNOLD: The action of ambernonium (win 8077) and related
    compounds in the mouse. J. Pharmacol. **119**, 541—549 (1957).
—, and A. G. KARCZMAR: Mechanism of *d*-tubocurarine antagonism of certain *bis* quaternary
    salts of basically substituted oxamides (win 8077 and analogs). Fed. Proc. **14**, 361 (1955).
— — J. W. HOWARD and A. ARNOLD: An evaluation of the pharmacologic action of some
    bis quaternary salts of basically substituted oxamides (win 8077) and analogs. J. Pharmacol.
    115, 185—198 (1955).
LANGEMANN, H.: 5-Oxy-Tryptamin als Anticholinesterase. Helv. physiol. pharmacol. Acta
    12, C 28 (1954).
LEHMANN, G.: Barrell Jubilee Vol., p. 314, Basle (1946).

LEMME, C. C., L. SOLLERO and B. HARGREAVES: In vitro activity of N-N'-bis (diethylamino-ethyl) oxamide bis benzyl-chloride (Mytelase) on the cholinesterase of the electric organ of electrophorus etetricus, L. Arch. int. Pharmacodyn. 121, 59—64 (1959).

LEVIN, A. P., and B. J. JANDORF: Inactivation of cholinesterase by compounds related to neostigmine. J. Pharmacol. 113, 206—211 (1955).

LÉVY, J.: Les cholinestérases. J. Physiol. (Paris) 39, 413—458 (1947).

—, and E. MICHEL-BER: Sur les propriétés gangliopléginnes, curarisantes et anticholin-estérasigues de quelques vinylogues des alcoyl-climéthyl-B-hydroxyéthylammonium. C. R. Soc. Biol. (Paris) 149, 1356—1358 (1955).

LINEWEAVER, H., and D. BURK: The determination of enzyme dissociation constants. J. Amer. Chem. Soc. 56, 658—666 (1934).

LONG, J. P., F. P. LUDUENA, B. F. TULLAR and A. M. LANDS: Stereochemical factors involved in cholinolytic activity. J. Pharmacol. 117, 29—38 (1956).

—, and F. W. SCHUELER: A new series of cholinesterase inhibitors. J. Amer. pharm. Ass. sci. Ed. 43, 79—86 (1954).

LULLMANN, H., W. FORSTER u. E. WESTERMANN: Über eine ,,Paradoxe" Atropinwirkung an isolierten Organen und ihre statistische Erfassung. Naunyn-Schmiedeberg's Arch. exp. Path. Pharmak. 215, 8—18 (1952).

MACFARLANE, D. W., E. W. PELIKAN and K. R. UNNA: Evaluation of curarizing drugs in man. V. Antagonism to curarizing effects of d-tubourarine by neostigmine, m-hydroxy-phenyltrimethylammonium and m-hydroxyphenyldimethylethylammonium. J. Phar-macol. 100, 382—392 (1950).

MARSHALL, F. N., and J. P. LONG: Pharmacologic studies on some compounds structurally related to the hemicholinium (HC-3). J. Pharmacol. 127, 236—240 (1959).

MATTHES, K.: The action of blood on acetylcholine. J. Physiol. (Lond.) 70, 338—348 (1930)

MICHEL, H. O., and S. KROP: The reaction of cholinesterase with diisopropyl fluorophosphate. J. biol. Chem. 190, 119—125 (1951).

MIKHEL'SON, M. Y.: The influence of narcotics on cholinesterase activity. Fiziol. Zhur. U.S.S.R. (Russian) (J. Physiol.) 32, 745—756 (1946). C. A. 43, 7142d.

MINOT, A. S.: Comparison of the actions of prostigmine and guanidine on the activity of cholinesterase in blood serum. J. Pharmacol. 66, 453—458 (1939).

MIQUEL, O.: The effect of chloroform and ether on the activity of cholinesterase. J. Pharmacol. 88, 190—193 (1946).

MORAND, P., and J. L. GAY: Sur l'inhibition de la cholinestérase sérique humaine par le bleu de crésyl brillant. C. R. Soc. Biol. (Paris) 147, 1090—1091 (1953).

MOUNTER, L. A., and V. P. WHITTAKER: Effect of thiol and other group-specific reagents on erythrocyte and plasma cholinesterases. Biochem. J. 53, 167—173 (1953).

NACHMANSOHN, D.: Sur l'action de la strychnine. C. R. Soc. Biol. (Paris) 129, 941—943 (1938).

NAESS, K., and K. H. SKRAMSTAD: Action of hydrallazine and the relation between hydrallazine and 5-hydroxytryptamine. Acta Pharmacol. (Kbh.) 10, 178—198 (1954).

PARTENI, L., and M. CORNEANU: Anticholinesterase effect of some compounds. Comun. Acad. Rep. Populare Romane. (Rumanian) 4, 161—166 (1954). C. A. 50, 10265e.

PATON, W. D. M., and E. J. ZAIMIS: The pharmacological actions of polymethylene bis-trimethylammonium salts. Brit. J. Pharmacol. 4, 381—400 (1949).

PAULESU, F.: Cholinesterase activity from different biological origin. (Italian.) Arch. int. Pharmacodyn. 105, 366—380 (1956).

—, L. VARGIU and G. GIBERTONI: Cholinesterase activity measured from different biological sources as measured with CT 3318. (Italian.) Arch. int. Pharmacodyn. 104, 11—18 (1955).

PULVER, R.: Über die Hemmung des enzymatischen Abbaus von Pharmaka durch Butazolidin. Arch. int. Pharmacodyn. 98, 437—442 (1954).

RANDALL, L. D., and G. LEHMANN: Pharmacological properties of some neostigmine analogs. J. Pharmacol. 99, 16—32 (1950).

SCHACTER, M., and S. DVORKIN: The cardiovascular action of bile salt with regard to inhibition of cholinesterase. Amer. J. Physiol. 137, 599—605 (1942).

SCHUELER, F. W.: Two cyclic analogs of acetylcholine. J. Amer. pharm. Ass., sci. Ed. 45, 197—199 (1956).

SCHWEITZER, A., E. STEDMAN and S. WRIGHT: Central action of anticholinesterases. J. Physiol. (Lond.) 96, 302—336 (1939).

SERLIN, I., and D. J. FLUKE: The size and shape of radiosensitive acetylcholinesterase unit. J. biol. Chem. 223, 727—736 (1956).

SKOU, J. C.: Local anesthetics. VII. Local anesthetic potency and inhibition of acetylcholin-esterase. Acta pharmacol. (Kbh.) 12, 109—114 (1956a).

— Local anesthetics. VIII. Potency and inhibition of acetylcholinesterase in erythrocytes. Acta pharmacol. (Kbh.) 12, 115—125 (1956b).

SLAUGHTER, D., and R. W. LACKEY: Effect of morphine sulfate on serum cholinesterase. Proc. Soc. exp. Biol. (N.Y.) 45, 8—10 (1940).

SMITH, C. M., S. L. COHEN, E. W. PELIKAN and K. R. UNNA: Mode of action of antagonists to curare. J. Pharmacol. 105, 391—399 (1952).

—, E. W. PELIKAN, L. R. MARANBA and K. R. UNNA: Relation between structure and activity in a series of bisisoquinolinium compounds. J. Pharmacol. 108, 317—329 (1953).

STEDMAN, E.: Studies on the relationship between chemical constitution and physiological action. I. Position isomerism in relation to miotic activity of synthetic urethanes. Biochem. J. 20, 719—734 (1926).

— Studies on the relationship between chemical constitution and physiological action. II. The miotic activity of urethanes derived from the isomeric hydroxybenzyldimethylamines (HBDM). Biochem. J. 23, 17—24 (1929).

— Chemical constitution and miotic action. Amer. J. Physiol. 90, 528—529 (1929a).

—, and G. BARGER: Physostigmine (ererine). Part III. J. chem. Soc. 127, 247—258 (1925).

—, and E. STEDMAN: Studies on relationship between chemical constitution and physiological action. III. The inhibitory action of certain synthetic urethanes on the activity of liver esterases. Biochem. J. 25, 1147—1167 (1931).

— — Studies on relationship between chemical constitution and physiological action. IV. The inhibitory activity of certain synthetic urethanes on the activity of esterases. Biochem. J. 26, 1214—1222 (1932).

STEMPEL, A., and J. A. AESCHLIMANN: Esters of basically substituted 3-pyridols with physostigmine-like activity. J. Amer. chem. Soc. 74, 3323—3326 (1952).

STOVNER, J.: The effect of choline on the action of anticholinesterases. Acta pharmacol. (Kbh.) 12, 175—186 (1956).

STUMPF, CH., and E. HERZFELD: Zur Frage der Cholinesterase-Hemmwirkung der Polymethylen-Dicarbaminsäure-Bischolinester. Naunyn-Schmiedeberg's Arch. exp. Path. Pharmak. 225, 119—121 (1955).

TAYLOR, I. M., J. M. WELLER and A. B. HASTINGS: Effect of cholinesterase and choline acetylase on the potassium concentration gradient and potassium exchange of human erythrocytes. Amer. J. Physiol. 168, 658—665 (1952).

THOMPSON, R. H. S.: The action of chemical vesicants on cholinesterase. J. Physiol. 105, 370—381 (1947).

TODRICK, A.: The inhibition of cholinesterase by antagonists of acetylcholine and histamine. Brit. J. Pharmacol. 9, 76—83 (1954).

—, K. P. FELLOWS and J. P. RUTLAND: Effect of alcohols on cholinesterase. Biochem. J. 48, 360—368 (1951).

TORDA, C.: The effect of chloroform and ether on the activity of cholinesterase. J. Pharmacol. 77, 50—53 (1943).

— Effect of hormones on contraction of striated muscle and cholinesterase. Proc. Soc. exp. Biol. (N. Y.) 53, 121—125 (1943a).

—, and H. G. WOLFF: Effect of convulsant and anticonvulsant agents on acetylcholine metabolism (activity of choline acetylose, cholinesterase) and on sensitivity to acetylcholine of effector organs. Amer. J. Physiol. 151, 345—354 (1947).

VANDERMEER, C., and H. TH. M. NIEUWERKERK: Influence of vitamin E on liver esterase and cholinesterase. Biochem. biophys. Acta 7, 263—271 (1951).

VINCENT, D.: Acétylcholine et entihistaminiques de synthèse. Essais expérimentaux sur le chien. C. R. Soc. Biol. (Paris) 144, 148—150 (1950).

—, and R. LAGREN: Action comparée de quelques dérivés al caloidiques puriques (caféine, théobromine, theophylinne et theophylline-ethylenediamine) sur les cholinestérase. C. R. Soc. Biol. (Paris) 144, 925—927 (1950).

—, and M. PARANT: Etude de l'action du chloramphenicol (chloromycetine) sur les cholinesterases. C. R. Soc. Biol. (Paris) 144, 1660—1663 (1950).

— — De l'action de la caféine sur les pseudocholinesterase. C. R. Soc. Biol. (Paris) 148, 1078—1080 (1954).

— — Atropine, apo-atropine et cholinestérases. C. R. Soc. Biol. (Paris) 150, 444—447 (1956).

— — and R. LAGREN: Essai de l'action de la streptomycine sur les cholinestérases in vitro. C. R. Soc. Biol. (Paris) 143, 228—230 (1949).

WAELSCH, H., and H. RACKOW: Natural and synthetic inhibitors of cholinesterase. Science 96, 386 (1942).

—, and D. NACHMANSOHN: Toxicity of atebrin. Proc. Soc. exp. Biol. (N. Y.) 54, 336—338 (1943).

WELS, P., u. K. PEPKE: Über den Einfluß der Sulfhydrilgruppe auf die Cholinesterase. Naunyn-Schmiedeberg's Arch. exp. Path. Pharmak. 204, 323—325 (1947).

WESCOE, W. C., W. F. RIKER and V. L. BEACH: Studies on the inter-relationship of certain cholinergic compounds. III. The reaction between 3-acetoxy phenyltrimethylammonium methylsulfate, 3-hydroxy phenyltrimethylammonium bromide and cholinesterase. J. Pharmacol. **99**, 265—276 (1950).

WHITE, A. C., and E. STEDMAN: On the physostigmine-like action of certain synthetic urethanes. J. Pharmacol. **41**, 259—288 (1931).

WILSON, I. B., and C. QUAN: Acetylcholinesterase studies on molecular complementariness. Arch. Biochem. **73**, 131—143 (1958).

WRIGHT, C. I.: The inactivation of choline esterase by morphine and derivatives. J. Pharmacol. **72**, 45—46 (1941).

—, and J. C. SABINE: Inactivation of cholinesterase by morphine, dilaudid, codeine and desomorphine. J. Pharmacol. **78**, 375—384 (1943).

— — Cholinesterases of human erythrocyte and plasma and their inhibition by antimalarial drugs. J. Pharmacol. **93**, 230—239 (1948).

WUEST, H. M., and E. H. SAKAL: Some derivatives of 3-pyridol with para-sympathomimetic properties. J. Amer. chem. Soc. **73**, 1210—1216 (1951).

YOUNG, D. C., R. A. VANDER PLOEG, R. M. FEATHERSTONE and E. G. GROSS: Interrelationships among the central, peripheral and anticholinesterase effects of some morphinan derivatives. J. Pharmacol. **114**, 33—37 (1955).

Chapter 9

Structure-Activity Relationships of the Organophosphorus Anticholinesterase Agents

By

Bo Holmstedt

With 8 Figures

Contents

A. Historical development of organophosphorus cholinesterase inhibitors*

Organic chemists have the habit of tasting new compounds. Useful drugs like local anaesthetics have been discovered in this way. On the other hand, it is amazing that so few scientists have met a premature death as a result. It is remarkable, for example, that the French nobleman and organic chemist PHILIPPE DE CLERMONT did not succumb to tetraethyl pyrophosphate (TEPP) poisoning in 1854. If this had happened, the toxicity of the anticholinesterase (anti-ChE) agents of the organophosphorus type would have been discovered much earlier than it actually was.

There is not the slightest doubt that DE CLERMONT tasted the compound he synthetized because he stated so in his first account of August 14, 1854, given before the French Academy of Sciences with professors DUMAS, PELOUSE, and BALARD as presidium. PHILIPPE DE CLERMONT at that time worked in the laboratory of the great chemist WURTZ who encouraged him to carry out these studies (DE CLERMONT 1854).

---

* This historical account has been compiled by the author on the basis of data available in the open literature. To follow the chronological sequence of scientific events during wartime activities is a delicate task, particularly because military security regulations make assessment difficult, and quite apart from the fact that the inability to publish may be a source of discomfort to the people involved. The author has tried to render justice to scientists who in different countries have worked with the organophosphorus compounds in industries, universities, and military research institutes.

«M. WURTZ *m'ayant engagé à étudier l'action de l'iodure d'éthyle sur différents sels d'argent, j'ai obtenu les résultats suivants:*»

The general account of his synthetic product reads:

«*L'éther pyrophosphorique est un liquide visqueux, d'une saveur brûlante, d'une odeur particulière, se dissolvant dans l'eau, l'alcool et l'éther; il devient promptement acide au contact de l'air humide. Une petite portion de cet éther, exposée pendant quelques jours à l'air, a absorbé jusqu'à 14 pour 100 de son poids d'eau.*»

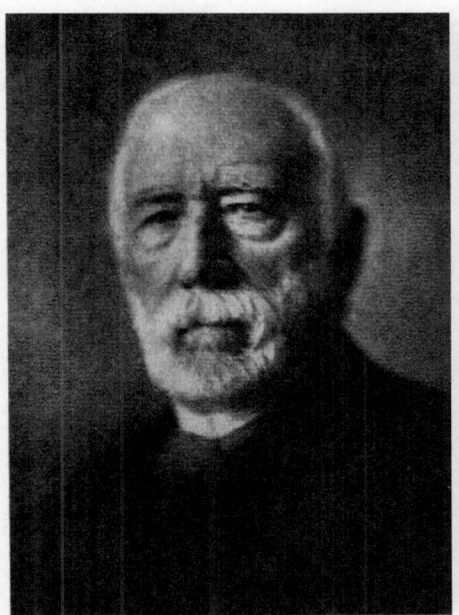 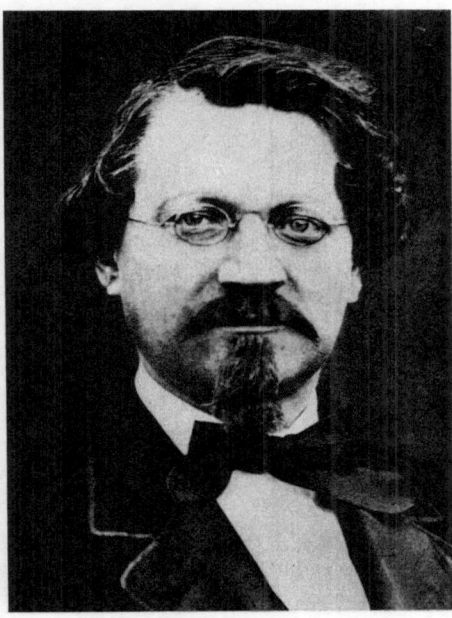

Fig. 1. PHILIPPE DE CLERMONT 1830—1921   Fig. 2. A. W. VON HOFMANN 1818—1892

A full account was given a year later (DE CLERMONT 1855). It is to be noted that TEPP had been synthetized before in WURTZ' laboratory.

«*Cet éther avait d'abord été obtenu au laboratoire de* M. WURTZ *par* M. MOSCHNINE.»

Nobody knows who Moschnine was.

It is difficult to explain why DE CLERMONT did not succumb to the TEPP he tasted. His method of synthesis certainly produces the toxic product, albeit in impure form. Maybe he diluted it before tasting. In any case there is nothing in the family record to indicate that he even became sick. On the contrary, PHILIPPE DE CLERMONT, one of the first generation of organic chemists, enjoyed a long and prosperous life, saw an immense part of his science grow up, including phosphorus chemistry, and died in 1921 at the respectable age of ninety.

The synthesis of tetraethyl pyrophosphate and analogues was repeated half a dozen times up to 1930 with no untoward effect observed on the chemists occupying themselves with the products. It must be mentioned, however, that compounds of greater volatility are more liable to cause harmful effects.

From the point of view of our present knowledge of organophosphorus anti-ChE agents it is easy to distinguish the important incidents in the past bearing upon the present synthetic and pharmacological work. Thus, in 1873 A. W. VON HOFMANN (1818—1892) synthetized methylphosphoryl dichloride. This occurred upon the return of this famous chemist to Germany after the many years he spent in London, and was his last contribution to the field of organophosphorus chemistry, most of which had been carried out in England. Methylphosphoryl dichloride constitutes the first example of the C-P linkage. This compound, unnoticed for many years, is one of the important steps in the synthesis of modern C-P compounds, although produced in other ways. Among these are insecticides and the nerve gas, Sarin.

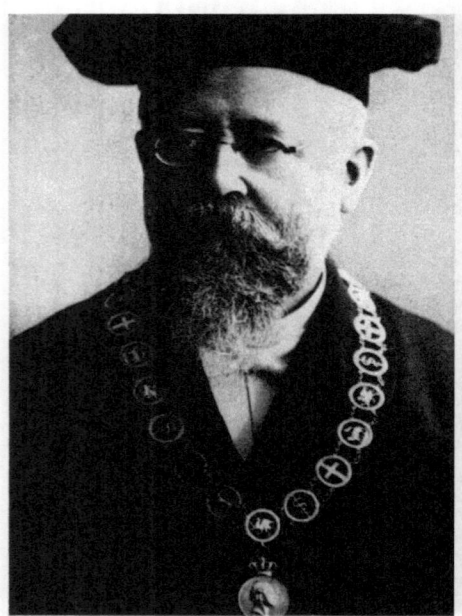 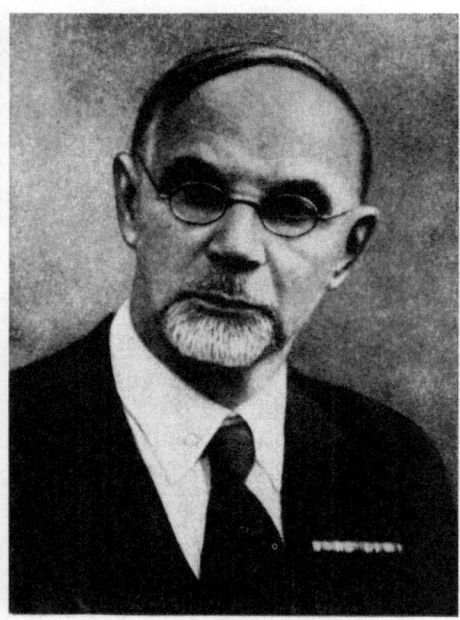

Fig. 3. C. A. A. MICHAELIS 1847—1916   Fig. 4. A. E. ARBUSOW born in 1877

In the latter part of the nineteenth century the synthesis of organophosphorus compounds was closely linked with the work of CARL ARNOLD AUGUST MICHAELIS (1847—1916), professor at the University of Rostock. All his own investigations and those of his pupils were collected in monographs devoted to various parts of the field. One of these bears notably upon the present subject, namely the one describing substances containing the N—P bond (MICHAELIS 1903). In this monograph is also reported a compound with a P—CN bond, diethylamidoethoxy phosphoryl cyanide. MICHAELIS gave no detailed description of how he made this compound, but he got it from a product obtained in a reaction worked out by one of his pupils (SCHALL 1898). This account later led to the synthesis of a number of important insecticides and the nerve gas, Tabun.

In Russia important work in organophosphorus chemistry was also being carried out at about the same time. This was and still is linked to the Kazan School of Chemistry which dates back to 1806, when it was founded by F. L. EVEST (A. E. ARBUSOW 1940). Of special importance is the publication printed in 1906 by professor ALECSANDR ERMININGEL'DOVICH ARBUSOW about the isomerization or reaction still bearing his name (A. E. ARBUSOW 1906). This constitutes one of the most commonly used ways of forming the stable C—P bond. Professor A. E. ARBUSOW's work has been continued by his son B. A. ARBUSOW, who is still active as head of the Institute in Kazan, and is a frequent contributor in the field of organophosphorus chemistry.

In general, the first decades of our century did not witness as much work on organophosphorus compounds as the last part of the 19th century. Indeed, the first item of importance to this account was the obtaining of TEPP in a pure distilled form by NYLÉN in Uppsala (NYLÉN 1930). The synthesis of TEPP in two ways, together with that of numerous other organophosphates, was published in NYLÉN's thesis which constitutes one of the fundamental works for present day studies. NYLÉN had no knowledge of the toxicity of his compounds when told of this by the present author 18 years afterwards.

TEPP was again synthetized the year after by the ARBUSOWS who also produced tetraethylmonothiono pyrophosphate (ARBUSOW and ARBUSOW 1931).

The following year witnessed the most important discovery in the field from a toxicological point of view. WILLY LANGE, at that time Privatdozent in chemistry at the university of Berlin, and his graduate student GERDA VON KRUEGER synthetized some compounds containing the P—F linkage. LANGE was originally an inorganic chemist. At this time fluorine had become generally available for chemical synthesis and LANGE introduced it for the first time into organophosphorus compounds. During the synthesis of dimethyl and diethyl phos-

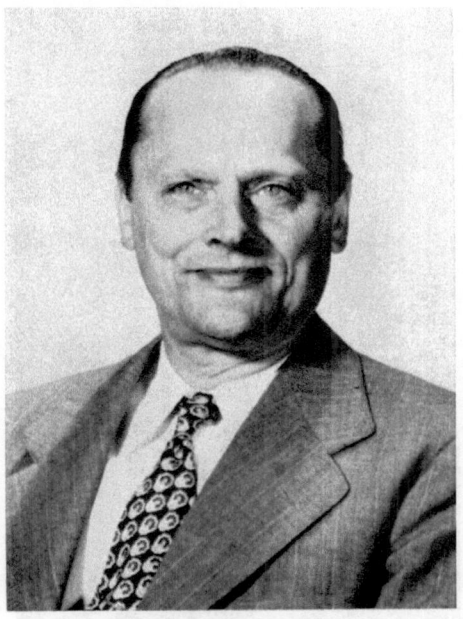

Fig. 5. WILLY LANGE born in 1900

phorofluoridate, the workers noticed the toxic effects of the vapor on themselves. Their short account of this included at the end of a purely chemical paper is astonishing in its pharmacological correctness (LANGE and KRUEGER 1932).

„Interessant ist die starke Wirkung der Monofluorphosphorsäurealkylester auf den menschlichen Organismus. Die Dämpfe dieser Verbindungen riechen angenehm und kräftig aromatisch. Doch schon einige Minuten nach dem Einatmen stellt sich ein starker Druck auf den Kehlkopf ein, verbunden mit Atemnot. Dann treten leichte Bewußtseins-Trübungen auf und Blendungs-Erscheinungen mit schmerzhafter Überempfindlichkeit des Auges gegen Licht. Erst nach mehreren Stunden klingen diese Erscheinungen ab. Sie werden anscheinend nicht von sauren Zersetzungsprodukten der Ester verursacht, sondern sie sind wahrscheinlich den Dialkylmonofluorphosphaten selbst zuzuschreiben. Die Wirkungen werden von sehr kleinen Mengen ausgeübt."

LANGE had an interest in synthetic insecticides as witnessed by the following passage in a letter (LANGE 1952).

"I started work on fluorophosphoric acid derivatives because I was interested in finding new types of organic insecticides. After my first observations with monofluorophosphoric acid esters, their action on myself and later on co-workers, and their insecticidal properties I offered these compounds to the I. G. Farbenindustrie for

evaluation in pest control; however, no one was interested in this field at that time. My interest in the insecticide field is hinted at in a brief review on progress in the preparation and use of fluoro derivatives, which appeared in Chem. Ztg."

The copy of the Chem. Ztg. in question contains a preface to LANGE's paper by the editor Dr. HERMAN STADLINGER in Köthen:

„Herr Dr. LANGE hat übrigens eine Reihe von neuen anorganischen Fluorosäure-Verbindungen nach den einfachsten Methoden dargestellt, mit dem Ziele, um weiteres Material für Untersuchungen der Wirksamkeit als Schädlingsbekämpfungsmittel in die Hand zu bekommen. Auch die von ihm gewonnenen, physiologisch stark wirkenden, neuen Ester von Fluorosäuren verdienen besondere Aufmerksamkeit."

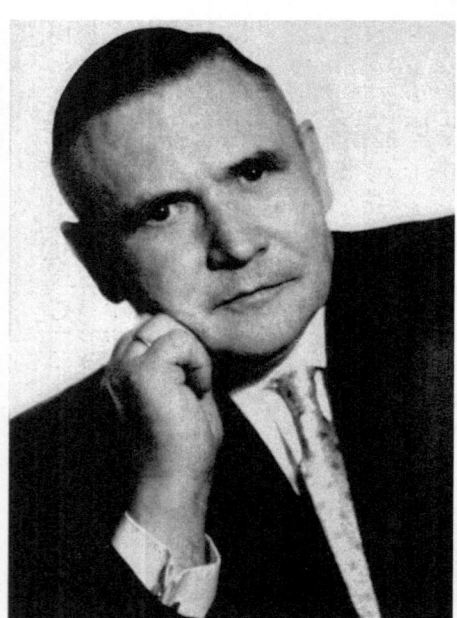

And in LANGE's paper are to be found the following sentences (LANGE 1935).

„Ob von den Fluoriden komplizierter organischer Ringsysteme oder den Estern der Fluorsäuren einige größere Bedeutung bei der Bekämpfung von Schädlingen erlangen werden, ist noch nicht entschieden. Ebenso ist die fungicide Wirkung der neueren Verbindungen noch wenig untersucht worden."

Later on the I. G. Farbenindustrie developed an interest in synthetic insecticides, then a completely undeveloped field. The scientific leader of the company, OTTO BAYER, appointed the chemist GERHARD SCHRADER for this work in 1934. It was not until 1936, however, that he turned his interest to the phosphorus compounds. At the

Fig. 6. GERHARD SCHRADER born in 1903

turn of the year (1936—1937) SCHRADER also noticed miosis and discomfort during his synthetic work. At that time he was repeating the synthesis of MICHAELIS' pupil SCHALL, previously mentioned. This occurrence led directly to the long sequence of synthetic organophosphates with insecticidal and toxic properties. It also led to the synthesis in Germany of chemical warfare agents of up till then unknown toxicity. In March 1937 SCHRADER patented the general formula for contact insecticides of this type (SCHRADER 1952) (see section B). The subsequent development of the organophosphate insecticides is thoroughly treated in SCHRADER's monograph (SCHRADER 1952). In the ensuing years 1938 to 1941 he developed the fluorine-containing compounds including DFP (WIRTH 1949) and the pyrophosphorus derivatives including TEPP. The systemically insecticidal OMPA and related compounds were patented together with H. KÜKENTHAL. In 1940 came Bladan, the active principle of which probably is TEPP. SCHRADER then turned to the thio- and thionophosphorus compounds. Paraoxon (E 600) and its sulphur analogue Parathion (E 605) were ready in 1944. The insecticidal value of the latter compound was elucidated at the end of the war. Up till then SCHRADER is said to have synthetized around 2000 organophosphorus compounds.

From 1935 onwards the German Government required that information about new toxic products of any importance should be submitted for investigation. Until 1944 around 200 compounds were considered sufficiently toxic by the Ministry of Defence to be classified as secret. This sometimes could be a great discomfort to commercial firms. Among these compounds was TEPP as witnessed by SCHRADER.

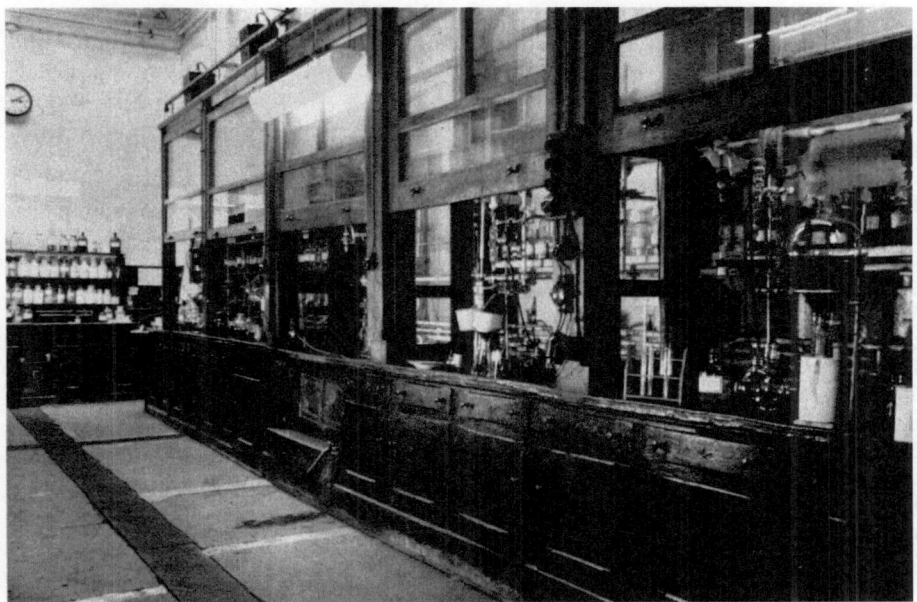

Fig. 7. The laboratory in which G. SCHRADER started the syntheses which led to the development of the modern organophosphorus insecticides

„Zu einer Verwendung des Pyrophosphorsäure-tetraäthylesters als Pflanzen-schutzmittel kam es nicht, da die eingereichte Verwendungsanmeldung 1939 vom Heereswaffenamt als „Geheim" erklärt wurde. Alle Bemühungen der I. G. Farben-industrie, den Tetraäthylester der Pyrophosphorsäure vom Heereswaffenamt für die Zwecke der gewerblichen Verwendung als Pflanzenschutzmittel freizubekommen, schlugen bis zum Kriegsende fehl." (SCHRADER 1952.)

Among these secret compounds were also ethyl-N,N-dimethyl phosphor-amidocyanidate prepared by SCHRADER in 1937 and bearing the code name Tabun, Gelan, Trilon 83 or D 7, and isopropyl methylphosphonofluoridate, Sarin or T 144. Numerous chemists studied the military properties of these compounds which were considered sufficiently interesting for immediate manufacture on an industrial scale.

In 1937, 1 kg of Tabun and also a small amount of Sarin were given to the Ministry of Defence. Around 5 kg of the latter product was submitted between 1938 and 1942. In 1938, laboratories and a small pilot plant were established for the study of these compounds. In the same year the Ministry of Defence decided to build a sizeable factory and the construction of this was started in January 1940 at a place called Dühernfurt, 40 kilometers north of Breslau and 1 km from the river Oder. This factory covered a surface of 1 km² and was camouflaged against air-raids by trees planted on the roofs of the buildings.

Because of the time required for the installation of the new equipment, the production of the necessary intermediary products could not start until 1942. Furthermore, the factory was also to produce its own starting products, such as chlorine, phosphorus oxychloride, phosphorus pentachloride, and dimethylamine. It employed 3,000 workers, all of whom lived in barracks in the neighbouring wood. It is to be noted that this factory was intended after the war to be the most important European plant for the manufacture of chlorine.

The first lot of Tabun was manufactured in May 1943 and small quantities of Sarin in June 1944. The rapid advancement of the Russian army prevented the destruction and evacuation of the factory. The allies did not know about it and never attacked it by air. It fell into the hands of the Russians with a stock of primary and intermediary products for the manufacture of Tabun and Sarin, and is said to have been dismounted and removed.

It is estimated that 10,000 to 12,000 tons of Tabun were manufactured at Dühernfurt. The estimated manufacture of Sarin was 600 tons at the same place, out of which only about 30 tons seem to have been manufactured in 1944. A third agent, Soman (pinacolyl-methylphosphonofluoride), was only at the laboratory stage at the end of the war.

The investigations of the pharmacological and toxicological properties of the organophosphorus compounds in Germany were carried out both by the industrial firms working with insecticides and laboratories belonging to the armed forces. The first pharmacological experiments with these agents were carried out independently at Farbenfabriken Bayer in Elberfeld by EBERHARD GROSS, and at the Militärärztliche Akademie in Berlin where the department was headed by WOLF-GANG WIRTH, who had as his co-worker J. SEXTEL. This was started in 1937. Later on, after the beginning of the war, the group at the Militärärztliche Akademie was joined by other prominent German pharmacologists, by then drafted. Among these were L. LENDLE, W. KOLL, H. GREMELS, and O. GRINDT.

H. GREMELS is said to have recognized the anti-ChE properties of Tabun at an early stage in 1940. Among other things he observed the potentiating effect of Tabun injection on the drop in the cat's blood pressure evoked by constant doses of acetylcholine (ACh) (LENDLE 1959). According to SCHRADER (1952) the enzyme-inhibiting properties of TEPP were recognized by EBERHARD GROSS in 1939. It is not stated whether this was done by biochemical or pharmacological investigations. In any event the parasympathomimetic effects of the nerve gases were clearly recognized by the German workers and atropine established as an antidote (COLLOMP 1949). The symptomatology was also well recognized both from experiments in animals of various species and by the exposure of volunteers to low concentrations of the compounds.

At the end of the war, military, and non-military investigating teams followed closely the advancing allied armies to get information from scientists about work of civilian or military interest. Thus, GERHARD SCHRADER, together with a great deal of the material from his investigations on insecticides, was taken to the castle Krantzberg where he was interrogated by British scientists. This subsequently resulted in a much read report about insecticides (SCHRADER 1947).

Through these interrogations of German scientists not only did the insecticides become known to the rest of the world but the existence of the nerve gases was disclosed to the allies. The latter compounds, however, were kept as military secrets.

Long before the interrogation of German scientists and the publication of reports about the work carried out in Germany during World War II, similar activities were carried out in England. KILBY (1949) has told how this came about:

"In England, soon after the beginning of the war, teams were set up by the Ministry of Supply to seek new or improved types of chemical warfare agents as a precaution against surprise should the enemy initiate this form of warfare. Teams at Cambridge were asked to pay special attention to fluorine compounds, and early in 1940 the author prepared samples of dimethyl and diethyl fluorophosphonate and carried out toxicity tests, in view of LANGE *and* KRUEGER's *published remarks."*

It is tempting to speculate why the teams at Cambridge were asked to pay special attention to fluorine compounds! A provocative thought is that information about the German activities had leaked out in one way or another. Strangely enough the Germans at about the same time feared that the allies had the nerve gases, due to the lack of information of compounds of similar structure in the patent literature.

„... daß mir von Herrn WIRTH *immer wieder versichert worden sei, daß man von deutscher Seite nicht daran dachte, diese Kampfstoffe einzusetzen, daß aber die Bearbeitung der Therapie deshalb so dringend notwendig sei, weil man auf Grund von Lücken in der Patentliteratur den dringenden Verdacht haben mußte, daß auf Seiten der Alliierten die Entwicklung von organischen Phosphorverbindungen als Kampfstoff im Gange wäre"* (W. KOLL 1960).

KILBY's survey of the open literature led him to the passage in LANGE and KRUEGER's paper about the toxic effects. This initiated the first synthetic and toxicological work with these compounds in England. Exposure of volunteers, including the investigators themselves, was carried out with the compounds but reported only after the war (KILBY and KILBY 1947).

Later on, many homologues and related compounds were synthetized by a team under H. McCOMBIE and B. C. SAUNDERS. Among these compounds was diisopropyl phosphorofluoridate (DFP), one of the most commonly used of the organophosphorus anticholinesterases in scientific investigations to-day. The synthesis of this compound was reported by B. C. SAUNDERS at a Ministry of Supply Meeting in London, December 11, 1941 (SAUNDERS 1957).

The pharmacological effects of the new compounds were studied by a team under Lord ADRIAN, which included W. FELDBERG and B. A. KILBY. The long-lasting miosis led these investigators to think that the organophosphates were enzyme-inhibitors like eserine. This was borne out by experiments on isolated organs including the frog rectus in 1942. The same year a biochemical team consisting of DIXON, MACKWORTH and WEBB compared DFP to eserine in Warburg experiments and found it to be a strong inhibitor of horse serum ChE. All the chemical, pharmacological, and biochemical experiments were published only after the war.

Diisopropyl phosphorofluoridate (DFP) is no doubt also the substance mentioned in an account of the American activities in this field during the war (BODANSKY 1945):

"At the beginning of this war, the British chemical warfare investigators began to study the physiological properties of a group of compounds which had been described by German chemists in the open literature in 1932. The British investigators found that these agents possessed an anticholinesterase action. In 1943, the Medical Division at Edgewood Arsenal became interested in this group of compounds, and comprehensive programs were initiated to study fully their toxicity and the mechanism of action and, if possible, to devise therapy against their injurious effects. One of these compounds appeared at first to be promising as a chemical warfare agent and, although it did not finally qualify in this respect, studies on the mechanism of its action revealed very interesting anticholinesterase properties.

"In contrast to the action of such substances as prostigmine and physostigmine, this compound decreased the activity of cholinesterases in tissues and in blood in an apparently irreversible manner."

When at the end of the war the existence of the German nerve gases was disclosed to the allies it was still kept a secret for military reasons. The greater toxicity of Tabun and Sarin outweighs that of a compound like DFP. The following passage from a talk given by A. GILMAN most certainly refers to one of the nerve gases.

"The third agent (i.e., Tabun — Ed.) will be discussed only very briefly. It shares with diisopropyl-fluorophosphate the ability irreversibly to inactivate cholinesterase. It differs from diisopropyl-fluorophosphate in possessing a more outstanding action on the nervous system. Certain species in particular cats and dogs, exhibit severe convulsions, which have their onset within a few minutes after the intravenous injection of the drug and which persist until death. The fact that an anticholinesterase agent possesses such extreme convulsant action could possibly be attributed to coincidence. However, there is one finding which points to an intimate relationship between convulsions and the chemical mediation of central synaptic transmission. If the animals receive a therapeutic dose of atropine, before the administration of this anticholinesterase, no convulsions are observed, and complete protection is afforded from what would, otherwise, be a lethal dose" (GILMAN 1946).

The formulas of Tabun and Sarin were published in 1948 by BONNAUD and by VALADE and SALLÉ who also reported some preliminary pharmacological experiments in the same year (VALADE and SALLÉ 1948). The first full account of the synthesis and pharmacology of Tabun was given in 1951 (HOLMSTEDT 1951).

During the nineteen-fifties, an enormous development took place in this field. This is well-known even to those remotely connected with work in toxicology, pharmacology, or field protection. Important events are the advent of Malathion, an insecticide with very low toxicity to man (CASSADAY 1950), the introduction of Systox (SCHRADER and LORENZ 1951), and the finding that a new type of sulfur-containing organophosphates was of extreme potency (GHOSH and NEWMAN 1955). To this may be added the synthesis of a series of pharmacologically interesting compounds related to choline esters and thiocholine esters (TAMMELIN 1958).

B. Chemistry

The cholinesterase inhibitors of the organophosphorus group can be denoted with the general formula which was given as early as 1937 by SCHRADER as the general formula for derivatives of phosphorus acids with insecticidal properties. It implies that biologically active compounds are obtained when in addition to oxygen or sulfur two similar or dissimilar substituents are bound to the phosphorus atom and an organic or inorganic acid residue is also present.

$$R_1 \diagdown P \diagup O(S)$$
$$R_2 \diagup \diagdown X$$

R_1 and R_2 are capable of almost infinite variation. They may represent alcohols, phenols, mercaptans, amides, or alkyl or aryl groups attached directly to the phosphorus, etc. Common X radicals are from fluorine (e.g., in DFP), paranitrophenol (e.g., in Paraoxon), and phosphates (in a "pyrophosphate," e.g., in TEPP), but in other inhibitors X may be cyanide, thiocyanate, carboxylate, chloride or almost any phenoxy or thiophenoxy group.

A large number of organophosphorus ChE-inhibitors have been collected in tables A to E, where references to synthesis and biochemistry are also given. Although it is possible to group the compounds according to strictly chemical rules, it has been found advantageous to utilize a "pharmacological method" of classification. The general chemical structure of the compounds is preferably discussed in connection with their structure-activity relationships. Here only a few facts about the stereochemistry will be mentioned

The stereoisomers of the anti-ChE agents of the phosphorus group in which the phosphorus alone is an asymmetric centre have been investigated very little, although it is well recognized that enzymes exhibit stereospecificity in their reactions with asymmetric carbon compounds (HOSKIN and TRICK 1955). Such specificity is likely to be a consequence of the asymmetric structure of the enzyme surface. In recent years the *d*- and *l*-enantiomorphs of asymmetric organic phosphorus inhibitors of ChE's have been synthetized. It was found that the *levo*-isomer of one such compound, O-ethyl S-(2-ethylthioethyl) ethylphosphono-thioate, reacted from 10 to 20 times faster than the *dextro*-isomer in the irreversible inactivation of four cholinesterase preparations studied (AARON, MICHEL, WITTEN and MILLER 1958).

$$H_5C_2O \diagdown \underset{\underset{C_2H_5}{|}}{\overset{\overset{O}{\|}}{P}} \diagdown SCH_2CH_2SC_2H_5 \qquad\qquad C_2H_5SCH_2CH_2S \diagdown \underset{\underset{H_5C_2}{|}}{\overset{\overset{O}{\|}}{P}} \diagdown OC_2H_5$$

Similar results have been reached with optically active phosphorothioates. HILGETAG and LEHMANN (1959) synthetized the optically active isomers of O,S-dimethyl O-(4-nitrophenyl)phosphorothioate:

$$H_3CO \diagdown \underset{\underset{SCH_3}{|}}{\overset{\overset{O}{\|}}{P}} \diagdown O\!\!-\!\!\langle\!\!\rangle\!\!-\!\!NO_2 \qquad\qquad O_2N\!\!-\!\!\langle\!\!\rangle\!\!-\!\!O \diagdown \underset{\underset{H_3CS}{|}}{\overset{\overset{O}{\|}}{P}} \diagdown OCH_3$$

In experiments on mammals with this compound, the LD_{50} perorally to rats was found to be 135 mg/kg for the *dextro*-isomer and 25 mg/kg for the *levo*-isomer which thus is roughly five times as toxic. When comparing the I_{50} of the isomers with rat brain as the source of enzyme, a difference was also noted in favour of the levo compounds. The I_{50} for the *levo*-isomer was $10^{-6.82}$ and for the *dextro*-isomer $10^{-6.08}$. Interestingly enough no differences in toxicity were found when the toxicities of the isomers were compared on a strain of *Drosophila*.

An example of the effect of a change in the structure of an organophosphorus substrate upon the stereospecificity of (in this case) enzymic hydrolysis may be found in evidence presented to show that a phosphorylphosphatase selectively hydrolyzes one of the stereoisomers of Tabun (HOSKIN and TRICK 1955), but apparently shows little or no specificity for those of Sarin (ADIE, HOSKIN and TRICK 1956).

C. Comparison of chemical structure with biological activity

For reasons thoroughly discussed and exemplified in another part of this volume (Chapter 7), the inhibition of the ChE enzymes by most organophosphorus ChE-inhibitors is thought to consist in a primary attachment of the organophosphate to the enzyme, and a secondary phosphorylation of the so called esteratic site of the enzymic protein molecule. It is immediately apparent that two factors especially are of importance in the chemistry of the inhibitors, their chemical configuration (likeness to the natural substrate determines the fit of the inhibitor) and the reactivity of the P—X bond (determining the rate of phosphorylation).

I. Reactivity

The inherent reactivity of the organophosphorus derivatives is of course affected by the structure of the R-groups as well as by that of the X-group. Alterations in this structure of the organophosphorus derivatives do not always have the expected effect on the activity of these compounds as esterase inhibitors or pharmacological agents.

Considering first the phosphorylating power of the compounds, inferences may be drawn to biochemical and pharmacological premises from the kinetic experiments performed by LARSSON in non-biological systems (LARSSON 1958).

According to this author, the reactivity of the phosphorus compounds is characterized mainly by the strength of the P—X bond and the electronic density of the phosphorus atom, which is controlled by the electron distribution of the substituents. Concerning the influence of the P—X bond, it seems reasonable to suppose that there is a relationship between the reaction rate and the basicity of the displaced X-group, i.e., the stronger the base produced the slower is the reaction. Several exceptions to this rule can be found, e.g., the cyano group in Tabun would be expected to be hydrolytically stable, but the high reactivity of the compound may probably be ascribed to the ready polarizability of this group. LARSSON pointed out that in principle this relationship can be applied to predict the influence of the X-group on the reactivity of an organic phosphorus compound.

The inhibition of acetylcholinesterase (AChE) of sheep erythrocytes by various analogues of Paraoxon has been studied by ALDRIDGE and DAVISON (1952). They found that the rate of the inhibitory reaction was directly proportional to the rate of spontaneous hydrolysis with 9 of the 11 compounds investigated. Examples have, however, also been cited to show that the rate of aqueous hydrolysis not always gives a reliable indication of the electrophilic character of the phosphorus atom concerned (MYERS 1954).

Despite certain divergencies, the general relationship between the innate reactivity and the inhibitory properties of the neutral phosphate esters thus seems to be fairly well established.

II. Chemical structure

The working out of a pharmacological structure-activity relationship for a group of organic compounds is hampered by many facts inherent in such a comparison. Generally, such relationships have been successfully worked out only for a fairly small number of intimately related compounds such as, for example, neuromuscular blocking agents or choline esters. In these cases, comparisons have usually been based on one pharmacologically determined parameter, such as head drop, frog rectus assay, or blood pressure experiments. Concerning groups of compounds believed to act wholly or partially through interference with known enzyme systems, biochemical determinations of enzyme activity also enter the picture.

1. Reasons for divergencies in structure-activity relationship

The reasons for the difficulties in determining the structure-activity relationship are borne out by many of the chapters in this volume. For the sake of convenience, the most important ones will be summarized briefly and exemplified, where this has not been done previously.

Purity of compounds used. A frequently overlooked fact is that impurities of the compounds used may be strong inhibitors of ChE's (ALDRIDGE and BARNES 1952). It is difficult to assess how many investigations have been invalidated due to this inadvertence. It is also well recognized that compounds used commercially as insecticides may vary considerably in their toxicity from one batch to another. It is therefore highly questionable whether pharmacological experiments with an "80% pure preparation of Parathion" are worth anything at all outside the applied toxicological aspects.

Physico-chemical properties of inhibitors. Possible loss of activity due to non-enzymic hydrolysis must not be overlooked. In numerous experiments TEPP has been used as inhibitor. The half-life of this compound in water is around 8 hours, and there is consequently a rapid loss of activity in such solutions. The importance of the stability of the compounds has been stressed in a paper by VANDEKAR and HEATH 1957.

Other physico-chemical properties of the inhibitors may be equally important as non-enzymic hydrolysis. The most commonly studied is the lipid solubility. Compounds highly soluble in lipids are prone to produce effects in the central nervous system, while more water-soluble inhibitors predominantly give rise to peripheral effects, striking examples of which BURGEN and CHIPMAN (1952) and KOELLE and STEINER (1956) have given. In the case of protolytic inhibitors, the dissociation constant determines the quotients between base and acid, forms which may have entirely different inhibitory and pharmacological properties (TAMMELIN 1958).

Reaction rate with cholinesterase. The reaction rate with cholinesterase is of course the most important of the factors determining the toxicity of the compounds. This has been treated in Chapter 7.

Workers in the field of organophosphorus ChE-inhibitors, when evaluating a new compound, are usually interested in the I_{50} and the LD_{50}, the first mentioned being the molar concentration of the inhibitor causing 50% inhibition of the enzyme activity. The I_{50} values for phosphorylating inhibitors are not simply an expression of their affinity for, or reaction velocity with, the enzyme. It has been pointed out by JANDORF et al. (1955) and GREEN (1958) that side-reactions are the reason why organophosphorus inhibitors do not give complete inhibition at all concentrations above the molar concentration of active enzyme groups. JANDORF et al. pointed out also that hydrolysis of the inhibitor is one side-reaction to be considered; others are reactions with groups in the proteins other than the active one. Inhibitors are used in considerable excess in most I_{50} determinations published (pI_{50} seldom passes 10), which diminishes the influence of side-reactions and enzyme concentration. However, the most potent inhibitors are used in concentrations close to the enzyme concentration, in which case the I_{50} values are strongly dependent on side-reactions, the enzyme concentration used, or both.

I_{50} values seem to be a better basis for a rough prediction of toxicity than the reaction velocity with the enzyme, mainly because the experimental situation in an I_{50} determination on an impure enzyme preparation has a closer resemblance to the situation *in vivo* than kinetic experiments where side-reactions are avoided as much as possible. It has been demonstrated by TAMMELIN (1958) that high toxicities are found both among the highly reactive methylfluorophosphoryl-cholines and among the slowly reacting thiocholine compounds. The first group of compounds is toxic due to their reactivity, and the second due to stability against side-reactions.

In comparing toxicity *in vivo* with antiesterase activity *in vitro*, it has been found that in small homologous series and where the enzymic and mortality determinations are made by the same investigator under identical conditions, such an approach yields useful information, and that an increased enzyme-inhibiting activity is associated with greater toxicity. However, discrepancies from the straight-line relationship between results *in vivo* and *in vitro* are not unusual (HOLMSTEDT 1951).

The source of enzymes is also prone to affect the results of these experiments. In many cases the ChE-inhibiting activities are determined with preparations from species other than those used for the toxicity tests.

Metabolism. The metabolism of organophosphorus anticholinesterase agents has been treated extensively in Chapter 10. It is by now clearly recognized that metabolism of the compounds may result in both more toxic agents (toxification) and less toxic agents (detoxification). The liver probably plays the greatest role in both processes. Some results suggest, e.g., that Paraoxon is detoxicated by the liver so quickly that only a small fraction of the injected amount becomes effective, and that the "toxification" of Parathion in the liver takes place more quickly than the detoxification of the Paraoxon formed (HOLTZ and WESTERMANN 1959).

Species. A considerable difference in susceptibility to organophosphorus ChE-inhibitors exists among various species. Enzymic detoxification may at least partly explain this. Low toxicity may be due to the ease of hydrolysis of the compounds by mammalian enzymes (CASIDA 1956). This is a major consideration in the evaluation of modern insecticides. By studying the metabolism in insects and in mammals it has recently been possible to produce tailor-made insecticides (ARTHUR and CASIDA 1958).

It should also be pointed out that in the complex pharmacodynamics of the poisons under discussion some species may be primarily "cardiovascular" and others primarily "respiratory" reactors. DIRNHUBER and CULLUMBINE (1955) observed a rise in blood pressure in rats after intravenous injection of Sarin, a reaction evidently peculiar to this species. They suggested that this rise is due mainly to constriction of the skin arterioles by a central action of Sarin on the vasomotor centre.

Sex difference. DUBOIS et al. (1949) working with Parathion observed a marked sex difference in the susceptibility of rats. This sex difference could be narrowed by predosing males and females with oestrogens and androgens, respectively. Since then, such differences have been observed repeatedly. In Table 1 are given the results of one series of experiments (DURHAM 1957). It will be seen that these sex differences occur predominantly with compounds that are rapidly metabolized in the body, some of which become ChE-inhibitors only after having been metabolized. For still other compounds, like OMPA, sex differences in toxicity are debatable (DUBOIS et al. 1950; FRAWLEY et al. 1957).

Table 1. *Acute oral LD_{50} values of selected phosphorus insecticides for white rats* (based on DURHAM 1957)

Compound	Oral LD_{50} mg/kg	
	Male	Female
Malathion . .	1375	1000
Chlorothion .	880	980
Diazinon . .	108	76
DDVP . . .	80	56
EPN	36	7.7
Parathion . .	15	3.6

Actual measurements of differences in the activities of the metabolizing enzymes in the male and female have been observed, at least for some compounds and in some species (MURPHY and DUBOIS 1958).

Animal experimental technique. Even such a simple consideration as the way in which the animal experiments are performed is frequently overlooked in considering the pharmacodynamics and toxicity of the inhibitors. An important item here is that narcosis considerably influences the results.

In unanaesthetized animals there is usually a decrease in pulse rate, an increase in pulse amplitude, a decrease in arterial oxygen tension, an increase in arterial carbon dioxide tension, and a fall in arterial blood pH before there are any evident signs of respiratory failure. In anaesthetized animals the effects on blood pressure and pulse rate are reduced and retarded, while the respiratory signs are as a rule more conspicuous (FREDRIKSSON et al. 1960). Attention has also been drawn to the fact that a sublethal degree of respiratory depression may, in certain instances, be made lethal by associated cardiovascular depression (DE CANDOLE 1956).

The means of administration also determines the toxicity of a compound, as pointed out among others by BOMBINSKI and DUBOIS (1958) and by HOLTZ and WESTERMANN (1959).

Receptor effects. Finally, attention may be drawn to pharmacological effects unrelated to ChE-inhibition. This is worthy of treatment in a separate part of this chapter.

2. Comments on Tables A — D

In spite of the above-mentioned difficulties, certain general rules concerning structure and activity may be drawn from the organophosphates listed in the tables. One such is that when R_1 = alkyl and R_2 = alkoxy, this results in more toxic compounds than when they are both alkoxy. Thus, Sarin and analogous compounds (Table A 1) have a greater toxicity than compounds like DFP. If in both types of compounds fluorine is substituted by iodine, cyanide, or thiocyanate, this inevitably results in a decrease of toxicity and ChE-inhibiting potency (Table A 2).

Also, substitution of the alkyl chain in the compounds of Table A 1—A 2 by, e.g., chloride reduces the toxicity. On the other hand branched chains in the alkyl groups give greater potency (Sarin, Soman, DFP). It may be noted that among compounds where $R_1 = R_2 = iso$propyl are to be found selective inhibitors of BuChE (DFP, *iso*-OMPA, and Mipafox). Aryl groups in R_1 and R_2 reduce the toxicity.

Considering Table A 3 and A 4, which contain compounds with an N-P bond, it appears that dialkylamido-alkoxy compounds, like Tabun, are generally more toxic than *bis*-dialkylamido compounds, like Dimefox. Tabun is a direct inhibitor of ChE, whereas Dimefox is transformed by mammals into one or several highly active ChE-inhibitors. Among the compounds selected for Table A 3 and A 4, those where X = cyanide are the most potent ones. Thus, the analogue of Tabun where X = F is only about one-fourth as toxic as the parent compound. Cyanates and thiocyanates are again less toxic.

Compounds with a great variety in the X radical are depicted in Tables B 1 and B 2. This also produces great variation in the toxicity. It is surprising that some of the compounds should have any activity at all. This pertains for example to diethyl trichloromethylphosphonate:

$$\begin{array}{c} C_2H_5O \\ \diagdown \\ P \diagup O \\ C_2H_5O \diagup \diagdown CCl_3 \end{array}$$

This and related substances have been studied biochemically by MYERS (1954), who stated that none of them is very active ($I_{50} \geqq 10^{-5}$ M). The strong electron-attraction by the three chlorine atoms produces a labile P-C bond, analogous to the P-CN bond. Apparently the ChE's are capable of hydrolyzing a labile C-P bond of this type, the end-product being presumably chloroform. By contrast, the C-P bond in Sarin and similar compounds is very stable.

The syntheses of a number of chlorovinyl phosphates have been published by PERKOW (1956), and the pharmacology studied by MEYER (1955). The metabolism of these and allied compounds has been extensively studied by CASIDA and co-workers (ARTHUR and CASIDA 1957, ARTHUR and CASIDA 1958, CASIDA 1956) and also by others (ROBBINS et al. 1956) (Table B 1—B 2). The best known of the compounds in this general group is Dipterex (Table B 1), for which it has been shown that a cleavage of the carbon-phosphorus bond occurs instead of a dehydrochlorination and rearrangement to form the vinyl derivative. The toxicity of the compound 0,0-dimethyl-2,2,2-trichloro-1-acetoxy-ethylphosphate to rats and several insect species appears to be due to enzymic hydrolysis of the acetyl group to form the more potent anti-ChE agent, Dipterex. In this case, the hydrolysis of the carboxylic ester produces a more potent inhibitor.

The presence of cyclic components in the X-group usually decreases toxicity (Table B 1). Notable exceptions to this rule are, however, Paraoxon and the Russian compound Armin. It is seen that here again the introduction of an alkyl instead of alkoxy to form the Russian analogue of Paraoxon increases the toxicity.

Compounds containing a thiol sulfur are listed in Table C 1. These compounds are directly acting ChE-inhibitors, some of which have a remarkably high toxicity, for example Amiton. Before the arrival of these compounds, any substitution of sulfur for oxygen in a molecule complying to the general formula was thought to decrease toxicity. This no longer holds true in general, but is still true where a phosphoryl group is changed to a thionophosphoryl group. Among the thiolo-series are found some extremely toxic ones. One reason for the high toxicity may be that these compounds are not attacked by phosphorylphosphatase.

The thiono-compounds in Table C 2 are fairly non-toxic. Also, a direct action on ChE's without previous metabolization is an exception; usually, the compounds have to be transformed into thiol isomers or oxidized to be inhibitors of appreciable potency.

Most I_{50}'s for thionates have been obtained on impure compounds, and inhibition may well have been due to oxidation products or isomers. The methods of determination published only ruled out these possibilities in one instance, and gave the pI_{50} of Parathion as 3.7 (ALDRIDGE and DAVISON 1953). There is no way of obtaining a pI_{50} for Methyldemeton, since it is converted too rapidly in water to other compounds.

Chloro-substituted compounds have also recently attracted much interest. SCHRADER, in his systematic variation of the Parathion molecule, also introduced chlorine as a substituent in the ring. He noticed that this reduced mammalian toxicity but also reduced the insecticidal activity (SCHRADER 1952; SCHRADER 1954). In the search for new compounds with lower mammalian toxicity, interest has returned to chlorinated derivatives of Parathion or Methylparathion. Of these the 2-chloro-(American Cyanamid 4124) and the 3-chloro-(Chlorothion) analogues have much lower mammalian toxicity than Parathion and also slightly less insect toxicity. It is believed that this is due to differences in breakdown and excretion.

Another group of compounds the metabolism of which has recently received much attention are the Systox and Thimet derivatives (see Tables C 1, C 2). The oxidation products of these compounds have been extensively investigated by FUKUTO et al. (1955). In a wide variety of biological tissues the Systox isomer was oxidized, first to the sulfoxide and then to further oxidation products, probably the sulfones. Usually more toxic compounds are produced. The same thing occurs with Metasystox, Disystox, and Thimet. For detailed references see the tables. Similarly Gusathion (Guthion, DBD) is converted to an anti-ChE agent by an oxidative reaction which occurs in the livers of mammals (MURPHY and DuBois 1957, 1958).

Metabolization to produce toxic compounds is necessary also for the compounds n Table C 3, the thiol-thiono compounds. Malathion, at present an insecticide of extreme importance, has the advantage of being much less toxic to mammals than to insects. Its breakdown in the hen, mouse, and roach has been studied by MARCH et al. (1956). The mouse and hen, to both of which Malathion is almost non-toxic, appeared to degrade the insecticide through similar intermediates, involving hydrolysis in two stages of the diethylsuccinate and hydrolysis of the P-S-C link. Each of these changes can occur with or without prior oxidation of the thiono-phosphoryl group. The extensive metabolism in the hen and mouse as well as the rapid excretion may well account for the low toxicity of Malathion in these animals in contrast to the roach, where metabolism is not extensive.

The cases of Malathion intoxication reported so far have been due to both percutaneous absorption and ingestion (for references see Malathion, Table C 3). The observations corroborate the assumption that man responds as other mammals in having an extensive metabolism as well as rapid excretion of the compound. Up to the time of writing, no lethal cases have been reported. The symptomatology of the cases described in the literature differs partially from that following other anti-ChE agents like Sarin, TEPP, and Parathion, especially with regard to the repeated loss of consciousness, the strong action upon the gastrointestinal system, the type of miosis, and the occurrence of paralysis. All symtoms are readily over-come by small doses of atropine, judging by the scanty data available. It must be remembered that commercial Malathion may contain a mixture of unknown substances.

Pyrophosphates and related compounds have been collected in Table D, which also contains the thiono-analogues. Derivatives of this kind have received compara-tively little attention in recent years, which is surprising in view of the fact that both highly toxic compounds and systemic insecticides are found in the group. Among the oxygen compounds TEPP, first synthetized in 1854, is still the most toxic; it is about 16 times as toxic as the corresponding tetra*iso*propyl derivative. Introduction of nitrogen in the structure decreases toxicity as evidenced by OMPA and *iso*-OMPA.

The introduction of thiono-sulfur also decreases toxicity, with one notable exception. Tetraethyl monothionopyrophosphate is among the most toxic of the organophosphorus ChE-inhibitors. This compound, first synthetized by the ARBUSOWS in 1931, has received comparatively little attention as an insecticide. FISZER in 1953 reported a startling high toxicity figure for this derivative. Given intramuscularly to mice and rats, the compound was said to have an LD_{50} of 0.05 mg/kg. Later investigators have found it considerably less toxic [LD_{50} mice 0.7 mg/kg (route not stated), SHUGAEV 1955; LD_{50} mice intraperitoneally 0.94 mg/kg, intramuscularly 0.5 mg/kg, McIVOR et al. 1956]. The latter authors described also the toxicity of analogous and related compounds in the monothiono series. None of these is as toxic as the tetraethyl derivate.

The reason for the differences in the toxicities found is difficult to explain. Apart from a mistake in calculation one has to be aware of the fact that isomeriza-tion products with transformation of thiono-sulfur to thiol-sulfur gives rise to considerably more toxic derivatives among Parathion-like compounds. The iso-mers among the sulfur-containing pyrophosphates largely remain to be prepared in pure form and studied (McIVOR et al. 1956).

III. Compounds resembling the substrate. Receptor effects

Table E lists compounds containing a quaternary atom in the labile group. These compounds demand special interest because of their special physical-chemical properties and because of the well-known pharmacological activity of quaternary ammonium bases. The "phosphostigmines" (Table E) are highly active inhibitors of ChE, and the quaternary salts are more active than the tertiary compounds (ANDREWS et al. 1952, BURGEN and HOBBIGER 1951, HOBBIGER 1954a, b).

From pharmacological and enzymological investigations it has been suggested repeatedly that AChE is located both inside and outside the cell membrane. Such suggestions have been based upon comparisons of the effects of tertiary and quaternary ammonium bases with anti-ChE activity. It is known that the quaternary nitrogen compounds penetrate less readily due to their lipid insolubility (BURGEN and CHIPMAN 1953, KOELLE and STEINER 1956).

Equipotent doses of phosphoryl compounds containing tertiary and quaternary nitrogen groups, respectively, gave very different degrees of inhibition when sympathetic ganglia were used as test objects and subsequently homogenized. It was shown with a histochemical technique that with the quaternary compound inactivation occurred predominantly at preganglionic terminations and peripheries of ganglion cells, whereas internal cytoplasmic AChE was relatively unaffected. This suggests that the latter, representing only a portion of the total AChE, is not immediately involved in the hydrolysis of ACh during cholinergic transmission (McIsAAC and KOELLE 1959).

Another striking example of the difference in action is given by SCHAUMANN and JOB (1958) who compared the quaternary ChE-inhibitor, echothiophate (Table E), and its tertiary analogue (217 AO, Table C1), the same compounds as employed in the foregoing study. Low doses of echothiophate which did not penetrate into the central nervous system inhibited neuromuscular transmission; even large amounts had no central effect on respiration. Because of its higher lipoid solubility, the tertiary analogue inhibited respiration by direct central action without visibly impairing neuromuscular transmission. However, neuromuscular block was observed when the central effects were prevented by atropine, and the tertiary compound then acted like echothiophate.

In past years a number of studies have indicated that anti-ChE agents have actions independent of their ChE-inhibiting power. The details of these experiments have been discussed by HOLMSTEDT (1959). Arguments in favour of such a concept are, e.g., that neostigmine has a direct excitatory action on a neuromuscular preparation after complete inactivation of ChE by DFP, that anti-ChE agents potentiate the blocking action on the neuromuscular junction of choline esters the enzymic hydrolysis of which is extremely slow, and above all that compounds, the chemical structures of which preclude hydrolysis by ChE's, are often potentiated by anti-ChE agents.

All the above experiments refer to the neuromuscular junction, where it has been possible to study such receptor effects in more detail. It must be observed here that quaternary ammonium bases are often inhibitors of ChE's. Several of these reversible inhibitors are also potent neuromuscular blocking agents; less active drugs are far less efficient inhibitors.

An idea which seems to be implicit from the above quoted results is that the active centre of AChE resembles anionic sites of the end-plate receptor. This was first suggested in rather general terms by ROEPKE, 1936 (cf. WESCOE and RIKER 1951). The hypothesis has been elaborated further by COHEN, VAN DER MEER, MEETER and co-workers (COHEN and POSTHUMUS 1958, COHEN and POSTHUMUS 1957, COHEN et al. 1955, VAN DER MEER and MEETER 1956, MEETER 1958). In their opinion the receptor possesses at least three varieties of molecular patterns:

1) A-groups, supposed to be specific anionic sites which, in combination with the cationic heads of drugs, initiate depolarization.

2) So-called B-groups, which could combine with DFP and similar compounds; this group is probably identical with a structure occurring in most esterases but is not necessarily capable of endowing the neuroreceptor with esterase activity.

3) C-groups, which are non-specific anionic sites. These are capable of combining with cationic drugs but in such an event no depolarization is evoked although the receptor might be blocked.

One bit of evidence which seems to make untenable the idea that the receptors resemble the active surface of ChE is the finding that β,β-dimethylbutylacetate, the carbon analogue of ACh, is an excellent substrate for AChE but is devoid of significant pharmacological action (BANISTER and WHITTAKER 1951). However important the positive charge of a quaternary nitrogen atom is in the depolarization processes, evidently it is of less importance in enzymic hydrolysis.

In view of the above-mentioned theories, the pharmacology of the so-called organophosphorylcholines and thiocholines attracts special interest because of both their strong inhibitory power and their extreme likeness to the substrate molecules (Table E). Methylfluorophosphoryl homocholine seems to be the most potent inhibitor so far described (TAMMELIN 1957). It may be mentioned here that sulphonium compounds are also highly active. Methylation of Systox and iso-Systox to produce the sulphonium derivative increases the inhibitory power 100-fold (FUKUTO et al. 1955).

Of the compounds in Table 2, the three quaternary nitrogen analogues are extremely toxic and have a high affinity for AChE, as suggested due to their attraction both to the "esteratic" and the "anionic site" of the enzyme (TAMMELIN 1957, 1958). The compounds evoke in low doses effects on the cat's blood pressure similar to those produced by choline esters, i.e., a rapid decrease followed by a rapid return to the normal level, and it has therefore been suggested that they have direct effects on the ACh receptors in addition to their potent indirect activity due to their inhibition of the enzyme (FREDRIKSSON 1957, 1958). This interpretation is supported also by the fact that the compounds show the same differences in effect as the corresponding choline esters. Thus, the choline analogue gives both muscarinic and nicotinic responses, the β-methylcholine analogue has predominantly muscarinic effects, the homocholine analogue has both muscarinic and nicotinic effects, and the carbocholine analogue evokes only weak muscarinic responses.

Recently, TAMMELIN (1957, 1958) showed that compounds of this type react extremely rapidly with AChE, and suggested that the blood pressure effects also might be due to the accumulation of ACh subsequent to the rapid inhibition of the enzyme.

It is scarcely possible to judge whether these compounds have any receptor effects from experiments on the cat's blood pressure, given in Table 2. More ideal experimental conditions are obtained when the frog rectus assay is used (FREDRIKSSON and TIBBLING 1959 b). If instead of eserine, Sarin 5×10^{-5} M is utilized for the pretreatment of the rectus muscle, complete enzyme inhibition is obtained. Graded responses to both ACh and the methylfluorophosphoryl cholines can be obtained on such a preparation. That the latter compound gives responses in spite of complete inhibition of ChE's, produced by a compound known to give a very slowly reversible inhibition, shows that the immediate effects are due to direct and not indirect cholinergic activity. Not only the enzyme activity determinations but also the fact that the response to the ACh standard was unaltered throughout the experiments show that there was complete inhibition of the enzyme activity. The responses can hardly be explained by releases of cholinergic transmittors from the tissues, since repeated doses of the test substances always give the same response. Thus, in the experiments by FREDRIKSSON and TIBBLING (1959 b) there was no

Table 2. *Comparison between Sarin and various fluorophosphorylcholines*

Name	Formula	Number of molecules equivalent to one molecule of acetylcholine			Toxicity				Enzyme inhibition pI_{50}	
		Frog rectus	Cat blood pressure		LD_{50} Intraperitoneal inj. Mice		LD_{50} Intravenous inj. Rabbits			
			Depressor response	Pressor response (after atropine)	mg/kg	μmol/kg	mg/kg	μmol/kg	Erythrocytes	Plasma
(I) Methylfluorophosphorylcholine	CH_3—P(=O)(F)—O—CH_2CH_2—$N^+(CH_3)_3$	18	90	20	0.10	0.32	0.010	0.032	10.0	8.4
(II) Methylfluorophosphoryl-β-methylcholine	CH_3—P(=O)(F)—O—CH(—CH_3)—CH_2—$N^+(CH_3)_3$	>4000	110	—	0.07	0.22	0.008	0.025	8.4	8.4
(III) Methylfluorophosphorylhomocholine	CH_3—P(=O)(F)—O—CH_2—CH_2—CH_2—$N^+(CH_3)_3$	550	150	60	0.05	0.15	0.006	0.019	11.0	8.4
(IV) Methylfluorophosphorylcarbocholine	CH_3—P(=O)(F)—O—CH_2—CH_2—$C(CH_3)_3$	>4000	400	—	0.80	4.4	0.100	0.550	9.0	8.3
Sarin	CH_3—P(=O)(F)—OC_3H_7-i				0.42	3.0	0.028	0.2	8.8	8.4

decrease in the response, even after more than ten repeated doses of the compounds. The immediate effects of the substances thus seem to be due to activity on cholinergic receptors, which is reasonable in view of the compounds' structural similarity to ACh.

The compounds have different relative potencies on the cat's blood pressure and on the frog rectus preparations (Table 2). Such species differences are to be expected. Furthermore, the two types of experiments are not directly comparable: in the frog rectus there was complete inhibition of the enzyme activity, whereas this certainly was not the case in the cat.

Table E also contains alkoxy-alkyl (alkoxy) -phosphorylthiocholines. These thiocholine esters in the experiments of TAMMELIN (1957) yielded inhibited AChE which showed reactivation curves (activity/time) identical with those from the corresponding organophosphoryl fluoride or anhydride, when pyridine-2-aldoxime methiodide (P-2-AM) was used as a reactivator. From this it can be concluded that the thiocholines, as well as the halogenides, phosphorylate the enzyme as exemplified in Figure 8 B (isopropoxy-methylphosphorylthiocholine or isopropyl methylphosphonofluoridate, Sarin). On the contrary, it has been found that a series of reactivators, including P-2-AM, fail to reactivate AChE inhibited with the methylfluorophosphoryl cholines in Table 2. (ENANDER 1958).

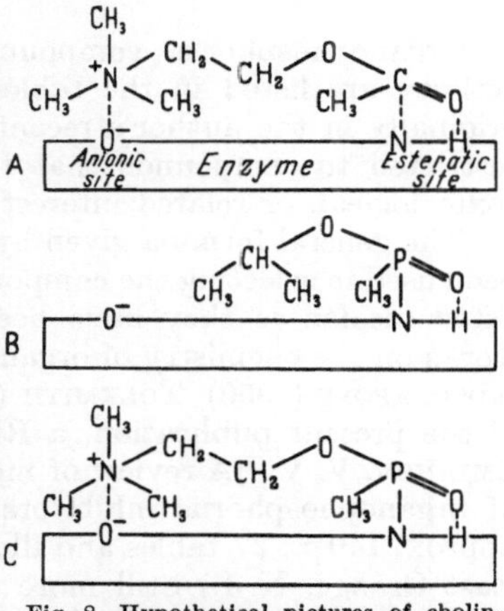

Acetylcholinesterase of the diaphragm of rats inhibited by fluorophosphorylcholines is impossible to reactivate detectably by P-2-AM, but strangely enough, motor activity is restored when P-2-AM is added to the isolated nerve-diaphragm preparation (FREDRIKSSON and TIBBLING 1959 a). No definite explanation for this is available at present, although it is possible that it is based on (a) restoration of an indetectable amount of AChE activity, or (b) direct pharmacological effect of P-2-AM.

Fig. 8. Hypothetical pictures of cholinesterase surface and choline esters. A. Dotted lines show points of attraction between choline esters and the enzyme. The methyl groups directed against the enzyme surface contribute to the formation of the complex. B. Inhibited cholinesterase after contact whith isopropoxy-methyl-phosphorylthiocholine or isopropoxy-methyl-phosphoryl fluoride. C. Inhibited cholinesterase after contact with methyl-fluorophosphorycholine

An ionic bond in the inhibited enzyme, analogous to that postulated in the substrate-enzyme complex (WILSON et al. 1950), and a shielding of the anionic site from the reactivator seem to explain the obstructed reactivation in the experiments in vitro (Fig. 8 C). The ionic bond increases the attraction of the organophosphoryl residue to the enzyme, which alone may be a sufficient explanation in the case of a reactivator like DINA. In the case of P-2-AM, which contains a positively charged ion, the shielding of the anionic site is likely to contribute.

However, studies of the spontaneous reactivation of enzymes inhibited with the above mentioned compounds at least partly contradict what has been said (FREDRIKSSON and TIBBLING 1960). When the spontaneous reactivation of enzymes inhibited with the compounds in Table 2 was investigated, it was found that reactivation occurs rapidly with the fluorophosphorylcholines, whereas, as is well known, it occurs very slowly after inhibition with Sarin. The differences in the spontaneous return of enzyme activity most likely mean that the phosphorylcholines produce a phosphorylated enzyme of different structure, possibly the one exemplified in Fig. 8 C. In this case a weaker linkage to the enzyme would explain the comparatively rapid spontaneous return of enzyme activity, and also the fact that fluorophosphorylcholines produce symptoms of considerably shorter duration than other organophosphorus ChE-inhibitors.

The dual qualities of the organophosphorylcholines of being both cholinesterase inhibitors and choline esters is unique. It is likely that the study of
this interesting group of compounds will yield even more profitable results in the
future. In the efforts to elucidate the action of drugs at a cellular and subcellular
level, their property of being positively charged irreversible ChE-inhibitors should
make them suitable for intracellular application through microiontophoresis.

D. Tables

Organophosphorus compounds with demonstrable or supposed anti-ChE
activity are listed in the tables, which are a modification of those published
originally in the author's recent review (HOLMSTEDT 1959). The listing has been
restricted to compounds that the author considers to be of pharmacological,
toxicological, or related interest.

The general formula given by SCHRADER and mentioned under Chemistry has
been used in selecting the compounds; however, some allied compounds have been
listed insofar as they have been investigated biologically. For comprehensive
works on the chemistry of organophosphorus compounds the reader is referred to
KOSOLAPOFF (1950), TOLKMITH (1959), and VAN WAZER (1958). During the course
of the present publication, a Russian review has appeared: LOSHADKIN, N. A.,
SMIRNOV, V. V. "A review of modern literature on the chemistry and toxicology
of organophosphorus inhibitors of cholinesterase" (Transl. from the Russian;
approx. 140 p., 27 tables and illustrations. Associated technical services, Box 271,
East Orange, N. J.) Still more recently, a monograph was published by D. F.
HEATH, entitled "Organophosphorus Poisons. Anticholinesterases and Related
Compounds" (403 pages, Pergamon Press, Oxford, 1961).

The nomenclature of phosphorus compounds has been extensively treated by
LARSSON, HOLMSTEDT and TJUS (1954) to which publication the reader is referred.
The tables include both the commonly used names, built around phosphoryl or
phosphine, and the Anglo-American names.

For reasons mentioned on page 439, values of pI_{50} and LD_{50} have been included
under Remarks. Unless otherwise stated, RBC refers to human red blood cells, and
the figure under LD_{50} to mg/kg body weight. The LD_{50} values have been restricted,
with few exceptions, to injection experiments in white mice and peroral administration to rats. They have as far as possible been collected from the literature, but in
some cases have been obtained by the author.

The abbreviations under the References columns denote Chemistry, Biochemistry, and Pharmacology, respectively. A key to the tables is given below.

Key to tables.

General formula: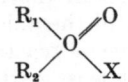

A. Compounds where X = halogen or CN, CNS, etc.
    1. R_1 = alkoxy, R_2 = alkyl   2. R_1 and R_2 = alkoxy   3. R_1 = alkylamido,
    R_2 = alkoxy (and similar compounds)   4. R_1 and R_2 = mono- or dialkylamido.
B. Compounds where X = alkyl, alkoxy, or aryloxy
    1. alkoxydialkyl or dialkoxyalkyl compounds   2. trialkoxy compounds and
    dialkoxy, aryloxy compounds.
C. Thiol- and thiono-phosphorus compounds
    1. thiol-compounds   2. thiono-compounds   3. thiolthiono-compounds
D. Derivatives of pyrophosphorous acid and similar compounds
E. Compounds containing a quaternary nitrogen. Phosphorylcholines, etc.

Table A1 (X = halogen; R_1 = alkoxy; R_2 = alkyl)

Chemical Formula	Name	References C*	References B*	References Ph*	Remarks
i-C₃H₇O, P(=O)(F), CH₃	*Iso*propoxy-methyl-phosphoryl fluoride	(45, 48, 50, 246, 247, 289)	(4, 5, 6, 7, 8, 43, 205, 212)	(61, 62, 87, 91, 92, 93, 94, 135, 163, 164, 191, 240, 309, 345, 378)	LD₅₀ mice i.p. 0.42 mg/kg pI₅₀ (RBC) 8.8 Experiments in human volunteers (164, 165)
C₃H₇CHO(CH₃), P(=O)(F), CH₃	*Iso*propyl methylphosphono-fluoridate (SARIN) (GB)				
CH₃, C₃H₇CHO, P(=O)(F), CH₃	2-Pentoxy-methyl-phosphoryl fluoride 2-Amyl-methylphosphono-fluoridate			(135)	
(CH₃)₃CCH₂CH₂O, P(=O)(F), CH₃	3,3-Dimethylbutoxy-methyl-phosphoryl fluoride 3,3-Dimethylbutyl methyl-phosphonofluoridate Methylfluorophosphoryl carbocholine	(247)	(140)	(138 139)	LD₅₀ mice i.p. 0.8 mg/kg pI₅₀ (RBC) 9.0
CH₃, (CH₃)₃CCHO, P(=O)(F), CH₃	Pinacolyloxy-methyl-phosphoryl fluoride Pinacolyl-methylphosphono-fluoridate (SOMAN)	(80, 289)		(61)	
CH₃, C₅H₁₁CHO, P(=O)(F), CH₃	2-Heptoxy-methyl-phosphoryl fluoride 2-Heptyl-methylphosphono-fluoridate			(135)	
i-C₃H₇O, P(=O)(F), C₂H₅	*Iso*propoxy-ethyl-phosphoryl fluoride *Iso*propyl-ethylphosphono-fluoridate	(246)			LD₅₀ mice i.p. 0.69 mg/kg pI₅₀ (RBC) 8.1

* C = Chemistry; B = Biochemistry; Ph = Pharmacology.

Table A2 (X = halogen, CN, SCN; R_1 and R_2 = alkoxy)

Chemical formula	Name	References			Remarks
		C*	B*	Ph*	
CH_3O–P(=O)(CH_3O)–F	Dimethoxy-phosphoryl fluoride Dimethyl phosphorofluoridate	(173, 320, 338)	(257, 369)	(225)	pI$_{50}$ (horse serum) 7.0
C_2H_5O–P(=O)(C_2H_5O)–F	Diethoxy-phosphoryl fluoride Diethyl phosphorofluoridate	(68, 244, 320, 321, 336, 338)	(10, 257, 369)	(225)	pI$_{50}$ (RBC horse) 6.1 pI$_{50}$ (horse serum) 8.1
n-C_3H_7O–P(=O)(n-C_3H_7O)–F	Di-n-propoxy-phosphoryl fluoride Di-n-propyl phosphorofluoridate	(68, 338)	(257, 369)		pI$_{50}$ (horse serum) 8.25
i-C_3H_7O–P(=O)(i-C_3H_7O)–F	Diisopropoxy-phosphoryl fluoride Diisopropyl phosphorofluoridate (DFP)	(226, 227, 320, 321, 338)	(10, 30, 31, 234, 257, 320, 369)	(204, 210, 235, 279, 320, 321)	LD$_{50}$ mice i.p. 4 mg/kg pI$_{50}$ (RBC horse) 5.75 pI$_{50}$ (horse serum) 8.9
(phenoxy)–P(=O)(phenoxy)–F	Diphenoxy-phosphoryl fluoride Diphenyl phosphorofluoridate	(68, 338)	(257, 369)		pI$_{50}$ (horse serum) 7.2
FCH_2CH_2O–P(=O)(FCH_2CH_2O)–F	Di-(2-fluoroethoxy)-phosphoryl fluoride Di-2-fluoroethyl phosphoro-fluoridate	(68, 320)		(68, 320)	
$ClCH_2CH_2O$–P(=O)($ClCH_2CH_2O$)–F	Di-(2-chloroethoxy)-phosphoryl fluoride Di-2-chloroethyl phosphoro-fluoridate	(68, 83, 320, 338)		(68, 320)	

Structure	Name				Notes
$(i\text{-}C_3H_7O)_2P(=O)I$	Diisopropoxy-phosphoryl iodide Diisopropyl phosphoroiodidate	(264)			
$(C_2H_5O)_2P(=O)CN$	Diethoxy-phosphoryl cyanide Diethyl phosphorocyanidate	(198)	(198)	(198)	LD$_{50}$ i.p. mice 1.4 mg/kg pI$_{50}$ (RBC) 7.1 For other references see (198)
$(C_2H_5O)_2P(=O)SCN$	Diethoxy-phosphoryl thio-cyanate Diethyl phosphorothiocyana-tidate	(320, 322)			

* See Table A 1.

Table A3 (X = halogen, CN, SCN, etc.; R_1 = alkylamido; R_2 = alkoxy, etc.)

Chemical formula	Name	References C*	References B*	References Ph*	Remarks
$(CH_3)_2N$–P(=O)–F, C_2H_5O	Dimethylamido-ethoxy-phosphoryl fluoride / Ethyl-N,N-dimethyl phosphor-amidofluoridate	(82, 320, 338)		(82)	LD_{50} i.p. mice 2.5 mg/kg
$(CH_3)_2N$–P(=O)–CN, CH_3O	Dimethylamido-methoxy-phosphoryl cyanide / Methyl-N,N-dimethyl phosphor-amidocyanidate	(198)	(27, 198)	(198)	LD_{50} i.p. mice 1.9 mg/kg pI_{50} (RBC) 7.8
$(CH_3)_2N$–P(=O)–CN, C_2H_5O	Dimethylamido-ethoxy-phosphoryl cyanide / Ethyl-N,N-dimethyl phosphor-amidocyanidate (TABUN)	(80, 198, 245)	(27, 198, 206)	(61, 191, 198, 201, 240)	LD_{50} mice i.p. 0.6 mg/kg pI_{50} (RBC) 8.4
$(CH_3)_2N$–P(=O)–CN, $i\text{-}C_3H_7O$	Dimethylamido-isopropoxy-phosphoryl cyanide / Isopropyl-N,N-dimethyl phosphoramidocyanidate	(198)	(27, 198)	(198)	LD_{50} mice i.p. 0.5 mg/kg pI_{50} (RBC) 8.9
$(C_2H_5)_2N$–P(=O)–CN, C_2H_5O	Diethylamido-ethoxy-phosphoryl cyanide / Ethyl-N,N-diethyl phosphoramidocyanidate	(198)	(27, 198)	(198)	LD_{50} i.p. mice 4 mg/kg pI_{50} (RBC) 7.5
$(CH_3)_2N$–P(=O)–OCN, C_2H_5O	Dimethylamido-ethoxy-phosphoryl cyanate / Ethyl-N,N-dimethyl phosphor-amidocyanatidate	(336, 338)			
$(CH_3)_2N$–P(=O)–SCN, C_2H_5O	Dimethylamido-ethoxy-phosphoryl thiocyanate / Ethyl-N,N-dimethyl phosphor-amidothiocyanatidate	(239)			Several other thiocyanates described in (239)
$(C_2H_5)_2N$–P(=O)–OC$_2$H$_5$, CH_3	Diethylamino-ethoxy-methyl-phosphine oxide / Ethyl-N,N-diethyl-P-methyl-phosphonamidate	(76, 311)			For toxicity of similar compounds see (76, 311)

* See Table A1.

Table A 4 (X = halogen; R_1 and R_2 = mono- or dialkylamido)

Chemical formula	Name	References C*	B*	Ph*	Remarks
$i\text{-}C_3H_7NH$—P(=O)(—F)—$i\text{-}C_3H_7NH$	Di(isopropylamido)-phosphoryl fluoride N,N′-Diisopropylphosphorodiamidic fluoride Mipafox. Isopestox. Pestox XV (Pest Control Ltd.)	(199, 268, 338)	(10, 32, 89 199, 251)	(89, 252)	pI$_{50}$ (RBC) 4.6, (purified plasma) 7.3 LD$_{50}$ rats i.p. 90 mg/kg Rabbits orally 100 mg/kg Selective inhibitor of BuChE
$(CH_3)_2N$—P(=O)(—F)—$(CH_3)_2N$	Bis(dimethylamido)-phosphoryl fluoride Tetramethylphosphorodiamidic fluoride Dimefox. BFPO. Hanane	(54, 82, 174, 181, 198, 268, 338)	(23, 198)	(109, 121, 181, 198, 297)	LD$_{50}$ mice i.p. 1.2 mg/kg pI$_{50}$ (RBC) 3.6 Transformed by plants, insects and mammals into one or several highly active cholinesterase inhibitors
$(C_2H_5)_2N$—P(=O)(—F)—$(C_2H_5)_2N$	Bis(diethylamido)-phosphoryl fluoride Tetraethylphosphorodiamidic fluoride	(181, 320, 336, 338)		(181, 320)	LD$_{50}$ mice s.c. 160 mg/kg

* See Table A1.

Table B 1 (*Alkoxydialkyl or dialkoxyalkyl compounds*)

Chemical formula	Name	References			Remarks
		C*	B*	Ph*	
CH_3, CH_3 P=O $OCH_2CH_2N(CH_3)_2$	2-Dimethylaminoethoxy-dimethyl-phosphine oxide 2-Dimethylaminoethyl dimethyl-phosphinate	(214)			For synthesis of similar compounds see (214)
C_2H_5O, C_2H_5O P=O CCl_3	Diethoxy-trichloromethyl-phosphine oxide Diethyl trichloromethylphosphonate Ro 3-0658	(238)		(288)	For biochemistry of similar compounds see (288)
C_2H_5O, C_2H_5O P=O $CCl_2COOC_2H_5$	Diethoxy-carbethoxydichloro-ethyl-phosphine oxide Diethyl carbethoxydichloro-ethylphosphonate Forstenon	(72)			
CH_3O, CH_3O P=O $CHCCl_3$ OH	Dimethoxy-2,2,2-trichloro-1-hydroxyethyl-phosphine oxide Dimethyl 2,2,2-trichloro-1-hydroxyethylphosphonate Dipterex, tested under code name Bayer L 13/59 (Farbenfabriken Bayer)	(38, 39, 158, 254, 255)	(22, 101, 269, 271, 285, 314)	(96, 110, 177, 377)	LD_{50} mice i.p. 500 mg/kg Rats orally 450 mg/kg pI_{50} rat brain 5.7 For pharmacology of similar compounds see (277)
CH_3O, CH_3O P=O $CHCCl_3$ $OCCH_2CH_3$ =O	Dimethoxy-2,2,2-trichloro-1-*n*-butyryl-oxy-ethyl-phosphine oxide Dimethyl-2,2,2-trichloro-1-*n*-butyryl-oxy-ethylphosphonate Butonate	(24)	(24)		LD_{50} rats s.c. 3000 mg/kg pI_{50} (RBC bovine) 5.0 For synthesis, toxicity and metabolism of a number of similar compounds see (24)

* See Table A1.

Table B 2 (*Trialkoxy and dialkoxy, aryloxy compounds*)

Chemical formula	Name	References			Remarks
		C*	B*	Ph*	
CH_3O, CH_3O—$P(=O)$—$OCHCl$—CCl_3	Dimethyl 1,2,2,2-tetrachloroethyl phosphate	(86)	(277)	(277)	LD$_{50}$ mice i.p. oil 5 mg/kg Most toxic of a series of compounds tested by MEYER (277)
C_2H_5O, C_2H_5O—$P(=O)$—$OCH=CHCl$	Diethyl 2-chlorovinyl phosphate Compound OS 1836 (Shell Chem. Corp.)		(280)	(233)	LD$_{50}$ mice orally 32 mg/kg pI$_{50}$ (RBC) 4.8 For other toxicity data see (233)
CH_3O, CH_2O—$P(=O)$—$OCH=CCl_2$	Dimethyl 2,2-dichlorovinyl phosphate DDVP	(38, 154, 262)	(24, 101, 118, 154, 271)	(118, 119, 232, 277, 377)	LD$_{50}$ rats orally 56 mg/kg (females), 80 mg/kg (males), mice i.p. 29 mg/kg A number of similar compounds synthetized by PERKOW (303) and investigated by MEYER (277)
CH_3O, CH_3O—$P(=O)$—O—$C(CH_3)=CH$—$COOCH_3$	Dimethyl 1-methyl-2-carbomethoxyvinyl phosphate Phosdrin. OS 2046 (Shell Chem. Corp.)	(66, 86, 154, 359)	(66, 154, 280)	(233)	LD$_{50}$ mice orally 8.9 mg/kg Isomers of different toxicity LD$_{50}$ rats i.p. α-phosdrin 0.35 mg/kg, β-phosdrin 35 mg/kg pI$_{50}$ (RBC) 5.6 For similar compounds see (154, 338)
CH_3O, CH_3O—$P(=O)$—$OC(CH_3)(Cl)=C$—$CON(C_2H_5)_2$	Dimethyl 1-chlorodiethylcarbamoyl-2-propen-1-yl phosphate Phosphamidon (Ciba)	(33)		(231)	
n-C_3H_7O, n-C_3H_7O—$P(=O)$—$OCH=CCl_2$	Di-n-propyl 2,2-dichlorovinyl phosphate DDP	(38, 338)	(209)		The pharmacology of several similar compounds described by MEYER (277)

* See Table A1.

Table B 2 (Continuation)

Chemical formula	Name	References			Remarks
		C*	B*	Ph*	
CH_3O, CH_3O —P(=O)—O— (4-NO_2 phenyl)	Dimethyl 4-nitrophenyl phosphate Paraoxon-ME	(338)	(186, 272)	(186)	LD_{50} mice s.c. 1.4 mg/kg pI_{50} (horse serum) 6.9
C_2H_5O, C_2H_5O —P(=O)—O— (4-NO_2 phenyl)	Diethyl 4-nitrophenyl phosphate E 600. Mintacol. Paraoxon	(133, 336, 337, 338, 352)	(12, 26, 90, 144, 149, 150, 272)	(26, 36, 37, 125, 309, 317, 372)	LD_{50} mice s.c. 0.6-0.8 mg/kg pI_{50} (RBC) 7.2 For biochemistry of several analogues see (144)
C_2H_5O, C_2H_5O —P(=O)—O— (4-Cl phenyl)	Diethyl 4-chlorophenyl phosphate	(144)	(12, 13, 144, 217, 272)	(217)	LD_{50} mice i.p. 138 mg/kg pI_{50} rat brain 4.8 For synthesis of a number of similar compounds see (144)
C_2H_5O, C_2H_5O —P(=O)—O—CH—C(CH$_3$)=N—NH (pyrazolyl)	Diethyl 3-methyl-5-pyrazolyl phosphate. G 24483 (J. R. Geigy, S.A.)	(167, 168)	(288)	(152)	LD_{50} mice orally 4 mg/kg
i-C_3H_7O, i-C_3H_7O —P(=O)—O— (2-OH phenyl)	Diisopropyl 2-hydroxyphenyl phosphate	(213)	(213)		
C_2H_5O, C_2H_5 —P(=O)—O— (4-NO_2 phenyl)	Ethoxy-4-nitrophenyloxy-ethyl-phosphine oxide Ethyl-4-nitrophenyl ethylphos-phonate Armin			(342)	LD_{50} mice 0.54 mg/kg (route of administration not stated) Medical use (342)

* See Table A1.

Table C 1 (*Thiol-compounds*)

Chemical formula	Name	References C*	References B*	References Ph*	Remarks
C_2H_5O — P(=O)(CH_3) — $SCH_2CH_2N(CH_3)_2$	Ethoxy-2-dimethylamino-ethyl-thio-methylphosphine oxide O-Ethyl S-(2-dimethylamino-ethyl) methylphosphonothioate	(346, 348)	(346, 348)		pI_{50} (RBC) 8.8 (346)
C_2H_5O — P(=O)(C_2H_5) — $SCH_2CH_2SC_2H_5$	Ethoxy-2-ethylthioethylthio-ethyl-phosphine oxide O-Ethyl S-(2-ethylthioethyl) ethylphosphonothioate	(1)	(1)		The *l*-enanthiomorph reacts 10—20 times faster than the *d*-enanthiomorph in four ChE prep. studied (1)
CH_3O — P(=O)(CH_3O) — $SCH_2CH_2SC_2H_5$	Dimethyl S-(2-ethylthioethyl) thiophosphate O,O-Dimethyl S-(2-ethylthio-ethyl) phosphorothioate P = O. Methylsystox. Isomethyl-systox. Isometaasystox. Iso-methyldemeton	(187, 338)	(182, 185)	(228, 287)	LD_{50} rats orally 60 mg/kg pI_{50} (RBC) 5.6, (rat brain) 5.8
CH_3O — P(=O)(CH_3O) — $SCH_2CH_2S(=O)C_2H_5$	Dimethyl S-(2-ethylsulphinyl-ethyl) thiophosphate O,O-Dimethyl S-(2-ethylsul-phinylethyl) phosphorothioate Isomethylsystox sulfoxide		(185, 374)	(374)	LD_{50} rats orally 30 mg/kg pI_{50} (RBC) 4.9, (rat brain) 5.2
CH_3O — P(=O)(CH_3O) — $SCH_2CH_2S(=O)(=O)C_2H_5$	Dimethyl S-(2-ethsulfonylethyl) thiophosphate O,O-Dimethyl S-(2-ethylsulfonyl-ethyl) phosphorothioate Isomethylsystox sulfone		(185, 374)	(374)	LD_{50} rats orally 40 mg/kg pI_{50} (RBC) 4.6, (rat brain) 4.9
C_2H_5O — P(=O)(C_2H_5O) — $SCH_2SC_2H_5$	Diethyl S-ethylthiomethyl thio-phosphate O,O-Diethyl S-ethylthiomethyl phosphorothioate		(185, 374)	(374)	LD_{50} rats orally 0.25 mg/kg pI_{50} (RBC) 5.5, (rat brain) 5.7

* See Table A1.

Table C 1 (Continuation)

Chemical formula	Name	References C*	References B*	References Ph*	Remarks
C_2H_5O–P(=O)(=O)–$SCH_2SC_2H_5$	Diethyl S-ethylsulphinylmethyl thiophosphate O,O-Diethyl S-ethylsulphinyl-methyl phosphorothioate		(185, 374)	(374)	LD_{50} rats orally 1 mg/kg pI_{50} (RBC) 6.0, (rat brain) 6.0
C_2H_5O–P(=O)(=O)–$SCH_2SC_2H_5$(=O)	Diethyl S-ethylsulfonylmethyl thiophosphate O,O-Diethyl S-ethylsulfonyl-methyl phosphorothioate		(185, 374)	(374)	LD_{50} rats orally 0.5 mg/kg pI_{50} (RBC) 6.0, (rat brain) 6.0
C_2H_5O–P(=O)–$SCH_2CH_2SC_2H_5$	Diethyl S-(2-ethylthioethyl)-thiophosphate O,O-Diethyl S-(2-ethylthioethyl) phosphorothioate Isodemeton. PO-Systox. Iso-Systox.	(270, 338, 340)	(115, 146, 148, 270, 275, 373, 374)	(98, 99, 115, 373, 374)	LD_{50} mice i.p. 5.6—5.9, s.c 6 mg/kg rats orally 1.5 mg/kg pI_{50} (RBC) 6.0, (rat brain) 7.0
C_2H_5O–P(=O)–$SCH_2CH_2SC_2H_5$(=O)	Diethyl S-(2-ethylsulphinylethyl) thiophosphate O,O-Diethyl S-(ethylsulphinyl-ethyl) phosphorothioate P=O-Systox sulfoxide. Isosystox Sulfoxide. Thiol Systox sulfoxide	(146, 330)	(115, 146, 148, 270, 275, 373)	(115)	LD_{50} mice i.p. 5.6—5.9 mg/kg rats orally 2.0 mg/kg pI_{50} (RBC) 5.6, (rat brain) 5.6
C_2H_5O–P(=O)(=O)–$SCH_2CH_2SC_2H_5$(=O)	Diethyl S-(2-ethylsulfonylethyl) thiophosphate O,O-Diethyl S-(2-ethylsulfonyl-ethyl) phosphorothioate P=O-Systox sulfone. Iso-Systox sulfone. Thiol Systox sulfone	(146, 330)	(115, 146, 148, 270, 275, 373)	(115)	LD_{50} mice i.p. 5.6—5.9 mg/kg rats orally 2.0 mg/kg pI_{50} (RBC) 5.8, (rat brain) 5.7

Structure	Name				LD₅₀ / pI₅₀ data
C_2H_5O, C_2H_5O, $P{=}O$, $SCH_2CH_2N(CH_3)_2$	Diethyl S-(2-dimethylaminoethyl) thiophosphate O,O-Diethyl S-(2-dimethylamino-ethyl) phosphorothioate 217 AO	(348)	(236, 348)	(202, 236, 265, 325, 348)	LD₅₀ mice i.p. 0.41 mg/kg pI₅₀ (RBC) 7.9 For pharmacology of corresponding quaternary compound see (236, 325)
C_2H_5O, C_2H_5O, $P{=}O$, $SCH_2CH_2N(C_2H_5)_2$	Diethyl S-(2-diethylaminoethyl) thiophosphate O,O-Diethyl S-(2-diethylamino-ethyl) phosphorothioate Amiton. Chipman. R-6199. Tetram. DSDP	(147, 155, 156, 276)	(276, 323)		Compound available as hydrogen oxalate LD₅₀ mice i.p. 0.5 mg/kg rats orally 3—7 mg/kg pI₅₀ (rat brain) 8.3
CH_3O, CH_3S, $P{=}O$, O-(4-NO_2-phenyl)	O,S-Dimethyl O-(4-nitrophenyl) thiophosphate O,S-Dimethyl O-(4-nitrophenyl) phosphorothioate	(192, 338)	(186, 192)	(186)	LD₅₀ rats orally Dextro-isomer 135 mg/kg Levo-isomer 25 mg/kg pI₅₀ (rat brain) D-isomer 6.08 L-isomer 6.82
CH_3O, CH_3O, $P{=}O$, S-(4-NO_2-phenyl)	O,O-Dimethyl S-(4-nitrophenyl) thiophosphate O,O-Dimethyl S-(4-nitrophenyl) phosphorothioate	(338)	(186)	(186)	LD₅₀ mice s.c. 7.5 mg/kg pI₅₀ (horse serum) 7.0
C_2H_5O, C_2H_5S, $P{=}O$, O-(4-NO_2-phenyl)	O,S-Diethyl O-(4-nitrophenyl) thiophosphate O,S-Diethyl O-(4-nitrophenyl) phosphorothioate	(338)	(13, 102, 186)	(186)	LD₅₀ mice s.c. 20 mg/kg pI₅₀ (horse serum) 6.0
C_2H_5O, C_2H_5O, $P{=}O$, S-(4-NO_2-phenyl)	O,O-Diethyl S-(4-nitrophenyl) thiophosphate O,O-Diethyl S-(4-nitrophenyl) phosphorothioate	(338)	(13, 102, 186)	(186)	LD₅₀ mice s.c. 1.25 mg/kg pI₅₀ (horse serum) 9.0
CH_3O, CH_3O, $P{=}O$, SCH_2-(5-methoxy-pyrone-4)	2-(Dimethoxy-phosphorylthio)-methyl-5-methoxy-pyrone-4 O,O-Dimethyl (2-methoxy-5-pyrone-4) methyl phosphoro-thioate Endothione 7175 RP		(128, 129)		LD₅₀ mice i.p. <20 mg/kg

* See Table A 1

Table C 2 (*Thiono-compounds*)

Chemical formula	Name	References			Remarks
		C*	B*	Ph*	
n-C₄H₉O S P OCH₂COOC₂H₅ / C₂H₅	n-Butoxy-carbethoxymethoxy-ethyl-phosphine sulfide / O-n-Butyl O-carbethoxymethyl ethylphosphonothioate			(312)	Prolonged effect on peristalsis (207)
CH₃–C(CH₃)(H)–CH₂O S P OCH₂COOC₂H₅ / C₂H₅	Isobutoxy-carbethoxymethoxy-ethyl-phosphine sulfide / O-Isobutyl O-carbethoxymethyl ethylphosphonothioate			(207, 312)	
C₂H₅O S P O–C₆H₄–NO₂	Ethoxy-4-nitrophenoxy-phenyl-phosphine sulfide / O-Ethyl O-(4-nitrophenyl) phenyl-phosphonothioate / EPN (du Pont)	(357)	(84, 195, 284, 316)	(104, 131, 195)	LD₅₀ rats orally 142 mg/kg (male) 14 mg/kg (female) } crystalline EPN; rats i.p. 64 mg/kg (male) mice i.p. 48 mg/kg (female) } technical EPN
CH₃O S P OCH₂CH₂SC₂H₅ / CH₃O	Dimethyl 2-ethylthioethyl thionophosphate / O,O-Dimethyl O-(2-ethylthio-ethyl) phosphorothioate / P = S-Methylsystox. Metasystox. Methyldemeton	(187, 340, 358)	(182, 185, 366, 374)	(228, 287, 374)	LD₅₀ rats orally 250 mg/kg For toxicity of related compounds see (365)
CH₃O S P OCH₂CH₂SC₂H₅ / CH₃O	Dimethyl 2-ethylsulphinyl-ethyl thionophosphate / O,O-Dimethyl O-(2-ethylsulphinylethyl) phosphorothioate		(374)	(374)	LD₅₀ rats orally 600 mg/kg pI₅₀ (RBC) 4.4, (rat brain) 5.2

Structure	Name				
CH_3O, CH_3O — $P(=S)$ — $OCH_2CH_2SO_2C_2H_5$	Dimethyl 2-ethsulfonylethyl thionophosphate O,O-Dimethyl O-(2-ethylsulfonyl-ethyl) phosphorothioate Methylsystox sulfone		(374)	(374)	LD_{50} rats orally 500 mg/kg pI_{50} (RBC) 4.4, (rat brain) 4.5
C_2H_5O, C_2H_5O — $P(=S)$ — $OCH_2CH_2SC_2H_5$	Diethyl 2-ethylthioethyl thionophosphate O,O-Diethyl O-(2-ethylthioethyl) phosphorothioate Demeton. Systox. E 1059	(176, 188, 271, 334, 338, 340)	(130, 146, 148, 270, 374)	(95, 98, 99, 373, 374)	LD_{50} rats orally 30 mg/kg pI_{50} (RBC) 5.3, (rat brain) 5.4 For transformation of the compound see (146, 148, 270, 374)
C_2H_5O, C_2H_5O — $P(=S)$ — $OCH_2CH_2S(=O)C_2H_5$	Diethyl 2-ethylsulphinylethyl thionophosphate O,O-Diethyl O-(2-ethylsulphinyl-ethyl) phosphorothioate Systox sulfoxide	(334)	(185, 374)	(374)	LD_{50} rats orally 100 mg/kg pI_{50} (RBC) 5.2, (rat brain) 5.3
C_2H_5O, C_2H_5O — $P(=S)$ — $OCH_2CH_2SO_2C_2H_5$	Diethyl 2-ethsulfonylethyl thionophosphate O,O-Diethyl O-(2-ethylsulfonyl-ethyl) phosphorothioate Systox sulfone	(334)	(185, 374)	(374)	LD_{50} rats orally 90 mg/kg pI_{50} (RBC) 4.3, (rat brain) 4.3
CH_3O, CH_3O — $P(=S)$ — O—C_6H_4—NO_2	Dimethyl 4-nitrophenyl thiono-phosphate O,O-Dimethyl O-(4-nitrophenyl) phosphorothioate Methylparathion	(222, 223)	(186, 274)	(97, 161, 186, 208)	LD_{50} mice s.c. 30 mg/kg rats orally 25 mg/kg pI_{50} (horse serum) 4.0
CH_3O, CH_3O — $P(=S)$ — O—$C_6H_3(NO_2)(Cl)$	Dimethyl 1-chloro-4-nitrophenyl thionophosphate O,O-Dimethyl O-(2-chloro-4-ni-trophenyl) phosphorothioate Dicapthon Experimental Insecticide 4124 (American Cyanamid)	(15, 339)	(308)		Of comparatively low mammalian toxicity, the acute oral LD_{50} to albino mice being 400 mg/kg (cf. 31.5 mg/kg for the diethyl analogue)

* See Table A1.

Table C2 (Continuation)

Chemical formula	Name	References			Remarks
		C	B	Ph	
	Dimethyl 3-chloro-4-nitrophenyl thionophosphate O,O-Dimethyl O-(3-chloro-4-nitrophenyl) phosphorothioate Chlorothion. Bayer 22/190	(331, 339)	(112, 308, 316)	(34, 113, 229, 230)	LD$_{50}$ rats i.p. 750 mg/kg rats orally 1500 mg/kg pI$_{50}$ (rat brain) 2.3 The low mammalian toxicity is ascribed to slow absorption by animal tissue
	Dimethyl 2,4,5-trichlorophenyl thionophosphate O,O-Dimethyl O-(2,4,5-trichlorophenyl) phosphorothioate Ronnel. Korlan Dow. ET 57	(261, 281, 307, 310)	(307, 308)	(263)	LD$_{50}$ rats orally male 1740 mg/kg, female > 2000 mg/kg. No measurable ChE inhibition *in vitro* Oxygen analogue 1000 times as active (263); see also (307)
	Diethyl 4-nitrophenyl thionophosphate O,O-Diethyl O-(4-nitrophenyl) phosphorothioate Parathion. E 605. Thiophos.	(28, 127, 336, 337, 338)	(12, 13, 102, 114, 130, 149, 150, 186, 272)	(3, 11, 81, 114, 121, 123, 124, 125, 142, 186, 221, 299)	LD$_{50}$ mice s.c. 10—12 mg/kg pI$_{50}$ (horse serum) 4.6, (mouse brain) 5.6 For conversion to analogues see (102, 268, 269, 338)
	Diethyl 2,4-dichlorophenyl thionophosphate O,O-Diethyl-O-(2,4-dichlorophenyl) phosphorothioate V-C 13, Nemacide	(361)			LD$_{50}$ rats orally 270 mg/kg
	Diethyl 4-methylumbelliferyl-(7) thionophosphate O,O-Diethyl O-(4-methylumbelliferyl)phosphorothioate Potasan, E 838 (Farbenfabriken Bayer)	(329, 337, 338, 340)	(13, 109, 132)	(42, 109, 132)	LD$_{50}$ mice s.c. 25 mg/kg rats i.p. 15 mg/kg pI$_{50}$ (rat brain) 8.3 (109)

Structure	Name				Notes
	Diethyl 3-chloro-4-methylumbelliferyl thionophosphate O,O-Diethyl O-(3-chloro-4-methylumbelliferyl)phosphorothioate Resitox. Co-Ral	(330)	(16, 241, 250, 296)	(220, 230)	LD$_{50}$ rats orally 90 to 110 mg/kg
	Diethyl 2-isopropyl-6-methyl-4-pyrimidyl thionophosphate O,O-Diethyl O-(2-isopropyl-6-methyl-4-pyrimidyl) phosphorothioate Diazinon. G. 24480 (J. R. Geigy)	(152, 168, 169, 170, 256)	(29, 55, 71, 84, 153, 308, 315)	(44, 55, 120, 153)	LD$_{50}$ mice i.p. 65 mg/kg LD$_{50}$ rats orally 108 mg/kg (male); 76 mg/kg (female) pI$_{50}$ (purified human plasma) 4.9 For metabolism of this and similar compounds see (29, 250)
	Diethyl 3-methyl-5-pyrazolyl thionophosphate O,O-Diethyl O-(3-methyl-5-pyrazolyl) phosphorothioate Pyrazothion. G. 23027 (J. R. Geigy)	(167)	(153)		Acute oral LD$_{50}$ (as 20% emulsion) 12 mg/kg mice 36 mg/kg rats
	Diethyl 8-quinolyl thionophosphate O,O-Diethyl O-(8-quinolyl) phosphorothioate		(9, 13)		
	Diethyl p-methylsulphinylphenyl thionophosphate O,O-Diethyl-O-(p-methylsulphinylphenyl) phosphorothioate Bayer 25141	(40, 326)	(40, 41)		For metabolism of this and related compounds see (40, 41)
	Dimethylamino-ethoxy-ethyl-thioethoxyphosphine sulfide O-Ethyl O-(2-ethylthioethyl) N,N-dimethylphosphoramido-thioate	(219)			For chemistry of related compounds see (219)

Table C 3 (*Thiolthiono-compounds*)

Chemical formula	Name	References			Remarks
		O*	B*	Ph*	
CH₃O, CH₃O–P(=S)(–O)–SCH₂CNHCH₃	O,O-Dimethyl S-(N-methyl-carbamylmethyl) thiothiono-phosphate. O,O-Dimethyl S-(N-methyl-carbamylmethyl) phosphoro-dithioate. Dimethoate. Rogor. American Cyanamid 12,880		(88)	(190, 318, 319)	LD_{50} mice orally 140 mg/kg (190). For toxicity of related compounds see (190)
CH₃O, CH₃O–P(=S)–S·CHCOOC₂H₅, CH₂COOC₂H₅	O,O-Dimethyl S-(1,2-dicarb-ethoxyethyl) thiothiono-phosphate. O,O-Dimethyl S-(1,2-dicarb-ethoxyethyl) phosphoro-dithioate. Malathion. Experimental insecticide 4049 (American Cyanamid)	(67, 196, 216)	(84, 85, 109, 113, 216, 258, 259, 284, 291, 292, 293)	(34, 109, 113, 131, 160, 172, 179, 216, 282, 285, 300, 364)	LD_{50} rats i.p. 750 mg/kg pI_{50} (rat brain) 4.0. Acute oral LD_{50} to mice and rats ranges from 480 to 5800 mg/kg. For synthesis and data about similar compounds see (141, 216). For isomerization and metabolism of Malathion see (85, 258, 291, 292, 293, 379). For malathion intoxications see (160, 180, 300, 304, 364)
CH₃O, CH₃O–P(=S)–SCH₂–N ... (benzotriazinone structure)	O,O-Dimethyl S-(4-oxo-1,2,3-benzotriazino(3)-methyl) thiothionophosphate. O,O-Dimethyl S-(4-oxo-3-H-1,2,3-benzotriazine-3-methyl) phosphorodithioate. Gusathion. Bayer 17147. Guthion. DBD	(253, 375, 376)	(283, 286)		LD_{50} mice i.p. 5 mg/kg (male) and 3 mg/kg (female). LD_{50} orally rats 16 mg/kg

Structure	Compound names	Ref.	Ref.	Ref.	Data
C_2H_5O—P(=S)—$SCH_2SC_2H_5$	O,O-Diethyl S-ethylthiomethyl thiothionophosphate O,O-Diethyl S-ethylthiomethyl phosphorodithioate Thimet	(50, 51, 143, 270, 335, 340)	(50, 51, 270, 313)	(374, 377)	LD$_{50}$ rats orally 2.1 mg/kg Mice i.p. 2.1 mg/kg No appreciable inhibition in vitro For metabolism and inhibition of ChE see (270, 313, 374)
C_2H_5O—P(=S)—$SCH_2SC_2H_5$ (sulfoxide, =O)	O,O-Diethyl S-ethylsulphinyl-methyl thiothionophosphate O,O-Diethyl S-ethylsulphinyl-methyl phosphorodithioate Thimet sulfoxide		(374)	(374)	LD$_{50}$ rats orally 2.1 mg/kg pI$_{50}$ (RBC) 3.8, (rat brain) 3.3
C_2H_5O—P(=S)—$SCH_2SC_2H_5$ (sulfone, O=, =O)	O,O-Diethyl S-ethylsulfonyl-methyl thiothionophosphate O,O-Diethyl S-ethylsulfonyl-methyl phosphorodithioate Thimet sulfone		(374)	(374)	LD$_{50}$ rats orally 1.7 mg/kg pI$_{50}$ (RBC) 4.5, (rat brain) 4.7
C_2H_5O—P(=S)—$SCH_2CH_2SC_2H_5$	O,O-Diethyl S-(2-ethylthioethyl) thiothionophosphate O,O-Diethyl S-(2-ethylthioethyl) phosphorodithioate Dithiosystox. Disystox. (Disyston. Bayer 19 639)	(270, 332, 340, 360)	(47, 270, 313, 374)	(47, 374)	LD$_{50}$ mice i.p. 5—6 mg/kg rats orally 5 mg/kg pI$_{50}$ rat brain 3.9 For metabolism and inhibition of ChE see under B
C_2H_5O—P(=S)—$SCH_2CH_2SC_2H_5$ (sulfoxide, O=)	O,O-Diethyl S-(2-ethylsulphinyl-ethyl) thiothionophosphate O,O-Diethyl S-(2-ethylsulphinyl-ethyl) phosphorodithioate Disyston sulfoxide		(374)	(374)	LD$_{50}$ rats orally 6.5 mg/kg No appreciable inhibition in vitro
C_2H_5O—P(=S)—$SCH_2CH_2SC_2H_5$ (sulfone, O=, =O)	O,O-Diethyl S-(2-ethylsulfonyl-ethyl) thiothionophosphate O,O-Diethyl S-(2-ethylsulfonyl-ethyl) phosphorodithioate Disyston sulfone		(374)	(374)	LD$_{50}$ rats orally 7.5 mg/kg No appreciable inhibition in vitro

* See Table A1.

Table C 3. (Continuation)

Chemical formula	Name	References C	B	Ph	Remarks
C_2H_5O S P SCH_2COCH_3 O	O,O-Diethyl S-(carbomethoxy-methyl) thiothionophosphate O,O-Diethyl S-(carbethoxy-methyl) phosphorodithioate Azethion			(218)	LD_{50} orally rats 1000 mg/kg (413)
C_2H_5O S P $SCH_2COC_2H_5$ O	O,O-Diethyl S-(carbethoxy-methyl) thiothionophosphate O,O-Diethyl S-carbethoxy-methyl phosphorodithioate Acethion	(295)	(295)		LD_{50} mice i.p. 1280 mg/kg pI_{50} (serum) 5.4 Description of several related compounds see (295)
C_2H_5O S P SCH_2 —⟨ ⟩— Cl	O,O-Diethyl S-(p-chlorophenyl-thiomethyl) dithiophosphate O,O-Diethyl S-(4-chlorophenyl-thio) methyl phosphoro-dithioate Trithion Stauffer R-1303	(343)	(166)		
C_2H_5O S P dioxane C_2H_5O S P	2,3-Bis-(diethoxy-thiophos-phorylthio)p-dioxane 2,3-p-dioxanedithiol-S,S-bis-(O,O-diethyl phosphoro-dithioate) Delnev. Hercules AC-528	(25, 105, 106, 116, 362)	(25)		LD_{50} male rats orally 110 mg/kg Present in cis-and trans-isomers
i-C_3H_7O S H P S—C—N^+ C_2H_5 C_2H_5 i-C_3H_7O S HS^-	O,O-Diisopropyl S-(diethylthio-carbamyl) thiothionophos-phate (hydrosulfide) O,O-Diisopropyl S-(diethylthio-carbamyl) phosphorodithioate hydrosulfide Compound 325 (Holcomb Manufacturing Co.)				LD_{50} orally mice 290 mg/kg rats 320 mg/kg

Table D (*Derivatives of pyrophosphorus acid and similar compounds*)

Chemical formula	Name	References			Remarks
		C*	B*	Ph*	
CH_3O—P(=O)(—OCH_3)—O—P(=O)(—OCH_3)—OCH_3	Tetramethyl pyrophosphate	(353)	(53)	(353)	LD_{50} mice i.p. 1.7 mg/kg pI_{50} (mouse brain) 7.7
C_2H_5O—P(=O)(—OC_2H_5)—O—P(=O)(—OC_2H_5)—OC_2H_5	Tetraethyl pyrophosphate (TEPP)	(171, 290, 327, 336, 338, 353)	(30, 31, 56)	(59, 61, 70, 92, 93, 94, 107, 301, 302, 341, 378)	LD_{50} mice i.p. 0.7 mg/kg pI_{50} (RBC) 7.5
i-C_3H_7O—P(=O)(—OC_3H_7-i)—O—P(=O)(—OC_3H_7-i)—OC_3H_7-i	Tetra*iso*propyl pyrophosphate (TIPP)	(353)	(10, 109, 273)	(109, 353)	LD_{50} mice i.p. 16 mg/kg pI_{50} (RBC horse, and mouse brain) 5.9
CH_3O—P(=O)(—OC_2H_5)—O—P(=O)(—OC_2H_5)—OCH_3	Dimethyl diethyl pyrophosphate *asym.*	(338)	(109)	(109)	LD_{50} mice i.p. 1.1 mg/kg pI_{50} (mouse brain) 8.1
CH_3O—P(=O)(—OC_3H_7-i)—O—P(=O)(—OC_3H_7-i)—OCH_3	Dimethyl diisopropyl pyrophosphate *asym.*	(338)		(109)	LD_{50} mice i.p. 2.5 mg/kg pI_{50} (mouse brain) 6.7
	Tetraorthocresyl pyrophosphate			(189)	

* See Table A1.

Table D (Continuation)

Chemical formula	Name	References C	References B	References Ph	Remarks
i-C$_3$H$_7$NH—P(O)—O—P(O)—NHC$_3$H$_7$-i, with NHC$_3$H$_7$-i	Tetramonoisopropyl pyrophosphortetramide DPDA. Iso-OMPA.	(175)	(10, 32, 288)		pI$_{50}$ (RBC) 3.5 (purified plasma) 5.9 Selective inhibitor of BuChE (10, 32)
C$_2$H$_5$O—P(O)—O—P(O)—OC$_2$H$_5$, (CH$_3$)$_2$N / N(CH$_3$)$_2$	Diethyl *bis*-dimethyl pyrophosphordiamide *sym.*	(198)	(198)	(198)	LD$_{50}$ mice i.p. 22 mg/kg LD$_{50}$ rats i.p. 11.5 mg/kg pI$_{50}$ (RBC) 6.4 pI$_{50}$ (rat brain) 6.3
(CH$_3$)$_2$N—P(O)—O—P(O)—OC$_2$H$_5$, (CH$_3$)$_2$N / OC$_2$H$_5$	Diethyl *bis*-dimethyl pyrophosphordiamide *asym.*	(338)	(109)	(109)	LD$_{50}$ rats i.p. 2.7 mg/kg pI$_{50}$ (rat brain) 6.5
(CH$_3$)$_2$N—P(O)—O—P(O)—N(CH$_3$)$_2$, (CH$_3$)$_2$N / N(CH$_3$)$_2$	Octamethyl pyrophosphortetramide OMPA, Schradan	(65, 157, 183, 184, 305, 306, 328, 333, 336, 338, 355)	(63, 64, 69, 151, 344, 355)	(111, 112, 121)	LD$_{50}$ mice i.p. 17 mg/kg LD$_{50}$ rats i.p.8 mg/kg, rats orally 8—10 mg/kg pI$_{50}$ (rat brain) 2.0
C$_2$H$_5$O—P(S)—O—P(O)—OC$_2$H$_5$, C$_2$H$_5$O / OC$_2$H$_5$	Tetraethyl monothionopyrophosphate	(21, 126, 266, 336, 338)	(75)	(342)	LD$_{50}$ mice 0.7 mg/kg Metabolization (676)
C$_2$H$_5$O—P(S)—O—P(S)—OC$_2$H$_5$, C$_2$H$_5$O / OC$_2$H$_5$	Tetraethyl dithionopyrophosphate Sulfotepp. E 393. Bladafum.	(336, 338, 354)	(53, 75, 115, 272, 354)	(354)	LD$_{50}$ mice s.c. 8 mg/kg
n-C$_3$H$_7$O—P(S)—O—P(S)—OC$_3$H$_7$-n, n-C$_3$H$_7$O / OC$_3$H$_7$-n	Tetra-n-propyl dithionopyrophosphate NPD. E-8573	(338, 354)	(113, 273)	(34, 108, 113)	LD$_{50}$ rats i.p. 1100 mg/kg pI$_{50}$ (rat brain) 5.3

			Acute toxic dose mice orally > 200 mg/kg pI$_{50}$ (mouse brain) 2.8
Tetra*iso*propyl dithionopyro-phosphate	(338)	(273)	
Bis-(diethoxy-thiophosphoryl-thio) methane *O,O,O,*-Tetraethyl S,S'-methylene *bis*phosphorodi-thioate Ethion, Nialate		(100)	LD$_{50}$ rats orally 208 mg/kg
Bis-(diethoxyphosphoryl)-ethylamine		(207, 342)	LD$_{50}$ mice 13.9 mg/kg Used in glaucoma (342)

Structures:

i-C$_3$H$_7$O, i-C$_3$H$_7$O — P(=S)—O—P(=S)—OC$_3$H$_7$-i, OC$_3$H$_7$-i

C$_2$H$_5$O, C$_2$H$_5$O — P(=S)—SCH$_2$S—P(=S)—OC$_2$H$_5$, OC$_2$H$_5$

C$_2$H$_5$O, C$_2$H$_5$O — P(=O)—N(C$_2$H$_5$)—P(=O)—OC$_2$H$_5$, OC$_2$H$_5$

Table E (Compounds containing a quaternary nitrogen)

Chemical formula	Name	References C*	References B*	References Ph*	Remarks
$(CH_3)_3\overset{+}{N}CH_2CH_2O$ —P(=O)(CH₃)F I⁻	Methyl-fluoro-phosphoryl-choline iodide 2-Trimethylammoniumethyl methylphosphonofluoridate iodide	(347, 348)	(122, 140, 348, 349)	(134, 139)	LD₅₀ mice i.p. 0.1 mg/kg pI₅₀ (RBC) 10.0
$(CH_3)_3\overset{+}{N}CH_2CH_2CH_2O$ —P(=O)(CH₃)F I⁻	Methyl-fluoro-phosphoryl-homo-choline iodide 3-Trimethylammoniumpropyl methylphosphonofluoridate iodide	(348)	(122, 138, 348, 349)	(136, 138, 139)	LD₅₀ mice i.p. 0.05 mg/kg pI₅₀ (RBC) 11.0
$(CH_3)_3\overset{+}{N}CH_2\overset{\underset{\textstyle CH_3}{\,}}{C}HO$ —P(=O)(CH₃)F I⁻	Methyl-fluoro-phosphoryl-β-methyl-choline iodide 2-Trimethylammonium-1-methyl-ethyl methylphosphono-fluoridate iodide	(347, 348)	(122, 348, 349)	(136, 138, 139)	LD₅₀ mice i.p. 0.07 mg/kg pI₅₀ (RBC) 8.4
C_2H_5O —P(=O)(CH₃)$SCH_2CH_2\overset{+}{N}(CH_3)_3$ I⁻	Ethoxy-methyl-phosphoryl-thio-choline iodide O, Ethyl-S-trimethylammonium-ethyl methylphosphonothioate iodide	(348)	(348, 349)		LD₅₀ mice i.p. 0.03 mg/kg pI₅₀ (RBC) 9.1
C_2H_5O —P(=O)(C₂H₅)$SCH_2CH_2\overset{+}{N}(C_2H_5)_3$ I⁻	Ethoxy-(2-triethylammonium-ethylthio)-ethyl-phosphine oxide iodide O-Ethyl S-(2-triethylammonium-ethyl) ethylphosphonothioate iodide		(203)		

Structure	Compound	Ref.	Ref.	Ref.	Notes
$(C_2H_5O)_2P(=O)O$–phenyl–$\overset{+}{N}(CH_3)_3$ $CH_3SO_4^-$	3-(Diethoxy-phosphoryloxy)-N-trimethylanilinium methyl sulfate (17) 3-(Diethylphosphato)-N-trimethyl-yl-anilinium-methyl sulfate Ro 3-0340. Diethylphospho-stigmine	(17)	(58, 288)	(58)	LD$_{50}$ mice i.p. 7.5 mg/kg pI$_{50}$ (RBC) 8.1 For synthesis, biochemistry, and pharmacology of similar compounds see (17, 58)
$(i\text{-}C_3H_7O)_2P(=O)O$–pyridinium–$CH_3$ $CH_3SO_4^-$	3-(Diisopropoxy-phosphoryloxy)-N-methylpyridinium-methyl sulfate (57) 3-(Diisopropylphosphato)-N-methyl-pyridinium methyl sulfate	(57)	(57)	(57)	For synthesis of the corresponding tertiary compound see (18)
$(C_2H_5O)_2P(=O)O$–quinolinium–CH_3 $CH_3SO_4^-$	3-(Diethoxy-phosphoryloxy)-N-methylquinolinium methyl sulfate (18) 3-(Diethylphosphato)-N-methyl-quinolinium methyl sulfate Ro 3-0422.	(18)	(288)	(288)	Several similar quaternary and tertiary compounds synthesized and tested biochemically (288)
$(C_2H_5O)_2P(=O)SCH_2CH_2\overset{+}{N}(CH_3)_3$ I^-	Diethoxyphosphoryl-thiocholine iodide O,O-Diethyl-S-2-trimethylam-monium-ethyl phosphoro-thioate iodide. 217 MI. Phospholine. Echothiophate	(348)	(236, 348, 349)	(215, 236, 325, 349)	LD$_{50}$ mice i.p. 0.14 mg/kg pI$_{50}$ (RBC) 8.4 Compared pharmacologically with corresponding tertiary compound (236, 325)
$(C_2H_5O)_2P(=O)SCH_2CH_2\overset{+}{N}(C_2H_5)_3$ I^-	O,O-Diethyl S-(2-triethylammoniumethyl) thiophosphate iodide O,O-Diethyl S-(2-triethylammoniumethyl) phosphorothioate iodide		(294)	(294)	LD$_{50}$ mice i.p. 0.17 mg/kg pI$_{50}$ (RBC) 9.5

* See Table A 1

Table E (Continuation)

Chemical formula	Name	References C	References B	References Ph	Remarks
C_2H_5O—P(=O)(CH_3)—$SCH_2CH_2N^+(C_2H_5)_2$　$CH_3SO_4^-$	O,O-Diethyl S-(2-diethylmethyl-ammoniumethyl) thiophosphate methylsulphate / O,O-Diethyl-S-2-diethyl-methyl-ammoniummethyl phosphoro-thioate methylsulfate	(269)			
(diphenylphosphine oxide)—$NHCH_2CH_2N^+(CH_3)_3$　I^-	Phenoxy-(2-trimethylammonium-ethylamino)-phenyl-phosphine oxide iodide / O-Phenyl-N-2-dimethylamino ethyl 4-phenylphosphon-amidate methiodide	(260)			The racemic methiodide and the two enantio-morphs tested pharma-cologically (260)
(diphenoxyphosphoryl)—$OCH_2CH_2N^+(CH_3)_3$　Br^-	Diphenoxy-phosphorylcholine bromide / Diphenyl-2-trimethylammonium-ethyl phosphate bromide	(178)		(178)	
$(CH_3)_3\overset{+}{N}CH_2CH_2O$—(phenoxyphosphoryl)—$OCH_2CH_2\overset{+}{N}(CH_3)_3$　2 Br^-	Phenoxy-phosphoryl dicholine dibromide / Phenyl-di(2-trimethylammonium ethyl) phosphate dibromide	(178)		(178)	
NH—(phosphoryl)—NH—$OCH_2CH_2\overset{+}{N}(CH_3)_3$　Br^-	Bis(phenylamido)phosphoryl-choline bromide / N,N'-Diphenyl-phosphordiamidic-choline bromide	(214)			

References

1. AARON, H. S., H. O. MICHEL, B. WITTEN and J. I. MILLER: Stereochemistry of asymmetric phosphorus compounds. II. Stereospecificity in the irreversible inactivation of cholinesterases by the enantiomorphos of an organophosphorus inhibitor. J. Amer. chem. Soc. 80, 456—458 (1958).
2. ADAMS, D. H., and V. P. WHITTAKER: The cholinesterase of human blood. II. The forces acting between enzyme and substrate. Biochim. biophys. Acta 4, 543—558 (1950).
3. ADEBAHR, G.: Nierenveränderungen bei der E 605-Vergiftung des Menschen. Arch. Toxikol. 18, 107—120 (1960).
4. ADIE, P. A.: The effect of the sarinase levels of liver on the survival of rabbits injected with sarin. Canad. J. Biochem. 34, 654—659 (1956).
5. — The purification of sarinase from bovine plasma. Canad. J. Biochem. 34, 1091—1094 (1956).
6. — Studies on the enzymatic hydrolysis of sarin and tabun. Canad. J. Biochem. 36, 15—20 (1958).
7. —, S. C. K. HOSKIN and G. S. TRICK: Kinetics of the enzymatic hydrolysis of sarin. Canad. J. Biochem. 34, 80—82 (1956).
8. —, and J. TUBA: The intracellular localization of liver and kidney sarinase. Canad. J. Biochem. 36, 21—24 (1958).
9. ALDRIDGE, W. N.: Some properties of specific cholinesterase with particular reference to the mechanism of inhibition by diethyl-p-nitrophenyl thiophosphate (E 605) and analogues. Biochem. J. 46, 451—459 (1950).
10. — The differentiation of true and pseudo cholinesterase by organo-phosphorus compounds. Biochem. J. 53, 62—67 (1953).
11. —, and J. M. BARNES: Some problems in assessing the toxicity of the "Organophosphorus" insecticides towards mammals. Nature (Lond.) 169, 345—352 (1952).
12. —, and A. N. DAVISON: The inhibition of erythrocyte cholinesterase by tri-esters of phosphoric acid. 1. Diethyl p-nitrophenyl phosphate (E 600) and analogues. Biochem. J. 51, 62—70 (1952).
13. — —The inhibition of erythrocyte cholinesterase by tri-esters of phosphoric acid. 2. Diethyl p-nitrophenyl thionphosphate (E 605) and analogues. Biochem. J. 52, 663—671 (1952).
14. — — The mechanism of inhibition of cholinesterases by organophosphorus compounds. Biochem. J. 55, 763—766 (1953).
15. American Cyanamid Co. U.S. Pat. 2,664,437.
16. ANDERSON, C. A., J. M. ADAMS and D. MacDOUGALL: Photofluorimetric method for determination of Co-Ral residues in animal tissues. J. Agric. Food Chem. 7, 256—259 (1959).
17. ANDREWS, K. J. M., F. R. ATHERTON, F. BERGEL and A. L. MORRISON: The synthesis of neurotropic and musculotropic stimulators and inhibitors. Part V. Derivatives of aminophenyl phosphates as anticholinesterases. J. chem. Soc. 1952, 780—784.
18. — — — Hydroxypyridine and hydroxyquinoline phosphates as anticholinesterases. J. chem. Soc. 1954, 1638—1640.
19. ARBUSOW, A. E.: Über die Struktur der phosphorigen Säure und ihre Derivate. IV. Isomerisation und Übergang der Verbindungen des dreiwertigen Phosphors in solche des fünfwertigen. Chem. Zbl. 2, 1640 (1906).
20. — The Kazan school of chemists. Uspekhi Khim. 9, 1378—1394 (1940).
21. —, u. B. A. ARBUSOW: Über die Ester der pyrophosphorigen, der Unterphosphor- und der Pyrophosphorsäure. J. prakt. Chem. 238, 103—132 (1931).
22. ARTHUR, B. W., and J. E. CASIDA: Metabolism and selectivity of O,O-dimethyl 2,2,2-trichloro-1-hydroxyethyl phosphonate and its acetyl and vinyl derivatives. J. Agric. Food Chem. 5, 186—191 (1957).
23. — — Biological and chemical oxidation of tetramethyl phosphordiamidic fluoride (dimefox). J. econ. Ent. 51, 49—56 (1958).
24. — — Pesticide toxicity. Biological activity of several O,O-dialkyl alpha-acyloxyethyl phosphonates. J. Agric. Food Chem. 6, 360—365 (1958).
25. — — Biological activity and metabolism of Hercules AC-528 components in rats and cockroaches. J. econ. Ent. 52, 20—27 (1959).
26. AUGUSTINSSON, K.-B.: Mintacol (diethyl p-nitrophenyl phosphate). Svensk farm. Tidskr. 57, 261—267 (1953).
27. — Biochemical studies with Tabun and allied compounds. Ark. Kemi 6, 331—350 (1953).
28. — The chemical determination of parathion and its application to biological material. Acta agric. Scand. 7, 165—189 (1957).
29. —, and G. JONSSON: Biochemical studies on the degradation products of diazinone. Experientia (Basel) 13, 438—443 (1957).

30. —, and D. NACHMANSOHN: Studies on cholinesterase. VI. Kinetics of the inhibition of acetylcholine esterase. J. biol. Chem. **179**, 543—559 (1949).

31. — — Distinction between acetylcholine-esterase and other choline ester-splitting enzymes. Science **110**, 98—99 (1949).

32. AUSTIN, L., and W. K. BERRY: Two selective inhibitors of cholinesterase. Biochem. J. **54**, 695—700 (1953).

33. BACHMANN, F.: Phosphamidon, ein neuer Phosphorsäureester mit systemischer Wirkung. Summary of Communications, IVth International Congress of Crop Protection 1957, p. 164.

34. BAGDON, R. F., and K. P. DUBOIS: Pharmacologic effects of chlorthion, malathion and tetrapropyl dithiono pyrophosphate in mammals. Arch. int. Pharmacodyn. **103**, 192—199 (1955).

35. BANISTER, J., and V. P. WHITTAKER: Pharmacological activity of the carbon analogue of acetylcholine. Nature (Lond.) **167**, 605 (1951).

36. BARNES, J. M., and J. I. DUFF: The role of cholinesterase at the myoneural junction. Brit. J. Pharmacol. **8**, 334—339 (1953).

37. — — Acetylcholine production in animals poisoned by diethyl-p-nitrophenyl phosphate (paraoxon). Brit. J. Pharmacol. **9**, 153—158 (1954).

38. BARTHEL, W. F., B. H. ALEXANDER, P. A. GIANG and S. A. HALL: Insecticidal phosphates obtained by a new rearrangement reaction. J. Amer. chem. Soc. **77**, 2424—2427 (1955).

39. — P. A. GIANG and S. A. HALL: Dialkyl α-hydroxyphosphonates derived from chloral. J. Amer. chem. Soc. **76**, 4186—4187 (1954).

40. BENJAMINI, E., R. L. METCALF and T. R. FUKUTO: The chemistry and mode of action of the insecticide O,O-diethyl O,-p-methylsulfinylphenyl phosphorothionate and its analogues. J. econ. Ent. **52**, 94—98 (1959).

41. — — — Contact and systemic insecticidal properties of O,O-diethyl O-p-methylsulfinylphenyl phosphorothionate and its analogues. J. econ. Ent. **52**, 99—102 (1959).

42. BERG, S., E. KUCHINKE u. K. FISCHER: Zur Kenntnis der Vergiftung mit dem Schädlingsbekämpfungsmittel Potasan G. Arch. Toxikol. **16**, 105—117 (1956).

43. BERRY, W. K.: Biochemical mechanism after poisoning with anticholinesterase. Proc. roy. Soc. Med. **46**, 801—802 (1953).

44. BOCKEL, P.: Vergiftung mit einem Phosphorsäureesterpräparat der Diazinon-Gruppe „Basudin". Dtsch. med. Wschr. **82**, 1230—1231 (1957).

45. BOCQUET, J. R.: Contribution à l'étude de la synthèse des halogenophosphates d'alkyle radioactifs et de l'inhibition de la cholinestérase par ces toxiques organophosphones. Les Editions Acta med. Belg. Bruxelles 1956.

46. BODANSKY, O.: Contributions of medical research in chemical warfare to medicine. Science **102**, 517—521 (1945).

47. BOMBINSKI, T. J., and K. P. DUBOIS: Toxicity and mechanism of action of di-syston. A. M. A. Arch. industr. Hlth **17**, 192—199 (1958).

48. BONNAUD: L'arme chimique est-elle périmée? Protar **14**, 113—115 (1948).

49. BOURRET, J., L. DEROBERT u. M. GUENIOT: Intoxications volontaires par insecticides organo-phosphorés (Parathion). Ann. Méd. lég. **38**, 160—164 (1958).

50. BOWMAN, J. S.: Further studies on the metabolism of Thimet by plants, insects, and mammals. J. econ. Ent. **51**, 838—843 (1958).

51. —, and J. E. CASIDA: Metabolism of the systemic insecticide O,O-diethyl S-ethylthiomethyl phosphorodithioate (Thimet) in plants. J. Agric. Food Chem. **5**, 192—197 (1957).

52. BOYD, G. R.: Determination of residues of O-2,4-dichlorophenyl O,O-diethyl phosphorothioate (V-C 13 Nemacide) by cholinesterase inhibition. J. Agric. Food Chem. **7**, 615—617 (1959).

53. BRAUER, R. W.: Inhibition of the cholinesterase activity of human blood plasma and erythrocyte stromata by alkylated phosphorus compounds. J. Pharmacol. **92**, 162—172 (1948).

54. Brit. Pat. 688, 760.

55. BRUCE, R. B., J. W. HOWARD and J. R. ELSEA: Toxicity of O,O-diethyl O-(2-isopropyl-6-methyl-4-pyrimidyl) phosphorothioate (Diazinon). J. Agric. Food Chem. **3**, 1017—1021 (1955).

56. BURGEN, A. S. V.: The mechanism of action of anticholinesterase drugs. Brit. J. Pharmacol. **4**, 219—228 (1949).

57. —, and L. M. CHIPMAN: The location of cholinesterase in the central nervous system. Quart. J. exp. Physiol. **37**, 61—74 (1952).

58. —, and F. HOBBIGER: The inhibition of cholinesterases by alkylphosphates and alkylphenolphosphates. Brit. J. Pharmacol. **6**, 593—605 (1951).

59. — C. A. KEELE and D. SLOME: Pharmacological actions of tetraethylpyrophosphate and hexaethyltetraphosphate. J. Pharmacol. **96**, 396—409 (1949).

60. DE CANDOLE, C. A.: Successful use of pressor drugs in paraoxon poisoning. Rev. canad. Biol. 15, No. 3 (1956).
61. — W. W. DOUGLAS, C. LOVATT EVANS, R. HOLMES, K. E. V. SPENCER, R. W. TORRANCE and K. M. WILSON: The failure of respiration in death by anticholinesterase poisoning. Brit. J. Pharmacol. 8, 466—475 (1953).
62. —, and M. K. MCPHAIL: Sarin and paraoxon antagonism in different species. Canad. J. Biochem. 35, 1071—1083 (1957).
63. CASIDA, J. E.: Metabolism of organophosphorus insecticides in relation to their antiesterase activity, stability, and residual properties. J. Agric. Food Chem. 4, 772—785 (1956).
64. — T. C. ALLEN and M. A. STAHMANN: Mammalian conversion of octamethyl-pyrophosphoramide to a toxic phosphoramide-N-oxide. J. biol. Chem. 210, 607—616 (1954).
65. — R. K. CHAPMAN, M. A. STAHMANN and T. C. ALLEN: Metabolism of schradan by plants and insects to a toxic phosphoramide oxide. J. econ. Ent. 47, 64—71 (1954).
66. CASIDA, J., P. GATTERDAM, L. GETZIN and R. CHAPMAN: Residual properties of the systemic insecticide O,O-dimethyl 1-carbomethoxy-1-propen-2-yl phosphate. J. Agric. Food Chem. 4, 236—243 (1956).
67. CASSADAY, J. T.: U.S. Pat. 2,578,652 v. 2. 3. 1950.
68. CHAPMAN, N. B., and B. C. SAUNDERS: Esters containing phosphorus. Part VI. Preparation of esters of fluorophosphonic acid by means of phosphorus oxydichlorofluoride. J. chem. Soc. 1948, 1010—1014.
69. CHENG, K. K.: A technique for total hepatectomy in the rat and its effect on toxicity of octamethyl pyrophosphoramide. Brit. J. exp. Path. 32, 444—447 (1951).
70. CHENNELLS, M., W. F. FLOYD and S. WRIGHT: Action of condensed alkyl phosphates on the nerve-muscle preparation and the central nervous system of the cat. J. Physiol. 108, 375—397 (1949).
71. CHOUTEAU, J., J. P. VIGNE, A. KARAMANIAN et R. L. TABAU: Sur l'activité antiestérasique de certain esters organophosphoriques complexes à propriétés insecticides. C. R. Soc. Biol. (Paris) 150, 1773—1777 (1956).
72. CIBA/Schweiz, DBP. 845,226.
73. DE CLERMONT, PH.: Note sur la préparation de quelques éthers. (Séance du lundi 14 août 1854.) C. R. 39, 338—340 (1854).
74. — Mémoire sur les éthers phosphoriques. Ann. Chim. Phys. 44, 330—336 (1855).
75. COATES, H.: Chemistry of phosphorus insecticides. Ann. appl. Biol. 36, 156—159 (1949).
76. COE, D. G., H. HURTIG, B. J. PERRY and E. S. SHERLOCK: Some new organophosphorus compounds with insecticidal properties. J. Agric. Food Chem. 7, 251—255 (1959).
77. COHEN, J. A., P. J. WARRINGA and I. INDORF: Relationship between the pharmacological action of neuromuscular drugs and their capacity to inhibit esterases. Acta physiol. pharm. néerl. 4, 187—200 (1955).
78. —, and C. H. POSTHUMUS: The mechanism of action of anticholinesterases. III. The action of anticholinesterases on the phrenic nerve-diaphragm preparation of the rat. Acta physiol. pharm. néerl. 5, 385—397 (1957).
79. — — The mechanism of action of anticholinesterases. Acta physiol. pharm. néerl. 4, 17—36 (1958).
80. COLLOMP: Les Trilons. Bull. d'Information technique et Scientifique. Numéro 23/G, Janvier 1949. Ministère de la Guerre. Section technique de l'armée.
81. CONLEY, B. E.: Antagonism of lethal action of parathion by 3-pyridine acetohydroxamic acid methyl iodide. Fed. Proc. 17, 360 (1958).
82. COOK, H. G., J. D. ILETT, B. C. SAUNDERS, G. J. STACEY, H. G. WATSON, I. G. E. WILDING and S. J. WOODCOCK: Esters containing phosphorus. Part IX. J. chem. Soc. 1949, 2921—2927.
83. — B. C. SAUNDERS and F. E. SMITH: Esters containing phosphorus. Part VIII. Structural requirements for high toxicity and miotic action of esters of fluorophosphonic acid. J. chem. Soc. 1949, 635—638.
84. COOK, J. W., J. R. BLAKE and M. W. WILLIAMS: The enzymic hydrolysis of malathion and its inhibition by EPN and other organic phosphorus compounds. J. Ass. off. agric. Chem. Wash. 40, 664—665 (1957).
85. — — G. YIP and M. WILLIAMS: Malathionase. I. Activity and inhibition. II. Identity of a malathion metabolite. J. Ass. agric. Chem. 41, 399—411 (1958).
86. COREY, R. A., S. C. DORMAN, W. E. HALL, L. C. GLOVER and R. R. WHETSTONE: Diethyl 2-chlorovinyl phosphate and di-methyl 1-carbo-methoxy-1-propen-2-yl phosphate. Science 118, 28—29 (1953).
87. CRAIG, F. N., P. D. BALES and H. M. FRANKEL: Lethality of sarin in a warm environment. J. Pharmacol. 127, 35—38 (1959).

476 References

88. DAUTERMAN, W. C., J. E. CASIDA, J. B. KNAAK and T. KOWALCZYK: Bovine metabolism of organophosphorus insecticides. Metabolism and residues associated with oral administration of dimethoate to rats and three lactating cows. J. Agric. Food Chem. **7**, 188—193 (1959).
89. DAVIES, D. R.: Cholinesterases and the mode of action of some anticholinesterases. J. Pharm. (Lond.) **6**, 1—26 (1954).
90. DAVISON, A. N.: Return of cholinesterase activity in the rat after inhibition by organophosphorus compounds. Biochem. J. **54**, 583—590 (1953).
91. DE BURGH DALY, M.: The effects of anticholinesterases on the bronchioles and pulmonary blood vessels in isolated perfused lungs of the dog. Brit. J. Pharmacol. **12**, 504—512 (1957).
92. — The cardiovascular effects of anticholinesterases in the dog with special reference to haemodynamic changes in the pulmonary circulation. J. Physiol **139**, 250—272 (1957).
93. —, and P. G. WRIGHT: The effects of anticholinesterases upon pulmonary vascular resistance in the dog. J. Physiol. **139**, 273—293 (1957).
94. — — The effects of anticholinesterases upon peripheral vascular resistance in the dog. J. Physiol. **133**, 475—497 (1956).
95. DEICHMANN, W. B., P. BROWN and C. DOWNING: Unusual protective action of a new emulsifier for the handling of organic phosphates. Science **116**, 221 (1952).
96. —, and K. LAMPE: Dipterex: Its pharmacologic action and an appraisal of the hazard associated with its use. Univ. Miami School Med. Bull. **9**, 7—12 (1955).
97. — W. PUGLIESE and J. CASSIDY: Effects of dimethyl and diethyl paranitrophenyl thiophosphate on experimental animals. A.M.A. Arch. industr. Hyg. **5**, 44—51 (1952).
98. —, and R. RAKOCZY: Buscopan in treatment of experimental poisoning by parathion, methyl parathion and systox. A.M.A. Arch. industr. Hyg. **7**, 152—156 (1953).
99. — — Toxicity and mechanism of action of Systox. A.M.A. Arch. industr. Hlth **11**, 324—331 (1955).
100. DICKINSON, B. C.: Ethion, a promising new acaricide and insecticide. J. econ. Ent. **51**, 354—357 (1958).
101. DIE, J. VAN: Inhibition of serum cholinesterase by O,O-dimethyl-2,2,2-trichloro-1-hydroxyethyl phosphonate and O,O-dimethyl O-2,2-dichlorovinyl phosphate. Koninkl. Ned. Akad. Wetenschap Proc. Ser. B **60**, 227—233 (1957).
102. DIGGLE, W. M., and J. C. GAGE: Cholinesterase inhibition in vitro by O,O-diethyl O-p-nitrophenyl thiophosphate (Parathion, E 605). Biochem. J. **49**, 491—494 (1951).
103. DIRNHUBER, P., and H. CULLUMBINE: The effect of anticholinesterase agents on the rats blood pressure. Brit. J. Pharmacol. **10**, 12—15 (1955).
104. DI STEFANO, V., L. HURWITZ, W. F. NEUMAN and H. C. HODGE: Coramine (Nikethamide) as an adjuvant to atropine in treatment of poisoning by EPN (ethyl p-nitrophenyl thionobenzene-phosphonate. Proc. Soc. exp. Biol. (N. Y.) **78**, 712—713 (1951).
105. DIVELEY, W. R., A. H. HAUBEIN, A. D. LOHR, and P. B. MOSELEY: Two new organophosphorus derivatives of p-dioxane with excellent insecticidal and acaricidal activity. J. Amer. chem. Soc. **81**, 139—144 (1959).
106. —, and A. D. LOHR: 2,3-p-dioxanedithiol S,S-bis(O,O-dialkyl phosphorodithioate). U.S. Patent No. 2,725,328, Nov. 20, 1955.
107. DOUGLAS, W. W., and P. B. C. MATTHEWS: Acute tetraethylpyrophosphate poisoning in cats and its modification by atropine or hyoscine. J. Physiol. (Lond.) **116**, 202—218 (1952).
108. DOULL, J., and K. P. DUBOIS: Toxicity and anticholinesterase action of tetra-n-propyl dithionopyrophosphate. J. Pharmacol. **106**, 382 (1952).
109. DUBOIS, K. P., and J. M. COON: Toxicology of organic phosphorus-containing insecticides to mammals. Arch. industr. Hyg. **6**, 9—13 (1952).
110. —, and G. J. COTTER: Studies on the toxicity and mechanism of action of dipterex. A.M.A. Arch. industr. Hlth **11**, 53—60 (1955).
111. — J. DOULL and J. M. COON: Studies on the toxicity and pharmacological action of octamethyl pyrophosphoramide (OMPA; Pestox III). J. Pharmacol. **99**, 376—393 (1950).
112. — — — The cholinergic action of octamethyl pyrophosphoramide (OMPA). J. Pharmacol. **98**, 6—7 (1950).
113. — — J. DEROIN and O. K. CUMMINGS: Studies on the toxicity and mechanism of action of some new insecticidal thionophosphates. A.M.A. Arch. industr. Hyg. **8**, 350 to 358 (1953).
114. — — and J. M. COON: Studies on the toxicity and mechanism of action of p-nitrophenyl diethyl thionophosphate (parathion). J. Pharmacol. **95**, 79—91 (1949).
115. — S. D. MURPHY and D. R. THURSH JR.: Toxicity and mechanism of action of some metabolites of Systox. A.M.A. Arch. industr. Hlth **13**, 606—612 (1956).

116. DUNN, C. L.: Determination of 2,3-p-dioxanedithiol S,S-bis(O,O-diethyl phosphoro-dithioate). J. Agric. Food Chem. 6, 203—209 (1958).
117. DURHAM, W. F.: The toxicity of chemicals used in mosquito control. Proc. of the Forty-fourth Ann. Meeting of the New Jersey Mosquito Extermination Ass. Held at Atlantic City March 13, 14 and 15, 1957, pp. 155—160.
118. — T. B. GAINES, R. H. McGAULEY, V. A. SEDLAK, A. M. MATTSON and W. J. HAYES: Studies on the toxicity of O,O-dimethyl-2,2-dichlorovinyl phosphate (DDVP). A.M.A. Arch. industr. Hlth 15, 340—349 (1957).
119. — W. J. HAYES JR.,and A. M. MATTSON: Toxicological studies of O,O-dimethyl-2,2-di-chlorovinyl phosphate (DDVP) in tobacco warehouses. A.M.A. Arch. industr. Hlth 20, 202—210 (1959).
120. DYBING, O., and E. SOGNEN: Hyperglycaemia in rats after diazinon and other cholin-esterase inhibitors. Acta pharmacol. 14, 231—235 (1958).
121. EDSON, E. F.: Threshold effects of organic phosphorus insecticides in the diet of the rat, pig and humans. Summary of communications. IVth International Congress of Crop Protection 1957, 221.
122. ENANDER, I.: Experiments with methyl-fluoro-phosphorylcholine-inhibited cholin-esterase. Acta chem. scand. 12, 780—781 (1958).
123. ERDMANN, W. D., H. D. KEMPE u. W. LÜHNING: Über die Wirkung von Esterase-blockern (E 605, Eserin und Prostigmin) auf das Atemzentrum von Katze und Hund. Naunyn-Schmiedeberg's Arch. exp. Path. Pharmak. 225, 359—368 (1955).
124. —, u. L. LENDLE: Vergiftungen mit esteraseblockierenden Insecticiden aus der Gruppe der organischen Phosphorsäure-Ester (E 605 und Verwandte). Ergebn. inn. Med. Kinder-heilk., new ser. 10, 104—184 (1958).
125. —, u. F. SAKAI: Analyse der unspezifisch lähmenden Wirkung einiger Alkylphosphate (E 600 und E 605). Naunyn-Schmiedeberg's Arch. exp. Path. Pharmakol. 236, 205—207 (1959).
126. FISZER, B., J. MICHALSKI and J. WIECZORKOWSKI: Roczniki Chem. 27, 482 (1953).
127. FLETCHER, J. H., J. C. HAMILTON, I. HECHENBLEIKNER, E. J. HOEGBERG, B. J. SERTL and J. T. CASSADAY: Preparation of O,O-diethyl O-p-nitrophenyl thiophosphate (Parathion). J. Amer. chem. Soc. 70, 3943—3944 (1948).
128. FOURNEL, J.: Action antidote de l'iodométhylate de l'α-pyridylaldoxime vis-à-vis des intoxications expérimentales provoquées par les insecticides organophosphorés. C. R. Soc. Biol. (Paris) 151, 1373—1377 (1958).
129. — J. DESMORAS, P. DUBOST, R. DUCROT et. L. JULOU: Toxicité d'un nouvel ester phosphorique à action endothérapique: le 7175 R.P. ou Endothion. Summary of com-munications. IVth International Congress of Crop Protection 1957, 221—222.
130. FRAWLEY, J. P., and H. N. FUYAT: Effect of low dietary levels of Parathion and Systox on blood cholinesterase of dogs. J. Agric. Food Chem. 5, 346—348 (1957).
131. — — E. C. HAGAN, J. R. BLAKE and O. G. FITZHUGH: Marked potentiation in mamma-lian toxicity from simultaneous administration of two anticholinesterase compounds. J. Pharmacol. 121, 96—106 (1957).
132. — E. C. HAGAN and O. G. FITZHUGH: A comparative pharmacological and toxicological study of organic phosphate-anticholinesterase compounds. J. Pharmacol. 105, 156—165 (1952).
133. FREAR, D. E. H.: Chemistry of the pesticides, p. 82. New York: D. van Nostrand Co. Inc. 1955.
134. FREDRIKSSON, T.: Pharmacological properties of methylfluorophosphorylcholines. Two synthetic cholinergic drugs. Arch. int. Pharmacodyn. 113, 101—113 (1957).
135. — Studies on the percutaneous absorption of sarin and two allied organophosphorus cholinesterase inhibitors. Acta derm.-venereol. (Stockh.) 38, 1—83, Suppl. 41 (1958).
136. — Further studies on fluoro-phosphorylcholines. Pharmacological properties of two new analogues. Arch. int. Pharmacodyn. 115, 474—482 (1958).
137. — C.-H. HANSSON and B. HOLMSTEDT: Effects of sarin in the anaesthetized and un-anaesthetized dog following inhalation, percutaneous absorption and intravenous in-fusion. Arch. int. Pharmacodyn. 126, 288—302 (1960).
138. —, and G. TIBBLING: Reversal of effects on the rat nerve-diaphragm preparation pro-duced by methylfluorophosphorylcholines. Biochem. Pharmacol. 2, 63—67 (1959).
139. — — Demonstration of direct cholinergic receptor effects of methylfluorophosphoryl-cholines. Biochem. Pharmacol. 2, 286—289 (1959).
140. — — Inhibition of cholinesterase with methylfluorophosphorylcholine and — carbo-choline, spontaneous return of activity. J. Biochem. Pharmacol. 3, 184—189 (1960).
141. *French patent* 1096341.
142. FUKUHARA, A.: Parathion poisoning. III. Effect of sulfhydryl compounds and 2-pyridine aldoxime methiodide on parathion poisoning. Okayama Igakkai Zasshi 69, 945—958 (1957).

143. FUKUTO, T. R., and R. L. METCALF: Manuscript submitted to J. Agric. Food Chem. 1954. See Agr. Chem. **9**, 130 (1954).
144. — — Structure and insecticidal activity of some diethyl substituted phenyl phosphates. J. Agric. Food Chem. **4**, 930—935 (1956).
145. — — R. B. MARCH and M. MAXON: A water soluble systemic insecticide O,O-diethyl S-2-ethylmercaptoethyl phosphorothiolate methosulfate. J. Amer. chem. Soc. **77**, 3670 to 3671 (1955).
146. — — — — Chemical behavior of Systox isomers in biological systems. J. econ. Ent. **48**, 347—354 (1955).
147. —, and E. M. STAFFORD: The isomerization of O,O-diethyl O-2-diethylaminoethyl phosphoro thionate. J. Amer. chem. Soc. **79**, 6083—6085 (1957).
148. — J. P. WOLF III, R. L. METCALF and R. B. MARCH: Identification of the sulfone plant metabolite of the thiono isomer of Systox. J. econ. Ent. **50**, 399—401 (1957).
149. GAGE, J. C.: A cholinesterase inhibitor derived from O,O-diethyl O-p-nitrophenyl thiophosphate in vivo. Biochem. J. **54**, 426—430 (1953).
150. —, and J. PAYTON: The action of diethyl-p-nitrophenyl thiophosphate (Parathion, E 605) in vivo. Résumé des communications IIe Congr. int. Biochimie, Paris, 1952.
151. GARDINER, J. E., and B. A. KILBY: I. The mammalian metabolism of bis(dimethyl-amino)phosphorous anhydride (Schradan). Biochem. J. **51**, 78—85 (1952).
152. GASSER, R.: Expériences dans la lutte contre les araignées rouges avec de nouveaux acaricides. III. Int. Congr. Phytopharmacy, Paris, 1952, p. 51.
153. — Über ein neues Insektizid mit breitem Wirkungsspektrum. Z. Naturforsch. 8 B, 225 to 232 (1953).
154. GATTERDAM, P. E., J. E. CASIDA and D. W. STOUTAMIRE: Relation of structure to stability, antiesterase activity and toxicity with substituted-vinyl phosphate insecticides. J. econ. Ent. **52**, 270—276 (1959).
155. GHOSH, R.: Phosphorodithioates. Brit. Pat. 783,281, Sept. 18, 1957.
156. —, and J. F. NEWMAN: A new group of organophosphorus pesticides. Chem. & Ind. **1955**, p. 118, Jan. 1929.
157. GIANG, P. A.: A bibliography of systemic insecticides. U.S. Dept. of Agriculture, Agricultural Research Service Ent. Research Branch E-874, 1954.
158. —, and R. L. CASWELL: Polarographic determination of O,O-dimethyl 2,2,2-tri-chloro-1-hydroxy-ethylphosphonate (Bayer L 13/59). J. Agric. Food Chem. **5**, 753—754 (1957).
159. GILMAN, A.: The effects of drugs on nerve activity. Ann. N. Y. Acad. Sci. **47**, 549—558 (1946).
160. GOLDMAN, H., and M. TEITEL: Malathion poisoning in a 34 month-old child following accidental ingestion. J. Pediat. **52**, 76—81 (1958).
161. GOTHELF, B., A. G. KARCZMAR and K. BLACHUT: Interaction of bisquaternary and phosphonate anticholinesterases. Fed. Proc. **17**, 372 (1958).
162. GREEN, A. L.: The kinetic basis of organophosphate poisoning and its treatment. Biochem. Pharmacol. **1**, 115—128 (1958).
163. GROB, D.: The manifestations and treatment of poisoning due to nerve gas and other organic phosphate anticholinesterase compounds. A.M.A. Arch. intern. Med. **98**, 221—239 (1956).
164. —, and A. M. HARVEY: The effects and treatment of nerve gas poisoning. Amer. J. Med. **14**, 52—63 (1953).
165. — — Effects in man of the anticholinesterase compound sarin (isopropyl methyl phosphonofluoridate). J. clin. Invest. **37**, 350—368 (1958).
166. GUNTHER, F. A., G. E. CARMAN, L. R. JEPPSON, J. H. BARKLEY and R. C. BLINN: Residual behavior of S-(p-chlorophenylthio)methyl O,O-diethyl phosphorodithioate (Trithion) on and in mature lemons and oranges. J. Agric. Food Chem. **7**, 28—30 (1959).
167. GYSIN, H.: Sur un nouveau groupe de substances insecticides. III. Int. Congr. Phytopharmacy, Paris, 1952, p. 40.
168. — Some new insecticides. Chimia 8, 205—210, 221—228 (1954).
169. —, u. A. MARGOT: DBP. 910,652 v. 20. 4. 1952.
170. — — Chemistry and toxicological properties of O,O-diethyl-O-(2-iso-propyl-4-methyl-6-pyrimidinyl) phosphorothioate (Diazinon). J. Agric. Food Chem. **6**, 900—903 (1958).
171. HALL, S. A., and M. JACOBSON: Hexaethyl tetraphosphate and tetraethyl pyrophosphate. Industr. Engng. Chem. **40**, 694—699 (1948).
172. HANZAL, R. F., H. J. HORN and L. W. HAZLETON: Anticholinesterase activity of parathion and malathion. Fed. Proc. **13**, 363—364 (1954).
173. HARDY, E. E., and G. M. KOSOLAPOFF: U.S. Pat. 1946. 2, 409,039.
174. HARTLEY, G. S.: Unpublished experiments. Pest Control, Ltd., Cambridge.
175. — Brit. Pat. 688,766, 1949.
176. — Congress abstracts, III. Int. Congr. Phytopharmacy Paris 1952.

177. HASIK, A., and M. BARGÁR: Prispevok k. farmakodynamike Dipterex (Beitrag zur Pharmakodynamik des Insektizids Dipterex). Biologia (Bratislava) 13, 428—439 (1958).
178. HAZARD, R., J. CHEYMOL, P. CHABRIER et A. CARAYON-GENTIL: Sur de nouveaux esters phosphorylés de la choline. C. R. Acad. Sci. (Paris) 243, 2180—2186 (1956).
179. HAZLETON, L. W., and E. G. HOLLAND: Toxicity of Malathion. A.M.A. Arch. industr. Hyg. 8, 399—405 (1953).
180. HEALY, J. K.: Ascending paralysis following malathion intoxication: a case report. Med. J. Aust. 46, 765 (1959).
181. HEAP, R., and B. C. SAUNDERS: Esters containing phosphorus. Part VII. Substituted diaminofluorophosphine oxides. J. chem. Soc. 1948, 1313—1316.
182. HEATH, D. F.: Reactions of ethylthioethyl O,O-dimethyl phosphorothioates in water. J. chem. Soc. 1958, 1643—1651.
183. — D. W. J. LANE and M. LLEWELLYN: Commercial octamethylpyrophosphoramide. III. Decomposition of the insecticide in plants using phosphorous as a tracer. J. Sci. Food Agric. 3, 60—69 (1952).
184. — — — Commercial octamethylphosphoroamide. IV. Decomposition of pyrophosphoric acid tetra (dimethylamide) and orthophosphoric acid tri(dimethylamide) in the living plant. J. Sci. Food Agric. 3, 69—73 (1952).
185. —, and M. VANDEKAR: Some spontaneous reactions of O,O-dimethyl S-ethylthioethyl phosphorothiolate and related compounds in water and on storage, and their effects on the toxicological properties of the compounds. Biochem. J. 67, 187—201 (1957).
186. HECHT, G., u. W. WIRTH: Zur Pharmakologie der Phosphorsäureester. Naunyn-Schmiedeberg's Arch. exp. Path. Pharmak. 211, 264—277 (1950).
187. HENGLEIN, A., u. G. SCHRADER: Zur Kenntnis der Isomerie-Erscheinungen bei den System-Insektiziden „Systox" und „Metasystox". Z. Naturforsch. 10 b, Heft 1 (1955).
188. — — u. R. MÜHLMANN: Quantitative infrarotspektroskopische Bestimmung des Isomerenverhältnisses in dem System-Insecticid „Systox". Z. analyt. Chemie 141, 276—281 (1954).
189. HENSCHLER, D., u. H.-H. BAYER: Toxikologische Untersuchungen über Triphenylphosphat, Trixylphosphate und Triarylphosphate aus Mischungen homologer Phenole. Naunyn-Schmiedeberg's Arch. exp. Path. Pharmak. 233, 512—517 (1958).
190. HEWITT, R., A. BREBBIA and E. WALETSKY: Carbamoyl alkyl phosphorodithioates as chemotherapeutic agents. J. econ. Ent. 51, 126—131 (1958).
191. HEYMANS, C., A. POCHET et H. VAN HOUTTE: Contributions à la pharmacologie du Sarin et du Tabun. Arch. int. Pharmacodyn. 104, 293—332 (1956).
192. HILGETAG, G., u. G. LEHMANN: Optisch aktive Thiophosphate. J. prakt. Chem. 8, 224 bis 234 (1959).
193. HOBBIGER, F.: The inhibition of cholinesterases by 3-(diethoxyphosphinyloxy)-N-methylquinolinium methylsulphate and its tertiary base. Brit. J. Pharmacol. 9, 159—165 (1954a).
194. — Anticholinesterases. A comparison between the in vitro activity and the in vivo action of certain organic phosphates. Chem. & Ind. 1954b, p. 1574.
195. HODGE, H. C., E. A. MAYNARD, L. HURWITZ, V. DISTEFANO, W. L. DOWNS, C. K. JONES and H. J. BLANCHET JR.: Studies of the toxicity and of the enzyme kinetics of ethyl p-nitrophenyl thionobenzene phosphonate (EPN). J. Pharmacol. 112, 29—39 (1954).
196. HOEGBERG, E. I., and J. T. CASSADAY: The reaction of O,O-dialkyl thiophosphoric acid salts with some α-haloacyl derivatives. J. Amer. chem. Soc. 73, 557—559 (1951).
197. HOFMANN, A. W.: Weitere Beobachtungen über die Phosphinsäuren. Ber. 6, 303—308 (1873).
198. HOLMSTEDT, B.: Synthesis and pharmacology of dimethylamidoethoxy-phosphoryl cyanide (Tabun) together with a description of some allied anticholinesterase compounds containing the N—P bond. Acta physiol. scand. 25, 1—120, Suppl. 90 (1951).
199. — A modification of the thiocholine method for the determination of cholinesterase. I. Biochemical evaluation of selective inhibitors. Acta physiol. scand. 40, 322—330 (1957).
200. — Pharmacology of organophosphorus cholinesterase inhibitors. Pharm. Rev. 11, 567 to 688 (1959).
201. —, and C. R. SKOGLUND: The action on spinal reflexes of dimethyl-amido-ethoxy-phosphoryl cyanide. "Tabun," a cholinesterase inhibitor. Acta physiol. scand. 29, 410—427 (1953).
202. HOLTZ, P., u. E. WESTERMAN: Giftung und Entgiftung von Parathion und Paraoxon. Naunyn-Schmiedeberg's Arch. exp. Path. Pharmak. 237, 211—221 (1959).
203. HOPF, H. S., and R. T. TAYLOR: Role of cholinesterase in insecticidal action. Nature (Lond.) 182, 1381—1382 (1958).
204. HORTON, R. G., G. B. KOELLE, B. P. MCNAMARA and H. J. PRATT: The acute toxicity of di-isopropyl fluorophosphate. J. Pharmacol. 87, 414—420 (1946).

480   References

205. HOSKIN, F. C. G.: The enzymatic hydrolysis products of sarin. Canad. J. Biochem. 34, 75—79 (1956).
206. —, and G. S. TRICK: Stereospecificity in the enzymatic hydrolysis of tabun and acetyl-β-methylcholine chloride. Canad. J. Biochem. 33, 963—969 (1955).
207. IL'YUCHENOK, T. YU.: Effect of organophosphorus compounds on salivation and intestinal secretion. Khim. i Primenenie Fosfororg. Soedinenii, Akad. Nauk S.S.S.R., Trudy 1-oi Konferents, 1955, pp. 318—323.
208. IWAMOTO, T., and M. TAGA: Effects of methylparathion on the cow and its distribution in the body. Igaku to Seibutsugaku 50, 54—57 (1956).
209. JANDORF, B. J.: Mode of action of pesticides. Mechanism of reaction of di-n-propyl-2,2-dichlorovinyl phosphate (DDP) with esterases. J. Agric. Food Chem. 4, 853—858 (1956).
210. —, and P. D. MCNAMARA: Distribution of radiophosphorus in rabbit tissues after injection of phosphorus-labeled diisopropyl fluorophosphate. J. Pharmacol. 98, 77—84 (1950).
211. — H. O. MICHEL, N. K. SCHAFFER, R. EGAN and W. H. SUMMERSON: General discussion on the physical chemistry of enzymes. Faraday Soc. (Oxford, 10—12 August) 12, 4808 (1955).
212. — — — — — The mechanism of reaction between esterases and phosphorus-containing anti-esterases. Disc. Faraday Soc. 20, 134—142 (1955).
213. — T. WAGNER-JAUREGG, J. J. O'NEILL and M. A. STOLBERG: The reaction of phosphorus-containing enzyme inactivators with phenols and polyphenols. J. Amer. chem. Soc. 74, 1521—1523 (1952).
214. JEAN, H.: Esters et sels de la choline et de quelques acides dérivés du phosphore. Bull. Soc. chim. Fr. 1957, 783—786.
215. JEWELL, H. A., and R. A. LEHMAN: Pharmacology of phospholine iodide-an alkyl phosphothiocholine. Fed. Proc. 17, 381 (1958).
216. JOHNSON, G. A., J. H. PLETCHER, K. G. NOLAN and J. T. CASSADAY: Decreased toxicity and cholinesterase inhibition in a new series of dithiophosphates. J. econ. Ent. 45, 279—283 (1952).
217. JONES, H. W., B. J. MEYER and L. KAREL: The relationship of cholinesterase inhibiting activity to the toxicity of some organic phosphorus compounds. J. Pharmacol. 94, 215 to 220 (1948).
218. JUNG, O.: Toxikologie des Dithiophosphorsäureesters Azethion. Arch. Tox. 16, 341—345 (1957).
219. KABAČNIK, M. E., N. A. GODOVIKOV, D. M. PAJKIN, A. M. P. SABANOV, L. F. EFIMOVA and N. M. GAMPER: Organophosphorus insecticides (in Russian) Žurnal obščej chimii, T. 29, 7, 2182—2190 (1959).
220. KAPLANIS, J. N., D. E. HOPKINS and G. H. TREIBER: Dermal and oral treatments of cattle with phosphorus-32-labeled Co-Ral. J. Agric. Food Chem. 7, 483—486 (1959).
221. KAY, K., L. MONKMAN, J. P. WINDISH, T. DOHERTY, J. PARÉ and C. RACICOT: Parathion exposure and cholinesterase response of Quebec apple growers. A.M.A. Arch. industr. Hyg. 6, 252—262 (1952).
222. KETELAAR, J. A. A.: Abstr. II. Int. Congr. Crop Protection, 1949.
223. —, and J. E. HELLINGMAN: Chemical studies on insecticides. Analyt. Chem. 23, 646—650 (1951).
224. KILBY, B. A.: Alkyl Fluorophosphonates and Related Compounds. Research 2, 417—422 (1949).
225. —, and M. KILBY: The toxicity of alkyl fluorophosphonates in man and animals. Brit. J. Pharmacol. 2, 234—240 (1947).
226. KILPATRICK, M. L., and M. KILPATRICK: The hydrolysis of diisopropyl fluophosphate. J. phys. Chem. 53, 1371—1384 (1949).
227. — — A mechanism for the hydrolysis of diisopropyl fluophosphate. J. phys. Chem. 53, 1385—1397 (1949).
228. KLIMMER, O. R., u. W. PFAFF: Untersuchungen über die Toxicität des neuen Kontaktinsekticides O,O-Dimethyl-thiophosphorsäure-O-(β-S-äthyl)-äthylester („Metasystox"). Arzneim.-Forsch. 5, 584—587 (1955).
229. — — Vergleichende Untersuchungen über die Toxicität organischer Thiophosphorsäureester. Arzneim.-Forsch. 5, 626—630 (1955).
230. KLOTZSCHE, C.: Zur Toxikologie neuerer insektizider Phosphorsäureester. Arzneim.-Forsch. 5, 436—439 (1955).
231. — Neue Insektizide Phosphor- und Phosphorsäureester. Nachrbl. deutsch. Pflanzenschutzdienst 10, 60 (1958).
232. KODAMA, J. K., H. H. ANDERSON, M. K. DUNLAP and C. H. HINE: Toxicity of organophosphorus compounds. A.M.A. Arch. industr. Hlth 11, 487—493 (1955).

233. KODAMA, J. K., M. S. MORSE, H. H. ANDERSON, M. K. DUNLAP and C. H. HINE: Comparative toxicity of two vinyl-substituted phosphates. A.M.A. Arch. industr. Hyg. 9, 45—61 (1954).

234. KOELLE, G. B., and A. GILMAN: The relationship between cholinesterase inhibition and the pharmacological action of di-isopropyl fluorophosphate (DFP). J. Pharmacol. 87, 421—434 (1946).

235. — — The chronic toxicity of diisopropyl fluorophosphate (DFP) in dogs, monkeys and rats. J. Pharmacol. 87, 435—448 (1946).

236. —, and E. C. STEINER: The cerebral distributions of a tertiary and a quaternary anticholinesterase agent following intravenous and intraventricular injection. J. Pharmacol. 118, 420—434 (1956).

237. KOLL, W.: Personal communication. In letter to the author, March 3, 1960.

238. KOSOLAPOFF, G. M.: Organophosphorus compounds. New York: John Wiley & Sons, Inc.; New York: Chapman & Hall, Ltd., 1950.

239. KOVACHE, H., H. JEAN and G. GARNIER: Étude de quelques composés organiques du phosphore. Chim. et Industr. 64, 287—299 (1950).

240. KROP, S., and A. M. KUNKEL: Observations on the pharmacology of the anticholinesterases sarin and tabun. Proc. Soc. exp. Biol. (N. Y.) 86, 530—533 (1954).

241. KRUEGER, H. R., J. E. CASIDA and R. P. NIEDERMEIER: Bovine metabolism of organophosphorus insecticides. Metabolism and residues associated with dermal application of Co-ral to rats, a goat, and a cow. J. Agric. Food Chem. 7, 182—188 (1959).

242. LANGE, W.: Fortschritte auf dem Gebiete der Darstellung und Verwendung von Fluorverbindungen. Chem. Ztg. 59, 393 (1935).

243. — Personal letter to the author. April 7, 1952.

244. —, u. G. VON KRUEGER: Über Ester der Monofluorphosphorsäure. Ber. dtsch. chem. Ges. 65, 1598—1601 (1932).

245. LARSSON, L.: The hydrolysis of dimethylamido-ethoxyphosphoryl cyanide (Tabun). Acta chem. scand. 7, 306—314 (1953).

246. — The alkaline hydrolysis of isopropoxy-methyl-phosphoryl fluoride (Sarin) and some analogues. Acta chem. scand. 11, 1131—1142 (1957).

247. — Studies on the chemical reactivity of organic phosphorus compounds. Diss. Svensk kem. Tidskr. 70, 405—427 (1958).

248. — B. HOLMSTEDT and E. TJUS: Some considerations regarding the nomenclature of organic phosphorus compounds. Acta chem. scand. 8, 1563—1569 (1954).

249. LENDLE, L.: Personal communication (1959).

250. LINDQUIST, D. A., E. C. BURNS, C. P. PANT and P. A. DAHM: Fate of P^{32}-labeled Bayer 21/199 in the white rat. J. econ. Ent. 51, 204—206 (1958).

251. LOCKER, A., u. H. SIEDEK: Über Aktivierung von Cholinesterasen durch Alkylphosphate in vivo. Experientia (Basel) 8, 146—148, 302—303 (1952).

252. — — Die Wirkung von Alkylphosphaten auf Gewebsatmung und Cholinesteraseaktivität. Z. ges. exp. Med. 119, 314—326 (1952).

253. LORENZ, W.: Farbenfabriken Bayer. DBP. 927,270.

254. — Insecticidal phosphonic ester. U.S. Pat. 2,701,225.

255. — A. HENGLEIN and G. SCHRADER: The new insecticide, O,O-dimethyl 2,2,2-trichloro-1-hydroxy-ethylphosphonate. J. Amer. chem. Soc. 77, 2554—2556 (1955).

256. LOULOUDES, S. J., J. N. KAPLANIS and C. C. ROAN: The synthesis of radioactive Diazinon using P^{32}. J. org. Chem. 21, 685—686 (1956).

257. MACKWORTH, J. F., and E. C. WEBB: The inhibition of serum cholinesterase by alkyl fluorophosphonates. Biochem. J. 42, 91—95 (1948).

258. MARCH, R. B., T. R. FUKUTO, R. L. METCALF and M. G. MAXON: Fate of P^{32}-labeled malathion in the laying hen, white mouse, and American cockroach. J. econ. Ent. 49, 185—195 (1956).

259. — R. L. METCALF, T. R. FUKUTO and F. A. GUNTHER: Fate of P^{32}-labeled malathion sprayed on Jersey heifer calves. J. econ. Ent. 49, 679—682 (1956).

260. MARSI, K. L., C. A. VANDERWERF and W. E. McEWEN: The synthesis and resolution of compounds of tetracovalent phosphorus. J. Amer. chem. Soc. 78, 3063—3066 (1956).

261. MARTIN, H.: Guide to chemicals used in crop protection. Canad. Dept. agric. Bull., 3rd Ed., October 1957, p. 136.

262. MATTSON, A. M., J. T. SPILLANER and G. W. PEARCE: Dimethyl 2,2-dichlorovinyl phosphate (DDVP), an organic phosphorus compound highly toxic insects. J. Agric. Food Chem. 3, 319—321 (1955).

263. McCOLLISTER, D. D., F. OYEN and V. K. ROWE: Toxicological studies of O,O-dimethyl-O-(2,4,5-trichlorophenyl) phosphorothioate (Ronnel) in laboratory animals. J. Agric. Food Chem. 7, 689—693 (1959).

264. McCOMBIE, H., B. C. SAUNDERS and G. J. STACEY: Esters containing phosphorus. Part III. J. chem. Soc. **1945**, 921—922.
265. McIsAAC, R. J., and G. B. KOELLE: Comparison of the effects of inhibition of external, internal and total acetylcholinesterase upon ganglionic transmission. J. Pharmacol. **126**, 9—20 (1959).
266. McIvOR, R. A., G. D. McCARTHY and G. A. GRANT: Preparation and toxicity of some alkyl thiopyrophosphates. Canad. J. Chem. **34**, 1819—1832 (1956).
267. MEETER, E.: The relation between end-plate depolarization and the repetitive response elicited in the isolated rat phrenic nerve-diaphragm preparation by DFP. J. Physiol. **144**, 38—51 (1958).
268. METCALF, R. L.: Organic insecticides. Their chemistry and mode of action. New York and London: Interscience Publishers 1955.
269. — ed.: Advances in pest control research. Vol. 1. New York and London: Interscience Publishers 1957.
270. — T. R. FUKUTO and R. B. MARCH: Plant metabolism of dithio-Systox and Thimet. J. econ. Ent. **50**, 338—345 (1957).
271. — — — Toxic action of Dipterex and DDVP to the house fly. J. econ. Ent. **52**, 44—49 (1959).
272. —, and R. B. MARCH: Studies of the mode of action of parathion and its derivatives and their toxicity to insects. J. econ. Ent. **42**, 721—728 (1949).
273. — — Properties of acetylcholine esterases from the bee, the fly and the mouse and their relation to insecticide action. J. econ. Ent. **43**, 670—677 (1950).
274. — — The isomerization of organic thionophosphate insecticides. J. econ. Ent. **46**, 288—294 (1953).
275. — — T. R. FUKUTO and M. G. MAXON: The nature and significance of Systox residues in plant materials. J. econ. Ent. **48**, 364—369 (1955).
276. — E. M. STAFFORD, T. R. FUKUTO and R. B. MARCH: The systemic behavior of O,O-diethyl S-2-(diethylamino) ethyl phosphorothiolate and its salts. J. econ. Ent. **50**, 205 to 210 (1957).
277. MEYER, F.: Untersuchungen über 17 neue Dialkyl-dihalogenvinyl- und tetrahalogenäthyl-phosphate. IV. Mitteilung: Kreislauf- und Atemwirkung der übrigen Dialkyl-dichlorvinyl- und tetrachloräthylphosphate. Arzneimittel-Forsch. **5**, 646—654 (1955); and previous papers in the same series.
278. MICHAELIS, C. A. A.: Über die organischen Verbindungen des Phosphors mit Stickstoff. Liebigs Ann. Chem. **326**, 129—258 (1903).
279. MODELL, W., S. KROP, T. HITCHCOCK and W. F. RIKER jr.: General systemic actions of di-isopropyl fluorophosphate (DFP) in cats. J. Pharmacol. **87**, 400—413 (1946).
280. MORSE, M. S., J. K. KODAMA and C. H. HINE: Cholinesterase-inhibiting properties of two vinyl-substituted phosphates. Proc. Soc. exp. Biol. (N. Y.) **83**, 765—768 (1953).
281. MOYLE, C. L. (to The Dow Chemical Co.): U.S. Patent 2,599,516 (June 3, 1952).
282. MURPHY, S. D., R. L. ANDERSON and K. P. DuBOIS: Potentiation of toxicity of Malathion by triorthotolyl phosphate. (24668). Proc. Soc. exp. Biol. (N. Y.) **3**, 483—487 (1959).
283. —, and K. P. DuBOIS: Enzymatic conversion of the dimethoxy ester of benzotriazine dithiophosphoric acid to an anticholinesterase agent. J. Pharmacol. **119**, 572—583 (1957).
284. — — Quantitative measurement of inhibition of the enzymic detoxification of malathion by EPN (ethyl p-nitrophenyl thionobenzenephosphonate). Proc. Soc. exp. Biol. (N. Y.) **96**, 813—818 (1957).
285. — — Inhibitory effect of dipterex and other organic phosphates on detoxification of malathion. Fed. Proc. **17**, 397 (1958).
286. — — The influence of various factors on the enzymatic conversion of organic thiophosphates to anticholinesterase agents. J. Pharmacol. **124**, 194—202 (1958).
287. MÜHLMANN, R., u. H. TIETZ: Das chemische Verhalten von Methylisosystox in der lebenden Pflanze und das sich daraus ergebende Rückstandsproblem. Höfchen-Briefe, Bayer (Leverkusen, Germany) Pflanzenschutz-Nachr. **9**, 116—140 (1956).
288. MYERS, D. K.: Studies on selective esterase inhibitors. Thesis, pp. 97. Amsterdam 1954.
289. *Neue chemische Kampfstoffe.* Protar **16**, 131—135 (1950).
290. NYLÉN, P.: Studien über organische Phosphorverbindungen. Diss., Uppsala 1930.
291. O'BRIEN, R. D.: The inhibition of cholinesterase and succinoxidase by malathion and its isomer. J. econ. Ent. **49**, 484—490 (1956).
292. — Properties and metabolism in the cockroach and mouse of malathion and malaoxon. J. econ. Ent. **50**, 159—164 (1957).
293. — The effect of malathion and its isomer on carbohydrate metabolism of the mouse, cockroach and house fly. J. econ. Ent. **50**, 79—84 (1957).
294. — Effect of ionization upon penetration of organophosphates to the nerve cord of the cockroach. J. econ. Ent. **52**, 812—816 (1959).

295. O'BRIEN, R. D., G. D. THORN and R. W. FISHER: New organophosphate insecticides developed on rational principles. J. econ. Ent. 51, 714—718 (1958).
296. —, and L. S. WOLFE: The metabolism of Co-ral (Bayer 21/199) by tissues of the house fly, cattle grub, ox, rat, and mouse. J. econ. Ent. 52, 692—695 (1959).
297. OKINAKA, A. J., J. DOULL, J. M. COON and K. P. DUBOIS: Studies cn the toxicity and pharmacological actions of bis(dimethylamido) fluorophosphate (BFP). J. Pharmacol. 112, 231—245 (1954).
298. OOSTERBAAN, R. A., M. G. P. J. WARRINGA, H. S. JANSZ, F. BERENDS and J. A. COHEN: The reaction of pseudocholinesterase with diisopropyl-phosphorofluoridate (DFP). IV. Int. Congr. Biochem., Wien, 1.—6. Sept. 1958. Suppl. to Int. Abstr. Biol. Sci., p. 38.
299. PANKASKIE, J. E., F. C. FOUNTAINE and P. A. DAHM: The degradation and detoxication of parathion in dairy cows. J. econ. Ent. 45, 51—60 (1952).
300. PARKER, G. F. jr., and W. R. CHATTIN: A case of malathion intoxication in a ten year old girl. J. Ind. med. Ass. 48, 491—492 (1955).
301. PAULET, G.: Nouvelle contribution à l'étude de l'action pharmacologique du tétraéthyl-pyrophosphate (TEPP). Arch. int. Pharmacodyn. 97, 157—185 (1954).
302. — Activité cholinestérasique et fonctionnement des centres respiratoires. J. Physiol. (Paris) 48, 915—936 (1956).
303. PERKOW, W.: Die Insektizide. 1. Aufl. Heidelberg: Alfred Hüthig 1956.
304. PETTY, C. H.: Organic phosphate insecticide poisoning. Residual effects in two cases. Amer. J. Med. 24, 467 (1958).
305. PIANKA, M.: Organophosphorus compounds. I. Interaction of organic phosphorohalogenides with solid alkalis: A new synthesis of Schradan. J. appl. Chem. 5, 109—120 (1955).
306. —, and B. D. OWEN: Organophosphorus compounds. II. Interaction of dimethylphosphoramidic dichloride with hexamethyl-phosphoramide: Adduct formation and radical exchange. J. apppl. Chem. 5, 525—535 (1955).
307. PLAPP, F. W., and J. E. CASIDA: Animal metabolism of insecticides. Bovine metabolism of organophosphorus insecticides. Metabolic fate of O,O-dimethyl O-(2,4,5-trichlorophenyl) phosphorothioate in rats and a cow. J. Agric. Food Chem. 6, 662—667 (1958).
308. — — Hydrolysis of the alkylphosphate bond in certain dialkyl aryl phosphorothioate insecticides by rats, cockroaches, and alkali. J. econ. Ent. 51, 800—803 (1958).
309. PUNTE, C. L., E. J. OWENS, E. H. KRACKOW and P. L. COOPER: Influence of physical activity on the toxicity of aerosols and vapors. A. M. A. Arch. industr. Hlth 17, 34—37 (1958).
310. RADELEFF, R. D., and G. T. WOODWARD: Toxicological studies of Dow ET-57 in cattle and sheep. J. econ. Ent. 50, 249—251 (1957).
311. RAZUMOV, A. I., O. A. MUKHACHEVA and E. A. MARKOVICH: Biologically active alkylated amide esters and mixed esters of alkylphosphonic acids. Khim. i. Primenic Fosfororg. Soedinenii, Akad. Nauk S.S.S.R., Trudy 1-oi Konferents, 1955, 194—204 (publ. 1957).
312. REUT, N. A.: Pharmacological and toxicological properties of thiophosphorus compounds. Khim. i. Primenenie Fosfororg. Soedinenii, Akad. Nauk S.S.S.R., Trudy 1-oi Konferents, 1955 pp. 313—317.
313. REYNOLDS, H. T., T. R. FUKUTO, R. L. METCALF and R. B. MARCH: Seed treatment of field crops with systemic insecticides. J. econ. Ent. 50, 527—539 (1957).
314. ROBBINS, W. E., T. L. HOPKINS and G. W. EDDY: The metabolism of P^{32}-labeled Bayer L 13/59 in a cow. J. econ. Ent. 49, 801—807 (1956).
315. — — — Metabolism and excretion of phosphorus-32-labeled diazinon in a cow. J. Agric. Food Chem. 5, 509—513 (1957).
316. ROSENBERG, P., and J. M. COON: Potentiation between cholinesterase inhibitors. Fed. Proc. 17, 406 (1958).
317. SAKAI, F., H. DALRI, W. D. ERDMANN u. G. SCHMIDT: Über die Atemlähmung durch Parathion oder Paraoxon und ihre antagonistische Beeinflußbarkeit. Naunyn-Schmiedeberg's Arch. exp. Path. Pharmak. 234, 210—219 (1958).
318. SANDERSON, D. M., and E. F. EDSON: Oxime therapy in poisoning by six organophosphorus insecticides in the rat. J. Pharm. (Lond.) 11, 721—729 (1959).
319. SANTI, R., and P. DE PIETRI-TOUELLI: Mode of action and biological properties of the S-(methylcarbamyl)methyl O,O-dimethyl-dithiophosphate. Nature (Lond.) 183, 398 (1959).
320. SAUNDERS, B. C.: Phosphorus and fluorine. The chemistry and toxic action of their organic compounds. Cambridge: University Press 1957.
321. —, and G. J. STACEY: Esters containing phosphorus. Part IV. Diisopropyl fluorophosphonate. J. chem. Soc. 1948, 695—699.
322. — — F. WILD and J. G. E. WILDING: Esters containing phosphorus. Part V. Esters of substituted phosphonic and phosphonous acids. J. chem. Soc. 1948, 699—703.

484   References

323. Scaife, J. E., and D. H. Campbell: The destruction of O,O-diethyl-S-2-diethylamino-
     ethyl phosphorothiolate by liver microsomes. Canad. J. Biochem. **37**, 297—305 (1959).
324. Schall, A.: Über die Einwirkung von Phosphoroxybromid auf sek. a liphatische Amine.
     Dissert. Rostock 1898; Liebigs Ann. Chem. **326**, 182 (1903).
325. Schaumann, W., and C. Job: Differential effects of quaternary cholinesterase inhibitor,
     phospholine, and its tertiary analogue, compound 217-AO, on central control of respira-
     tion and on neuromuscular transmission. The antagonism by 217-AO the respiratory
     arrest caused by morphine. J. Pharmacol. **123**, 114—120 (1958).
326. Schrader, G.: Belgian Patent 556,009.
327. — DBP. 720,577.
328. — DBP. 918,603.
329. — DBP. 814,297 v. 2. 10. 1948.
330. — DBP. 881,194 v. 31. 7. 1951.
331. — DBP. 921,870 v. 3. 5. 1952.
332. — DAS. 10,101,960 v. 13. 10. 1955.
333. — and H. Kükenthal: DBP. 918,603 v. 5. 8. 1941.
334. — and W. Lorenz: DBP. 876,692 v. 7. 7. 1951; DBP. 876,691 v. 6. 7. 1951; DBP. 871,448
     v. 31. 7. 1951.
335. — — DBP. 917,668 v. 2. 8. 1952.
336. — BIOS Final Report, 1947, p. 714.
337. — Organische Phosphor-Verbindungen als neuartige Insektizide (Auszug). Angew. Chem.
     62, 471—473 (1950).
338. — Die Entwicklung neuer Insektizide auf Grundlage von organischen Fluor- und Phos-
     phorverbindungen. Monographie No. 62, 2. Aufl. Weinheim: Verlag Chemie 1952.
339. — Chlorothion, a new relatively nontoxic insecticide from the series of the thiophosphoric
     acid esters. Angew. Chem. **66**, 265—267 (1954).
340. — Die insektiziden Phosphorsäureester. Angew. Chem. **69**, 86—90 (1957).
341. Scott, M. J.: The effects of anticholinesterases upon the spleen of the dog. J. Physiol.
     139, 489—496 (1957).
342. Shugaev, B. B.: Alkyl pyrophosphates, their pharmacological and toxicological pro-
     perties. Khim. I Primenenie Fosfororg. Soedinenii, Akad. Nauk S.S.S.R., Trudy 1-oi
     Konferents, 1955, pp. 301—309.
343. *South African Patent* 1748/55.
344. Spencer, E. Y., R. D. O'Brien and R. W. White: Permanganate oxidation products of
     Schradan. J. Agric. Food Chem. **5**, 123—127 (1957).
345. Stewart, W. C.: The effects of sarin and atropine on the respiratory center and neuro-
     muscular junctions of the rat. Canad. J. Biochem. **37**, 651—660 (1959).
346. Tammelin, L.-E.: Dialkoxy-phosphorylthiocholines, alkoxy-methyl-phosphorylthio-
     cholines and analogous choline esters. Acta chem. scand. **11**, 1340—1349 (1957).
347. — Methyl-fluoro-phosphorylcholines. Acta chem. scand. **11**, 859—865 (1957).
348. — Choline esters; substrates and inhibitors of cholinesterases. Svensk kem. Tidskr. **70**,
     157—181 (1958).
349. — Organophosphorylcholines and cholinesterases. Ark. kemi **12**, 287—298 (1958).
350. Tibbling, G.: Unpublished.
351. Tolkmith, H.: Electron group polarizability and molecular properties of organophos-
     phorus compounds. Ann. N. Y. Acad. Sci. **79**, 187—231 (1959).
352. Topley, B.: Insecticidal phosphorus compounds. Chem. & Ind. **1950**, Dec. 30, 859—868.
353. Toy, A. D. F.: The preparation of tetraethyl pyrophosphate and other tetraalkyl pyro-
     phosphates. J. Amer. chem. Soc. **70**, 3882—3886 (1948).
354. — Tetraethyl dithionopyrophosphate and related tetraalkyl dithionopyrophosphates.
     J. Amer. chem. Soc. **73**, 4670—4674 (1951).
355. Tsuyuki, H., M. A. Stahmann and J. E. Casida: Preparation, purification, isomerization
     and biological properties of octamethylpyrophosphoramide N-oxide. J. Agric. Food Chem.
     3, 922—932 (1955).
356. Tuthill, J. W. G.: Malathion poisoning. New Engl. J. Med. **258**, 1018—1019 (1958).
357. *U.S. Pat.* 2,503,390.
358. *U.S. Pat.* 2,640,847; 2,597,534.
359. *U.S. Pat.* 2,685,552.
360. *U.S. Pat.* 2,759,010; D.B.P. 947,369.
361. *U.S. Pat.* 2,761,806.
362. *U.S. Pat.* 2,833,805 and 2,725,328; 2,815,350.
363. Valade et Sallé: Apercu sur les nouveaux toxiques de guerre. Rev. vét. Milit. **3**,
     377—385 (1948).
364. Valters, M. N. I.: Malathion intoxication. Med. J. Aust. **44**, 876—880 (1957).

365. VANDEKAR, M.: The toxic properties of demeton-methyl (Metasystox) and some related compounds. Brit. J. Ind. Med. 15, 158—167 (1958).
366. —, and D. F. HEATH: The reactivation of cholinesterase after inhibition *in vivo* by some dimethyl phosphate esters. Biochem. J. 67, 202—208 (1957).
367. VAN DER MEER, C., and E. MEETER: The mechanism of action of anticholinesterases. II. The effect of diisopropylfluorophosphonate (DFP) on the isolated rat phrenic nerve-diaphragm preparation. Acta physiol. pharm. néerl. 4, 454—471 (1956).
368. VAN WAZER, J. R.: Phosphorus and its compounds. Interscience publ. New York 1958.
369. WEBB, E. C.: The biochemical reactions of chemical warfare agents. Biochem. Soc. Symp., No. 2, pp. 50—60. Cambridge 1948.
370. WESCOE, W. C., and W. F. RIKER jr.: The pharmacology of anti-curare agents. Ann. N. Y. Acad. Sci. 54, 438—459 (1951).
371. WILSON, I. B., F. BERGMANN and D. NACHMANSOHN: Acetylcholinesterase. IX. Structural features determining the inhibition by amino acids and related compounds. J. biol. Chem. 186, 693 (1950).
372. WIRTH, W.: Zur Pharmakologie der Phosphorsäureester. Diäthyl-p-nitrophenylphosphat. ("Mintacol"). Naunyn-Schmiedeberg's Arch. exp. Path. Pharmak. 207, 547—568 (1949).
373. — Zur Pharmakologie der Phosphorsäureester. Diäthylthiophosphorsäureester des Äthylthioglykol (,,Systox-Wirkstoff"). Naunyn-Schmiedeberg's Arch. exp. Path. Pharmak. 217, 144—152 (1953).
374. — Zur Wirkung System-insecticider Phosphorsäure-Ester im Warmblüter-Stoffwechsel. Naunyn-Schmiedeberg's Arch. exp. Path. Pharmak. 234, 352—363 (1958).
375. WOLLENBERG, O.: Kolorimetrische Bestimmung des Insektizides ,,Gusathion"-,,Bayer 17147". Angew. Chem. 68, 581 (1956).
376. —, u. G. SCHRADER: Neuer spezifischer Nachweis des Insektizides ,,Bayer 17147" (,,Gusathion"). Angew. Chem. 68, 41 (1956).
377. VRBOVSKY, L., FR. V. SELECKY u. L. ROSIVAL: Toxikologische und pharmakologische Studien der Phosphorsäureester-Insectiziden. Naunyn-Schmiedeberg's Arch. exp. Path. Pharmak. 236, 202—205 (1959).
378. WRIGHT, P. G.: An analysis of the central and peripheral components of respiratory failure produced by anti-cholinesterase poisoning in the rabbit. J. Physiol. 126, 52—70 (1954).
379. YIP, G., and J. W. COOK: Malathionase. III. Substrate specificity studies. J. Ass. off. agric. Chem. 42, 405—407 (1959).

Chapter 10

Metabolism of Organophosphorus Anticholinesterase Agents

By

L. A. MOUNTER

With 1 Figure

Contents

Introduction

The growth of the chemical industry has brought a large number of new compounds into common use. Technological developments are sometimes attended by toxicological problems, the study of which in certain cases has led to significant advances in biochemical knowledge. An example of this has been provided by the development of a group of organic derivatives of phosphoric acid, some of which are among the most poisonous substances known. Many of these compounds, originally developed as pesticides, are also useful tools in physiology and biochemistry and may provide new drugs for medicine. A number of organophosphorus compounds have been considered as potential chemical warfare agents, and other related substances are finding new uses in chemical industries. BALLS and JANSEN (1953) have pointed out that any extensively toxic substance is to be suspected *a priori* of being an inhibitor of some vitally important enzyme system, and the physiological process characteristic of a number of organophosphorus compounds was found to be the inhibition of cholinesterases (ChE's).

The toxicity of a substance is usually manifest through the development of physiological signs and symptoms; from a study of these effects some indication of the nature of the biochemical disorders producing intoxication may be derived. Yet, it must be emphasized that physiologically important actions other than those responsible for primary effects may result from the presence of the toxic agent. This may be illustrated by the physiological reactions of trivalent arsenic derivatives, where the principle cause of death is believed to be inhibition of the pyruvate oxidase system. This interaction is probably the primary cause of neurological symptoms, yet many other enzymes are affected by these substances, the specific reaction of which is with the thiol groups of proteins. In intoxication by esters of organophosphorus compounds a similar complexity of action appears to exist. The first clinical symptoms, similar to those observed in acetylcholine (ACh) poisoning, are due to an accumulation of ACh following the inhibition of the enzymes effecting its breakdown. The marked physiological response and the sensitivity of ChE's to inhibition by these agents is such that originally it was thought the reagents were specific for ChE's. The term anticholinesterase (anti-ChE) agent is applied commonly to organophosphorus compounds possessing neurotoxic properties. Although rapid manifestation of cholinergic blockade is the most striking effect *in vivo* of intoxication by organophosphates, several other enzyme systems are affected.

The recognition of the anti-ChE action of di*iso*propyl phosphorofluoridate (DFP) prompted investigations of the reaction mechanisms of organophosphorus compounds. The inhibition process is due to phosphorylation of the esteratic sites, and this reaction is the dominant factor in the mediation of toxic effects. In the course of extensive studies, the following conclusions were reached: (1) anti-ChE effects were shown by a number of different types of organophosphorus compounds; (2) enzymes other than ChE's could be inhibited by organophosphorus esters; (3) several of the most active enzyme inhibitors were susceptible to enzymatic hydrolysis. (4) A number of organophosphorus compounds that had little anticholinergic activity *in vitro* were very toxic *in vivo*. The last phenomenon (4) was shown to be caused by metabolic conversion to new, highly toxic derivatives. It follows that reactivity with isolated enzyme systems does not always parallel the toxicity *in vivo*. The latter property is governed by several factors including enzymatic hydrolysis to nontoxic products and the ability of the organism to convert less reactive compounds to active inhibitors. Examination of the chemical structures of the organophosphorus esters shows the features common to those substances possessing anti-ChE activity *in vitro*. A general formula (modified from SCHRADER 1952) is as follows:

$$\begin{array}{c} R_1O \\ \diagdown \\ O{=}P{-}X \\ \diagup \\ R_2 \end{array}$$

where R_1 is an alkyl group, R_2 is alkyl, alkoxy or dialkylamino, and X is F, CN, aryl, or pyrophosphate. The phosphorus atom must possess electrophilic character and the P—X bond in the above formula has anhydride characteristics. The highly reactive chlorophosphates have little biological activity, and their anti-ChE effects are greatly reduced by the replacement of the *p*-nitrophenyl groups by less powerful electron attracting groups in a series of dialkyl-arylphosphates (METCALF and MARCH 1949).

MAZUR (1946) observed that 10^{-2} M DFP in the presence of serum or plasma produced a considerable CO_2-evolution from a bicarbonate medium, and that similar results could be obtained when plasma was replaced by tissue extracts. He showed that this reaction was due to DFP-hydrolyzing enzymes. ALDRIDGE (1951) also reported the hydrolysis of diethyl-*p*-nitro-phenyl phosphate (Paraoxon, E 600) by an esterase of rabbit serum. Further studies of the enzymatic hydrolysis of organophosphorus anti-ChE compounds indicated that there are a number of similarities between the chemical properties of the enzymes that are inhibited by and those that hydrolyze these compounds, although in the latter case there is no irreversible phosphorylation of the active center.

Several investigations have shown that this type of enzymatic hydrolysis influences toxicity. JANDORF and MCNAMARA (1950) pointed out that although

DFP was known as a powerful anti-ChE agent and was used clinically when prolonged depression of ChE activity was desired, relatively little was known about
the metabolism of DFP in the animal body. Due to the high toxicity of the substance to be studied, the doses administered could not exceed a few hundred μg/kg
body weight; it was impossible to use standard analytical procedures for determination of the traces of *iso*propyl groups or fluoride in the tissues. Labelled DFP[32] provided a convenient method of following the distribution of phosphorylated products in
tissues after the administration of the inhibitor to rabbits. As a control experiment,
P[32]-labelled sodium di-*iso*propylphosphate, a nontoxic substance except in high
dosage levels which produces none of the symptoms characteristic of DFP intoxication, was injected intravenously. It was found that the radioactive phosphorus
of DFP is retained in relatively large amounts by kidney, liver, and lung. Only
small amounts of radioactivity were detected in other organs. The specific retention of P[32] depended on the dose administered and on the time of survival. No
specific retention of P[32] was observed when sodium di-*iso*propylphosphate was
administered. No correlation appeared to exist between the ChE activities of the
rabbit organs and their ability to retain DFP-derived phosphorus.

The results of these experiments demonstrate clearly that despite the failure
of DFP to react with proteins (other than certain enzymes) *in vitro*, a considerable
proportion of the phosphorus derived from injected DFP remains bound to tissue
proteins *in vivo*. The fate of DFP in the human body has also been studied by
COHEN and WARRINGA (1954). These authors followed the excretion of P[32] and
the inhibition of blood ChE after DFP[32] injection. They concluded that the metabolism of DFP involved both protein binding and detoxication: about 80% of
the P[32] was excreted in the urine as di-*iso*propyl phosphoric acid and about 20%
remained bound in the tissue. COHEN represented the fate of DFP by the following
scheme:

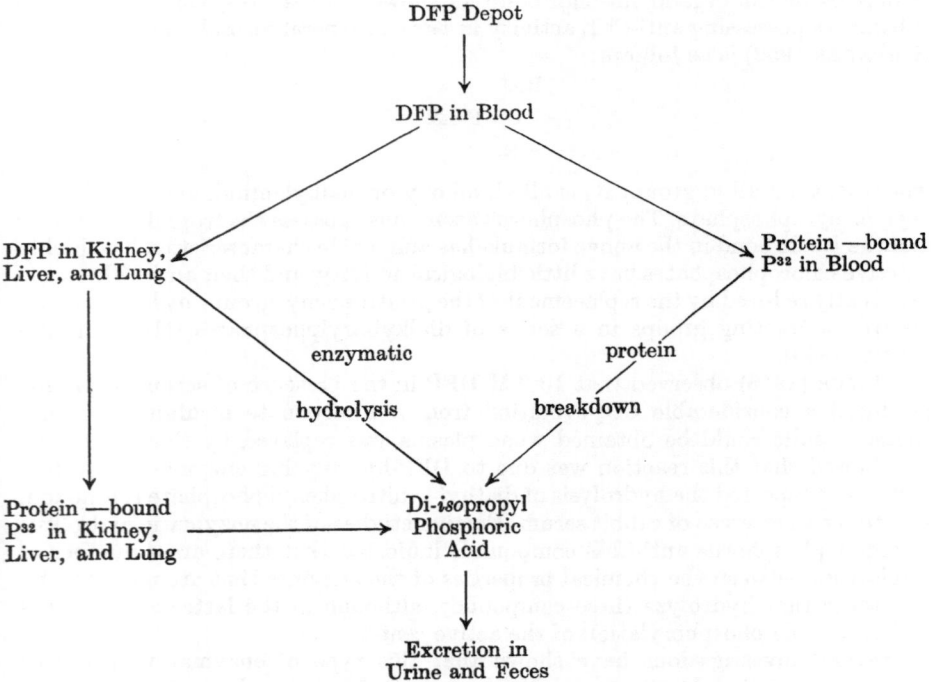

These experiments suggest the existence of other significant biochemical reactions in addition to the inhibition of ChE's by toxic phosphorus compounds. The importance of enzymatic hydrolysis in detoxication was shown by the work of HOBBINGER (1951) who observed a reduction in the effective concentration of tetraethyl pyrophosphate (TEPP) incubated with tissues. HARVEY et al. (1947) found that if the brachial artery was excluded from the general circulation and DFP injected, there was no systemic effect of DFP if a short time elapsed before removal of the occlusion.

MAZUR (1946) showed that considerable detoxication of DFP occurred in the liver. Immediately after the observation of the hydrolysis of DFP by rabbit plasma, MAZUR (1946) investigated the nature of this reaction. He showed that the hydrolytic agent was thermolabile and had all the characteristics of an enzyme reaction. A number of tissue extracts could also hydrolyze DFP; the greatest contribution to the detoxication occurred in the liver, but the kidney was also very active per unit weight of tissue. MAZUR carried out some purification of the enzyme from kidney and studied its properties. Since no natural function of these enzymes was known, no attempt was made to assign a name to them, but for convenience the term DFPase was sometimes applied.

By ethanol fractionation of kidney extracts, MAZUR obtained a purified preparation that was shown to be devoid of ChE's and to have a greatly reduced alkaline phosphatase activity. The DFP-hydrolyzing enzyme could not be identified with any known enzyme. When the properties and specificities of the rabbit kidney and plasma enzymes were recorded, some variations were noted, although there was little evidence for a clear distinction between the two reactions. ALDRIDGE (1951) reported the hydrolysis of diethyl-p-nitrophenylphosphate by sera. Rabbit blood was particularly rich in this enzyme, which was identified as an esterase capable of hydrolyzing aromatic esters such as p-nitrophenyl acetate. The distribution and properties of this esterase differed from those reported by MAZUR for hydrolysis of DFP by tissue extracts, and it seemed probable that different enzymes might be involved in the breakdown of toxic organophosphorus compounds.

The suggestion that there might be more than one type of enzyme involved in the degradation of toxic organophosphorus compounds has been confirmed, and a summary of our knowledge of these enzymes is given below. It must be stressed however that this is very incomplete.

The majority of the early work on detoxication of phosphorus compounds was carried out with substances that had been considered for use as chemical warfare agents and different investigators seldom employed the same range of potential substrates in their studies. In later years, the major emphasis in this field has been on toxicological problems associated with the development of pesticides. Many of these compounds in the latter category are of more complex structure and can undergo hydrolysis at different portions in the molecule. In some cases, metabolic changes may be demonstrated by the isolation of new products from studies *in vivo*. Investigations of this type do not permit an evaluation of the enzymes which may be involved in the reactions and contribute little to knowledge of their properties. The studies carried out to date have revealed a complexity of distribution and overlapping specificity; consequently, tabulation of substrate specificity, properties, and distribution is impossible. The situation is further complicated by problems of nomenclature. The chemical names of many organophosphorus compounds have undergone several revisions in recent years. Thus, DFP was first known as di-*iso*propyl fluorophosphonate, followed by di-*iso*propyl fluorophosphate, and currently as di-*iso*propoxy-phosphoryl fluoride, or di-*iso*propyl phosphorofluoridate. The natural substrates for enzymes which hydrolyze this compound are not known; some esterases hydrolyze DFP but there are other metal-activated tissue enzymes which do not appear to be simple esterases, nor can they be identified with existing phosphatases. For convenience such terms as DFPase are used to describe enzymes which catalyze its hydrolysis, but it must be born in mind that these terms do not have the desirable connotation of specificity and function which are sought in enzyme nomenclature.

In the following sections some of the enzymes known to be involved in the metabolism of toxic organophosphorus compounds are discussed.

A. Enzymatic hydrolysis of organophosphorus compounds by tissue enzymes

Following the original observation that DFP was hydrolyzed by serum and aqueous tissue extracts, MAZUR (1946) attempted to purify the enzyme from kidney, which was found to be rich in the enzyme. Using ethanol precipitation, he obtained a preparation 15 times more active than the kidney homogenate. The enzyme was sensitive to heavy metals, particularly Cu^{++} and Hg^{++}, in quite low concentrations. A later study of the DFP-hydrolyzing enzyme of hog kidney was made by MOUNTER and CHANUTIN (1953a, 1953b, 1954). Improved ethanol fractionation yielded a preparation approximately 50 times more active than the original kidney extract. This preparation was used for further studies of properties and specificity. Although most metals inhibited the enzymatic hydrolysis of DFP, it was observed that Mn^{++} and Co^{++} had pronounced activating effects (Fig. 1). A further potentiation of activity was observed when certain nitrogenous compounds, particularly imidazole and pyridine derivatives, were added together with the metal ion (Table 1). It was concluded that the enzyme activation involved the formation of a chelate complex between groups in the protein molecule and the

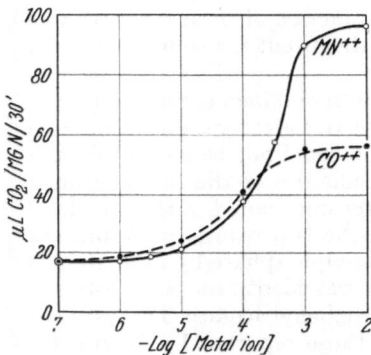

Fig. 1. Effects of Mn^{++} and Co^{++} on DFPase activity. Manganous chloride or cobaltous sulfate of varying concentrations incubated in side arm of Warburg flask for 20 min before adding to substrate in main compartment

Table 1. *Effect of activators on DFPase activity*
Activator concentration, 10^{-3} M. Activity, ml of CO_2 per mg N per 30 minutes.

Activator	No Metal Ion			+ Co++			+ Mn++		
	Control	+ Act.	Effect %	Control	+ Act.	Effect %	Control	+ Act.	Effect %
Cysteine	18	27	50	40	52	30	66	110	67
Histidine	18	19	6	40	42	5	61	139	113
Proline	23	25	10	57	75	32	70	81	16
Imidazole.	17	20	18				64	64	0
Imidazole 4,5-dicarb-oxylic acid	17	32	88				64	128	100
2,2'-Dipyridyl	15	22	47				15	56	274

From MOUNTER et al. (1953a).

metal ion. The enzyme-metal complexes bind the organo-nitrogen activator, and these systems have characteristic dissociation constants. It was possible to predict the effect of certain potential inhibitors, and the activating metal could be replaced by other metals of high affinity with resulting inhibition (MOUNTER and CHANUTIN 1953 b, 1954). These observations are similar to reports of activation of phosphatases by Mg^{++} and histidine (BODANSKY 1946, AEBI and ABELIN 1948), but recovery data and specific activity measurements made at different stages of precipitation clearly distinguish the DFP-hydrolyzing enzyme of hog kidney from any of the known phosphatases. In later studies, the same degree of potentiation of DFPase by metals and cofactors was not observed when titrimetric methods instead of manometric methods were used for the measurement of activity

Table 2. *Hydrolysis of phosphorus esters by hog kidney DFPase*

Compound	μmoles hydrolyzed per 30 min per mg N (substrate concentration, 0.01M)
Diethyl phosphorofluoridate	1150
Di-n-propyl phosphorofluoridate	870
Di*iso*propyl phosphorofluoridate	36
Di-n-butyl phosphorofluoridate	470
Di*iso*butyl phosphorofluoridate	250
Di-n-amyl phosphorofluoridate	90
Di*iso*amyl phosphorofluoridate	10
Di-n-octyl phosphorofluoridate	0
Bis(dimethylamino)fluorophosphine oxide	0
Tetraethyl pyrophosphate	240
Tetra-n-propyl pyrophosphate	130
Tetra*iso*propyl pyrophosphate	10
Tetrakis(dimethylamino) pyrophosphate	0
Diethyl cyanophosphate	35
Diethyl-p-nitrophenyl phosphate (Paraoxon)	0
Diethyl-p-nitrophenyl thionophosphate (Parathion)	0

From MOUNTER and DIEN (1956).

(O'NEILL et al. 1954). On the other hand, COHEN and WARRINGA (1957) also observed the pronounced activating effects of Mn^{++} and dipyridyl, and in addition obtained a naturally occurring activator in the course of precipitation studies. The activating fraction in the presence of Mn^{++} gave preparations several times more active then the Mn^{++}-dipyridyl complex; the nature of these phenomena has not yet been explained.

Kinetic and specificity studies were made of the hog kidney enzyme. A number of different types of organophosphorus compounds were hydrolyzed, in each case the acid anhydride link being the one attacked. Phosphorofluoridates, cyanophosphates, and tetraalkyl pyrophosphates yielded anionic products which were non-toxic (MOUNTER 1955). It appeared that kidney DFPase might be responsible for the hydrolysis of certain amino acid esters, and MOUNTER (1956) suggested that the enzyme was identical with hog kidney Acylase I. Despite the close similarity in many properties, in later studies the two types of activity were partially separated and the hypothesis thus appears to be untenable (BELL and MOUNTER 1958). COHEN and WARRINGA (1957) also separated DFPase and Acylase I activities and made specificity studies using highly purified preparations. When the preparations were studied an added complexity was involved: metal ions, in particular Mn^{++}, appeared to show different effects with different substrates; the pattern of activation was considerably altered by the addition of the activating fraction (obtained in their purification procedure, Fraction G). By other criteria, it would seem that the kidney preparations of "DFPase" are homogeneous, and a single enzyme is responsible for the hydrolysis of the various

Table 3. *Distribution of DFPase*

The results are expressed in *microl* of CO_2 per gm wet weight tissue per 30 minutes, and in activity ratios equal (activity with 10^{-3} *M* metal ion in the side arm)/(activity with no added metal ion).

Organ	Rat			Human			Cat			Guinea pig			Pigeon			Turtle		
	Per gm	Ratios		Per gm	Ratios		Per gm	Ratios		Per gm	Ratios		Per gm	Ratios		Per gm	Ratios	
		Mn++	Co++		Mn++	Co++		Mn++	Co++		Mn++	Co++		Mn++	Co++		Mn++	Co++
Kidney	2,550	4.3	2.3	7,000	1.3	1.3	4,800	1.6	2.0	1,300	1.4	0.9	4,500	1.5	1.2	2,400	3.2	2.0
Liver	4,200	1.9	1.2	5,200	1.2	1.1	3,300	1.5	1.6	950	2.1	0.9	2,400	1.1	1.0	700	2.7	1.1
Intestinal mucosa	2,300	2.2	1.4				7,700	1.9	2.0	2,200	3.1	1.3	540	7.3		1,700	4.2	2.8
Brain	1,300	2.6	1.5							520	3.1	0.8	340	4.4	2.9	450	3.3	1.6
Heart	1,450	3.4	1.8							350	3.6		240	2.5	1.4	670	1.5	1.2
Lung	670	4.0	2.2	175	5.0	3.0	2,000	2.3	2.1	620	4.0	2.1	200	2.6	1.8	330	3.0	2.0
Testis	2,700	2.9	1.4	1,100	2.4		1,250	5.1	7.0	420	3.2	0.7						
Bone marrow	2,350	3.3	1.6				630	3.3	3.5	1,020	3.8	3.7						
Pancreas				1,900	1.7	1.5												

From MOUNTER, DIEN and CHANUTIN (1955).

compounds. A possible exception is the case of DFP and dimethyl-amido-ethoxyphosphoryl cyanide (Tabun), where the hydrolysis of a mixture of the two substrates gave a greater activity than either alone. It is apparent that considerably more work must be done before the complexities of the specificity and activities of kidney DFPase can be elucidated. It is quite possible that a metal-activated complex reacts somewhat differently with different substrates, although only a single apoenzyme is involved. A summary of specificity data is presented in Table 2.

Many potential substrates have been tried with kidney DFPase preparations, and in the course of purification studies comparison of the activities of several known enzymes has been made. Investigations have shown that the known proteases, several peptidases, phosphatases, and esterases are not identical with DFPase (MOUNTER and DIEN 1956, O'NEILL 1955, COHEN and WARRINGA 1957). It is improbable that substances so different from normal metabolites as are the phosphorofluoridates and related compounds are hydrolyzed by enzymes specific for their degradation. Although MAZUR (1946) had shown that several tissue extracts would hydrolyze DFP and its homologues, it is now of interest to see if enzymes of this type are generally distributed in the tissue of various species. The hydrolysis of DFP was effected by all tissues studied, the highest activity being shown by kidney, liver and tissues such as testis and intestinal mucosa which have a high metabolic activity and a high rate of proliferation. The results of this study are presented in Table 3.

The effects of Mn^{++} and Co^{++}, which had been shown to activate kidney DFPase, were tested on the tissue extracts. As a result of this study (MOUNTER et al. 1955) and the use of other homologous phosphorofluoridates (MOUNTER 1955), it was found that more than one enzyme capable of hydrolyzing DFP might be present in a single tissue; these enzymes are distinct from the A-esterases to be discussed in the following section. In liver a soluble enzyme may be extracted that hydrolyzes DFP more rapidly than the di-n-butyl phosphate and is activated by Mn^{++} and Co^{++}. The insoluble fraction from this same preparation hydrolyzed di-n-butyl phosphorofluoridate more rapidly than DFP; this latter enzyme was inhibited by Mn^{++} and Co^{++} but was activated by Ca^{++} (Table 4). ADIE and TUBA

Table 4. *Effect of metal ions on DFPase activity of kidney and liver fractions*

Enzyme Source	Fraction	Metal Ions*			
		Mn^{++}	Co^{++}	Mg^{++}	Ca^{++}
Hog kidney	Soluble	490	190	110	100
Hog kidney	Insoluble	150	100	100	—
Rat kidney	Soluble	480	21	110	100
Rat kidney	Insoluble	140	110	100	—
Hog liver	Soluble	320	180	110	—
Hog liver	Insoluble	45	50	80	150
Rat liver	Soluble	760	380	110	100
Rat liver	Insoluble	40	40	40	200

* Metal ions, 10^{-3} M. Figures represent number of times control value (= 100%) with no added divalent ion.

From MOUNTER (1955).

(1958) studied the hydrolysis of Tabun and Sarin (*iso*propyl methylphosphono-fluoridate) by various enzyme preparations. In rat serum, human plasma, and monkey liver it appears that a single enzyme is responsible for the hydrolysis of both substrates; the ratios of activities of other tissue extracts towards the two substrates differ considerably, indicating that more than one enzyme may be involved.

The activities of only the liver and kidney have been studied in the various cytological fractions obtained by gradient density centrifugation. The greatest activity was found in the supernatant fraction; some activity was present in microsomes, but little in mitochondria or nuclei. The distribution pattern differed among species. It is interesting in this respect to consider observations of optical specificity in regard to rates of hydrolysis by various enzyme extracts. Tabun exists in two sterioisometric forms, and it was shown that rat serum hydrolyzed the *dextro*-rotary form more rapidly than the *levo*-rotary form (HOSKIN and TRICK 1955). The latter isomer is of very low toxicity. AUGUSTINSSON (1957)-extended these studies to other enzyme extracts; he found that hog kidney preparations obtained by ethanol fractionation hydrolyzed the d-isomer of Tabun aproximately 10 times as rapidly as the l-isomer, whereas purified human plasma Tabunase showed negligible stereospecificity. Since tissue such as liver has been shown to contain more than one enzyme capable of hydrolyzing toxic phosphorus compounds, stereospecificity might provide a means of determining whether (a) the varied results of measurements of activities in cell fractions, and (b) the distribution of activity among cell fractions from different species are due to mixtures of enzymes.

Studies of the distribution of DFP-hydrolyzing enzymes have been extended by a survey of the enzymatic activities of a number of species of microorganisms

(MOUNTER et al. 1955, MOUNTER and TUCK 1956). DFP was hydrolyzed by all the organisms studied, with the exception of two types of micrococci (Table 5). The highest activities were observed in gram-negative organisms, and the effects of Mn^{++}, Co^{++}, and Mg^{++} on the different preparations suggest species differences between the enzymes. This is also evidenced by the relative rates of hydrolysis

Table 5. *Hydrolysis of DFP by microorganisms*
Substrate concentration, 10 mM.

Species	Activity, μl CO_2 per 100 mg per hr	Effect of metal ions*		
		Mn^{++}	Co^{++} $(10^{-3} M)$♀	Mg^{++}
Proteus vulgaris (—)	1,400	+	—	0
Pseudomonas aeruginosa (—)	1,100	+	—	0
Serratia marcescens (—)	900	0	—	
Salmonella pullorum (—)	650	+	—	+
Pasteurella avicida (—)	470	+	—	—
Escherichia coli (—)	400	+	—	
Shigella alkalescens (—)	270	+	—	0
Aerobacter aerogenes (—)	260	+	—	—
Staphylococcus albus (+)	180	—	—	0
Clostridium sporogenes (+)	170	—	+	0
Corynebacterium xerose (+)	100	+	±	+
Hemophilus pertussis (—)	60			
Bacillus subtilis (+)	50	+	+	+
Neisseria sicca (—)	30	+	+	+
Mycobacterium phlei (+)	< 25			
Streptococcus faecalis (folic acid var.) (+) . . .	< 25			
Streptococcus faecalis (+)	< 25			
Micrococcus pyogenes (+)	Negligible			
Micrococcus citreus (+)	Negligible			

From MOUNTER, BAXTER and CHANUTIN (1955).

The symbols in parentheses indicate Gram-negative or Gram-positive staining.

* + = activation; — = inhibition; 0 = negligible effect.

♀ Concentration in the side arm; final concentration after mixing with substrate, 10^{-4} M.

of different substrates (Table 6), although these variations may be due to the presence of more than one enzyme. It has been stated that ChE's are absent from most microorganisms (GOLDSTEIN and GOLDSTEIN 1953), so that the marked ability of many species to hydrolyze DFP re-emphasizes the belief that the activities of ChE's and DFPase are not related functionally to one another.

The assay methods for the enzymatic degradation of DFP and related compounds are based upon the formation of acid groups resulting from hydrolytic action. Direct titrimetric assay may be employed, or alternatively a manometric assay is provided by formation of the acid which, in turn, liberates CO_2 from a bicarbonate buffer media. MAZUR (1946) concluded that the hydrolytic cleavage of DFP by kidney extracts was at the P—F link, with hydrofluoric and di*iso*propyl phosphoric acids as the products of hydrolysis. This was later confirmed by MOUNTER and DIEN (1954) who showed that there was a stoichiometric liberation of inorganic fluoride when DFP and its homologues were hydrolyzed. It is presumed that the hydrolysis of other substrates by this enzyme also occurs at the anhydride-like bond. In the case of the dialkyl-dichlorovinyl phosphates, dialkyl-phosphoric acid is formed, while the other product is probably dichloroacetalde-hyde; the latter substance has been shown to be produced when chymotrypsin is inhibited by dialkylchlorovinyl phosphate (JANDORF 1956). The enzymatic hydrolysis of a substituted chlorovinylphosphate by plasma and liver extracts has also been described by HERMANN and PULVER (1958).

Table 6. *Hydrolysis of organophosphorus compounds by microorganisms*
The rate of hydrolysis = microl of CO_2 per 100 mg of organism per hr. Substrate concentration, $10^{-2} M$. All the determinations were made in the presence of $10^{-4} M$ Mn^{++}. The figures in parentheses represent the percentage of the rate of DFP hydrolysis.

Compound	Rate with organism			
	E. coli	P. fluorescens	P. pentosaceum	S. faecalis
Di*iso*propyl phosphorofluoridate (DFP)	3100 (100)	980 (100)	800 (100)	50 (100)
Diethyl phosphorofluoridate (DEFP)	3800 (120)	900 (90)	600 (75)	100 (200)
Di-*n*-butyl phosphorofluoridate (DBFP)	2150 (55)	960 (100)	460 (60)	50 (100)
Bis(dimethylamino) phosphorofluoridate.	0 (0)	0 (0)	0 (0)	
Tetraethyl pyrophosphate (TEPP)	1300 (40)	390 (40)	130 (15)	20 (40)
Dichlorovinyl dimethyl phosphate (DCVMP).	610 (40)*	250 (50)*	190 (45)*	
0,0-Diethyl-0-4-nitrophenyl phosphate (Paraoxon)	50	0 (0)	20	0 (0)

From MOUNTER and TUCK (1956).

* Percentage rate times 2, since hydrolysis of 1 mole of substrate liberates 1 *mole* of acid (MOUNTER and DIEN 1954).

It is apparent that other sites of hydrolytic cleavage of organophosphate triesters and their derivatives are theoretically possible. Some evidence for these reactions has been obtained *in vivo* and is mentioned below. The hydrolytic enzymes which have been most widely studied and characterized are those which effect the anhydride-like bond cleavage. These are the tissue enzymes, described in this section, and some esterases.

B. The hydrolysis of organophosphorus compounds by esterases

The first recorded observation of the enzymatic hydrolysis of DFP was by rabbit serum (MAZUR 1946); a second type of compound, 0,0-diethyl-*p*-nitrophenylphosphate, was also found (ALDRIDGE 1951) to be hydrolyzed by sera, particularly by that of rabbit (ALDRIDGE 1953). This enzymatic hydrolysis was due to the action of nonspecific esterases that can be distinguished from the enzymes discussed in the preceding section by their kinetics, distribution, and specificity. Despite the facts that (a) a considerable amount of work has been carried out on the breakdown of phosphorus compounds by serum fractions and (b) the same enzymes are capable (in certain instances, at least) of hydrolyzing esters containing no phosphorus, in some respects less is known of the specificity and properties of these enzymes than of the tissue enzymes for which no natural substrates are known.

MAZUR (1946) in his original work noted some differences between the properties of plasma and of tissue enzymes which hydrolyzed DFP, but did not have the opportunity to elucidate them or to differentiate the enzymes. In his later study, ALDRIDGE (1951, 1953b) found an enzyme in rabbit serum which hydrolyzed diethyl-*p*-nitrophenyl phosphate, *p*-nitrophenyl acetate, and other aromatic esters. He showed that plasma contained at least two esterases, distinct from ChE's, which are capable of hydrolyzing aromatic esters. The first group, the A-esterases, were not inhibited by toxic phosphorus compounds and hydrolyzed acetates more readily than butyrates; the second group, the B-esterases, hydrolyzed butyrates more readily than acetates and were very sensitive to inhibition by DFP and related compounds. It must be emphasized that not all esterases classified as A-esterases, on the basis of their sensitivity to inhibition by phosphorus compounds and other properties, are capable of effecting the hydrolysis of phosphate ester anti-ChE agents. Esterases that hydrolyze DFP are also found in certain tissues.

Blood contains several hydrolytic enzymes of overlapping specificities. AUGUSTINSSON and HEIMBURGER (1954b) studied the hydrolysis of Tabun by the sera of eight different species. They all contained a Tabun-hydrolyzing enzyme; activity was particularly high in rabbit blood. It was obviously of interest to decide if these different phosphorus compounds were hydrolyzed by a single enzyme. Studies which indicated that one enzyme in rabbit serum hydrolyzed both diethyl-p-nitrophenyl phosphate and DFP were reported by ALDRIDGE (1951). MOUNTER (1954) concluded that the same enzyme in rabbit sera was responsible for the hydrolysis of DFP, tetraethyl pyrophosphate (TEPP), diethyl-p-nitrophenyl phosphate, and p-nitrophenyl acetate. The evidence was based upon data obtained in experiments employing mixed substrates, inhibition studies, and determination of relative rates of hydrolysis of the various substrates by different enzyme preparations and fractions. It should be pointed out that no activation of these serum enzymes by Mn^{++}, Co^{++}, other divalent metal ions, or by cofactors was observed, as in the case of the enzymes discussed in the preceding section.

In the study of Tabun hydrolysis by plasma, AUGUSTINSSON (1954) suggested that his "Tabunase" is not identical with ALDRIDGE's A-esterase but is an enzyme of overlapping specificity. Although the greater part of AUGUSTINSSON's work on the enzymatic hydrolysis of organophosphorus compounds was carried out using Tabun as substrate, some specificity studies were made with other compounds (AUGUSTINSSON and HEIMBURGER 1954d). The hydrolysis of Tabun by sera and a number of tissue extracts was investigated. The relative rates of hydrolysis of a number of organophosphates by rabbit plasma and human serum fractions showed differences between the enzyme from the two sources. AUGUSTINSSON has published a series of reports of his studies of enzymatic hydrolysis of organophosphorus compounds (AUGUSTINSSON and HEIMBURGER 1954a, 1954b, 1954c, 1954d, 1955a, 1955b). It is unfortunate that it is not known whether a single enzyme or mixture of enzymes hydrolyzed different phosphate esters. The ambiguities that remain to date are particularly apparent in the studies of the A-esterases. ALDRIDGE's (1951) work on the reaction of esterases with Paraoxon, which were carried out ten years ago, comprises perhaps one of the most complete reports of enzymatic degradation of organophosphorus compounds, but relatively few of the compounds later studied by other workers were available for his use. ALDRIDGE was unable to purify serum A-esterase by ammonium sulfate fractionation; he obtained some separation by ethanol fractionation using a modification of COHN's plasma fractionation procedure. The highest A-esterase activity was obtained in the fraction corresponding to COHN's Fractions I + II + III, precipitated with 19% (v/v) ethanol at pH 5.8. The esterase was present also in other fractions, but with lower specific activity. With human serum fractions, AUGUSTINSSON and HEIMBURGER (1954b) found that Tabun was hydrolyzed most rapidly by Fraction IV—I, a globulin fraction; when it was compared to the original serum, this represented only a four-fold purification. ADIE (1956) studied the hydrolysis of Tabun and Sarin with a highly purified plasma fraction obtained from ox blood;

in this case the activity was present in an electrophoretically homogeneous fraction corresponding to a subfraction of COHN's Fraction VI. Thus, different workers have found the serum esterase activity to be present in entirely different fractions and have assayed the enzyme or enzymes with different substrates. These results may be due to (a) species differences or (b) the fact that the enzyme present in small amounts co-precipitates with other fractions and this co-precipitation is dependent upon the components of the system and the conditions of the experiment.

The properties of the A-esterase of rabbit serum were studied by ALDRIDGE (1951, 1953a, 1953b). He showed that the enzyme readily hydrolyzed p-nitrophenyl acetate and diethyl-p-nitrophenyl phosphate; butyrates were only slightly hydrolyzed. The pH optimum was approximately 7.5; while there was some reduction of activity in the presence of barbital (veronal), the same rates of hydrolysis were found in phosphate, borate, or bicarbonate buffers. The addition of thiol reagents such as p-chloromercuribenzoate and heavy metal ions inhibited the enzyme; the reaction was reversed by incubation with thiol compounds such as cysteine and glutathione. Cholinesterase inhibitors such as physostigmine (eserine) have no effect on A-esterase. Using human serum fractions, AUGUSTINSSON and HEIMBURGER (1955b) found that Sr^{++} or Ba^{++} activated the hydrolysis of Tabun but not of DFP.

Enzymes that hydrolyze Paraoxon are widely distributed with considerable species variation. There is no correlation between their distribution and that of other hydrolytic enzymes, such as proteases, lipases, and other esterases. Purified hog kidney extracts of DFPase did not hydrolyze Paraoxon significantly (MOUNTER and DIEN 1956).

C. Other esterases

It is apparent that in addition to the primary hydrolysis of toxic organophosphorus esters at the most electrophilic bond, cleavage of other bonds might be anticipated. In studies of the metabolism of organophosphorus insecticides, many products have been isolated from tissue extracts after reactions in vivo. These products include those derived by dealkylation of alkoxy groups attached to the phosphorus atom. Thus, in the metabolism of dialkyl-aryl phosphorothioates by cow, rat, and insect tissues, both hydrolysis of the alkyl phosphate and of aryl phosphate bonds have been shown to take place (PLAPP and CASIDA 1958a, 1958b). Similar dealkylation may occur with other less complex phosphate esters, but little study has been made in vitro of the enzymes which may be involved. Probably one reason for this is that detoxication by the formation of anionic products is largely confined to the cleavage of electrophilic bonds. Some reactions of organophosphorus compounds that involve carboxylic ester hydrolysis are discussed in the following section.

D. Reactions involved in the metabolism of organophosphorus compounds

Following the elucidation of the anti-ChE action of toxic organophosphates, it was generally assumed that the various phosphorus compounds exert their action by direct reaction as potent enzyme inhibitors. The investigations reported in the previous section have described work which has shown that other enzymes can convert toxic phosphate esters to relatively non-toxic products. By contrast, the results of other studies led to the conclusion that toxicity in vivo may be considerably greater than would be anticipated from the anti-ChE activity measured in vitro. Whenever such observations have been adequately investigated, it has been found that metabolism *in vivo* is responsible for the formation of new and more active toxic agents. Anticholinesterase activity may therefore be decreased or enhanced by reaction with various enzyme systems; an understanding of the course of these reactions is of significance in determining the pharmacological effects of phosphate esters. The interrelationship of the various enzyme systems is of particular importance in the development of insecticides, since by making use of knowledge of differences in metabolic pathways selective toxicity against insect pests may be attained concomitantly with low mammalian toxicity. Studies of the differential toxicity and the metabolic pathways involved are expanding rapidly as more potential pesticides are tested. The subject has been reviewed by METCALF (1955), CASIDA (1956), and more recently by O'BRIEN (1960). CASIDA (1956) has discussed the experimental approaches available for investigating the metabolism of organophosphates. He has pointed out that to validate proposed mechanisms, conversion of phosphorus compounds to more active antiesterases, several approaches should be used concurrently. The four general methods are as follows:

a) Correlation of anti-ChE activity *in vitro* with toxicity *in vivo*.

b) Comparison of ChE inhibition *in vivo* with the inhibition of the same tissue enzyme *in vitro* at the same concentration of inhibitor. (This method includes also studies of antiesterase specificity differences between the chemical applied and its active metabolite.)

c) Incubation of organophosphates with tissue preparations, and comparison of antiesterase activity before and after incubation.

d) Physicochemical separation of organophosphate metabolites from tissues. (This is particularly useful where radioactively labelled substances are used.)

CASIDA (1956) stated that a good organophosphate insecticide requires a suitable balance of group specificity, anti-ChE activity, and stability, and that this balance varies with each new economic use of an antiesterase agent. Several reviews exist describing the development of contact and systemic insecticides (HALL 1950, METCALF 1955, SCHRADER 1952); knowledge is accumulating so that it may soon be possible to predict the structure required to fulfill specific functions in insect control problems (O'BRIEN 1959b). A large part of the work in this field during the last decade has been essentially empirical and only a small fraction of the compounds synthesized and tested has come into general use in biological studies. During the course of this work certain general metabolic pathways have been found which may increase or decrease biochemical activity. In addition to the hydrolytic cleavage described in the preceeding section, the following types of reactions have been widely reported.

I. Phosphorothioate oxidation

DIGGLE and GAGE (1951) pointed out that although pure diethyl-*p*-nitrophenyl phosphorothioate (Parathion) is a poor ChE inhibitor *in vitro*, it is a potent inhibitor *in vivo*. These observations led to the hypothesis that activation resulted from action *in vivo*, and they showed that incubation of Parathion with liver slices produced a potent inhibitor. By contrast, liver homogenate was unable to activate Parathion. DAVISON (1955) later showed that the addition of Mg^{++}, DPN, and nicotinamide to liver homogenates provided a system which was capable of oxidizing the phosphorothioate to a potent antiesterase. The metabolic products of Parathion from both animal (GAGE 1953) and insect tissue (METCALF and MARCH 1953) has been shown to be the corresponding 0,0-diethyl-*p*-nitrophenyl phosphate (Paraoxon).

A considerable amount of work has been carried out on the oxidative activation of phosphorothioates by tissues. In certain instances, it is possible that rapid hydrolytic cleavage of the parent compound, or its metabolic product, precludes the isolation of a toxic metabolite. There are also several individual reports regarding the precise intracellular localization of the oxidative system, its cofactor requirements, and activity differences associated with sex and species. O'BRIEN (1959a) showed TPNH was more effective in providing the activating reaction than TPN, and this, in turn, was better than DPNH or DPN. Further studies of phosphorothioate activation are in progress, as an increasing number of these compounds is being tested for insecticidal activity. It is not yet clear whether all these compounds are activated by the same enzyme system, particularly since studies are complicated by the fact that they do not all seem to require metabolic activation; thus 0,0-diethyl phosphorofluorothioate appears to react directly with the esteratic site (JANSEN et al. 1951). Furthermore, certain of the more complex organophosphorus compounds are susceptible to enzymatic attack at various positions in the molecule. As a general rule, it appears that the phosphorothioates are oxidized to the corresponding phosphates, and that activation of anti-ChE activity occurs when the stability of the original compound is such that it is not sufficiently reactive to manifest a direct effect as an inhibitor. However, this rule is not without exception, for it appears that 0,0-diethyl-0-ethyl-2-mercaptoethylphosphorothionate (Systox) is oxidized to a sulfoxide or sulfone, which is the active insecticide.

II. Oxidation of phosphoramides

0-Ethyl-N-(*bis*-dimethylamido)-phosphorocyanide and the corresponding phosphorofluoridate are among the most toxic compounds of the present series. Their toxicity exceeds that of DFP and in both cases they appear to phosphorylate the active centers of esterases directly. By contrast, certain dialkyl phosphoramides, e.g., Dimefox and OMPA (Schradan).

$$[(CH_3)_2N]_2P(O)F \text{ and } [(CH_3)_2N]_2P(O)OP[N(CH_3)_2]_2$$

are poor inhibitors of ChE's *in vitro* but show a high toxicity *in vivo* with attendant manifestations of anti-ChE activity. OMPA was one of the first of the organophosphorus compounds which was shown to be activated *in vivo* by biological oxidation (DUBOIS et al. 1950, GARDINER and KILBY 1950). Its metabolism has been investigated by several groups of workers; liver slices contain the activating system which is present also in several insect tissues. The ability to activate phosphoramides is lowest in homogenates but may be restored on the addition of nicotinamide, magnesium, and either diphospho- or triphosphopyridine nucleotide. The reaction shows many similarities to the oxidation of phosphorothioates, but it is not known whether the same enzyme systems are responsible for the activation of the sulfur compounds and the phosphoramides. The cofactor requirements and the observation that mixtures of microsomal fractions together with the particle-free supernatant solution from high speed centrifugation are required to effect optimal conversion of OMPA to an active inhibitor suggest there may be several stages of enzymatic action involved in the metabolism. These have been discussed by O'BRIEN (1960) and by FENWICK (1958). The active metabolite of a phosphoramide may be either the N-oxide or the isomeric hydroxy-methyl compound. The product is a potent anti-ChE agent but is of relatively low stability (TSUYUKI et al. 1955) and isomerizes to the corresponding N-methoxide which has a relatively low anti-ChE action. The actions may be represented as follows:

$$\begin{array}{ccc}
\mathrm{CH_3} & \mathrm{CH_3}\quad\mathrm{O} & \mathrm{CH_3O} \\
\diagdown & \diagdown\quad\nearrow & \diagdown \\
\mathrm{N{-}P}\!\!\equiv\;\longrightarrow & \mathrm{N}\quad\longrightarrow & \mathrm{N} \\
\diagup & \diagup\quad & \diagup \\
\mathrm{CH_3} & \mathrm{CH_3}\quad\mathrm{P}\!\!\equiv & \mathrm{CH_3}\quad\mathrm{P}\!\!\equiv
\end{array}$$

There is no evidence that this type of oxidation occurs with the monoalkyl phosphoramides. It has also been pointed out that the species specificity of the insecticidal action of OMPA does not correlate directly with the ability of the individual species to oxidize the material to the N-oxide (CASIDA 1956).

III. Thioether oxidation

Certain organophosphate compounds contain the thioether link C-S-C. The systemic insecticide "Dimeton," or "Systox," contains this group and comprises a mixture of thio compounds — 0,0-diethyl-0-ethyl-2-mercaptoethyl phosphoro-thionate and 0,0-diethyl-S-ethyl-2-mercaptoethyl phosphorothiolate. Studies *in vitro* of the mechanisms of action of these compounds have been limited, but it appears that oxidation of the phosphorothionate to a phosphate is relatively insignificant. The active compounds in this case are the sulfoxides and sulfones. Thus, the reactions may be represented as:

$$\overset{\displaystyle S}{\underset{\diagup}{}}$$
$$(\mathrm{C_2H_5O})_2\mathrm{P{-}OCH_2CH_2SC_2H_5}\ \ (\text{Thionate isomer})\ \rightarrow$$

$$(\mathrm{C_2H_5})\mathrm{O_2P{-}OCH_2CH_2{-}\overset{\uparrow}{S}\,C_2H_5}\ (\text{Thionate sulfoxide})\ \rightarrow$$

$$(\mathrm{C_2H_5O})_2\mathrm{P{-}OCH_2CH_2{-}\underset{\downarrow}{\overset{\uparrow}{S}}\,C_2H_5}\ \ (\text{Sulfone})$$

These products and those derived from the thiolate are susceptible also to hydrolysis. It appears that the phosphorothiodate sulfoxides are more stable than those of the phosphorothionates, although the sulfones are of similar stability (FUKUTO et al. 1955).

IV. Carboxylic ester hydrolysis

Certain potential insecticides are organophosphates containing a carboxylic ester group. These ester groups may be hydrolyzed *in vivo* to yield products of either reduced or increased anti-ChE activity. Detoxication of Malathion (0,0-dimethyl-S-[1,2-dicarboxyethyl] phosphorothionate) involves enzymatic hydrolysis of the carboxylic ester groups. Other degradation products are found, and the overall metabolic pictures differ considerably in insects and mammals (MARCH et al. 1955c). A number of studies of these reactions has been made, generally by the chromatographic isolation of the degradation products. A particular point of interest in the studies of Malathion, which is an important insecticide because of its low mammalian toxicity, is the fact that its toxicity is greatly increased in the presence of other compounds, especially other organophosphates. It has been shown that the enzyme or enzymes responsible for the cleavage of the ester linkages of Malathion are inhibited by a number of compounds, including Parathion. When an animal or tissue is treated with Parathion, or EPN, the pattern of Malathion degradation products changes so that the predominant products are those derived from the hydrolysis of the P-C bond rather than the ester bond. Such changes in metabolism probably provide a basis for the synergistic effects frequently observed in studies of pesticidal or drug actions (see Chapter 18).

The action of esterases upon Malathion is involved in the detoxication of this compound. By contrast, hydrolysis of an ester bond may result in increased antiesterase activity. An example of this is the deacylation of 0,0-dimethyl-2,2,2-trichloroacetoxyethyl phosphonate to yield 0,0-dimethyl-2,2,2-trichloro-1-hydroxyethyl phosphonate which in turn rearranges to a highly toxic chlorovinyl phosphate (ARTHUR and CASIDA 1957).

Conclusions

With the further development of organophosphorus compounds as drugs, pesticides, and pharmacological tools it is to be anticipated that considerably more information will be obtained pertaining to the metabolism of the various types of compounds. It will be particularly interesting to ascertain if the same enzymes are responsible for the oxidative activities of various thiolates and phosphoramides. Other systems now appearing as particular isolated examples of metabolism, e.g., the oxidative degradation system of the insecticide 'Amiton' (SCAIFE and CAMPBELL 1959), may later prove to be of more general interest when a larger number of compounds has been investigated thoroughly. The brief summary given above of the main types of reaction so far encountered emphasizes the complexity of the biological reaction of toxic phosphorus compounds and the influence that these reactions may have on the mediation of anti-ChE responses.

Although the practical importance of these biochemical studies is clear, there are additional facets of these problems that should not be ignored. Frequently it is observed that there are certain similarities between various individual reactions; studies of the similarities of mechanism and differences in specificity may contribute to the understanding of basic biochemical problems. In this respect, it will be interesting to observe the results of subsequent work in the microsomal oxidative activation of organophosphates; perhaps here is an opportunity to use a variety of synthetic materials to evaluate the complexity and specificity of oxidative mechanisms. In the field of study of hydrolytic enzymes, the use of specific labelling of the active centers of enzymes that are inhibited by anti-ChE organophosphates has provided a valuable and unique tool. As pointed out by FRANKEL-CONRAT (1954), the ability to obtain a specific labelling of a position in a macromolecule, and the concomitant association of this position with biological function, has provided an entirely new prospect for the study of enzymatic mechanisms. The value of this method is illustrated by the elucidation of the amino acid sequence in peptides obtained as degradation products of the active sites of several hydrolases (COHEN et al. 1959). As yet no unequivocal results or theories may be presented; however it is difficult to conceive of the interest and attention that is being paid to certain current speculations on the manner in which enzymes function without the assumption of the near availability of results. The recent reports of KOSHLAND et al. (1958), of NEURATH and HARTLEY (1959) and HARTLEY (1959) are examples of these provocative discussions.

Specific labelling of enzymes that hydrolyze organophosphate inhibitors without their being affected by them is of course impossible. From kinetic and inhibition studies it is evident that resemblances in properties and specificity cannot be fortuitous (MOUNTER et al. 1957a, b). A number of proteases that contain a thiol group in their active center are not inhibited by DFP, although the structures may be analogous to those of DFP-inhibited enzymes. If a serine group be replaced by the analog cysteine then there would be no hydroxyl for group phosphorylation by organophosphate esters. Amplification of these discussions is beyond the scope or purpose of this chapter, but these ideas are not the least significant of those deriving from the explosive growth of the biochemistry of toxic phosphate esters.

Literature

ADIE, P. A.: The purification of sarinase from bovine plasma. Canad. J. Biochem. **34**, 1091 to 1094 (1956).
— The intracellular localization of liver and kidney sarinase. Canad. J. Biochem. **36**, 21—24 (1958).
AEBI, H., and I. ABELIN: Die Wirkungsweise verschiedener Effektoren auf die Aktivit-t der alkalischen Nierenphosphatase. Helv. chim. Acta **31**, 1943—1958 (1948).
ALDRIDGE, W. N.: Some observations on the characteristics of serum esterases with special reference to the hydrolysis of diethyl p-nitrophenyl phosphate (E 600). Ph. D. Thesis, London University (1951).
— Serum esterases. I. Two types of esterase (A and B) hydrolyzing p-nitrophenyl acetate, propionate, butyrate and a method for their determination. Biochem. J. **53**, 110—117 (1953a).
— Serum esterases. II. An enzyme hydrolyzing diethyl p-nitrophenyl phosphate (E 600) and its identity with the A-esterase of mammalian sera. Biochem. J. **53**, 117—124 (1953b).
ARTHUR, B. W., and J. E. CASIDA: Metabolism and selectivity of 0,0-dimethyl 2,2,2-trichloro-1-hepteoxethyl phosphonate and its acetyl and vinyl derivatives. J. Agric. Food Chem. **5**, 186—191 (1957).
AUGUSTINSSON, K.-B.: The enzymic hydrolysis of organophosphorus compounds. Biochim. biophys. Acta **13**, 303—304 (1954).
— Enzymatic hydrolysis of organophosphorus compounds. I. Occurrence of enzymes hydrolyzing dimethyl-amido-ethoxy-phosphoryl cyanide (Tabun). Acta chem. scand. 8, 753 to 761 (1954a).
— Enzymatic hydrolysis of organophosphorus compounds. II. Analysis of reaction products in experiments with tabun and some properties of blood plasma tabunase. Acta chem. scand 8, 762—767 (1954b).
— Enzymatic hydrolysis or organophosphorus compounds. III. Effect of cholinesterase inhibitors and inhibition of cholinesterase in the presence of tabunase. Acta chem. scand. 8, 915—920 (1954c).
— Enzymatic hydrolysis of organophosphorus compounds. IV. Specificity studies. Acta chem. scand. 8, 1533—1541 (1954d).
— Enzymatic hydrolysis of organophosphorus compounds. VII. The stereospecificity of phosphorylphosphatases. Acta chem. scand. **11**, 1371—1377 (1957).
—, and G. HEIMBURGER: Enzymatic hydrolysis of organophosphorus compounds. V. Effect of phosphoryl phosphatase on the inactivation of cholinesterases by organophosphorus compounds *in vitro*. Acta chem. scand. **9**, 310—318 (1955a).
— Enzymatic hydrolysis of organophosphorus compounds. VI. Effect of metallic ions on the phosphorylphosphatases of human serum and swine kidney. Acta chem. scand. **9**, 383—392 (1955b).
BALLS, A. K., and E. F. JANSEN: Stoichiometric inhibition of chymotrypsin. Advanc. Enzymol. **13**, 321—343 (1952).
BELL, F. E., and L. A. MOUNTER: Studies of hog kidney acylase I. I. Comparison with hog kidney dialkylfluorophosphatase. J. biol. Chem. **233**, 900—902 (1958).
BODANSKY, O.: Mechanism of inhibition of phosphatase activity by glycine. J. biol. Chem. **165**, 605—613 (1946).
CASIDA, J. E.: Metabolism of organophosphorus insecticides in relation to their antiesterase activity, stability and residual properties. J. Agric. Food Chem. **4**, 772—785 (1956).
COHEN, J. A., R. A. OOSTERBAAN, H. S. JANSZ and F. BEREND: The active site of esterases. J. Cell. Comp. Physiol. **54**, Suppl. 1, 231—244 (1959).
—, and M. G. P. J. WARRINGA: The fate of P[32] labelled diisopropyl fluorophosphonate in the human body and its use as a labelling agent in the study of the turnover of blood plasma and red cells. J. clin. Invest. **33**, 459—467 (1954).

COHEN, J. A.: Purification and properties of dialkylfluorophosphatase. Biochim. biophys. Acta **26**, 29—39 (1957).

DAVISON, A. N.: The conversion of Schradan (OMPA) and parathion into inhibitors of cholinesterase by mammalian liver. Biochem. J. **61**, 203—209 (1955).

DIGGLE, W. M., and J. C. GAGE: Cholinesterase inhibition *in vitro* by 0,0-diethyl-0-p-nitrophenyl thiophosphate (parathion, E 605). Biochem. J. **49**, 491—494 (1951).

DUBOIS, K. P., J. DOULL and J. M. COON: Studies on the toxicity and pharmacological action of octamethyl pyrophosphoramide (OMPA, Pestox III). J. Pharmacol. exp. Ther. **99**, 376—393 (1950).

FENWICK, M. C.: The production of an esterase inhibitor from Schradan in the fat body of the desert locust. Biochem. J. **70**, 373—381 (1958).

FRANKEL-CONRAT, H.: Chemical studies of enzymes and other proteins. J. cell. comp. Physiol. **47**, Suppl. 1, 133—149 (1956).

FUKUTO, T. R., R. L. METCALF, R. B. MARCH and M. G. MAXON: Chemical behavior of systox isomers in biological systems. J. Econ. Entmol. **48**, 347—354 (1955).

GAGE, J. C.: A cholinesterase inhibitor derived from 0,0-diethyl-0-p-nitrophenyl thiophosphate *in vivo*. Biochem. J. **54**, 426—430 (1953).

GARDINER, J. E., and B. A. KILBY: Some observations on the fate of bis(dimethylamino)-phosphorus anhydride in the rabbit. Biochem. J. **46**, xxxii—xxxiii (1950).

GOLDSTEIN, D. B., and A. J. GOLDSTEIN: An adaptive bacterial cholinesterase from a pseudomonas species. J. gen. Microbiol. **8**, 8—17 (1953).

HALL, S. A.: Organic phosphorus insecticides. Advances in Chem. Ser. No. I, 150—159 (1950).

HARVEY, A. M., J. L. LILIENTHAL jr., D. GROB, B. F. JONES and S. A. TALBOT: The admivistration of diisopropyl fluorophosphate to man. IV. Johns Hopkins Hosp. Bull. **81**, 267 to 292 (1947).

HERRMAN, B., and R. PULVER: Der enzymatische Abbau des Insectizids Chlorophan (Dimethyl-(1-Methoxy-2,2-dichlorovinyl)Phosphat] als. Entgiftungsreaktion. Arch. Int. Pharmacodyn. **117**, 223—231 (1957).

HOBBIGER, F.: Inhibition of cholinesterases by irreversible inhibitors *in vitro* and in vivo. Brit. J. Pharmacol. **6**, 21—36 (1951).

HOSKIN, F. C. G., and G. S. TRICK: Stereospecificity in the enzymatic hydrolysis of tabun and acetyl-methylcholine chloride. Canad. J. Biochem. **33**, 963—969 (1955).

JANDORF, B. J.: Mechanism of reaction of di-n-propyl-2,2-dichlorovinyl phosphate (DDP) with esterases. J. Agric. Food Chem. **4**, 853—858 (1956).

—, and P. D. McNAMARA: Distribution of radiophosphorus in rabbit tissues after injection of phosphorus-labelled diisopropyl fluorophosphate. J. Pharmacol. **98**, 77—84 (1950).

JANSEN, E. F., A. L. CURL and A. K. BALLS: Reaction of -chymotrypsin with analogues of diisopropyl fluorophosphate. J. Biol. Chem. **190**, 557—562 (1951).

KOSHLAND, D. E., jr., W. J. RAY, jr. and M. J. ERWIN: Protein structure and enzyme action. Fed. Proc. **17**, 1143—1150 (1958).

MARCH, R. B., T. R. FUKUTO, R. L. METCALF and M. G. MAXON: Fate of P^{32}-labeled malathion in the laying hen, white mouse and american cockroach. J. Econ. Entmol. **49**, 185—195 (1956).

MAZUR, A.: An enzyme in animal tissues capable of hydrolyzing the phosphorusfluorine bond of alkyl fluorophosphates. J. biol. Chem. **164**, 271—289 (1946).

METCALF, R. L.: Organic Insecticides. Their Chemistry and Mode of Action. New York and London: Interscience Publ. 1955.

—, and R. B. MARCH: Studies of the mode of action of parathion and its derivatives and their toxicity to insects. J. Econ. Entmol. **42**, 721—728 (1949).

— Further studies on the mode of action of organic thionophosphate insecticides. Ann. Entomol. Soc. Am. **46**, 63—74 (1953).

MOUNTER, L. A.: Some studies of enzymatic effects of rabbit serum. J. biol. Chem. **209**, 813 to 817 (1954).

— The complex nature of dialkylfluorophosphatases of hog and rat liver and kidney. J. biol. Chem. **215**, 705—711 (1955).

— Dialkylfluorophosphatase of kidney. IV. Dissociation constant of active groups. J. biol. Chem. **219**, 677—683 (1956).

— Identity of diisopropylfluorophosphatase and acylase. Fed. Proc. **15**, 317 (1956).

—, H. C. ALEXANDER, K. D. TUCK and L. T. H. DIEN: The pH dependence and dissociation constants of esterases and proteases treated with diisopropyl fluorophosphate. J. biol. Chem. **226**, 867—872 (1957a).

—, R. F. BAXTER and A. CHANUTIN: Dialkylfluorophosphatases of microorganisms. J. biol. Chem. **215**, 699—704 (1955).

—, and A. CHANUTIN: Dialkylfluorophosphatase of kidney. II. Studies of activation and inhibition by metals. J. biol. Chem. **204**, 837—846 (1953b).

MOUNTER, L. A., and A. CHANUTIN: Dialkylfluorophosphatase of kidney. III. Studies of activation and inhibition by cofactors. J. biol. Chem. **210**, 219—226 (1954).
—, and L. T. H. DIEN: Dialkylfluorophosphatase of kidney. V. The hydrolysis of organophosphorus compounds. J. biol. Chem. **219**, 685—690 (1956).
— — and A. CHANUTIN: The distribution of dialkylfluorophosphatases in the tissues of various species. J. biol. Chem. **215**, 691—697 (1955).
—, C. S. FLOYD and A. CHANUTIN: Dialkylfluorophosphatase of kidney. I. Purification and properties. J. biol. Chem. **204**, 221—232 (1953a).
—, and K. D. TUCK: Dialkylfluorophosphatases of microorganisms. II. Substrate specificity studies. J. biol. Chem. **221**, 537—541 (1956).
— — H. C. ALEXANDER and L. T. H. DIEN: The reactivity of esterases and proteases in the presence of organophosphorus compounds. J. biol. Chem. **226**, 873—879 (1957b).
NEURATH, H., and B. S. HARTLEY: The hydrolysis of peptide and ester bonds by proteolytic enzymes. J. cell. comp. Physiol. **54**, Suppl. 1, 179—202 (1959).
O'BRIEN, R. D.: Activation of thionophosphates by liver microsomes. Nature (Lond.) **183**, 121—122 (1959a).
— Comparative toxicology of some organophosphorus compounds in insects and mammals. Canad. J. Biochem. **37**, 1113—1122 (1959b).
— Toxic Phosphorus Esters. New York: Academic Press 1960.
O'NEILL, J. J.: Ph.D. Thesis, University of Maryland (1954).
—, T. WAGNER-JAUREGG, Y. SNIDER, C. CASTLE and M. STROLBERG: Purification and properties of kidney phosphofluorase. Fed. Proc. **14**, 261 (1954).
PLAPP, F. W., and J. E. CASIDA: Hydrolysis of the alkyl-phosphate bond in certain dialkyl aryl phosphorothioate insecticides in rats, cockroaches and alkali. J. Econ. Entmol. **51**, 800—803 (1958a).
— Bovine metabolism of organophosphorus insecticides. II. Metabolic fate of 0,0-dimethyl-0(2,4,5-trichlorophenyl)phosphorothioate in rats and cows. J. Agric. Food. Chem. **6**, 662—667 (1958b).
SCAIFE, J. F., and D. H. CAMPBELL: The distruction of 0,0-diethyl-S-2-diethyl aminoethyl phosphorothiolate by liver microsomes. Canad. J. Biochem. **37**, 297—305 (1959).
SCHRADER, G.: Die Entwicklung neuer Insektizide auf Grundlage von organischen Fluor- und Phosphorverbindungen. Monographie No. 62, 2. Aufl., Weinheim: Verlag Chemie 1952.
TSUYUKI, H., M. A. STAHMANN and J. E. CASIDA: Preparation, purification, isomerization and biological properties of octamethylpyrophosphoramide N-oxide. J. Agric. Food Chem. **3**, 922—932 (1955).

Chapter 11

Actions at Autonomic Effector Sites

By

Harry Cullumbine

Contents

A. Introduction

The autonomic nervous system is concerned with the regulation of the involuntary mechanisms of the body. It has afferent, central, and efferent nervous components, including specialized sensory areas responsive to chemical or pressure changes. Functionally, it is an elaborate system of reflexes designed to control automatically the responses of the smooth muscles, the blood vessels, the heart, and the glands of the body. The efferent nerves supplying these latter structures have been classified as "adrenergic" or "cholinergic," according to the nature of the supposed chemical mediator released at their effector sites. Even the adrenergic efferent pathways, however, have a cholinergic component, the sympathetic preganglionic nerves, and cholinergic mechanisms have been suggested as being involved in the functioning of some central and afferent parts of the autonomic nervous system. It is obvious, therefore, that the anticholinesterase (anti-ChE) agents, by interference with these cholinergic phenomena, may produce profound and widespread changes in the function of the autonomic nervous system. All these changes will be manifested by effects produced in the organs and tissues supplied by the autonomic effector nerves. For example, general intoxication with an anti-ChE agent may produce miosis, lacrimation, salivation, tightness of the chest, respiratory distress, and cardiovascular embarrassment (see Chapters 18, 20, and 22 for details).

This chapter is concerned solely with those effects of the anti-ChE agents which are *initiated* at the autonomic effector sites. Some reference to effects originating centrally to these sites must inevitably be made, but the detailed discussion of such effects will be found in subsequent chapters.

B. Actions on the secretory glands

The lacrimal, sweat, bronchial, salivary, gastric, and pancreatic gland cells all have a cholinergic innervation, and so would be expected to be influenced by anti-ChE agents.

I. Salivary glands

The humoral transmitter of parasympathetic stimuli for salivary secretion has been shown to be acetylcholine (ACh) (BEZNÁK 1932, GIBBS and SZELÖCZEY 1932), and there is a considerable cholinesterase (ChE) activity in the submaxillary gland (MACINTOSH 1937, RIKER and WESCOE 1949, DIRNHUBER and LOVATT EVANS 1954). In both the cat and the dog this gland contains more acetylcholinesterase (AChE) than butyrocholinesterase (BuChE).

1. Potentiated secretion

HEIDENHAIN (1872) observed that physostigmine (eserine) caused increased salivary secretion even after the ganglia were paralyzed with nicotine, and also that it increased the effectiveness of stimulation of the chorda tympani after atropine. This work has been confirmed many times by different authors; especially informative is the work of DIRNHUBER and LOVATT EVANS (1954) and EMMELIN and STRÖMBLAD (1958).

DIRNHUBER and LOVATT EVANS found that the close arterial injection of an anti-ChE agent into the submaxillary gland of the dog or cat results in the potentiation of the effect of ACh or chorda tympani stimulation. The anti-ChE agent is retained by the gland tissues and the potentiating effect can be satisfactorily explained by the resultant inactivation of the ChE's in the gland or in its ganglia.

2. Spontaneous secretion

When repeated or larger doses of an anti-ChE agent are administered, a spontaneous secretion of saliva occurs. In order to produce a spontaneous flow, at least 60% of the AChE has to be inhibited; selective inactivation of even 80% of the BuChE does not lead to spontaneous flow. These observations are in general agreement with those of RIKER and WESCOE (1949), who reported that spontaneous secretion begins when about 90% of the total ChE of the gland has been inhibited by di*iso*propyl phosphorofluoridate (DFP), at which level the maximal decrease of threshold of chorda stimulation occurs also; reduction to 50% had no physiological effects.

It would appear that the AChE has the more important physiological function in the submaxillary gland. This receives further support from the observation that relatively large doses of selective BuChE-inhibitors are required to produce even a potentiation of the action of ACh or of chorda tympani stimulation.

The spontaneous flow of saliva following a sufficient dose of an anti-ChE agent is probably not due to the accumulation of ACh in the circulating blood because the onset of such secretion following intraarterial injection seems to be too prompt, and both EMMELIN and MUREN (1950a) and DIRNHUBER and LOVATT EVANS (1954) have reported a continuous secretion of saliva from a gland perfused with eserinized blood or plasma. Nor, as first suggested by HEIDENHAIN (1872), can it be due to a central action of the drug upon the salivary centers in the medulla, because the secretion rate is unaffected by section of all the nerves to the gland.

Even large doses of ganglion-blocking agents only slow but do not otherwise affect the salivary flow unless the blood pressure is profoundly affected; therefore, an action upon the ganglion cells on the course of the chorda fibers would not seem to be responsible. It is more probable that the action is upon ChE in or near the secreting cells. This ChE could be situated near the parasympathetic nerve endings. The gland contains much ChE; CHANG and GADDUM (1933) have shown that the dog's submaxillary gland contains from 1.5 to 3.3 μg ACh/g, while EMMELIN and MUREN (1950a) found the cat's chorda tympani nerve to contain about 1.5 μg ACh/g.

It seems likely that ACh is constantly being set free in the salivary glands. BEZNÁK (1932) and GIBBS and SZELÖCZEY (1932) could find no ACh in the effluent from perfused glands prior to chorda stimulation, but HENDERSON and ROEPKE (1933) and EMMELIN and MUREN (1950b) demonstrated its presence, the amount being greatly increased by chorda stimulation. After poisoning with an anti-ChE agent, the small amounts of ACh liberated would be expected to accumulate, and ultimately to reach a threshold concentration so that secretion would ensue. Atropine in quite small doses at once checks this spontaneous secretion, presumably by acting peripherally to the site of liberation of the ACh, i.e., at the secretory cells.

3. Augmented secretion

The submaxillary gland has both a parasympathetic and a sympathetic nerve supply, and stimulation of either will cause a secretion of saliva. BRADFORD (1888) was the first to show that the secretory response to stimulation of either the chorda or the sympathetic supply was augmented if the chorda had been stimulated a few seconds beforehand. LANGLEY (1889) called this "augmented secretion". BABKIN (1950) later showed that stimulation of either nerve gave an augmented secretion if the other nerve had been previously stimulated. DIRNHUBER and LOVATT EVANS (1954) found that ACh could replace chorda stimulation, and epinephrine sympathetic stimulation in this sequence and, further, that the response to sympathetic stimulation or to epinephrine was augmented after poisoning by an anti-ChE agent. SECKER (1934) made a similar observation, but inferred that ACh acted as the mediator of both sympathetic and parasympathetic impulses. FELDBERG et al. (1935) and DIRNHUBER and LOVATT EVANS (1954) preferred to consider it as merely another instance of augmented secretion, i.e., that the accumulation of sufficient ACh in or near to the gland cells after an anti-ChE agent causes an enhanced response after either sympathetic stimulation or the injection of epinephrine. (Large doses of epinephrine, when injected intra-arterially, stop the spontaneous flow for long periods; this effect can be attributed to local vasoconstriction and anoxia, enhanced by raised metabolism.)

4. Reduced secretion

There is an optimal rate of stimulation of the chorda tympani; very rapid stimulation gives a slower rate of secretion than a slow one (WILLS 1941). This is analogous to the phenomenon of Wedensky inhibition seen in neuromuscular conduction, where it is readily evident following poisoning with anti-ChE agents

(LOVATT EVANS 1951). Similarly, in the salivary gland, following a large dose of ACh, stimulation of the chorda is much less effective than it was immediately before. Also, after an anti-ChE agent, the injection of a large dose of ACh or prolonged chorda stimulation may have a reduced effect. Both at the neuro-muscular junction and in the salivary gland, these "block" phenomena can be attributed to the presence of excess ACh. This illustrates the similarity of the cholinergic mechanisms at two very dissimilar anatomical sites.

5. Supersensitivity

EMMELIN and STRÖMBLAD (1958a) have studied the action of anti-ChE agents on the cat's parotid gland, which can be either pre- or postganglionically denervated. When anti-ChE agents, such as physostigmine (eserine), tetraethyl pyrophosphate (TEPP), and diethyl 4-nitrophenyl phosphate (Paraoxon, E 600) were injected into the parotid duct, they caused a secretion of saliva. After chronic preganglionic parasympathetic denervation, the effects of the agents were increased above normal. This was attributed by EMMELIN and STRÖMBLAD to the development in the gland cells of a supersensitivity to ACh. A similar supersensitivity was pro-duced in the submaxillary gland by daily subcutaneous injections of the anti-cholinergic drug, diphenyl-piperidinoethyl-acetamide (EMMELIN and STRÖMBLAD 1957). It was presumed from these results that there is a liberation of ACh from the postganglionic endings which is not due to impulses from the central nervous system. Acute pre- or post-ganglionic denervation does not alter the response to anti-ChE agents (DIRNHUBER and EVANS 1954, EMMELIN et al. 1954, EMMELIN and STRÖMBLAD 1958), therefore, the ACh-release apparently is not initiated from the cell body of the postganglionic neurone.

After chronic parasympathetic post-ganglionic denervation, the secretory effect of anti-ChE agents is much smaller, although the gland is even more sensitive to ACh and methacholine. Such a gland still contains ACh (CHANG and GADDUM 1933), although in reduced quantity; therefore, there may be a small non-nervous production of ACh. This could account for some of the aforementioned actions of the anti-ChE agents. They could be due also to a direct effect on the super-sensitive gland cells. A third possibility is that section of the auriculo-temporal nerves does not remove all the cholinergic fibers in the parotid gland, especially because not only atropine but also cocaine abolishes the effect of anti-ChE agents. The small secretory response, however, was still obtained by EMMELIN and STRÖM-BLAD after section of the facial nerve or extirpation of the superior cervical ganglion.

The nature of the supersensitivity of the parotid gland after chronic denerva-tion is not clear. MACINTOSH (1937) found no change in the ChE content of the submaxillary gland after chorda section, whereas STRÖMBLAD (1955) reported that preganglionic denervation of the parotid or submaxillary gland resulted in a 30% decrease in ChE activity in the gland, and postganglionic denervation of the parotid gland resulted in a 60% decrease. STRÖMBLAD (1957) later compared the percentage decrease in ACh activity of homogenates of denervated salivary glands with that found following the injection of anti-ChE agents into the glands via the secretory duct in amounts sufficient to cause supersensitivity. He concluded that the supersensitivity found after denervation cannot be wholly due to a decrease in ChE activity.

6. Paroxysmal secretion

EMMELIN and STRÖMBLAD (1958b) described also the influence of physostig-mine on the phenomenon known as "paroxysmal" secretion, i.e., the intermittent flow of saliva from the parotid glands of cats which occurs during the early stages of degeneration of its postganglionic parasympathetic fibers. This secretion was abolished by intravenous injection of or by cocaine injected into the salivary duct. Physostigmine injected into the duct provoked a period of increased paroxysmal secretion. It was thought that the paroxysmal secretion is the result of paroxysmal release of ACh from the endings of the degenerating postganglionic nerve fibers.

It can be seen that there is strong presumptive evidence from the work of several investigators that there is a continuous, small production of ACh in the salivary glands, and that this may not be under nervous control.

II. Salivary in comparison with bronchial secretion

The practical importance of the glandular secretions caused by anti-ChE agents is that in acute anti-ChE poisoning there is a profuse secretion of fluid from the mouth, nose and eyes, and its accumulation in the airway may aggravate the respiratory distress produced by other mechanisms. In order to obtain quantitative information, CULLUMBINE and DIRNHUBER (1955) collected fluids flowing from the cannulated trachea and also from the mouth and nose of anesthetized rabbits, cats, and monkeys before and after the administration of anti-ChE agents. To facilitate the free flow of bronchial fluid, the animals were allowed to breathe warm, moist air, but rebreathing with accumulation of carbon dioxide was avoided. It was found that all the anti-ChE agents tried—*iso*propoylmethylphosphono-fluoridate (Sarin), N-*p*-chlorophenyl-N-methyl carbamate of *m*-hydroxy phenyl-trimethylammonium bromide (Nu 1250), and DFP—had a much greater effect on the oral than on the bronchial flow. The fluid flow rates increased in parallel with the severity of the general signs of anti-ChE poisoning. If the dose was not large enough to cause skin twitching, flow rates remained at pretreatment levels. Similarly, in conscious dogs, subcutaneously injected Sarin usually provoked intense salivary secretion only at doses which caused generalized convulsions. A slightly increased flow of saliva appeared shortly before the onset of the convulsions, but the animal could usually swallow this secretion. As the convulsions became more intense, copious saliva escaped from the animal's mouth. Extrapolation from these data indicates that in severe cases of anti-ChE poisoning in man, total volumes of oral fluid of the order of 1.75 litres could be formed if therapeutic counter-measures were not available.

III. Other secretory glands

In addition to producing salivation and increased bronchial secretion, the anti-ChE agents can cause lacrimation and may augment sweating (LOVATT EVANS and SMITH 1956). Gastric secretion (acid and pepsin) is also increased (PEWSNER 1906), while the intestinal secretion is apparently enhanced (UVNÄS 1948) and the secretion from the pancreas may be raised (GOTTLIEB 1894). None of these effects has been studied in sufficient detail to enable any precise statement as to how they are produced.

HOKIN and HOKIN (1953) have studied enzyme secretion and the uptake of p^{32} into phospholipids in slices of pigeon pancreas. They found that ACh with physostigmine, carbamylcholine, or, less effectively, pilocarpine stimulated the secretion of amylase and, at the same time, the incorporation of P^{32} into the phospholipid faction of the stimulated slices was greatly increased. Neither respiration nor the incorporation of P^{32} into acid-soluble phosphate esters was increased, and the stimulant effects of the cholinomimetic drugs were abolished by atropine. Later, SCHUCHER and HOKIN (1954) showed that ACh or carbamyl-choline stimulated the secretion by pigeon pancreas slices of lipase and ribonuclease in addition to amylase. This stimulation was not accompanied by increased enzyme synthesis, which suggests that the variation in enzyme content of pancreatic cells following ingestion of food or cholinergic stimulation "may merely reflect a constant rate of enzyme synthesis with superimposed variations in the secretory rate".

In possible conformity with the observed lack of correlation between enzyme synthesis and enzyme secretion, are the additional observations that stimulation of enzyme secretion in either pigeon pancreas or in rabbit parotid slices was not accompanied by any significant changes in the ribonucleic acid (RNA) concentration (HOKIN and HOKIN 1954b), and stimulation of enzyme secretion in pigeon pancreas slices with ACh and physiostigmine, or with casbamylcholine, was not accompanied by any increase in the rate of incorporation of P^{32} into RNA (HOKIN and HOKIN 1954c).

Although cholinomimetic drugs stimulate both enzyme secretion and the incorporation of P^{32} into phospholipids, the latter two phenomena are not directly related. Thus, enzyme secretion and the incorporation of P^{32} into phospholipids *in vitro* did not parallel each other as the concentration of ACh was increased or when choline or physostigmine was added. Again, the incorporation of P^{32} *in vivo* into phospholipids was found to be the same in the pancreas of fed and fasted mice, and in both this incorporation was stimulated by cholinomimetic drugs (HOKIN and HOKIN 1954a). It is possible that the quantities of ACh liberated in the pancreas under normal physiological conditions are too small to have a detectable effect on the phospholipids.

Acetylcholine with physostigmine stimulated the incorporation of P^{32} into the choline-containing phospholipids, into the non-choline-containing phospholipids, and into the glycerophosphatides of pancreas slices, but the incorporation of glycerol-1-C^{14} into the glycerophosphatides was not stimulated. This indicates that ACh stimulates the independent turnover of phosphate (and presumably the base attached to it) in preformed phospholipids (HOKIN and HOKIN 1954a). It was postulated that ACh acts at the molecular level by splitting certain susceptible lipoproteins into free phospholipids and proteins, thus rendering the phosphate-base moiety of the phospholipids accessible to enzymes which could catalyze its independent turnover. HOKIN and HOKIN suggested that such a mechanism of action, i.e., dissociation of lipoproteins, of ACh could possibly be true for all types of cells responsive to ACh; changes in the lipoproteins of the cell membrane could affect permeability and so produce physiological changes. On the other hand, HOKIN and HOKIN (1953) stated that cholinomimetic drugs had little or no effect on the incorporation of P^{32} into the phospholipids of pigeon and guinea-pig liver, guinea-pig heart ventricle, pigeon gizzard (smooth muscle) or guinea-pig kidney cortex. A relatively slight stimulation of P^{32} uptake into phospholipids was observed in slices of pigeon brain and guinea-pig brain cortex, and some stimulation (not quantitated, see HOKIN and HOKIN 1954a) in the rabbit parotid and submaxillary glands. There would have to be "specific receptor lipoproteins" to account for the high physiological specificity of ACh, and the different tissues could vary widely in their content of this type of lipoprotein. An account of the present status of these interesting studies will be found in the recent publications (HOKIN and HOKIN 1959, M. R. HOKIN et al. 1960) and an extensive review (HOKIN and HOKIN 1960); their possible physiological significance is also discussed in Chapter 6.

C. Actions on smooth muscle

I. Bronchi

One salient feature of anti-ChE poisoning in experimental animals is a lessened distensibility of the lungs which is generally attributed to the occurrence of bronchoconstriction. The effect has been observed in a variety of species with such compounds as DFP (MODELL et al. 1946, HEYMANS and JACOB 1947), "Hexaethyltetraphosphate" (HETP) (DAYRIT et al. 1948), TEPP (VERBEKE 1949a), and ethyl-NN-dimethyl-phosphoramidocyantidate (Tabun) HOLMSTEDT (1951), and is often of such severity as to be suggested as the cause of death (KOELLE and

GILMAN 1949). The degree of bronchoconstriction produced by Sarin, Tabun, Paraoxon, DFP, and TEPP does vary, however, with the species examined, being at the time of respiratory failure slight in rabbits, severe in dogs and cats, and insignificant in monkeys (KROP and KUNKEL 1954, DE CANDOLE et al. 1953). This variation between species has been related to the relative amount of peribronchial smooth muscle (JOHNSON et al. 1958). Therefore, the failure of ventilation after intoxication with an anti-ChE agent cannot always be attributed solely to the production of bronchoconstriction.

Probably DIXON and BRODIE (1903) were the first to suggest that an anti-ChE agent, physostigmine, could constrict bronchial muscles and increase the effect of vagal stimulation. TRENDELENBURG (1912) also showed that physostigmine constricted isolated bronchial muscle. Bronchoconstriction has been demonstrated in the decapitated cat, in the dog heart-lung preparation (with ACh added to the circulating blood), and radiographically in the rabbit following administration of anti-ChE agents (DE CANDOLE et al. 1953). In the rabbit, evidence of narrowing of the bronchi and of all sizes of bronchioles was obtained at all intravenous dosage levels of Sarin.

The explanation of the bronchoconstriction produced by anti-ChE agents has been disputed. It has been attributed to an action on the vagal ganglion cells (VERBEKE 1949a, HEYMANS 1949), or to the accumulation of ACh at the vagal postganglionic nerve endings (KOELLE and GILMAN 1949). DE CANDOLE et al. (1953), using twin preparations of guinea-pig trachea in order to obtain the necessary control observations demanded in the examination of slow, prolonged, and sometimes irreversible effects, have shown that Sarin, DFP, and TEPP in high dilutions not only sensitize the isolated muscle to ACh, but throw it into spasm. The tracheal spasmogenic potencies of these compounds parallel their ability to inhibit ChE (KOPPANYI et al. 1947), and the tracheal contractions induced show features, namely, long latency and slow development, which have been held to characterize drugs acting indirectly by permitting accumulation of ACh (ADRIAN et al. 1947).

HAWKINS and SCHILD (1951), using an isolated preparation consisting of a chain of human bronchial rings, found that physostigmine, in a concentration of 10^{-7}, potentiated the contraction response to ACh. Larger doses of physostigmine themselves caused slowly developing contractions which took a long time to reverse.

II. Cilia

Although the classification of cilia with smooth muscle can hardly be justified on morphological grounds, certain functional similarities, as well as convenience, have dictated this procedure. Ciliary movement has been studied in the mucous membrane of the frog esophagus, both *in situ* and when isolated, and also in the isolated mucous membrane of the rabbit trachea (KORDIK, BÜLBRING and BURN 1952). In both preparations it was found that low concentrations of ACh increased the rate of movement and high concentrations depressed it. Similarly, low concentrations of physostigmine increased and high concentrations depressed ciliary movement. These observations suggest that the ciliary movement is controlled by the production of ACh, and the fact that ciliary movement is depressed or arrested by atropine and by *d*-tubocurarine adds further support to this view. KORDIK et al. also demonstrated the presence of choline acetylase, AChE, and ACh in the mucous membrane of the rabbit trachea, but the site of synthesis of the ACh could not be stated with certainty. The isolated tracheal mucous membrane preparation did not contain ganglion cells, but a few nerve fibers were present in the submucosa so that the ACh could have been liberated from the nerve endings. This appeared unlikely when it was shown that cocaine in 2% concentration had no effect on ciliary movement, but the decisive evidence in favor of the non-nervous origin of ACh in ciliated tissues came from further experiments using the gill plates of the sea mussel, *Mytilis edulis* (BÜLBRING, BURN and SHELLEY 1953). These gill plates represent a ciliated tissue which contains no nerve fibers. BÜLBRING et al. found that the plates contained choline acetylase, AChE, and ACh and, also, that their ciliary movement was accelerated by low concentrations and slowed by high concentrations of ACh and of physostigmine. Atropine reduced the action of ACh, and *d*-tubocurarine slowed the rate of movement. Therefore, ACh can be produced locally in a nerve-free and muscle-free structure, and it controls the ciliary movement.

BURN (1956) cited this function of ACh as being that of a "local hormone," which he defined as "an exciting substance which acts locally."

GUNTHER and ALLEN (1959) have studied human ciliated tissue. They have reported that perfusion of explants of human respiratory ciliated epithelium with physostigmine markedly enhanced the stimulant action of ACh on ciliary activity. (See Chapter 6 for further discussion.)

III. Gastro-intestinal tract

HARNACK and WITKOWSKI (1876) first showed that physostigmine causes contraction and increased peristalsis in the stomach and small and large intestines. These actions were confirmed by SCHÜTZ (1886), using the isolated stomach, by BATTELLI (1897) for the stomach in man, by SUBBOTIN (1869) and JACOBI (1891) for the intestine in animals, and by UNGER (1907) on isolated gut strips. GASSER (1926) and v. ESVELD (1928) showed that occasional plexus-free strips might react, but that plexus-containing strips were more sensitive. Small doses given to the cat or the dog increased the responsiveness of the gut to vagal stimulation (DIXON and RANSOM 1924).

The duodenum is very susceptible to the action of anti-ChE agents; it shows increased tonus and rhythmicity following doses that produce no discernible effects on respiration or circulation (KROPP and KUNKEL 1954). Doses of Tabun or Sarin producing respiratory and circulatory effects produce rapid, intense spastic contraction of the duodenum.

The effect of anti-ChE agents on the tone of isolated intestine preparations from several species has been studied by many investigators (HEATHCOTE 1932, FELDBERG and SOLANDT 1942, BACQ 1947, FELDBERG and LIN 1949, KOELLE et al. 1950, SHELLEY 1955). With low concentrations of anti-ChE agents there is an increase in tone and sometimes an increase in the amplitude of the pendular movements. As the concentration increases, the pendular movement diminishes, and at high concentrations it may cease altogether. BACQ (1947) found that isolated cat or rabbit intestine would not respond to a second dose of physostigmine or DFP, and KOELLE et al. (1950) were unable to obtain a direct quantitative relationship between DFP concentration and the response of isolated cat intestine. SHELLEY (1955), however, expressing responses as a percentage of the maximum response and testing each dose of physostigmine or DFP on a different piece of rabbit duodenum in order to avoid the effects of previous doses, did find a quantitative agreement between different experiments.

KOELLE (1953), using histochemical methods, found AChE in nervous tissue throughout the intestinal wall of the rabbit, and in low concentrations in the interstitial cells of the muscle layers; BuChE was demonstrable in the ganglion cells, the interstitial cells, and the mucosa. SHELLEY (1955) employed manometric methods and reported a similar distribution in the different layers of the intestinal wall.

KOELLE et al. (1950) made manometric and histochemical determinations of the residual ChE activities of the cat intestine after exposure to DFP, and found that concentrations of DFP which produced large increases in tone had caused almost complete inhibition of the BuChE, whereas the AChE had been hardly affected. From this and the observed distribution of BuChE, they concluded that intestinal motility is closely related to BuChE activity. Evidence in support of this comes from the work of BURN et al. (1952), who found that intestinal loops from rats previously exposed to X-rays were more sensitive than usual to ACh; the BuChE activity of these loops was less than half of that of controls, while the AChE activity was not changed. The results of SHELLEY (1955), however, do suggest that AChE may also be important. She found that maximum increase in tone of isolated rabbit duodenum treated with DFP coincided with complete inhibition of AChE activity, whereas complete BuChE inhibition occurred at a much lower concentration of DFP.

The high sensitivity of the gut to anti-ChE agents is illustrated by the fact that SHELLEY (1955) found regularly an increase in tone of the rabbit intestine with physostigmine, 2.7×10^{-7} M, or with DFP, 10^{-7} M, concentrations sufficient to produce only 10 to 20% inhibition of AChE activity. The significance of these observations will be discussed later.

The increase in tone and motility of the intestine produced by anti-ChE agents can be prevented by atropine, pyridine-2-aldoxime methiodide (P-2-AM) and other reactivators, and by ganglion-blocking agents. The last mentioned observation suggests that the effects are due at least in part to accumulation of ACh at the autonomic ganglia in the intestinal wall (ERDMANN and HEYE 1958). Large doses of anti-ChE agents produce a reduced gut response, and even inhibition of motility (SHELLEY 1955, HEATHCOTE 1932). This paralytic effect is reversible by washing, and is not prevented or reversed by atropine or P-2-AM, (ERDMANN and HEYE 1958); therefore, it is probably a direct effect of the anti-ChE agent on the smooth muscle.

HUGHES (1955) reported that the *muscularis mucosae* of the cat, rabbit, and rat contracts under the influence of ACh or physostigmine, and this response can be blocked with atropine.

The great susceptibility of the smooth muscle of the gastro-intestinal tract to anti-ChE agents is also seen in man. Following toxic doses of these compounds, especially when administered by mouth or through the skin, gastrointestinal symptoms, such as abdominal cramps, increased intestinal movements and diarrhea, occur early and are severe (GROB et al. 1947).

The work of BRUNAUD and DUSSARDIER (1951) on sheep and cow stomachs should be mentioned. They found that vagal stimulation, in addition to causing bradycardia, also caused contraction of the stomach, but whereas physostigmine sensitized the heart to this vagal stimulation it did not sensitize the stomach. Atropine blocked both vagal effects. Intravenous ACh in these species also caused bradycardia but it inhibited the tone of the stomach. Both these effects of ACh were potentiated by physostigmine and inhibited by atropine. Following further experiments, DUSSARDIER (1954) believed that the stomach contraction produced by intravenous ACh was due to a stimulation of the bulbar center controlling gastric motility in ruminants. Intra-arterial injection of ACh or intravenous injection of large doses of ACh in atropinized animals did produce stomach contractions.

IV. Spleen

SCOTT (1957) found that intravenous injection of TEPP in the anesthetized dog causes a considerable contraction of the spleen with a co-incidental increase in hematocrit value. A similar contraction is obtained in the perfused denervated spleen, suggesting that the contraction is due to an agent carried in the blood. In adrenalectomized dogs with normally innervated spleens, however, TEPP still causes a reduction in splenic volume. A contraction is seen also in the innervated spleen cross-perfused from a donor dog. No contraction occurs in adrenalectomized preparations with the spleen denervated. Section of the vagi does not alter this response to TEPP, which is probably due to two factors: an increased sympathetic discharge and an increased secretion of suprarenal medullary hormones. Atropine reverses the contraction of the spleen caused by TEPP provided pulmonary ventilation is restored to its resting value.

V. Eye

The anti-ChE agents can cause constriction of the pupil, spasm of accommodation, twitching of the eyelid, and a lowering of the intra-ocular pressure. These full effects are usually seen only after direct exposure of the eye to droplets or vapors. The degree of miosis has been used as a measure of the ChE inhibitory activity of these compounds (SANDERSON 1957). The spasm of accommodation usually occurs slightly later, and lasts a shorter time than does the miosis. Because of contraction of the ciliary muscle, the lens becomes more spherical and fixed for near vision.

The anti-ChE agents produce other effects on vision besides those due to miosis. They can cause an increase in near and far accommodation, and a decrease in light perception (UPHOLT et al. 1956). The absolute visual threshold in the dark adapted eye is elevated, and this elevation of threshold is independent of the production of miosis (RUBIN and GOLDBERG 1957, RUBIN et al. 1957). It is believed that this effect upon the visual threshold is due to an extra-ocular action of the agent (Sarin). It may involve the central nervous system, since whereas intra-muscularly injected atropine sulfate significantly lowers the elevated visual threshold, an intramuscular injection of atropine methyl nitrate, which does not penetrate the blood-brain barrier, has no marked effect (RUBIN and GOLDBERG 1958).

Actions of anti-ChE agents on the normal and glaucomatous eye are described fully in Chapter 24.

D. Actions on the cardiovascular system

I. Variations in response

All anti-ChE agents can cause, in most species, a slowing of the heart and a marked fall in the systemic blood pressure, but the detailed picture varies with the species studied, the depth and nature of the anesthesia, the amount of agent administered, and the presence and degree of hypoxia (VERBEKE 1949b, HOLM-STEDT 1951, DE CANDOLE et al. 1953, KROP and KUNKEL 1954, DALY and WRIGHT 1956, DELGA 1957, ERDMANN and LENDLE 1958). The fall in blood pressure may be preceded by a rise, especially if smaller doses are given to lightly anesthetized animals.

While the above statement is generally true, many exceptions to it have been reported. In the rat, Sarin, DFP, physostigmine, TEPP, and Paraoxon cause an increased heart rate and a sustained rise in blood pressure (DIRNHUBER and CULLUMBINE 1955, VARAGIC 1955). Physostigmine in the spinal cat, and Parathion, physostigmine, and neostigmine in decerebrate cats, all produce a blood pressure increase (VON EICKSTEDT et al. 1955). Sublethal doses of TEPP have been said to have a pressor effect in the dog (PAULET 1954), while HEYMANS et al. (1956) reported that Tabun and Sarin intravenously administered to chloralose-anesthetized dogs may induce either arterial hypotension or hypertension.

These diverse responses to anti-ChE agents described by different workers suggest that these compounds may produce a variety of effects at different sites, central, reflex, and peripheral. To appreciate the importance of actions at autonomic effector sites, the responses of the heart and the peripheral circulation will be considered separately.

II. Heart

1. Bradycardia

As stated, the most common effect of anti-ChE agents on the heart is a slowing of the rate. HEYMANS et al. (1956) have shown that this is due to a peripheral action. Thus, in the dog after administration of Sarin or Tabun, the bradycardia persists after section of the cervical vagus nerves, and it is seen following injection in the surviving decapitated trunk. Furthermore, injection into the circulation of the perfused isolated head, connected to its trunk only by the vagus nerves, does not induce bradycardia (HEYMANS 1950). Therefore, these anti-ChE agents, unlike ACh, apparently do not stimulate directly the vagal cardioinhibitory center. Also, unlike ACh, they do not cause a reflex bradycardia by stimulation of the chemoreceptors of the carotid body, since injection into the circulation of the carotid body does not induce bradycardia; likewise, it is not influenced by denervation of the carotid sinus (HEYMANS 1951).

Ganglioplegic agents, such as tetraethylammonium, Pendiomide (azamethonium), and hexamethonium, given in doses sufficient to block the intracardiac vagal synapses diminish the response, but some degree of bradycardia still persists. This residual bradycardia can be abolished by atropine (HEYMANS et al. 1956, HOLMSTEDT 1951) and by P-2-AM (ERDMANN and LENDLE 1958). Therefore, the bradycardia is due, in part, to a nicotinic stimulant action on the parasympathetic ganglia and, in part, to a peripheral muscarinic effect.

2. Role of butyrocholinesterase (BuChE)

BURN and WALKER (1954) suggested that it is inhibition of BuChE which leads to slowing of the heart rate. Using the heart-lung preparation of the dog, they found that the dimethylcarbamate of (2-hydroxy-5-phenylbenzyl)-trimethyl-ammonium bromide (Nu 683), a specific inhibitor of BuChE, was active but that the dimethobromide of 1:5-di (p-N-allyl-N-methyl-aminophenyl)-pentan-3-one (284.C.51), a specific inhibitor of AChE, was not. Other anti-ChE agents, such as physostigmine, neostigmine, and DFP, were also active in this preparation, and the rate could be restored to normal by injecting small amounts of atropine. These results led BURN and WALKER to conclude that ACh is formed continuously in the heart-lung preparation and that the pacemaker is under its control. The ACh apparently does not come from the pre-ganglionic vagus nerve endings, since slowing by anti-ChE agents is seen also in preparations made in dogs in which the vagi have been cut 4 days before.

Further supporting evidence for the roles of ACh and BuChE has been supplied by BURN and his co-workers. Physostigmine usually decreases the rate of contraction of isolated rabbit auricles. Auricles kept in Locke's solution for 24 hours show an increased sensitivity to physostigmine (BURN and KOTTEGODA 1953), which is accompanied by a progressive loss in BuChE but no change in the AChE content. There is no change in the ChE's of auricles beating in Kreb's solution, and no change in sensitivity to physostigmine (BÜLBRING et al. 1954).

It should be remembered also that the enzyme in the atrial wall of the dog and cat is predominantly BuChE, and activity is present in the muscle fibers, walls of the blood vessels, ganglion cells, thick nerve fibers and their complex terminal formations, and in the fibers of the subendocardial network (HOLMES 1957).

As noted above, BURN and WALKER (1954) concluded that locally produced ACh controls the pacemaker, which agrees with the hypothesis of BÜLBRING and BURN (1949) that the activity of cardiac muscle is due to the local formation of ACh. Further evidence has appeared in support of this view. GLAESSER and TEDESCHI (1955) showed that low concentrations (about 10^{-6} g/ml) of physostigmine, neostigmine, and DFP behaved like ACh in increasing the maximum rate of stimulation which isolated rabbit auricles driven electrically would follow. This maximum rate was found to be decreased by higher concentrations of physostigmine, but still increased by higher concentrations of neostigmine and DFP. This effect of the high concentration of physostigmine is similar to that of quinidine on this preparation, and BRISCOE and BURN (1954, see below) have noted similarities between the effect of a high concentration of physostigmine and that of quinidine on auricles beating spontaneously.

KATSH (1957) has shown that anti-ChE agents inhibit or arrest spontaneously beating, isolated auricles of the guinea-pig, and MARSHALL and KATSH (1957) have found that anti-ChE agents shorten the duration of the action potential and diminish the developed tension of spontaneously beating isolated rabbit auricles. These effects were similar to those produced by ACh, and they could be reversed by atropine. They could be explained on the basis that the anti-ChE agents prevent the destruction of endogenously-produced ACh.

A further effect of ACh and of anti-ChE agents on pacemaker function has been described by MARSHALL and VAUGHAN WILLIAMS (1956) (v. i.).

The bradycardia produced by anti-ChE agents is accompanied by corresponding EKG changes, such as slowing of rate, prolongation of the P-R interval, later conduction defects, and finally complete heart-block (HOLMSTEDT 1951, KROP and KUNKEL 1954). In addition, there is a decrease in cardiac output and a decrease in oxygen consumption; both these changes can be reversed by atropine (HOLM-STEDT 1951, DALY 1957a).

3. Membrane permeability

MARSHALL and VAUGHAN WILLIAMS (1956) have described a means of separating the activity of the pacemaker region from that of the rest of the atrium. Isolated rabbit auricles were slowly cooled from 30° C. At 14 to 20° C., when all other electrical and mechanical activity had ceased, small rhythmical non-propagated potentials were observable in the region of the pacemaker. On rewarming, faster and larger action potentials appeared and were propagated across the whole auricle. These large potentials were associated with the development of contractions. When the auricles were kept at a temperature at which non-propagated pacemaker potentials only were observed, ACh, 10^{-6} to 10^{-8} g/ml, caused propagated action potentials and full auricular contractions. The effect of ACh at the lower temperatures was potentiated by physostigmine and abolished by atropine. Physostigmine and atropine alone had no effect on the pacemaker potentials.

Since the pacemaker potentials were distinguishable only at low temperatures, and since ACh in the extremely small amounts used had no effect on auricles at 30° C., there is no evidence whether ACh has any physiological function in linking the pacemaker with the rest of the atrium. Acetylcholine synthesis is greater in the pacemaker region than elsewhere, but the reason for this is again not known. MARSHALL and WILLIAMS (1956) tentatively suggested that in the cooled auricles the resting membrane potential was reduced to a level at which the rate of sodium entry, which WEIDMANN (1955) has shown to be a function of resting potential, was too slow to initiate conduction. Acetylcholine, by slightly increasing the resting membrane potential, could perhaps accelerate sodium entry so that a sufficient membrane potential would be initiated to discharge the membrane around the pacemaker. BURGEN and TERROUX (1953), HOFFMANN and SUCKLING (1953) and TRAUTWEIN and DUDEL (1958) have shown that ACh does increase the resting potential of cardiac muscle.

Acetylcholine also alters the membrane resistance or conductance, and the alteration is accentuated by physostigmine. TRAUTWEIN, KUFFLER and EDWARDS (1956) have studied the membrane characteristics in isolated muscle strands from auricles of frogs to which square pulses were applied. Acetylcholine in concentrations which slowed or stopped the heart beat produced a reduction of the length constant of the membrane and a shortened time constant. The effects were reversible and increased with ACh concentration. These effects of ACh were transient but could be prolonged by the addition of prostigmine. Therefore, the inhibition produced by ACh increased the conductance of the muscle membrane.

WEBB and HOLLANDER (1956), using electrically-driven (200/min) isolated rat atria, found that physostigmine, like ACh, caused an increase in resting potential, plus a marked decrease in the duration of the action potential (due to a more rapid rate of repolarization). There was hardly any change in the form of contraction and a slight decrease in the rate of conduction.

These changes in membrane potential and resistance produced by ACh and accentuated by anti-ChE agents have been considered as indications that ACh changes the permeability to specific ions. TRAUTWEIN and DUDEL (1958), in fact, concluded that the mechanism of action of ACh on cardiac muscle is "a specific increase of the membrane permeability to potassium ions."

Some workers have taken a somewhat different view, that membrane permeability is dependent upon the activity of AChE. HOLLAND, DUNN and GREIG (1952) have shown that alterations in the rate of metabolism of ACh by AChE may be correlated with changes in the permeability of isolated guinea-pig auricles to sodium and potassium. In media containing a low potassium ion concentration the hydrolysis of ACh was accompanied by a release of potassium from the auricles. The potassium lost was replaced by an equivalent amount of sodium. That this cation movement was dependent on AChE activity is supported by the observations that:

(a) the maximal movement occurred when the ACh concentration allowed the maximal rate of hydrolysis by AChE;

(b) a substrate which is readily hydrolyzed by AChE, e.g., acetyl-β-methylcholine, had an effect like ACh; a substrate which is only slightly hydrolyzed, e.g., benzoylcholine, had no effect;

(c) inhibitors, such as physostigmine and methylene blue, partially or completely reversed the release of potassium by ACh depending upon the concentration of substrate employed. ACh in all concentrations employed produced a prompt cessation of the auricular beat and this depression of activity was partially reversed by the inhibitors. Atropine promptly restored cardiac activity and also completely reversed the potassium liberation and sodium penetration produced by ACh.

It must be remembered that the amount of an ion in a tissue is the resultant of two flows, an influx and an efflux. Either flow may be affected alone or both may be differentially affected. These flows are dependent, *inter alia*, upon the ion concentration in the medium, the nature of the ions, the presence and concentration of ACh, the presence of anti-ChE agents, and the presence of atropine. In the isolated rabbit atria, both the efflux and the influx of potassium are increased by an increase of the K^+ in the medium, the effect on influx being the more marked

(HOLLAND, KLEIN and BRIGGS 1959). At an external concentration of 6.0 mM both fluxes were equal; below 6.0 mM efflux exceeded influx; above 6.0 mM influx was the greater. Temperature and anoxia studies indicated that at low external K^+ concentrations, the fluxes were mainly passive in nature; in media with high K^+ active transport was more evident.

Acetylcholine alters these relationships by lowering the external K^+ concentration for flux equilibrium to 4.0 to 4.5 mM. Acetylcholine increased both influx and efflux of K^+, but the effect on efflux was more or less independent of K^+ concentration, while that on influx was greatly enhanced as K^+ in the medium was increased. Atropine and, less effectively, physostigmine reversed this influence of ACh.

The concentrations of other cations in the medium also affected the K^+ fluxes. If the calcium concentrations in the media were normal, a decrease in Na^+ depressed both K^+ fluxes; if Ca^{++} was reduced, a decrease in Na^+ was without affect. HOLLAND, KLEIN and BRIGGS (1959) interpreted their findings as indicating that ACh affects only the passive movement of K^+ when the external K^+ is low, but that ACh stimulates active transport at higher external K^+ concentrations. They suggested, further, that Ca^{++} either increases passive movements of K^+ or it determines the degree of coupling between Na^+ and K^+ fluxes.

The concept of HOLLAND, DUNN and GREIG (1952) that the permeability of the auricular membrane is normally dependent upon the active hydrolysis of ACh by AChE has been elaborated in a provocative hypothesis of GOVIER, FREYBURGER, GIBBONS, HOWES and SMITS (1953). This was the suggestion that cardiac decompensation due to pentobarbital, penicillin G, physostigmine, or DFP is due to altered cell membrane integrity which, in turn, is the result of interference with the choline cycle. In the dog heart-lung preparation they showed that cardiac decompensation due to pentobarbital, physostigmine, and DFP was accompanied by a decrease in the ChE activity of the heart muscle. Ouabain reversed to a varying degree the decompensation produced by these substances and maintained or increased ChE activity. Failure due to penicillin G was poorly remediable by ouabain; penicillin can inhibit both choline acetylase and ChE. Choline in large doses also hindered or relieved the decompensation of atropinized preparations caused by these inhibitors, and it was suggested by GOVIER et al, that here choline may function as an ion, substituting for cations lost due to failure of the ChE-choline acetylase system.

The role of ions in another type of cardiac dysfunction has also been studied and should be mentioned because of the light the results shed on the mechanism of excitation of cardiac muscle. Using isolated rabbit atria, it was found that ACh-induced fibrillation was associated with an increase in both Na^+ influx (HOLLAND and BRIGGS 1959) and K^+ efflux (KLEIN and HOLLAND 1958). More Na^+ entered the tissues than K^+ was lost, and it was later found that chloride influx was also increased in this arrythmia (SEKUL and HOLLAND 1959). The K^+ efflux returned to control rates although fibrillation continued, but the increased chloride permeability remained above control levels. It was concluded that ACh-induced fibrillation resulted from a marked increase in Na^+ influx, and that this inward Na^+ movement was initially inactivated mainly as the result of K^+ leaving the tissue in exchange. It was further suggested that the increased chloride permeability may play an important role in maintaining fibrilllation.

A sudden increase (8 times normal) in the extracellular Ca^{++} concentration also induces fibrillation in isolated rabbit atria (BRIGGS and HOLLAND 1960). The Ca^{++} induced fibrillation was accompanied by increases in both K^+ efflux and chloride influx, but the K^+ movement was less and the chloride shift greater than in ACh induced fibrillation. Both types of fibrillation could be prevented by reducing the extracellular Na^+ concentration, which suggests that an increase in Na^+ movement is of prime importance in both arrythmias. In Ca^{++} induced fibrillation, however, increased chloride influx would seem to be important both in initiating and maintaining the fibrillation.

It is difficult to reconcile, at present, the views of HOLLAND and his co-workers, that anti-ChE agents reverse the effect of ACh on ion-movements across the cardiac muscle membrane, with the observations of others that the anti-ChE agents mimic or accentuate the changes in membrane potential and resistance produced by ACh. There is evidence from experiments with other tissues that, as HOLLAND et al. reported for cardiac muscle, the anti-ChE agents do reduce membrane permeability.

Using a preparation of isolated frog skin, KIRSCHNER (1953) found that TEPP and physostigmine completely inhibited the active transport of sodium ions when they were added to the inside of the skin. At the same time, the diffusion resistance (electrical D.C. resistance) increased markedly, which probably indicated that no structural damage to the skin had been produced. The inhibition of sodium transport was reversible with physostigmine but usually irreversible with TEPP. Similarly, KOCH (1953), using *Eriocheir* gills, found that the active transport of ions from the outside to the inside of the gills was inhibited by a number of anti-ChE agents, and ROTHENBERG (1950) reported that the transport of sodium in the squid axon was also decreased by anti-ChE agents. VAN DER KLOOT (1958) has studied the effect of ChE inhibitors on the resting potential and the sodium distribution of the frog's sartorius muscle. These muscles, when incubated in a Ringer's solution containing half of the normal concentration of sodium, responded by extruding sodium against the concentration gradient into the external medium. This sodium extrusion could be blocked by prior exposure of the muscle to HETP, and reversibly blocked by exposure to physostigmine. The inhibition of sodium extrusion by physostigmine was correlated with the inhibition of intracellular ChE. Neostigmine did not affect sodium extrusion, presumably because it did not penetrate into the muscle fiber to inhibit the intracellular ChE.

All the effects described above suggest that anti-ChE agents are inhibitors of sodium transport across cell membranes, but they are not in agreement with the results obtained from studies on ion transport and ChE activity using red blood cells or chicken brain. GREIG and HOLLAND (1949a) noted that physostigmine altered the fragility of dog erythrocytes, and in further studies (HOLLAND and GREIG 1950) they found that when the AChE of the erythrocyte was actively metabolizing ACh the cell remained intact for a considerable period of time. When the enzyme became inactive due to either lack of substrate (ACh) or to inhibition by physostigmine, then the cell lost its selective permeability and cations migrated to establish equilibrium with the surrounding medium. The qualitative changes observed varied with the species-type of erythrocyte. In the case of cat and dog erythrocytes, which have a high sodium and a low potassium content, the presence of ACh decreased the permeability to both sodium and potassium but had a greater effect on the permeability to potassium. Rabbit erythrocytes have a high potassium content and a low sodium content, and here ACh had the greater influence on sodium permeability. In each case physostigmine reversed the ACh effect.

Certain diazonium salts of sulfanilic acid and *p*-nitroaniline are rather potent inhibitors of ChE and they also increase the fragility of erythrocytes (HOLLAND and KLEIN 1956). The degree of hemolysis produced was more marked when the red cells were suspended in solutions of electrolytes than in non-electrolyte solutions, suggesting that the diazo compounds interfere with cation transport processes. There may not, however, be a direct causal relationship between ChE inhibition and red cell fragility. GREIG and GIBBONS (1956) have shown that 50 to 60% of the ChE of human erythrocytes can be removed by treatment with the lecithinase of snake venom without causing any great hemolysis. The active transport of potassium into and of sodium out of such venom-treated cells was impaired. In neither the experiments with the diazo compounds nor the experiments with lecithinase was there any evidence that the alteration of active transport was associated with any action on glycolysis in the cells.

In contrast with the results reported by HOLLAND and his co-workers, THOMPSON and WHITTAKER (1952) found that E 600 scarcely affected the active extrusion of sodium from the human red cell, and WAGLEY and LOWE (1956) could find no change in the mechanical fragility of human blood following marked inhibition of blood ChE by Sarin or physostigmine. VAN DER KLOOT (1958) criticised the experiments of THOMPSON and WHITTAKER on the grounds that the measurements of ChE activity were made on the extra-cellular enzyme, and concluded that in general the evidence is in favor of anti-ChE agents being able to increase the permeability of the erythrocyte membrane to cations.

There is also evidence that other membranes may show an increase in permeability under the influence of anti-ChE agents. GREIG and HOLLAND (1949b) found that physostigmine decreased the time required for the onset of convulsions produced in frogs by acid fuchsin. Physostigmine also caused procaine, which normally is not a surface anesthetic, to produce anesthesia of the rabbit's cornea (GREIG, HOLLAND and LINDVIG 1950). In addition, the administration of physostigmine to mice prior to the intravenous injection of barbital was found to reduce the anesthetic time-lag by about 50%, and this was accompanied by a measurable increase in the rate of penetration of the drug into the brain (GREIG and MAYBERRY 1950). The implication of these experiments is that physostigmine can increase the permeability of the hemoencephalic barrier and of the cornea. Is this increased permeability the result of ChE inhibition? In the latter experiment no estimations of ChE activity were made. Pertinent to this are the results of STRICKLAND and THOMPSON (1954) who studied the effects of DFP, physostigmine, and the neostigmine analogue, Nu 1250, upon the leakage of potassium from slices of chicken brain. All three anti-ChE agents were shown to increase the outflow of potassium from the slices, but the minimum concentrations required to cause potassium leakage were in every case much greater than the concentrations of inhibitors required to produce complete inhibition of AChE or BuChE activity in the brain slices. STRICKLAND and THOMPSON suggested, therefore, that the permeability of the nerve cell membrane is not dependent on ChE activity. Is increased potassium loss an indication of increased membrane permeability, and is it a measure of altered sodium transport?

The theory that membrane permeability varies with the rate of metabolism of ACh by AChE is intriguing. If true, then the ACh-AChE system must subserve a different function in different tissues. As noted, the permeability of the hemoencephalic, corneal, and erythrocyte membranes is increased by anti-ChE agents; the permeability of cardiac muscle, voluntary muscle, skin, nerve axon, and crab gill membranes is decreased by anti-ChE agents. This difference may be related to the different functions of the tissues. In those membranes concerned with maintaining osmotic or fluid balance, then an active ChE mechanism could be considered to assist this by opposing any increase in membrane permeability. In other tissues, and especially where the rapid initiation and propagation of activity is necessary, then an active ChE mechanism could be of value in maintaining a high membrane permeability. This subject is discussed further in Chapter 6.

4. Possible actions at non-esteratic sites

Low concentrations (10^{-7} M to 10^{-6} M) of most anti-ChE agents slow the rate of the contracting auricles, and this action is probably an uncomplicated anti-ChE action. This suggests that the contracting auricles form ACh, and that the formation controls the rate. Neither hexamethonium nor cocaine modifies this action, which suggests that the ACh is not of nervous origin.

BURN and his co-workers, however, have also produced evidence that all the effects of anti-ChE agents on the isolated auricle may not be due to ChE inhibition. If physostigmine is added to the bath containing contracting rabbit auricles, when the concentration reaches a point between 10^{-4} and 10^{-3} g/ml, the contractions cease (BRISCOE and BURN 1954). At this time the amount of ACh present in the auricles is not greater than that found in normal auricles. Moreover, if ACh is added to the bath, the contractions are resumed. (A further addition of ACh inhibits the contractions.) Therefore, it is unlikely that the arrest of the beat by physostigmine is caused by accumulation of ACh.

BRISCOE and BURN suggested that the arrest of the beat by physostigmine is perhaps related to a failure of conduction. Thus, quinidine and physostigmine appear to act as synergists in causing arrest of the auricles, and quinidine is known to depress conduction. Auricles arrested by physostigmine are electrically inexcitable (BURN and KOTTEGODA 1953), and physostigmine does diminish the rate of conduction in a strip of frog ventricle (ROTSCHUH and BAMMER 1952). The evidence, however, is not conclusive. Whereas BURGEN and TERROUX (1953) stated that ACh slows the rate of conduction in isolated cat auricles, VAUGHAN WILLIAMS (see BRISCOE and BURN 1954) observed that the rate of conduction in the rabbit auricle is increased by ACh.

High concentrations of neostigmine increase the rate and do not cause arrest of the beat; neostigmine does not modify the amplitude (BRISCOE and BURN 1954). Neostigmine is known to have a direct action in addition to its anti-ChE action at the neuromuscular junction (RIKER and WESCOE 1946). However, DFP, like physostigmine, depresses both rate and amplitude in high concentrations and causes arrest of the auricles (BRISCOE and BURN 1954).

Further evidence that the anti-ChE agents have other actions when they are present in high concentrations was provided by TEDESCHI (1954). When a low concentration of physostigmine (10^{-6} g/ml) was added to the bath in which isolated rabbit auricles were beating, the addition of a small amount of ACh arrested the contractions. A small amount of atropine caused them to beat again. This effect of atropine could be imitated by a high concentration of physostigmine (e.g., 4×10^{-4} g/ml), or of neostigmine, or of other anti-ChE agents (e.g., Nu 683, Nu 1250, 285.C.51). The organophosphorus ChE inhibitors (e.g., DFP, TEPP, Paraoxon, and tetramono*iso*propyl pyrophosphortetramide [Iso-OMPA]) did not have this atropine-like action.

In the rat those anti-ChE agents which penetrate the blood-brain barrier produce an increased heart rate, and it is implied that this is the result of an action on the medullary centers (DIRNHUBER and CULLUMBINE 1955).

5. Actions on the ventricles

Although it is generally accepted that the ventricles do not receive cholinergic innervation, the experiments of BENFORADO (1958) do suggest the presence of a receptor mechanism for ACh in the mammalian ventricle. In Langendorff preparations of the isolated rabbit heart, excision of the atria and severance of the atrio-ventricular bundle resulted in the onset of idio-ventricular rhythm at a rate much below the original sino-atrial rate. Acetylcholine perfusion decreased the rate still further. Physostigmine augmented this effect, while atropine prevented or abolished it. Similar results could be obtained with the rat heart.

III. Peripheral circulation
1. Systemic circulation

Hypotension is commonly seen after the administration of adequate doses of anti-ChE agents to most animal species. This could be due to a decreased cardiac output resulting from the bradycardia, to a decreased peripheral resistance, or to both.

VERBEKE and VOTAVA (1949) and VERBEKE (1949b), using HETP and TEPP, respectively, in the dog, attributed the resultant fall in blood pressure to peripheral vasodilatation. HOLMSTEDT (1951), on the other hand, reported an increased calculated total peripheral resistance following infusion of Tabun into the rabbit. PAULET (1954) concluded that the pressor action of small doses of TEPP in the dog is due to actions on sympathetic ganglia, adrenals, and medullary centers.

DALY and WRIGHT (1956) used alterations in arterial pressure in isolated, innervated dog organ preparations perfused at constant blood volume inflow, the perfusion being either from the same animal or from a donor dog, to indicate changes in peripheral vascular resistance. They reported that Sarin and TEPP invariably caused vasoconstriction in the limbs and the splanchnic area. This was due, partially at least, to an increase in sympathetic, tone, because it was reduced by nerve section or by blocking the autonomic ganglia with hexamethonium. [This increased vasoconstrictor discharge could be brought about by increased vasosensory reflexes, by central asphyxia, by a direct central action, or by an action on the sympathetic ganglia; these possibilities were fully discussed by DALY and WRIGHT (1956).] These workers also believed that the vasoconstrictive action of anti-ChE agents might be caused by an additional mechanism, namely, the liberation of a sympathomimetic substance from the adrenal glands. Such an action was first demonstrated by STEWART and ROGOFF (1921) using physostigmine in the cat.

When the vasoconstrictor mechanisms in the limb are excluded by division of the nerves to the limb and by removal of the suprarenals, a vasodilator effect of anti-ChE agents is unmasked. Thus, DALY andWRIGHT (1956) found that injection of Sarin caused vasodilatation in cross-perfusion experiments when the limb was perfused from an adrenalectomized donor. This effect must have been due to agents carried by the blood, and at least three possibilities must be considered. (1) Sarin may have a direct vasodilator action; for example, PAULET (1954) reported that small doses of TEPP injected into the femoral artery caused vasodilatation. (2) Again, Sarin, by impairing ventilation, may produce a local asphyxia which is known to cause vasodilatation (COHNHEIM 1872, ROY and BROWN 1879). (3) Perhaps, as is more likely, the effect is due to the accumulation of endogenous ACh, which also causes vasodilatation (DALE 1914).

The rat, as stated previously, appears to behave somewhat differently from other species; here, anti-ChE agents cause a rise in blood pressure (DIRNHUBER and CULLUMBINE 1955, VARAGIC 1955), which is probably due to a direct action on the vasomotor center. The pressor effect is not obtained with anti-ChE drugs containing quaternary nitrogen atoms.

The effect of anti-ChE agents on the systemic peripheral circulation is, thus, a complex one. Vasoconstriction may be produced by a variety of indirect mechanisms; vasodilatation may by caused by local actions. Uniformity of response under different experimental conditions, therefore, cannot be expected.

2. Pulmonary circulation

DALY (1957b) and DALY and WRIGHT (1957) have also studied the effects of Sarin and TEPP on the pulmonary circulation in the dog, and reported the production of an increased pulmonary vascular resistance. They concluded that this increased resistance is due in part to constriction of the pulmonary vascular bed proper. This constriction is probably largely caused by changes in alveolar gas tensions occurring in anti-ChE poisoning, and possibly also by nervous effects peripheral to the intrapulmonary ganglia.

E. Discussion

The anti-ChE agents have proved to be wonderful research tools for studying cholinergic phenomena in biological systems. By their use, some light has been thrown on the physiological roles of the various esterases, on the sites of origin and the metabolism of ACh, and on the physiological importance of cholinergic mechanisms in different tissues and in the whole organism.

I. Quantitative aspects of cholinesterase (ChE) inhibition

There is strong evidence that many tissues contain a great excess of ChE's, and that most of this has to be inhibited before effects are produced (GUNTER and MENDEL 1945, MAZUR and BODANSKY 1946, KOELLE and GILMAN 1946a, HAWKINS and MENDEL 1947, NACHMANSOHN and FELD 1947, HAWKINS and GUNTER 1949, HAWKINS and MENDEL 1949, RIKER and WESCOE 1949). More recent work suggests that this may not always be true, at least in some tissues.

SHELLEY (1955) found an increase in tone of the rabbit gut with doses of physostigmine or DFP sufficient to produce only 10 to 20% inhibition of AChE activity, although with the former drug quantitation of ChE inhibition is uncertain (see below), and with the latter considerably greater inhibition of BuChE occurs concomitantly (KOELLE et al. 1950). ADMIRAAL et al. (1955) gave the following relationship between ChE inhibition and pharmacological effect: 25% inhibition — increased motility of the longitudinal muscles; 40% inhibition — increased motility of the circular muscles; 80% inhibition — peristalsis appears.

BURN and KOTTEGODA (1953) observed changes in the rate and amplitude of beat of isolated rabbit auricles in the presence of a concentration of physostigmine sufficient to produce not more than 16% inhibition of ACh hydrolysis by auricle homogenates *in vitro*. DIRNHUBER and LOVATT EVANS (1954) reported that at least 60% of the AChE of the submaxillary gland must be inhibited in order to obtain a spontaneous flow of saliva, but their records of individual experiments indicate that with only half this degree of inhibition, potentiation of the effects of ACh or of chorda stimulation can be obtained.

As SHELLEY (1955) has indicated, one of the difficulties of attempting to correlate ChE inhibition with tissue response is that with a reversible inhibitor, such as physostigmine, the inhibition of ChE in the intact tissue is probably greater than that measured with homogenates. The difficulty of obtaining direct evidence of the degree of inhibition produced by reversible inhibitors *in vivo* has resulted in some of the cholinemimetic responses produced by such agents being attributed to a direct action at cholinoceptive effector sites (RANDELL and LEHMANN 1950, WESCOE et al. 1950). KOELLE (1957) has discussed this aspect of reversible anti-ChE action. The neuronal membrane probably separates the total AChE into external, functional enzyme, which is probably directly concerned with the hydrolysis of ACh involved in cholinergic transmission, and internal, reserve AChE, which may represent the more recently synthesized enzyme. The ease of penetration of membranes, the dose, the rate of administration and the absorption of the agent could all affect the relative proportions of functional or reserve enzyme inhibited. Therefore, and also because partial reversal of inhibition occurs on dilution of a reversible inhibitor-enzyme complex (STRAUSS and GOLDSTEIN 1943), the percentage inactivation of total AChE, as measured by the usual homogenate techniques, may be a poor indication of the actual inactivation of functional AChE (see Chapter 6 for further discussion).

SHELLEY (1955) has suggested that in those tissues with a low ChE activity and a high ACh content, such as the rabbit duodenum and the rabbit auricle, signs of ACh accumulation would appear with a relatively slight degree of ChE inhibition. In other words, the degree of inhibition of ChE needed to produce a response from a given tissue may be dependent on the relative dominance of the ACh-production mechanism or the ACh-destruction mechanism. We have seen that in at least three tissues, the heart, the gut and the salivary glands, the experimental results of some workers do suggest that there is a constant production of ACh which may not be neurogenic in origin (see further discussion of "local hormonal" role of ACh in Chapter 6). In two of these three tissues there is further evidence that BuChE may play an important role.

II. General role of butyrocholinesterase (BuChE)

The generally accepted view is that it is only the AChE which has the established physiological function of promoting the hydrolysis of endogenous ACh. The results described above indicate that this may not always be true at autonomic effector sites.

The work of BURN et al. suggests that BuChE may be the important enzyme in controlling the ACh level of atrial tissue. BÜLBRING and BURN (1949) have suggested that the rate and force of beat of the auricles is dependent upon the local formation of ACh. The evidence presented by BRISCOE and BURN (1954) would indicate a myogenic origin of this ACh; if so, the BuChE would act here as a general tissue enzyme to prevent excessive accumulation of ACh at the pacemaker, with consequent disturbance of the auricular rhythm.

Similarly, the results of KOELLE et al. (1950) and of BURN et al. (1952) suggest that BuChE controls the ACh level, and thereby the tone of the small intestine. Here too, as in the auricles, ACh is constantly being set free, all of which may not be nervous in origin (FELDBERG and LIN 1949). The work of SHELLEY (1955) does suggest that AChE is at least as important as BuChE in the rabbit intestine. Probably both enzymes have an essential role in this tissue. The richness of the innervation *via* AUERBACH's plexus would lead one to expect that AChE should be important, although it must be remembered that this plexus has a high content of both AChE and BuChE.

DIRNHUBER and LOVATT EVANS (1954) believe that AChE is the important enzyme in the submaxillary gland, with the BuChE having a "general mopping-up function of a subsidiary kind." They considered that the necessity for the latter is occasioned by the salivary glands', like the intestine and the auricles, being sites of constant production of ACh, and consequently there must be a mechanism for preventing ACh concentrations from passing a certain limit.

It could be suggested that in the heart, the gut and the salivary glands, a degree of "alertness," or basic functional level, is maintained by a constant production of non-neurogenic ACh, the degree of "alertness," or the level of ACh accumulation, being controlled by the activity of BuChE. Variations from the basic functional level of a tissue could normally be initiated by the liberation of neurogenic

ACh, the accumulation of which would be controlled by AChE. Whether this could be generally true in all tissues with an autonomic effector innervation is not known.

Literature

ADMIRAAL, J., D. K. MYERS and J. C. VAN HOUTEN: Effect of inhibition of cholinesterase on the motility of the small intestine. Nature (Lond.) 176, 468—469 (1955).

ADRIAN, E. D., W. FELDBERG and B. A. KILBY: The cholinesterase inhibiting action of fluorophosphonates. Brit. J. Pharmacol. 2, 56—58 (1947).

BABKIN, B. P.: Secretory Mechanisms of the Digestive Glands. New York: P. B. Hoeber 1950.

BACQ, Z. M.: Action du D.F.P. (duodopropyl-fluorophosphonate) sur le rectus isolé d'mphibien et l'intestin isolé de Mammifère. C. R. Soc. Biol. (Paris) 141, 857—859 (1947).

BATTELLI, F.: Action de diverses substances des mouvements de l'estomac. Arch. ital. biol. 27, 263 (1897).

BENFORADO, J. M.: A depressant effect of acetylcholine on the idioventricular pacemaker of the isolated perfused rabbit heart. Brit. J. Pharmacol. 13, 415—418 (1958).

BEZNAK, A. v.: Die autacoide Aktivität des venösen Blutes von sezernierenden Submaxillardrüsen. Pflügers Arch. ges. Physiol. 229, 719—729 (1932).

BRIGGS, A. H., and W. C. HOLLAND: K^{42} and Cl^{36} fluxes during ACh- and Ca-induced atrial fibrillation. Amer. J. Physiol. 198, 838—840 (1960).

BRISCOE, S., and J. H. BURN: Quinidine and anticholinesterases on rabbit auricles. Brit. J. Pharmacol. 9, 42—48 (1954).

BRUNAUD, M., and M. DUSSARDIER: Studies on the chemical mediator of the vagus nerve of ruminants. J. Physiol. (Lond.) 43, 281—302 (1951) (French).

BÜLBRING, E., and J. H. BURN: Action of acetylcholine on rabbit auricle in relation to acetylcholine synthesis. J. Physiol. (Lond.) 108, 508—524 (1949).

— — and H. SHELLEY: Acetylcholine and ciliary movement in the gill plates of Mytilus edulis. Proc. roy Soc., Ser B 141, 445—466 (1953).

—, S. R. KOTTEGODA and H. SHELLEY: Cholinesterase activity in the auricles of the rabbit's heart and their sensitivity to escrine. J. Physiol. (Lond.) 123, 204—213 (1954).

BURGEN, A. S. V., and K. G. TERROUX: On the negative inotropic effect in the cat's auricle. J. Physiol. (Lond.) 120, 449—464 (1953).

BURN, J. H.: Functions of Automatic Transmitters. p. 62. Baltimore: Williams and Wilkins 1956.

—, P. KORDEK and R. H. MOLE: The effect of x-ray irradiations on the response of the intestine to acetylcholine and on its content of "pseudo"-cholinesterase. Brit. J. Pharmacol. 7, 58—66 (1952).

—, and S. R. KOTTEGODA: Action of eserine on the auricles of the rabbit heart. J. Physiol. (Lond.) 121, 360—373 (1953).

—, and J. M. WALKER: Anticholinesterases in the heart-lung preparation. J. Physiol. (Lond.) 124, 489—501 (1954).

CHANG, H. C., and J. H. GADDUM: Choline esters in tissue extract. J. Physiol. (Lond.) 79, 255—285 (1933).

COHNHEIM, J.: Untersuchungen über die embolischen Prozesse. Berlin: Hirschwald 1872.

CULLUMBINE, H., and P. DIRNHUBER: Oral and bronchial fluids in poisoning with anticholinesterases. J. Pharm. (Lond.) 7, 580—585 (1955).

DALE, H. H.: The action of certain esters and ethers of choline and their relation to muscarine. J. Pharmacol. exp. Ther. 6, 147—190 (1914).

DAYRIT, C., C. H. MANRY and M. H. SEEVERS: On the pharmacology of hexaethyl tetraphosphate. J. Pharmacol. exp. Ther. 92, 173—186 (1948).

DE BURGH, DALY M.: The effects of anticholinesterases on the bronchioles and pulmonary blood vessels in isolated perfused lungs of the dog. Brit. J. Pharmacol. 12, 504—512 (1957b).

— The cardiovascular effects of anticholinesterases in the dog with special reference to haemodynamic changes in the pulmonary circulation. J. Physiol. (Lond.) 139, 250—272 (1957a).

—, and P. G. WRIGHT: The effects of anticholinesterases upon peripheral vascular resistance in the dog. J. Physiol. (Lond.) 133, 475—497 (1956).

DE CANDOLE, C. A., W. W. DOUGLAS, C. LOVATT EVANS, R. HOLMES, K. E. V. SPENCER, R. W. TORRANCE and K. M. WILSON: The failure of respiration in death by anticholinesterase poisoning. Brit. J. Pharmacol. 8, 466—475 (1953).

DELGA, J.: Les anticholinestérasiques organophosphorés. J. Pharm. Chim. (Paris) 10, 47—87 (1957).

DIRNHUBER, P., and H. CULLUMBINE: The effect of anti-cholinesterase agents on the rat's blood pressure. Brit. J. Pharmacol. 10, 12—15 (1955).
—, and C. LOVATT EVANS: The effects of anticholinesterases on humoral transmission in the submaxillary gland. Brit. J. Pharmacol. 9, 441—458 (1954).
DIXON, W. E., and T. G. BRODIE: Contributions to the physiology of the lungs. Part I. The bronchial muscles, their innervation, and the action of drugs upcn them. J. Physiol. (Lond.) 29, 97—173 (1903).
DIXON, W. E., and F. RANSOM: Physostigmin. Heffter's Handbuch 2, 786—812 (1924).
DUSSARDIER, M.: In vivo actions of acetylcholine and adrenaline on gastric motility in ruminants. J. Physiol. (Lond.) 46, 777—797 (1954) (French).
EICKSTEDT, K. W. v., W. D. ERDMANN u. K. P. SCHAEFER: Über die blutdrucksteigernde Wirkung von Esteraseblockern (E 605, Eserin und Prostigmin). Naunyn-Schmiedeberg's Arch. exp. Path. Pharmak. 226, 435—441 (1955).
EMMELIN, N., and A. MUREN: Acetylcholine release at parasympathetic synapses. Acta physiol. scand. 20, 13—32 (1950a).
— — "Paralytic" secretion of saliva. Acta physiol. scand. 21, 362—379 (1950b).
— — and R. STRÖMBLAD: Secretory and vascular effects of various drugs injected into the submaxillary duct. Acta physiol. scand. 32, 325—338 (1954).
—, and B. C. R. STRÖMBLAD: Sensitization of the submaxillary gland above the level reached after section of the chorda tympani. Acta physiol. scand. 38, 319—330 (1957).
— — The effect of anticholinesterases on the parotid gland after parasympathetic decentralization or denervation. Brit. J. Pharmacol. 13, 193—196 (1958a).
— — "Paroxysmal" secretion of saliva following parasympathetic denervation of parotid gland. J. Physiol. (Lond.) 143, 506—514 (1958b).
ERDMANN, W. D., u. D. HEYE: Analyse der erregenden und lahmenden Wirkung von Alkylphosphaten (Parathion, Paraoxon, Systox) am isolierten Kaninchendarm. Naunyn-Schmiedeberg's Arch. exp. Path. Pharmak. 232, 507—521 (1958).
—, u. L. LENDLE: Vergiftungen mit esteraseblockierenden Insecticiden aus der Gruppe der organischen Phosphorsäure-Ester (E 605 und Verwandte). Ergebn. inn. Med. Kinderheilk. 10, 104—184 (1958).
ESVELD, L. W. v.: Verhalten von plexushaltigen und plexusfreien Darmmuskelpräparaten. Naunyn-Schmiedeberg's Arch. exp. Path. Pharmak. 134, 347—386 (1928).
EVANS, C. LOVATT: Neuromuscular block by anticholinesterases. J. Physiol. (Lond.) 114, 6 P (1951).
—, and D. F. G. SMITH: Sweating responses in the horse. Proc. roy. Soc. Edinb. 145, 61—63 (1956).
FELDBERG, W., and J. A. GUIMARAIS: Some observations on salivary secretion. J. Physiol. (Lond.) 85, 15—36 (1935).
—, and R. C. Y. LIN: Acetylcholine release and synthesis in the wall of the small intestine. J. Physiol. (Lond.) 109, 32 P (1949).
—, and O. M. SOLANDT: The effects of drugs, sugars and allied substances on the isolated small intestine of the rabbit. J. Physiol. (Lond.) 101, 137—171 (1942).
GASSER, H. S.: Plexus-free preparations of the small intestine. A study of their rhythmicity and of their response to drugs. J. Pharmacol. exp. Ther. 27, 395—410 (1926).
GIBBS, O. S., u. J. SZELÖCZEY: Die humorale Übertragung der Chorda Tympani-Reizung. Naunyn-Schmiedeberg's Arch. exp. Path. Pharmak. 168, 64—88 (1932).
GLAESSER, A., and R. E. TEDESCHI: Action of anticholinesterases on isolated auricles driven electrically. Arch. int. Pharmacodyn. 101, 200—204 (1955).
GOTTLIEB, R.: Beiträge zur Physiologie und Pharmakologie der Pankreassecretion. Naunyn-Schmiedeberg's Arch. exp. Path. Pharmak. 33, 261—285 (1894).
GREIG, M. E., and A. J. GIBBONS: Cation transport in erythrocytes treated with lecithinase A. Arch. Biochem. 61, 343—347 (1956).
—, and W. C. HOLLAND: Increased permaability of the hemoencephalic barrier produced by physostigmine and acetylcholine. Science 110, 237 (1949b).
— — The relationship between cholinesterase activity and permeability of dog erythrocytes. Arch. Biochem. 23, 370—384 (1949a).
— — and P. E. LINDVIG: The anesthetization of the rabbit's cornea by non-surface anesthetics. Brit. J. Pharmacol. 5, 461—464 (1950).
—, and T. C. MAYBERRY: The relationship between cholinesterase activity and brain permeability. J. Pharmacol. exp. Ther. 102, 1—4 (1951).
GROB, D., J. L. LILIENTHAL jr., A. M. HARVEY and B. F. JONES: The administration of di-isopropyl fluorophosphate (DFP) to man. Johns Hopk. Hosp. Bull. 81, 217—244 (1947).
GUNTER, C., and C. R. ALLEN: Acetylcholine: its significance in controlling ciliary activity of human respiratory epithelium in vitro. J. appl. Physiol. 14, 901—904 (1959).

GUNTER, J. M., and B. MENDEL: The inhibition of cholinesterase in vivo. Canad. Chem. Proc. 29, 136 (1945).

HARNACK, E., u. L. WITKOWSKI: Pharmakologische Untersuchungen über das Physostigmin und Calabarin. Naunyn-Schmiedeberg's Arch. exp. Path. Pharmak. 5, 401—454 (1876).

HAWKINS, D. F., and H. O. SCHILD: The action of drugs on isolated human bronchial chains. Brit. J. Pharmacol. 6, 682—690 (1951).

HAWKINS, R. D., and J. M. GUNTER: Studies on cholinesterase. 5. The selective inhibition of pseudo-cholinesterase in vivo. Biochem. J. 40, 192—197 (1946).

—, and B. MENDEL: Selective inhibition of pseudo-cholinesterase by di-isopropyl fluorophosphonate. Brit. J. Pharmacol. 2, 173—180 (1947).

— — Studies on cholinesterase. 6. The selective inhibition of true cholinesterase in vivo. Biochem. J. 44, 260—264 (1949).

HEATHCOTE, R. ST. A.: The action of physostigmine with special reference to the circulatory system and the intestine. J. Pharmacol. exp. Ther. 44, 95—108 (1932).

HEIDENHAIN, R.: Über die Wirkung einiger Gifte auf die Nerven der glandula submaxillaris. Pflügers Arch. ges. Physiol. 5, 309—318 (1872).

HENDERSON, V. E., u. M. H. ROEPKE: Über den lokalen hormonalen Mechanismus der Parasympathikusreizung. Naunyn-Schmiedeberg's Arch. exp. Path. Pharmak. 172, 314—324 (1933).

HEYMANS, C.: Les antidotes du di-isopropylfluorophosphonate (DFP). Arch. int. Pharmacodyn. 81, 230—234 (1950).

— Les substances anticholinéstérasiques. Expos. ann. Biochim. méd. 12, 21—53 (1951).

—, and J. JACOB: Sur la pharmacologie du di-isopropyl-fluorophosphonate (DFP) et le rôle des cholinestérases. Arch. int. Pharmacodyn. 74, 233—252 (1947).

—, A. POCHET and H. VAN HOUTTE: Contributions à la pharmacologie du sarin et du tabun. Arch. int. Pharmacodyn. 104, 293—332 (1956).

HOKIN, M. R., and L. E. HOKIN: Enzyme secretion and the incorporation of P^{32} into phospholipides of pancreas slices. J. biol. Chem. 203, 967—977 (1953).

— — Effects of acetylcholine on phospholipides in the pancreas. J. biol. Chem. 209, 549 to 558 (1954a).

— — Ribonucleic acid content of pancreas and parotid glands during enzyme synthesis and secretion. Biochim. biophys. Acta 13, 236—240 (1954b).

— — The incorporation of ^{32}P into the nucleotides of ribonucleic acid in pancreas slices during enzyme synthesis and secretion. Biochim. biophys. Acta 13, 401—412 (1954c).

— — Studies of pancreatic tissue in vitro. Gastroenterology 36, 368—376 (1959).

— — The role of phosphatidic acid and phosphoinositide in transmembrane transport elicited by acetylcholine and other humoral agents. Int. Rev. Neurobiology 2, 99—136 (1960).

— — and W. D. SHELP: The effects of acetylcholine on the turnover of phosphatidic acid and phosphoinositide in sympathetic ganglia, and in various parts of the central nervous system in vitro. J. gen. Physiol. 44, 217—226 (1960).

HOLLAND, W. C., and A. H. BRIGGS: Fibrillation and potassium influx. Science 129, 212 (1959).

—, C. E. DUNN and M. E. GREIG: Studies on permeability VII.: The effect of several substrates and inhibitors of acetyl cholinesterase on permeability of isolated auricles to Na and K. Amer. J. Physiol. 168, 546—556 (1952).

—, and M. E. GREIG: Studies on the permeability of erythrocytes. III. The effect of physostigmine and acetylcholine on the permeability of dog, cat and rabbit erythrocytes to sodium and potassium. Amer. J. Physiol. 162, 610—615 (1950).

—, and R. L. KLEIN: Effects of diazonium salts on erythrocyte fragility and cholinesterase activity. Amer. J. Physiol. 187, 501 504 (1956).

— — and A. H. BRIGGS: Factors affecting action of acetylcholine on transmembrane flux of K in isolated rabbit atria. Amer. J. Physiol. 196, 478—482 (1959).

HOLMES, R. L.: Cholinesterase activity in atrial wall of dog and cat heart. J. Physiol. (Lond.) 137, 421—426 (1957).

HOLMSTEDT, B.: Synthesis and pharmacology of dimethylamido-ethoxy-phosphoryl cyanide (Tabun) together with a description of some allied anticholinesterase compounds containing the N-P bond. Acta physiol. scand. 25, 1—120, Suppl. 90 (1951).

HUGHES, F. BARBARA: Muscularis mucosae of oesophagus of cat, rabbit and rat. J. Physiol. (Lond.) 130, 123—130 (1955).

JACOBI, C.: Beiträge zur physiologischen und pharmakologischen Kenntnis der Darmbewegungen mit besonderer Berücksichtigung der Beziehung der Nebenniere zur denselben. Naunyn-Schmiedeberg's Arch. exp. Path. Pharmak. 29, 171—211 (1891).

JOHNSON, R. P., A. J. GOLD and G. FREEMAN: Comparative lung-airway resistance and cardiovascular effects in dogs and monkeys following parathion and sarin intoxication. Amer. J. Physiol. 192, 581—584 (1958).

KATSH, S.: Inhibition of isolated auricles by anticholinesterases and reactivation with atropine and epinephrine. Amer. J. Physiol. **188**, 538—542 (1957).

KIRSCHNER, L. B.: Effect of cholinesterase inhibitors and atropine on active sodium transport across frog skin. Nature (Lond.) **172**, 348—349 (1953).

KLEIN, R. L., and W. C. HOLLAND: Na^{24} and K^{42} exchange in atrial fibrillation. Amer. J. Physiol. **193**, 239—243 (1958).

KOCH, H. J.: Cholinesterase and active transport of sodium chloride through the isolated gills of the crab *Eriocheir Sinensis* (M. Edw.), Colston Papers **6**, 15 (1953).

KOELLE, G. B.: Cholinesterases of the tissues and sera of rabbits. Biochem. J. **53**, 217—226 (1953).

— Histochemical demonstration of reversible anticholinesterase action at selective cellular sites *in vivo*. J. Pharmacol. exp. Ther. **120**, 488—503 (1957).

—, and A. GILMAN: Anticholinesterase drugs. J. Pharmacol. exp. Ther. **95** (Part II, Pharmacol. Rev.), 166—216 (1949).

— — The relationship between cholinesterase inhibition and the pharmacological action of of di-isopropyl fluorophosphate (DFP). J. Pharmacol. exp. Ther. **87**, 421—434 (1946a).

—, E. S. KOELLE and J. S. FRIEDENWALD: The effect of inhibition of specific and nonspecific cholinesterase on the motility of the isolated ileum. J. Pharmacol. exp. Ther. **100**, 180—191 (1950).

KOPPANYI, T., A. G. KRACZMAR and T. O. KING: Effect of tetraethyl pyrophosphate on sympathetic ganglionic activity. Science **106**, 492—493 (1947).

KORDIK, P., E. BÜLBRING and J. H. BURN: Ciliary movement and acetylcholine. Brit. J. Pharmacol. **7**, 67—79 (1952).

KROP, S., and A. M. KUNKEL: Observations on the pharmacology of the anticholinesterases sarin and tabun. Proc. Soc. exp. Biol. (N. Y.) **86**, 530—533 (1954).

LANGLEY, J. N.: On the physiology of the salivary secretion. Part V. The effect of stimulating the cerebral secretory nerves upon the amount of saliva obtained by stimulating the sympathetic nerve. J. Physiol. (Lond.) **10**, 291—328 (1889).

MACINTOSH, F. C.: Choline-esterase content of normal and denervated submaxillary gland of the cat. Proc. Soc. exp. Biol. (N. Y.) **37**, 248—251 (1937).

MARSHALL, J. M., and S. KATSH: Inhibition by anticholinesterases of the electrical and mechanical activity of isolated rabbit auricles *in vitro*. Amer. J. Physiol. **190**, 495—499 (1957).

—, and E. M. VAUGHAN WILLIAMS: Pacemaker potentials. The excitation of isolated rabbit auricles by acetylcholine at low temperatures. J. Physiol. (Lond.) **131**, 186—199 (1956).

MAZUR, A., and O. BODANSKY: The mechanism of *in vitro* and *in vivo* inhibition of cholinesterase activity by di-isopropyl fluorophosphate. J. biol. Chem. **163**, 261—276 (1946).

MODELL, W., S. KROP, P. HITCHCOCK and W. F. RIKER: General systemic actions of di-isopropyl fluorophosphate (DFP) in cats. J. Pharmacol. exp. Ther. **87**, 400—413 (1916).

NACHMANSOHN, D., and E. A. FELD: Studies on cholinesterase. IV. On the mechanism of di-isopropyl fluorophosphate action *in vivo*. J. biol. Chem. **171**, 715—724 (1947).

PAULET, G.: Nouvelle contribution à l'étude de l'action pharmacologique du tetraethyl pyrophosphate (TEPP). Arch. int. Pharmacodyn. **98**, 157—185 (1954).

PEWSNER, M.: Der Einfluß des Physostigmins, Dionins and Euphthalmins auf die Magensaftbildung. Biochem. Z. **2**, 339—349 (1906).

RANDALL, L. O., and G. LEHMANN: Pharmacological properties of some neostigmine analogs. J. Pharmacol. exp. Ther. **99**, 16—32 (1950).

RIKER, W. F., and W. C. WESCOE: The relationship between cholinesterase inhibition and function in a neuroeffector system. J. Pharmacol. exp. Ther. **95**, 515—527 (1949).

ROTHENBERG, M. A.: Studies on permeability in relation to nerve function. II. Ionic movements across axonal membranes. Biochim. biophys. Acta **4**, 96—114 (1950).

ROTHSCHUH, K. E., u. H. BAMMER: Über positiv dromotrope Wirkungen von Acetylcholin am Froschherzstreifen. Z. ges. exp. Med. **119**, 327—337 (1952).

ROY, C. S., and J. G. BROWN: The blood pressure and its variations in the anterioles, capillaries and smaller veins. J. Physiol. (Lond.) **2**, 323—359 (1879).

RUBIN, L. S., and M. N. GOLDBERG: Effect of sarin on dark adaptation in man: threshold changes. J. appl. Physiol. **11**, 439—444 (1957).

— — Effect of tertiary and quaternary atropine salts on absolute scotopic threshold changes produced by an anticholinesterase (Sarin). J. appl. Physiol. **12**, 305—310 (1958).

—, S. KROP and M. N GOLDBERG: Effect of sarin on dark adaptation in man: Mechanism of action. J. appl. Physiol. **11**, 445—449 (1957).

SANDERSON, D. M.: Assessment of direct cholinesterase inhibitory activity by pupillary niosis. J. Pharm. (Lond.) **9**, 600—604 (1957).

SCHUCHER, R., and L. H. HOKIN: The synthesis and secretion of lipase and ribonuclease by pigeon pancreas slices. J. biol. Chem. **210**, 551—557 (1954).

SCHÜTZ, E.: Über die Einwirkung von Arzneistoffen auf die Magenbewegungen. Naunyn-Schmiedeberg's Arch. exp. Path. Pharmak. 21, 341—372 (1886).
SCOTT, MARY J.: Effects of anticholinesterases on the spleen of the dog. J. Physiol. (Lond.) 139, 489—496 (1957).
SECKER, J.: The humoral control of the secretion by the submaxillary gland of the cat following sympathetic stimulation. J. Physiol. (Lond.) 82, 293—304 (1934).
SEKUL, A. A., and W. C. HOLLAND: Cl^{36} and Ca^{45} exchange atrial fibrillation. Amer. J. Physiol. 197, 752—756 (1959).
SHELLEY, H.: A correlation between cholinesterase inhibition and increase in muscle tone in rabbit duodenum. Brit. J. Pharmacol. 10, 26—35 (1955).
STEWART, G. N., and J. M. ROGOFF: The action of drugs upon the output of epinephrin from the adrenals. VII. Physostigmine. J. Pharmacol. exp. Ther. 17, 227—248 (1921).
STRAUS, O. H., and A. GOLDSTEIN: Zone behavior of enzymes. Illustrated by the effect of dissociation constant and dilution on the system cholinesterase-physostigmine. J. gen. Physiol. 26, 559—585 (1943).
STRICKLAND, K. P., and R. H. S. THOMPSON: The effect of cholinesterase inhibitors on the leakage of potassium from brain slices. Biochem. J. 58, XX (1954).
STRÖMBLAD, B. C. R.: Supersensitivity caused by denervation and by cholinesterase inhibitors. Acta physiol. scand. 41, 118—138 (1957).
STRÖMBLAD, R.: Acetylcholine inactivation and acetylcholine sensitivity in denervated salivary glands. Acta physiol. scand. 34, 38—58 (1955).
SUBBOTIN, V.: Über die Anwendung des Extr. semin. physostigmatis venenosi beim atonischen Zustande des Darmkanals. Arch. Pat. Clin. med. 6, 285—288 (1869).
TEDESCHI, R. E.: Atropine-like activity of some anticholinesterases on the rabbit atria. Brit. J. Pharmacol. 9, 367—369 (1954).
THOMPSON, E. H., and V. P. WHITTAKER: Cholinesterase activity and sodium transport in the human red cell. Biochim. biophys. Acta 9, 700—701 (1952).
TRAUTWEIN, W., u. J. DUDEL: Mechanism of action of acetylcholine on heart muscle. Pflügers Arch. ges. Physiol. 266, 324—334 (1958) (German).
—, S. W. KUFFLER and C. EDWARDS: Changes in membrane characteristics of heart muscle during inhibition. J. gen. Physiol. 40, 135—145 (1956).
TRENDELENBURG, P.: Physiologische und pharmakologische Untersuchungen an der isolierten Bronchialmuskulatur. Naunyn-Schmiedeberg's Arch. exp. Path. Pharmak. 69, 79—107 (1912).
UNGER, M.: Beiträge zur Kenntnis der Wirkungsweise des Atropins und Physostigmins auf auf den Dünndarm von Katzen. Pflügers Arch. ges. Physiol. 119, 373—403 (1907).
UPHOLT, W. M., G. E. QUINBY, G. S. BATCHELOR and J. P. THOMPSON: Visual effects accompanying TEPP-induced miosis. Arch. Ophthal. (Chicago) 56, 128—134 (1956).
UVNÄS, B.: The effect of atropine, acetylcholine, eserine and di-isopropylfluorophosphate on the gastric secretion of the cat. Acta physiol. scand. 15, 427—437 (1948).
VAN DER KLOOT, W. G.: The effect of enzyme inhibitors on the resting potential and on the ion distribution of the sartorius muscle of the frog. J. gen. Physiol. 41, 879—900 (1958).
VARAGIC, V.: The action of eserine on the blood pressure of the rat. Brit. J. Pharmacol. 10, 349—353 (1955).
VERBEKE, R.: Nouvelles contributions à la pharmacologie du di-isopropylfluorophosphonate (DFP). Arch. int. Pharmacodyn 79, 1—31 (1949a).
— De l'action pharmacologie du tetraethylpyrophosphate (TEPP). Arch. int. Pharmacodyn. 80, 19—27 (1949b).
—, and Z. VOTAVA: Contribution à la pharmacologie du hexaéthyltetraphosphate (HETP). Arch. int. Pharmacodyn. 79, 367—380 (1949).
WAGLEY, P. F., and H. J. LOWE: Observations on mechanical fragility of human erythrocytes. I. Effect of cholinesterase inhibition. Bull. Johns Hopk. Hosp. 99, 87—90 (1956).
WEBB, J. L., and P. B. HOLLANDER: Action of acetylcholine and adrenaline on the cellular membrane potentials and contractility of rat atrium. Circulat. Res. 4, 332—336 (1956).
WEIDMANN, S.: The effect of the cardiac membrane potential on the rapid availability of the sodium-carrying system. J. Physiol. (Lond.) 127, 213—224 (1955).
WESCOE, W. C., W. F. RIKER and V. L. BEACH: Studies on the inter-relationships of certain cholinergic compounds. III. The reactions between 3-acetoxy phenyltrimethyl ammonium methylsulfate, 3-hydroxy phenylmethyltanium bromide and cholinesterase. J. Pharmacol. exp. Ther. 99, 265—276 (1950).
WILLS, J. H.: Electrolyte changes in submaxillary glands during stimulation. Amer. J. Physiol. 135, 164—174 (1941).

Chapter 12

Actions at Autonomic Ganglia

By

Eleanor Zaimis

With 13 Figures

Contents

Introduction

For the maintenance of smooth function at the periphery, the co-ordination which takes place at the various levels of the central nervous system as well as the processes that go on in the autonomic ganglia appear to be of the utmost importance. Because of this, the relation of pre- and postganglionic fibers is very critical, and the ganglionic synapse is provided with elaborate mechanisms for the regulation of its activity.

For many years, during which both the electrical and chemical theories of synaptic transmission had their staunch supporters, the mechanism of transmission across the ganglionic synapse was a matter of controversy. To-day, however, as a result of an impressive amount of data, it is almost generally accepted that transmission at this site is chemical and that the transmitter substance is acetylcholine (ACh). Many substances have been proposed as chemical transmitters at various sites but none has been so firmly established, or has had the enzymatic systems involved in its synthesis and destruction so fully character- ized, as has ACh. During this work a great amount of fundamental information about the transmission processes was made possible only because of anticholin- esterase (anti-ChE) drugs. In return, the phenomena of chemical transmission have helped to clarify understanding of the actions of these drugs and to guide the search for new ones.

A survey of the literature, however, makes it clear that there are still many important gaps in our knowledge of both the various physiological functions taking place at the ganglionic synapse and the pharmacology of the anti-ChE drugs. Of the two, the pharmacology of the anti-ChE drugs suffers from the disadvantage that there have been only a few studies directly concerned with the problem. Most of the information is indirect and comes from their use as experimental tools in the analysis of physiological events at the ganglionic synapse.

The space devoted to each section and the choice of the papers to be discussed have been dictated by the amount of pertinent information, which it is hoped will bring out not only what knowledge is available at present, but also the weaknesses and the aspects on which more work is required.

Additional information may be obtained from reviews by KOELLE and GILMAN (1949), HEYMANS (1951), MITCHELL (1953), PATON (1954), PERRY (1956), PERRY (1957), PATON (1958), HOLMSTEDT (1959), and CAUSEY (1960).

A. Anatomical considerations

The sympathetic and parasympathetic ganglia of the autonomic nervous system are peripheral structures which contain synapses between preganglionic and postganglionic neurons. Most parasympathetic ganglion cells are either scattered diffusely throughout the effector tissues or congregated in anatomically recognisable ganglia close to the structures they innervate, whereas the sym- pathetic ganglia are larger and, as a rule, situated at some distance from the effector organs. *Postganglionic* sympathetic neurons, however, can be found at numerous places along the sympathetic chains and the rami communicantes, splanchnic nerves, and plexuses.

In contrast to the parasympathetic, the sympathetic preganglionic neuron effects con- nections with more than one ganglion cell. BILLINGSLEY and RANSON (1918) found in cats that the superior cervical sympathetic ganglion contains on an average 120,000 cells, whereas the preganglionic trunk possesses about 3,800 myelinated nerve fibers, giving a ratio of approximately 1 preganglionic fibre to 32 ganglion cells. WOLF (1941) reinvestigated the prob- lem and estimated that the ratio in the superior cervical sympathetic ganglion varied between 1:1 and 1:17, whereas in the ciliary (parasympathetic) ganglion the ratio between pre- ganglionic and postganglionic cells was only 1:2. MITCHELL (1953), however, in his excellent account of the anatomy of the autonomic nervous system, pointed out that a direct comparison of histological counts gives no indication of what may be called the "physiological divergence" between preganglionic and postganglionic elements, and furthermore, that it would be a mistake to generalise from the particular samples that the disparity between sympathetic and parasympathetic ratios is always in the same proportion.

Such a preganglionic-postganglionic relationship has been considered functionally equiva- lent to a nerve-branching of the preganglionic fiber. This is, however, an incorrect view because all the available evidence strongly suggests that a ganglion is not only a transmitting and distributing but also a co-ordinating centre. While a preganglionic neuron makes con- nections with several ganglion cells, the latter receive branches from a number of different preganglionic fibers. This overlapping distribution of pre- and postsynaptic elements, together with the fact that the component parts of the individual neuron have different properties, empowers the ganglion to modulate the fluctuating patterns of nervous activity while *en route* from the central nervous system to the peripheral effector cells.

The *preganglionic* neurons, some of which, according to DE CASTRO (1932), end as small loops *("boutons")*, are myelinated, but as they approach their terminations they lose the myelin sheath and the Schwann cells become spread over, separating the axon terminal from the surrounding tissues in the extracellular space. The Schwann cell, however, is absent at the junctional regions between the nerve endings and the ganglion cell. The *postganglionic* neuron is a typical ganglion cell with its three main parts: the dendrites, the cell body, and the axon which transmits excitation away from the cell body.

In most ganglia the cell body (cyton or perikaryon) of the postganglionic neuron is enveloped by a thin, nucleated capsule which is perforated by the axon and longer dendrites and which is continuous with the neurilemma around the axon. The postganglionic fibers are unmyelinated, although according to MAXIMOW and BLOOM (1948) most apparently naked fibers possess traces of myelin. The dendrites of the ganglion cells vary in size and distribution; the longer ones penetrate the cell capsules and ramify in the intercellular spaces, but many break up within the capsules. The preganglionic fibers ending in the ganglia split up and form synaptic connections with both intracapsular and extracapsular dendrites (MITCHELL 1953). Various writers have studied dendritic forms and patterns in extreme detail and have distinguished various types of ganglion cells (DE CASTRO 1932, 1951). MITCHELL (1953), however, considers such classifications as exercises which "delight ardent neurohistologists, but merely heap useless burdens on the memories of others as they provide no significant information of compensatory value."

B. Development of the concept of chemical transmission

In 1904, T. R. ELLIOT, while a research student of physiology at Cambridge, demonstrated that denervation does not prevent the action of adrenaline on various structures and moreover, that the chronically denervated plain muscle of the dilator pupillae "will respond to adrenaline with greater rapidity and longer persistence than does the iris whose nervous relations are uninjured." Because of this finding and the previous assumption that adrenaline did "not evoke any reaction from muscle that has at no time of its life been innervated by the sympathetic" he put forward the brilliant suggestion that "adrenaline might be the chemical stimulant liberated on each occasion" when sympathetic nerve impulses arrive at the periphery. This discovery is undoubtedly one of the foundation stones which led finally to the formulation of the theory of chemical transmission.

Ten years later SIR HENRY DALE (1914), in a detailed pharmacological study, presented evidence that acetylcholine (ACh) not only mimics the responses to stimulation of parasympathetic nerves but also stimulates directly autonomic ganglia. One of his fundamental observations was the "biochemical similarity between the ganglion cells of the whole involuntary system and the terminations of voluntary nerve-fibres in striated muscle, on the one hand, and the mechanism connected with the peripheral termination of craniosacral involuntary nerves on the other." Furthermore, in the same paper SIR HENRY DALE pointed out the extraordinary evanescence of the action of ACh, suggesting that an esterase probably contributed to its rapid removal from the blood. One cannot help being impressed by the elegance of thought with which SIR HENRY DALE discussed his findings. Finally, OTTO LOEWI (1921) described his beautiful experiments, showing that stimulation of the vagus nerve produced its inhibitor effects on the frog's heart by the liberation of ACh. Thus the transmission of the effects of nerve impulses by the release of chemical agents became, for the first time, an experimental reality.

A few years later, FELDBERG and MINZ (1933) demonstrated that in the presence of physostigmine (eserine) a substance "pharmacologically indistinguishable" from ACh could be detected in the venous blood collected from the suprarenal glands during splanchnic stimulation. And, indeed, one year later FELDBERG et al. (1934) provided supporting evidence that the substance was ACh. At the same time they demonstrated that the adrenaline discharge from the adrenal glands caused by splanchnic stimulation was increased by eserine. This effect of eserine was first reported by STEWART and ROGOFF (1921) who found that in cats the administration of eserine, either intravenously or subcutaneously, increased the "epinephrin" output of the adrenals by tenfold, and that after denervation the eserine potentiation disappeared. FELDBERG and his colleagues (1934) found the same potentiation in experiments in which the adrenaline discharge was elicited by intra-arterially injected ACh, and they concluded that ACh was the humoral transmitter of splanchnic impulses to the suprarenal medulla and that the preganglionic sympathetic fibres were cholinergic. Following this first demonstration of transmission of preganglionic impulses by liberation of ACh, evidence was produced that the preganglionic fibers of a sympathetic ganglion are also cholinergic (FELD-BERG and GADDUM 1934). Using KIBJAKOW's method (1933), FELDBERG and GADDUM found that stimulation of the preganglionic fibers of a ganglion perfused with eserinized Locke's solution caused the liberation of ACh. They were, however, unable, in the absence of eserine, to detect any ACh in the perfusate. The same year, FELDBERG and VARTIAINEN (1934) produced more evidence concerning the site and the conditions of liberation of ACh. For example, they found that eserine added to the perfusing fluid in a concentration of $1 \times 10^{-6} M$ strongly sensitized the ganglion cells to the effects of preganglionic impulses and to injected ACh, lowering the threshold dose 8 to 20 times. Under their experimental conditions, in the absence of eserine the threshold dose of ACh injected into the perfusing fluid was 1 to 3 μg. The most effective conditions for this demonstration were found in recording contractions of the nictitating membrane caused by equal periods of submaximal stimulation applied to the cervical sympathetic trunk at a frequency of about 2/sec. With periods of stimulation at 10 to 30/sec, the potentiation, although definite, was less pronounced. These findings were in contrast with those of ECCLES (1934), who detected only a depressant effect of eserine when recording the action potentials set up in the ganglion and its postganglionic branches by single and repeated volleys in the preganglionic nerve. Such a depressant effect was seen by FELDBERG and VARTIAINEN but only with stronger concentrations of eserine ($1 \times 10^{-4} M$) which completely abolished the response of the ganglion cells to nervous impulses or chemical stimulants but left the release of ACh by preganglionic impulses unaffected. The authors were also able to show that if a relatively large dose of ACh (20 to 100 μg) was injected into the perfusing fluid, the ganglion cells, after a brief stimulating period became, for the time, completely unresponsive to preganglionic impulses or to further injections of ACh. Finally, choline, like ACh, was found to exhibit both a stimulant and a paralysing effect, but of a lower order. The threshold dose for stimulation varied in different experiments from 25 to 100 μg, but with 1 mg or more stimulation of the ganglionic cells was followed by paralysis of their response to preganglionic impulses, to choline itself, or to other stimulant substances.

Quite obviously the fundamental discovery that ACh is the substance released by the preganglionic nerve endings, which stems from the work of FELDBERG and his colleagues, would have been impossible without eserine. Since then a number of workers, notably MACINTOSH and his colleagues, have confirmed and extended these observations and throughout their work, eserine and other anti-ChE drugs have proved of the utmost importance.

MACINTOSH (1941) studied the distribution of ACh in various autonomic nerves and ganglia in the cat.

To each animal eserine sulphate (1 mg/kg) was given intravenously before the removal of the various structures. He found that cholinergic fibers may contain about as much ACh as ganglia; for example, there was little difference between the ACh content of the preganglionic cervical sympathetic trunk and that of the superior cervical ganglion. Certainly it is wrong to conclude from these results that ACh is not concentrated at ganglionic synapses. As MACINTOSH pointed out, the preganglionic synaptic endings form only 1% of the ganglion's volume, and as they account for most of the ganglion's ACh, their ACh content must be far higher than that of the axon. The first evidence that ACh is concentrated at the synaptic endings was presented by BROWN and FELDBERG (1936a), who found that the ganglion loses nearly all its ACh when the preganglionic fibers degenerate. Later, MACINTOSH (1938) demonstrated that 3 days following preganglionic section the ACh content was reduced by 74%, and transmission across the ganglionic synapse was nearly abolished at a time when the ganglion cells could still be stimulated effectively by potassium ions. In parallel experiments, COPPÉE and BACQ (1938) showed that during the same period conduction in the preganglionic fibers was still maintained. These results together show that both the preganglionic fibers and the ganglion cells were still functionally active at a stage when ACh had almost disappeared from the ganglion and transmission across the synapse was abolished.

C. Minute structure

There had been a good many indications in the past that ACh is present inside the nerve endings, not in free solution but possibly chemically combined or encapsulated within minute intracellular structures. And indeed, during the last few years, with the help of the enormous resolving capabilities of the electron microscope, anatomists have reported the presence of minute particles of about 0.05 μ diameter concentrated, usually in large numbers, in the presynaptic axoplasm of all junctions so far examined (DE ROBERTIS and BENNETT 1954, PALADE 1954, PALAY 1954, ROBERTSON 1956). These particles, named "synaptic vesicles", were suggested as possible depots of synaptic transmitters.

When ganglionic synapses were examined under the electron microscope they were found to possess several features in common with other synapses. For example, the presynaptic nerve fiber terminal was found to contain mitochondria and a large number of vesicles densely packed at the places where the presynaptic membrane is closest to the postsynaptic one. Only a few such vesicles were found in the axon above the ending or in the other cellular structures around the synapse; as a matter of fact, their high concentration at the nerve endings helps to distinguish the axonal cytoplasm from that of the surrounding Schwann cells, (CAUSEY 1960). Both the presynaptic and postsynaptic membranes are about 60 Å thick and are separated by an intervening space — the synaptic cleft — of about 120 to 200 Å, which reqresents the real discontinuity of cell cytoplasm at the level of the junction. Electron micrographs of the synaptic region in autonomic ganglia have been discussed by CAUSEY and his colleagues in a series of papers (CAUSEY and HOFFMAN 1956, CAUSEY and BARTON 1958, BARTON and CAUSEY 1958). These authors strongly emphasized the exceedingly intimate relationship between neurons and Schwann or satellite cells. According to them, the entire ganglion cell is invested by a capsule formed of satellite cells. In the immediate vicinity of the postsynaptic membrane, all the component elements appear to be present in their normal relationships, in contrast to the tendency for aggregations of mitochondria and small vesicles in the presynaptic axons. The presynaptic axons, which vary in diameter from 0.2 to 2 μ, are all contained within the cytoplasm of what may be considered as their last Schwann cell. Furthermore, CAUSEY and HOFFMAN (1956) found that when the preganglionic fibers are severed and therefore the presynaptic nerve endings degenerate, both the Schwann cells of the nerve fibers and the satellite cells of the neuron are mobilized, in preparation possibly for the active reception of the new nerve fibers. This is a finding similar to that of MILEDI (1960) who demonstrated that several days after cutting the motor nerve of the frog sartorius muscle, the Schwann cell replaces the axon in its synaptic position. Possibly the Schwann and the satellite cells play a very active part in the functions of the synaptic region. Up to the present, however, very little is known of either their metabolism or their pharmacology. Because of the similarity between Schwann cell and satellite cell, CAUSEY and HOFFMAN (1956) inferred that they are, in fact, modulations of a common cell type — a cell which intimately envelops the entire neuron from cell body to termination. Furthermore, CAUSEY (1960) suggested that it might be useful to adopt the term "satellite" for all cells that enfold or enclose axons or nerve cells. According to him, one of the advantages of using the term satellite to cover the whole of perineuronal cells is that it immediately draws attention to the possibility of a metabolic interrelation between the satellite cell and the nerve cell and its axon.

D. Choline acetylase and acetylcholinesterase

Besides ACh, cholinergic neurons contain choline acetylase (ChAc), the specific enzyme for the synthesis of ACh, and acetylcholinesterase (AChE), the enzyme which hydrolyzes the transmitter. All three are found in significant amounts along the whole length of every cholinergic neuron, but the concentration is highest at the nerve endings. According to MacINTOSH (1959), the most likely explanation for the presence of ACh and the two enzymes in the proximal parts of the neurons is that the enzymes are synthesized in the cell body and from there are carried to the nerve endings by the axoplasmic current streaming down each fiber.

The intracellular distribution of ChAc was studied by HEBB and SMALLMAN (1956) who found that after differential centrifugation of rabbit brain homogenates most of the enzymes present could be recovered in the granule fraction which included the bulk of the mitochondria. Later, HEBB and WHITTAKER (1958) produced evidence that ACh and ChA reside in the same subcellular particles and that the release of enzyme and ACh from their stores occurs in the same proportions under widely varying treatments, for example, freezing and thawing, dilution, and mixing with ether. But their evidence this time indicated that the particles which contain ACh and its synthesizing enzyme are different from mitochondria.

GLICK (1938) and NACHMANSOHN (1940) demonstrated that autonomic ganglia contain sufficient cholinesterase (ChE) to inactivate, within the refractory period of the system, the ACh liberated by stimulating preganglionic fibers, provided the ChE is concentrated at the preganglionic endings. SAWYER and HOLLINSHEAD (1945), immediately after MENDEL and RUDNEY's demonstration (1943) that there are two distinct enzymes which hydrolyze ACh, reinvestigated in the cat the enzyme content of the superior cervical ganglion and of its preganglionic fibers by a microchemical method and found that the ganglion contains significant amounts of AChE ("true" ChE) and BuChE (butyro- or "pseudo" ChE). Furthermore, they reported that both enzymes are most active in the region where preganglionic endings and ganglion cells are most concentrated.

The exact site of ChE activity in relation to the structural elements of various tissues is of great importance to both pharmacologists and physiologists. Such details of localization have been learned by the use of a microscopic histochemical technique introduced by KOELLE and FRIEDENWALD (1949), which is based on the fact that thiocholine esters are split by the enzymes as effectively as choline esters. Subsequent modifications of this method (KOELLE 1951) together with the use of selective inhibitors of AChE and BuChE (KOELLE 1955) allowed a more accurate localization of the two groups of enzymes. Furthermore, from a comparison of the effects produced by several anti-ChE drugs with varying lipoid-solubility, KOELLE and his colleagues concluded that the enzyme is separated by the cell membrane into external and internal fractions and that transmission in the cat's superior cervical ganglion is affected by the inhibition of only the external one (KOELLE and STEINER 1956, KOELLE 1957, MCISAAC and KOELLE 1959). In order to determine whether the external AChE is distributed at the pre- or post-synaptic site, KOELLE and KOELLE (1959) compared, in the cat, the effect of various anti-ChE substances in normal and preganglionically denervated ganglia. The results showed that in the stellate and superior cervical ganglia essentially all the external AChE is presynaptic. On the other hand, in the ciliary ganglion the enzyme was observed both pre- and postsynaptically (see Chapter 6).

Release of acetylcholine

A. Spontaneous release of acetylcholine

During the last few years evidence has been produced that ACh is released spontaneously from nerve endings "at rest". FATT and KATZ (1952), recording with intracellular electrodes from the endplate region of a resting amphibian muscle, detected a local spontaneous activity which was going on all the time in an intermittent random fashion and at an intensity well below the firing threshold of the muscle fiber. Because of their size, about 1% of that of the normal endplate response, these discharges were called "miniature" endplate potentials. Simple pharmacological tests convinced KATZ and his co-workers (KATZ 1958) that these spontaneous discharges are the result of a random impact of ACh on the endplate region.

While curarine reduced their size, both amplitude and duration were increased by neostigmine. In other words, the effects of these drugs on the miniature endplate potentials were similar to their known effects on the endplate response produced by a nerve impulse, or on the depolarization elicited by the local application of ACh. A statistical test indicated that the events were quantal in nature; in other words, that ACh was released in "packets" made of an equal number of ACh molecules.

Similar events apparently take place at the ganglionic synapse; MacINTOSH (1959) showed that in ganglia perfused with an eserinized fluid, a resting discharge of ACh, amounting to about 0.3 mμg/min, can be detected. Long before, BROWN and FELDBERG (1936a) and MacINTOSH (1938) had observed that when a ganglion was perfused with eserinized Locke's solution, the venous effluent quite often contained some ACh at the beginning of the perfusion. Calculations showed that the concentration of ACh in such samples was about 5% of the concentration found during preganglionic stimulation. It is rather amusing that, because at that time a discharge of ACh at rest was not considered a physiological event, the authors felt rather apologetic about their findings and tried to devise means of lessening this "spontaneous" initial output.

According to MacINTOSH (1959), a *resting* superior cervical ganglion from a cat, with its normal blood supply, contains about 0.25 μg of ACh and this content is not much changed during synaptic activity. The same is true of a perfused ganglion provided normal heparinized plasma is used as the perfusion fluid. However, although the ACh content stays the same, ACh turnover occurs, slowly during rest and briskly during activity. At the same time MacINTOSH measured the ACh content of the unstimulated ganglion in the presence of an anti-ChE drug. The experiments were performed in anesthetized cats maintained on artificial respiration and protected with atropine and a neuromuscular blocking drug. The preganglionic cervical sympathetic trunk was sectioned and either TEPP (tetraethyl pyrophosphate) or eserine was administered intravenously every 5 minutes in a dose of 1 mg/kg. Under this treatment the ACh content of the ganglion rose steadily over an hour or two and eventually reached more than double the initial value (Fig. 1). All these results put together demonstrate that ACh is continuously being made and destroyed at a slow rate in resting nerve endings.

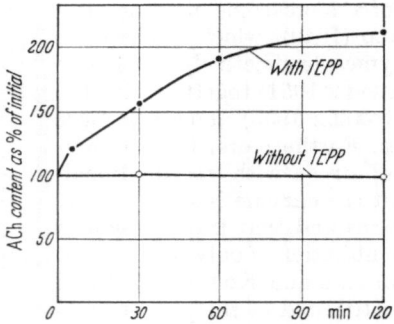

Fig. 1. ACh content of unstimulated ganglia (expressed as percentage of ACh in control ganglia excised at start of each experiment). Above: data from experiments in which TEPP was given by vein (1 mg/kg every 5 min); the preganglionic trunk had been sectioned and the animals were maintained on artificial respiration and protected with atropine and gallamine. Below: data from experiments on animals similarly treated except for the administration of TEPP (from MacINTOSH 1959)

B. Acetylcholine released during activity

I. Ganglia in vivo

Attempts have been made to study ganglia with their natural blood supply (FELDBERG and VARTIAINEN 1934, MacINTOSH 1938). In such a preparation, and in the presence of eserine, stimulation of preganglionic fibers yielded a smooth contraction of the nictitating membrane without any sign of the "inhibitory" phase; unfortunately, under these conditions release of ACh in substantial quantity, by preganglionic stimulation, occurred irregularly or not at all. EMMELIN and MACINTOSH (1956) suggested that these negative results were due to incomplete inhibition of ChE's. They repeated the experiments with larger doses of eserine but even then evidence of ACh release following sympathetic stimulation was obtained only in three out of nine animals. A rough estimate showed that only about 10% of the ACh set free in the ganglia was able to reach the distant vessels and produce a fall of blood pressure. Moreover, even the largest doses of eserine that could be given without excessively lowering the blood pressure were inadequate to preserve ACh from destruction by ChE's. For example, blood was taken from a cat 10 min after the injection of 25 mg of eserine sulphate per kg; when ACh was added to this blood, the final concentration being 10^{-8} M and the temperature 35°, 50% of it was destroyed within 30 min. EMMELIN and MACINTOSH concluded, therefore, that it was impracticable to determine the true output of ACh from a ganglion with its natural circulation. The same conclusion was reached by DALE et al. (1936) who failed to detect any ACh in the venous blood of animals, pretreated with eserine, when the skeletal muscle retained its natural circulation; in contrast, ACh always appeared in the venous effluent with saline perfusion.

II. Perfused ganglia

LOCKE's solution can hardly be considered a complete physiological medium and the ganglia perfused with it usually show signs of abnormal function. For example, the connective tissue surrounding the ganglia rapidly becomes distended with fluid, and transmission of impulses with prolonged stimulation is not well maintained. MACINTOSH (1938) found that ganglia perfused with a tenfold dilution of the cat's own heparinized blood in normal LOCKE's solution containing eserine sulphate (1 in 250,000) showed no sign of edema even after perfusion had continued for several hours. Some of the ganglia were examined histologically and there was no recognisable difference between the perfused and the control ganglia. This observation was followed up by a series of fundamentally important studies which led eventually to many outstanding advances in the knowledge of the mechanisms involved in the metabolism of ACh at the ganglionic synapse and of the factors concerned with its release from the preganglionic nerve endings.

Together with EMMELIN, MACINTOSH (1956) compared the following perfusion fluids: (a) LOCKE's solution as used in most of the earlier studies (bicarbonate-Locke), (b) a solution of the same tonicity containing phosphate buffer at pH 7.4 instead of bicarbonate (phosphate-Locke), (c) heparinized plasma, (d) blood, and finally, (e) defibrinated blood. Heparinized plasma proved to be a very satisfactory perfusion fluid. There was no edema and the flow was better maintained than with the saline fluids. Heparinized blood was found to be unsuitable; its cells settled so rapidly within the cannulae and major vessels that the flow soon stopped. With defibrinated blood, perfusion was more satisfactory, but the flow was very slow. However, when the amount of ACh liberated under the various conditions of perfusion was calculated, it was found that within fairly close limits it was the same provided a ChE inhibitor was present in adequate concentration.

The same authors attempted to find out to what extent ACh output depended on the concentration of eserine in the perfusion fluid. Their results showed that the concentration could be varied within wide limits without any important effect on the ACh output, provided that enough drug was present to inactivate the enzyme. In the same series of experiments the authors studied three more anti-ChE drugs and found that with perfusion fluids containing DFP (diisopropyl phosphorofluoridate) ($5 \times 10^{-5} M$), TEPP ($2 \times 10^{-4} M$), or neostigmine methyl-sulphate ($1.7 \times 10^{-5} M$) the output of ACh was a little, but not significantly, below the average found in the experiments with eserine ($10^{-5} M$).

In these experiments the ACh output was expressed as the weight in pg ($g \times 10^{-12}$) of ACh chloride liberated per single maximal stimulus applied to the preganglionic trunk. The following are the mean values for each perfusion fluid based on the output obtained during the first 3-min period of stimulation at a frequency of 20 to 25/sec.

Perfusion fluid	ACh output per maximal volley (pg)
Bicarbonate-Locke (eserine sulphate 5×10^{-6})	28.5
Phosphate-Locke (eserine sulphate 5×10^{-6}) .	26
Plasma (eserine sulphate 10^{-5})	20.5
Blood (eserine sulphate 10^{-4})	21

Obviously, despite the considerable variation in the perfusion fluid, there was no significant variation in the quantity of ACh discharged at the preganglionic endings. In discussing their findings, EMMELIN and MACINTOSH pointed out that the earlier volleys of each period of stimulation release more ACh than the later ones, possibly because in a ganglion thus perfused and with prolonged stimulation the ACh output usually falls approximately exponentially to reach a steady low level. In this, they confirmed the observations of FELDBERG and VARTIAINEN (1934) and PERRY (1953) who calculated that in the sympathetic ganglion the initial output of ACh per volley is about 100 pg (100 $\mu\mu$g). Furthermore, Perry found that in experiments in which the preganglionic trunk was subjected to prolonged stimulation at varying frequencies, the ACh output eventually became constant at about 4 mμg/min, whatever the frequency of stimulation.

Under the same experimental conditions, EMMELIN and MACINTOSH (l. c.), found that 0.1 μg of ACh, dissolved in 0.2 ml of eserinized LOCKE's solution injected into the perfusion stream above the ganglion, regularly produced a discharge of impulses in the postganglionic fibers.

Assuming this amount of ACh to be equally distributed through the volume of the ganglion (approximately 12 μl), the final concentration of ACh would be at the most of the order of $5 \times 10^{-7} M$. BIRKS (1954), however, (mentioned by EMMELIN and MACINTOSH 1956) has found that when TEPP is used instead of eserine, the cells of the perfused ganglion regularly respond to only $5 \times 10^{-8} M$ ACh. A possible explanation for this difference, put forward by EMMELIN and MACINTOSH, is that the ganglion cells are not maximally responsive to ACh in the presence of eserine, a substance which has been shown to possess some ganglionic blocking action "of a competitive type" (FELDBERG and VARTIAINEN 1934, FELDBERG and HEBB 1948, PATON and PERRY 1953).

When no anti-ChE drug is added to the perfusion fluid, no ACh can be detected in the effluent collected during preganglionic stimulation but choline appears instead (BROWN and FELDBERG 1936b). EMMELIN and MACINTOSH (1956) repeated these experiments and in addition attempted to find out whether the quantity of choline released during synaptic activity in the absence of eserine agreed well with the quantity of ACh released when eserine was present. Their results clearly showed that in the absence of any esterase inhibitor, the perfused ganglion on stimulation liberates choline in an amount corresponding to that of ACh it releases when its ChE's are inhibited. Thus, it appears that eserine does not affect the liberation of ACh but only preserves it from destruction after it has been liberated.

That eserinized plasma is a more satisfactory perfusion fluid was further demonstrated by BIRKS and MACINTOSH (1957).

In a first group of experiments evidence was once more produced that ganglia stimulated at 20/sec during perfusion with Locke's solution cannot maintain their high initial rate of ACh output for a long time. In contrast, ganglia stimulated at the same frequency but perfused with eserinized plasma, release ACh at about the same rate initially, but the output is maintained at a high steady level (Fig. 2). Furthermore, they found that plasma dialysates support ACh release as well as plasma.

One of the most important observations that came out of BIRKS and MAC-
INTOSH's (1957) work was that in the presence of hemicholinium (α,α-dimethyl-
ethanolamino-4,4'-biacetophenone, HC-3) the ACh output rate falls off very
rapidly in ganglia perfused with either Locke solution or plasma. SCHUELER (1955)
has designated as "hemicholiniums" a series of quaternary bases which exhibit a
kind of toxicity suggestive of some interference with cholinergic mechanisms.
MACINTOSH et al. (1956) found that HC-3 was competing in some way with choline,
and therefore suggested that the drug might act as an inhibitor of choline transport, possibly by preventing the access of extracellular choline to the intracellular

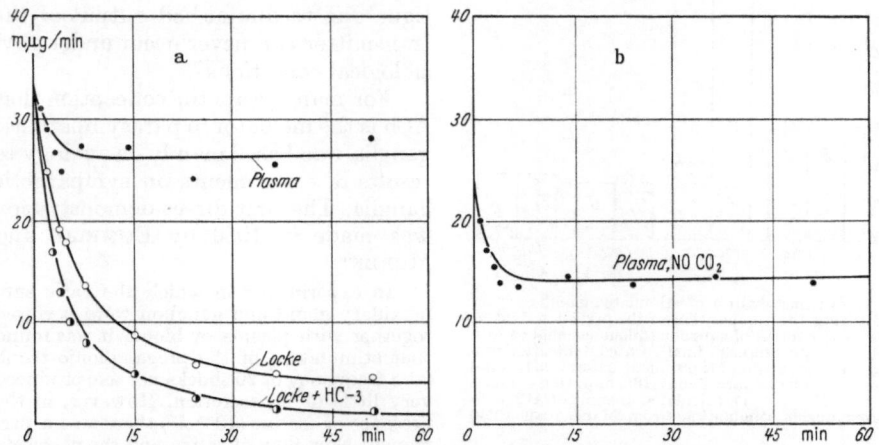

Fig. 2. a) ACh output from eserinized superior cervical ganglia during 1 hour's preganglionic stimulation at
20/second (each curve gives the mean values for five experiments). Perfusion fluids from above downward:
heparinized cat plasma equilibrated with 5% CO_2 in O_2, oxygenated Locke's solution, oxygenated Locke's solution
containing HC-3 (2×10^{-5} M). b) ACh output from ganglia similarly stimulated, during perfusion with eserinized
plasma equilibrated with CO_2-free oxygen (mean of five experiments) (from MACINTOSH 1959)

sites of acetylation. Therefore, the finding that in the presence of HC-3 plasma
loses its ability to maintain a steady output of ACh from the ganglion suggested
that plasma supports ACh synthesis better than Locke solution. BROWN and FELD-
BERG (1936b) observed that the addition of minute quantities of whole blood to the
fluid perfusing a ganglion which had been fatigued by prolonged preganglionic
stimulation, produced a partial restoration of the peripheral responses and an
increase of the ACh concentration of the venous effluent. Their conclusion was
that this improvement in function was due to the replenishing in the ganglion of
some material essential for ACh synthesis which was removed or not replenished
by the saline perfusion fluid during prolonged stimulation. Furthermore, they
attempted to determine the constituent of the injected blood which could be
responsible for the augmentation of ACh output; they found that in some experiments the addition of a solution of choline caused a marked increase in the ACh
output and an increase in the contraction of the nictitating membrane. It was the
strong accelerating action of choline on the synthesis of ACh which caused NACH-
MANSOHN and MACHADO (1943) to designate the enzyme responsible for the synthesis "choline acetylase" (ChAc).

In a second series of experiments, BIRKS and MACINTOSH (1957) compared the
ACh output of ganglia with the change that had occurred in their ACh content
during stimulation. As Fig. 3 shows, the Locke-perfused ganglia had synthesized
a considerable amount of ACh during one hour's activity but they had also lost

about half their initial stock. In contrast, the plasma-perfused ganglia had kept their ACh stock intact in spite of having released a great deal more of the transmitter, and furthermore, they had accumulated some surplus ACh that they could not release. On the other hand, ganglia under the influence of HC-3 had synthesized hardly any ACh and their ACh content was reduced to 15 to 20% of its initial level. This was a clear-cut demonstration that plasma contains some factor that promotes synthesis "so effectively indeed that it looks as if junctional fatigue due to diminished output of the transmitter can never occur under physiological conditions".

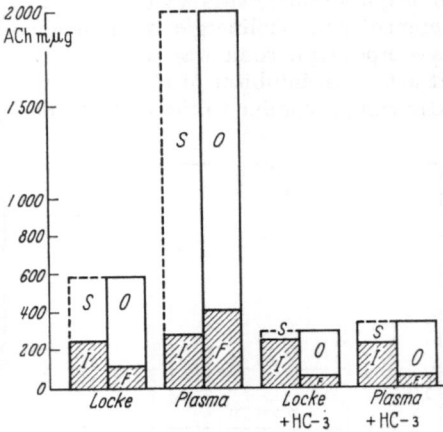

Fig. 3. ACh metabolism of stimulated ganglia: effect of changing the composition of the perfusion fluid. I, initial ACh content of ganglion (taken as equal to ACh in control ganglion). F, final ACh content after preganglionic stimulation for 60 min at 20/second. O, total amount of ACh discharged into effluent during stimulation S (= F + O − I), calculated amount of ACh synthesized during stimulation (from MacIntosh 1959)

For many years the conception that ACh is the mediator in parasympathetic ganglia was based mainly on analogy to results of experiments on sympathetic ganglia. The first direct demonstration was made in 1950 by EMMELIN and MUREN.

In experiments in which the cat's submaxillary gland and ganglion were perfused together with plasma or blood, it was found that stimulation of the preganglionic trunk (at a frequency of 20 shocks per sec) produced very little or no secretion. However, in the presence of eserine (10^{-5} M) there was a permanent slow flow of saliva and the perfusate contained ACh, the average content of the first three-minute control sample being 0.005 μg. Moreover, in the presence of eserine, ACh appeared in the perfusate without preganglionic stimulation. When the whole procedure was repeated with eserinized plasma containing curare, it was found that the blockade of ganglionic transmission did not prevent, but only reduced, the release of ACh by approximately 10%. The authors concluded, therefore, that the ACh output obtained in the presence of curare represented the amount of transmitter liberated by the preganglionic nerve endings.

III. Additional factors necessary for normal acetylcholine release

HARVEY and MACINTOSH (1940) demonstrated that the output of ACh from the superior cervical ganglion during stimulation of the preganglionic trunk is reduced when the perfusion fluid is deficient in calcium. This was confirmed by HUTTER and KOSTIAL (1954) who found also that by increasing the concentration of calcium ions in LOCKE's solution to 8 to 10 mM, twice the usual amount of ACh is liberated by preganglionic stimulation. Furthermore, they demonstrated that magnesium ions in concentrations causing block of ganglionic transmission (15 to 25 mM) reduced the output of ACh and that calcium ions (40 to 10 mM) relieved the block and restored the ACh output.

Undoubtedly calcium has an important role in controlling ACh release. MACINTOSH (1959) has put forward the suggestion that calcium ions entering the nerve terminals during the impulse release ACh by disrupting the ACh-retaining vesicles. The basis of this suggestion was the demonstration by HODGKIN and KEYNES (1957) that during activity in squid nerve fibers there is a sharp rise in calcium influx, while during rest the calcium that has entered is slowly pumped out. HARVEY and MACINTOSH (1940) observed also that when the perfusion fluid is free of calcium ions, yet contains the usual concentrations of the other salts of Locke's solution and eserine, the ganglion cells begin almost immediately to discharge, an effect accompanied by a corresponding failure of the output of ACh. This was in agreement with the results of BRINK et al. (1946) who showed that the absence of calcium ions causes a long, continued spontaneous activity of the cells of a sympathetic ganglion, in the form of a repetitive discharge of impulses along the postganglionic axons (Fig. 4) and a simultaneous failure of transmission of excitation from the nerve endings of the preganglionic fibers. Furthermore, under these conditions the ganglion cells become less sensitive to the paralysing as well as to the stimulating effect of ACh (HARVEY and MacINTOSH 1940).

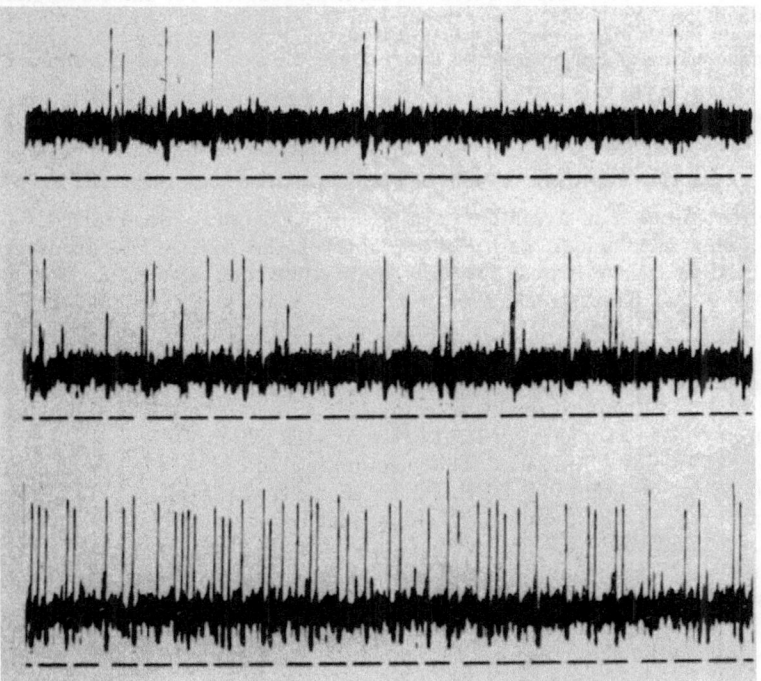

Fig. 4. Impulses discharged by a few sympathetic ganglion cells in response to stimulation of the preganglionic nerve at a frequency of 50 per second. The ganglion was perfused with a modified Ringer's solution containing various amounts of calcium chloride: Uppermost record, 4.4 mM; middle record, 2.2 mM; bottom record, 1.1 mM. The middle record represents the normal level of calcium. Time in 0.1 seconds (from BRINK et al. 1946)

Besides calcium, carbon dioxide is apparently necessary for optimal release (MacINTOSH 1959).

Plasma equilibrated with CO_2—O_2 mixture has a pH of 7.4. When CO_2 is left out and the plasma is gassed with O_2 alone, the pH rises above 8 and the results obtained are different. The output rate of ACh is lower from start to finish (Fig. 2), but this is not because there is any shortage of ACh in the nerve endings (as the final content is significantly higher than when CO_2 is present), but because each preganglionic volley sets free a smaller proportion of the ACh from the depots. According to MacINTOSH the effect of CO_2 on ACh release is probably due to increased ionization of plasma calcium. BIRKS and MacINTOSH (1957) have also shown that plasma dialysate supports ACh release as well as plasma because they both contain a heat-labile factor necessary for optimal ACh synthesis.

HUTTER and KOSTIAL (1955), studying the relationship between the sodium ion concentration and the release of ACh from the preganglionic nerve endings, found that so long as the perfusion fluid contained 30% of the normal sodium concentration, no change in the amount of ACh released could be detected.

BROWN (1954) showed that the release of ACh was susceptible to fluctuations in temperature.

The preparation used was the isolated superior cervical ganglion perfused with eserinized LOCKE's solution. A reduction in temperature from 39° to 20° caused an approximately tenfold decrease of the ACh output. Ganglionic transmission, however, as judged by the contractions of the nictitating membrane, continued apparently unimpaired. Later, KOSTIAL and VOUK (1956), under the same experimental conditions but using a lower frequency of stimulation (2/sec instead of 10/sec used by BROWN), found that within the range from 40° to 20°, the temperature was without appreciable effect. Below 20°, however, specifically in the range between 20° and 10°, the output of ACh was markedly reduced. The authors suggest that the apparent discrepancy between their results and those of BROWN can be explained by the difference in the frequency of stimulation used. It would be interesting to know whether this discrepancy occurs in ganglia perfused with eserinized plasma instead of eserinized LOCKE's solution.

Actions of anticholinesterase agents

A. Pharmacological effects based on indirect measurements

A great number of available data is concerned only with qualitative physiological, pharmacological, and toxic effects of the anti-AChE drugs resulting, undoubtedly, from actions affecting more than one structure. For example, systemic blood pressure changes have been extensively studied and varying effects have been reported. The finding, especially, that several anti-ChE drugs elicit a pressor response has given rise to many speculations, and many workers have attempted to find a correlation between the hypertensive effect and the ability of these drugs to facilitate ganglionic transmission. The following papers have been chosen as good representatives of such attempts.

KOPPANYI and KARCZMAR (1951) compared the effects of various anti-ChE drugs (eserine, neostigmine, DFP, HETP (hexaethyltetraphosphate, a mixture of organophosphorus compounds of which TEPP is the chief active component), TEPP, and Parathion (0,0-diethyl 0-[4-nitrophenyl]-phosphorothioate) on the pressor action of ACh in atropinized dogs and cats. The changes observed were considered a measure of the relative effects of these drugs on sympathetic ganglia. It is difficult to see how the authors reached such a conclusion; as a rule their experiments were performed in the presence of large doses of atropine (15 to 20 mg/kg), known to cause a nearly complete interruption of ganglionic transmission. A possible mechanism which might have contributed to the pressor effect of ACh under the conditions of these experiments, or in several of those described below, is the release by ACh of norepinephrine from stores associated with the terminals of postganglionic sympathetic adrenergic fibers, as postulated by BURN and RAND (1960).

MENDEZ and RAVIN (1941) demonstrated that in cats pretreated with relatively small doses of atropine, neostigmine produced a rise in blood pressure which lasted 4 to 5 min; this effect could be obtained repeatedly in the same animal and occurred in spinal, anesthetized, eviscerated, and adrenalectomized cats. Furthermore, large doses of nicotine did not prevent the effect. The authors concluded, therefore, that it was the constriction of peripheral vessels due to a direct effect of neostigmine, and not the stimulation of sympathetic ganglia, which played an important role in the rise in blood pressure. SALERNO and COON (1949) studied in cats and dogs the pharmacological actions of HETP and TEPP and compared them with those of eserine, neostigmine, and DFP. Under barbiturate anesthesia and under the influence of atropine (1 mg/kg), all drugs except DFP produced initially a rise in blood pressure which was followed by vasodepression. The effect was still present after adrenalectomy, evisceration, or paralysing doses of nicotine; large doses of Dibenamine, however, antagonized it. The authors concluded that any ganglionic effect was not nicotine-like, and that the ChE inhibitors produce the hypertensive effect either by a peripheral "sympathin-like" action, or by stimulating the ganglia through a mechanism which is not altered by large doses of nicotine. However, they pointed out that neither of these possible actions could be considered as resulting from ChE inhibition.

DIRNHUBER and CULLUMBINE (1955) found that in rats the usual hypertensive effect of Sarin (isopropyl methylphosphonofluoridate), DFP, eserine, TEPP, and Paraoxon (E 600, diethyl 4-nitrophenyl phosphate) was absent in the spinal animal or in the presence of atropine. Furthermore, in non-atropinized animals large doses of hexamethonium prevented the pressor response. The authors concluded that the rise in blood pressure was the result of peripheral vasoconstriction brought about by a central effect transmitted to the periphery through the sympathetic nervous system. Such a central action was also suggested by LANGLEY and KATO as early as 1915 when they found that the rise in blood pressure which eserine produced was much less in the spinal atropinized cat.

VARAGIĆ (1955) showed that in rats anesthetized with urethane or decerebrated small doses of eserine (about 50 μg/kg) caused an appreciable rise of blood pressure, but that neostigmine and other quaternary anti-ChE drugs were ineffective. The hypertensive effect was antagonized by atropine and nicotine; furthermore, after very large doses of hexamethonium (128 to 167 mg/kg) the pressor response to a small dose of eserine (30 to 90 μg/kg) disappeared but amounts of eserine such as 1.5 mg/kg were still active. He concluded that the hypertensive effects appeared to be mainly due to a discharge of impulses from the brain, causing, at the periphery, vasoconstriction. PAULET (1954) found that in dogs under chloralose anesthesia and after the administration of 0.1 to 1 mg of atropine, TEPP, injected intravenously in a dose range of 0.2 to 8 mg, produced a rise in blood pressure. The response was not prevented by large doses of nicotine (which blocked the effect of subsequent doses of nicotine), was reduced by adrenalectomy, and was blocked by antiadrenaline compounds only when administered in doses large enough to abolish responses to electrical stimulation of sympathetic nerves. PAULET concluded from his results that the hypertensive response is apparently due to a mechanism which affects the central nervous system and the sympathetic ganglia, but is independent of the anti-ChE activity of TEPP. HEYMANS (1951) supported the view that the hypertensive response is due to a mechanism independent of ChE inhibition, and denied any action of anti-ChE drugs on sympathetic ganglia. DALY and WRIGHT (1956) made direct measurements of the changes produced by anti-ChE drugs on the peripheral circulation. Their results, obtained from well-controlled experiments, showed that in the dog, Sarin and TEPP caused an increase in resistance to blood flow through the limbs and splanchnic vascular bed. Changes in peripheral vascular resistance were indicated by alterations in the arterial pressure in isolated innervated organ preparations perfused at constant blood volume inflow; perfusion was carried out either from the same animal or from a donor dog. The various constrictor responses were antagonized by atropine, and it was concluded that the vasoconstriction was due to an increased discharge in the sympathetic nervous system. In discussing their results the authors pointed out that an increased vasoconstrictor discharge could be brought about by several mechanisms: reflexes from the vasosensory zones of the carotid sinuses and arch of the aorta, central asphyxia, a central action, or an action on the sympathetic ganglia. Because of all these possibilities, they stated, quite rightly, that in the absence of information on the preganglionic activity, it is impossible to assess on an animal under the influence of the anti-ChE drugs to what extent facilitation of synaptic transmission in sympathetic ganglia contributes to the increased peripheral resistance.

The same is true for any results which are not based on measurements of events occurring at the ganglionic synapse. For example, several workers attempted to study interactions between ganglionic blocking and anti-ChE drugs through recordings of blood pressure changes. In some instances the conclusions reached were far apart, although the same species of animal and the same drugs were used. Obviously, blood pressure changes which, as a rule, are the result of a combination of actions on several sites are not adequate for the study of ganglionic effects. The following reports illustrate this point:

GROB and HARVEY (1950) found that the administration of neostigmine before or after pentamethonium, a quaternary drug which blocks ganglionic transmission by competition with ACh, did not antagonize the effects resulting from the autonomic blockade. On the other hand, REARDON et al. (1947) reported that neostigmine, in relatively small doses (0.5 to 1 mg intravenously), produced a rapid and dramatic relief of the circulatory effects of TEA (tetraethylammonium), a drug also known to block ganglionic transmission by competition with ACh. Furthermore, the antagonistic action was seen in both man and dog. Similarly, GRIMSON et al. (1955) found in dogs that the fall in blood pressure produced by chlorisondamine (Ecolid), yet another quaternary ganglionic blocking drug, was promptly reduced by the intravenous administration of 0.5 to 1 mg of neostigmine. LONG et al. (1960) reported that neostigmine and various other reversible ChE inhibitors produce a pressor response in animals that have been pretreated with hexamethonium, pentolinium, or other ganglionic blocking drugs. From an analysis of their results the authors reached the conclusion that this action of the ChE inhibitors is ganglionic in origin. Similarly, HILTON (1961) studied the blood pressure effects of neostigmine and eserine in dogs pretreated with various ganglionic blocking drugs, and found that both ChE inhibitors restored the blood pressure to preblockade levels. Adrenalectomy or the previous administration of small doses of anti-adrenaline drugs (phentolamine, Dibenamine, piperoxan) and TM-10 (choline 2,6-xylyl ether bromide), a substance which apparently blocks transmission in adrenergic neurons, (GEUS et al. 1959) did not interfere with this antagonism. The dose of the anti-adrenaline compounds used was sufficient to produce reversal of injected adrenaline but inadequate to produce a complete blockade of sympathetic stimulation. The response, however, was blocked by small doses of atropine (1 mg/kg) and phenoxybenzamine. Furthermore, he found that neostigmine administered before hexamethonium was unable to prevent the hexamethonium-induced fall in blood pressure. From these results, HILTON concluded that the ability of the ChE inhibitors to restore the blood pressure was not due to accumulation of ACh at either sympathetic ganglia or the adrenal medulla. He based this conclusion on two main points: a) that atropine blocked instead of potentiating the response, and b) that the response was still present after adrenalectomy. A true antagonism at the ganglionic synapse between the ganglionic blocking drugs and the ChE inhibitors could have been the cause of his findings if, according to HILTON, some of the postganglionic fibres mediated transmission, not by the usual sympathetic pathways or the usual sympathetic chemical mediator.

B. Pharmacological effects based on direct measurements

More direct information about the pharmacological effects of anti-ChE drugs at the ganglionic synapse has been obtained from experiments in which were recorded the responses of either postganglionic neurons or effector structures to preganglionic stimulation or injected ACh.

MARRAZZI and JARVIK (1947) found that DFP caused an increase in the number of postsynaptic fibers responding to submaximal preganglionic stimulation of the inferior mesenteric sympathetic ganglion of the cat. Atropine, on the other hand, had an inhibitory effect. CHENNELS et al. (1947), studying the effect of HETP in the same species, found that the response of the nictitating membrane to preganglionic stimulation was unchanged until 1 mg/kg of the drug was injected, when some potentiation occurred. BURGEN et al. (1949) demonstrated that in atropinized cats TEPP potentiated the response of the nictitating membrane to stimulation of the preganglionic fibers. After the intravenous administration of 2 mg/kg of TEPP, the effect of preganglionic stimulation at frequencies of 1 to 2/sec was equal to that obtained with control stimulation at 5 times these frequencies. Furthermore, they were able to show that the contraction of the nictitating membrane and the rise of blood pressure elicited in atropinized animals by large doses of ACh, injected intravenously, were potentiated by TEPP; HETP acted like TEPP but was 4 times less potent. A similar potentiating action was demonstrated for Tabun (ethyl-N,N-dimethyl phosphoramidocyanidate), again in atropinized cats. HOLMSTEDT (1951) studied the effect of this drug on the response of the nictitating membrane to various frequencies of stimulation of the cervical sympathetic trunk. Following an intravenous injection of 0.27 mg/kg of Tabun, preganglionic stimulation at 2 to 5 stimuli/sec elicited contractions larger than those previously obtained at a frequency of stimulation of 10/sec.

CHOU and DE ELIO (1948) found that eserine had a weak decurarizing effect on the superior cervical ganglion of the cat, but that neostigmine had none. In ganglia perfused with LOCKE's solution, tubocurarine was added to the perfusing fluid at a concentration of 1 to 4 μg/ml. When the contractions of the nictitating membrane, elicited by maximal stimulation of the preganglionic fibers at a rate of 8 stimuli/sec, had decreased by 30 to 40%, eserine was added. A dose of 0.1 to 0.4 μg of eserine antagonized the blockade, while doses of 1 to 5 μg had no effect, or occasionally caused a further depression. In contrast to eserine, repeated doses of 0.005, 0.4, 2 and 20 μg of neostigmine proved ineffective. Furthermore, the authors found that by changing the tertiary eserine into a quaternary salt, eserine methiodide, the anticurare activity of the compound markedly decreased. They attributed these results to the failure of quaternary compounds to penetrate the cell membrane adequately.

Results obtained from studies on the adrenal medulla, although they raise complex problems, complement those on synaptic transmission in autonomic ganglia. In order to study the effects of eserine, MALMÉJAC (1953) used simultaneously the coeliac plexus (an autonomic ganglion) and the adrenal gland in the same animal (dog) and under identical conditions. In experiments in which the organs were perfused *in vivo* with blood of a donor dog while retaining their innervation intact, MALMÉJAC demonstrated that eserine administered intra-arterially potentiated the responses to both splanchnic stimulation and injected ACh. Furthermore, he showed that denervation abolishes this effect.

C. Correlation of functional changes with inactivation of cholinesterase

The measurements just described, although adequate for demonstrating pharmacological events in autonomic ganglia, do not indicate the degree of responsibility of ChE inhibition in the phenomena observed. KOELLE and his colleagues undertook this difficult task in a series of fundamentally important studies, and succeded in establishing correlation of functional changes produced by anti-ChE drugs with varying degrees of inactivation of AChE and non-specific ChE.

To begin with, KAMIJO and KOELLE (1952) studied the effects of DFP a) on the contractions of the nictitating membrane elicited by supramaximal stimulation of the partially resected preganglionic cervical sympathetic trunk, and b) on the action of TEA, a substance known to interrupt ganglionic transmission by competition with ACh (PATON and PERRY 1953).

When the whole of the preganglionic sympathetic trunk is stimulated with supramaximal shocks, a maximal response of the effector organ is produced. Under such conditions it is difficult to demonstrate an effect produced by anti-ChE drugs. For this reason, KAMIJO and KOELLE reduced the response of the nictitating membrane by partial resection of the preganglionic trunk. The experiments were performed on cats under barbiturate anesthesia and in the presence of atropine, 5 mg/kg administered intravenously, a dose large enough to reduce by approximately 50%, the response of the nictitating membrane to preganglionic stimulation. The intravenous administration of DFP in a dose of 0.25 mg/kg produced complete inactivation of non-specific ChE and 44% inactivation of AChE activity, but had very little effect on the mechanical response of the nictitating membrane elicited by preganglionic stimulation or on the TEA effect. Following larger doses, ranging from 0.5 to 2 mg/kg, the effect of preganglionic stimulation was potentiated progressively and the TEA blockade antagonized. The effects were both definite and marked. Very little enzymatic activity was present after 1 mg/kg of DFP and finally, following 2 mg/kg, AChE could not be detected. At higher dose levels of DFP, however, the effects were clearly inhibitory; the height of the nictitating membrane contraction decreased, the antagonism to TEA diminished and moreover, the action of TEA appeared to be potentiated in the presence of these larger doses of DFP.

From these results the authors concluded that the potentiating effect of DFP was due to its anti-ChE activity, presumably through preservation of ACh liberated at the synapse. They pointed out, however, that the depressant effects were unlikely to be due to accumulation of inhibitory concentrations of ACh because the frequency of stimulation used in their experiments was low (2/sec), and suggested that they may have been the result of a direct effect of DFP. However, as the authors themselves admitted, some of their experimental conditions may have influenced the results obtained, especially the large doses of atropine (5mg/kg) and the barbiturate anesthesia.

In order to find out if any of the DFP effects were due to alterations of conduction in the preganglionic fibres, HOLADAY et al. (1954) repeated the study by recording simultaneously preganglionic and postganglionic action potentials over a wide range of doses of DFP. The experiments were performed *in vivo*, on the superior cervical ganglion of both atropinized and non-atropinized cats, and *in vitro* on the isolated superior cervical ganglion of the rat. Ganglionic action potentials were recorded with the aid of an electrode which supported the postganglionic nerve and a second electrode placed directly over the ganglion. Doses of DFP large enough (2 mg/kg) to inhibit all ganglionic ChE activity did not produce any appreciable effect on the postganglionic responses to *maximal* preganglionic stimulation. On the other hand, postganglionic activity elicited by *submaximal* stimulation was increased by doses of DFP (0.25 to 2 mg/kg) which inactivated completely the non-specific ChE and partially the AChE. In general, facilitation was more obvious in responses elicited by high frequency of stimulation. Following higher does of DFP (4 to 8 mg/kg), postganglionic responses to both maximal and submaximal stimulation were regularly depressed. With increasingly higher doses the height of the preganglionic action potentials decreased also but, as a rule, the depression of the postganglionic ones came first. Although the previous administration of 1 mg/kg of atropine had very little effect, a dose of 5 mg/kg caused a depression of ganglionic transmission which lasted for several hours. In such preparations, DFP restored the postganglionic action potentials to their control height or even produced a small increase. Furthermore, it was found that in the presence of atropine the dose of DFP required to cause depression of the postganglionic action potentials was greater than that required in non-atropinized animals. Almost invariably, DFP altered the form of the ganglionic action potentials. The early negative after-potential decreased in magnitude and duration and was replaced by a positive after-potential which appeared, as the doses became larger, progressively earlier and with increasing magnitude. These findings agree with those described by R.Eccles (1952a). Some differences were noted in the response of the isolated rat ganglia. First, the potentiating effect of DFP was more obvious at low frequencies of preganglionic stimulation, while the inhibitory effect of larger doses was facilitated by an increase in frequency. Second, in these preparations after-discharge followed, as a rule, the administration of DFP. It appeared usually in response to low frequency volleys, and was suppressed by either an increase in the frequency or in the duration of the stimulation. Holaday et al. concluded, therefore, that while facilitation of ganglionic transmission following DFP is due primarily to inactivation of AChE, the depressant effect of higher doses on both transmission and conduction is probably due to an action unrelated to its anti-ChE activity. Furthermore, it was concluded that dose ranges producing facilitation of transmission had no consistent effect on preganglionic conduction.

Koelle (1957) found that in cats the intravenous injection of ambenonium chloride, a slowly reversible quaternary anti-ChE drug, produced an inhibition of the AChE localized only in the preganglionic fibers and their nerve endings, and at the periphery of the cholinergic ganglion cells. This portion of the enzyme, readily accessible to a lipoid-insoluble quaternary compounds, was named *external or functional AChE*. The uninhibited portions, within the cytoplasm of the cholinergic neurons, was named *internal or reserve AChE*. From the pharmacological point of view the concept of a dual localization of the enzyme is of the utmost importance, and McIsaac and Koelle (1959), utilizing a variety of tertiary and quaternary inhibitors, investigated the effect of progressive inactivation of external and total AChE on ganglionic transmission. The experiments were performed in cats anesthetized with ether followed by chloralose, and the effects of graded doses of the drugs studied were determined upon the contraction of the nictitating membrane, and upon the preganglionic and ganglionic action potentials in response to supramaximal stimulation of the partially resected preganglionic cervical sympathetic trunk. For the inhibition of *overall* AChE or the selective inhibition of *external* AChE, the tertiary and quaternary analogues of a potent, irreversible anti-ChE drug were used. The tertiary member, 2-diethoxyphosphinylthioethyldimethylamine acid oxalate(217AO), penetrates lipoidal membranes much more readily than the quaternary analogue, 2-diethoxyphosphinylthioethyltrimethylammonium iodide (217MI, echothiophate, Phospholine), the ratio of the respective oil-water partition coefficients being 217:1. The effects of selective inhibition of *internal* AChE were studied by injecting a reversible, quaternary anti-ChE agent, B.W. 284 (1,5-bis-(4-allyldimethylammoniumphenyl)pentan-3-one dibromide) or edrophonium chloride (3-hydroxyphenyldimethylethylammonium chloride, Tensilon), followed after a brief interval by a high dose of the irreversible, readily penetrating anti-ChE agent, DFP.

In these experiments, after partial resection of the preganglionic trunk and the administration of atropine, control contractions of the nictitating membrane were obtained before the intravenous administration of B.W. 284 (1 to 25 μg/kg) or edrophonium (1 to 2 mg/kg); immediately afterward, the animal received 3.68 mg (20 μmol) DFP/kg, intravenously, and the nictitating membrane response was recorded every 5 minutes for 1 hour. Three ganglia were tested: the superior cervical, the stellate, and the ciliary. Acetylcholinesterase inhibition was measured manometrically, and the cytological distribution of the residual AChE was examined histochemically.

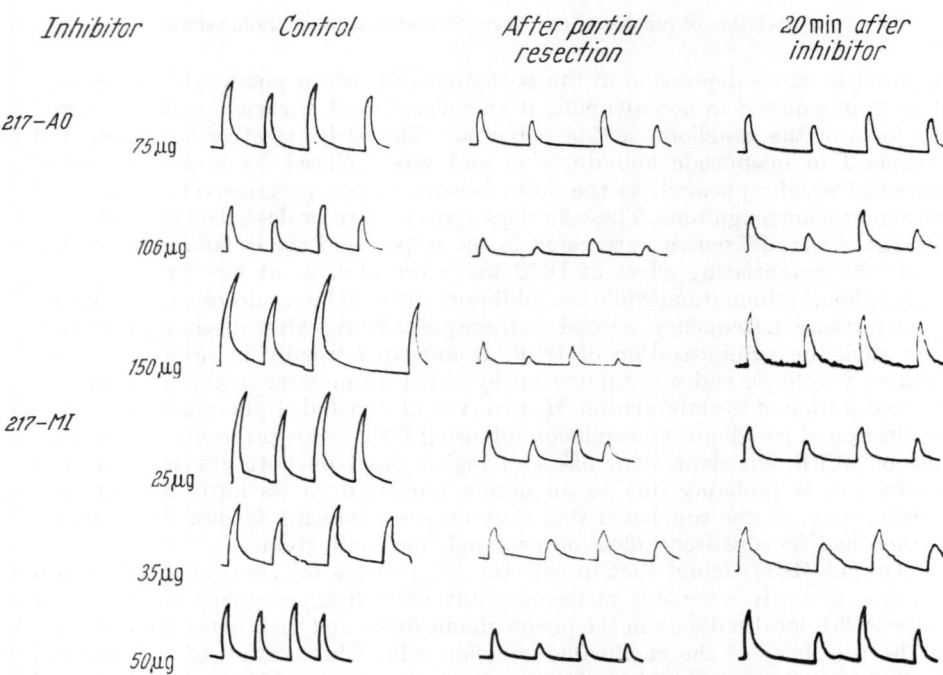

Fig. 5. Facilitation of contraction of the nictitating membrane in response to supramaximal stimulation of the partially resected preganglionic cervical sympathetic trunk at frequencies of 5 and 2 stimuli per sec following i.v. 217 AO and 217 MI (from McIsaac and Koelle 1959)

Table 1. *Effects of i.v. injection of 217 AO and 217 MI on ganglionic action potentials following supramaximal stimulation of the partially resected preganglionic trunk*
(from McIsaac and Koelle 1959)

Drug	Dose μg/kg	Ganglionic action potential % of control 20—60 min after drug	Ganglionic AChE Activity % of Control	
			Stellate	Superior cervical
None		107		
None		101	110	99
Atropine	500	98	105	98
217 MI	35	107	34	33
217 MI	35	152	11	6
217 MI	35	81	11	0
Average.		113 ± 21[1]	19 ± 8	13 ± 10
217 MI	50	195	1	11
217 MI	50	152	22	13
217 MI	50	113	28	23
Average.		153 ± 24	17 ± 8	16 ± 4
217 AO and	106	105	5	1
atropine	106	100	9	12
Average.		103	7	7
217 AO and	150	116	2	3
atropine	150	115	0	1
Average.		116	1	2
217 AO and	300	130	[2]	3
atropine	300	119	0	0
Average.		125		2

[1] Standard error of the mean.
[2] Sample lost.

Both the tertiary amine, 217 AO, and its quaternary analogue, 217 MI, were found to potentiate the reponse of the cat's nictitating membrane to supra-maximal stimulation of the partially resected preganglionic trunk (Fig. 5). Larger doses, however, of either drug reduced the response. Ganglionic potentials were similarly affected. The doses of the two compounds required for equivalent effects were inversely proportional to their anti-ChE potencies. However, the tertiary 217 AO produced a considerably greater degree of inhibition of the AChE of the superior cervical and stellate ganglia than did equally effective doses of the quaternary 217 MI. Table 1 illustrates these differences. The differences were even greater in the ciliary ganglion, which contains almost exclusively cholinergic ganglion cells and because of that a high proportion of intraneuronal AChE. Histochemical examination disclosed that in all ganglia following the administration of the tertiary agent the enzyme was inhibited nearly uniformly both at

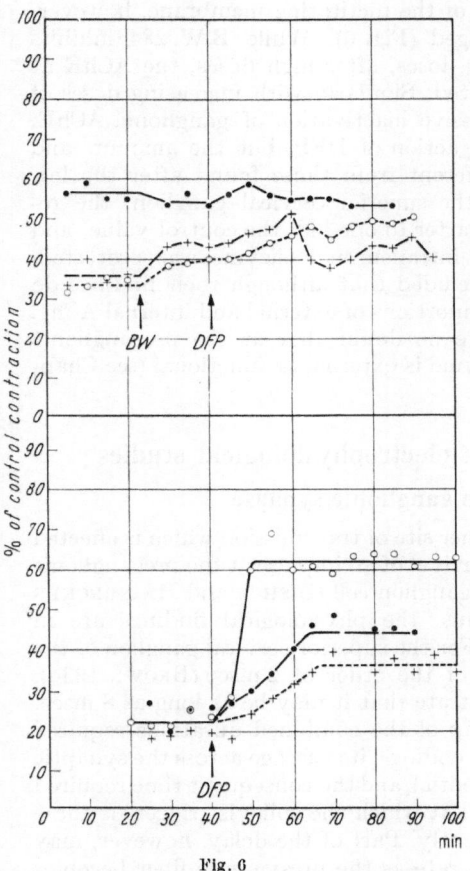

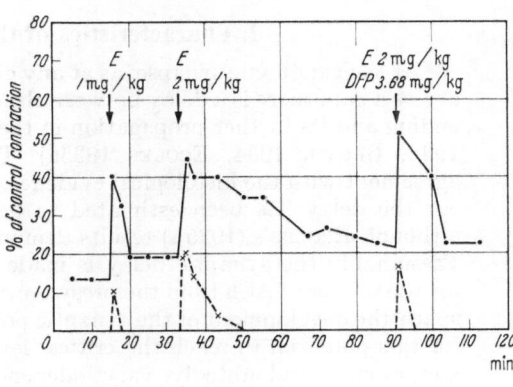

Fig. 6

Fig. 7

Fig. 6. Effects of DFP (3.68 mg/kg, i.v.) following B.W. 284 (3 μg/kg, i.v.) (upper chart), and DFP alone (lower chart) upon response of the nictitating membrane to supramaximal stimulation of the partially resected pre-ganglionic trunk. Experiments in upper chart identified in Table 4 as nos. 89 (+), 92 (○) and 99 (●), and in lower chart as nos. 96 (●), 85 (○) and 93 (+) (from McIsaac and Koelle 1959)

Fig. 7. Typical effect of edrophonium (E) alone and edrophonium followed in 10 sec by DFP on the response of the nictitating membrane to stimulation of the partially resected preganglionic nerve. Solid circles (●) represent contractions due to nerve stimulation, and crosses (X) represent spontaneous contractions (from McIsaac and Koelle 1959)

the preganglionic endings and within the cytoplasm of the cholinergic ganglionic neurons. In contrast, under the influence of the quaternary compound the enzyme was inhibited selectively at the preganglionic endings and was relatively unaffected at intra-neuronal sites (see p. 228). These findings strengthen the hypothesis that the pharmacological effects of anti-ChE drugs are due to inhibition of the enzyme only at external or functional sites which, in sympathetic ganglia, are represented chiefly by the preganglionic endings.

In a second series of experiments, McIsaac and Koelle demonstrated that in the presence of B.W.284, which protects the external AChE against irreversible inhibition by DFP, the latter compound, in doses large enough to inactivate practically all the internal enzyme, did not produce its usual potentiating effect. With 1 to 3 μg/kg of B.W. 284, followed by the administration of 3.6 mg/kg of DFP, no AChE activity was detected manometrically and only low concentrations were noted histochemically; the response of the nictitating membrane, however, to preganglionic stimulation was unchanged (Fig. 6). While B.W. 284 inhibits almost exclusively external AChE at low doses, after high doses, the AChE at intracellular sites was significantly protected. Similarly with increasing doses of the quaternary 217 MI, there was progressive inactivation of ganglionic AChE. Edrophonium prevented the potentiating action of DFP, but the amounts and sites of AChE protection were quite different from those found after the low protective dose of B.W. 284 (Fig. 7). In the superior cervical ganglion, the residual AChE activity ranged from one-quarter to one-half the control value, and in all ganglia a considerable amount of intraneuronal enzyme was protected. Because of these results, the authors concluded that although their findings do not permit quantitation of the absolute proportions of external and internal AChE in any of the ganglia studied, they leave no doubt that at the preganglionic cholinergic nerve endings most of the enzyme is external or functional (see Chapter 6).

D. Pharmacological effects based on electrophysiological studies

I. Characteristics of the ganglionic synapse

At the ganglionic synapse, as at any other site of transmission which is effected across a gap, there is a delay between the arrival of an impulse at the preganglionic ending and its further propagation in the ganglion cell (Bishop and Heinbecker 1932, Brown 1934, Eccles 1935a). Thus, the physiological findings are in agreement with the histological evidence. For the superior cervical ganglion of the cat the delay has been estimated to be of the order of 2 msec (Brown 1934), although Eccles's (1935a) results demonstrate that it may be as long as 8 msec. Presumably the synaptic delay is made up of the combined durations required for the release of ACh from the presynaptic endings, its passage across the synaptic space, the development of the synaptic potential, and the consequent time required for this potential to reach the critical level at which the spike is triggered; these factors may, undoubtedly, vary independently. Part of the delay, however, may be in the slowing down of the conduction rate as the presynaptic fiber becomes finer and finer towards its termination.

Another characteristic is that transmission across the synapse is essentially in one direction only. Thus, an antidromic discharge is not propagated from the postganglionic to the preganglionic fibers. However, it leaves the postganglionic neuron refractory, with the result that the effect of an immediately following preganglionic impulse may be extinguished at the synapse (Eccles 1936).

In the discussion of the anatomical arrangement in an autonomic ganglion, it was seen that a preganglionic fiber, through the great number of its nerve endings, may make connections with several postganglionic neurons and furthermore, that a single postganglionic neuron may have synaptic relations with endings belonging to various preganglionic fibers. Consequently, the simple case of a single fiber synapsing with a single ganglion cell is most unlikely to occur. Because of this multiple innervation of ganglion cells, impulses inadequate to stimulate were they to arrive alone may sum in their effects to produce a response in the postganglionic axon when arriving in several fibers almost simultaneously. Such an effect, due to convergence of impulses, is known as *spatial summation*. Another phenomenon characteristic of the ganglionic synapse is that of *facilitation* (temporal summation). This is brought about by the situation in which a series of impulses may induce, in several ganglion cells, a state of subliminal excitation, insufficient alone to initiate propagated impulses in the postsynaptic neurons. With the added effect, however, of further impulses impinging on the same ganglion cells, transmission across the synapse is now effected (Fig. 8). The response to this second set of impulses is said to be facilitated by the pre-established state of subliminal excitability. LARRABEE and BRONK (1947) showed that facilitation at a ganglionic synapse is clearly detectable after a single preganglionic volley; furthermore, that soon after a period of repetitive activity, many more ganglion cells respond to a volley of impulses travelling down a limited number of preganglionic fibers. For example, for many seconds, the amplitude of the postganglionic spike potential was found to be several-fold greater than the response to a similar preganglionic volley before the repetitive excitation. Following a detailed analysis of the

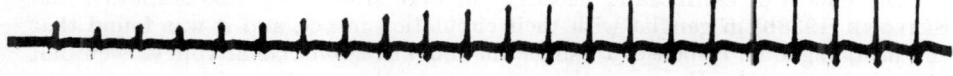

Fig. 8. Increase of postganglionic spike potentials during train of preganglionic volleys. Shows progressive recruitment of ganglion cells. Time: 0.5 sec (from BRONK 1939)

possible mechanisms involved in the facilitation process, LARRABEE and BRONK concluded that the prolonged facilitation is probably due to a persistent alteration of the terminals of the presynaptic fibers as a result of which the stimulating action of presynaptic impulses is increased. On the other hand, the branching and overlapping distribution of the preganglionic terminals makes possible not only summation, but also occlusion (SHERRINGTON 1929). When each of two or more active groups of terminals ending on the same ganglion cells can fire a response, a synchronous activation of the groups does not give simple addition of responses; in fact, some of the expected additive effect is lost, or occluded.

BRONK (1939), in his classical paper on synaptic mechanisms in sympathetic ganglia, gave an excellent account of the possible patterns of interaction. According to him, the ultimate response in the postganglionic nerve trunk is determined by the frequency of impulses arriving at each synapse and the number of synapses at which they arrive. Even subliminal excitations will ultimately affect the outcome if they persist long enough, for they will eventually summate provided the time relations are suitable.

II. Ganglionic potentials

For the study of ganglionic transmission, two sympathetic ganglia, the superior cervical and the stellate, and one parasympathetic, the ciliary, have been the preparations of choice. Unfortunately, in contrast to pharmacological analyses, the electrical investigations, so essential for knowledge of events taking place within seconds or milliseconds, have proved extremely difficult and will no doubt remain so until microelectrodes are used with more success in penetrating ganglion cells. Much of the present knowledge of electrical events has been obtained from extracellular recordings of the potentials generated by ganglia during activity.

1. Ganglia in vivo

The first attempt to record electrically the activity of a ganglion *in vivo* was apparently that made by FISCHER and LÖWENBACH (1933). They described an irregular series of spike potentials associated with the normal activity of the stellate ganglion and noticed at times slower potential changes as well. A more detailed analysis was made by ECCLES (1935a, b), recording with one electrode on the superior cervical ganglion and the other on the postganglionic trunk.

ECCLES (l.c.) demonstrated that the initial response is a spike potential during which the ganglion is, for a short period of time, strongly negative to its postganglionic trunk. Furthermore, he found that this first potential is followed by another slower negative potential during which the threshold of excitation is lowered, and later by a long-lasting positive one during which the threshold is raised. Similar slow potential waves were recorded by LLOYD (1937) from the inferior mesenteric ganglia. The normal action potential of a parasympathetic ganglion, the ciliary, was described by WHITTERIDGE (1937) who found that the complex was similar to that described by ECCLES for the superior cervical ganglion, and consisted of a rapid negative spike lasting some 5 to 10 msec, followed by a slow positive wave which lasted some 125 to 150 msec. A second spike component which followed the main spike and was usually smaller was observed and was attributed to a group of fibers with slower time relationships. According to WHITTERIDGE, the whole action potential complex of the ciliary ganglion lasts only about 150 msec and is thus much shorter than that in the superior cervical ganglion which lasts about 500 msec. Doubts, however, have been expressed as to whether the slow potential waves are cell body potentials or accentuated after-potentials due to local conditions (BRONK et al. 1938).

The effects of eserine and neostigmine were studied by ROSENBLUETH and SIMEONE (1938b) in ganglia with their circulation intact, and it was found that the postganglionic responses to single maximal or submaximal volleys were not altered significantly. However, the negativity of the ganglion with respect to the postganglionic trunk appeared to be increased, and the responses of the ganglion to two shocks applied, at short intervals, to the preganglionic trunk were usually greater. ECCLES, too (1944) found that the eserinized ganglion does not discharge repetitively in response to a single preganglionic volley, nor is the time course of of the slow potential waves much affected.

2. Isolated ganglia

In the superior cervical sympathetic ganglion, either isolated and perfused (BROWN and FELDBERG 1936a) or isolated and immersed in KREB's solution (R. ECCLES 1952a), a preganglionic volley produced an action potential which showed, in general, many of the features of the action potential recorded from a ganglion with its natural circulation.

R. ECCLES (1955), PASCOE (1955), and MALCOLM and PERRY (1955) attempted to insert microelectrodes into ganglion cells. This, however, proved a very difficult task and was met with partial success only. The main difficulty apparently lies in the tough, fibrous capsule which surrounds each individual cell. Using the rabbit's isolated superior cervical ganglion immersed in KREB's solution, R. ECCLES found that the majority of the recorded resting potentials fell in the range of 65 to 80 mV but remained at this value for a very short time, usually no more than several minutes; preganglionic stimulation elicited spikes up to 90 mV of 4 to 7 msec duration, with an inflection (identified as the synaptic potential) on the rising phase; finally, slow after-potentials were occasionally recorded following the main spike potential, but very often their time course was obscured by the cell injury caused by the insertion of the microelectrodes. In these experiments, just before the insertion of the microelectrodes the oxygen supply was cut down in order to prevent any movement. This reduction of O_2 supply might well have influenced some of the results. In PASCOE's experiments, the microelectrode was mounted on a piezoelectric crystal and moved forward by passing a direct current pulse through the crystal. With this technique, resting potentials from 20 to 60 mV were recorded for the superior cervical ganglion of the rat, *in vitro* and *in vivo*. The resting potentials, however, showed a rapid decay and preganglionic stimulation produced a synaptic potential which only occasionally showed a small superimposed spike. Finally, MALCOLM and PERRY, using the superior cervical ganglion of the rat immersed in LOCKE's solution, attempted to facilitate the entry of the microelectrode by "digesting the ganglion" with a mixture of trypsin and hyaluronidase. Resting potentials of the order of 40 to 85 mV were recorded but transmitted spikes were never seen.

III. Synaptic potential

In the presence of curare the ganglionic spike potential is abolished and replaced by a relatively prolonged local response, the synaptic potential, which is attributable to the depolarization of the ganglion cells by the transmitter. This was demonstrated by ECCLES (1943) in the cat's superior cervical ganglion, *in vivo*, and by R. ECCLES (1952a, b) in the rabbit's isolated superior cervical ganglion *in vitro*.

A synaptic potential is a non-propagated local response, an electrotonic potential that falls off exponentially with increasing distance from the postjunctional region. Its outstanding characteristic is that it is a graded response and therefore it can be modified; for example, the stronger the stimulus, the greater the degree of depolarization of the postsynaptic membrane leading to a greater synaptic potential. This is in contrast to the propagated response which is an all-or-nothing event and consequently can be blocked but not otherwise modified. Furthermore, the synaptic potential has no refractory period; thus, additional potentials can sum with it. The moment this summated effect reaches a critical level of depolarization, it triggers the electrically propagated all-or-nothing action potential which travels along the postganglionic neuron leaving a period of refractoriness behind it.

From experiments performed in the curarized cat's stellate ganglion with its circulation intact, ECCLES (1944) concluded that the only effect produced, even by the largest dose of eserine, on the synaptic potentials was a lengthening of their time course. When fully developed with large doses of eserine (6 or more mg/kg), the size of the prolonged potential was found to be approximately proportional to the number of preganglionic volleys, provided that the rate of stimulation was not below 20/sec, or above 140/sec when the impulse ceased to be fully effective.

The time course of the synaptic potential obtained by R. ECCLES in the curarized *isolated* superior cervical ganglion was considerably longer than that obtained by ECCLES in the ganglion with its normal circulation. For example, the synaptic potential in the *isolated* superior cervical ganglion decayed to a half at 80 to 110 msec from onset, while that in the ganglion *in vivo* had practically disappeared at 40 msec. Furthermore, R. ECCLES's (1952b) recordings in the presence of tubocurarine ($1.6 \times 10^{-5} M$) revealed a prolonged late negative wave, following the positive wave. With progressively increasing doses of tubocurarine (up to $8 \times 10^{-5} M$) and following a brief preganglionic tetanus at frequency rates ranging from 20 to 60/sec, the synaptic potential was greatly decreased and both the positive and the late negative waves were increased. The addition of neostigmine ($3 \times 10^{-8} M$) produced two widely differing effects; in the presence of just-blocking concentrations of tubocurarine, it lengthened the slow decay of the negative wave, while in the presence of larger concentrations of tubocurarine it increased and greatly prolonged the positive wave and it depressed, delayed, and eventually abolished the late negative wave.

From these experiments, R. ECCLES concluded that the effect of neostigmine in prolonging and increasing the positive wave indicates that high concentrations of curare do actually reverse the action of ACh from "the normal depolarizing to a polarizing action". However, changes in "shapes" of responses obtained from ganglia isolated and immersed in fluids (considered "physiological" by investigators, but possibly not so by the ganglia), under the influence of large quantities of active drugs may not represent physiological or pharmacological events of great importance.

IV. Repetitive stimulation

When the postganglionic action potential of a ganglion with its *normal circulation intact* is recorded during repetitive stimulation of a preganglionic nerve at frequencies below 5/sec, the successive responses are found to be relatively constant in height. At frequencies above 20/sec the successive volleys become smaller, the rate of failure depending upon the frequency of stimulation. For example, at frequencies above 40/sec there is a rapid decline of the successive spike potentials (ROSENBLUETH and SIMEONE 1938a, BRONK 1939, ECCLES 1944, LARRABEE and BRONK 1947). ECCLES (1944) found that eserine in doses up to 8 mg/kg had no significant effect on spike heights during tetanic stimulation with frequencies ranging from 12 to 130/sec. Similar results were obtained by BRONK et al. (1938). In contrast, ROSENBLUETH and SIMEONE (1938b) reported that both eserine and neostigmine modified strikingly the response to repetitive stimulation, causing a progressive decrease in spike height with frequencies at about 20/sec. ECCLES, discussing this discrepancy, suggested that the results obtained by ROSENBLUETH and SIMEONE were probably due to poor circulation through the ganglia.

V. After-discharge

Many ganglion cells which have been discharging impulses in response to a train of rapidly recurring preganglionic volleys continue in action for some time after the end of the preganglionic stimulation (Fig. 9). The duration of this after-discharge is graded by the frequency and duration of the previous excitation (BRONK 1939). According to ECCLES (1944) an after-discharge is invariably set up after short bursts of rapid preganglionic tetanization, for example, by 25 stimuli at 130/sec. Although the frequency of stimulation needs to be higher than would be found physiologically, this after-discharge is of particular interest since sympathetic ganglia certainly contain no interneurons and they therefore furnish an example of one type of prolonged excitatory state which cannot be due to activity in chains of interneurons.

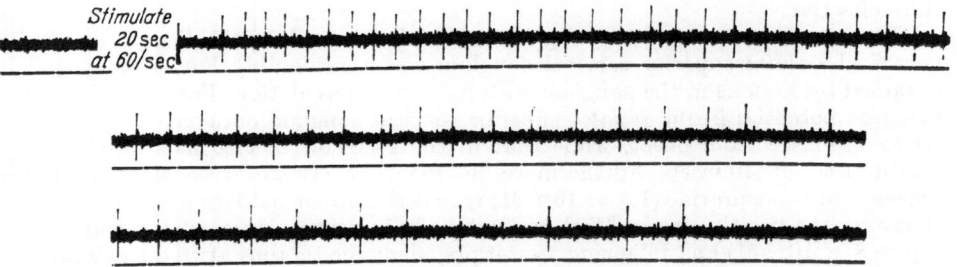

Fig. 9. Repetitive after-discharge from a ganglion cell following 20 sec of preganglionic stimulation at 60 per sec. Continuous record. Last impulse 27 sec after end of stimulation. Time: 0.5 sec (from BRONK 1939)

Eserine increases and prolongs the after-discharge set up by rapid repetitive stimulation, and furthermore it also causes it to occur with rates too slow to give after-discharges from the non-eserinized ganglion (ROSENBLUETH and SIMEONE 1938b, ECCLES 1944). For example, a very small and brief after-discharge is increased and prolonged by 0.1 mg/kg of eserine and is enormously affected by a further 0.2 mg/kg. According to ECCLES (1944), in the eserinized ganglion the important factor determining after-discharge is the number of preganglionic volleys and not the rate of stimulation, which is the criterion for the non-eserinized ganglion.

An interesting phenomenon, observed in perfused ganglia subjected to repetitive stimulation in the presence of an anti-ChE drug, was reported by EMMELIN and MACINTOSH (1956). By using the nictitating membrane responses as an indicator, it was found that at the end of a period of repetitive stimulation the nictitating membrane relaxed almost as rapidly and completely as if no anti-ChE drug had been present in the perfusion fluid; soon, however, it began to contract again and the recording rose slowly and smoothly to a maximum that was maintained for many minutes, and was sometimes not far below that seen with preganglionic excitation. The phenomenon was seen during perfusion with Locke's solution, plasma, or blood in the presence of eserine, neostigmine, DFP, or TEPP. According to EMMELIN and MacINTOSH, it was certainly due to discharge of ganglion cells, for it could be inhibited temporarily either by blocking the postganglionic trunk by cold or by the addition of a small dose of procaine HCl to the perfusion fluid. But it was not due to the persistence of free ACh in the ganglion, since it was not modified by the addition of tubocurarine or hexamethonium to the perfusion fluid. Moreover, no trace of ACh could be detected in the effluent obtained during even the most intense discharge of this type. The late onset of this response and its long duration made EMMELIN and MacINTOSH wonder if the mechanism behind it was similar to that which elicits an after-discharge in eserinized ganglia *in vivo*. The differences, however, may be only apparent and due to the fact that in ganglionic preparations with their normal blood supply, the time course of the various processes appears as a rule shorter than that in ganglia which are isolated and perfused, or are isolated and immersed in various fluids.

VI. Direct application of acetylcholine

The demonstration that the effects of nerve impulses can be reproduced by ACh applied directly to an autonomic ganglion has been one of the foundation stones on which the theory of chemical transmission was built.

In a masterly series of experiments, BRONK (1939) described the action of ACh added to the fluid perfusing an autonomic ganglion.

The stellate ganglion of the cat was prepared and the activity of its ganglion cells was recorded in the postganglionic fibres of the inferior cardiac nerve. It was found that ACh, in a concentration of 100 μg/ml of perfusion fluid, caused a vigorous discharge of impulses from the ganglion cells (Fig. 10). Moreover, when the discharge of impulses from a single cell was studied, it was found that ACh initiated rhythmically recurring impulses which continued as long as the level of ACh was maintained by the perfusion. There was no evidence, however, of adaptation or failure provided the concentration of ACh was below that which caused paralysis. The frequency of the discharge increased with increasing concentrations of ACh, but finally, with a large dose, the excitatory action ceased, the discharge of impulses was arrested, and the ganglion cells could no longer be stimulated by volleys of preganglionic impulses. BRONK concluded also that the sensitivity of the preganglionic nerve endings to ACh must be strikingly different from that of ganglion cells, as he was unable to find any evidence of stimulation of the preganglionic fibers even when as much as 500 μg of ACh was added to each ml of perfusion fluid (Fig. 10).

More recently, DOUGLAS et al. (1960) obtained similar results from a number of experiments on the isolated superior cervical ganglion of the rabbit. Eserine sulphate, $1 \times 10^{-5} M$, was added to the perfusion fluid and it was found that although ACh could now initiate discharges in the postganglionic nerves in concentrations ten times smaller than those effective before eserine, there were again no discharges in the preganglionic trunk. Furthermore, PASCOE (1956), in experiments on the isolated superior cervical ganglion of rats and rabbits, found that ACh produced a rapid depolarization which was restricted to the ganglion cells and did not involve the preganglionic nerve endings.

Recently, RIKER and SZRENIAWSKI (1959) found that ACh injected intra-arterially into the common carotid artery elicited repetitive activity in both the pre- and postganglionic nerves of the cat's superior cervical ganglion. From these results the authors concluded that the presynaptic nerve terminals are a significant site of drug action. Such an interpretation, however, was questioned by DOUGLAS et al. (1960) who carried out a similar study but demonstrated that the activity recorded in the preganglionic trunk was, in fact, postganglionic activity due to ACh stimulating aberrant ganglion cells. Apparently thousands of aberrant

ganglion cells may be present along the length of the cervical sympathetic trunk
between the stellate and the superior cervical ganglia. Therefore the postganglionic

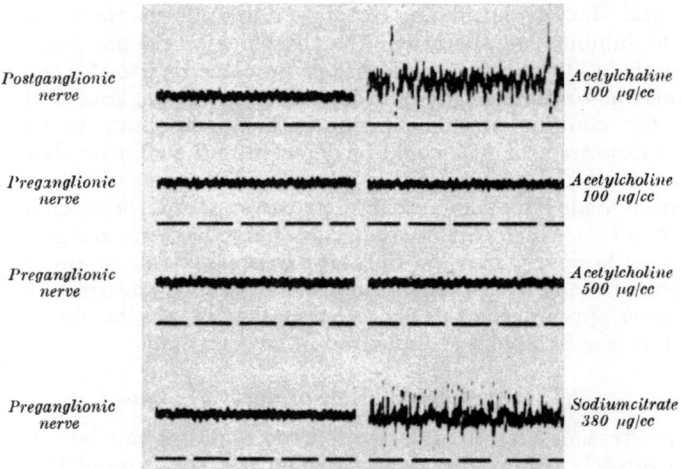

Postganglionic nerve — *Acetylcholine 100 µg/cc*

Preganglionic nerve — *Acetylcholine 100 µg/cc*

Preganglionic nerve — *Acetylcholine 500 µg/cc*

Preganglionic nerve — *Sodiumcitrate 380 µg/cc*

Fig. 10. Preganglionic and postganglionic responses to ACh and sodium citrate. Controls with Ringer's fluid in
left hand column. Time: 0.1 sec (from BRONK 1939)

fibers arising from these various cells intermingle with the preganglionic fibers
supplying the superior cervical ganglion. Moreover, in addition to these fibers,
there may be others which descend caudally from ganglion cells located in the

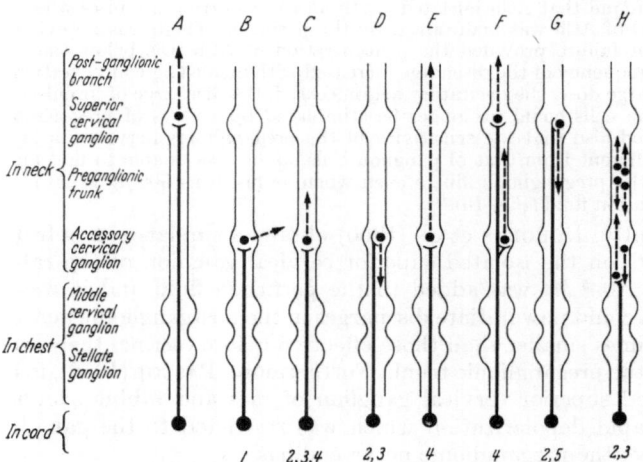

Fig. 11. Diagrams showing arrangements of pre- and postganglionic fibres in the cervical sympathetic trunk.
A, the conventional arrangement. *B-H*, Alternative arrangements known to occur. Preganglionic fibres are
indicated by the solid lines; postganglionic fibres by the interrupted lines. The numbers below each diagram
refer to the original papers and the animals studied: References: 1. LANGLEY, J. N., J. Physiol 14, i—ii (1893),
cat. 2. FOLEY, J. O., J. Comp. Neurol. 82, 77—92 (1945), cat. 3. BUTSON, A. R. C., Brit. J. Surg. 38, 223—239
(1950), cat, rabbit. 4. DOUGLAS, W. W., and J. M. RITCHIE, J. Physiol. 133, 220—231 (1956), rabbit. 5. DOUGLAS,
W. W., et al., J. Physiol. 153, 250—264 (1960), rabbit (from DOUGLAS et al. 1960)

superior cervical ganglion. Fig. 11 shows possible arrangements of pre- and
postganglionic fibers as schematized by DOUGLAS et al. (1960). The same conclusion

was reached by ECCLES (1944) from experiments on the cat's stellate ganglion *in vivo*. ECCLES noticed that in the presence of eserine, the after-discharge set up by a short burst of rapid preganglionic stimulation could be recorded both post- and preganglionically. However, various tests applied in order to analyze this phenomenon demonstrated that the after-discharge was, in fact, occurring in postganglionic fibers passing from the stellate ganglion to the upper thoracic spinal nerves. Quite obviously, activity recorded in the preganglionic trunk is not due to ACh setting up antidromic impulses in the preganglionic nerve fibers.

The preganglionic nerve endings appear also to be less sensitive to potassium, the potent paralysing effect of which on ganglion cells does not extend to the fine terminals of the preganglionic fibers until long after the ganglion cells have been seriously affected. This was demonstrated by BROWN and FELDBERG (1936a) on the perfused cervical sympathetic ganglion of the cat. In experiments in which a contraction of the nictitating membrane was maintained by prolonged preganglionic stimulation, the injection of a small volume of KCl solution inhibited the contraction. Nevertheless, throughout the continued stimulation, the output of ACh was maintained at a level as high as that during the full contraction of the nictitating membrane.

VII. Depolarization of ganglion cells by acetylcholine

PATON and PERRY (1953) were the first to produce evidence of a local electrical response of the ganglion cell to injected ACh. In cats anesthetized with chloralose, the superior cervical ganglion was prepared with its blood supply intact. Through recording electrodes, one looped around the body of the ganglion, the other placed at the point where the postganglionic trunk had been tied and cut, potential differences were measured. As Fig. 12 shows, a negativity of the ganglion relative to the cut postganglionic trunk was recorded as an upward deflexion, whether transiently due to an action potential, or as a relatively prolonged rise in base line due to a steady depolarization. Acetylcholine injected intra-arterially (1 to 10 μg) or intravenously (200 μg) gave rise to a transient depolarization of the ganglion. Larger doses of ACh, or small doses in the presence of 200 μg of eserine adminis-

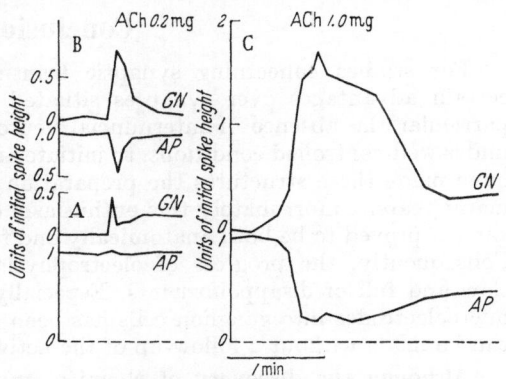

Fig. 12. The effect of acetylcholine on the spike height of the ganglionic action and the depolarization of the ganglion cells. *GN*, ganglionic negativity in terms of initial spike height; *AP*, spike height of action potential. *A*, effect of 200 μg acetylcholine after 200 μg eserine i.v.; *C*, effect of 1.0 mg acetylcholine i.v. (from PATON and PERRY 1953)

tered intravenously, produced a larger depolarization accompanied by a reduction in spike height (Fig. 12). From the fact that the ganglionic body became negative to the postganglionic trunk after treatment with ACh, PATON and PERRY concluded that the depolarization is a local response of the ganglion cells and spreads only decrementally down the postganglionic trunk. Thus, ACh at the ganglion, as at the neuromuscular junction, can cause a localized depolarization of the cell membrane, which is then capable of exciting the discharge in the postsynaptic fiber. From the short-lived depolarization and its considerable prolongation by eserine, the authors concluded that the ChE activity at the ganglion is considerable. An interesting finding was that large doses of eserine, in the absence of ACh, abolished the action potential without producing any depolarization of the ganglion. This type of eserine block was seen only after single shocks; tetani released sufficient ACh to produce a depolarization.

PERRY and TALESNIK (1953), using the same technique and the same animal species, studied the effect of ACh at the synapses of a parasympathetic ganglion. The ciliary ganglion was chosen, and it was found that the ganglion cells were depolarized by ACh and that, in general, the pattern of responses was closely similar to that described by PATON and PERRY (1953) for the superior cervical ganglion. Thus, direct evidence was produced that the postsynaptic parasympathetic ganglion cells are sensitive to ACh.

Depolarization of ganglion cells by ACh was demonstrated also by PASCOE (1956) in isolated ganglia from rats and rabbits. Recordings from the superior cervical ganglion immersed in LOCKE's solution containing $3 \times 10^{-6} M$ neostigmine methyl sulphate, showed that the addition of ACh in a concentration of $10^{-5} M$ produced a rapid depolarization which was restricted to the ganglion cells and did not involve the preganglionic terminals. Neostigmine, itself, depolarized the ganglion cells. However, with the concentration used in these experiments $(3 \times 10^{-6} M)$, the effect was small. On washing out ACh, the depolarization was replaced by a positive over-swing; in other words the ganglion became temporarily positive to the postganglionic trunk. In discussing these results, PASCOE pointed out, quite rightly, that with external recording it is very difficult to state with certainty the cause of this potential change.

Conclusions

For studies concerning synaptic transmission, autonomic ganglia present certain advantages over synapses situated in the central nervous system. In particular the absence of internuncial neurons and the ability of the ganglion, under well-controlled conditions, to initiate and conduct impulses for long periods, have made these structures the preparation of choice to electrophysiologists for many years. Unfortunately this enthusiasm did not last indefinitely because the ganglia proved to be both anatomically and functionally very complex structures. Consequently, the progress of electrophysiological studies has been relatively slow and full of disappointments. Especially the lack of success in introducing microelectrodes into ganglion cells has been a great handicap as no real analysis can be made without a follow-up of the activity of single neurons.

Although the discovery of chemical transmission occurred nearly simultaneously at both sites, the study of the ganglionic synapse lags behind that of the neuromuscular junction. Thus, very reluctantly we have to draw the conclusion today, that specific junctional changes taking place at the ganglionic synapse cannot be decided from the available information.

Because of these technical difficulties ganglionic and postganglionic potentials, elicited by electrical stimulation of the preganglionic trunk, have often been used as a measure of variations in the activity of the ganglion cells. However electrical stimulation of preganglionic fibers is very unlike the natural activity in the preganglionic nerve and the consequent sequence of events which follows at the synapse. Under normal conditions, the ganglion cell is subjected to trains of rhythmically recurring waves of activity conducted along some of the preganglionic fibers. Furthermore the rhythmic activity of the various fibers probably differs both in frequency and in phase. In contrast, when a maximal electrical stimulus is applied to the preganglionic trunk supplying the ganglion, all nerve fibers are induced to fire simultaneously. This in turn leads to a discharge, although not quite synchronous, of all the ganglion cells.

BROWN and MATTHEWS (1960) have shown in the cat that when a muscle is activated by a single maximal shock applied to its nerve, the resulting twitch is larger and lasts longer than that produced by slightly asynchronous activation of the same muscle fibers. Furthermore, when recording from the ventral roots they found that a synchronous nerve volley was followed by a "back-response", presumably due to restimulation of the same nerve fibers by the muscle action potential. They concluded, therefore, that the synchronized twitch is abnormal because it may include the response of some muscle fibers contracting tetanically, as a result of excitation circling from nerve to muscle and back again. Such an ephaptically induced "back-response" may be excited in the fine terminals of any motor axon, and spread from there to the other branches of the same axon; its demonstration, therefore, well emphasizes the dangers of investigating the function of the nervous system by initiating synchronous volleys of nerve impulses.

Potentials recorded from the ganglia and the postganglionic trunk depend on the amount of ACh liberated by the nerve terminals, on the activity of the ChE's, and on the sensitivity of the ganglion cell membrane.

KATZ and his colleagues (see KATZ 1958) have demonstrated that the quantum of ACh which is liberated from the nerve terminals is remarkably constant and unaffected by any experimental procedures whether they be drugs, changes in ionic environment, temperature, or osmotic differences. On the other hand, the frequency at which the quanta of ACh are liberated can be easily and markedly affected by factors which change the conditions of the nerve ending. Alterations in the chemical environment and the frequency of preganglionic stimulation appear to be important factors for the normal activity of the nerve endings.

LARRABEE and BRONK (1952) have studied the metabolism of sympathetic neurons *in vitro* and *in situ* under conditions of rest and of action. Their main measurements were concerned with rates of uptake of oxygen and of glucose, and with functional effects resulting from lack of oxygen and of glucose. Frequently during their experiments the metabolic requirements of the sympathetic neuron were compared with those of somatic nerves, and the results obtained revealed extremely interesting differences.

For example, they found that when glucose was withdrawn there was a failure of both the preganglionic and postganglionic responses, the latter falling more rapidly. Thus in the absence of glucose the capacity for function can be lost, not only by the intraganglionic structures but also by the axons of the sympathetic neurons. Furthermore, it was found that this axonal failure could be greatly accelerated by activity. This susceptibility of the sympathetic structures to lack of glucose contrasts strikingly with the well known resistance exhibited by certain somatic nerve fibers. A further interesting observation was that at rest, failure in the absence of glucose could be considerably delayed by reduction of temperature. In contrast, during stimulation at a frequency of 6/sec, the rate of failure appeared to be altogether independent of temperature. The postganglionic action potential fell to half its initial height in about 15 min at all temperatures from 21 to 39°. This implies that in activity, the frequency of action becomes the dominant regulator of the biological processes going on at the ganglionic synapse.

LARRABEE and BRONK demonstrated also that at rest, sympathetic ganglia consume oxygen several times faster than preganglionic, postganglionic, or somatic nerve trunks. During activity, however, percentage increases as great as those in ganglia were found in sympathetic trunks. Thus the increments in rate of oxygen uptake were very different during activity in somatic and in sympathetic nerve trunks, despite their similarities at rest. The rate of oxygen consumption increased with frequency of preganglionic stimulation up to 10 or 15/sec, but no further increase was seen at higher frequencies. According to LARRABEE and BRONK this appeared to be related to a failure of ganglion cells to respond to every volley of presynaptic impulses above 10 or 15/sec, because the height of the postganglionic potential declined when these frequencies were exceeded.

KRNJEVIČ and MILEDI (1959) have found that repetitive stimulation of rat muscle *in vitro* or *in situ* leads to presynaptic block of nerve conduction which may be intermittent or complete but which is reversed when the stimulation is stopped or continued at a lower rate. With an intracellular micro-electrode in the region of the endplate, presynaptic failures were easily recognised, since unlike the other types of block no local endplate potentials could be recorded. According to KRNJEVIČ and MILEDI the most likely sites for the presynaptic block seemed to be points of branching of the fiber where the safety factor of transmission is sharply reduced. In both *in vitro* and *in situ* preparations stimulation of the nerve at 50/sec usually caused intermittent failure of many fibers within 2 to 5 min. As a rule, however, the frequency needed for the appearance of failure was lower *in vitro* (very often 10 to 30/sec) than *in situ*. Furthermore, presynaptic block, especially *in vitro*, was precipitated by anoxia and found to be very sensitive to warming or cooling.

As the oxygen requirements of the autonomic nerve fibers during activity are greater than those of somatic nerves, and as the preganglionic nerve terminals are very fine and follow a long and elaborate course, it would be only too easy for conduction to fail along them. The influence of such variables must therefore be carefully considered as they can easily alter the results obtained from experiments in which either the output of ACh or the magnitude of the ganglionic potential is measured. In such experiments a steady frequency of stimulation is usually applied to the preganglionic trunk. However, very often, after a certain period of stimulation, the ACh output or the height of the ganglionic or postganglionic spike potential is reduced. Preganglionic failures of the type just described may be the cause of these reduced responses more often than it is generally realized.

Uncertainties of interpretation also arise because different effects have been observed under different experimental conditions; for example, it would appear that there are some fundamental differences between *in situ* and *in vitro* measurements.

Here the difficulty at once arises that there is no means of proving that the physiological properties of isolated tissues suffer no alteration through being separated from the body of which these tissues are an integral part. ECCLES (1935a) found that when the blood supply to the ganglion was interfered with by the division of its vessels, all the ganglionic processes exhibited a longer time course. For example, the latent period of the ganglionic action potential was more than double, its constituent waves became slower, and the refractory period showed a corresponding lengthening. However, a similar lengthening in the time course of the various processes appears, as we have already discussed, in ganglia which are isolated and perfused or are isolated and immersed in various fluids. Furthermore autonomic ganglia with their circulation intact respond much better and for longer periods of time to repetitive preganglionic stimulation than ganglia *in vitro*. And as a rule, even under the best possible experimental conditions, the margin of safety of an isolated preparation has proved to be lower than that of a ganglion in an essentially intact condition.

During the last few years information has slowly accumulated which indicates that there are considerable changes in the ionic content of isolated tissues following immersion in physiological saline solutions. CREESE and his colleagues (CREESE and NORTHOVER 1961, CREESE, D'SILVA and NORTHOVER 1958, CREESE, SCHOLES and WHALEN 1958) studied in detail some of the alterations produced.

For example, it was found that rat diaphragm muscle immersed in saline solution for 2 hr at 38° showed a substantial rise in sodium content when compared with normal values *in vivo*, and furthermore that in the presence of dialysed human serum the total sodium of the muscle and the fiber sodium were maintained at normal values. Functional alterations which may follow changes of ionic concentrations are well exemplified by the following results.

According to FATT (1954), in a curarized frog muscle at 20° the endplate potential recorded from a single endplate has a rising phase of 1 to 1.5 msec, and declines to one-half in a further 2 msec. In the presence of neostigmine or eserine the rising phase has a duration of about 2 msec after which the decay to one-half takes another 5 msec. This results, of course, from a prolongation of the active depolarizing phase. Furthermore, FATT showed that when curare is applied in progressively increasing doses, the duration of the endplate potential shortens and finally in higher concentrations the potential decreases without further change in time course. In a second series of experiments, however, in which a solution of low sodium content was used, FATT found that the rising phase of the endplate potential takes about 2 msec and the time to one-half decay is another 6 msec. Moreover, when neostigmine is added to a solution with low sodium content, it results in an endplate potential starting with the normal rate of rise, but which has a flattened summit lasting for 30 to 40 msec and decays to one-half in another 100 msec. Thus the duration of this endplate potential is of an entirely different order of magnitude from that obtained from the curarized, neostigmine-treated endplate immersed in a solution with normal sodium content.

From the results of MacINTOSH and his colleagues, discussed previously, it is obvious that ganglia perfused with heparinized plasma function much more satisfactorily than ganglia perfused with a physiological saline solution. It appears, therefore, that a ganglion *in vitro* may undergo considerable alterations which are brought to the surface especially when the activity is rapid or when the responses of the ganglion cells to various drugs are studied.

For efficient ganglionic activity, rapid elimination of ACh is very important because if the substance should persist for a long time in high concentrations, it would rapidly lead to a failure of transmission. This was clearly shown in PATON and PERRY's (1953) experiments which demonstrated that injected ACh produced a longlasting depolarization of the cell membrane during which transmission was blocked.

In contrast to the neuromuscular junction, at the ganglionic synapse most of the functional ChE exists in the presynaptic terminals and not at the post-synaptic membrane (KOELLE and KOELLE 1959). Because of this localization, the question has frequently arisen whether the presence of the enzyme is essential for the termination of the activity of ACh. In general, it is believed that although the enzyme plays an important role, there is probably another mechanism involved. It has even been suggested that diffusion alone may be adequate (OGSTON 1955, EMMELIN and MacINTOSH 1956). OGSTON has calculated that if ACh were suddenly liberated at the centre of a spherical aqueous volume of 1 μ radius and allowed to dissipate by diffusion alone, the mean concentration of ACh within the sphere would be lowered by 90% in 1.7 msec. Moreover, EMMELIN and MacINTOSH suggested that it may be unnecessary for the whole of the free ACh to be removed within the refractory period, for it is possible that ACh stimulates the ganglion cells most effectively when its concentration is rising steeply.

Accordingly, alternative or additional functions of the presynaptically local-ized ChE should be considered. One possibility is that the enzyme serves as an extra line of defense to prevent the activation of adjacent neurons. Recently, KOELLE (1961) put forward the suggestion that ACh, released at the presynaptic terminals by a nerve impulse, may have a dual role: a transmitter action at the postsynaptic site, and an action effecting the release of additional quanta of ACh from the nerve endings. Consequently, according to KOELLE, the primary function of the presynaptic ganglionic enzyme would be to limit the effect of ACh on the presynaptic terminals themselves (see Chapter 6).

Cholinesterases (both AChE and BuChE) are widely distributed in animal tissue. For example, all nerve fibers, whether or not they contain ACh and choline acetylase (ChAc), do contain AChE in relatively high concentrations. Unfortu-nately we do not know its function there, nor do we know its function in other tissues such as the red blood cells. Similarly the physiological meaning of BuChE remains a mystery. Furthermore it is difficult at present to assign a function for all the ACh and ChAc of non-nervous origin. Good examples of such tissues are the placenta of humans and primates or the spleen of oxen and horses.

During the last few years evidence has been produced that the various members of the cholinergic system may be involved in the active transport of materials across membranes. KIRSCHNER (1953) showed that anti-ChE drugs can inhibit the active sodium transport across isolated frog skin.

For example he found that TEPP added to the inside of the skin produced a transient rise in the net flux of sodium ions (inflow minus outflow) followed by an irreversible inhibition which was virtually complete in an hour (Fig. 13). Eserine on the other hand produced a reversible inhibition. Furthermore, he found that when the drugs were applied to the outside of the skin, eserine was more or less ineffective, and TEPP stopped the net movement of sodium at concentrations greater than $10^{-2} M$, possibly then because of structural damage. An interesting finding was that atropine applied to the outside of the skin produced a marked increase in the transport of the sodium ions.

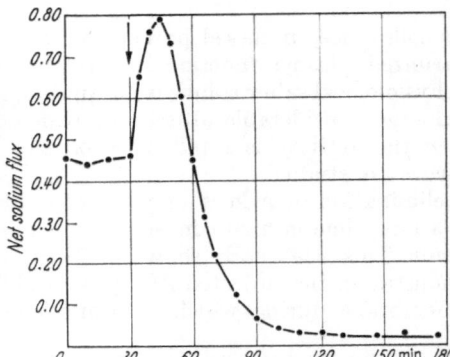

Fig. 13. Effect of tetraethylpyrophosphate on the active transport of sodium ions. The drug was added at the arrow to a concentration of $6 \times 10^{-3} M$. The net flux is in μM per cm² of skin per hr (from KIRSCHNER 1953)

VAN DER KLOOT (1956 and 1958) studied the role of ChE on the sodium transport of the sartorius muscle of the frog.

He placed the muscle in RINGER solution in which one half of the sodium chloride had been replaced by sucrose. Under these conditions, although the concentration of sodium in the solution still exceeded that within the muscle fiber, the muscle responded by actively transporting sodium ions into the external fluid, so that after 30 min the sodium content of the muscle had markedly decreased. This decrease in sodium content was prevented by the previous exposure of the muscle to HETP or by the addition of eserine to the RINGER solution. The eserine inhibition was reversible. In contrast, neostigmine was found to be ineffective. Apparently the substance must be able to penetrate into the muscle fiber. Furthermore, in experiments in which the effects of graded concentrations of eserine on the transport of sodium and on the activity of ChE were measured, it was found that the concentrations of eserine which inhibited sodium extrusion produced a comparable inhibition in the activity of the intracellular ChE.

From these and other experiments, VAN DER KLOOT put forward the suggestion that "cholinesterase is part of a cellular mechanism for ion regulation which, in the course of evolution has been adapted to serve the ever more complex needs of excitable tissues and of synaptic junctions."

KOCH (1954) studied the influence of anti-ChE drugs on the active transport of sodium through the isolated gills of the crab, *Eriocheir sinensis*.

The gills of this freshwater crab continue to absorb ions when isolated from the body. KOCH found that 1 g of fresh gill tissue is able to hydrolyse 43 mg of ACh per hour. This figure compares favourably with the figure of 5 to 50 mg given by NACHMANSOHN (1952) for nerve fibers. The blood of the crab itself contains a ChE which is inhibited by anti-ChE drugs. However, when the blood is washed out as completely as possible from the gills, a considerable ChE activity remains, and KOCH concluded that possibly this ChE is present in the gill epithelium itself. His results show that eserine, DFP, and TEPP inhibited sodium transport, but while the inhibition produced by eserine and DFP was reversible that by TEPP was irreversible. However, when choline was added ($10^{-3} M$) the inhibition produced by TEPP was reversed. In the same series of experiments, KOCH demonstrated that basic dyes inhibit both ChE activity and salt transport.

KOCH concluded from his results that ChE appears to play an important role in the mechanism which actively transports sodium ions through the gill epithelium of the crab. Furthermore, in discussing the well known actions of ACh and ChE, he made the suggestion that these widely different mechanisms appear to be dependent on some common basic cellular activity which "may turn out to be an active transport phenomenon."

That ACh and ChE play an important role in ion transport across the cell membranes during physiological activity has also been suggested by ROTHENBERG (1950), HOLLAND and AUDITORE (1956), and more recently by TOSCHI (1959) and HOKIN et al. (1960). On the other hand, a number of investigators have argued against this proposal (for references see VAN DER KLOOT 1958). However, VAN DER KLOOT pointed out that in the experiments which served as evidence against a relationship between ion transport and ChE, the measurements of ChE were made on the extracellular enzyme. This subject is discussed in detail in Chapters 6 and 11.

CAVANAGH and THOMPSON (1954), in discussing the problems concerned with the demyelination which certain anti-ChE drugs are known to cause in humans, suggested that the glial or Schwann cells may be involved in the development of myelin. We have already seen that these satellite cells, which intimately envelop the entire neuron from cell body to termination, are thought to play an important role in the metabolic requirements of the nerve cell and its axon. Furthermore, it is known that BuChE is present in relatively large amounts in the satellite cells. From the sum of all this evidence, one could draw the conclusion that anti-ChE drugs by inhibiting BuChE interfere with the active transport of important metabolites the absence of which may be responsible for the development of demyelination. This matter is treated fully in Chapter 19.

Anticholinesterase drugs are obviously pharmacologically active at the ganglionic synapse. The effects, however, which result from accumulation of ACh appear to be less prominent and more difficult to demonstrate than at the neuromuscular junction. At the motor endplate these drugs produce a marked and prolonged potentiation of locally liberated or injected ACh, and effectively antagonize substances competing with ACh. In contrast, at the ganglionic synapse special conditions are required in order to demonstrate a clear-cut potentiation of ACh, and substances competing with ACh are poorly antagonized. For this reason considerable doubt has been cast on the physiological importance of the ganglionic ChE's in terminating the action of ACh. The reviewer's impression is that the pharmacological effects of anti-ChE drugs which are due to accumulation of ACh are the same both at the ganglionic synapse and the neuromuscular junction, but that at the ganglia these effects are overshadowed by actions independent of ChE inhibition i.e., actions which may well be present at the neuromuscular junction but appear more prominent at the ganglionic synapse because of the rather unusual anatomical and functional conditions at the latter site.

Many criteria for effects of the anti-ChE drugs which are unrelated to ChE inhibition have been brought forward, particularly with regard to neuromuscular transmission. ZAIMIS (1953) reported that in cats after relatively small doses of neostigmine (50 to 75 μg/kg, injected intravenously), the voltage applied to the sciatic nerve in order to obtain a maximal response from a skeletal muscle sometimes had to be increased as much as ten times. Furthermore, the demonstration has been made repeatedly that compounds, the chemical structures of which preclude hydrolysis by ChE's are often potentiated by anti-ChE drugs (ZAIMIS 1951, RIKER 1953). BOWMAN (1955) found that neostigmine administered intraarterially was either without effect or produced a small degree of vasodilatation. However, when adrenaline or noradrenaline was administered immediately after neostigmine, its vasoconstrictor effect was markedly potentiated.

36*

Anticholinesterase drugs in high concentrations have been found to block conduction of nerve impulses along nerve fibers (BULLOCK, NACHMANSOHN and ROTHENBERG 1946). Because of this finding the hypothesis has been put forward that ACh is connected with the formation of the nerve impulse (NACHMANSOHN 1940, 1952). CRESCITELLI et al. (1946), however, demonstrated that such a conduction block requires very high concentrations of an anti-ChE drug and that there is no parallel relationship between the magnitude of the action potential and the cholinesterase activity. They concluded, therefore, that the block produced by the local application of an anti-ChE drug is not the result of the anti-ChE action of the compound. Furthermore, BROOKS et al. (1949) found that in a given species the concentration of DFP required to block conduction was approximately one hundred times that which interfered with central nervous system function, and that interference with cellular respiration paralleled interference with function better than did reduction of ChE activity. A nerve blocking action of DFP has also been reported by TOMAN et al. (1947) who concluded that it was the result of a direct action of the anti-ChE drug independent of inhibition of cholinesterases (see Chapters 6 and 15).

A direct action of eserine on the cervical sympathetic ganglion of the cat was reported by FELDBERG and HEBB (1948). In experiments on the perfused ganglion they found that eserine in very high concentrations could prevent the passage of a nerve impulse elicited by a variety of agents, e.g., citrate, phosphate, and ACh. This action could be demonstrated on the ganglion after degeneration of the preganglionic fibers as well as on the intact ganglion, although after denervation the ganglion no longer contained AChE or ACh. This is reminiscent of PATON and PERRY's (1953) finding that large doses of eserine, in the absence of ACh, abolished the action potential without producing any depolarization of the ganglion.

In discussing the various problems concerned with the physiology of ganglionic transmission, we have seen that ganglion cells are able to maintain their activity during repetitive preganglionic stimulation *in situ*, but that this ability decreases in isolated preparations. In the presence of anti-ChE drugs, however, the responses to tetanic stimulation of ganglia both *in situ* and *in vitro* fall off rapidly, and furthermore, failure is accelerated by these drugs at all frequencies of stimulation. The same phenomenon is seen at the neuromuscular junction but to a lesser degree. Moreover, in the hands of most workers the amount of ACh liberated in a ganglion perfused with eserinized LOCKE's solution in response to preganglionic stimulation falls off rapidly. PERRY (1953), however, has shown that perfusion with the same fluid but in the absence of stimulation does not reduce the amount of ACh liberated per volley. Furthermore, he was unable to demonstrate any reduction of ACh liberated by stimulation of a ganglion which had been perfused previously with LOCKE's solution containing eserine, 10^{-5} M, and ACh, 10^{-6} M, for 40 min in the absence of stimulation. It is, therefore, the two factors, anti-ChE drug and stimulation together, and not either alone, which causes the reduction in output.

If a dual function of the cholinesterases, hydrolysis of ACh in conjunction with synaptic transmission on the one hand, and participation in active transport mechanisms on the other, is accepted, a possible explanation can be offered for the rather acute failure of nerve activity in the presence of an anti-ChE drug. The important question, however, is whether these drugs so act in what might be called the "pharmacologically significant" range. Until the right answer is known, and until the physiological functions of the various members of the cholinergic system are understood in full, our doubts will continue to exist and our imagination will be allowed to flourish.

Literature

BARTON, A. A., and G. CAUSEY: Electron microscopic study of the superior cervical ganglion. J. Anat. (Lond.) **92**, 399—407 (1958).

BILLINGSLEY, P. R., and S. W. RANSON: On the number of nerve cells in the ganglion cervicale superius and of nerve fibers in the cephalis end of the truncus sympathicus of the cat and on the numerical relations of preganglionic and postganglionic neurones. J. comp. Neurol. **29**, 359—384 (1918).

BIRKS, R. I., and F. C. MACINTOSH: Acetylcholine metabolism at nerve-endings. Brit. med. Bull. **13**, 157—161 (1957).

BISHOP, G. H., and P. HEINBECKER: A functional analysis of the cervical sympathetic nerve supply to the eye. Amer. J. Physiol. **100**, 519—532 (1932).

BOWMAN, W. C.: Blood flow in relation to the effects of adrenaline on skeletal muscle. Ph. D. Thesis Univ. London 1955.

BRINK, F., D. W. BRONK and M. G. LARRABEE: Chemical excitation of nerve. Ann. N. Y. Acad. Sci. **47**, 457—485 (1946).

BRONK, D. W.: Synaptic mechanisms in sympathetic ganglia. J. Neurophysiol. **2**, 380—401 (1939).

— S. S. TOWER, D. Y. SOLANDT and M. G. LARRABEE: The transmission of trains of impulses through a sympathetic ganglion and in its postganglionic nerves. Amer. J. Physiol. **122**, 1—15 (1938).

BROOKS, V. B., R. E. RANSMEIER and R. W. GERARD: Action of anticholinesterases, drugs and intermediates on respiration and electrical activity of the isolated frog brain. Amer. J. Physiol. **157**, 299—316 (1949).

BROWN, G. L.: Conduction in the cervical sympathetic. J. Physiol. (Lond.) **81**, 228—242 (1934).

— The effect of temperature on the release of acetylcholine from sympathetic ganglia. J. Physiol. (Lond.) **124**, 26P (1954).

—, and W. FELDBERG: The action of potassium on the superior cervical ganglion of the cat. J. Physiol. (Lond.) **86**, 290—305 (1936).

— — The acetylcholine metabolism of a sympathetic ganglion. J. Physiol. (Lond.) **88**, 265—283 (1936/37).

BROWN, M. C., and P. B. C. MATTHEWS: The effect on a muscle twitch of the back-response of its motor nerve fibres. J. Physiol. (Lond.) **150**, 332—346 (1960).

BULLOCK, T. H., D. NACHMANSOHN and M. A. ROTHENBERG: Effects of inhibitors of choline esterase on nerve action potential. J. Neurophysiol. **9**, 9—22 (1946).

BURGEN, A. S. V., C. A. KEELE and D. SLOME: Pharmacological actions of tetraethylpyrophosphate and hexaethyltetraphosphate. J. Pharmacol. exp. Ther. **96**, 396—409 (1949).

BURN, J. H., and M. J. RAND: Sympathetic postganglionic cholinergic fibers. Brit. J. Pharmacol. **15**, 56—66 (1960).

CAUSEY, G.: The Cell of Schwann. Edinburgh & London: E. & S. Livingstone 1960.

—, and A. A. BARTON: Synapse in the superior cervical ganglion and their changes under experimental conditions. Exp. Cell. Res. Suppl. **5**, 338—346 (1958).

—, and H. HOFFMAN: The ultrastructure of the synaptic area in the superior cervical ganglion. J. Anat. (Lond.) **90**, 502—507 (1956).

CHENNELLS, M., J. DEL CASTILLO, W. F. FLOYD, D. SLOME and S. WRIGHT: Physiological effects of alkyl polyphosphates. Nature (Lond.) **160**, 760—761 (1947).

CHOU, T. C., and F. J. DE ELIO: The anticurare activity of eserine on the superior cervical ganglion of the cat. Brit. J. Pharmacol. **3**, 113—115 (1948).

COPÉE, G., et Z. M. BACQ: Dégénérescence, conduction et transmission synaptique dans le sympathique cervical. Arch. int. Physiol. **47**, 312—320 (1938).

CREESE, R., and J. NORTHOVER: Maintenance of isolated diaphragm with normal sodium content. J. Physiol. (Lond.) **155**, 343—357 (1961).

— J. L. D'SILVA and J. NORTHOVER: Effect of insulin on sodium in muscle. Nature (Lond.) **181**, 1278 (1958).

— N. W. SCHOLES and W. J. WHALEN: Resting potentials of diaphragm muscle after prolonged anoxia. J. Physiol. (Lond.) **140**, 301—317 (1958).

CRESCITELLI, F., G. B. KOELLE and A. GILMAN: Transmission of impulses in peripheral nerves treated with di-isopropyl fluorphosphate (DFP). J. Neurophysiol. **9**, 241—252 (1946).

DALE, H. H.: The action of certain esters and ethers of choline, and their relation to muscarine. J. Pharmacol. exp. Ther. **6**, 147—190 (1914).

— W. FELDBERG and M. VOGT: Release of acetylcholine at voluntary motor nerve endings. J. Physiol. (Lond.) **86**, 353—380 (1936).

DE BURGH DALY, M., and P. G. WRIGHT: The effects of anticholinesterases upon peripheral vascular resistance in the dog. J. Physiol. (Lond.) **133**, 475—497 (1956).

DE CASTRO, F.: Sympathetic ganglia, normal and pathological. In: W. PENFIELD, Ed., Cytology and Cellular Pathology of the Nervous System, Section VII, vol. I, 317—379. New York: Paul B. Hoeber 1932.
— Aspects anatomiques de la transmission synaptique ganglionnaire chez les Mammifères. Rapport no. 1. Arch. int. Physiol. **59**, 479—513 (1951).
DIRNHUBER, P., and H. CULLUMBINE: The effect of anticholinesterase agents on the rat's blood pressure. Brit. J. Pharmacol. **10**, 12—15 (1955).
DOUGLAS, W. W., D. W. LYWOOD and R. W. STRAUB: On the excitant effect of acetylcholine on structures in the preganglionic trunk of the cervical sympathetic: with a note on the anatomical complexities of the region. J. Physiol. (Lond.) **153**, 250—264 (1960).
ECCLES, J. C.: Synaptic transmission through a sympathetic ganglion. J. Physiol. (Lond.) **81**, 8P (1934).
— The action potential of the superior cervical ganglion. J. Physiol. (Lond.) **85**, 179—236 (1935a).
— Slow potential waves in the superior cervical ganglion. J. Physiol. (Lond.) **85**, 464—500 (1935b).
— The actions of antidromic impulses on ganglion cells. J. Physiol. (Lond.) **88**, 1—39 (1936).
— Synaptic potentials and transmission in sympathetic ganglion. J. Physiol. (Lond.) **101**, 465—483 (1943).
— The nature of synaptic transmission in a sympathetic ganglion. J. Physiol. (Lond.) **103**, 27—54 (1944).
ECCLES, R. M.: Action potentials of isolated mammalian sympathetic ganglia. J. Physiol. (Lond.) **117**, 181—195 (1952a).
— Responses of isolated curarized sympathetic ganglia. J. Physiol. (Lond.) **117**, 196—217 (1952b).
— Intracellular potentials recorded from a mammalian sympathetic ganglion. J. Physiol. (Lond.) **130**, 572—584 (1955).
ELLIOT, T. R.: On the action of adrenalin. J. Physiol. (Lond.) **31**, 20P (1904).
EMMELIN, N., and F. C. MACINTOSH: The release of ACh from perfused sympathetic ganglia and skeletal muscles. J. Physiol. (Lond.) **131**, 477—496 (1956).
—, and A. MUREN: Acetylcholine release at parasympathetic synapses. Acta. physiol. scand. **20**, 13—32 (1950).
FATT, P.: Biophysics of junctional transmission. Physiol. Rev. **34**, 674—710 (1954).
—, and B. KATZ: Spontaneous subthreshold activity at motor nerve endings. J. Physiol. (Lond.) **117**, 109—128 (1952).
FELDBERG, W., and J. H. GADDUM: The chemical transmitter at synapses in a sympathetic ganglion. J. Physiol. (Lond.) **81**, 305—319 (1934).
—, and C. HEBB: The stimulating action of phosphate compounds on the perfused superior cervical ganglion of the cat. J. Physiol. (Lond.) **107**, 210—221 (1948).
—, u. B. MINZ: Das Auftreten eines acetylcholinartigen Stoffes im Nebennierenvenenblut bei Reizung der Nervi splanchnici. Pflügers Arch. ges. Physiol. **233**, 657—682 (1933).
— — and H. TSUDZIMURA: The mechanism of the nervous discharge of adrenaline. J. Physiol. (Lond.) **81**, 286—304 (1934).
—, and A. VARTIAINEN: Further observations on the physiology and pharmacology of a sympathetic ganglion. J. Physiol. (Lond.) **83**, 103—128 (1934).
FISCHER, M. H., u. H. LÖWENBACH: Aktionsströme des Ganglion stellatum und des Nervus depressor. Pflügers Arch. ges. Physiol. **233**, 722—731 (1934).
GEUS, R. J., R. A. MCLEAN, J. PASTERNAK, P. A. MALTIS and G. E. ULLYOT: Pharmacology of trimethyl-(2-(2,6-xylyloxy)-propyl)-ammonium chloride, monohydrate; SKF No. 6890-A or β TM 10. Fed. Proc. **18**, 394 (1959).
GLICK, D.: Choline esterase and the theory of chemical mediation of nerve impulses. J. gen. Physiol. **21**, 431—438 (1938).
GRIMSON, K. S., A. K. TARAZI and J. W. FRAZER Jr.: A new orally active quaternary ammonium, ganglion blocking drug capable of reducing blood pressure, Su-3088. Circulation **11**, 733—741 (1955).
GROB, D., and A. McG. HARVEY: Observations on the effects of the autonomic blocking agent, bis-trimethylammonium pentane di-bromide (C_5) in normal subjects and in patients with peripheral vascular disease and hypertension, and comparison with tetraethylammonium chloride. Johns Hopk. Hosp. Bull. **87**, 616—639 (1950).
HARVEY, A. M., and F. C. MACINTOSH: Calcium and synaptic transmission in a sympathetic ganglion. J. Physiol. (Lond.) **97**, 408—416 (1940).
HEBB, C. O., and B. N. SMALLMAN: Intracellular distribution of choline acetylase. J. Physiol. (Lond.) **134**, 385—392 (1956).
—, and V. P. WHITTAKER: Intracellular distributions of acetylcholine and choline acetylase. J. Physiol. (Lond.) **142**, 187—196 (1958).

HEYMANS, C.: Les substances anticholinestérasiques. Expos. ann. Biochim. méd. **12**, 21—53 (1951).

HILTON, J. G.: The pressor response to neostigmine after ganglionic blockade. J. Pharmacol. exp. Ther. **132**, 23—28 (1961).

HODGKIN, A. L., and R. D. KEYNES: Movements of labelled calcium in squid giant axons. J. Physiol. (Lond.) **138**, 253—281 (1957).

HOKIN, M. R., L. E. HOKIN and W. D. SHELP: The effects of acetylcholine on the turnover of phosphatidic acid and phosphoinositide in sympathetic ganglia and in various parts of the central nervous system in vitro. J. gen. Physiol. **44**, 217—226 (1960).

HOLADAY, D. A., K. KAMIJO and G. B. KOELLE: Facilitation of ganglionic transmission following inhibition of cholinesterase by DFP. J. Pharmacol. exp. Ther. **111**, 241—254 (1954).

HOLLAND, W. C., and G. V. AUDITORE: Effect of acetylcholine on rate of uptake and equilibrium distribution of physostigmine in human erythrocytes. J. appl. Physiol. **9**, 147—152 (1956).

HOLMSTEDT, B.: Synthesis and pharmacology of dimethylamidoethoxy-phosphoryl cyanide (Tabun) together with a description of some allied anticholinesterase compounds containing the N-P bond. Acta physiol. scand. **25**, 1—120, Suppl. 90 (1951).

— Pharmacology of organophosphorous cholinesterase inhibitors. Pharmacol. Rev. **11**, 567 to 688 (1959).

HUTTER, O. F., and K. KOSTIAL: Effect of magnesium and calcium ions on the release of acetylcholine. J. Physiol. (Lond.) **124**, 234—241 (1954).

KAMIJO, K., and G. B. KOELLE: The relationship between cholinesterase inhibition and ganglionic transmission. J. Pharmacol. exp. Ther. **105**, 349—356 (1952).

KATZ, B.: Microphysiology of the neuro-muscular junction. A physiological 'Quantum of Action' at the myoneural junction. Johns Hopk. Hosp. Bull. **102**, 275—295 (1958).

KIBJAKOW, A. W.: Über humorale Übertragung der Erregung von einem Neuron auf das andere. Pflügers Arch. ges. Physiol. **232**, 432—443 (1933).

KIRSCHNER, L. B.: Effect of cholinesterase inhibitors and atropine on active sodium transport across frog skin. Nature (Lond.) **172**, 348—349 (1953).

KOCH, H. J.: Cholinesterase and active transport of sodium chloride through the isolated gills of the crab Eriocheir sinensis (M. Edw.). In: J. A. KITCHING, Ed., Recent Developments in Cell Physiology, 15—31. London: Butterworth (1954).

KOELLE, G. B.: The elimination of enzymatic diffusion artifacts in the histochemical localization of cholinesterases and a survey of their cellular distribution. J. Pharmacol. exp. Ther. **103**, 153—171 (1951).

— The histochemical identification of acetylcholinesterase in cholinergic, adrenergic and sensory neurons. J. Pharmacol. exp. Ther. **114**, 167—184 (1955).

— Histochemical demonstration of reversible anticholinesterase action at selective cellular sites *in vivo*. J. Pharmacol. exp. Ther. **120**, 488—503 (1957).

— A proposed dual neurohumoral role of acetylcholine: its functions at the pre- and post-synaptic sites. Nature (Lond.) **190**, 208—211 (1961).

—, and J. S. FRIEDENWALD: A histochemical method for localizing cholinesterase activity. Proc. Soc. exp. Biol. (N. Y.) **70**, 617—622 (1949).

—, and A. GILMAN: Anticholinesterase drugs. J. Pharmacol. exp. Ther. **95**, 166—216 (1949).

—, and E. C. STEINER: The cerebral distributions of a tertiary and a quaternary anticholinesterase agent following intravenous and intraventricular injection. J. Pharmacol. exp. Ther. **118**, 420—434 (1956).

KOELLE, W. A., and G. B. KOELLE: The localization of external or functional acetylcholinesterase at the synapses of autonomic ganglia. J. Pharmacol. exp. Ther. **126**, 1—8 (1959).

KOPPANYI, T., and A. G. KARCZMAR: Contribution to the study of the mechanism of action of cholinesterase inhibitors. J. Pharmacol. exp. Ther. **101**, 327—344 (1951).

KOSTIAL, K., and V. B. VOUK: The influence of temperature on the acetylcholine output from a sympathetic ganglion. J. Physiol. (Lond.) **132**, 239—241 (1956).

KRIVOY, W. A., E. R. HART and A. S. MARRAZZI: Further analysis of the actions of DFP and curare on the respiratory center. J. Pharmacol. exp. Ther. **103**, 351 (1951).

—, and J. H. WILLS: Adaptation to constant concentrations of acetylcholine. J. Pharmacol. exp. Ther. **116**, 220—226 (1956).

KRNJEVIĆ, K., and R. MILEDI: Some effects produced by adrenaline upon neuromuscular propagation in rats. J. Physiol. (Lond.) **141**, 291—304 (1958).

LANGLEY, J. N., and T. KATO: The physiological action of physostigmine and its action on denervated skeletal muscle. J. Physiol. (Lond.) **49**, 410—431 (1915).

LARRABEE, M. G., and D. W. BRONK: Prolonged facilitation of synaptic excitation in sympathetic ganglia. J. Neurophysiol. **10**, 139—154 (1947).

— — Metabolic requirements of sympathetic neurons. Cold Spr. Harb. Sym. quant. Biol. **17**, 245—266 (1952).

LLOYD, D. P. C.: The transmission of impulses through the inferior mesenteric ganglia. J. Physiol. (Lond.) **91**, 296—313 (1937).

LOEWI, O.: Über humorale Übertragbarkeit der Herznervenwirkung. Pflügers Arch. ges. Physiol. **189**, 239—242 (1921).

LONG, J. P., H. H. KEASLING and J. W. ECKSTEIN: Hypertensive response to intravenous neostigmine. Pharmacologist **2**, 88 (1960).

MACINTOSH, F. C.: L'effect de la section des fibres préganglionnaires sur la teneur en acétylcholine du ganglion sympathique. Arch. int. Physiol. **47**, 321—324 (1938).

— The distribution of acetylcholine in the peripheral and the central nervous system. J. Physiol. (Lond.) **99**, 436—442 (1941).

— Formation, storage, and release of acetylcholine at nerve endings. Canad. J. Biochem. **37**, 343—356 (1959).

— R. I. BIRKS and P. B. SASTRY: Pharmacological inhibition of acetylcholine synthesis. Nature (Lond.) **178**, 1181 (1956).

MALCOLM, J. L., and W. L. M. PERRY: A method for recording intracellular potentials from a sympathetic ganglion. J. Physiol. (Lond.) **128**, 29P (1955).

MALMÉJAC, J.: Pharmacodynamie du ganglion sympathique. Actualités pharmacol. **6**, 141—174 (1953).

MARRAZZI, A. S., and N. E. JARVIK: The differential effects on synaptic transmission and nerve conduction of DFP and atropine. Fed. Proc. **6**, 354 (1947).

MAXIMOW, A. A., and W. BLOOM: A Textbook of Histology, Ed. 5. Philadelphia: W. B. Saunders 1948.

MCISAAC, R. J., and G. B. KOELLE: Comparison of the effects of inhibition of external, internal and total acetylcholinesterase upon ganglionic transmission. J. Pharmacol. exp. Ther. **126**, 9—20 (1959).

MENDEL, B., and H. RUDNEY: Studies on cholinesterase; cholinesterase and pseudocholinesterase. Biochem. J. **37**, 59—63 (1943).

MENDEZ, R., and A. RAVIN: On the action of prostigmine on the circulatory system. J. Pharmacol. exp. Ther. **72**, 80—89 (1941).

MILEDI, R.: Properties of regenerating neuromuscular synapses in the frog. J. Physiol. (Lond.) **154**, 190—205 (1960).

MITCHELL, G. A. G.: Anatomy of the Autonomic Nervous System. Edinburgh & London: E. & S. Livingstone 1953.

NACHMANSOHN, D.: On the physiological significance of choline esterase. Yale J. Biol. Med. **12**, 565—589 (1940).

— Chemical mechanisms of nerve activity. In: Modern Trends in Physiology and Biochemistry. New York: Academic Press 1952.

—, and A. L. MACHADO: The formation of acetylcholine. A new enzyme, "choline acetylase." J. Neurophysiol. **6**, 397—403 (1943).

OGSTON, A. G.: Removal of acetylcholine from a limited volume by diffusion. J. Physiol. (Lond.) **128**, 222—223 (1955).

PALADE, G. E.: Electron microscope observations of interneuronal and neuromuscular synapses. Anat. Rec. **118**, 335 (1954).

PALAY, S. L.: Electron microscope study of the cytoplasm of neurons. Anat. Rec. **118**, 336 (1954).

PASCOE, J. E.: A technique for the introduction of intracellular electrodes. J. Physiol. (Lond.) **128**, 26P (1955).

— The effects of acetylcholine and other drugs on the isolated superior cervical ganglion. J. Physiol. (Lond.) **132**, 242—255 (1956).

PATON, W. D. M.: Transmission and block in autonomic ganglia. Pharmacol. Rev. **6**, 59—67 (1954).

— Central and synaptic transmission in the nervous system (Pharmacological aspects). Ann. Rev. Physiol. **20**, 431—470 (1958).

—, and W. L. M. PERRY: The relationship between depolarization and block in the cat's superior cervical ganglion. J. Physiol. (Lond.) **119**, 43—57 (1953).

PAULET, G.: Nouvelle contribution à l'étude de l'action pharmacologique du tétraéthylpyrophosphate (TEPP). Arch. int. Pharmacodyn. **97**, 157—185 (1954).

PERRY, W. L. M.: Acetylcholine release in the cat's superior cervical ganglion. J. Physiol. (Lond.) **119**, 439—454 (1953).

— Central and synaptic transmission (Pharmacological aspects). Ann. Rev. Physiol. **18**, 279—308 (1956).

— Transmission in autonomic ganglia. Brit. med. Bull. **13**, 220—226 (1957).

—, and J. TALESNIK: The role of acetylcholine in synaptic transmission at parasympathetic ganglia. J. Physiol. (Lond.) **119**, 455—469 (1953).

REARDON, M. J., F. A. MARZONI and J. P. HENDRIX: The effect of neostigmine (prostigmine) on the actions of tetraethylammonium (etamon) in dogs and man. Fed. Proc. **6**, 364 (1947).

RIKER, W. F. Jr.: Excitatory and anti-curare properties of acetylcholine and related quaternary ammonium compounds at the neuromuscular junction. Pharmacol. Rev. 5, 1—86 (1953).

—, and Z. SZRENIAWSKI: The pharmacological reactivity of presynaptic nerve terminals in a sympathetic ganglion. J. Pharmacol. exp. Ther. 126, 233—238 (1959).

ROBERTIS, E. DE, and H. S. BENNETT: Submicroscopic vesicular component in the synapse. Fed. Proc. 13, 35 (1954).

ROBERTSON, J. D.: Preliminary observations on the ultrastructure of a frog muscle spindle. Proc. Stockholm Cong. Electron Microscopy, 197—200. Stockholm: Almqvist & Wiksell 1956.

ROSENBLUETH, A., and F. A. SIMEONE: The responses of superior cervical ganglion to single and repetitive activation. Amer. J. Physiol. 122, 688—707 (1938a).

— — The action of eserine or prostigmin on the superior cervical ganglion. Amer. J. Physiol. 122, 708—721 (1938b).

ROTHENBERG, M. A.: Studies on permeability in relation to nerve function. Biochim. biophys. Acta 4, 96—114 (1950).

SALERNO, P. R., and J. M. COON: A pharmacologic comparison of hexaethyl tetraphosphate (HETP) and tetraethyl pyrophosphate (TEPP) with physostigmine, neostigmine and DFP. J. Pharmacol. exp. Ther. 95, 240—255 (1949).

SAWYER, C. H., and W. H. HOLLINSHEAD: Cholinesterases in sympathetic fibers and ganglia. J. Neurophysiol. 8, 135—153 (1945).

SCHUELER, F. W.: A new group of respiratory paralyzants. I. The hemicholiniums. J. Pharmacol. exp. Ther. 115, 127—143 (1955).

SHERRINGTON, C.: Some functional problems attaching to convergence (Ferrier lecture). Proc. roy. Soc. B. 105, 332—362 (1929).

STEWART, G. N., and J. M. ROGOFF: The action of drugs upon the output of epinephrin from the adrenals. VII. Physostigmine. J. Pharmacol. exp. Ther. 17, 227—248 (1921).

TOMAN, J. E. P., J. W. WOODBURY and L. A. WOODBURY: Mechanism of nerve conduction block produced by anticholinesterases. J. Neurophysiol. 10, 429—441 (1947).

TOSCHI, G.: A biochemical study of brain microsomes. Exp. Cell. Res. 16, 232—255 (1959).

VAN DER KLOOT, W. G.: Cholinesterase and sodium transport by frog muscle. Nature (Lond.) 178, 366—367 (1956).

— The effect of enzyme inhibitors on the resting potential and on the ion distribution of the sartorius muscle of the frog. J. gen. Physiol. 41, 879—900 (1958).

VARAGIĆ, V.: The action of eserine on the blood pressure of the rat. Brit. J. Pharmacol. 10, 349—353 (1955).

WHITTERIDGE, D.: The transmission of impulses through the ciliary ganglion. J. Physiol. (Lond.) 89, 99—111 (1937).

WOLF, G. A., Jr.: The ratio of preganglionic neurons to postganglionic neurons in the visceral nervous system. Anat. Rec. 79, 80, Suppl. 2 (1941).

ZAIMIS, E. J.: The action of decamethonium on normal and denervated mammalian muscle. J. Physiol. (Lond.) 112, 176—190 (1951).

— An effect of neostigmine on the sciatic nerve of the cat. XIX. Internat. physiol. Congr. 910—911 (1953).

Chapter 13

Actions at the Neuromuscular Junction

By

Gerhard Werner and Albert S. Kuperman

With 21 Figures

Introduction

The transmitter process at the neuromuscular junction is defined as the causal chain of events which relates two all-or-none excitatory processes, namely a conducted excitation of motor nerve axons and a propagated response of corresponding muscle fibres. The individual events constituting the transmitter process may be affected discretely by appropriate chemical agents, resulting in phenomena observable at different levels of experimental procedure. Consequently, a set of data is obtained which stands in a signal-event relationship to the transmitter process.

The first systematic investigations of pharmacological effects at the neuromuscular junction were carried out by CLAUDE BERNARD (1856) with the curare alkaloid. More than thirty years later, PAL (1900) and ROTHBERGER (1901) investigated the anticurare activity of another naturally occurring alkaloid, physostigmine. The recognition of an aspect of physostigmine's action which was not foreseen by these earlier investigations, relates to the discovery by ENGELHART and LOEWI (1930) that this substance inhibits an enzyme characterized by its ability to catalyse the hydrolysis of acetylcholine (ACh) and therefore termed "cholinesterase" (ChE), (LOEWI and NAVRATIL 1926; STEDMAN et al. 1932). Subsequently, other agents were found to inhibit ChE and these were shown to affect neuromuscular transmission in a manner similar to physostigmine.

The significance of pharmacologic studies with anticholinesterase (anti-ChE) agents goes beyond that of systematic enumeration of effects exerted at the myoneural junction by a class of agents. Such compounds are obviously useful as chemical tools in an examination of the nature of the causal link between nerve and muscle excitation. In fact, the modifying actions of some of these agents on neuromuscular transmission weighed heavily in the context of arguments which led to a humoral theory of junctional transmission (DALE 1934; DALE et al. 1936; BROWN 1937c). Clearly, there is an essential supposition implicit if actions of agents known to inhibit ChE are interpreted as evidence for preservation of a hydrolyzable substrate endowed with transmitter function; this supposition asserts that such modifying effects on neuromuscular transmission cannot be produced in any manner other than inhibition of ChE (KOELLE and GILMAN 1949). Much of the work on pharmacological actions of inhibitors of ChE's centers around this supposition and due emphasis will be placed on the evaluation of relevant evidence (cf. RIKER 1953).

A. Responses in populations of skeletal muscle fibres

The contractile response of skeletal muscle to motor nerve stimulation is frequently taken as a measure of the occurrence of transmission in a population of neuromuscular junctions. The reactivity of such a population to chemical agents may be evaluated as an effect on neurally evoked muscle contraction provided the agents do not alter non-decremental conduction in axon and muscle fibres or affect the contractile mechanism by any means other than reaction with junctional foci. It is thereby assumed that the contribution of each activated motor unit to the total tension developed remains constant. However, intermittent transmitter failure may occur. In the course of repetitive stimulation at frequencies exceeding 40 per sec, motor units which had remained quiescent for short periods of presynaptic transmission failure may intermittently contribute a multiple of the tension normally developed on indirect stimulation with single pulses (BROWN and BURNS 1949).

The interpretation of a population response to chemical agents may be complicated by the fact that the units are not synchronously activated. The factor of temporal dispersion is of great significance for excitation by drugs *in vitro* with diffusion as the limiting process (BRECHT and FENEIS 1950), whereas with close arterial injection, a minimal degree of temporal dispersion is approached (BROWN et al. 1936). Neural excitation of muscle with single maximal pulses produces significant asynchrony of activity only under special conditions, e.g., in post-tetanic potentiation (BERNHARD et al. 1941) or in the course of the curare and neostigmine action (LOCKE 1961; LOCKE and HENNEMAN 1960). A high degree of asynchrony and, in fact, dissociation of activity at different junctions of individual motor units develops in the course of repetitive indirect stimulation (KRNJEVIĆ and MILEDI 1958a). In the absence of such special situations, activity in muscle fibres constituting one motor unit is temporally dispersed only over several msec in accordance with the conduction time required for the nerve impulse to traverse the territory of a motor unit (BUCHTHAL et al. 1957). The degree of synchrony of muscle action potentials has a remarkable influence on the amount of tension developed: two almost identical action potentials, but differing slightly in synchrony, may give rise to contractions of as much as 30% difference in tension (MERTON 1956). Possibly, this apparent difference between synchronous and dispersed muscle action potentials is due to a slower conduction velocity of synchronous potentials, leading to more effective triggering of the contractile mechanism (MERTON 1954). Alternatively, a synchronous motor volley known to elicit a back response over motor nerve fibres (LLOYD 1942) might initiate a brief tetanic contraction in the muscle (BROWN and MATTHEWS 1960).

Muscle contraction in the nerve-muscle preparation is conventionally examined under conditions of maximal or supramaximal motor nerve stimulation with monophasic square waves at a recurrence rate of 5 to 15 per min. This frequency is at least 60 to 100 times lower than that which occurs during postural reflex activity in motor axons left in continuity with the center (ADRIAN and BRONK 1929). The recurrence rate of nerve impulses arriving at the neuromuscular junction greatly affects some of the physiologic manifestations and pharmacologic reactions of the transmitter process; data obtained with stimulation at low rates may not, without careful consideration, be extrapolated to higher stimulus frequencies. Also, the pulse duration on stimulation with single pulses is critical in that at pulse durations exceeding 0.2 to 0.5 msec repetitive activity may be set up in motor nerves. Drug evaluation proceeds, in that case, at conditions of stimulation with short bursts of nerve impulses, rather than at excitation with single nerve volleys (MOGEY and TREVAN 1948).

These considerations provide some methodologic and physiologic background for interpretation of pharmacologic studies of transmitter events through measurement of contractile or electrical responses of muscle fibre populations.

Kinetics of drug action

Drug-receptor (or drug-enzyme) interactions and dose-response relations are usually considered at equilibrium of the reactants; accordingly, the explicit consideration of time may be omitted from the formal description of such reactions. In these cases, the equilibrium of the drug-receptor interaction is ultimately determined by the free energy of formation of drug-receptor bonds. A different situation arises when duration of exposure of receptors to drug molecules is significantly shorter than the time required for establishment of equilibrium: only a kinetic formulation of drug-receptor reactions is capable of representing this situation adequately. In this case, the activation energy of drug-receptor reactions, rather than the free energy of the reaction, chiefly determines the apparent potency of an agent. Consequently, two entirely different aspects of the drug-receptor reaction may be evaluated, depending on the design of an experiment as equilibrium- or rate-assay.

This may be illustrated in a quantitative way: consider the kinetics of a bimolecular reaction, $[R] + [A] \overset{k_1}{\underset{k_2}{\rightleftharpoons}} [RA]$, where k_1 represents the reaction velocity constant of the forward reaction; also, assume the intrinsic activity of the drug-receptor complex, RA, equal to one. The time-effect relation is then described by:

$$\frac{E_{Ae} - E_{At}}{E_{Ae}} = \exp\left(-k_1 t_{(A)} \frac{E_A max}{E_{Ae}}\right)$$

(E_{At} = effect of a dose $[A]$ at the time t; E_{Ae} = effect of the dose $[A]$ at equilibrium; $E_A$max = effect of a very large dose of $[A]$ at equilibrium (ARIENS et al. 1956a, b).) This formula clearly indicates that the effect obtained with the dose $[A]$ at any instant before establishment of the equilibrium is a function of the rate constant of the forward reaction; if the time required for establishment of equilibrium is sufficiently long, and duration of drug exposure sufficiently short, the maximal effect obtainable with a given dose under rate conditions may fall far short of that obtained at equilibrium.

These reflections are important for the evaluation of results obtained with the method of "close arterial injection" (BROWN et al. 1936), since the duration of exposure of receptors to injected agents is limited by the velocity of blood circulation and by local barriers between the capillaries and the receptors. Deviations from results of equilibrium-assays will be considerable with those agents which approach equilibrium very slowly (BURGEN 1949). Conversely, if the drug-receptor reaction proceeds at sufficiently high velocity, attainment of equilibrium will be determined by diffusion as the rate-limiting process (HOLMES et al. 1951).

Also in a different context, time may represent a significant parameter of drug action. JENDEN et al. (1954) observed that decamethonium, or ACh in the presence of neostigmine, acts on the neuromuscular junctions in two distinct phases: the first consists in neuromuscular block of rapid onset, associated with diminished response to indirect stimulation, and followed by partial recovery in the presence of drug; the second phase is characterized by its similarity with a steady-state curare paralysis. In terms of membrane potential measurements at individual neuromuscular junctions, this transition from stage I to II is observable as transition from membrane depolarization to membrane stabilization (THESLEFF 1955a, b; 1956; AXELSSON and THESLEFF 1958). Assuming that both phases can be attributed to the drug reaction with one set of homogeneous receptors only, JENDEN et al. (1954) suggested that phase I reflects the initial drug-receptor reaction, whereas phase II stands for quasi-stationary receptor occupation. This is, of course, not the only possible interpretation; nevertheless, the phenomenon as such stresses the need for explicit consideration of time relations in drug-receptor reactions with respect to the kinetic or equilibrium situation of particular experimental procedures. More recently, PATON (1961) proposed a theory of drug action based on the assumption that excitation by a stimulant drug is proportional to the rate of drug-receptor combination, rather than to the proportion of receptors occupied by the drug.

I. Amphibian muscle

1. Tonic fibres

The heterogeneity of frog skeletal muscle with respect to many physiological and pharmacological properties was clearly shown by SOMMERKAMP (1928) and later by WACHOLDER and his colleagues (WACHOLDER and VON LEDEBUR 1930, 1931; WACHOLDER and NOTHMANN 1932). Some muscles, or even certain parts of a muscle, were found to respond with a slow and maintained shortening to mechanical, electrical, or chemical excitation; this was in distinct contrast to the rapid and transient contraction elicited by the "twitch" fibres (for distribution of slow and fast fibres, see: KUFFLER and VAUGHAN-WILLIAMS 1953b). Subsequently, the dual innervation of frog skeletal muscle was established, the tonic fibres being supplied by motor neurons averaging 5 μ in diameter (TASAKI and MIZUTANI 1944; TASAKI and TSUKA-GOSHI 1944). Small nerve fibre impulses produce junction potentials which are non-propagated, capable of gradation, and of a relatively long time course (KUFFLER and GERARD 1947; KUFFLER and VAUGHAN-WILLIAMS 1953a). The mechanical response of the slow muscle fibre is also confined to the junctional foci, but because of the dense multiple innervation of these fibres the local potentials can activate the contractile system over a large segment. Furthermore, the intensity of activity at each junction can be graded either by recruitment of new nerve fibres or by an increase in the frequency of nerve discharge; the slow fibre does not respond with propagated activity under any circumstances, and in this respect its behavior is sharply distinct from that of twitch fibres (KUFFLER and VAUGHAN-WILLIAMS 1953a, b).

In accordance with GASSER's (1930) definition of contracture as prolonged, non-propagating, and reversible muscle shortening, the activity of the tonic fibre may be viewed as contracture. However, KUFFLER and VAUGHAN-WILLIAMS (1953a, b) pointed out that twitch fibres are also under certain circumstances capable of reacting with contractures to catelectrotonus or chemical excitation; but twitch fibres appear to possess a mechanism, less pronounced in slow fibres, which results in a dissociation of the contractile process from membrane depolarization.

This ability of frog muscle fibres to conduct impulses, and consequently react to neural or chemical stimuli with a twitch response, appears correlated with a typical histological structure: in transverse sections, such fibres present myofibrils in uniform distribution ("Fibrillenstruktur"). Fibres of the tonic type, on the other hand, are histologically characterized by irregularly shaped areas of sarcoplasm containing myofibrils in small number ("Felderstruktur"). Also, the junctional formations appear morphologically different in tonic and twitch fibres. True endplates («terminaisons en plaque») are encountered only in the latter; however, synaptic formation with finely medullated nerves ending in «terminaisons en grappe» occur in muscle fibres of tonic reactivity (KRÜGER 1950).

Because of the coupling between contractile response and membrane depolarization in the small motor system, the degree of contraction of a tonic fibre represents an estimate of junctional excitation. Accordingly, the frog rectus muscle, consisting primarily of small-nerve innervated fibres, is suitable material for quantitative pharmacologic studies.

CHANG and GADDUM (1933) established that physostigmine potentiates the response of the frog rectus to the acetyl-, proprionyl-, butyryl-, valeryl-, glycollyl-, and pyruvyl-esters of choline. The response to choline or carbaminoylcholine is not enhanced by physostigmine. It is now pertinent to inquire whether this sensitization of response to choline esters can be accounted for solely by inhibition of enzymatic hydrolysis or by a more direct modification of the drug-receptor reaction.

a) Esterases of frog rectus abdominis muscle

The frog rectus contains at least three different esterases, each contributing in varying degree to the hydrolysis of choline esters (Table 1). JACOB and PECOT-DECHAVASSINE (1958) have shown that the hydrolysis of butyrylcholine (BuCh) is particularly susceptible to inhibition by diisopropyl phosphorofluoridate (DFP), and consequently the respective enzyme is assumed to be a BuChE. These same workers also found that ACh hydrolysis was specifically inhibited by the diiodo-methylate of bis-(piperidinomethyl-coumaranyl-5)-ketone (3318 CT); this agent is believed to be a relatively specific inhibitor of acetylcholinesterase (AChE) (FUNKE et al. 1953). Also, a third group of enzymes was revealed which catalyzed the hydrolysis of thiocholine esters.

JACOB and PECOT-DECHAVASSINE (1955) determined also the potentiation of the contractile response to choline esters by DFP, 3318 CT, and neostigmine. Several significant relations are revealed by comparing these results with measurements of enzyme inhibition in vitro.

Diisopropyl phosphorofluoridate potentiates specifically the contractile response to BuCh, an effect which could be attributed to inhibition of BuChE. An evaluation of the actions of 3318 CT is complicated by the appearance of a depressant effect at higher concentrations

(Jacob 1944). Nevertheless, 3318 CT potentiates the effects of ACh and propionylcholine (PrCh) to an extent that can be accounted for by inhibition of AChE. Accordingly, in a muscle initially treated with 3318 CT, DFP leads to an additional enhancement of the PrCh response in accordance with the 30% contribution which BuChE makes to its hydrolysis. Jacob (1955) showed that the time required for attainment of equilibrium between enzyme and 3318 CT, and the velocity of the reverse reaction on the addition of substrate, are fairly high. Consequently, estimates of enzyme inhibition *in vitro* at given substrate and inhibitor concentrations are probably applicable to the situation prevailing in the frog rectus assay even though exposure to substrate is limited to short intervals (see page 572).

Table 1. *Relative contribution of the different esterases of frog rectus muscle to the hydrolysis of choline and thiocholine esters*

Esters	Concentration M	Hydrolysis, in percent of total enzymatic hydrolysis, effected by:		
		AChE	BuChE	Other esterases
ACh	0.01	95—100	(5)**	—
PrCh	0.01	65—70	30	(5)**
AThCh	0.01	70	15	15
BuCh	0.03	0	100	—
BuThCh	0.01	0	70	30

** The values in brackets are within the limits of the experimental error.

(From: Jacob and Pecot-Dechavassine 1958.)

The potentiating effect of neostigmine for contractures elicited by ACh, PrCh, and BuCh is contrasted by the lack of sensitization of the contractile response to the amyltrimethylammonium ion; only in high concentrations does neostigmine cause a slight increase of response to the stable onium ion.

b) Sensitization by carbamate esters

Miquel (1946) showed that neostigmine and physostigmine potentiate the contractile response to ACh even after previous exposure of the muscle to DFP in concentrations which produce complete inactivation of ChE's. Thus, a direct action of carbamates on the rectus preparation was indicated. However, the manometric method used in this investigation may have been too insensitive to detect residual ChE activity, for these results have not been confirmed by other workers (Bacq 1947; Quilliam and Strong 1949).

The relationship between the direct action of carbamates and their ability to sensitize to ACh has been carefully studied by Hobbiger (1950).

The degree of maximal sensitization to ACh obtained with physostigmine, neostigmine, Nu 683 (dimethylcarbamic ester of 5-phenyl-2-hydroxybenzyl-trimethylammonium) and Nu 5130 (dimethylcarbamic ester of 3-hydroxymethylpyridine) was compared with that resulting from pretreatment of the muscle by tetraethyl pyrophosphate (TEPP). Neostigmine and Nu 5130 sensitize the rectus muscle to about the same extent as TEPP, but physostigmine and Nu 683 produce considerably lower ceiling values for maximal sensitization (Fig. 1); however, the inhibition of ACh hydrolysis by ground rectus muscle is approximately the same for each compound at maximally sensitizing concentrations. Doses of the carbamic esters, and of TEPP, which produce optimal sensitization to ACh are equipotent in antagonizing the depression of responses to ACh by *d*-tubocurarine. But the carbamates no longer act as anticurare agents if the rectus muscle is previously treated with TEPP to the point of complete inactivation of ChE's; furthermore, the carbamates in this circumstance do not counteract the depression of responses to carbaminoylcholine or nicotine by *d*-tubocurarine. In concentrations above those necessary for optimal sensitization, physostigmine and neostigmine produce a contracture by a direct action, which can be suppressed by *d*-tubocurarine.

The complex effects of carbamates on the rectus muscle become particularly obvious in preparations maximally sensitized to ACh by TEPP: neostigmine, in doses producing contracture in untreated muscles, augments the effect of small doses of ACh, but depresses the response to higher concentrations of ACh. The depressant effect on the ACh response of fully sensitized muscles is more marked with physostigmine; Nu 683 and Nu 5130 produce effects in such preparations which resemble closely those of *d*-tubocurarine.

HOBBIGER (1950) concluded from these observations that carbamic esters, in low concentrations, sensitize the frog rectus muscle to ACh by inhibition of ChE's; similarly, their anticurare action is related solely to inhibition of ChE's. The direct stimulating actions of carbamates in higher concentrations, and their curare-like blocking actions in fully ACh-sensitized muscles, were considered as qualitatively different actions, unrelated to sensitization and anticurare action. In muscles exposed to TEPP prior to the assay, depression of reactivity to ACh by physostigmine follows the quantitative relations characteristic for competitive inhibition (KIRSCHNER and STONE 1951).

RIKER (1953) emphasized the fact that different carbamates produced considerably different ceiling values for maximal sensitization to ACh, although ACh-hydrolysis was inhibited equally in all instances (see Fig. 1); this indicated the participation, in the sensitization of the rectus muscle to ACh, of mechanisms unrelated to inhibition of ChE's. Working with the dorsal muscle of the leech, KAHLSON and UVNÄS (1938) revealed the complex nature of the sensitization to choline esters by carbamates: ACh action was enhanced 500-fold by a concentration of physostigmine which completely inhibited the muscle ChE's. However, 10 times more physostigmine resulted in a 1500-fold sensitization to ACh, which persisted for many hours even during repeated washings of the preparation. These investigations, therefore, led to a distinction between the true and apparent sensitivity of the leech muscle for ACh, the former referring to the sensitivity prevailing at complete ChE-inhibition, the latter designating increments of sensitivity for ACh obtained by raising the physostigmine concentration above values required for complete ChE-inhibition. Curiously, some aliphatic alcohols also potentiate the response to ACh in physostigmine-sensitized rectus muscle (EMMELIN 1940).

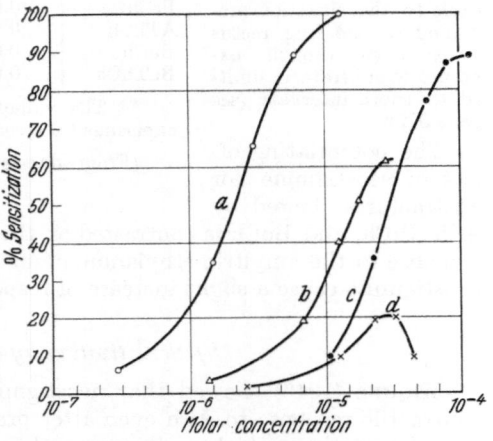

Fig. 1. Effect of carbamic esters on the sensitivity of the frog rectus to ACh. The action of each drug is expressed in per cent of the sensitization produced by TEPP on the same muscle (see text). Ordinates: Per cent sensitization (effect of TEPP = 100 per cent). Abscissae: molar concentration of the carbamic esters. (a) Neostigmine methylsulphate, (b) eserine salicylate, (c) Nu 5130, (d) Nu 683. (From: HOBBIGER 1950)

Pyridostigmine possesses about 1/3 of the potentiating potency of neostigmine (SMITH et al. 1957). With both agents, the maximal potentiating effect is attained in the course of 30 to 50 min, and at a rate characteristic for each dose level; the slow attainment of maximal effect parallels the time course of equilibration of enzyme-inhibitor, or enzyme-inhibitor-substrate systems *in vitro*. With purified bovine erythrocyte AChE, neostigmine exerts its maximal inhibitor effect only after contact with the enzyme for at least 10 min; pyridostigmine reaches an equilibrium after 30 min or more (SMITH et al. 1957). Addition of substrate after preincubation of these inhibitors with enzyme initiates a slow approach to a new equilibrium as evidenced by the progressive increase in the rate of hydrolysis. Also, dissociation of the physostigmine-enzyme complex after addition of substrate proceeds slowly and reaches the new equilibrium after some 40 to 50 min (BURGEN 1949).

From these measurements, it appears that the equilibrium value of ChE-inhibition by carbamates prevailing during measurement *in vitro* grossly underestimates the enzyme inhibition existing before addition of substrate (GOLDSTEIN 1944). Since, in experiments with the rectus muscle, duration of contact with ACh is short as compared with the slow dissociation rate of the inhibitor-enzyme complex, enzyme inhibition is virtually not altered during the test. Consequently, the potentiating effect of carbamates is determined at considerably higher degrees of ChE-inhibition than obtained with identical inhibitor concentrations in equilibrium with substrate. BURGEN (1949) estimated that a physostigmine concentration reducing the ACh hydrolysis by 40% at equilibrium with substrate would inhibit about 90% of the enzyme activity under non-competitive conditions; an equivalent degree of inhibition under competitive conditions would require about a forty times higher concentration of physostigmine.

Disregarding these considerations, and analyzing the potentiation by physostigmine of the contractile response to ACh in terms of the component rate processes of diffusion and enzymatic destruction of substrate, JENDEN (1958) arrived at an apparent dissociation constant, between ChE and physostigmine, of the magnitude $11.2 \times 10^{-7} \pm 0.7$; this value is about twenty times greater than estimates derived from the equilibrium between purified AChE of electric eel and physostigmine (NACHMANSOHN and WILSON 1951). JENDEN (l.c., 1958) attributed this discrepancy to the possibility that the attachment to cellular structures may considerably alter the specificity and affinity of the enzyme for agents. In any case, these quantitative studies do not indicate that the rectus muscle, during the period of exposure to ACh, is capable of lowering the concentration of this agent in the extracellular space by enzymatic hydrolysis. The potentiating effect of physostigmine was, therefore, attributed to an action on a barrier with hydrolyzing function, located in the immediate vicinity of the junctional elements.

AESCHLIMANN and STEMPEL (1946) examined a series of neostigmine analogs of the type listed in Table 2 and found that the inhibitory potency of some of these compounds (Nu-1250 and Nu-1197) on purified AChE exceeded that of neostigmine. Nevertheless, some of these agents depressed markedly the response of the frog rectus muscle to ACh. Thus, it becomes obvious that the optimal molecular requirements for inhibition of AChE and for potentiation of response to ACh, within the series of carbamates, are not identical.

Dicholine esters of aliphatic dicarboxylic acids were useful agents for the study of quantitative relations between enzymatic hydrolysis and potentiation of actions by inhibitors of ChE's.

Table 2. *Relation between relative cholinesterase inhibitor potency and anticurare activity in a series of neostigmine congeners*

$-OCON\begin{smallmatrix}R\\CH_3\end{smallmatrix}$ $^+N(CH_3)_3 X^-$	R	Anticholinesterase activity relative to that of neostigmine	"Curare-Like" action on frog rectus relative to Intocostrin (d-tubocurarine)
Neostigmine	CH_3	1	none
Nu-613	C_6H_5	1/20	none
Nu-1250	$4\text{-}ClC_6H_4$	5	1/5
Nu-1197	$4\text{-}CH_3C_6H_4$	1	1/4
Nu-1208	$3\text{-}CH_3C_6H_4$	1/5	1/8
Nu-1243	$3\text{-}ClC_6H_4$	> 1/5	1/6
Nu-1249	$2\text{-}ClC_6H_4$	> 1/5	2/5
Nu-1214	$2\text{-}CH_3C_6H_4$	> 1/100	1/8
Nu-1173	$3,4\text{-}(CH_3)_2C_6H_3$	1/5	> 1/2
Nu-658	$2,3\text{-}(CH_3)_2C_6H_3$	> 1/100	1

(From: AESCHLIMANN and STEMPEL, Jubilee Volume Emil BARRELL, Basle, 1946; page 309.)

The rate of hydrolysis by BuChE increases with increasing length of the dicarboxylic acid chain (BOVET-NITTI 1949; GINZEL et al. 1951b). Thus, the speed of hydrolysis of succinylcholine amounts to only about 2 to 5% of that for ACh, while the adipic acid dicholine ester is hydrolysed at about 1/2 of the rate of ACh; the sebacic acid dicholinester approaches closely the hydrolysis rate of ACh under comparable conditions. These compounds stimulate the frog rectus muscle, and their potency compares with that of ACh (= 100%) as follows:

$$\begin{array}{ll}
\text{Sebacic acid dicholine} & - \ 74\% \\
\text{Adipic acid dicholine} & - \ 15\% \\
\text{Succinic acid dicholine} & - \ 2\%
\end{array}$$

Exposure of the rectus muscle to physostigmine (10^{-5}) augments the stimulating potency of the sebacic acid dicholine ester about two-fold and that of adipic acid dicholine by about 1.25; the potency of succinic acid dicholine remains unaltered. Under the same conditions, the response to ACh is potentiated 4.4 times (GINZEL et al. 1951a, b). Obviously, the correlation between rate of hydrolysis by BuChE, and degree of potentiation by physostigmine, is not very good in quantitative terms, although the trend is indicated that the least hydrolyzable compound is also the least potentiated, and *vice versa*. Some limitations of these results should, however, be borne in mind: the enzyme used for measurement of hydrolysis was obtained from horse serum, and hydrolysis of these agents by frog muscle esterase may be different; succinyldicholine is the only compound of this series which was tested for hydrolysis by frog muscle, and it was found not to be hydrolyzed (COHEN and POSTHUMUS 1955). Furthermore, hydrolysis of the dicholine esters results in formation of the corresponding dicarboxylic acid monocholine esters (GINZEL et al. 1951a, b; WHITTAKER 1951; FRASER 1954), which may affect the muscle response, though they are in every respect considerably less potent than the dicholine esters.

On the normal unsensitized frog rectus muscle, decamethonium produces a contracture, different from that elicited by ACh by longer latency, slow rate of development, and delayed relaxation after removal of the drug; the contractile response is suppressed by *d*-tubocurarine and by the members of the homologous *bis*trimethylammonium compounds with shorter chain length (PATON and ZAIMIS 1949). Decamethonium, on the other hand, enhances the response to ACh, and also to succinyldicholine (LÜLLMANN and FÖRSTER 1953). The stimulating action of decamethonium, in turn, is slightly increased after complete inactivation of ChE's by TEPP (ZAIMIS 1951). There is no reason to assume that the stimulating and potentiating actions of decamethonium are in any way related to its weak anti-ChE activity *in vitro* (PATON and ZAIMIS 1952).

c) Sensitization by aryl quaternary ammonium compounds

SMITH et al. (1952) undertook an extensive study of the correlation between different pharmacologic actions of 3-hydroxy-phenyltrialkylammonium ions on the frog rectus muscle and their inhibitory potency on AChE of frog muscle, bovine erythrocytes, and electric eel. Some of these results are summarized in Table 3.

Of all the compounds tested, the trimethyl derivative is the most potent stimulating agent, although its activity amounts only to 1/30 of that of ACh. Increasing ethyl substitution on the nitrogen reduces the stimulating activity of the phenolic quaternary ammonium compounds. The potentiation of the contractile response to ACh, determined as concentration of the potentiating agent required to halve the ED_{50} of ACh, is most prominent with the diethylmethyl derivative: its potency amounts to 1/2 of the potency of neostigmine. The diethylmethyl compound is also the most potent anticurare agent of the series and a statistical analysis reveals for this, as well as for the other compounds listed, a satisfactory correlation between potentiation of the response to ACh in the presence, and in the absence, of *d*-tubocurarine.

From Table 3b it can be seen that statistically significant correlation coefficients can also be established between potentiation of ACh (with and without curare in the muscle bath) and inhibition of ACh hydrolysis by bovine erythrocytes and frog muscle homogenate. This certainly represents evidence compatible with the

Table 3a. *Comparison of stimulation, potentiation of ACh, and AChE inhibition*
(b = slope of dose effect curve; Sb = standard error of slope)

Compound	Stimulation		Potentiation of ACh			Anti-cholinesterase activity 50% inhibition		
	ED_{50} (M $\times 10^3$)	$ED_{50}/$ ACh ED_{50}	ED_{50} (M $\times 10^6$)	b	Sb	Electric eel (M $\times 10^5$))	Bovine RBC (M $\times 10^5$)	Frog rectus (M $\times 10^5$)
3-OH-phenyltrimethyl-ammonium	0.3	30	2.0	1.1	0.4	4.0	4.8	10.0
3-OH-phenyldimethyl-ethylammonium	4.1	216	2.8	1.3	0.2	1.3	3.4	5.0
3-OH-phenylmethyldi-ethylammonium	76.9	12,220	0.5	1.0	0.2	0.5	3.1	1.2
3-OH-phenyltriethyl-ammonium	80.2	10,700	13.0	1.3	0.3	2.5	20.0	13.0
Neostigmine	3.9	560	0.2	2.1	0.4	0.3	0.07	0.5
Physostigmine	61.7	75,000	0.5	1.0	0.2	0.04	0.08	1.4
Tetraethylpyrophos-phate	17.5	879	0.1	0.8	0.6	0.002	—	—

Table 3b. *Correlation coefficients of ACh potentiation, stimulation, and ChE inhibition obtained
with the 3-OH-phenyltrialkylammonium compounds, neostigmine, physostigmine,
and tetraethylpyrophosphate*

	Pot. of ACh	Anti-curare	Cholinesterase Inhibition		
			Frog muscle tissue	Bovine erythrocytes	Electric eel
Anti-curare frog rectus	0.97*				
AChE inhibition					
(1) frog muscle tissue	0.82*	0.83*			
(2) bovine erythrocytes	0.98*	0.95*	0.85*		
(3) electric eel	0.45	0.49	0.87*	0.52	
Direct stimulation frog rectus	—0.12	—0.28	—0.33	—0.24	—0.35

Significant (P < 0.05) correlation coefficients are marked with asterisk.
(From: SMITH et al. 1952.)

assumption of a causal relationship between anti-ChE and ACh-potentiating activity, as proposed by SMITH et al. (1952). The absence of a correlation between contractile effect and ACh potentiating potency conclusively eliminates an intimate relation between the mechanisms of these actions.

Some significance may be attributed to the lack of correlation between inhibitory potency of these compounds on the AChE of electric eel, and their ACh-potentiating and anticurare activities on the frog rectus muscle.

Curiously, SMITH et al. (1952) found also that inhibitory potencies on frog and eel AChE are significantly correlated with each other (Table 3). In other words, a molecular configuration suitable for inhibition of eel AChE can be expected to inhibit frog AChE, but is not likely to potentiate the contracture by ACh; conversely, a molecular structure endowed with high inhibitory potency on frog AChE is likely to potentiate the response to ACh and also to inhibit eel AChE. One can argue that these findings can only be reconciled by assuming that, to produce any one of these actions, different molecular characteristics are required which frequently, but not necessarily, occur in association with each other. Viewed this way, it becomes questionable whether the significant correlation coefficients listed in Table 3 are indeed indicative of causal relations, or whether they are merely a measure of the degree of overlap of classes of agents endowed with independently variable actions on the reactivity of frog muscle receptors and AChE.

SMITH et al. (1957) determined the potentiation of response to ACh in relation to time of exposure of the muscle to different concentrations of the *m*-hydroxy-phenyldimethylethylammonium ion (edrophonium, Tensilon). In contradistinction

37*

to observations with neostigmine and physostigmine, potentiation of response to ACh is maximal after an exposure to edrophonium for only two minutes, or less, and decreases subsequently over a period of 10 to 20 min until it reaches an equilibrium value (Fig. 2). This time course of potentiation was interpreted in terms of the kinetics of ChE inhibition. Indeed, by means of an automatic titration method, WILSON (1955) has been able to show for edrophonium that formation of the enzyme-inhibitor complex in the absence of substrate is virtually completed in 12 sec. Also, the reverse reaction proceeds at a fairly high rate: dissociation of the enzyme-edrophonium complex on dilution is completed in about 1—1/2 min; in comparison, neostigmine requires 12 min for half-dissociation. Consequently, it may be assumed that for edrophonium under experimental conditions of the frog rectus assay, essentially competitive conditions prevail on addition of substrate.

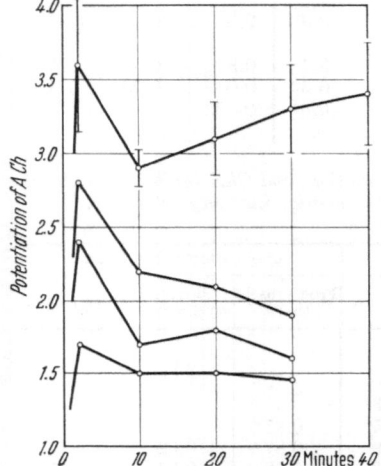

Fig. 2. Time course of potentiation of acetylcholine by edrophonium. Curves relating potentiation of acetylcholine with time of the exposure of the rectus abdominis muscle of the frog to edrophonium. Concentrations: Top curve, $9.9 \times 10^{-6} M$, 5.0, 2.5, and bottom curve, $1.25 \times 10^{-6} M$, respectively. Brackets on top curve denote standard deviation of the mean response. (The variability of responses at this concentration was greater than that obtained with any other concentration or drug in this preparation.) (From: SMITH et al. 1957)

The curve relating potentiation of response to ACh with the time during which the muscle was in contact with edrophonium (Fig. 2), suggested to SMITH et al. (1957) that there were two components involved in potentiation: an initial high potentiation explicable by the rapid establishment of an enzyme-inhibitor equilibrium, and a secondary depression of the muscle reactivity to ACh, with slower onset.

Rapid onset of action also characterizes the potentiation of response to ACh by some other N-trialkylammonium derivatives (HOBBIGER 1951). Besides edrophonium, the following ions were tested, and gave essentially similar results: 3-benzoxy-N-trimethyl-aniliniumbromide (Ro 2-2650), 3-acetoxy-N-methyl-diethyl-anilinium iodide (Ro 2-2651), and 3-m-toluyloxy-N-trimethyl-anilinium bromide (Ro 2-2783). However, maximal potentiation with the N-trimethylanilinium agents (Ro 2-2650 and Ro 2-2783) is less than that obtained with the ethyl-substituted compounds, and an increase in the concentration of the trimethyl-agents results in depression of response to ACh. All four neostigmine analogues, however, antagonize depression of response to ACh by d-tubocurarine.

The curves of potentiation by 3-hydroxy-phenyltrimethylammonium are similar to those of edrophonium (SMITH et al. 1957). WESCOE et al. (1950) obtained in the presence of the trimethyl analogue hydrolysis rates for ACh that remained constant over prolonged periods of time; therefore, equilibrium must have been reached within intervals too short to be measured by the manometric method. However, the triethyl derivative produced, in the experiments of SMITH et al. (1957), maximal potentiation of response to ACh only 10 to 30 min after its addition to the muscle bath. This compound, therefore, presents a curve of action reminiscent of that considered characteristic for carbamate esters (see page 576).

Edrophonium and some other N-trialkylanilinium compounds were tested for anticurare action on the frog rectus muscle by HOBBIGER (1951). These agents potentiate the response to ACh in the presence of depressant concentrations of d-turocurarine, but the curare antagonism of these agents cannot be demonstrated after ChE is inhibited by TEPP. Under these conditions, the N-trialkylanilinium compounds actually augment the existing depression by curare of the contractile response to ACh. HOBBIGER (1951) concluded from these observations that the anticurare action of edrophonium, and its congeners, is entirely explicable by their ChE-inhibiting function.

Different results, and a different interpretation, were reported by ARIENS et al. (1956a). In these experiments, edrophonium increased the response of the frog rectus muscle not only to ACh, but also to stable tetraalkylammonium ions; the quantitative relations were determined, and an example is presented in Fig. 3.

As a result of sensitization by edrophonium, the dose-response curve for butyltrimethylammonium is shifted towards lower concentrations of the stimulating ion; d-tubocurarine reduces the response to butyltrimethylammonium in the presence or absence of edrophonium. However, depression by curare is less marked in the sensitized than in the normal muscle. ARIENS et al. (1956a) arrived at the conclusion that edrophonium also potentiated the effect of d-tubocurarine, but to a lesser extent than it sensitized the muscle for butyltrimethyl- ammonium. In the particular experiment of Fig. 3, the inhibition indices of curare on contracture by butyltrimethylammonium are 1/15 and 1/40, with and without edrophonium, respectively. ARIENS and DE GROOT (1954) and ARIENS et al. (1955, 1956a, b) accounted for these and similar observations by assuming the existence of two interdependent receptor systems, R and R', such that in the presence of two drugs, A and B, dissociation constants or intrinsic activity of the receptor drug combination, AR, is influenced by a simultaneously occurring drug receptor reaction BR'.

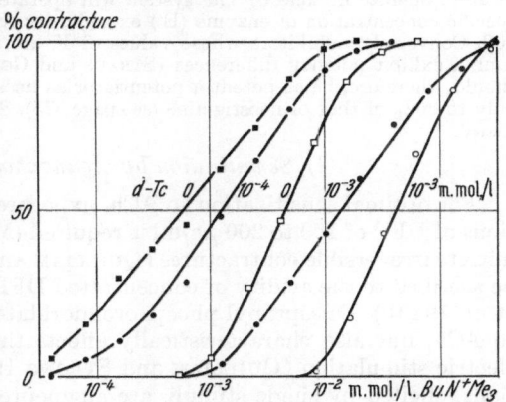

Fig. 3. Dose response curves for sensitization *to Bu-N+-Me₃* by *edrophonium*, in the absence and in the presence of constant concentrations d-tubocurarine. *Open points:* without edrophonium. *Black points:* with edrophonium *(0.01 m.mol/l)*. *Abscissae:* concentration of Bu-N+;Me₃in m.mol/l. *Ordinate:* effect as a fraction of the maximal effect by Bu-N+-Me₃. Owing to the fact that the sensitization by edrophonium is rather inconstant in its appearance, the dose-action curves represented were calculated from a group of six experiments, selected out of eighteen experiments. (From: ARIENS et al. 1956a)

The receptor systems R and R' may be viewed as two reactive sites at a protein molecule, or as reactive groups of different molecules constituting a reaction chain. This basic model can be extended in many different ways: e.g., the case of two agents, A and C, competing for R may be considered for the representation of the experiment of Fig. 3, whereby the simultaneous interaction BR' is assumed to alter the dissociation constants of the complexes, RA and RC. Obviously, this general model is extremely flexible and, therefore, permits formal description of a great variety of drug interactions under equilibrium conditions.

The intrinsic limitation of the singular view that the potentiating actions of the agents described in sections b and c may be related solely to inhibition of ChE's has previously been pointed out. This also became apparent in investigations on pharmacological actions of dicholine esters of aliphatic dicarbamic acids (CHEYMOL et al. 1954; KLUPP et al. 1953). The compounds of the general formula

$$Me_3\overset{+}{N}-CH_2-O-CO-NH-(CH_2)_n-NH-CO-O-CH_2-CH_2\overset{+}{N}-Me_3 \ (n=4, 6,$$

8, and 10) are powerful inhibitors of AChE and BuChE, and potent stimulating agents on the rectus muscle; curare depresses the contractile response to these agents. However, these agents in concentrations below those eliciting contracture, do not potentiate the response to ACh; moreover, on prolonged exposure they reduce the sensitivity to ACh.

Also, on purely theoretical grounds, arguments may be raised against the assumption of a direct relationship between inhibition of enzymatic hydrolysis

of stimulating agents and potentiation of their excitatory activity. It has been
stated repeatedly that the conditions of bioassay on the rectus muscle are such
that carbamates may, for all practical purposes, be considered as irreversible
inhibitors; the analysis of zone behavior of STRAUS and GOLDSTEIN (1943) can,
therefore, be applied.

The concentration of ChE at motor endplates has been estimated at 10^{-4} M (STRAUS and
GOLDSTEIN 1943). Assuming the same enzyme concentration at the junctional regions of the
rectus muscle, the enzyme-inhibitor system will, for inhibitors with dissociation constant (K)
of 10^{-6}, operate in zone C. The system will operate under zone C conditions as long as the
specific concentration of enzyme (E′) exceeds, for the inhibitor used, the boundary value of
200. Conversely, inhibitors whose values of K are such as to leave the system in zone C,
cannot exhibit potency differences (STRAUS and GOLDSTEIN, l.c.) Physostigmine (K = 10^{-8})
should, therefore, be as potent a potentiator as neostigmine; its potency amounts, however,
only to 60% of that of neostigmine (see page 575). Similar discrepancies exist for other carbamates.

d) Sensitization by organophosphorus compounds

For optimal sensitization to ACh, exposure for at least one hour to concentrations of DFP of 100 to 200 μg/ml is required (MIQUEL 1946); higher concentrations
initiate irreversible contractures (QUILLIAM and STRONG 1949), but this effect may
be ascribed to the acidity of concentrated DFP solutions (FINERTY 1947; BURGEN
et al. 1949b). Diisopropyl phosphorofluoridate does not only alter the sensitivity
to ACh, but also characteristically affects the response of the rectus muscle to
electric stimulation (QUILLIAM and STRONG 1949). Isotonically recorded contractions, elicited by single stimuli, are augmented by DFP in concentrations which
also increase the reactivity to ACh; fasciculation does not occur, but single stimuli
initiate repetitive muscle action potentials. In normal rectus muscles, brief tetanic
stimulation causes powerful contractions, usually followed by several succeeding
twitches. After treatment with DFP, short electric stimulation elicits contractures
of several minutes duration. Dissociation of chemical and electrical excitability,
on the other hand, was obtained by EMMELIN (1941) in the frog rectus after exposure to solutions of hexylbarbital (Evipal); selective depression of reactivity to
ACh was shown to be related to the presence of an N-methyl group in the barbiturate molecule.

In muscles fully sensitized by physostigmine, DFP did not cause any additional
potentiation of the response to ACh (QUILLIAM and STRONG 1949). But JACOB
and PECOT-DECHAVASSINE (1958) obtained with DFP in muscles suitably treated
with 3318 CT, an additional sensitization of response to PrCh which may have
been related to the proportional contribution of BuChE to the hydrolysis of this
substrate (see page 574).

In an attempt to examine the validity of the alleged causal relationship between inhibition of ChE's and potentiation of response to ACh, COHEN and
POSTHUMUS (1955) measured the sensitization by DFP for different choline esters.
DFP, in a concentration of 1.1 to 1.4 × 10^{-4} W/V, increased the sensitivity to ACh
about 12-fold, whereas the maximal sensitization to BuCh was only 2- to 5-fold;
curiously, optimal potentiation of response to BuCh occurred at strikingly low
concentrations of DFP, namely 2 to 4 × 10^{-7} W/V. The relatively small degree of
sensitization to BuCh may be related to the slow rate of its hydrolysis by frog
muscle enzymes, i.e., about 1/4 of the rate of ACh hydrolysis (COHEN and POSTHU-
MUS 1955). However, the response to succinylcholine is also potentiated by DFP,
although hydrolysis of this agent by frog muscle cannot be demonstrated. Furthermore, DFP potentiates the contractile responses of the rectus muscle to
decamethonium, choline, and edrophonium. This, COHEN and POSTHUMUS (1955)
considered as crucial evidence against the view that potentiating effects on the

frog rectus are solely explicable in terms of inhibition of ChE's. These authors were also impressed by the partial reversibility of the potentiating effect of DFP. Reversibility of ChE inhibition during the first few hours of exposure to DFP has been demonstrated by BULLOCK et al. (1946). To account for potentiation of responses to hydrolyzable and stable quaternary ammonium ions by DFP, COHEN and POSTHUMUS (1955) and COHEN et al. (1955) suggested that the receptor of striated muscle contains at least two kinds of reactive groups: the B-groups, essentially resembling the sites of ChE's which react with DFP, and anionic (A) groups, which, on reaction with certain cations, initiate membrane depolarization. Reaction of B-groups with DFP enhances, in this view, the reactivity of A-groups with hydrolyzable or stable cations. The assumption of two reactive and inter-dependent groups in one receptor molecule forms also part of ARIEN's receptor model (see page 581). In extension of this hypothesis, COHEN et al. (1955) stated that essentially all drugs which are capable of modifying neuromuscular trans-mission, also inhibit AChE and BuChE; furthermore, depolarizing drugs (as far as they have been investigated) inhibit preferentially AChE, whereas curare-like agents apparently do not exhibit such relative specificity. It was, therefore, suggested that reactivity of agents with the molecular species of BuChE *in vitro* is equivalent, *in vivo*, to reactivity with junctional receptors; agents which *in vitro* inhibit preferentially AChE cause, as result of the receptor-drug reaction, membrane depolarization. A somewhat different correlation between pharma-cologic action and anti-ChE specificity was suggested by TODRICK (1954), in that the majority of neuromuscular blocking agents appeared to inhibit preferentially AChE, whereas antimuscarinic agents seemed to be relatively more effective inhibitors of BuChE.

2. Twitch fibres

The discovery by LANGLEY (1905, 1907) of the distinct reactivity of the neural region in frog skeletal muscle to nicotine was decisive in the development of the concept of "receptive substance". In fact, a considerable part of the subsequent experimental work to be described in this section was, in design and interpretation, greatly influenced by this concept. It has, thereby, become possible to attribute to it a more definite meaning in terms of morphological structure and functional relations.

a) Contractile response

Injection of 0.1 to 1.0 μg ACh into the sciatic artery supplying the gastrocne-mius muscle of the frog causes very striking effects: the muscle abruptly contracts, and the tension attained may be greater than that of the twitch response to maximal indirect stimulation. This contractile response is accompanied by an outburst of asynchronous diphasic muscle action potentials (BROWN 1937b). With larger doses (1 to 10 μg ACh), the quick contraction is followed by a contracture which terminates the outburst of electrical activity; during the contracture the indirect excitability and, to a smaller degree, the direct excitability of the muscle remain depressed. Obviously, the muscle fibres of the frog gastrocnemius are capable of a dual mode of reaction to ACh. Similarly, BREMER (1932) argued that the contractural response obtained with the frog gastrocnemius muscle by pairs of indirect stimuli at an interval of 2 to 4 msec is expressive of a dual reactivity of its muscle fibres and different from SOMMERKAMP's phenomenon in the *M. ileofibularis* (see page 573).

Compared to its effect in mammalian preparations, physostigmine is exceed-ingly ineffective in altering the response of frog muscle to indirect stimulation and to ACh. Brown (1937b) did not observe any effect on the twitch response; the slow contractural response to ACh and the concomitant depression of indirect excitability were only slightly exaggerated in the eserinized preparations. However, chronic denervation increased the sensitivity of the preparations to ACh by about 10 times without altering the general pattern of response. This, in conjunction with the failure of physostigmine to sensitize, led Brown (1937b) to the conclusion that the sensitization after denervation is not (or at least not in its entirety) due to a reduction of junctional ChE activity. Although the correctness of this conclusion was substantiated by later findings (Meng 1940; Miledi 1960a), the premise on which it was based can no longer be considered valid since physostigmine, apart from being a weak inhibitor of frog ChE (Hawkins and Mendel 1946), suppresses the excitatory activity of ACh at higher concentrations (Fatt 1950).

From this, as well as from an earlier series of experiments by Brown (1937a), a fundamental and generally accepted concept emerged: maintenance of repetitive activity in single muscle fibres is assumed to be a result of the sustainance of appropriate concentrations of ACh at the endplate region. However, this assumption was not supported by evidence available from the earlier work of Gasser and Dale (1926) who had found, in the rectus muscle of the frog, that relaxation of the contracted muscle and return of electric excitability occur during continued immersion of the muscle in solutions of ACh. Admittedly, these latter results refer to equilibrium conditions, but the occurrence of relatively rapid adaptive membrane changes to stimulating agents has now been demonstrated by Thesleff (1955a, b).

Shortly after Brown (1937a) had published these results, Raventos (1937b) communicated observations in the frog gastrocnemius which led him to different conclusions.

It was found that low doses of ACh (0.05 to 0.25 μg) caused contracture only, whereas the initial twitch was seen only with doses between 0.5 and 10.0 μg ACh. Raventos was impressed also by the insensitivity of indirect excitability and twitch response to physostigmine, while contracture and concomitant depression of excitability were exaggerated. The contracture was specifically suppressed by atropine (1 to 10 μg), but low doses of curarine abolished only the twitch response to ACh without reducing the contractural phase or diminishing indirect excitability. On the basis of these findings, two sites of action for ACh were proposed: the twitch response to ACh was thought to be initiated from the motor nerve terminals; consequently, the blocking action of curarine was also attributed to this site of action. The atropine-sensitive contracture, on the other hand, was believed to originate from muscle fibres directly.

Soon after Dale and Feldberg (1934) had suggested that ACh might be a chemical transmitter at nerve endings, Cowan (1936a, b, c; 1938), examined this proposition by pharmacological means. His experiments were carefully designed on the basis of the following premises: (1) liberation of ACh from frog hind limbs during nerve stimulation is not impeded by the presence of curarine in the perfusion fluid (Brinkman and Ruiter 1924, 1925); (2) paralysis of neuromuscular transmission by quaternary ammonium cations involves a permutite-like ion-exchange reaction at the myoneural junction (Ing and Wright 1931; Ing 1936); (3) both ACh and curarine (Boehm 1920; King 1935) are quaternary ammonium cations; (4) physostigmine (Rothberger 1901) and miotine (White and Stedman 1931) are curare antagonists and cholinesterase inhibitors.

Cowan reasoned that pharmacologic reversal of curare paralysis could be explained in two ways: either these agents protect the liberated ACh from hydrolysis and allow for more efficient competition with curare for the part of the muscle juxtaposed to the nerve endings; or these drugs lower the threshold of the whole muscle to ACh, or at least of the part juxtaposed to the nerve endings. Cowan did not consider the possibility of drug interactions at the level of nerve terminals as was done by Raventos (1937b).

The major assumption made by BRINKMAN and RUITER (1924, 1925) and DALE et al. (1936) in their studies concerning the effects of curare on neuromuscular transmission was that most of the ACh liberated into the perfusate had its origin in the nerve endings. Indeed, such an assumption was compatible with the finding that stimulation of chronically denervated mammalian muscle produces no trace of ACh in the venous effluent (DALE et al. 1936). It was later reported that many organs, including resting frog skeletal muscle, contain a labile complex compound having ACh as an integral component (ABDON and HAMMARSKJOLD 1944). This discovery prompted the study of ACh liberation within the organ itself, instead of into the perfusate, by determining the breakdown of the so-called ACh precursor and the corresponding formation of free ACh (ABDON and LJUNGDAHL-OSTBERG 1944). Tetanization of the frog anterior roots did produce an easily detectable accumulation of free ACh in the muscle, and it was assumed that under normal conditions of transmission this ACh is rapidly resynthesized into its bound form (ABDON and BJARKE 1945). The significant observation of ABDON and BJARKE (1945) was that curare, in concentrations which completely blocked neuromuscular transmission, also abolished the formation of free ACh in the muscle after nerve stimulation; but direct muscle stimulation still produced normal concentrations of ACh. Accordingly, it was concluded that the locus of curare's action must be central to the site of ACh liberation. These experiments left it an open question whether the process of ACh liberation from its bound form belongs more to muscle metabolism than to neuromuscular transmission. Also important in this connection was the finding that denervation does not produce a significant decrease in the concentration of ACh precursor until after the period of time required for endplate destruction (ABDON 1945); this decrease may, therefore, be merely part of the generalized muscle degeneration which ultimately succeeds sectioning of the motor nerve.

Besides physostigmine and neostigmine, COWAN (1938) examined several other carbamates and the m-hydroxy-phenyltrimethylammonium ion with respect to effects on transmission in normal and curarized nerve-muscle preparations.

In normal preparations, these agents altered characteristically the mechanical response to repetitive stimulation. For instance, at a stimulation frequency of 150 per sec, development of tension during the initial phase of stimulation was depressed, the minimum which followed was made smaller, and the secondary rise of tension was augmented (Fig. 4). The relative activities of the compounds used did not parallel their inhibitory activity in vitro on Stedman's ChE concentrate (STEDMAN and STEDMAN 1935). But their relative activities in reversing paralysis due to curarine were of the same order of magnitude as were their activities on the responses of the Ringer-soaked preparations. The simple m-hydroxy-phenyltrimethylammonium ion was about 10,000 times more potent as an anticurare agent than expected from its weak ChE inhibiting potency. COWAN, as well as JACOBSOHN and KAHLSON (1938), noted that physostigmine is a much weaker anticurare agent in the frog than neostigmine.

The lack of correlation between anti-ChE activity and curare antagonism in the frog was particularly disturbing to COWAN, since MARNAY and NACHMANSOHN (1938) had demonstrated the presence of high concentrations of an ACh-splitting enzyme in the neural region of the frog sartorius. Also, on examination of a series of compounds with anti-ChE activity in the cat nerve-muscle preparation, BACQ and BROWN (1937) had found a fairly good parallelism between anti-ChE potency and the minimal dose necessary to cause augmentation of the indirectly elicited twitch tension. While granting the proposition that inhibitors of ChE reverse curare depression by virtue of protection of ACh, COWAN had to admit two additional possibilities: agents may counteract curare by mechanisms other than inhibition of ChE; alternatively, because of adsorption to impurities in ChE concentrates, agents may not manifest their true ChE inhibiting potency in vitro. The first alternative is equivalent to the statement that the class of anticurare agents includes, as a subclass, the ChE inhibitors; the second alternative indicates that negative correlations between ChE inhibition in vitro and effects in vivo cannot be clearly interpreted. COWAN's data give evidence for an additional complicating factor encountered if chemically heterogeneous agents are selected for comparison since, in the absence of complete dose-response studies, the possibility cannot be excluded that different mechanisms of action are involved. Indeed, COWAN's results established that the lack of correlation was due primarily to the fact that the tertiary agents used were, in contrast to the quaternary agents, uniformly low in potency at the neuromuscular junction.

The phenomenon of latent summation at the neuromuscular junction was the subject of a penetrating study in the course of which important evidence on pharmacological actions of physostigmine and neostigmine was obtained. BREMER and KLEYNTJENS (1937) determined the tension developed in curarized gastrocne-

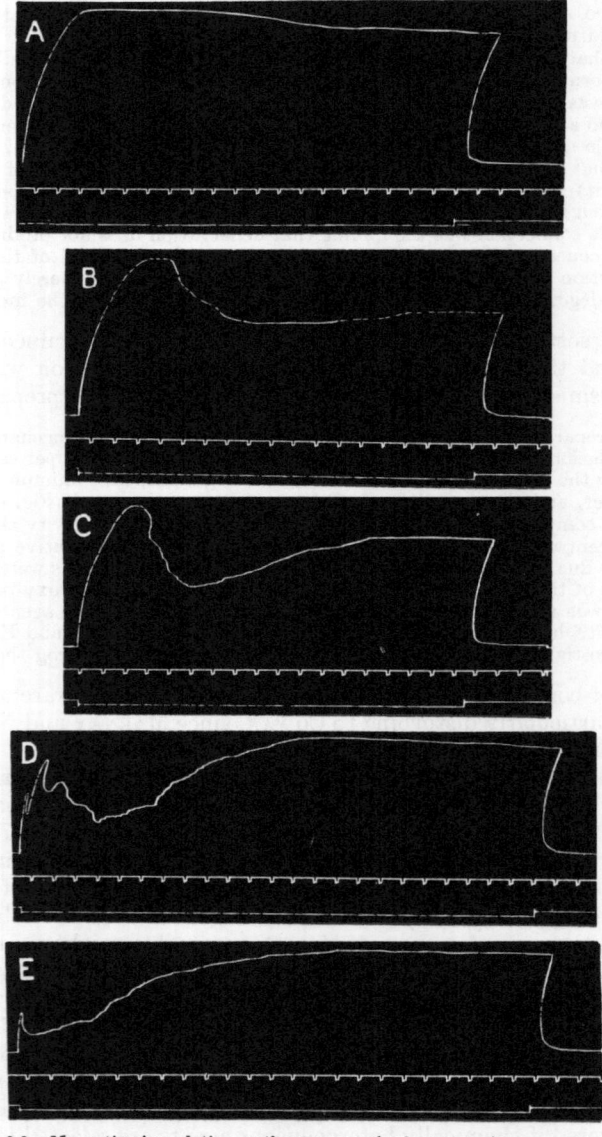

Fig. 4. The effect of 0.3 μ M neostigmine solution on the response of a frog sartorius nerve-muscle preparation to stimulation with 150 shocks per sec. A: Stimulation of pelvic end of Ringer soaked muscle with maximal shocks of time constant 1450 μsec. B: Nerve stimulation with shocks of time constant 109 μsec. C: 27 min after replacement of Ringer by neostigmine solution; stimulation of nerve as in B. D: 37 min after addition of neostigmine solution; stimulation of nerve as in B. E: 68 min after addition of neostigmine solution; stimulation of nerve as in B. The time markings are seconds. (From: COWAN 1938)

mius muscles of frogs when pairs of indirect stimuli were applied at different stimulus intervals; maximal tension was obtained at stimulus intervals of about 5 msec, and the tension decreased exponentially as the stimulus interval increased. At about a 60 msec interval, summation was no longer observable. These curves were viewed as measures of the dissipation of a latent excitatory event at the neuromuscular junction which was set up by the first stimulus in each pair of stimuli, the residual value of which at any one instant was capable of summation with the excitatory state initiated by the subsequent stimulus. Interestingly, the half-time of exponential decay of the subliminal excitatory state was not at all affected by physostigmine or neostigmine; the only effects produced by these agents were a shortening of the stimulus interval for optimal summation and an increase of the maximal muscle tension that could be developed (Fig. 5). These effects occurred within 5 to 10 min after intravenous injection of the agents to spinal frogs and could be followed only until decurarization prevailed, i.e., until only the first stimulus in each pair elicited a contraction. In view of these observations, BREMER and KLEYNTJENS (1937) arrived at a curious dilemma: either the summation curves of

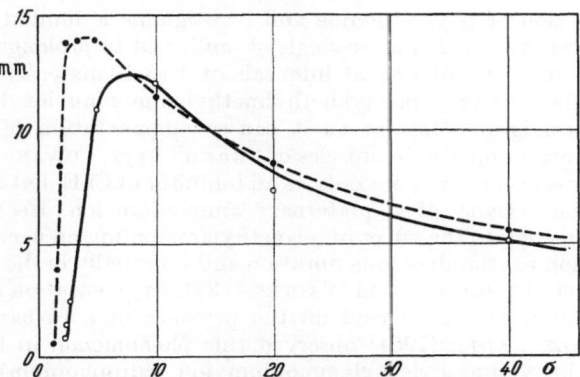

Fig. 5. Summation of twitch height in incompletely curarised frog gastrocnemius muscle on stimulation of motor nerves with paired shocks at various intervals. Ordinate: twitch height, in mm; abscissa: stimulus interval, in msec. The dotted line represents summation curve in control period; the continuous line was obtained 15 min after injection of 200 μg physostigmine into the abdominal vein. Note the shortening of the minimal stimulus interval resulting in summation, and the absence of changes at longer stimulus intervals.
(From: BREMER and KLEYNTJENS 1937)

latent excitation in curarized preparations were not related to liberation and dissipation of ACh, provided physostigmine or neostigmine acted solely as inhibitors of ChE; or, assuming ACh to be the agent liberated and dissipated, anticurare action of these agents had to be a pharmacologic action unrelated to ChE-inhibition. In non-curarized preparations, however, physostigmine and neostigmine prolonged the minimum interval between successive stimuli, leading to summation of tension; curare abolished this prolonging action (COWAN 1940b).

BREMER's work on latent summation was based on the assumption that the entire population of junctional regions in the curarized frog gastrocnemius muscle behaves alike with respect to activation by nerve volleys. However, SAMOJLOFF (1908) found that the second nerve volley of paired stimuli in non-curarized frog muscles caused a considerably larger muscle action potential; ADRIAN and LUCAS (1912) obtained evidence that under certain vaguely defined conditions, when a single nerve volley fails to excite some fibres of the frog muscle, a second volley, 20 to 40 msec later, becomes effective. BROWN and HARVEY (1938a) analyzed the same phenomenon in the leg muscles of the hen; here it was found to be due to recruitment by the second nerve volley of muscle fibres which did not respond to the first. Indeed, the occurrence of incomplete transmission at neuromuscular junctions of frogs on activation by single indirect stimuli was conclusively demonstrated by KUFFLER (1952); he showed also that in cases of incomplete transmission, repetitive stimulation is capable of increasing the "transmitter ratio" to a one-to-one correspondence between nerve and muscle action potentials. Therefore, it is conceivable that the curves of "latent addition", as determined by BREMER, cannot be attributed only to residual changes in a homogeneous population of individual junctions, but that they reflect also recruitment of additional muscle fibres by the second nerve volley.

In addition to twitch augmentation, COWAN (1940a) observed that physostigmine and neostigmine induced irregular twitching for several seconds after each stimulus (or pair of stimuli) which was superimposed on a smoothly declining curve of residual tension. These effects are seen only in muscles of frogs kept at low temperature (0 to 5° C) for some 40 hours prior to experiment; otherwise, the action of physostigmine and neostigmine is limited to the development of some residual tension after single stimuli, and to prolongation of residual tension after double stimulation at intervals of 3 to 10 msec. The dimethyl-carbamic ester of the 3-hydroxy-phenyldiethylmethylammonium ion differs from physostigmine and neostigmine insofar as it causes augmentation of twitch response and after-fibrillation also in muscles of "warm" frogs. COWAN considered the possibility that this agent acted not only as an inhibitor of ChE, but also by virtue of its possessing the activity of a quaternary ammonium ion. He was impressed by a possible analogy to the effect of tetraethylammonium on nerve, which consists in sensitization to stimuli of long duration and eventually in the establishment of spontaneous activity (COWAN and WALTER 1937). Augmentation of twitch response was indeed found not to depend on the presence of a carbamate grouping; NASTUK and ALEXANDER (1954) observed this phenomenon in frog muscles with the 3-OH-phenyldimethylethylammonium ion (edrophonium). This increased mechanical response was found to be associated with the occurrence of repetitive muscle action potentials in single muscle fibres. The time course of this potentiating action is distinctly different from that of neostigmine in that the peak value of twitch tension is reached earlier and maintained for shorter periods with the phenolic compound. The transience of the potentiating action despite continuous exposure of the muscle to edrophonium may be indicative of a dual action of this agent.

The apparent duality of action of hydroxyanilinium ions was the subject of a subsequent study by NASTUK and ALVING (1958).

It has frequently been suggested that the brevity of the potentiating action of intra-arterially injected ammonium phenolates in mammalian muscle is merely an artifact, created by the absence of equilibrium conditions. Experiments with the indirectly stimulated frog sciatic nerve-sartorius muscle preparation under equilibrium conditions revealed that the rapidity of decline of augmentor activity was greatest with the 3-OH-phenyltrimethyl-ammonium ion; stepwise replacement of methyl by ethyl groups led to prolongation and increase of the augmentative phase of action. In accordance with the earlier results of NASTUK and ALEXANDER (1954), the augmentative action on twitch tension was attributed to the ChE inhibitor action of these agents; however, the subsequent decline of facilitatory action and the transition, with the trimethyl or dimethylethyl analogue, into muscle depression was interpreted as a sign of a direct receptor-drug interaction with subsequent "receptor-inactivation." This assumption was based on the finding of THESLEFF (1955a) and KATZ and THESLEFF (1957b) that reaction of junctional receptors with depolarizing quaternary ammonium ions is followed by loss of their reactivity. However, this attempt to explain the transience of potentiating action on continuous exposure to ammonium phenolate ions fails to account for the loss of augmentative effect that also takes place with the triethyl analogue; there is no reason to assume "receptor inactivation" with this non-depolarizing agent. NASTUK and ALVING (1958) also noted the relative persistence of potentiating action of neostigmine on continuous exposure as compared with the phenolate compounds. The diethylmethylammonium analogue of neostigmine, however, was even more enduring in its augmentative effect. It is, therefore, apparent that in both the phenolic and carbamate series of agents, the nature of the alkyl substituent on the quaternary nitrogen atom greatly influences the persistence of drug action.

The *meta*-substituted hydroxy group in the 3-OH-phenyltriethylammonium ion is apparently not essential for the augmentative action, since phenyltriethylammonium is also capable of potentiating the twitch tension of the indirectly stimulated muscle, although to a lesser extent. However, it remains to be determined whether this effect of the unsubstituted ion is qualitatively identical to that of the *meta*-substituted aromatic quaternary ammonium ions.

Interestingly, the anticurare action of the hydroxyanilinium ions, which becomes manifest at concentrations below those required for twitch potentiation, does not decline with duration of exposure to these agents.

The records of NASTUK and ALVING (1958) indicate that in the presence of curare in the muscle bath, ammonium phenolate ions do not exert an augmentative effect in excess of restoration of transmission. Therefore, one may question the validity of these authors' contention that a preparation in which neuromuscular transmission is partially blocked by *d*-tubocurarine is a more sensitive indicator of potentiation by these agents than is a noncurarized preparation. It appears rather that neuromuscular facilitation, i.e., augmentative action on transmission in excess of normal, cannot be obtained with ammonium phenolate ions in the presence of curare. In mammalian muscle it is also necessary to distinguish between the anticurare and twitch potentiating actions of facilitatory ions (see page 630).

The inhibitory actions of physostigmine, although studied by several investigators, were of particular interest to FENG. With the term "junctional inhibition", FENG (1936) connoted the occurrence of different degrees of block at the neuromuscular junction with progressive increase of frequency of tetanic nerve stimulation. This inhibitory state is characterized not only by block of passage of impulses from nerve to muscle, but also by interference with the propagation of excitation along the muscle fibre itself. The term "junctional inhibition" was considered to fulfill the defining criteria of WEDENSKY inhibition, as stated by KATO et al. (1929). FENG (1937a) also obtained evidence that the inhibitory state at the junctional region is accompanied by a localized contraction of muscle fibres in the neighborhood of nerve endings.

Inhibition and local contraction at the neuromuscular junction were greatly intensified by physostigmine (FENG 1941); following tetanic stimulation at higher frequencies, the local contraction even assumed the appearance of contracture. FENG stressed the special nature of this post-tetanic physostigmine-induced contracture, which could not be elicited from the nerve-free endings of the sartorius muscle, and the extent and duration of which were directly related to the degree of WEDENSKY inhibition established during the tetanic stimulation.

The interpretation of the post-tetanic physostigmine contracture as the result of ACh accumulation in the junctional region appeared obvious at first, although FENG and SHEN (1937) considered also the possibility that repetitive discharges in nerve endings were involved. FENG (1937c) then proceeded to search for other relevant evidence, and established the conditions under which physostigmine potentiates the frog muscle twitch response to single indirect stimuli.

BROWN (1937a) and KRUTA (1935) had not been able to demonstrate this phenomenon which was so impressive in mammalian muscles (BROWN et al. 1936). However, it was discovered that potentiation of the twitch response by physostigmine occurs only at extremely low rates of stimulation (e.g., 1 stimulus every 2 min). The case for ChE-inhibition by physostigmine as cause for junctional inhibition and facilitation was strengthened by the demonstration of both phenomena subsequent to intra-arterial injection of ACh in suitable doses (FENG 1937b). However, FENG (1938) observed also that barium ions were capable of altering the response of frog muscles to indirect stimuli in the same way as physostigmine. A barium-treated muscle responded with tetanic contractions to single indirect stimuli, and when tetanized through its nerve, gave the characteristic response consisting of WEDENSKY inhibition and subsequent prolonged contracture. Since the barium ion does not inhibit ChE in the concentration used, FENG felt that the explanation of the physostigmine-induced effects in terms of ChE inhibition could now be questioned; for if the anti-ChE action plays no part in the production of barium contracture, it may likewise not be the important factor in the development of the physostigmine contracture. Repetitive activity in muscle fibres after single-shock stimulation of the nerve also occurred in muscles soaked with guanidine solutions (FENG 1938), and peculiarly, all the signs of physostigmine action on the neuromuscular junction could even be obtained with aliphatic alcohols and ketones of short chain length (FENG and LI 1941 c).

In summary, there exists a group of events originating at the neuromuscular junction which are apparently intimately related to each other; these are WEDENSKY inhibition, post-tetanic contracture, and potentiation of twitch responses by conversion of nerve volleys into repetitive firing of muscle fibres. These phenomena occur under the influence of some agents (barium ion, guanidine) which do not inhibit ChE *in vitro*. On the other hand, even if it is granted that physostigmine acts by virtue of ChE inhibition, it is difficult to understand why repetitive muscle activity occurs only under the very special condition of extremely slow rate of stimulation; mere accumulation of ACh does not, therefore seem to be the only factor responsible for the phenomenon of drug-induced twitch potentiation in the frog.

A totally new aspect of drug action arose when DUN and FENG (1940 b) discovered that the repetitive activity in guanidine- and barium-treated muscles was accompanied by antidromically conducted impulses in motor nerves; but, surprisingly, this effect could not be seen in frogs treated with physostigmine, although it was subsequently shown to be prominent in mammalian nerve-muscle preparations (FENG and LI 1941 a). The possible implications of the retrograde activity in motor nerves as a sign for a presynaptic action of twitch potentiating agents are discussed on page 635.

b) Local potential ("endplate potential") in populations of myoneural junctions

The electromyogram of indirectly stimulated striated muscle contains a component which becomes prominent in the course of tetanic stimulation leading to transmission block, or after curarization (GOPFERT and SCHAEFER 1937; ECCLES and O'CONNOR 1938). This component exhibits the characteristics of a graded, local response, capable of summation, and apparently lacking refractoriness (ECCLES and O'CONNOR 1939); it is restricted to the region of motor endplates and has, therefore, been referred to as the endplate potential (EPP). Its magnitude and time course are considered a reliable measure of the intensity of transmitter action at the neuromuscular junction. More directly, it is an estimate of the current flow in a volume conductor with a population of myoneural junctions acting as a sink. However, if recorded from the surface of isolated nerve muscle junctions (cf. KUFFLER 1948), the EPP reflects the time course of membrane current.

The junctional negativity has been shown to represent a significant and primary event in the transmission of impulses from motor nerve to muscle; its modifications by anti-ChE drugs have, therefore, been extensively studied. Reciprocally, these drugs have been used to ascertain the nature of the transmitter process with respect to the possible role of the ACh-AChE system. In the following descriptions of such experiments, two factors will receive primary consideration: (1) substances which inhibit ChE *in vitro* may *in vivo* exert important effects other than ChE-inhibition; (2) activity in the nerve fibres and terminals may be altered during drug effects on neuromuscular transmission.

α) d-Tubocurarine as a tool for studies of the transmitter process. *d*-Tubocurarine (*d*TC) is an important chemical tool in studies on the relation of ChE-inhibiting agents to the transmitter process.

In fact, such investigations are frequently designed to evaluate the action of ChE inhibitors on transmission modified by *d*TC; consequently, such observations and their interpretations are stated in terms of assumptions regarding the nature of this agent. Pharmacologically, *d*TC is characterized by its antagonism of the depolarization of the endplate and muscle membrane produced by quaternary ammonium ions (COWAN 1936c; FATT 1950; FLECKENSTEIN et al. 1951; AXELSSON and THESLEFF 1959); this antagonism has been described as a competitive one (VAN MAANEN 1950b). The depression of the transmitter process by curare is commonly associated with this property since BRINKMAN and RUITER (1925) and DALE et al. (1936) had obtained evidence that liberation of a humoral transmitter agent, supposedly identical with ACh, is not affected by dTC.

The work of GÖPFERT and SCHAEFER (1937) revealed that the curve of action of dTC presents two aspects even prior to the onset of transmission block: (1) dTC shortens the minimal stimulus interval with which complete transmission from nerve to muscle can occur (see also: KOSTYUK 1958); (2) the onset of WEDENSKY inhibition during prolonged tetanic stimulation is delayed. Even if the restoring action of dTC on transmission block by WEDENSKY inhibition should be due to protection of the endplate region from persistent depolarization by accumulated ACh, one is still left without explanation for the facilitatory influence of dTC on transmission of short bursts of high frequency nerve volleys. Furthermore, LI and TING (1941) found that the sensitivity for intra-arterially injected ACh in cats remained unaltered during high-frequency tetanization and nearly complete Wedensky inhibition; ROSENBLUETH and CANNON (1940) even found that the contractile response to ACh increased after short periods of indirect stimulation.

The initial facilitatory action of dTC on transmission of closely spaced nerve volleys has its counterpart in the potentiation of junctional negativity by conditioning nerve volleys during deep curarization (ECCLES et al. 1941b). Similarly, there exists a reciprocal relation between dTC and Wedensky inhibition; transmission of single nerve volleys can be restored in fully curarized preparations after periods of high frequency tetanic nerve stimulation (BOEHM 1895) which would otherwise produce Wedensky inhibition.

In partially curarized preparations, transmission can be restored by applying, in addition to a single nerve volley, a subthreshold catelectrotonic current to the receptive region of the muscle. This procedure is not effective in restoring transmission during a state of WEDENSKY inhibition at the neuromuscular junction (KATZ 1939). Partial or complete restoration of transmission can be achieved in curarized preparations by short periods of tetanic conditioning of the muscle nerve (LILEY and NORTH 1953), and by stretch of the muscle (HUTTER and TRAUTWEIN 1956).

The existence of different stages of curare action, and the complicated diversity of reciprocal relations between curare and transmitter activity under various conditions of neural activation cannot be accounted for entirely by a postsynaptic action of curare. These considerations obviously complicate the interpretation of effects of ChE inhibitors on the transmitter process in curarized preparations; their neglect, on the other hand, has led to "circular arguments."

β) **Effects of physostigmine on the endplate potential.** FENG (1940, 1941) undertook the first comprehensive study of the effects of physostigmine on junctional negativity.

In toad sartorius muscles which had been soaked in solutions containing curare and physostigmine, the endplate negativity was consistently larger and more prolonged than in the absence of physostigmine. FENG suggested that such effects were obtained only on exposure to physostigmine in concentrations, and for periods of time, which exceeded those required for inhibition of ChE; but this claim was not verified directly. In the absence of curare and physostigmine, similar prolonged negative junctional potentials accompanied the transmission block produced by high frequency tetanic nerve stimulation; these local potentials of WEDENSKY inhibition were not as well maintained in the presence of curare. In eserinized and uncurarized preparations, large persistent negative potentials accompanied by repetitive muscle discharges were recorded from the region of the nerve endings. The negative local potential and the repetitive muscle activity were exaggerated further by application of two nerve shocks in close succession, or after high frequency tetanic stimulation. The prolonged negative potential also accompanied the post-tetanic physostigmine contracture. Curiously, the afterdischarges in Ba^{++}- or guanidine-treated muscles were not associated with prolonged junctional negativity; but these agents, in distinction from physostigmine, initiated retrograde activity in motor nerve fibres and thereby revealed a presynaptic site of action.

FENG concluded that the simultaneous occurrence of prolonged junctional potentials and muscle repetition, as seen after physostigmine administration, is indicative of postsynaptic facilitation of neuromuscular transmission; conversely, muscle repetition in the absence of prolonged junctional negativity was believed to be of presynaptic origin.

The prolongation of endplate negativity by physostigmine was also observed by ECCLES et al. (1942); with a sufficient dose, and on repetitive stimulation, the junctional negativity can be lengthened to several seconds (Fig. 6). With a moderate dose of physostigmine, prolongation of endplate negativity is prominent only with two or more volleys following one another at short intervals; at intervals exceeding 20 msec, a second volley produces less junctional negativity than the first. The prolonged and large junctional potential in eserinized preparations after repetitive stimulation is associated with transmission block. FENG (1941) also was impressed with the simultaneous occurrence in eserinized muscles of large junctional negativity and WEDENSKY inhibition. The prolongation of the endplate

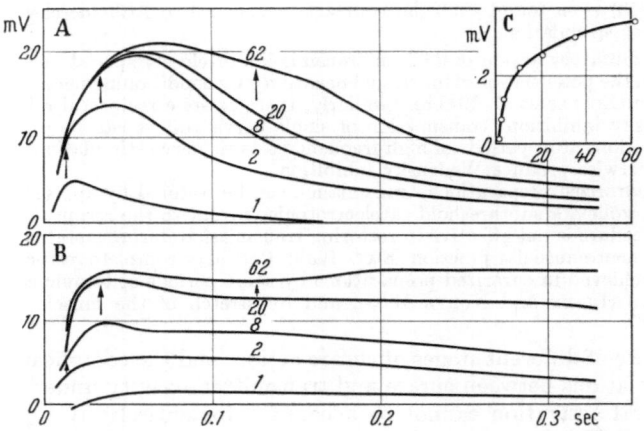

Fig. 6. Endplate negativity in frog sartorius muscle, resulting from repetitive nerve stimulation at a frequency of 250 per sec. The number of stimuli are shown in fig.; arrows indicate end of stimulation periods with 8, 20 and 62 stimuli. The curves are smoothed by disregarding small diphasic spikes; amplifier distortion is negligible. A: Physostigmine, 10^{-5} M. B: Physostigmine, 3×10^{-5} M. C: Plot of potential height, measured at 0.4 sec after the middle of the stimulation periods (ordinate) versus number of stimuli (abscissa). The results were obtained in the presence of physostigmine, 3×10^{-5} M. (From: ECCLES et al. 1942)

negativity by physostigmine does not occur at low environmental temperatures. Similarly, FENG and SHEN (1937) noted that the localized contracture in eserinized muscle disappears at low temperatures.

A detailed study of the reciprocal antagonism between curare and physostigmine in the frog sartorius muscle, with respect to amplitude and duration of the endplate negativity, revealed important relations (ECCLES et al. 1941a, b). In eserinized muscle curare primarily obliterates the "slow-wave" component of the endplate potential (see page 593). Conversely, physostigmine results in a marked increase of the peak amplitude of curare-endplate potentials and prolongs decay. With respect to the peak amplitude, curare and physostigmine behave competitively, i.e., peak amplitudes in the presence of low curare concentrations approximate the peak potential values in the simultaneous presence of physostigmine and higher curare concentrations; but the high peak potentials in curare solutions of reduced concentrations always decline faster than the equivalent amplitudes of muscles exposed to properly matched curare-physostigmine mixtures (Fig. 7).

ECCLES et al. (1941b) demonstrated that the endplate potential has properties characteristic of a local catelectrotonic potential: (1) the negativity spreads with a decrement of about 50% per mm and with progressive slowing of its time course; (2) the time factor of decay is of the same order of magnitude as that of a catelectrotonic potential (SCHAEFER

1939); (3) on passage of a propagated muscle spike, the junctional negativity is built up to a smaller potential and decays more rapidly; (4) upon reaching a certain critical amplitude, the local negativity triggers a muscle impulse. In consequence of this conception of the junctional negativity, most of its declining phase must be viewed as passive electrotonic decay; only a small fraction of its total time course is related to the transmitter action proper which results in establishment of the catelectrotonus. ECCLES et al. (1941b) calculated on the basis of HILL's (1936) local potential theory that the transmitter action in frogs at 20° does not occupy more than the initial 2 to 3 msec of the junctional negativity. Extending this reasoning to the physostigmine experiments, ECCLES et al. (1942) showed that this agent more than doubles the duration of the transmitter action.

The effects of physostigmine and curare on transmitter action were viewed as evidence for the identity of the transmitter process with liberation of ACh from nerve terminals. In this context, the effects of physostigmine on the junctional negativity were associated with its anti-ChE activity. However, even in the presence of large doses of ChE inhibitor, transmitter action is still relatively brief and some additional physostigmine-resistant mechanism of ACh-removal has to be supposed.

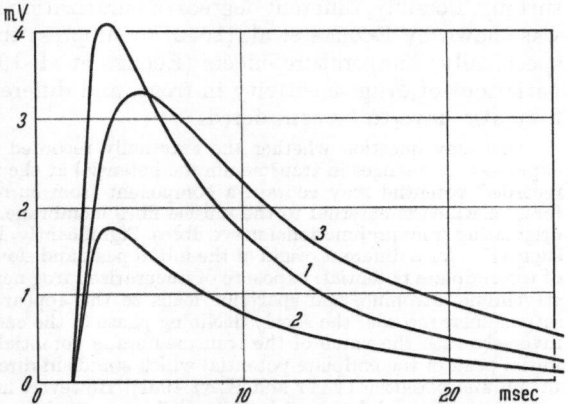

Fig. 7. Endplate potentials of curarised frog muscle. 1: after 6 µmol curarine; 2: after 9 µ mol curarine; 3: after 9 µmol curarine *and* physostigmine, 10⁻⁵ M. (From: ECCLES et al. 1942)

γ) **The two components of the externally recorded endplate potential.** From experiments in frogs and cats, ECCLES et al. (1942) obtained evidence that the endplate negativity in heavily eserinized muscles consists of two successive and distinct waves of depolarization, i.e., a lengthened potential exponentially decaying within 50 to 100 msec, and a separate wave of delayed rise and extremely slow decay (see Fig. 6). In the cat, but not in the frog, the "slow-wave" is associated with repetitive discharges in motor nerve fibres (see page 634). The "slow-wave" is easily suppressed by curare. It was postulated that under the influence of physostigmine, there occurs a separate delayed transmitter action while the stimulus-evoked transmitter action subsides. In an attempt to reconcile this phenomenon with the assumed transmitter role of ACh, consideration was given to a possible spread of ACh over larger areas while its enzymatic destruction was inhibited by physostigmine. Extrajunctional receptors for ACh exist, however, only in the immediate vicinity of the junction (MILEDI 1960b; KATZ and MILEDI 1961).

The two components of decay of the electrical event at the junctional region were also studied by COPPÉE (1943) who arrived at a completely different interpretation.

COPPÉE assumed the myoneural junction to function as a zone of decremental conduction. The initial phase of the junctional negativity was attributed to a local action potential, and the subsequent "slow wave" was assigned to a negative after potential of the decrementally conducted action potential. Like SCHAEFER (1939), COPPÉE did not observe any increase by physostigmine of the junctional negativity in curarized preparations; nor did ACh, in curarized preparations, produce an electrical event equivalent to the slow wave potential. However, phenolic agents induced a conspicuous exaggeration of the slow potential without altering the sensitivity of the muscle to ACh. In view of these findings, COPPÉE suggested two different mechanisms of anticurare action: one, based on augmentation of the slow electrical event at the neuromuscular junction (phenolic agents like sympathomimetic amines, local catelectrotonus, veratrine); the other, consisting in a facilitation of excitation of the muscle fibre by the junctional electrical event (e.g., physostigmine). Only in the latter step of transmission was ACh supposed to intervene as transmitting agent. In continuation of COPPÉE's work, GOUTIER (1949a, b) concluded that the anticurare action of methylxanthines is based on prolongation of the slow component of the junctional negativity, and apparently not related to ChE-inhibition.

It is doubtful whether COPPÉE's hypothesis regarding the nature of the endplate negativity provides a satisfactory concept to account for the physiology and pharmacology of neuromuscular transmission. Also, the conflicting results obtained with physostigmine by ECCLES et al. (1942) and COPPÉE (1943) are disturbing. Possibly, different degrees of curarization may be responsible, since curare was shown by ECCLES et al. (1942) to suppress the slow wave component rather specifically; temperature effects (ECCLES et al. 1942; COWAN 1940a, b), seasonal variations of drug sensitivity in frogs, and differences in the curare preparations may also have to be considered.

One may question whether the externally recorded "slow wave" is, in its entirety, an expression of changes in transmembrane potential at the postsynaptic site. Alternatively, the recorded potential may contain a component from current flow, the driving electromotive force of which is external to the muscle fibre membrane, as would be the case for a current originating from prejunctional nerve fibres. Significantly, FURUKAWA (1957) obtained evidence suggestive for a different origin of the initial peak and slow wave ("second hump") component of the endplate potential: exposure of uncurarized frog nerve-muscle preparations to procaine, strychnine, atropine, and sparteine leads to the appearance of a slow wave component in intracellular records; the slowly declining phase of the endplate potential varies in magnitude inversely with the value of the transmembrane potential, and is, thereby, distinct from the initial peak of the endplate potential which stands in direct relation to the magnitude of the membrane potential (FATT and KATZ 1951). However, measurements of transmembrane potentials at the endplate region of partially curarized frog muscles revealed for phenolic compounds, like epinephrine and norepinephrine, an increase of height of the junctional potential by 10%, but delayed decay or appearance of an additional slow component was not noted (HUTTER and LOWENSTEIN 1955).

δ) Effects of neostigmine and analogues on the endplate potential. ECCLES and MACFARLANE (1949) realized that physostigmine might not have been the optimal agent to ascertain the significance of ChE inhibition to the transmitter process, since its inhibitory potency on the ACh-hydrolyzing enzymes of frog is relatively weak (HAWKINS and MENDEL 1946). Therefore, a systematic investigation was undertaken with neostigmine and some other carbamic acid esters (Table 4). In the presence of d-tubocurarine (1:10,000), neostigmine prolongs the rising phase of the junctional potential in concentrations of 2×10^{-7} M; this effect becomes more marked with increasing concentrations. Duration of decay is also prolonged, and this effect is more apparent in the first half of the decay period than in the second. The steepness of the rising phase increases at lower drug concentrations, but higher concentrations may result in a slowing of the potential rise. The increase of duration and steepness of the rising phase results in augmentation of the maximal height of junctional negativity.

In the curarized frog muscle, the second of two volleys at a short interval evokes an endplate potential of about double the amplitude of the first, but the time course shows no significant alteration (FENG 1940; ECCLES et al. 1941b); from such data, curves were plotted which relate the time course of diminution of potentiation to increasing volley intervals. Neostigmine does not alter the course of these potentiation curves. This conforms with results reported by FENG (1940) for physostigmine, and may be related to the negligible effects of physostigmine and neostigmine on the facilitation curves determined for the mechanical response of curarized muscle (see Fig. 5) (BREMER and KLEYNTJENS 1937).

The response of curarized muscle to repetitive stimulation consists in an initial rise, and subsequent stabilization at a plateau of the junctional potential. In the presence of neostigmine, the maximum height of the summated potentials is increased. More conspicuous is the effect of neostigmine on the decay of the summated junctional potential after discontinuation of the repetitive stimulus. Normally, this proceeds in two distinct steps, one with a time constant of 20 msec, the second with a half-decay time of 1 sec or more. In the presence of neostigmine the fast component of decay is little altered, but the slow component is greatly increased and still further prolonged (FILLENZ and HANAFIN 1947).

The agents listed in Table 4 altered the junctional negativity in essentially the same way as neostigmine, irrespective of their being tertiary or quaternary amines; DFP induced similar changes. ECCLES and MACFARLANE (1949), therefore, argued that these agents must act by some common mechanism; indeed, these agents are all inhibitors of ChE's *in vitro*. Their inhibitory potencies on electric eel AChE do not parallel their activity in altering rise and decay of the junctional potential (see also Table 2; Nu-1250 and Nu-1197), but this discrepancy may be accounted for by differences in solubility at the junctional region, or by different susceptibility of frog ChE. Assuming that the observed changes of the junctional negativity were due solely to protection of ACh from enzymatic hydrolysis, the duration of active depolarization by ACh in the presence of neostigmine was estimated not to exceed 10 msec.

Table 4. *Effect of different carbamates and DFP on the externally recorded endplate potential of curarised frog nerve-muscle preparations*

Anti-ChE substance	Summit-time of 5 msec for EPP*		Half-decay time of 20 msec for EPP*		Potential slow component/maximum potential = 0.18		Half-time decay slow component of 1.5 sec		Depressant action on EPP* to about 5 μV	
	Molar conc.	Activity relative to neostig.	Molar conc.	Activity relative to neostig.	Molar conc.	Activity relative to neostig.	Molar conc.	Activity relative to neostig.	Molar conc.	Activity relative to neostig.
1	2	3	4	5	6	7	8	9	10	11
Neostigmine	3.2×10^{-6}	100	2.3×10^{-6}	100	6.1×10^{-6}	100	7.6×10^{-6}	100	2.5×10^{-3}	100
Dimethyl carbamate of 3-hydroxy-2-dimethyl aminomethyl pyridine dihydrochloride (Nu-2126)	3.6×10^{-6}	89	2.8×10^{-6}	82	1.1×10^{-5}	55	1.1×10^{-5}	69	6.0×10^{-3}	40
p-Chlorphenylmethyl carbamate of m-dimethylaminophenol methyl bromide (Nu-1250)	5.0×10^{-5}	6.4	3.0×10^{-5}	7.7	4.0×10^{-5}	15	$> 1.0 \times 10^{-4}$	< 7.6	1.7×10^{-4}	1500
Dimethyl carbamate of 3-hydroxy-1-methylpyridinium bromide (Nu-1317)	1.3×10^{-4}	2.5	7.0×10^{-5}	3.3	3.6×10^{-5}	17	3.0×10^{-4}	2.5	1.3×10^{-3}	200
Physostigmine	1.6×10^{-4}	2.0	1.0×10^{-4}	2.3	1.8×10^{-4}	3.4	2.3×10^{-4}	3.3	7.0×10^{-4}	350
p-Tolylmethyl carbamate of m-dimethylaminophenolmethyl bromide (Nu-1197)	3.2×10^{-4}	1.0	1.4×10^{-4}	1.6	$> 1.3 \times 10^{-4}$	< 4.7	$> 2.6 \times 10^{-4}$	< 2.9	5.0×10^{-4}	500
DFP	5.3×10^{-4}	0.6	4.8×10^{-4}	0.5	1.5×10^{-4}	4.1	$> 7.0 \times 10^{-4}$	< 1.1	1.0×10^{-3}	250

* EPP: endplate potential. (From: ECCLES and MACFARLANE 1949.)

By plotting the relative changes of amplitude or duration of endplate negativity in relation to the logarithms of doses of the agents used, ECCLES and MACFARLANE (1949) obtained sigmoid curves. It was suggested that these sigmoid curves represent dissociation curves of drug-ChE complexes at the receptor site; for neostigmine, an apparent dissociation constant of approximately 5×10^{-6} M was derived. Clearly, the similarity of shape of these curves with dissociation curves of enzyme-inhibitor complexes is of a purely formal nature, since dissociation curves, in general, have a sigmoid shape; their slopes are determined only by the molar ratios of the reacting constituents at equilibrium. The observed sigmoid curves may also stand for receptor-drug equilibria not related to ChE. One is not bound, therefore, to accept the conclusion of ECCLES and MACFARLANE (1949) that the apparent magnitude of the estimated dissociation constant places the system, with respect to ChE, in zone A of STRAUS and GOLDSTEIN (1943). If, however, the system operates in zone C, — as it would on the basis of the magnitude of the known enzyme-inhibitor dissociation constants — it is difficult to account for potency differences of various carbamates purely on grounds of an inhibitory action on ChE (see page 582).

II. Avian muscle

In avian muscle, the characteristic effect of substances with nicotine-like action consists in an initial quick development of tension followed by a contracture which becomes more evident as the dose of the nicotinic agent is increased (BROWN and HARVEY 1938b). In its reaction to ACh, avian muscle closely resembles normal amphibian tonic muscle, and mammalian muscle after degeneration of its motor nerve supply (GASSER and DALE 1926). Transmission in avian muscle differs from that in mammalian muscle in that, in the former, a considerable proportion of fibres (25%) fails to respond to a single stimulus; the ineffective stimulus, however, is followed by a period of raised excitability for 150 msec, during which a second stimulus causes the recruitment of fibres. A tetanus is followed by a similar but longer period of facilitation with recruitment (BROWN and HARVEY 1938a).

The effect of physostigmine on avian muscle differs from its effect on mammalian muscle in several respects (BROWN and HARVEY 1938b); it induces potentiation of the contractile response to maximal motor nerve stimuli to a lesser extent, and more transiently, than in mammalian muscle; the potentiation is primarily due to an increase in the number of muscle fibres responding to a single nerve volley, whereas small repetitive discharges occur, if at all, only transiently. However, repetition can be produced in eserinized avian muscle subsequent to tetanic stimulation of the motor nerve. BROWN and HARVEY (1938b) suggested that these differences between avian and mammalian muscle could be accounted for by assuming that the amount of ACh liberated by a single impulse at a motor nerve ending in avian muscle is only slightly above a critical threshold level for most fibres, and is subliminal for some. However, the presence in avian skeletal muscle of two types of muscle fibres with structurally different nerve endings may also have to be considered (KRÜGER and GUNTHER 1958). The spontaneous activity at neuromuscular junctions of chick muscle provides evidence of two types of muscle fibres: one with a focal endplate, the other with multiple junctional regions distributed along the muscle fibre (GINSBORG 1960).

The avian gastrocnemius muscle possesses the convenient property of reacting with contraction and contracture to agents of the nicotine type, and with flaccid paralysis to agents of the curare type (BUTTLE and ZAIMIS 1949; GINZEL et al. 1951c; THESLEFF and UNNA 1954). This was utilized by PELIKAN et al. (1954) to study the excitatory and anticurare action of some hydroxy-phenyltrialkylammonium compounds. Neostigmine and the m-hydroxy-phenyltrialkylammonium ions are effective antagonists of d-tubocurarine. As in the mammalian muscle, antagonism of curare by neostigmine is slow in onset but increases continuously;

the anticurare action of the m-hydroxy-phenyltrialkylammonium ion, on the other hand, is prompt in onset. After attaining its maximum, however, there is frequently a recurrence of paralysis but to a lesser degree than was present immediately before administration of the anticurare agent. There is no correlation between the ability to restore transmission blocked by curare, and the ability to elicit contractures; this is particularly obvious with neostigmine which does not cause contractures at all but is at the same time the most powerful anticurare agent of this series (Table 5).

From the apparent lack of correlation between excitatory and anticurare action, PELIKAN et al. (1954) inferred that the restoring action on transmission of these agents cannot be causally related to their direct excitatory action. Indeed, anticurare and excitatory action are manifest at different dose levels and stimulation in the absence of curare — with the exception of the phenyltrimethylammonium ion — requires considerably higher doses than restoration of transmission in the presence of curare (Table 5). Moreover, some bisquaternary ammonium compounds may set up submaximal contractures during complete transmission block by curare without restoring indirect excitability (GINZEL et al. 1951 c). Conversely, contractures may be suppressed by anodic polarization of

Table 5. *Comparison of potency of anticurare agents in inducing contracture of the chicken gastrocnemius and antagonizing tubocurarine*

Drugs	Number of experiments	Dose (μg/kg) to produce 25% of maximum contracture	Dose (μg/kg) reversing PD*$_{75-90}$ of d-tubocurarine	μg of d-tubocurarine antagonized per μg of anticurare agent
3-Hydroxy-phenyltrimethyl-ammonium	9	350	150—250	1.69 ± 0.17
3-Hydroxy-phenyldiethyl-methylammonium	8	1000	150—250	1.78 ± 0.30
3-Hydroxy-phenylmethyldi-ethylammonium	7	> 3000	150—250	1.35 ± 0.10
3-Hydroxy-phenyltriethyl-ammonium	8	none with 5000	150—250	0.44 ± 0.12
Neostigmine.	1	none with 250	25	ca. 25
Phenyltrimethylammonium . .	3	150	1000	ca. 0.24
Phenol	2	clonic convulsions	—	0

* PD = Paralytic dose. (From: PELIKAN et al. 1954.)

muscle without affecting the occurrence of transmission (GINZEL et al. 1952). These observations certainly reveal an independence of contractural effects from transmission. It appears, therefore, that neostigmine and the hydroxyanilinium compounds exert their antagonism of curariform blockade independently of their contractural effects. PELIKAN et al. (1954) suggested that this idea was compatible with the assumption that anticurare action is a result of ChE-inhibition at the junctional region. This contention was apparently strengthened by the fact that prior administration of TEPP abolished the anticurare action of these agents. Neostigmine and some simple m-hydroxy-phenyltrialkylammonium ions are capable of increasing the twitch contraction height on stimulation with single pulses, and of decreasing contraction height of muscles stimulated tetanically (PELIKAN et al. 1954).

Normal chick plasma has a BuChE activity of about 1/18 of that of human plasma. Whereas some potentiation of the contractural effect of succinylcholine was noted in eserinized animals, inactivation of AChE by 284C51 (see page 624) had no effect on the sensitivity to succinylcholine (FRASER 1954).

III. Mammalian muscle

Cholinesterase of neuromuscular junction

From the relative rates of hydrolysis by rat muscle homogenate of benzoylcholine and acetyl-β-methylcholine (methacholine, Mecholyl), ORD and THOMPSON (1950) concluded that AChE is the principal ChE enzyme. This contention was also supported by the high concentrations of DFP required to inhibit ACh hydrolysis by rat muscle homogenates. By means of histochemical methods, KOELLE (1950) and DENZ (1953) conclusively identified the enzyme at the neuromuscular junction of striated muscle as chiefly AChE; the rat diaphragm, however, also contains some BuChE (DENZ 1953; DAVISON 1953; GIACOBINI 1959). KOELLE (1957a) has developed the histochemical approach into a powerful tool to determine directly the relation between ChE inhibition at an effector site and effects produced *in vivo* by reversible anti-ChE agents: the method is based on KOSTER's (1946) observation that a reversible inhibitor can prevent the lethal action of DFP by transient competitive combination with the enzyme (KOELLE 1946). By administration of DFP to animals which had previously received a dose of a reversible inhibitor, N,N'-*bis*-(diethyl-2-chlorobenzylammonium ethyl)-oxamide dichloride (ambenonium chloride, Mytelase chloride; LANDS et al. 1955), KOELLE (1957a) histochemically estimated the degree of AChE inhibition at effector sites which prevailed *in vivo* just prior to the administration of DFP; the AChE activity at various effector structures, including striated muscle, was indeed reduced after treatment of the animals with ambenonium in pharmacologically active doses. However, KOELLE (1957a) was careful to point out that this correlation between *in vivo* actions and histochemically demonstrated enzyme inhibition at selective sites does not necessarily exclude the possibility of a direct drug-receptor interaction as well. These investigations also revealed significant facts regarding the distribution of AChE at effector sites: the histochemically determined degree of AChE inhibition by ambenonium was not paralleled by significant inhibition of total AChE activity of tissue homogenates. KOELLE (1957a) interpreted this divergence on the basis of a possible separation, by a lipoid-like membrane, of "external" from "internal" AChE (BURGEN and CHIPMAN 1952). Only the former is thought to be functionally important, whereas the latter supposedly serves as "reserve" (KOELLE and STEINER 1956; McISAAC and KOELLE 1959). Equal degrees of inhibition of "functional" esterase may, therefore, be associated with largely divergent degrees of inhibition of total esterase activity in homogenates, depending only on the permeability of the separating membrane for the inhibitor used.

CREVIER and BÉLANGER (1956) attempted to determine histophotometrically the inhibition of AChE at the neuromuscular junction of rats sacrificed after physostigmine administration: lethal doses of physostigmine were required to reduce the enzyme activity by 50%. However, this procedure may have underestimated the true enzyme inhibition at the time of death of the animal; the enzyme-inhibitor complex is likely to have partly dissociated during incubation of the tissue specimens.

Most of the AChE activity can apparently be attributed to the subneural apparatus which represents invaginations of the sarcolemma into the sarcoplasm; however, the terminal axoplasmic membrane is so intimately opposed to the grooved (postsynaptic) sarcolemma that it is difficult to decide whether enzymatic activity can also be recognized in terminal axonal branches (COUTEAUX 1958). This question is discussed further in Chapter 6.

1. Potentiation of contractile response and anticurare action under equilibrium conditions

a) Carbamate esters

The essential argument of most studies on anticurare action relates to the part played by AChE inhibition at the neuromuscular junction; specifically, the issue is whether or not, for series of homologous agents, a direct proportionality exists between AChE inhibiting potency and anticurare activity. However, there is no doubt about the existence of mechanisms of anticurare action which are unrelated to AChE inhibition. The curare-receptor reaction may be described in terms of a chemical equilibrium, the equilibrium constant of which is temperature-dependent (HOLMES et al. 1951). Furthermore, the degree of transmission block varies in accordance with the concentration of K-ions, to the extent that QUILLIAM and TAYLOR (1947) postulated that for curare to produce block, it must first displace K-ions from receptor sites (see also CREESE et al. 1961).

In extension of previous work of Bülbring and Chou (1947), Blaschko et al. (1949) compared the inhibitory potency of neostigmine and other carbamate esters on dog nucleus caudatus AChE with anticurare activity in the rat diaphragm. The results, summarized in Table 6, reveal a statistically significant correlation between these two independent series of measurements; no correlation exists between anticurare activity and inhibitor potency against BuChE.

Several points of interest are apparent from Table 6. Amongst the congeners of neostigmine, the diethylmethyl derivative is by far the most potent ChE inhibitor and anticurare agent. Introduction of another ethyl group decreases the activity in both respects below that of neostigmine. Blaschko et al. (1949) were impressed also by the lack of potency of the amine oxide homologue of neostigmine; this was related to the fact that amine oxides of the general structure {R₃NOH} OH (where R is an alkyl or aromatic radical) are bases with very small dissociation constants. It was, therefore, believed that the strongly basic character of the phenolic nitrogen radical is a requirement for anti-ChE and anticurare activity.

Riker (1953), in reviewing the data of Blaschko et al. (1949), pointed out that there are some exceptions to the alleged parallelism of anti-ChE and anticurare potency which do not become apparent when considering only the correlation coefficient of the series as a whole: physostigmine and substance 38, although equal with respect to their anti-ChE potency, differ markedly in anticurare potency; also, the triethyl-homologues of neostigmine and miotine, although equipotent with respect to inhibition of AChE, differ in anticurare activity.

In the rat diaphragm, neostigmine antagonizes not only the neuromuscular paralysis by *d*-tubocurarine, but also paralysis by decamethonium and amyltrimethylammonium (Brand 1952). Secher (1951) devoted a special study to the quantitative aspects of the neostigmine action on the rat diaphragm depressed, *in vitro*, by ether: in small doses, neostigmine and physostigmine restore the etherdepressed neuromuscular transmission, but in higher doses, both agents potentiate the paralyzing effect of ether.

Physostigmine and neostigmine, in suitable doses and at low frequency of stimulation, augment the contractions of the indirectly stimulated rat diaphragm preparation (Bülbring 1946). Characteristically, this augmenting action reaches its maximum gradually in the course of several minutes of exposure to the agents. Brown et al. (1936) first observed the twitch potentiation by physostigmine in the cat; the slow onset of action was attributed to gradual accumulation of ACh with the arrival of each nerve volley at the neuromuscular junction. However, this

Table 6. *Relation between anticurare- and anti-ChE activity in a series of carbamate esters*

Compounds	Anticurarine activity pD_{20} value	Anti-ChE activity pI_{50} value	
		AChE	BuChE
Neostigmine (RNMe₃)*	7.60	7.4	7.2
RNMe₂Et*	8.19	8.0	7.3
RNMeEt₂*	8.57	8.2	8.0
RNEt₃*	6.59	7.2	7.4
Miotine HCl	7.85	7.2	6.4
Physostigmine sulfate	7.21	7.1	7.7
No. 38**	6.23	7.1	7.6
Nu 1250 (see Table 4 and 2) . .	7.26	7.4	7.9
Nu 1197 (see Table 4 and 2) . .	7.31	6.9	7.1
Nu 683***	5.44	6.2	8.5
5130****	5.26	6.4	5.8
5220/5 (RNMe₂OH)*	4.77	4.5	4.4

* R = *m*-(CH₃)₂N · CO₂C₆H₄⁻

** =

(CH₃)₂N · CO · O — N⁺ SO₄CH₃⁻ / CH₃

*** = CH₂N₊(CH₃)₃ Br⁻ / O · CO · N(CH₃)₂

**** = O · CO · N(CH₃)₂ / N⁺ Br⁻ / CH₃

(From: Blaschko et al. 1949.)

supposition is not corroborated by the observations of TAUGNER and FLECKEN-STEIN (1950): in parallel assays of the two halves of rat diaphragms, equal degrees of augmentation of twitch tension were obtained at any given time after addition of physostigmine to the bath, irrespective of whether the muscle was stimulated throughout this period or not; therefore, the characteristic time-action curve of physostigmine in this preparation is not related to recurrent nerve activity. TAUGNER and FLECKENSTEIN (1950) were not satisfied with the alternative assumption of continuous accumulation of spontaneously liberated ACh at the neuromuscular junction in the presence of neostigmine or physostigmine; it was considered more likely that the augmenting effect reflected a direct action on receptors. The curve of onset of augmentation may, in this case, be viewed as a measure of the kinetics of a drug-receptor reaction; it would speak for the essential similarity of AChE and receptor structures, that maximal augmentation is attained at a rate similar to that with which equilibrium between physostigmine and ChE is established *in vitro* in the presence of substrate (BURGEN 1949).

Table 7. *Effect of neostigmine on contraction of rat diaphragm at different frequencies of nerve stimulation*

Dose of neostigmine (μg per 100 ml)	Rate of stimulation per minute			
	5—8	9—12	14—16	18—24
0.1 —0.2	no effect or increase	increase	increase	increase
0.25—0.3	increase	increase	uncertain	—
0.4 —0.5	increase	uncertain	increase followed by depression	—
1.0 —2.0	uncertain	increase followed by depression	depression	depression
10.0	depression	—	—	—

(From: BÜLBRING 1946.)

Potentiation of the twitch response of the rat diaphragm by neostigmine depends critically on the dose and stimulation frequency (BÜLBRING 1946). Table 7 clearly shows that the potentiating effect of increasing doses of neostigmine is converted into depression at higher rates of stimulation; also, the upper frequency limit at which augmentation occurs is shifted towards lower frequencies as the neostigmine dose increases. Qualitatively identical results are obtained with physostigmine, but the threshold dose for potentiation is about 10 times lower than that of neostigmine, and as little as 0.1 μg per 100 ml leads to reversible depression at a stimulus frequency of 5 per min (BÜLBRING 1946). High doses of physostigmine and neostigmine diminish both direct and indirect excitability of the muscle preparation. Addition of appropriate doses of curare or Ca-ions restores transmission and excitability (RUMMEL and SCHULZ 1954).

In diaphragm preparations of rats treated with botulinum toxin, reduction of ACh output on motor nerve stimulation was observed (BURGEN et al. 1949a). At the same time, miniature endplate activity diminishes (BROOKS 1954) or ceases, and ACh sensitivity spreads from the endplate to the entire muscle membrane in a similar manner and with the same time course as in chronically denervated muscle (THESLEFF 1960; see also: AXELSSON and THESLEFF 1959). Neostigmine and physostigmine cause, in preparations partially paralyzed by this toxin, small temporary increases in tension; as in normal muscles, these agents produce depression of neuromuscular transmission in higher concentrations. However, if this depression were a consequence of excessive ACh accumulation, one would expect the toxin-treated preparations to be less susceptible to paralysis by these drugs.

The mechanism of transmission failure for nerve tetani in the presence of neostigmine or physostigmine is open to speculation. THESLEFF (1959) demonstrated that periods of tetanic stimulation of the phrenic nerve are followed by reduced sensitivity of motor endplates to electrophoretically applied ACh. Accordingly, transmission failure on tetanic stimulation may be ascribed to accumulation of ACh and consequent 'desensitization' of junctional receptors (c.f., AXELSSON and THESLEFF 1958). However, the work of KRNJEVIĆ and MILEDI (1958a, 1959) revealed the establishment of presynaptic conduction block at stimulus frequencies exceeding about 20 per sec. This presynaptic block is presumably related to changes in the intramuscular portion of motor nerve fibres occasioned by anoxia. Thus, it seems likely that the junctions are, under a variety of experimental conditions, activated at frequencies below those of nerve trunk stimulation; consequently, transmitter accumulation to the extent of "receptor desensitization" may not be attained. With this precaution in mind, KRNJEVIĆ and MITCHELL (1960; 1961) designed experiments to determine the amount of ACh liberated at single nerve endings of eserinized rat diaphragm preparation: the mean value obtained (i.e., 1.1×10^{-17} mole ACh per impulse and ending) is of the same order as the amount of ACh that elicits an EPP on electrophoretic application to an individual junction.

Pertinent findings were also reported by STRAUGHAN (1960a): ACh release from guinea pig nerve-diaphragm preparations increased with raising the stimulus frequency from 6 to 50 stimuli per sec, and declined at higher rates of nerve stimulation. The sensitivity of the endplate to locally applied ACh remained unchanged during depression of the EPP evoked by repetitive nerve stimulation (OTSUKA and ENDO 1960b). From studies of the quantum content of neurally evoked EPP's, THIES (1960) concluded that neither presynaptic conduction block nor depression of postsynaptic sensitivity to transmitter will ordinarily occur during physiologic activity, but ACh release per impulse will be submaximal during all natural activity.

In addition to potentiating the indirectly developed twitch tension, physostigmine causes the appearance of an "after-contracture" in some skeletal muscles of the rabbit (RIESSER 1921): single twitch responses of the *semitendinosus* muscle are followed by residual muscle shortening of several seconds duration. Such "after-contractures" do not, however, occur in the *extensor communis* muscle, and RIESSER (1921) generalized that this phenomenon is characteristic only for eserinized "red" (tonic) muscle.

The morphologic distinction between tonic and tetanic muscle, as originally proposed for the frog (see page 574), has been established for mammalian skeletal muscle (KRÜGER 1950). Evidence was obtained that different skeletal muscles contain, in various proportions, tetanic muscle fibres with "fibrillar" structure, and tonic muscle fibres with "field" structure: e.g., in the diaphragm of rat and rabbit, the two fibre types occur in approximately equal number (GUNTHER 1952). Measurements of membrane resting and action potentials in a large number of muscle fibres of the rat diaphragm did not reveal any differences between the two groups of muscle fibres (MUSCHOLL 1957). Whatever physiologic or pharmacologic differences may exist between tonic and tetanic muscles cannot, therefore, be due to membrane characteristics of the muscle fibres. Such differences may, however, be related to the occurrence of two types of synaptic formations, i.e., «terminaisons en plaque» with heavily myelinated preterminal motor fibres in tetanic ("white") muscles, and «terminaison en grappe» with very fine nerve branches in tonic ("red") muscles.

The rat diaphragm has been conveniently used to study the potentiation, by physostigmine and neostigmine, of the paralyzing action of some aliphatic dicholine esters (GINZEL et al. 1951a). Potentiation was maximal for adipyldicholine (2 to 20 times, depending on the concentration of the ChE inhibitor), while homologous compounds with shorter, and longer, chain-lengths were potentiated to a lesser extent. Potentiation was negligible, or absent (LÜLLMANN and FÖRSTER 1953), with succinyldicholine. Isoboles for 50% paralysis, resulting from combinations of appropriate concentrations of physostigmine and dicholine esters of dicarboxylic acids, were constructed; there was no correlation between the degree of potentiation and the velocity of enzymatic hydrolysis of these agents by BuChE or AChE of the *nucleus caudatus* (GINZEL et al. 1951b).

The choline ester of carbamic acid (carbaminoylcholine, carbachol) has strong muscarinic and nicotinic properties (KREITMAIR 1932) and is a potent neuromuscular blocking agent in mammalian striated muscle (BACQ and BROWN 1937). Doubling of the carbaminoylcholine molecule led to a substance with diminished muscarinic and muscle-paralyzing potency (BOVET et al. 1951). However, by increasing the chain-length through interposition of 6 to 10 methylene groups between the carbamic acid residues, compounds with very remarkable pharmacologic properties were obtained (CHEYMOL et al. 1954; KLUPP et al. 1953; KRAUPP et al. 1954). Although these agents are potent inhibitors of ChE's (e.g., I_{50} of the octamethylene homologue for BuChE = 10^{-6} M; for AChE = 2×10^{-7} M), they do not exert any anticurare action on the isolated rat diaphragm (KOBINGER and KRAUPP 1955). Moreover, paralysis by the octamethylene homologue, which is the most potent ChE inhibitor of this series can be at least partly reversed by physostigmine. Curiously, addition of a small dose of d-tubocurarine to a preparation which had been exposed for some time to a paralyzing concentration of this agent facilitates the restoring activity of physostigmine. Measurements of endplate potentials in the cat *gracilis* muscle also revealed that transmission block by octamethylene-dicarbaminoylcholine is best antagonized by combined administration of d-tubocurarine and physostigmine in appropriate doses (PILLAT et al. 1955).

This unusual observation may indicate that the octamethylene homologue and d-tubocurarine compete for the same receptors, and that conditions for antagonism by physostigmine become more favorable as an increasing proportion of receptors is occupied by curare (KOBINGER and KRAUPP 1955). The dicholine esters of aliphatic dicarbamic acids possess, however, some depolarizing activity and it is not certain whether the interaction with curare could not thereby be complicated; but the absence of any anticurare action of the agent on the rat diaphragm, and the partial reversibility by physostigmine of its paralyzing action, may be indicative of rapid transition of initial depolarization into competitive (curare-like) block.

b) Hydroxyanilinium ions

In 1950, RANDALL and LEHMANN (1950), RIKER and WESCOE (1950), and MACFARLANE et al. (1950) reported studies on a number of neostigmine analogues which possessed striking anticurare action *in vivo*, but were relatively weak inhibitors of ChE *in vitro*. These agents were either hydroxyanilinium salts, or their esters (esters of carbamic acid are not considered in this section). It was also found that these substances reached the peak of anticurare action *in vivo* much more quickly than neostigmine, and that they could be administered repeatedly without loss of anticurare potency or decrease in sensitivity of transmission to d-tubocurarine. These findings prompted a detailed study by HOBBIGER (1952) of some neostigmine analogues under equilibrium conditions in the rat diaphragm. Besides edrophonium, HOBBIGER used the 3-benzoxy- and 3-m-toluyloxy-phenyltrimethylammonium ion (Ro 2-2650 and Ro 2-2783, respectively) and the 3-acetoxy-phenyldiethylmethylammonium ion (Ro 2-2651). In accordance with their action on the contractile force of the diaphragm upon stimulation with single pulses, these agents could be classified into two categories. The compounds containing a dimethylethyl- or methyldiethyl-group (edrophonium and Ro 2-2651) potentiated the twitch tension in concentrations of 1 μg per ml, and higher; they were in this respect about 50 times less potent than neostigmine. On the other hand, twitch potentiation could not be obtained at any concentration with the N-trimethyl agents, Ro 2-2650 and Ro 2-2783. But all four neostigmine analogues antagonized the action of curare on the diaphragm. The onset of anticurare action was much more rapid with the neostigmine analogues than with neostigmine. For the ethyl derivatives (Ro 2-2651 and Ro 2-3198), the ratio of stimulant to anticurare activity was the same as that for neostigmine.

From observations on the frog rectus muscle (see page 580), HOBBIGER (1952) inferred that the trimethyl analogues possess some depolarizing activity, and it was suggested that this could explain the absence of twitch potentiation by these agents in the non-curarized diaphragm. In the presence of curare, however, the endplate would be protected from the depolarizing action of the trimethyl derivatives, and their potential capacity to facilitate transmission could then become manifest as anticurare action. Indeed, HOBBIGER (1952) showed that agents with presumably pure depolarizing activity (like C_{10}) exert only insignificant curare antagonism in the rat diaphragm. This explanation assumes, therefore, that curare suppresses depolarization of endplates more specifically than facilitatory actions of drugs on neuromuscular transmission. However, MOGEY and YOUNG (1949), VAN DER MEER and MEETER (1956a) and WERNER (1959) found that curare suppresses facilitatory drug actions in concentrations far lower than those affecting transmission of single nerve volleys.

In diaphragm preparations exposed for one hour to DFP (20 μg/ml), neostigmine and its analogues did not exert any anticurare action (HOBBIGER 1952). The assay was performed after exchange of the DFP-containing Tyrode solutions for DFP-free solutions. These preparations were not able to sustain a tetanus (EVANS 1951; BURGEN and HOBBIGER 1951). Also, the concentrations of d-tubocurarine required to block neuromuscular transmission exceeded the equally effective curare concentrations in normal preparations by about two and one-half times. The only effect that could be obtained in such preparations after paralysis by d-tubocurarine consisted in depression of twitch height by high doses of neostigmine and some of its analogues; catechol and KCl, on the other hand, were as effective anticurare agents as on normal diaphragm. HOBBIGER (1952) concluded from these observations that the neostigmine analogues did not produce their anticurare action by virtue of free phenolic groups (either present in the original compound, or freed by enzymatic hydrolysis of the esters). Furthermore, the absence of curare antagonism in DFP-treated preparations was considered evidence that the anticurare action of neostigmine and its analogues was solely due to ChE-inhibition. The AChE-inhibitory potency of the agents used was 1/100 to 1/400 of the inhibitory potency of neostigmine. This interpretation of the results is complicated by the fact that assay of anticurare action was carried out in diaphragm preparations which were unable to maintain tetanic contractions. This fact appears important in view of the observation by BERRY and EVANS (1951) that transmission of tetanic stimuli (even if tested at a stimulus frequency of 80 per sec) can be restored after treatment with DFP, although the ChE of the diaphragm preparations remains completely inhibited within the limits of error of measurement. Therefore, it is questionable whether the diminution by DFP of the anticurare action of neostigmine and its analogues is a consequence of ChE inhibition per se, or whether it is attributable only to that aspect of DFP action which results in inhibition of repetitive excitability. The latter effect is easily reversible and is apparently unrelated to ChE inhibition. Indeed, direct actions of DFP on synaptic receptors have been inferred by several authors (BARSTAD 1956a, b; NAESS 1956; AXELSSON et al. 1957).

c) Aliphatic mono- and bisquaternary ions

Some polymethylene bis-onium salts are capable of augmenting the twitch tension of the rat diaphragm (BARLOW and ING 1948); this action is particularly prominent with the bis-triethylammonium compounds of short chain length, and with the decamethylene-bis-quinolinium ion (BQ_{10}). BARLOW and ING (1948) determined also the inhibitory potency of these compounds on the AChE of the nucleus caudatus and found a "rough correlation" between AChE inhibition and augmentative effect. However, BARLOW and ING (1948) were reluctant to explain augmentative activity solely in terms of ChE inhibition and admitted that other mechanisms of facilitatory action should be explored.

It was recognized early that the anticurare action of physostigmine extends over a limited dosage range of curare; this limitation of anticurare action was shown also for edrophonium and neostigmine in the rat (VAN MAANEN 1950a). Under equilibrium conditions in the rat diaphragm, the tetraethylammonium ion (TEA, NEt$_4$) produces an additional anticurare effect when the amount of curare that can be antagonized by neostigmine is exceeded (KENSLER 1950). The reverse of this was also shown to be true, thereby revealing a limited anticurare action for

NEt$_4$. Tetraethylammonium increases the height of the endplate potentials in curarized rat diaphragm (STOVNER 1958b) and in preparations exposed to high concentrations of Mg-ions (STOVNER 1957). This effect of NEt$_4$ on the Mg^{++}-blocked diaphragm is specific, insofar as neither its β-hydroxy derivative nor choline restores transmission. Since NEt$_4$ lacks significant anti-ChE action (KENSLER and ELSNER 1951), and also since the time course of the EPP is not altered by it, STOVNER (1957, 1958b) concluded that this ion restores transmission by acting on preterminal motor nerves. More specifically, STOVNER considered the evidence to be compatible with the assumption that NEt$_4$ increases the liberation of ACh from the nerve endings.

In the rat, paralysis of neuromuscular transmission by d-tubocurarine, C$_{10}$, and duodecyltrimethylammonium is antagonized by NEt$_4$ and propyltriethylammonium, i.e., agents that lack any depolarizing activity. Conversely, butyl- and amyl-trimethylammonium, known to be strong depolarizing agents in the cat (PHILIPPOT and SCHLAG 1956), summate their paralyzing action with that of curare. In view of these findings, PHILIPPOT (1956) proposed that the variety of ways in which chemical agents affect neuromuscular transmission cannot adequately be accounted for solely on the basis of depolarization and drug competition at postsynaptic structures.

d) Organophosphorus compounds

In the rat phrenic nerve-diaphragm, TEPP in concentrations of about 0.02 to 0.2 μg/ml produces twitch potentiation and restores transmission in curarized preparations. Higher doses of TEPP, in the absence of curare, depress transmission (BURGEN et al. 1949b).

Evidence has been obtained that organophosphates inhibit ChE by phosphorylation of the active enzyme center (BURGEN 1949; WILSON and BERGMANN 1950). This type of inhibition is commonly called "irreversible," but GROB (1950) and HOBBIGER (1951) demonstrated marked differences in the duration of action between different agents of this group. BURGEN and HOBBIGER (1951) reasoned that, if organophosphates inhibit ChE by attachment of an alkylphosphate group to the enzyme, the rate of enzyme recovery should be determined only by the nature of the alkyl group. Also, variation in the alkyl group of a series of such agents permitted an examination of the relation between kinetics of enzyme inhibition *in vitro* and actions obtained on nerve-muscle preparations. The compounds studied by BURGEN and HOBBIGER (1951) are listed in Table 8.

In accordance with expectations, the kinetics of inhibition by dialkylphosphostigmines differed with different alkyl groups. The dimethylester resembled neostigmine insofar as the addition of substrate to the preincubated enzyme-inhibitor mixture was followed by an increase of enzyme activity during the first 30 min, by which time a new state of equilibrium had been reached. Phosphorylation of the enzyme by this compound probably does not occur at all and the agent may thus be considered a truly reversible inhibitor. However, no enzyme reactivation by addition of substrate was observed with the diethyl-, di*iso*propyl-, or di*sec*-butylester. Only the former showed some reactivation within a time course similar to that after treatment of enzyme with TEPP; the esters with the larger radicals resembled DFP, since, after removal of uncombined inhibitor, reactivation did not take place *in vitro*.

Similarly, the time course of recovery of neuromuscular transmission in the rat diaphragm was determined after removal of inhibitor; the interference by ChE inhibitors with the ability of the nerve-muscle preparation to sustain a tetanic contraction was chosen as a criterion of measurement (BURGEN and HOBBIGER 1951; EVANS 1951). After temporary exposure to neostigmine or dimethylphosphostigmine, recovery of sustained tetanic contraction at frequencies of 25, 50, and 100 stimuli per sec, was completed within 30 to 40 min. After diethyl-phosphostigmine and TEPP, recovery of tetanic response was incomplete at the lower, and absent at the highest stimulus frequency; however, after exposure to DFP or di*sec*butyl-phosphostigmine, no significant recovery to stimulation at 50 or 100 per sec took place within the observation period of 90 min.

Table 8. *Inhibitor potency of some alkylphosphates on red cell AChE and serum BuChE*

$$O{-}P{<}^{OR}_{OR}$$
$$\downarrow$$
$$O$$
$$N^+$$
$$H_3C\ CH_3CH_3\ [CH_3SO_4]^-$$

Code No.	R	Chemical name	Short title	Molar conc. required for 50% inhibition of	
				Red cell AChE	Serum BuChE
Ro 3-0412	—CH₃	*m*-(dimethylphosphato)-N-trimethylanilinium methylsulphate	Dimethylester	7.5×10^{-8}	6.3×10^{-9}
Ro 3-0340	—CH₂CH₃	*m*-(diethylphosphato)-N-trimethylanilinium methylsulphate	Diethylester	8×10^{-8}	1.2×10^{-9}
Ro 3-0411	—CH$<^{CH_3}_{CH_3}$	*m*-(diisopropylphosphato)-N-trimethylanilinium methylsulphate	Diisopropylester	2.1×10^{-7}	3×10^{-9}
Ro 3-0397	—CH$<^{CH_3}_{CH_2CH_3}$	*m*-(disecbutylphosphato)-N-trimethylanilinium methylsulphate	Disecbutylester	1.6×10^{-7}	9×10^{-9}
Neostigmine	—	—	—	1.14×10^{-7}	6.9×10^{-7}
TEPP	—	—	—	1.2×10^{-8}	8×10^{-10}

(From: BURGEN and HOBBIGER 1951.)

These experiments strongly support the theory that the dialkylphosphoryl residue of the ChE inhibitor molecule determines duration of enzyme inhibition. In addition, they show that recovery time of tetanic excitability depends on the dialkylphosphoryl groups of the inhibitor agents used. However, it is striking that the ability of the nerve-muscle preparation to sustain a tetanus at 25 per sec recovered within 90 min after removal of DFP or the disecbutylester, although, *in vitro*, no measurable enzyme reactivation occurred within 48 hours. Also, BERRY and EVANS (1951) found no evidence for enzyme reactivation in rat diaphragms after exposure to TEPP or DFP at a time when the response to single and tetanic stimulation was fully restored. Consequently, they proposed two alternatives: either the AChE at the neuromuscular junction is not essential for junctional transmission at low frequency of transmission, or a very low activity of AChE — within the error of estimate — will suffice for transmission.

BARNES and DUFF (1953) attempted to analyze the time course of action of several alkylphosphates in the rat diaphragm preparation; diethyl-*p*-nitrophenyl phosphate (Paraoxon) was used as the principal agent.

The kinetics of its enzyme inhibition and reactivation are known from studies of ALDRIDGE (1950) and DAVISON (1953, 1955). Acetylcholinesterase and BuChE are phosphorylated by this inhibitor; the reaction is bimolecular, i.e., the time for 50% inhibition is inversely proportional to the inhibitor concentration. Reactivation of AChE occurs slowly (60% in 4 days) and is apparently incomplete, whereas reactivation of BuChE is completed in about 24 hours.

If Paraoxon is added to give a final concentration of 4×10^{-7} M in the organ bath, there is a latent period of 2 min before the contractions begin to increase (Fig. 8). The tension then increases rapidly for 3 to 4 min and fasciculation occurs during this period of augmented contractions. However, within 10 min of the addition of the inhibitor, the contractions return to their original size even though the diaphragm may be left in the solution containing the inhibitor for several hours: nevertheless, the ability to sustain a tetanic contraction is lost throughout this period. Concomitantly, the sensitivity to paralysis by addition of ACh to the bath is increased. This sequence of events takes place at a greater rate with higher concentrations of inhibitor in the bath. Removal of Paraoxon by repeated washing usually does not affect the twitch tension, but the response to a tetanus recovers in the course of some 30 to 40 min, and the sensitivity to ACh decreases concomitantly. Addition of a second dose of Paraoxon to the preparation after removal of the initial dose does not result in fasciculation or twitch potentiation; its only effect is a reduction of tetanic excitability and enhanced sensitivity to the depressant action of ACh.

Inhibition of rat diaphragm ChE by Paraoxon proceeds at a rate similar to that of ChE inhibition in red cells or tissue homogenates. BARNES and DUFF (1953), therefore, considered it permissible to calculate how much AChE and BuChE activity would be present in the diaphragm at different times after adding or removing Paraoxon. For this purpose, the rate constants of Paraoxon for inhibition and reactivation as determined *in vitro* by DAVISON (1953) were utilized. In Table 9, the results of such calculations are summarized for different times after the addition of Paraoxon to a final concentration of 1×10^{-7} M. Accordingly, enhancement of twitch response to single stimuli takes place when ChE activity is reduced from 50% to 10% of normal, but this effect disappears when the ChE activity decreases still further.

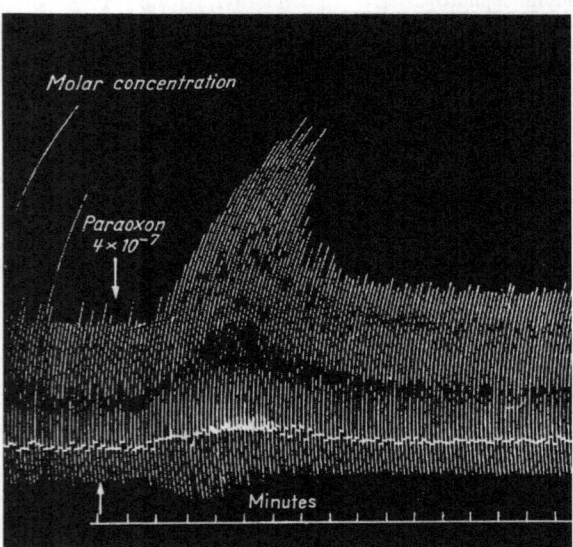

Fig. 8. Effect of *p*-nitrophenyl diethyl phosphate (Paraoxon) on indirectly elicited contraction of rat diaphragm. Frequency of phrenic nerve stimulation: 8 per min. At arrow: addition of Paraoxon, 4×10^{-7} M. Marks of irregular twitching can be seen at base line during the period of enhanced contractions. (From: BARNES and DUFF 1953)

The ability to sustain a tetanus is abolished only when less than 10% of the normal ChE activity remains. However, during recovery from complete inhibition, the power to sustain a tetanus is restored at a time at which less than 5% of the BuChE and virtually none of the AChE has been reactivated (BARNES and DUFF 1953).

These considerations corroborate the contention that alkylphosphates affect the transmitter process in a manner which is not solely explicable on the basis of ChE inhibition. The same conclusion was also reached by BARSTAD (1956a, b), who designed experiments on the basis of the premise that the early phase of neuromuscular block by depolarizing agents (e.g., ACh) can be antagonized by *d*-tubocurarine in appropriate concentrations. Accordingly, if transmission block by DFP were due solely to accumulation of excessive concentrations of ACh at the junctional regions, curare should restore transmission. BARSTAD (1956a) found, however, that the restoring effect of *d*-tubocurarine on transmission is limited to moderate depression by low doses of DFP, and that blockade of single nerve volleys by DFP in concentrations of 2 to 5×10^{-4} M or higher is enhanced by

Table 9. *Calculated activity of AChE and BuChE, and indirect excitability of rat diaphragm at different times after addition and removal of Paraoxon*

Time after addition of Paraoxon (min)	Condition of diaphragm	Calculated enzyme activity, % of normal	
		AChE	BuChE
6	Beginning of enhanced contraction	42	60
18	Failure of tetanus	8	22
20	End of enhanced contraction	5	17
60	50% inhibition by 5×10^{-6} M ACh	0.1	0.5

Time after removal of Paraoxon (min)	Condition of diaphragm	Calculated return of enzyme activity, % of normal	
		AChE	BuChE
30	Ability to hold tetanus	—	3
60	50% inhibition by 6×10^{-5} M ACh	—	11
120	50% inhibition by 1.2×10^{-4} M ACh	—	21
180	50% inhibition by 2×10^{-4} M ACh	1.5	30

(From: BARNES and DUFF 1953.)

curare. On the other hand, this transmission block is easily reversible on exchange of the bath fluid for DFP-free Tyrode solutions, even if exposure of the muscle to inhibitor extends for one hour; BARSTAD (1956b), like BERRY and EVANS (1951), did not find any indication for reactivation of ChE in the diaphragm preparation under these circumstances. More recently, BARSTAD (1960) found that about two-thirds of the total ChE activity must be inhibited by DFP for enhancement of single contractions to occur; maximal augmentation of contraction on single shock stimulation corresponds to about 90% ChE inhibition. Nerve stimulation at a rate of 60 per sec can lead to sustained muscle contraction in the presence of enzyme inhibition to 10 to 15% of normal activity.

From observations on the frog rectus muscle, COHEN and POSTHUMUS (1955) suggested that the action of DFP was due to its combination with a reactive site (B-group) of AChE, and also to its combination with a similar reactive site of neuroreceptors; the latter reaction was supposed to augment the outcome of inter-action of suitable agents with type A reactive groups of the same neuroreceptor (see page 583). This model was applied also to studies with DFP on the phrenic nerve-diaphragm preparation (COHEN and POSTHUMUS 1957). It could, indeed, be shown that DFP increased the sensitivity of the diaphragm preparation for trans-mission block not only by ACh (BARNES and DUFF 1953) and other hydrolyzable esters, but also by such stable agents as decamethonium, edrophonium, or choline. This is analogous to the potentiation by DFP, in the frog rectus muscle, of response to stable ions. COHEN and POSTHUMUS (1957), therefore, suggested that their ex-planatory model is applicable to the mammalian neuromuscular junction, and proposed that DFP in this case acts also with reactive sites that occur both in AChE and neuroreceptors (B-group); depending on the location of the reactive site, irreversible ChE inhibition or reversible sensitization would result.

The demonstration of partially reversible sensitization to ACh in preparations in which ChE was completely inactivated, with small additional doses of DFP (VAN DER MEER and MEETER 1956b), provides a further clue as to the possible dual mode of action of DFP at the neuromuscular junction. On the other hand, partial inactivation of ChE by short exposure to DFP is followed by fasciculation and by the appearance of repetitive muscle action potentials in response to single nerve volleys. Antidromically conducted nerve impulses may simultaneously be recorded from motor nerve fibres to which the single stimuli are applied. Enhanced contraction, fasciculation, and antidromic nerve activity are present when the

ChE activity in the diaphragm is reduced to about 20% of normal; these signs disappear with complete enzyme inhibition. When the DFP-containing solution is removed from the muscle preparation during the initial phase of enhanced mechanical and electrical response, a prolonged period of spontaneous fasciculation of the diaphragm may follow (VAN DER MEER and MEETER 1956a).

During the phase of augmentation of twitch tension on stimulation with single pulses, a prolonged local negative potential may be recorded from the junctional region. This is particularly marked in the course of, and immediately after, tetanic stimulation (MEETER 1958). In the later stage of DFP action, the depolarization of the junctional region results in conduction block and decreased muscle excitability following each nerve volley, but repetitive activity in muscle fibres may persist; this may appear strange in view of the simultaneous decrease in excitability of the muscle fibres, but MEETER (1958) suggests that the repetitive muscle response is caused by the gradient of muscle membrane potential between normal and adjacent depolarized regions (BURNS et al. 1955). However, the astonishingly high potency of d-tubocurarine, and Ca, or Mg ions, in suppressing the DFP-induced muscle repetition and fasciculation (VAN DER MEER and MEETER 1956a) cannot easily be accounted for. A similar suppression of repetition and fasciculation may be brought about by a second dose of DFP.

MEETER (1958) attributed the persistent junctional negativity and accompanying depression of muscle excitability to ACh accumulation. However, botulinum toxin, which is known to diminish the output of transmitter substance from pre-junctional nerve fibres during stimulation (BURGEN et al. 1949a; BROOKS 1954), is unable to oppose the inhibition of tetanic contraction produced by DFP. NAESS and SÖGNER (1958), therefore, concluded that this inhibition cannot be due solely to accumulation of ACh at the motor endplate. Facilitation of transmitter release from nerve terminals, on the other hand, is supposed to be induced by NEt_4 (see page 604). This view is based on the twitch-potentiating affect of NEt_4 in nerve-muscle preparations pretreated with DFP or neostigmine in low concentration. Administration of the same dose of NEt_4 to normal muscle preparations does not significantly affect twitch height or muscle action potentials; in preparations treated with DFP, it does not alter the muscle twitches elicited by direct stimulation. However, NEt_4 antagonized the blockade of transmission of single and repetitive nerve impulses which is produced by high concentrations of DFP (STOVNER 1958a).

Different oximes, like di*iso*nitrosoacetone (DINA) and mono*iso*nitrosoacetone (MINA), were tested for their ability to reverse the action of organophosphorus anti-ChE agents on neuromuscular transmission in the rat diaphragm. Both DINA and MINA readily abolished twitch potentiation and block of tetanic excitability by TEPP, DFP and *iso*propyl methylphosphonofluoridate (Sarin). When MINA or DINA was added to a final concentration of 10^{-2} M, complete recovery of contractile response to stimulation at a frequency of 100 per sec was achieved in periods as short as 2 to 5 min. Also, the prolongation of junctional negativity by the anti-ChE agents was reversed. The speed of action of the oximes was independent of the duration of previous contact of the organophosphorus compound with the diaphragm (HOLMES and ROBINS 1955).

During prolonged exposure of the diaphragm to MINA or DINA, a reduction of indirect and direct excitability develops. Direct actions on the nerve-muscle preparations are more pronounced with pyridine-2-aldoxime methiodide (P-2-AM), one of the most potent *in vitro* ChE reactivators known; its blocking action on neuromuscular transmission is easily reversible upon washing of the preparation. The method employed to demonstrate the restoring action of P-2-AM on transmission blocked by organophosphates was, therefore, to remove the P-2-AM from the muscle bath after a few minutes of contact with the inhibited preparation, and to test subsequently for indirect excitability. The reversal of neuromuscular block by oximes in these experiments was specific, insofar as only paralysis by organophosphates was reversed, but not transmission block by curare or decamethonium (HOLMES and ROBINS 1955). The restoring action of oximes on transmission blocked by organophosphates is accompanied by moderate increase of ChE activity in the nerve-muscle preparations. KEWITZ (1957) observed *in vivo* partial reactivation of ChE in the diaphragm of rats when P-2-AM was injected 1 to

$1^1/_2$ hrs after the administration of Paraoxon or DFP. Treatment of DFP-intoxicated cats with P-2-AM, MINA, or diacetylmonoxime (DAM) resulted in histochemically verifiable reactivation of junctional and ganglionic AChE (KOELLE 1957b; RAJAPURKAR and KOELLE 1958). For a complete coverage of reactivation, see the contributions of HOBBIGER (Chapter 21) and GROB (Chapter 22) in this volume.

e) Catechols

BURN (1945) has reviewed the evidence that epinephrine augments the activity of ACh in a number of different effector organs. In the isolated diaphragm of the kitten, for instance, epinephrine potentiates ACh so that it causes a larger contracture (DALE and GADDUM 1930). In the cat gastrocnemius muscle, epinephrine markedly increases, at low stimulus frequencies, the potentiating action of neostigmine on twitch tension; but the opposite effect appears at higher rates of stimulation (BÜLBRING and BURN 1942). Moreover, the dose of neostigmine is critical: the facilitation by epinephrine and norepinephrine is best obtained after doses of neostigmine which are subthreshold for twitch potentiation (BURN and HUTCHEON 1949). BURN (1945) discussed the possibility that these actions of epinephrine might be related to its ChE inhibitory activity. Inhibition of AChE and BuChE by epinephrine was later determined by BENSON (1948) and BENSON and MEEK (1949): with ACh as substrate, epinephrine in a concentration of 6×10^{-3} M reduced the activity of AChE and BuChE only to about one-half.

The potentiation of the contractile response resulting from combined administration of neostigmine, or physostigmine, and epinephrine can be convincingly demonstrated in the rat diaphragm preparation at appropriate stimulus frequencies (BÜLBRING 1946; TAUGNER and FLECKENSTEIN 1950). In this preparation, epinephrine facilitates the contractile response to stimulation with single pulses even in the absence of neostigmine or physostigmine; fatigue seems to favor the appearance of the epinephrine effect. In the rat, epinephrine partially restores transmission after paralysis with d-tubocurarine, decamethonium, or amyltrimethylammonium (BRAND 1952).

A state of refractoriness to direct electrical and chemical excitation can be produced in the chronically denervated diaphragm by repeated administration of ACh in small doses; epinephrine, norepinephrine, isopropyl-norepinephrine, and ephedrine are effective in restoring the electric excitability, but the muscle remains refractory to stimulation by ACh (McDOWALL and WATSON 1951). This finding obviously indicates that the sympathomimetic amines are capable of acting on the muscle fibre directly, rather than at the endplate region. Indeed, this was also the conclusion reached by BROWN et al. (1948). The absence of repetitive action potentials in muscle, the twitch tension of which has been increased by epinephrine (GOFFART 1952), and the apparent prolongation of the active state in indirectly as well as directly stimulated muscle also favor this view (GOFFART and RITCHIE 1952). However, in the frog, epinephrine and norepinephrine increase twitch tension by recruitment of muscle fibres, and the anticurare action of these agents is associated with increase of amplitude of the endplate potential (HUTTER and LOEWENSTEIN 1955; KRNJEVIĆ and MILEDI 1958b). On the basis of some work with the rat diaphragm, MONTAGU (1955) came to the conclusion that epinephrine affects neuromuscular transmission in mammalian nerve-muscle preparations in addition to its action on the duration of the active state in the muscle fibre; the indirect excitability was very critically affected by epinephrine when the Ca-ion content of the Ringer solution was reduced. It has also been established that epinephrine relieves at least in some degree the intermittent presynaptic failure of conduction caused by tetanic stimulation of the motor nerve. More regularly, epinephrine also induces an acceleration of the discharge rate of miniature endplate potentials without affecting their amplitude (KRNJEVIĆ and MILEDI 1958b).

The anticurare action on the rat diaphragm of catechol and a series of phenolic agents was the object of a study by MOGEY and YOUNG (1949).

At a given dose of *d*-tubocurarine, the antagonism by catechol and related agents is limited to partial restoration of transmission, no matter how high a concentration of catechol is used. On the other hand, the concentration of *d*-tubocurarine may be increased over a large range, and partial antagonism by catechol can still be demonstrated. In other words, it appears that catechol antagonism of curare paralysis is not limited by a stoichiometric relationship of the two agents, but rather that catechol is capable of reversing only some aspect of the curare action. Indeed, TREVAN (1948) had suggested that *d*-tubocurarine may act at two sites, but that it is reversible by decurarizing agents at only one of the two.

With respect to repetitive activity, there is a sharp distinction between the actions on the neuromuscular junction of catechol, and those of physostigmine or neostigmine.

MOGEY and TREVAN (1948) found that stimulation of the phrenic nerve with single shocks of 6 to 7 msec duration leads to tetanic responses of the diaphragm muscle. This repetitive activity on stimulation with pulses of long duration can be exaggerated by physostigmine. Minute doses of *d*-tubocurarine suppress the augmentative action of physostigmine on repetitive activity, but do not diminish tetanic responses occurring before physostigmine administration. Catechol, instead of facilitating the repetitive activity, abolishes it. Another point of difference consists in the failure of catechol to improve transmission in fatigued preparations. This also is unlike the action of epinephrine on such preparations.

The ChE inhibitory potency of the phenolic agents used by MOGEY and YOUNG (1949) is relatively insignificant and there is no reason to assume that their anti-curare effect is related to enzyme inhibition. Instead, MOGEY and YOUNG (1949) suggested that attachment of the phenolic groups to proteins may result in steric hindrance of the interaction of the receptor with curare molecules. It is, however, remarkable that phenolic agents in the curarized frog muscle prolong the endplate potential considerably (see page 594). COPPEE (1943) related this phenomenon to the anticurare action of phenols, and stated that this effect is not associated with increase in sensitivity of the junctional region to ACh.

2. Potentiation of contractile response and anticurare action under rate conditions

Data obtained from experiments *in vitro* indicate the existence of considerable variation in the velocity with which drugs react with ChE *in situ*. When small doses of drug are injected into the arterial circulation of muscle, the contact of drug with enzyme or receptor is limited in time; a rate situation thus prevails, and chemical equilibrium between reactants may never be achieved. The fact that anti-ChE agents with extremely low velocity constants (e.g., carbamates and organophosphates) produce marked effects after intra-arterial injection of small doses suggests that these effects are unrelated to AChE inhibitor potency *in vitro*. However, it is conceivable that the kinetics of drug reaction with sessile ChE molecules is not comparable to the situation *in vitro*. It then becomes a question of semantics whether the term "cholinesterase" can legitimately be used for designating a receptor structure.

a) Carbamate esters

α) Physostigmine. Until 1936, pharmacologic studies of neuromuscular transmission were concerned primarily with direct stimulatory and depressant actions of quaternary ammonium ions on skeletal muscle.

Furthermore, most experiments of this kind were performed on frog muscle, particularly the rectus abdominis, a muscle which differs considerably in its physiological properties from mammalian skeletal muscle. The introduction of the now classical cat nerve-muscle preparation by BROWN et al. (1936) provided an appropriate technique for investigating neuro-muscular pharmacology and physiology in mammals. Using this preparation in conjunction with the intra-arterial injection technique, it was demonstrated that ACh produces a twitch-like contraction of skeletal muscle, thus supporting the hypothesis that this agent is the chemical transmitter at the neuromuscular junction (DALE et al. 1936).

The early contributions of Brown et al. (1936) and Brown (1937a) described a phenomenon which serves as a point of departure in studies concerning the facilitation of neuromuscular transmission. Physostigmine was observed to increase the isometric tension developed by cat muscle in response to single maximal nerve shocks (Fig. 9); this increase was promptly associated with the conversion of single nerve impulses into repetitive discharges in muscle.

Using belly-to-tendon leads, Brown (1937a) showed that during potentiation of the contractile response, the initial spike is followed by lower amplitude waves

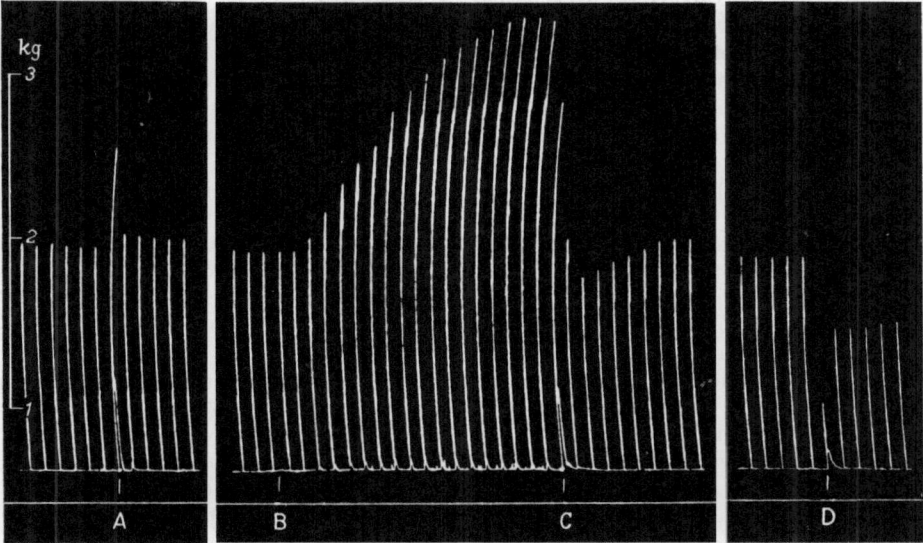

Fig. 9. Effect of acetylcholine and physostigmine on isometric twitch tension of cat's gastrocnemius muscle. Stimulation of sciatic nerve with maximal break shocks, one every 10 sec. At A, C and D: 25 μg ACh in 0.5 ml by close arterial injection, during intermission of one shock to nerve. At B: 0.8 mg Physostigmine, intravenously. (From: Brown et al. 1936)

which last for another 60 msec. The successive deflections diminish progressively in size, the base broadens, and the interval between consecutive discharges gradually lengthens. This indicates temporal dispersion of activity in individual units which are initially relatively synchronized. The same conclusion was reached from records obtained with concentric needle electrodes which restricted the pickup to a smaller number of muscle fibres. During the synchronous phase of muscle repetition the potential deflections follow each other in time intervals of 2 to 4 msec. These measurements, although of limited precision because of temporal dispersion of discharges in groups of muscle fibres, conclusively showed that physostigmine gives a transient, waning, tetanic response of the muscle to a single maximal nerve volley.

Close range intra-arterial injection of ACh (Brown 1937a) also initiates a highly asynchronous tetanic activity in the muscle. From electrical records of small groups of fibres, Brown (1937a) ascertained that individual muscle fibres discharge repetitively for short periods of time after injection of ACh. Synchronous repetition appeared when ACh was injected into a preparation which had been treated several hours earlier with physostigmine.

Physostigmine increases the contractile response produced in normal muscle to intravenously injected ACh. However, in the indirectly stimulated eserinized preparation, ACh reduces the response to nerve impulses after its stimulant effect is over (Fig. 9). During this depressant after-action of ACh, another similar injection has a greatly reduced contractile effect. It appeared impossible at first to obtain significant augmentation of indirectly developed twitch tension with ACh. This was finally observed, however, in an eserinized preparation at a time when the potentiating action of physostigmine had largely worn off (BROWN 1937a).

BROWN et al. (1936) postulated that the physostigmine-induced twitch potentiation was mediated through its anti-ChE action. This would allow for suprathreshold concentrations of ACh to persist at the endplate longer than the muscle refractory period and thus initiate repetitive discharges. No direct action of physostigmine on motor nerve was detected during the facilitatory action. The possibility was considered, however, that in the presence of physostigmine, a single nerve impulse could be converted into repetitive activity at the nerve endings; but such an action had no relation to any known effect of physostigmine or to any known manner of conduction in nerve. The chemical transmission theory seemed to be the only one which embraced all of the known facts at that time. Essentially, these facts were (1) ACh is released at the motor nerve endings by the arrival of nerve impulses, (2) ACh produces contractile responses in skeletal muscle, (3) ACh is rapidly destroyed in the presence of ChE, (4) physostigmine is a potent ChE inhibitor, and (5) physostigmine potentiates the neurally-elicited contractile response.

Important confirmatory evidence for the proposed mechanism of physostigmine's facilitatory action was produced shortly afterwards by BACQ and BROWN (1937). They compared the twitch-potentiating potencies and anti-ChE potencies in vitro of several carbamate esters, including physostigmine, and found a perfect correlation between these two parameters.

It seemed logical and proper during these initial studies of the actions of physostigmine on neuromuscular transmission to view the twitch potentiating effect solely within the context of the ACh-AChE theory. But even then evidence was already accumulating which questioned the validity of this view and which continues to serve as the basis for further inquiry. Some of this evidence will now be reviewed.

After a suprathreshold dose of physostigmine has attained its maximum effectiveness, the application of a second nerve shock produces no response in the muscle at all; as the interval between two nerve volleys is increased to about 30 msec, there appears a muscle action potential of reduced size in response to the second volley, but this is not followed by repetitive activity. In order for a second nerve volley to produce repetitive activity after its primary muscle action potential, a stimulus interval of at least 200 msec is required. After a subthreshold dose of physostigmine has been given, there is no occlusion of the second of two nerve shocks given at short intervals; rather, the two summate to produce augmentation of tension and muscle repetition similar to that elicited by one volley after an effective dose of physostigmine (BROWN 1937a) (Fig. 10).

Although BROWN et al. (1936) had noted the complete suppression of physostigmine-induced twitch potentiation by ether, no explanation of this effect was offered. Indeed, it still remains difficult to reconcile this phenomenon with the generally accepted mechanism of physostigmine's facilitatory action. The dismissal of this effect of ether as curariform in nature is not warrented because the ether concentrations required do not depress transmission per se, only the drug-induced facilitation of transmission.

The inverse relationship between physostigmine potentiation and stimulus frequency was first recognized by BACQ and BROWN (1937), and they even attributed an earlier failure to observe physostigmine's effect (ROSENBLUETH et al. 1936) to the use of an excessive rate of nerve stimulation. In the amphibian nerve-muscle preparation, the frequency of nerve stimulation is an even more critical parameter than in the mammal; the maximal rate of nerve stimulation which can be used in the frog to demonstrate physostigmine potentiation is two per minute (FENG 1937c).

In summary, there were three lines of evidence which indicated that the physostigmine-induced twitch potentiation was not solely the result of ChE inhibition at the motor endplate. These were, (1) the blockade of transmission to a single nerve volley at a time when the contractile response is maximally potentiated by physostigmine, (2) the suppression of physostigmine potentiation by ether, and (3) the suppression of physostigmine potentiation by high-frequency nerve stimulation.

Important clues to the nature of the physostigmine action may be derived from its time-action curve after intravenous injection of 0.2 to 1.0 mg/kg; maximum potentiation of contractile response is obtained within 5 to 10 min; residual action may be followed for as long

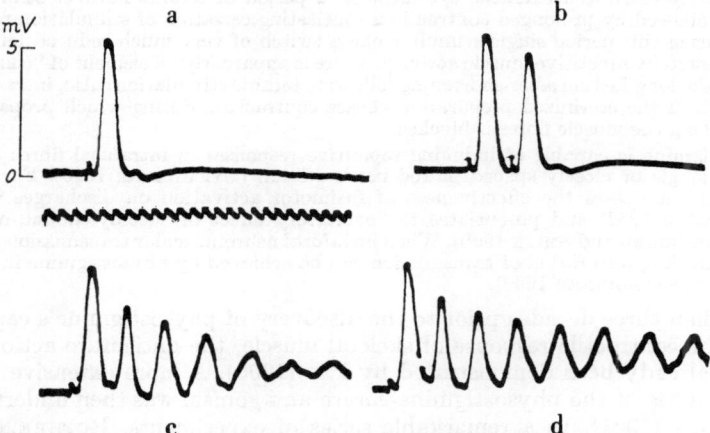

Fig. 10. Effect of physostigmine on action potentials of indirectly stimulated inferior oblique muscle of the cat. a and b: Responses of normal muscle to single and paired nerve volleys, respectively; the latter at stimulus interval 3.4 msec. c and d: Responses after 2 mg physostigmine, intravenously. c: Single nerve volley. d: Two nerve volleys, 2.4 msec apart. (From: BROWN and HARVEY 1941)

as one to two hours after injection, particularly on stimulation with double nerve volleys. This time course of action compares well with the estimated recovery from serum ChE inhibition after the intravenous administration of a single dose of physostigmine (KRAYER et al. 1944). However, the period of onset of action is shortened considerably when the intra-arterial route of administration is used. In this case, the maximal potentiating effect of a dose of only 1 to 5 µg/kg is established within 1 to 3 min after injection. This time interval is relatively short as compared with the time required for reaching *in vitro* equilibrium of enzyme-inhibitor association. It is difficult, therefore, to view the effect of physostigmine *in vivo* under these conditions as analogous to the enzyme-inhibition *in vitro*, unless the kinetics of inhibition for enzyme located in tissue are very different from that occurring *in vitro*. Furthermore, duration of action of small intra-arterial doses is of the same magnitude as that of initially equi-effective intravenous doses, and residual effects in both cases can be followed for one to two hours by using paired stimuli (WERNER 1960a). This indicates that the equilibrium of the physostigmine reaction with whatever group it interacts with in tissue is considerably different from the equilibrium with ChE in blood.

Additional information on the effects of physostigmine was obtained by BROWN and HARVEY (1941) using mammalian extrinsic ocular muscles. The immediate effect of physostigmine on the muscles, when given intravenously or by intra-carotid injection, consisted in the appearance of highly synchronized twitches resulting at times in development of tension equal to, or greater than, that caused by a maximal nerve volley. The twitching was further increased by stimulation of the nerve: in this case, the initial muscle spike was followed by a regular series of action potentials which underwent a constant logarithmic decrementation (Fig. 10). An increase in amplitude of successive muscle action potentials could be recorded from eserinized extrinsic ocular muscles when paired stimuli at intervals of 1 to 1.4 msec were applied to the nerve. But the second spike in a repetitive series evoked by a single nerve volley in eserinized muscles occurred 0.7 to 1.0 msec later than a response to a second nerve volley could occur in untreated muscle. There were reasons for assuming that the earliest possible repetitive muscle spike occurring on single stimulation in eserinized muscle could not be advanced in time by an additional nerve volley; this second volley could, however, augment subsequent repetitive responses. BROWN and HARVEY (1941) were, therefore, led to suspect that physostigmine prolongs the refractory period of muscle and interferes with the conduction in nerve of the second of two closely spaced volleys.

In the fully eserinized extrinsic eye muscles, a period of tetanic indirect stimulation is frequently followed by prolonged contractions, outlasting cessation of stimulation for several minutes; during this period single stimuli evoke a twitch of very much reduced tension, but one still followed by repetitive muscle activity. There is apparently an element of "contracture" involved in the long-lasting after-shortening following tetanic stimulation; also, intra-arterially injected ACh in the eserinized preparation causes contracture during which propagation of excitation along the muscle fibres is blocked.

Physostigmine is capable of inducing repetitive responses in intrafusal fibres of muscle spindles to single or closely spaced paired nerve stimuli (EYZAGUIRRE 1960). Furthermore, physostigmine increases the effectiveness of fusimotor activation on discharges in muscle afferents (HUNT 1952) and potentiates the excitatory effect of succinylcholine on spindle afferents (BRINGLING and SMITH 1960). When intrafusal neuromuscular transmission is blocked by d-tubocurarine, restoration of transmission can be achieved by physostigmine in an all-or-none fashion (EYZAGUIRRE 1960).

More than three decades prior to the discovery of physostigmine's capacity to increase the contractile response of skeletal muscle, the anticurare action of this drug had already been demonstrated by PAL (1900). A more extensive pharmacologic analysis of the physostigmine-curare antagonism was then undertaken by ROTHBERGER (1901). In a remarkable series of experiments, ROTHBERGER succeeded in localizing the anticurare action of physostigmine to the periphery. He further concluded that the site of action of physostigmine must be at the same point at which curare acts, a locus specified as the intramuscular motor nerve terminations. ROTHBERGER also recognized the difficulty of demonstrating physostigmine's anticurare action in the frog as compared to the mammal. In passing, it should be noted that these early studies were accomplished without the awareness of either physostigmine's anti-ChE activity or of the significance of ChE to neuromuscular transmission.

The anticurare action of physostigmine was later confirmed on mammalian nerve-muscle preparations by ROSENBLUETH et al. (1936) and still later by KOP-PANYI and VIVINO (1944) using a much purer curare alkaloid. Still more recently, BURKE et al. (1948) and WESCOE and RIKER (1951) have stressed the slow time course of this effect. Even following a close intra-arterial injection of physostigmine into the blood supply of the cat gastrocnemius, recovery from total curare paralysis required at least several minutes for completion (WESCOE and RIKER 1951) (Fig. 11). In both of these investigations, neostigmine was found to produce a much more prompt curare antagonism. This disparity between the time course of neostigmine's and physostigmine's anticurare action in mammals, is apparently related to the fact that in the frog physostigmine has only a negligible anticurare effect compared to neostigmine (JACOBSOHN and KAHLSON 1938). As previously suggested by RIKER (1953), it seems as if the mechanism of neostigmine's anticurare action differs qualitatively, at least in part, from that of physostigmine.

By 1936, there had also been several investigations concerned with the structural requisites for physostigmine-type action. Following the work of STEDMAN and BARGER (1925) on the molecular structure of physostigmine, STEDMAN (1926) suggested that all pharmacological actions of this alkaloid were associated with the carbamate group. This idea was supported by the finding that physostigmine and a number of carbamate analogues produced miosis after instillation into cats' eyes (STEDMAN and STEDMAN 1929, STEDMAN 1929). Some of these agents were later submitted to more detailed pharmacologic examination, particularly the methyl carbamic ester of *m*-hydroxy-phenylethyldimethylamine (miotine) (WHITE and STEDMAN 1931). Like physostigmine, this agent produced muscle fasciculations and possessed anticurare activity. In 1937, BACQ and BROWN demonstrated that miotine also produced a physo-

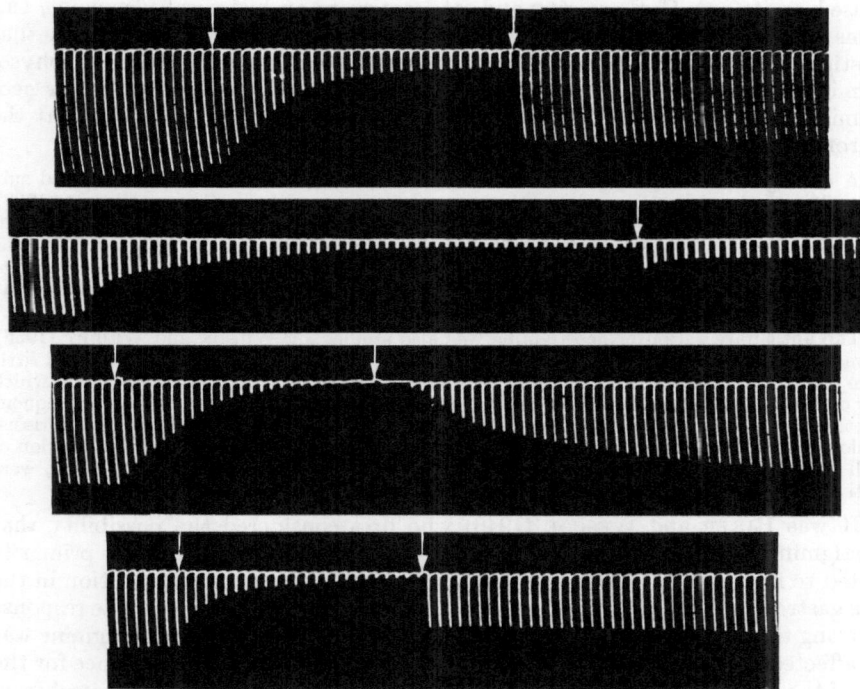

Fig. 11. Anticurare action of drugs in cat gastrocnemius muscle. Muscle stimulated indirectly at rate of 10 per min. All injections intra-arterial; circulation restricted to gastrocnemius muscle; pentobarbital anesthesia. Top: *d*-tubocurarine, 60 µg/kg, followed by 3-OH-PNMe₃, 50 µg/kg. Below: *d*-tubocurarine, 60 µg/kg, followed by PNMe₃, 50 µg/kg. Below: *d*-tubocurarine, 60 µg/kg, followed by physostigmine, 50 µg/kg. Bottom: *d*-tubocurarine, 60 µg/kg, followed by decamethonium, 10 µg/kg. (From: WESCOE and RIKER 1951)

stigmine-like potentiation of isometric tension. Additionally, BACQ and BROWN (1937) tested the methyl carbamic esters of hordenine and of the *m*-hydroxy- and *p*-hydroxy-phenyltrimethylammonium ion; all these carbamates were seen to potentiate the indirectly developed isometric tension of cat muscle. The structural feature common to all of these compounds was the carbamate group, and this group had earlier been shown to be primarily responsible for the anti-ChE activity resident in these compounds (STEDMAN 1926). But ELLIS et al. (1943) later found that breakdown products of physostigmine lacking the carbamate group produced potentiation of the neurally elicited isometric tension. These products possessed about one-fifth the twitch potentiating potency of physostigmine and about one-hundredth the anti-BuChE potency. On the basis of this and other observations to be reported on subsequent pages, it now seems obvious that a structural feature common to most twitch potentiating compounds is the amine nitrogen, and that other substituents in the molecule, like the carbamate group, serve primarily to enhance potency.

β) **Neostigmine and other carbamate analogues of physostigmine.** The synthesis of neostigmine (Prostigmin) and demonstration of its anticurare activity by AESCHLIMANN and REINERT (1931) was a contribution to the pharmacology of neuromuscular transmission the importance of which has not been generally appreciated. The significance of this contribution resides in the ultimate recognition of the quaternary ammonium ion as a primary structural requirement for curare antagonism and twitch potentiation. In fact, there are many such ions, lacking in substituents such as the carbamate or phenolic hydroxyl, which are now known to facilitate neuromuscular transmission (KUPERMAN et al. 1961a, b). The presence of the carbamate group in the neostigmine molecule has obviously served to direct attention away from its onium center; instead, interest has been focused on its anti-ChE activity and, at least from an historical viewpoint, this seems appropriate. However, evidence has already been cited which suggests that neostigmine cannot be viewed simply as another carbamate analogue of physostigmine which merely happens to contain a quaternary nitrogen atom; for neostigmine appears to possess a qualitatively different mechanism of action at the neuromuscular junction.

A neostigmine analogue synthesized by AESCHLIMANN and REINERT (1931), called substance 36, was also shown to possess anticurare activity along with neostigmine (BRISCOE 1937). These experiments of BRISCOE were actually inspired by the finding that both neostigmine (PRITCHARD and BLACK 1933, WALKER 1934) and substance 36 (LAURENT 1935) were beneficial in the treatment of myasthenia gravis. Around this time, the capacity of neostigmine to potentiate the neurally evoked contractile response of cat muscle was also observed (WILSON and WRIGHT 1936, ROSENBLUETH et al. 1936).

The anticurare action of neostigmine was also studied by WILSON and WRIGHT (1936). It was found that ACh, intra-arterially injected into curarized preparations, produced little or no effect; but if the curarized muscle was first treated with a dose of neostigmine, which may or may not have caused an effect (depending on the depth of curarization), subsequent injections of a larger dose of ACh gave rise to considerable and sustained restoration of transmission. Similarly, the anticurare action of K^+ ions was increased by prior administration of small doses of neostigmine. However, K^+ and neostigmine, singly or in combination, were relatively ineffective in improving transmission in fatigued preparations.

It was RIKER and WESCOE (1946) who first considered the possibility that neostigmine exerted a direct action at the neuromuscular junction, not primarily related to its anti-ChE action. Supporting evidence was the demonstration in the cat's gastrocnemius muscle preparation of a rapidly developed contractile response following the intraarterial injection of neostigmine. This action of neostigmine was not affected by prior inactivation of ChE by large doses of DFP. Evidence for the role of the methonium center in the direct action of neostigmine was derived from stepwise simplification of its molecular configuration (WESCOE et al. 1949, RIKER and WESCOE 1950). The muscle stimulating activity of neostigmine was, thereby, conclusively traced to the phenyltrimethylammonium ion. Neither the carbamate configuration nor the presence of an ester linkage was essential for the contractile effect. Significantly, removal of the carbamate ester link reduced the anti-ChE activity to about 1/100 of that of neostigmine, but the muscle stimulant activity remained practically unaltered.

The work of RIKER and WESCOE (1946) conclusively showed that the methonium group of the neostigmine molecule is responsible for its contractile effect on innervated or denervated muscle. Obviously, this action is similar to that produced by ACh (BROWN et al. 1936) and a variety of other choline esters and stable quaternary ammonium ions (BACQ and BROWN 1937, RANDALL and LEHMANN 1950). A methonium center is not absolutely required for this direct stimulatory action on muscle; analogues in which one or more methyl groups are replaced by ethyl groups also act in this way, albeit with reduced potency. Since the researches of ING and WRIGHT (1931) it has been recognized that quaternary ammonium ions, in addition to their direct contractile effect, also depress neuromuscular transmission. In the case of an unstable molecule like ACh, this depression is exceedingly brief in contrast to the more enduring effect of the stable ions. However, when ACh is injected during the course of a physostigmine-induced potentiation of isometric tension, a marked and prolonged depression of transmission is then produced (BROWN et al. 1936; BACQ and BROWN 1937) (Fig. 9). These observations led to the supposition that the depression of transmission by high doses of carbamates, or by lower doses in the presence of high-frequency nerve volleys, is attributable to the accumulation and persistence of depressant concentrations of ACh.

In 1946, LEHMANN studied the effects of a large number of carbamates containing the onium center.

Some of these agents produced muscle paralysis only in the presence of low rates of nerve stimulation (one stimulus every 15 sec), even though they were relatively potent inhibitors of ChE; others blocked transmission only at higher rates of stimulation. An increase of the muscle paralyzing potency was brought about by a variety of changes in the molecule; e.g., transfer of the carbamate group in phenyl-benzyl compounds from position 4 to position 2 greatly enhanced depressant potency, and hydrogenation of the phenyl group further augmented this activity. Attachment of cyclic onium groups greatly increased neuromuscular paralyzing potency without altering ChE inhibitor activity. Surprisingly, a change from the onium salt to the tertiary amine sometimes resulted in an increase of depressant activity without any appreciable alteration of anti-ChE potency. LEHMANN (1946) pointed out that, on the whole, strong muscle paralyzing activity tended to be associated with less anti-ChE potency.

Two conclusions may be derived from these data: first, that carbamates with onium groups represent a molecular configuration suitable to react directly with receptor structures at the neuromuscular junction; second, that the muscle paralyzing potency of these agents — if compared in a large enough series of compounds — is not correlated with anti-ChE potency. One is left without any cogent reason to assume that transmission block by neostigmine, for instance, is a result of ACh accumulation in the presence of inhibited ChE, since transmission block by closely related congeners definitely cannot be interpreted in this way.

γ) **Drug effects in the presence of bursts of nerve volleys and prolonged tetani.** BACQ and BROWN (1937) clearly showed that an important parameter for determining whether physostigmine would produce potentiation or depression of isometric tension is the frequency with which nerve volleys impinge on the neuromuscular junction. The investigations of BRISCOE (1936a, b; 1937) also emphasized this point for other carbamate-type potentiating agents, and a later report by BRISCOE (1938) analyzed the problem in more detail. It was found that the first stage of change induced by agents of the "eserine-group" consists in an alteration of the normal grading between stimulus frequency and tetanic tension, e.g., the optimum rate of stimulation for the gastrocnemius muscle shifts from 100/sec in the control period to about 50/sec after drug administration. Also, the response to tetanic stimulation at low frequency is affected: the initial contraction may or may not be diminished in size; this is followed by a brief period of depression which is then succeeded by a rise of tension; thereby, a notch appears in the myogram (Fig. 12). The identical sequence of events was shown by COWAN (1938) to occur in frog muscles. BRISCOE (1938) further discovered that the potentiating effects of carbamates on twitch tension are frequency-sensitive. With decreasing intervals between nerve shocks, drug-induced twitch potentiation becomes less prominent and ultimately inhibition prevails.

The characteristic pharmacologic alteration of response to tetanic stimulation is abolished by curare in subparalyzing doses. Clearly, it is not easy to choose the dose of curare which will prevent this effect of physostigmine-like agents and yet not produce its own depressant action; but BRISCOE (1938) demonstrated that this is, in principle, possible. A point of considerable interest was also raised by BRISCOE (1938) with respect to the action of curare: in mild curare poisoning there is no reversal of grading between stimulus frequency and tetanic tension, but the intensity of the tetanic contraction is reduced. Apparently, the nature of the transmission failure induced by carbamates at high stimulus frequencies is different from that caused by partial curarization; indeed, agents of the carbamate groups are capable of restoring transmission in presence of curare. Reciprocally, small doses of curare restore transmission impaired by carbamates (BRISCOE 1936b, 1937; COWAN 1936a, ROSENBLUETH and MORISON 1937). It is for this reason that ROSENBLUETH and MORISON (1937) criticized the indiscriminate use of the term "Wedensky Inhibition" to designate such seemingly heterogeneous processes as partial transmission failure for repetitive volleys caused by agents of the carbamate group on the one hand, and by curare-like agents on the other (ROSENBLUETH 1950).

The degree of transmission block with curare, in doses subparalytic for transmission of single nerve volleys, also depends, within limits, on the stimulus frequency (BREMER and TITECA 1935). In fact, BROWN (1938) demonstrated that after a subparalytic dose of curarine,

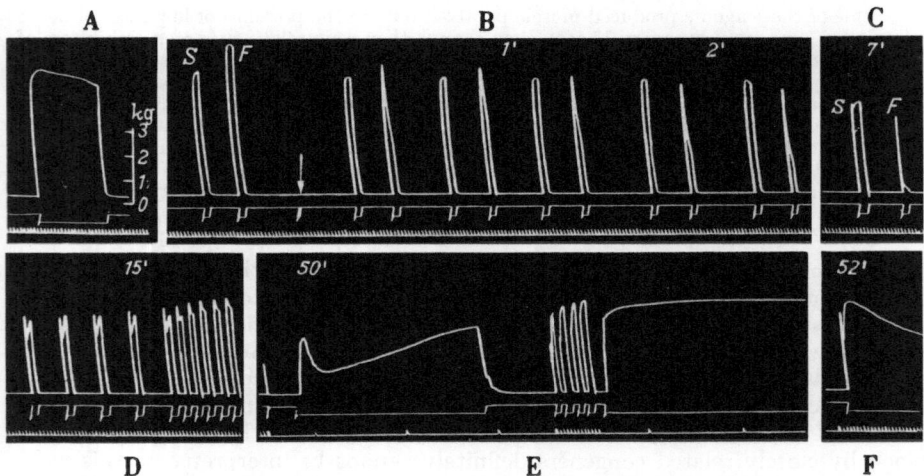

Fig. 12. Isometric tension records of indirectly stimulated cat's quadriceps muscle. A: Effect of prolonged stimulation (20 sec) at fusion rate, normal muscle. B: Slow and fast (50 and 125 per sec) rates alternated in two-second spells. At arrow 0.5 mg/kg substance 36 injected intravenously. In the second minute grading is reversed. C: In seventh minute notch in slow rate response. Lower line all at slow rate of stimulation. D: Effect of decreasing interval between spells of stimulation. E: After 8 min inactivity; notched curve on fast drum. The second curve on the fast drum taken immediately after the four contractions shown on slow drum. F: One min later, curve notched. Effect of prolonged stimulation. Inserted figures give interval after injection. Time, seconds. (From: BRISCOE 1938)

the muscle action potential in response to the second of two nerve volleys spaced 50 msec apart is about 10% larger than the first; as the stimulus interval increases, depression of the second muscle action potential prevails, the effect reaching a maximum between 200 to 400 msec. This inhibitory after-effect is capable of being summated (ROSENBLUETH and MORISON 1937).

To inquire whether facilitation of transmission by a conditioning motor nerve volley can be attributed to summation of ACh quanta, MAASKE et al. (1938) performed experiments in partially curarized preparations treated with physostigmine. These experiments were analogous to those of BREMER and KLEYNTJENS (1937), designed for the study of latent summation in the frog (see page 587).

Curare or magnesium was administered until a single stimulus to the nerve evoked a barely visible twitch; while this degree of paralysis was maintained with constant infusion of appropriate concentrations of curare solution or magnesium, pairs of supramaximal stimuli were applied, and complete curves of facilitation were determined repeatedly. The same procedure was then repeated after administration of 0.5 mg physostigmine/kg, and additional curare. In a few instances, the period of effective summation was found to be shorter after physostigmine than before; usually, the curves before and after physostigmine nearly coincided, but the descending portion of the curve was never prolonged. On the other hand, physostigmine decurarized with respect to transmission of single nerve volleys. Accordingly, MAASKE et al.

(1938) argued that if this decurarizing action were due to ChE inhibition, it should be possible for physostigmine to prolong the period of facilitation, unless destruction of each quantum of ACh even in the presence of physostigmine is so rapid that summation is impossible.

Considerable attention has been devoted to the study of transmission in the course of prolonged periods of tetanic stimulation, and this work has led to the distinction of different "stages" of neuromuscular transmission: the schematic representation of the sequence of changes is shown in Fig. 13.

When 300 to 500 maximal stimuli per second are applied to the motor nerve of leg muscles in the cat, vigorous and brief contraction follows; subsequently, a sequence of rises and falls of tension during continuous stimulation occurs (ROSENBLUETH and CANNON 1940). Stage 2 and 3 b were attributed to transmission failure. After administration of carbamates, stage 3 b is augmented, and occurs at notably lower stimulus frequencies; injection of ACh acts, at that stage, similarly. It has been postulated that transmission failure of stage 3 b is indicative of excessive depolarization consequent to accumulation of ACh. At stimulus rates of 60 to 120 per second applied for several hours, a different series of changes takes place in normal cat muscles (CANNON and ROSENBLUETH 1940): the initial rise of tension (Stage 1) is followed by a gradual decline leading to almost complete transient relaxation of muscle (Stage 4: see Fig. 13);

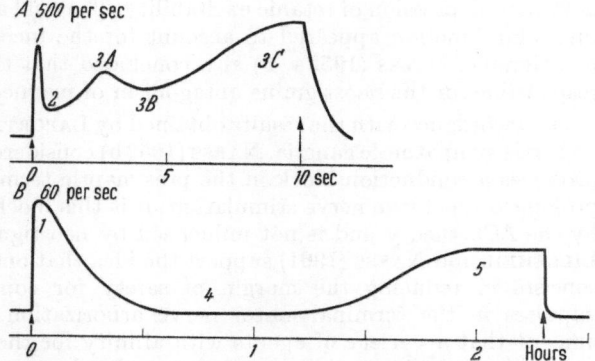

Fig. 13. Diagrams of mechanograms obtained from leg muscles of cats upon stimulation of their motor nerves at rapid frequencies. (From: ACHESON 1948)

in this phase, transmission can be improved by administration of ACh or ChE inhibitors. Failure at Stage 4 was ascribed to decrease of ACh output from motor nerve endings; restorative synthesis of ACh in Stage 5 was invoked to account for the spontaneous restoration of transmission when stimulation continues (ROSENBLUETH 1950).

Tetanic stimulation of motor nerves leads to transient depolarization at the endplate region which is intensified and prolonged by neostigmine, causing neuromuscular block and depression of direct excitability of the muscle. These effects are reversed by the passage of anodal current into the junctional region (BURNS and PATON 1951). The same changes are induced in the absence of tetanic stimulation by decamethonium (BURNS and PATON 1951) and by some dicholine esters of aliphatic dicarboxylic acids (GINZEL et al. 1952). The depression of direct excitability in the presence of neostigmine may be the consequence of a conduction block for the muscle action potential in a depolarized zone of the muscle fibre (GJONE 1955).

In his investigations of neuromuscular transmission in the rabbit, NAESS (1952 b) observed that failure of transmission for tetani of 200 to 300 impulses per second prevailed at a point of the curve of action of neostigmine where responses to single nerve stimuli were potentiated. He confirmed also what had been indicated by many previous studies, i.e., curare paralyzes transmission of high frequency volleys to a greater degree than it does at low stimulus frequency. A corollary to these observations is the fact that the small "twitch" contractions evoked by high frequency tetanic stimulation during deep curarization, although considerably increased by neostigmine, still maintain the character of "twitch" responses. Thus, neostigmine has little anticurare action at higher stimulus frequencies. NAESS (1952 b) therefore suggested that the interaction between curare and neostigmine at the neuromuscular junction cannot be completely described solely in terms of a postsynaptic action of curare and the anti-ChE action of neostigmine.

BUCHTHAL and LINDHARD (1942) and ENGBAEK (1948) had previously obtained evidence that the action of curare on the lizard and frog neuromuscular junction proceeds in two discrete steps: (1) low concentrations of curare blocked the transmission from nerve to muscle without affecting the response of the endplate to ACh; (2) the threshold of the endplate response increased at 300 to 400 times higher concentrations of curare. Similarly, NAESS (1952c) described two distinct phases of curare action in rabbits: (1) reduction of single and tetanic contractions with predominant depression of single twitches, followed by (2) predominant depression of tetanic excitability. The dual action of curare at the neuromuscular junction appeared to account for the incomplete anticurare action of neostigmine. NAESS (1952a, b) also concluded that the preservation of ACh was responsible for the neostigmine antagonism of magnesium paralysis.

In accordance with the results obtained by LAPORTE and LORENTE DE NO (1950) on turtle sympathetic ganglia, NAESS (1952b) considered the possibility that curare produces a conduction block in the presynaptic terminals which is reinforced by prolonged repetitive nerve stimulation; it is this block which cannot be explained by the ACh theory and is not influenced by neostigmine. More recent studies of LILLEHEIL and NAESS (1961) support the idea that one aspect of the curare action consists in reducing the margin of safety for conduction of trains of nerve impulses in the terminal motor nerve arborization. In this context, it is significant that a variety of agents with affinity for the neuromuscular junction — e.g., gallamine triethiodide, neostigmine, edrophonium, decamethonium — behave like curare at increasing frequencies of nerve stimulation. PRESTON and VAN MAANEN (1953) found that these agents have dose-response curves with identical slopes, that the slopes do not vary at different stimulus frequencies, and that with all agents tested the dose necessary to produce 50% paralysis decreased considerably when the stimulus frequency was raised from one stimulus every 15 sec to 5 stimuli per sec.

Clearly then, the abundance of evidence from many laboratories and several approaches indicates that all agents with junctional affinity are capable of producing a transmission block through modification of some frequency-sensitive process at the neuromuscular junction. An important structural requisite for this affinity, and hence for the blocking action, appears to be the presence in the molecular configuration of a tricovalent nitrogen atom, quaternization of which enhances potency.

δ) Post-tetanic phenomena. After repetitive nerve stimulation of suitable frequency and duration the neurally-evoked twitch response is increased, a phenomenon usually called post-tetanic potentiation (GUTTMAN et al. 1937; v. PIRQUET 1938; BROWN and v. EULER 1938). When physostigmine is administered prior to nerve tetanization, post-tetanic potentiation is markedly exaggerated (FENG et al. 1938). This effect of physostigmine is obtained with doses that produce only very slight twitch potentiation by themselves. After larger doses, which cause more pronounced increases in twitch tension, the additional increase in the size of the twitches after tetanization becomes relatively less; when the physostigmine potentiation reaches a maximum, no additional post-tetanic increase is apparent. In both normal and physostigmine-treated preparations, curare completely abolishes post-tetanic potentiation (FENG et al. 1939a; STANDAERT 1961).

The foregoing observations were made on decerebrate cats or cats anesthetized with chloralose. In cats under diallyl barbituric acid (Dial) anesthesia, ROSEN-

BLUETH and MORISON (1937) also found that physostigmine (or neostigmine) enhanced post-tetanic potentiation. But these results were not consistently obtained, and sometimes even a transient post-tetanic depression was produced in the presence of these facilitatory agents. In the *soleus* muscle, post-tetanic twitch augmentation is accompanied by repetitive action potentials in muscle fibres. Post-tetanic twitch potentiation in the normal *gastrocnemius* or *tibialis* muscle occurs in the absence of muscle repetition (BROWN and v. EULER 1938; ROSENBLUETH and CANNON 1940); however, physostigmine is capable of inducing repetitive activity in these muscles during the post-tetanic period (FENG et al. 1939a; WERNER 1960a). Moreover, each facilitated response (in the absence of physostigmine) is followed by a period of junctional inhibition that may last 70 to 100 msec, during which the response to a second nerve volley is greatly diminished (FENG et al. 1939b). A physostigmine-potentiated response is also followed by a prolonged phase of inhibition (BROWN 1937a). This inhibitory after-effect of either physostigmine or nerve tetanization was regarded by FENG et al. (1939b) as another aspect of the same process at the neuromuscular junction which leads to the facilitation of transmission. The possible involvement of K^+ in post-tetanic augmentation (BROWN and v. EULER 1938; FENG et al. 1939a; ROSENBLUETH and MORISON 1937) was ruled out, since K^+ — although increasing the twitch tension and the amplitude of the muscle action potential — does not cause repetitive activity in muscle fibres nor does it induce retrograde activity in motor nerve fibres; in fact, K^+ only diminishes post-tetanic repetition in both muscle and nerve (FENG and LI 1941a; WERNER, unpublished observations).

These observations strongly suggest that the increase in contractile response seen either post-tetanically or after physostigmine is identical in all essential characteristics (FENG et al. 1939b). This idea receives further support from the striking finding that repetitive antidromic after-discharge occurs in motor axons supplying the *soleus* muscle after either nerve tetanization or physostigmine administration (FENG and LI 1941a; WERNER 1960a). Moreover, not only do a variety of twitch-potentiating drugs in addition to physostigmine augment the post-tetanic increase in twitch tension (KUPERMAN, unpublished observations), but also drug-induced twitch potentiation is augmented by tetanic conditioning (KUPERMAN and WERNER 1960) (Fig. 14). Especially significant is the fact that many of the agents, twitch potentiating effects of which were increased by nerve tetanization, could not be considered as AChE inhibitors, e.g., tetraethylammonium and phenyltriethylammonium ions (KUPERMAN et al. 1961a) (see page 628).

Post-tetanic decurarization has also been viewed by FENG and LI (1941a) as still another aspect of the same junctional process which leads to post-tetanic and physostigmine-induced twitch potentiation. HUTTER (1952b) showed that post-tetanic decurarization could not be accounted for by an increased sensitivity of the endplate region to ACh, and he therefore postulated a presynaptic locus for this effect. LILEY and NORTH (1953) found that post-tetanic decurarization is accompanied by an increase in amplitude of endplate potentials, suggesting an increase in the amount of transmitter released from the nerve terminals by each nerve volley. That nerve tetanization does indeed induce some alteration of the nerve terminals is indicated by the increase in discharge frequency of miniature potentials seen immediately following a tetanus (BROOKS 1956). The increase in discharge frequency of miniature potentials has also been obtained with the twitch potentiating agents neostigmine (BOYD and MARTIN 1956a) and m-hydroxy-phenyldiethylmethylammonium ion and its non-hydroxy analogue (VAN DER KLOOT and KUPERMAN, unpublished observations on frog muscle).

All the foregoing results are pertinent to the hypothesis that the post-tetanic and drug-induced twitch potentiation, and decurarization are manifestations of similar alterations at the neuromuscular junction, and that such alterations occur at least in part at the motor nerve terminals. Accordingly, the effects of repetitive nerve stimulation, twitch potentiating agents, and anticurare drugs (including physostigmine) are interchangeable and additive.

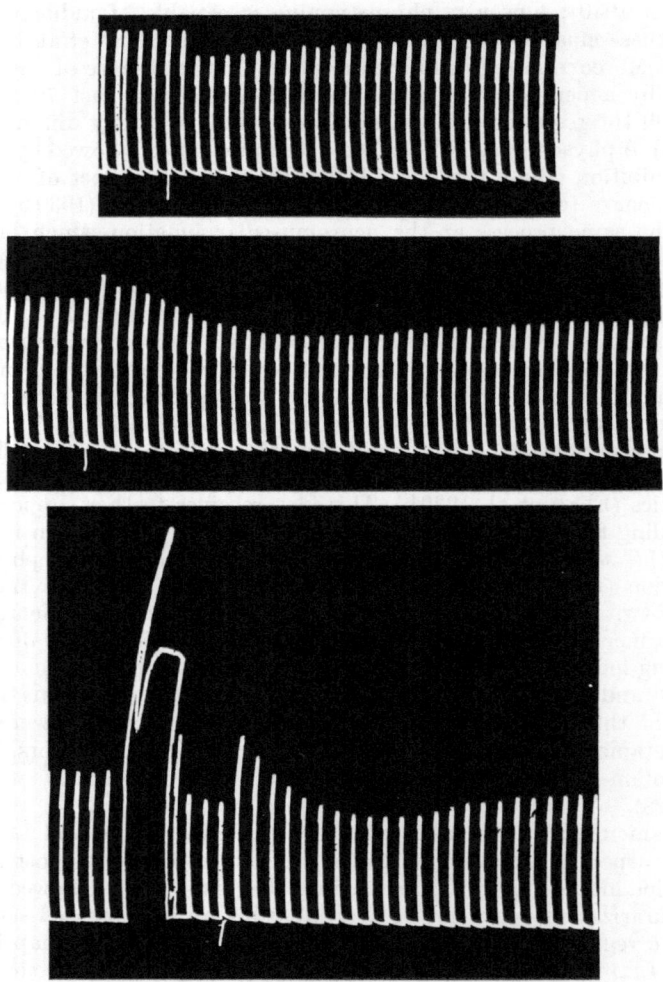

Fig. 14. Effect of tetanic conditioning on response to 3-OH-PNMe₃ in cat gastrocnemius muscle. Muscle stimulated indirectly with supramaximal square wave pulses at rate of 1 every 7 sec; all injections into popliteal artery; circulation restricted to gastrocnemius muscle; chloralose anesthesia. Top: 3-OH-PNMe₃, 1 µg/kg. Middle: 3-OH-PNMe₃, 5 µg/kg. Bottom: 3-OH-PNMe₃, 1 µg/kg injected at signal after nerve tetanization (400/sec for 20 sec). (From: KUPERMAN and WERNER 1960)

ε) **Interaction with neurotropic agents.** That the presence of anesthesia is detrimental to the production of twitch potentiation by physostigmine and related agents has already been discussed. BROWN et al. (1936) and BACQ and BROWN (1937) had first established that the twitch potentiating effect of physostigmine and related agents is easily observed in decerebrate cats or in cats under chloralose anesthesia; ether and tribromoethanol (Avertin) diminished or abolished this action of the carbamates. During ether anesthesia, a larger dose of neostigmine is necessary to cause an augmentative effect, and a depressant effect of neostigmine appears at a lower dose than in the absence of anesthesia (NAESS 1950; SECHER 1951). Intra-arterially injected thiopental, in doses of several mg/kg, abolishes twitch potentiation by neostigmine; but thiopental exerts a restorative action on neuromuscular transmission if, for reasons of dose or high stimulation frequency, depression by neostigmine prevails (KRAATZ et al. 1953). Other barbiturates usually deepen the depression of transmission produced by high doses of carbamates or DFP (SIRNES 1954).

In the absence of a carbamate, thiopental and pentobarbital may elicit slight potentiation of the maximal twitch; this is possibly due to a slowing of the contractile process in the muscle fibres, rather than to an action on neuromuscular transmission. Both agents diminish the ability of muscles to maintain tetanic contractions (KRAATZ et al. 1953) and also augment the blocking action of curare on neuromuscular transmission (PICK and RICHARDS 1947). The impairment of transmission by barbiturates is particularly pronounced at stimulus frequencies exceeding 200 per sec.

Of considerable interest is the fact that appropriate doses of procaine abolish the increase in twitch tension produced by physostigmine (HARVEY 1939a) or neostigmine (JACO and WOOD 1944). In this respect, procaine acts like small doses of d-tubocurarine (WERNER et al. 1959). Concomitantly, procaine reduces the ACh output from the neuromuscular junction during tetanic nerve stimulation (STRAUGHAN 1960b). In higher doses, procaine also depresses the twitch tension developed by maximal nerve volleys. Transmission of single volleys may temporarily be restored after a brief period of tetanic stimulation of the nerve. Like curare, procaine reduces the contractile response to ACh in these higher doses. It may be noted in passing that procaine, applied locally to motor nerves, selectively blocks conduction in small motor fibres (MATTHEWS and RUSHWORTH 1957).

In the foregoing experiments and in those with barbiturates, it may be assumed that the doses of the neurotropic agents used do not, by virtue of the route of administration employed, alter axonal properties significantly (HEINBECKER and BARTLEY 1940; TOMAN 1949; LARRABEE and POSTERNAK 1952). From this, and from the absence of effects of barbiturates on denervated muscle, it appears that the depression of twitch potentiation by these neurotropic agents is attributable to a site of action intermediate between motor nerve axons and postsynaptic muscle structures (RIKER et al. 1959a; WERNER et al. 1959).

In eserinized muscle, quinine prevents the repetitive responses evoked by single nerve volleys and the transmission paralysis of tetanic stimulation (HARVEY 1939b; OESTER and MAASKE 1939); indeed, quinine appears even more effective than curare in this respect (RAVIN 1940). Quinine also produces a decrease in post-tetanic potentiation and inhibition of spontaneous twitching elicited by physostigmine. At slow rates of stimulation, quinine may induce potentiation of the contractile response, but this occurs also on direct stimulation (in curarized muscle) and is, therefore, probably related to its prolonging effect on the muscle action potential, rather than to its anti-ChE potency *in vitro* (VAHLQUIST 1935).

ζ) **Potentiation of response to dicholine esters of α-ω-dicarboxylic acids.** In a report on the neuromuscular blocking actions of succinyldicholine and related esters of α-ω-dicarboxylic acids, BOVET-NITTI (1949) and BOVET et al. (1951) described a synergism of these agents with physostigmine. Similarly, treatment of animals with TEPP increased the neuromuscular paralyzing potency of succinyldicholine (LOW and TAMMELIN 1951). CASTILLO and DE BEER (1950) also studied this potentiation of response, and they initially presumed it to be due to the prevention of esteratic hydrolysis of the dicholine ester. However, DE BEER et al. (1951) subsequently made a significant observation with the *bis*-succinylamide of choline: this compound has no effect by itself on neuromuscular transmission and does not possess any anti-ChE activity; but, like physostigmine, it is nevertheless capable of prolonging the paralyzing action of succinyldicholine. This finding, and the fact that enzymatic hydrolysis of succinyldicholine by BuChE is exceedingly slow, make it highly improbable that the potentiating effect of physostigmine on the action of succinyldicholine is related to its ChE-inhibitory potency. Moreover, a potent inhibitor of AChE, namely the compound 284C51 (1 : 5-*bis*(4-allyl dimethyl-ammonium-phenyl)-*n*-pentan-3-one-dibromide), does not alter the response to succinyldicholine (FRASER 1954).

Succinyldicholine (SOMERS 1953) and dicholine esters of homologous dicarbamic acids (GINZEL et al. 1951 b) produce physostigmine-like potentiation of neurally-evoked twitches. It is, therefore, conceivable that the synergism between these agents at the neuromuscular junction is an expression of a common site of direct action rather than the result of ChE inhibition by the carbamate. In fact, physostigmine and neostigmine also potentiate the initial twitch potentiating response to stable agents like decamethonium (see page 649).

In an homologous series of dicholine esters of α-ω-dicarboxylic acids, no correlation was found to exist between the degree to which physostigmine prolonged their neuromuscular blocking action in cats, and their rates of hydrolysis by AChE and BuChE. However, potentiation of the contractural action on frog rectus and avian muscle and of the twitch response of mammalian muscle was more marked with compounds of higher rates of hydrolysis (GINZEL et al. 1951 b, d).

η) Dicholine esters of aliphatic dicarbamic acids. Mono- and dialkyl-*bis*-carbaminates are potent inhibitors of BuChE and erythrocyte AChE (KLUPP et al. 1953; KRAUPP et al. 1955a). These agents inhibit AChE relatively more than BuChE, and this conforms with the general postulate of JACOB and FUNKE (1953) according to which a dibasic configuration represents an essential condition for agents inhibiting AChE selectively. The activity of the mono-alkyl-*bis*-carbaminates of the general configuration:

$$(CH_3)_3 \equiv \overset{+}{N} \text{—}\bigcirc\text{—}O \cdot CO \cdot HN\text{—}(CH_2)n NH \cdot CO \cdot O\text{—}\bigcirc\text{—}N \equiv (CH_3)_3 \quad 2\,X^-$$

$(n = 4,6,8)$;

can be compared with the activity of the *m*-trimethylammonium-phenylcarbamate structure, from which the former are derived by twinning two symmetrical configurations: ChE inhibitory potency increases with the number of methylene groups between the neostigmine residues, and potency is further increased by methylation of the carbamate nitrogen (i.e., dialkyl-*bis*-carbamates); for the most potent agent of this series ($n = 10$), decamethylene-bis-(N-methyl-carbaminoyl-*m*-trimethylammonium phenol), the I_{50} value for AChE amounts to 10^{-10} (KRAUPP et al. 1955a).

On intravenous administration to rats, these compounds increase the twitch tension evoked by single stimuli, abolish the ability of skeletal muscles to maintain tetanic contractions, and exert a prolonged anticurare action. With regard to inhibitory actions on neuromuscular transmission, these agents are considerably more potent than neostigmine. There is no correlation between ChE inhibitory potency *in vitro* and the neuromuscular blocking activity in the presence of tetanic stimulation. In fact, N-methylation diminishes the latter activity and also leads to augmentation of enzyme inhibitory action. Neuromuscular paralysis with single nerve volleys can be obtained in the rat, but not in the cat, with doses exceeding those required for twitch potentiation and blockade of tetanic contraction (KRAUPP et al. 1955a).

FUNKE and DEPIERRE (1950) reported the high anticurare potency of some derivatives of aminophenol: the diiodomethylate of *bis*-(*m*-dimethyl-aminophenoxy)-1,3-propane (2842 CT) was more potent than neostigmine; its activity could further be increased by introducing into the molecule one or two urethane functions (3152 CT and 3113 CT) (FUNKE et al. 1952). These agents are also potent reversible inhibitors of erythrocyte AChE (LEVIN and JANDORF 1955).

ϑ) **Aminoalkylamides of dicarboxylic acids.** Potent inhibition of AChE has been demonstrated with some quaternary salts of aminoalkylamides of dicarboxylic acids (ARNOLD et al. 1954; KARCZMAR and HOWARD 1955). LANDS et al. (1955) investigated the neuromuscular effects of N,N-*bis*(2-diethylaminoethyl) oxamide *bis*-2-chlorobenzyl chloride (WIN 8077, Mytelase, ambenonium) and of its 2-methoxy analog (WIN 8078, Methoxyambenonium). Ambenonium and its methoxy congener are effective antagonists of *d*-TC, but only ambenonium facilitates the response to indirect stimulation of skeletal muscle. The methoxy compound is about 100 times less potent as an inhibitor of the ChE of cat tibialis muscle homogenate than is ambenonium (BLABER 1960). Thus, there is no correlation between the relative potency of these agents to antagonize *d*-TC paralysis and their ChE inhibitor potency *in vitro*.

Both ambenonium and methoxyambenonium elicit twitch responses on close arterial injection. However, while ambenonium augments on the cat's tibialis muscle the excitatory and paralyzing action of ACh, succinylcholine and decamethonium, methoxyambenonium diminishes these effects (KARCZMAR 1957). Since methoxyambenonium antagonizes paralysis by *d*-TC and depolarizing agents as well, KARCZMAR questioned the validity of the current views that *d*-TC and depolarizers cause paralysis in the cat's tibialis muscle by entirely different modes of action. BLABER (1960), while confirming most of KARCZMAR's observation, arrived at the conclusion that larger doses than those required to antagonize *d*-TC are needed to restore transmission from paralysis by decamethonium; it was claimed that, at these higher doses, oxamides produce a neuromuscular block resembling in many ways that caused by *d*-TC. Accordingly, this curare like action was considered responsible for the decamethonium antagonism. The complexity of the detailed mechanism of action of oxamides is apparent: while the neuromuscular block by oxamides resembles that by *d*-TC in that it is antagonized by tetanic stimulation and depolarizing agents, it is unlike that produced by *d*-TC in that it is not antagonized by neostigmine or edrophonium (BLABER 1960).

b) Hydroxyanilinium ions

The indications that neostigmine possessed a qualitatively different mechanism of facilitatory action from physostigmine and the demonstration of its direct excitatory action on muscle (RIKER and WESCOE 1946) led to an investigation of neostigmine analogues which lacked the carbamate group but retained the onium center. Initially, 3-acetoxy-phenyltrimethylammonium ion was studied because of its structural similarity to both ACh and neostigmine (RIKER et al. 1949).

Actually, this compound can be viewed as an ACh analogue in which a phenyl ring has replaced the aliphatic chain connecting the acetoxy and trimethylammonium groups. Thus, it was not surprising that this agent produced twitch-like muscle contraction following its rapid intra-arterial injection into innervated or chronically denervated muscle just as do ACh and neostigmine; physostigmine, lacking the methonium center, also lacks this pharmacologic action (LANGLEY and KATO 1915). In addition to this contractile effect, the 3-acetoxy analogue produced also a physostigmine- or neostigmine-like potentiation of neurally-evoked isometric tension accompanied by repetitive muscle discharge; this effect is observed with ACh only under special conditions (see page 612). The 3-acetoxy compound also was found to exert a potent anticurare action. There was a striking difference between the time-action curves of the 3-acetoxy ester on the one hand and the carbamate esters on the other; the twitch potentiating effect of the 3-acetoxy analogue was immediately maximal following intra-arterial injection and decayed rapidly over a period of about four minutes irrespective of dose. The anticurare action of this agent also reached a maximum immediately following injection, but the effect was prolonged. In contrast, the carbamate esters achieve their maximal pharmacologic effect only after the passage of several twitches (Figs. 9 and 11), and their twitch. potentiating action endures for twenty minutes to one hour or more, depending on dose. It is important to note, however, that neostigmine's facilitatory effects are achieved more rapidly than are physostigmine's (WESCOE and RIKER 1951). Also, ACh itself possesses an immediate, maximal, and permanent anticurare action under certain conditions (BRISCOE

1936b, WILSON and WRIGHT 1936) (see page 616). Accordingly, the onium center seems to be a structural requisite for the rapid development of pharmacologic effects; moreover, the carbamate moiety appears to inhibit this property of the quaternary grouping.

Simplification of the molecular structure of the 3-acetoxy ester was achieved by synthesis of 3-hydroxy-phenyltrimethylammonium ion (3-OH-PNMe$_3$) (RIKER and WESCOE 1950). Previously, COWAN (1938) had demonstrated the physostigmine-like properties of this ion in the frog, and RANDALL and LEHMANN (1950) discovered its potent anticurare action in cats. After intra-arterial injection, this agent also evoked an immediate and maximal twitch potentiation which lasted for several minutes (RIKER and WESCOE 1950). The demonstration of this effect of 3-OH-PNMe$_3$ required careful selection of doses, for like all methonium ions, this agent is also a potent depressant of neuromuscular transmission. The depressant action of 3-OH-PNMe$_3$ occurs in the same dose range in which potentiation appears; consequently the potentiation is diminished and ultimately obscured by the blocking action as the dose is increased (RIKER et al. 1957). For comparison, the depressant effects of 3-OH-PNMe$_3$ and neostigmine appear at about five times and forty times the minimal potentiating doses, respectively (RIKER et al. 1957; RANDALL and LEHMANN 1950). The simple phenyltrimethylammonium ion (PNMe$_3$) rarely produces any potentiation, and depression of isometric twitch tension predominates over its entire dose range (RIKER et al. 1957).

The discovery of the physostigmine-like properties of non-carbamate agents led to a comparison of ChE inhibitor potencies of these various compounds.

Acetylcholinesterase is reversibly inhibited 50% by 3-OH-PNMe$_3$ at a concentration of 2.5×10^{-5} M; the equally effective concentration for BuChE is 8×10^{-4} M (WESCOE et al. 1950). The 3-acetoxy-PNMe$_3$ ion is an approximately equipotent reversible inhibitor. Hence, the anti-AChE potency of either of these ions is about 1/100 that of physostigmine.

The relatively weak anti-ChE activities of 3-OH-PNMes and its acetyl ester, and the speed of onset of their facilitatory actions on neuromuscular transmission indicated to WESCOE and RIKER (1951) that these effects are related to direct interactions of the agents with receptors at the neuromuscular junction, not to inhibition of ChE. Also, there was no cogent reason to attribute the anticurare action of these agents to anything other than direct and competitive antagonism with curare at receptor sites. It was also stated that a division of quaternary ammonium ions into those acting by ChE inhibition and those acting by direct receptor interaction is largely arbitrary; in accordance with ROEPKE's view (1937), emphasis was placed on a concept according to which reactivity *in vivo* of agents with synaptic receptors must, for reasons of essential similarity of structure, be associated *in vitro* with some degree of ChE inactivation (WESCOE and RIKER 1951). MACFARLANE et al. (1950) also suspected that the anticurare action of 3-OH-PNMe$_3$ and its congeners is not related to anti-ChE activity.

This interpretation was challenged by the finding of HOBBIGER (1952) that pretreatment of cat *tibialis* muscle with TEPP abolished the anticurare action of hydroxyanilinium ions and their esters without affecting the curare antagonism by decamethonium. Thus, it was thought that the anticurare action of hydroxy anilinium agents — in distinction from that of a true "depolarizer" — can manifest itself only if active ChE is present at the neuromuscular junction. However, this conclusion is based on the assumption that TEPP cannot react with any receptor structures except those exhibiting ChE activity. Furthermore, the interrelation between these agents appears more complicated than one would expect if their action on ChE activity were the only determining factor for their effects on neuromuscular transmission. HALL and PARKES (1953) observed that neostigmine and edrophonium do not, after pretreatment with large doses of DFP and TEPP, antagonize the transmission block produced by decamethonium or succinyldicholine, as they do in the absence of such pretreatment; rather, they actually intensify the neuromuscular paralysis.

The argument that 3-OH-PNMe$_3$ and 3-acetoxy-PNMe$_3$ cannot be acting through ChE inhibition loses strength in view of the finding that edrophonium (3-OH-PNMe$_2$Et) reaches equilibrium with AChE *in vitro* within twelve seconds (WILSON 1955). This ion is also known to cause twitch potentiation and antagonize curare-induced depression with a time-action curve similar to that of 3-OH-PNMe$_3$ (RANDALL 1950; RANDALL and LEHMANN 1950). Although no data are available on this point, it may be presumed that 3-OH-PNMe$_3$ is also characterized by exceedingly rapid reactivity with AChE *in vitro* and accordingly, rapid reactivity with junctional AChE.

The considerable variation in both magnitude and pattern of response to the intra-arterial administration of a homologous group of hydroxyanilinium ions is illustrated in Fig. 15 (KUPERMAN, unpublished observations).

The twitch potentiation produced by 3-OH-PNEt$_3$ is monophasic, but the response to the other methyl-ethyl analogues in this series is biphasic, i.e., transmission block is produced in a certain population of muscle fibres. The size of the population affected in this way depends on the particular drug used and its dose. The presence of only one N-methyl group, as in the diethylmethyl analogue (3-OH-PNEt$_2$Me), is sufficient to yield the biphasic response. A comparison of potencies, however, reveals the especially marked increase in depressant effect with the transition from -$\overset{+}{N}$-Et$_2$Me to -$\overset{+}{N}$-Me$_2$Et, a phenomenon similar to that found for the ethylmethyl congeners of ACh (HOLTON and ING 1949). These structure-activity correlations, and also the evidence obtained by RIKER et al. (1957) on denervated muscle, indicate the blocking phase of this mixed response to be the consequence of methonium ion depolarizing action. Obviously, the depressant action limits the range within which the peak potentiating response is a linear function of dose. In any homologous series of quaternary ammonium ions which are twitch potentiating agents, this range would be most restricted for the methonium ion and expand sharply with the replacement of N-methyl by ethyl radicals. Outside the upper limit of this dose range, dose and response are inversely related, and with sufficiently large doses only depression appears.

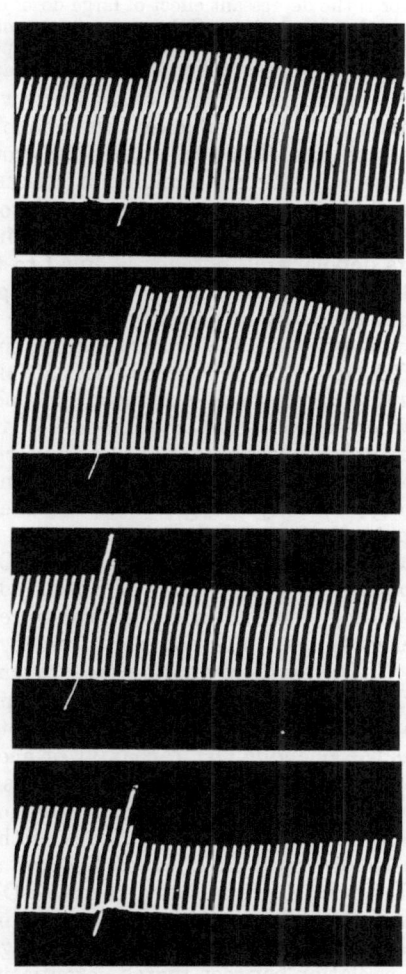

Fig. 15. Effects of hydroxyanilinium ions on the isometric twitch tension of cat *gastrocnemius* muscle. Muscle stimulated indirectly with supramaximal square pulses at a rate of 1 every 7 sec; all agents injected into the popliteal artery; circulation restricted to gastrocnemius muscle; spinal transection at T-12; dose 25 μg/kg in each case. Top: 3-OH-PNEt$_3$. Below: 3-OH-PNEt$_2$Me. Below: 3-OH-PNMe$_2$Et. Bottom: 3-OH-PNMe$_3$.
(From: KUPERMAN, unpublished record)

It has been found that the ability to produce neuromuscular depression is a property of many twitch potentiating agents, irrespective of their depolarizing capacity. The intra-arterial injection of these agents in doses just below those required to produce augmentation of the indirectly developed twitch tension usually elicits a depression which never exceeds 30% of the control (Fig. 14) (KUPERMAN 1960). This response has been obtained with appropriate doses of the *meta*-hydroxyanilinium, tetraalkylammonium, phenyltrialkylammonium, and aromatic tertiary amine compounds; it was less frequently observed with physostigmine and DFP. Significantly, tetanic conditioning converts this depressant response into one of twitch potentiation (Fig. 14) (KUPERMAN and WERNER 1960). In contrast, the threshold depression produced by a depolarizing ion like $PNMe_3$ is not significantly altered by tetanic conditioning, nor is the depressant effect of large doses of $3\text{-}OH\text{-}PNMe_3$ and other facilitatory agents which are also depolarizers. Subsequent to the monophasic potentiating effect produced by an agent like $3\text{-}OH\text{-}PNEt_3$, or to the biphasic response to an ion like $3\text{-}OH\text{-}PNMe_3$, there frequently appears a prolonged depression of twitch amplitude (Fig. 15).

Since the $PNMe_3$ ion has no twitch potentiating and only weak anticurare activity, it is possible that the phenolic OH specifically conveys facilitatory action on this ion. Alternatively, the OH group may serve merely to lessen the depolarizing potency of the methonium ion (RIKER et al. 1954), thus diminishing the depressant activity and unmasking a facilitatory component. However, the tolyl-*iso*stere, $3\text{-}CH_3\text{-}PNMe_3$, was found to be lacking in facilitatory effects despite the fact that its depolarizing potency is equal to that of the *meta*-OH analogue (RIKER et al. 1957). Other *meta*-substituted analogues of $3\text{-}OH\text{-}PNMe_3$ have been tested; each has a depressant potency equal to or less than that of the phenolic compound, but none possesses facilitatory action; these ions include meta-CH_3O-, C_2H_5O-, C_2H_5-, CH_2OH-, Cl-, NO_2- and NH_2-$PNMe_3$ (KUPERMAN et al. 1961 b). These *meta*-substituents have also been incorporated into the $PNEt_2Me$ and $PNEt_3$ ions; whereas the *meta*-OH analogues of these ions have potent facilitatory effects on transmission, none of the other derivatives has. These results support the view that a phenolic OH group, or a similar structure containing an anionic oxygen (e.g., carbonyl oxygen of carbamate group) is a specific requirement for twitch potentiating and anticurare action. Evidence has been presented that with increasing ionization of the phenolic OH in $3\text{-}OH\text{-}PNEt_3$, there is increased twitch potentiating activity in the isolated rat phrenic nerve-diaphragm preparation; binding between the OH group and receptor can thus be attributed to the unshared electron pair in the oxygen atom (STANDAERT 1959).

The results of another recent structure-activity investigation, however, reveal that twitch potentiation can be produced by compounds which contain an appropriate onium configuration but which lack a second functional group such as the phenolic OH, carbamyl, or acetoxy (KUPERMAN et al. 1961 a). Representatives of this type of facilitatory ions are $PNEt_3$, $PNEt_2Me$ and NEt_4. In Fig. 16, the dose-twitch potentiation regression lines for a series of quaternary ammonium ions are illustrated. The slopes of these lines divide the ions into a steeper and a lesser sloped class, called Group I and Group II, respectively, for convenience. In Group I are included the *meta*-OH, *para*-OH, and *meta*-carbamyl aniliniums; in Group II are the unsubstituted anilinium ions, *ortho*-substituted anilinium ions, and aliphatic ions (not shown in Fig. 16). Within Group I there exists a perfect correlation between twitch potentiating potency and anti-AChE activity, but such correlation is absent in Group II.

These observations affirm the view that affinity of quaternary ammonium ions for AChE is related to their capacity to facilitate neuromuscular transmission. But molecular requirements not associated with such an affinity are also important determinants of facilitatory action; these requirements relate to the onium center and, in fact, the common structural basis for twitch potentiation resides with the onium grouping. On this basis, it is probable that the second functional group in the Group I ions, e.g., phenolic OH, enhances interaction between the quaternary nitrogen and receptor, and in this way greater potency and ceiling effect are achieved. For optimal facilitatory activity the second functional group must be a carbamyl group, *meta* oriented to the onium center; the onium center which provides optimal activity is diethylmethylammonium (-NEt₂Me). Accordingly, the most potent twitch potentiating agent in the homologous series of *meta*-substituted anilinium ions is 3-(CH₃)₂NCOO-PNEt₂Me. Similarly, the most potent hydroxy-anilinium ion is 3-OH-PNEt₂Me; 4-OH-PNEt₂Me is more effective than its -NEt₃ analogue; PNEt₂Me is more potent than PNEt₃. It has been suggested that these functional groups either facilitate transport of the effective onium center to the receptor or that they change the steric configuration of the receptor, so that a better fit between onium center and receptor is achieved (KUPERMAN et al. 1961 a).

From still another point of view, the second functional group gives the molecule the capacity to act as a ChE inhibitor in addition to whatever other pharmacological properties are already inherent in the onium configuration. Thus, WILSON

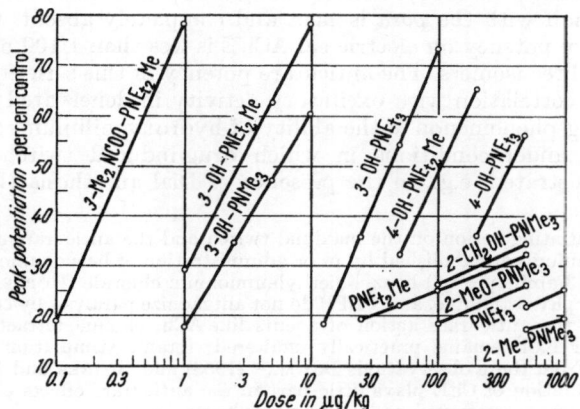

Fig. 16. Dose-response regression lines for potentiation of the isometric twitch tension in cat's *gastrocnemius* muscle by various aromatic quaternary ammonium ions. 3-Me₂NCOO-PNEt₂Me: *m*-dimethylcarbamyl-phenyl-diethylmethylammonium. 3-OH-PNEt₂Me: *m*-hydroxy-phenyldiethylmethylammonium. 3-OH-PNMe₃: *m*-hydroxy-phenyltrimethylammonium. 3-OH-PNEt₃: *m*-hydroxy-phenyldiethylmethylammonium. 4-OH-PNEt₂Me: *p*-hydroxy-phenyldiethylmethylammonium. 4-OH-PNEt₃: *p*-hydroxy-phenyltriethylammonium. 2-CH₂OH-PNMe₃: *o*-hydroxymethyl-phenyltrimethylammonium. PNEt₂Me: phenyldiethylmethylammonium. 2-MeO-PNMe₃: *o*-methoxy-phenyltrimethylammonium. PNEt₃: phenyltriethylammonium. 2-Me-PNMe₃: *o*-methyl-phenyltrimethyl-ammonium. (From: KUPERMAN et al. 1961 a)

and QUAN (1958) have presented evidence to indicate that the phenolic OH group engages in hydrogen bonding to the esteratic site of AChE and that the electrophilic carbon of the carbamyl group binds to some nucleophilic center also at the esteratic site. This view is distinctly opposite to that which focuses on the anionic oxygen and is difficult to reconcile with two facts: (1) the twitch potentiating potency of 3-OH-PNEt₃ increases with greater acidic dissociation of the OH group (STANDAERT 1959); (2) 3-NH₂-PNEt₃, 3-NH₂-PNEt₂Me, and 3-NH₂-PNMe₃ have no facilitatory activity whatsoever despite the fact that the amino group is approximately equivalent to the phenolic OH with respect to hydrogen bonding, solubility properties, and spatial distribution.

Among the isomeric forms of the hydroxy-phenyltrimethylammonium ion, depressant activity on cat muscle is most marked when the OH group is located in the position *para* to the -NMe₃ grouping (DEPIERRE and FUNKE 1950); the *ortho* isomer is about 40 times less muscle-depressant, and the *meta* isomer assumes an intermediate position. Also, anticurare potency is considerably more marked with the *meta* and *para* isomers than with the *ortho* compound. In dogs under chloralose anesthesia, RANDALL (1950) could not demonstrate twitch potentiation for the *ortho* and *para* isomers. In chronically denervated muscle, the *ortho* isomer possesses only 1/40 of the excitatory activity of the *meta* isomer (RANDALL 1950).

Apparently, 4-OH-PNMe$_3$ possesses a facilitatory component of action which manifests itself also as a potent anticurare effect. In fact, both 4-OH-PNEt$_2$Me and 4-OH-PNEt$_3$ potentiate the isometric twitch response (KUPERMAN et al. 1961a). It is only the *ortho* position of the OH group which is unfavorable for anticurare, twitch potentiating, paralyzing (in innervated muscle), and excitatory (in denervated muscle) actions. Nevertheless, other *ortho*-substituted anilinium ions (e.g., 2-CH$_3$O-PNMe$_3$) exist which facilitate neuromuscular transmission. Thus, the *ortho*-OH group may serve to attenuate the onium charge density through a direct field interaction and consequently reduce ionic interaction between the quaternary nitrogen and a negatively charged receptor grouping (RIKER 1953).

In a series of benzoic acid esters, the position of substitution on the phenyl-trimethylammonium ion is also of critical importance for anticurare potency (RANDALL and LEHMANN 1950): activity is again optimal with the *meta* isomer, reduced to one-half with the *para* isomer, and completely absent with the *ortho* isomer. Inhibitory potency on electric eel AChE is less than 1/100 of that of neostigmine for all three isomers. The anticurare potency of this series of agents does not exhibit any correlation with excitatory activity in denervated muscle.

An interesting phenomenon is the ability of hydroxyaniliniums to antagonize curare paralysis under conditions in which drug-induced twitch potentiation cannot be demonstrated, e.g., in the presence of Dial anesthesia (RANDALL and LEHMANN 1950).

Both the potentiating action on the maximal twitch and the anticurare action of 3-OH-PNMe$_2$Et (edrophonium) are abolished by prior administration of benzoquinonium (*p*-benzo-quinone-2,5-*bis*-N-(3-aminopropyl)-benzyl-diethylammonium chloride (HOPPE 1951); furthermore, neostigmine, physostigmine, and TEPP do not antgaonize paralysis by curare after such pretreatment, but the anticurare action of agents like ACh, choline, tetraethylammonium, decamethonium, or KCl remains practically unaltered; tetanic stimulation restores transmission as usual. From these observations BOWMAN (1958) and BLABER and BOWMAN (1959) concluded that inhibition of ChE plays little part in the anticurare effects of compounds of the hydroxyanilinium, neostigmine, and organophosphorus types.

After the antagonism of a curariform paralysis by a hydroxyanilinium ion, a second injection of the same dose of curare produces the same degree of transmission block as before administration of the antagonist; conversely, the hydroxy-anilinium ions can be administered repeatedly in alternation with *d*-tubocurarine without any signs of cumulative effects on muscle (RANDALL 1950, 1951). It has, therefore, been suggested that the hydroxyanilinium compounds manifest anti-curare activity by virtue of an ability to displace curare from its site of attachment to the receptor. Indeed, the fact that a powerful depolarizing agent like butyl-trimethylammonium antagonizes curare paralysis very effectively (DALLEMAGNE et al. 1951) appears to suppoert this view. However, this hypothesis does not account for the prolonged abolition by curare of drug-induced twitch potentiation. Curare antagonism by these drugs and also by physostigmine is obvious only with respect to restoration of transmission of single nerve impulses; but these agents do not restore the ability of curarized muscle to respond to single nerve impulses with repetitive activity unless the preparation is subjected to a short conditioning tetanus (WERNER 1959). In contrast to the "partial" antagonism of the actions of *d*-tubocurarine by drugs, tetanic nerve stimulation always restores the capacity of the muscle to respond with twitch potentiation to the injection of facilitatory agents (WERNER and KUPERMAN, unpublished observations). These facts necessitate a re-evaluation of the conclusions of FENG et al. (1939b) that a physostigmine-potentiated response and post-tetanic twitch augmentation are identical in all their essential characteristics. This may, indeed, be the case with respect to twitch potentiation, but it cannot be further deduced that this equivalence extends also to curare antagonism.

c) Organophosphorus compounds

During DFP intoxication in cats, impairment of neuromuscular transmission was observed which sometimes outlasted the period of drug administration by 6 to 10 days (MODELL et al. 1946); when stimulated to activity, the animals ran a few yards and then sprawled out on the floor unable to stand until they had rested for a few minutes. During that phase of intoxication, tetanic contractions could not be maintained. Similar neuromuscular effects and sporadic muscle fasciculation were also seen in dogs and monkeys (KOELLE and GILMAN 1946). Also, in man, localized fasciculation and muscle weakness were noted after intra-arterial injection of DFP. Characteristically, the second of two successive stimuli at short intervals evoked a muscle action potential of considerably reduced height (HARVEY et al. 1946). However, when DFP was administered to cats over several days, an additional phenomenon occurred: the response to close intra-arterial injection of ACh resembled the response normally obtained in muscles after chronic denervation. HUNT and RIKER (1947) therefore suggested that protracted exposure to DFP resulted in the development of an injury at the mammalian neuromuscular junction related to the change induced by chronic denervation. Transmission of single nerve volleys was unimpaired, but tetanic contractions could not be maintained.

On close arterial injection, DFP causes a slowly developing potentiation of the isometric twitch tension (HUNT 1947; BROWN et al. 1947) in the course of which spontaneous twitches of the muscle may occur; ACh or neostigmine, injected during the phase of potentiation, depresses the muscle response. During and after the potentiation, stimulation of the nerve at a frequency of 50 to 200 per sec produces a poorly sustained contraction which is followed by a transient depression of the response to single nerve volleys. In subfacilitating doses, DFP causes ACh to potentiate the maximal twitch tension.

Like DFP, TEPP (CHENNELS et al. 1949), dimethylamidoethoxyphosphoryl cyanide (Tabun) (HOLMSTEDT 1951), and fluorophosphorylcholine derivatives (FREDRIKSSON 1957, 1558) also potentiate the twitch response in appropriate doses and at low stimulus frequencies. The potentiated mechanical response to TEPP is accompanied by repetitive muscle action potentials, but at higher stimulus frequencies (10 to 50/sec) the peripheral after-discharges disappear. Repetitive after-discharges do not occur in directly stimulated denervated muscle. In innervated muscle, they are easily abolished by small doses of d-tubocurarine (CHENNELS et al. 1949). In man, GROB and HARVEY (1949) were impressed by the appearance of myriads of fasciculations after intra-arterial injection of TEPP. Single nerve stimuli are followed by repetitive muscle action potentials, but if the stimulation frequency is raised to 12 to 50 per sec, the amplitude of the successive muscle action potentials declines progressively. A long-lasting inhibitory process at the neuromuscular junction also becomes apparent when two maximal motor nerve stimuli are applied at varying intervals: the second nerve volley is not followed by repetition of the muscular response unless the volley interval exceeds about 250 msec. Obviously, following treatment with TEPP, passage of an impulse across the neuromuscular junction is depressed for a considerable period of time after a conditioning stimulus. Repetitive muscle activity in cats after physostigmine administration also remained suppressed at stimulus intervals shorter than 200 msec (BROWN and HARVEY 1941; WERNER 1960a). GROB and HARVEY (1949) thought that this phenomenon is compatible with the assumption of accumulation and slowness of dissipation of ACh in the presence of TEPP. However, the work of ECCLES and MACFARLANE (1949) and ECCLES et al. (1942) led to results which, if interpreted on the basis of the ACh theory, could not account for more than a doubling or tripling of the normal period of ACh action (maximally, some 10 msec) at the junctional region (see page 593). It is, therefore, difficult to understand how an inhibitory process of 200 or more msec duration could be related to persistence of transmitter substance for only some 10 msec.

After intraveneous administration of TEPP and during tetanic stimulation, a prolonged negativity was established in the region of the neuromuscular junction (DOUGLAS and PATON 1954); curare reversed this potential change. With higher doses of TEPP, a fluctuating depolarization of the endplate region occurred in the absence of nerve stimulation, but this was ascribed to the presence, in recently tied and cut nerves, of injury discharges. By increase of dose to 2 to 20 mg/kg, intraveneously, a steady depolarization took place in the absence of any nerve activity, spontaneous or evoked; this response was reduced in magnitude and developed slowly in chronically denervated muscle. This residual effect was ascribed to increased circulating ACh in the blood. The greater effect in innervated muscle, and its immediate onset, were attributed to activity of nerve endings in the muscle. These effects of TEPP were reversible within one hour after intraveneous injection, and complete cycles of depolarization and repolarization could, even with the largest doses, be obtained at hourly intervals. Also, recovery from neuromuscular paralyzing actions of high doses of TEPP took place within one hour (DOUGLAS and MATTHEWS 1952). This is a remarkably fast recovery in view of the fact that in rats following administration of single doses of TEPP, sensitivity of the lacrymal glands for injected ACh returns to normal in the course of about six days (HOBBIGER 1951); but hydrolysis of the enzyme-inhibitor complex can occur, and the enzymes of different organs vary greatly in sensitivity for TEPP (HOBBIGER 1951).

More direct evidence on the relation between inhibition of ChE at the myoneural junction and changes of neuromuscular transmission after administration of DFP or TEPP, was obtained by MCNAMARA et al. (1954). Depression of the contractile response to single stimuli in denervated (directly stimulated) and normal (indirectly stimulated) muscle was not regularly and invariably associated with the histochemically verifiable reduction of ChE activity; conversely, recovery from depression of the contractile response could occur in innervated and denervated muscle when cholinesterase was not detectable by histochemical means at the neuromuscular junction. MCNAMARA et al. (1954) and MURTHA et al. (1955) emphasized the depression of conduction in sciatic nerves of poisoned animals, which was neither in time course nor in degree related to the residual ChE activity in the nerve. However, the failure after single doses of TEPP and DFP to maintain indirectly evoked tetanic contractions was irreversible within periods of observation extending over ten hours, and could, in the view of MCNAMARA et al. (1954) be ascribed to ChE inhibition. Nevertheless, the lack of correlation between recovery of transmission and restoration of ChE activity seemed to indicate some additional actions of these agents.

Transmission block in the cat *tibialis anterior* muscle resulting from intravenous or intra-arterial injection of TEPP is slowly reversed by intravenous administration of pyridine-2-aldoxime methiodide (P-2-AM) (HOLMES and ROBINS 1955). The abruptness of improvement of respiratory movements by P-2-AM in Sarin- or Tabun-poisoned animals stands in contrast to the slowness of recovery of transmission in leg muscles; indeed, BROWN et al. (1957) felt that the speed of onset of respiratory improvement militates against the view that this effect could be a consequence of reactivation of junctional ChE. Furthermore, a number of agents containing a quaternary ammonium group were found to restore to normal the twitch height of the cat gastrocnemius muscle after depression by Sarin; quaternary derivatives of atropine, as well as *d*-tubocurarine and gallamine, markedly increased the rate of return (KUNKEL et al. 1956). Also, some oxamide derivatives, e.g., WIN 12306 (N-N'-*bis*-(N-di-propyl, N-chlorobenzyl ammonoethyl) oxamide dichloride), promoted the recovery of the Sarin-inhibited twitch, but did not affect the recovery of tetanic response (WILLS et al. 1957). Interestingly, WIN 12306 conferred on the muscle a high degree of resistance to a second dose of Sarin, but the other agents used did not protect from subsequent doses of the inhibitor. For these and other reasons, KUNKEL et al. (1956) did not believe that ChE is the sole point of attack of Sarin and related compounds at the neuro-muscular junction. In fact, Sarin, DFP, and other organophosphates and phos-phorofluoridates injected intra-arterially cause contracture of denervated skeletal muscle (GROBLEWSKI et al. 1956).

Respiratory failure in mammals intoxicated with organophosphorus compounds can be attributed to at least three different principal actions (DE CANDOLE et al. 1953): broncho-constriction, neuromuscular block, and central respiratory failure. Depending on the compound, dose, and species, one or another component of action predominates. When atropine is ad-ministered before Sarin, larger doses of the latter are required to depress respiration; under these conditions, respiratory depression seems due to neuromuscular transmission block (STEWART 1959).

3. The endplate potential

In the completely curarized mammalian nerve-muscle preparation, physo-stigmine (eserine) causes the rise of the endplate potential to continue to a higher and later peak from which it decays a little more slowly than in the non-eserinized

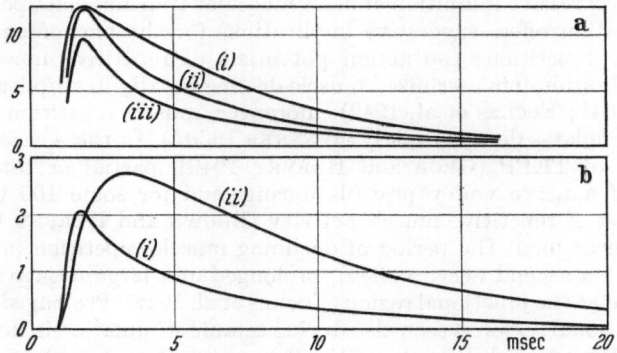

Fig. 17. Effect of physostigmine and curare on endplate potential of soleus muscle of cat. a: Endplate potentials added to the decaying negativity of a preceding endplate potential, with the nerve volleys for 1st and 2nd endplate potential separated by 1.6 msec. i: normal muscle; ii and iii: after successive doses of curare. b: Endplate potential produced by single nerve volley in same experiment. i: in curarised muscle; ii: in fully eserinised muscle to show delayed summit and slowed decay. The rate of rise is slower than in (i) on account of deeper curarisation. Ordinate: percentage of maximum spike potential. Abscissa: time from nerve stimulus. (From: ECCLES et al. 1941a)

control (ECCLES et al. 1941a, b; 1942) (Fig. 17). The more prolonged rise may indicate that the active phase of the transmitter process is increased in duration by about three-fold. There is no reason to assume that the small slowing in decay is indicative of an alteration by physostigmine of the electric constants of the muscle membrane. In non-curarized preparations, physostigmine causes consider-able prolongation of the junctional negativity set up by a single nerve volley. The negativity may outlast the recovery period of the muscle membrane after triggering a propagated muscle spike and may reappear, after the muscle spike, with an amplitude of as much as 1/3 or more of the spike height. After administra-tion of higher doses of physostigmine, a secondary persistent negative potential is set up by a nerve volley which usually can be distinguished from the endplate potential proper by its discrete rising phase. An identical secondary slow wave can be obtained at low doses of physostigmine, when paired nerve volleys at close interval (2 msec) are fired. Subparalytic doses of curare abolish the slow wave without affecting the initial component of the junctional potential. During per-sistence of the slow wave, which may continue for a second or more, a second nerve volley fails to induce any further potential change at the neuromuscular junction (ECCLES et al. 1941a, b; 1942).

In curarized frog muscles, a nerve volley evokes a larger endplate potential if it is preceded by a conditioning stimulus at a short interval; the time course of facilitation of the junctional potential is identical with that of neuromuscular facilitation by subthreshold cathodal pulses. Furthermore, electric excitability of muscle fibres remains unaltered in the presence of curare in concentrations which block neuromuscular transmission and the response to locally applied ACh (KUFFLER 1945). It was, therefore, assumed that facilitation of transmission is due to local subthreshold depolarization of muscle fibres (KATZ 1939; ECCLES et al. 1941 a). Mammalian muscle is, however, different in that the amplitudes of successive endplate potentials decrease progressively on repetitive stimulation at high frequencies (LUNDBERG and QUILISCH 1953). Facilitation of transmission occurs only in the post-tetanic period and may last for 100 sec or more (LILEY and NORTH 1953). To make this sequence of events plausible within the immediate frame of the humoral theory of transmission, it was necessary to postulate corresponding changes of the release of ACh during and after tetanic stimulation. The occurrence of progressive inhibition of neuromuscular transmission upon repetitive indirect stimulation offers suggestive implications for the phenomenon of drug-induced muscle repetition: the action potentials of repetitive muscle activity evoked by single stimuli in eserinized muscle decline rapidly in amplitude (BROWN and HARVEY 1941; ECCLES et al. 1942); moreover, muscle repetition induced by ammonium phenolates decays rapidly (WERNER 1960a). In these cases, and after administration of TEPP (GROB and HARVEY 1949), partial or total block of transmission of a nerve volley prevails during, and for some 100 to 200 msec after, each burst of repetitive muscle activity (BROWN and HARVEY 1941; WERNER 1960a). Throughout the period of declining muscle repetition (and block of transmission for a second nerve volley), prolonged and large negative potentials may be recorded at the junctional region (ECCLES et al. 1942). Prolonged depolarization of the junctional region is seen also during tetanic stimulation in non-curarized preparations (BURNS and PATON 1951). Thus, stimulation with single shocks appears in drug-conditioned preparations to be equivalent to repetitive nerve stimulation in the absence of potentiating agents; drugs with facilitatory effects on neuromuscular transmission act as if they converted a single nerve volley into tetanic nerve activity.

Thus, a remarkable paradox characterizes the action of ChE-inhibiting agents and their structural congeners on neuromuscular transmission: development of tension on excitation by single nerve volleys increases, while, at the same time, transmission for subsequent nerve volleys is curtailed. Apparently, the temporal dispersion of the partially blocked repetitive muscle action potentials results in increase of the contractile forces of single twitches (BERNHARD et al. 1941). The designation of such agents as potentiators or facilitatory drugs refers, therefore, only to the mechanical manifestation of twitch contractions and to the occurrence of some repetitive activity; with respect to junctional transmission, such agents are endowed with marked inhibitory actions which become more apparent with increasing stimulus frequencies.

4. Antidromic activity in motor nerves and its relation to the mechanism of potentiating and anticurare action

After administration of neostigmine, MASLAND and WIGTON (1940) observed the occurrence in ventral root fibres of antidromically conducted activity subsequent to an orthodromic nerve volley; this phenomenon was interpreted to indicate a presynaptic action of the agent at the neuromuscular junction. At about the same time, FENG and LI (1941a, b) observed the appearance of anti-dromically conducted activity in motor nerve fibres during irrigation of cat leg muscles with physostigmine solution. In the frog, DUN and FENG (1940b) could not evoke such retrograde activity with physostigmine, although barium ions, guanidine, and veratrine (DUN and FENG 1940a) were very active in this respect. Realizing the implications of this discovery, FENG and LI (1941a) proceeded to test their hypothesis (see page 630), according to which facilitation of neuro-muscular transmission by physostigmine is identical in nature to post-tetanic facilitation; indeed, in ventral root filaments of the cat *soleus* muscle under chlo-ralose anesthesia, retrograde nerve activity and muscle repetition occurred simul-taneously when single test volleys were applied during the post-tetanic period. Post-tetanic and physostigmine-induced repetitive activity are also alike insofar as a second nerve volley fired within some 45 or more msec after a conditioning volley does not elicit nerve repetition (cf., WERNER 1960a).

The occurrence of repetitive retrograde activity in motor nerve fibres of eserinized cats was readily confirmed by ECCLES et al. (1942). These authors stressed the lack of synchrony of nerve and muscle repetitive volleys which one might anticipate if retrograde nerve activity is assumed to reflect the occurrence of transmission in a precise one-to-one correspondence. It was essentially because of the variability of association of nerve and muscle repetitive volleys that ECCLES et al. (1942) did not accept the claim of MASLAND and WIGTON (1940) and FENG and LI (1941a) of a presynaptic site of action of neostigmine and physo-stigmine. Moreover, LLOYD (1942) was led to the conclusion that activity in normal and eserinized muscle is capable of eliciting centripetal volleys in motor nerves through retrograde excitation of nerve terminations.

However, it may be noted that the back response observed by LLOYD (1942) originates at the distal end of motor nerve fibres contemporaneously with, or immediately after transmission of the nerve volley to the muscle. On the other hand, the first spike in a train of repetitive back responses characteristics of facilitatory agents originates at the distal end of the motor nerve with a delay of several msec (WERNER 1960b). Furthermore the latter back response is far more susceptible to suppression by d-tubocurarine than is the former (WERNER 1961a). These are reasons to believe that antidromic after-discharge in motor nerves can be initiated in different ways, distinguishable by latency and pharmacologic reactivity.

RIKER et al. (1959a, b) also observed in motor nerve and muscle the variability of association of post-activation repetitive activity when hydroxyanilinium ions were used as facilitatory agents. But, significantly, retrograde nerve activity was obtained with 3-OH-PNMe$_3$ in doses which produced complete block of trans-mission for the orthodromic test volley. From this evidence, it was inferred that the repetitive antidromic nerve discharges are not secondary to muscle activity, and that the reactivity of receptors involved in the antidromic nerve response is not dependent on the occurrence of transmission. Contrariwise, a separation of muscle and motor axon repetitive response to 3-OH-PNEt$_3$ could be achieved in decerebrate or chloralose-anesthetized cats by administration of small doses of pentobarbital or by cyclopropane anesthesia; these neurotropic agents readily diminished or abolished the repetitive antidromic nerve response without affecting axonal conduction. However, muscle repetition and twitch potentiation were only slightly or not at all reduced, depending on the dose of the neurotropic agent.

The separation of nerve and muscle repetitive responses suggested to RIKER et al. (1959b) that a structure intermediate between the motor axon and endplate is capable of generating repetitive activity subsequent to its invasion by nerve volleys. This generating function was attributed to the motor nerve terminals, viewed as a distinct functional unit in which a local potential could develop. The primary action of drugs that induce facilitation at the neuromuscular junction was postulated to consist in augmentation of this local generating activity, so that repetitive excitation of the postsynaptic structure occurs. This event may, under suitable circumstances, be signalled by the initiation of propagated antidromic spikes in the motor axon. On the basis of the experiments in which dissociation of "forward" and "backward" response was seen, it appeared that the safety margin for axonal excitation by terminal activity is narrower than that for transmission to the postsynaptic unit (RI-KER et al. 1959a, b). The capacity of motor nerve terminals to respond with graded local activity points to an analogy with the excitatory process in dendrites in which, essentially, a train of "all-or-none" impulses can be converted into a relatively steady state (BISHOP 1956).

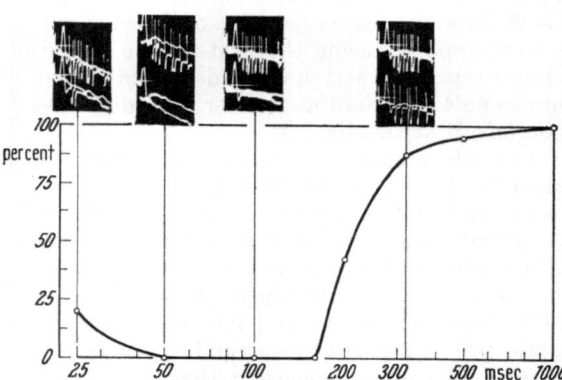

Fig. 18. Intensity of retrograde nerve activity in relation to interval between paired stimuli, after intra-arterial injection of 25 μg 3-hydroxy-phenyldiethylmethylammonium; *gastrocnemius* muscle; chloralose anesthesia (80 mg/kg, i.v.). The number of nerve spikes following the second of a pair of stimuli (in percent of the control response on stimulation with single volley) is plotted against the volley interval (in msec, logarithmic scale). The points represent mean values of 4 to 6 consecutive sweeps. Representative records are inserted at 25 msec, 50 msec, 100 msec, and 320 msec. Upper sweep in each record shows muscle action potential and retrograde nerve activity following the conditioning stimulus; lower sweep in each record shows activity following the test stimulus at the specified intervals. Note the complete absence of retrograde nerve activity at volley intervals of 50 and 100 msec. From: WERNER 1960a)

In nerve-muscle preparations treated with physostigmine (ECC-LES et al. 1942), or with hydroxyanilinium agents (WERNER 1960a), transmission of a second nerve volley is curtailed when it is fired at an interval of 10 to 100 msec after the initiation of repetitive muscle activity by a conditioning volley. During an interval of 20 to 160 msec after the conditioning volley, a second nerve volley also fails to elicit a burst of antidromic nerve spikes (FENG and LI 1941a;

WERNER 1960a; Fig. 18). Partial or total transmission block also prevails for the repetitive nerve volleys which appear in the motor nerve axon (Fig. 18). This finding illustrates clearly the point discussed on page 634, that repetitive muscle activity following invasion by single volleys of drug-conditioned nerve terminals is associated with some degree of transmission block. Indeed, the commonly observed lack of regular one-to-one correspondence of repetitive nerve and muscle volleys can be understood as the necessary consequence of a certain degree of functional autonomy of the motor nerve terminal. On the other hand, there exists an interval of 1 to 4 msec after arrival at the neuromuscular junction of an orthodromic volley during which a second nerve volley greatly augments repetitive activity in muscle and nerve. The cumulative result of orthodromic stimulation with paired volleys at short intervals is such that doses of the potentiating agents, subthreshold at single stimulation, may become highly effective in inducing nerve and muscle repetition, indistinguishable in appearance and duration from that obtained with single volleys, after larger priming doses of the drugs; conversely, this cumulative effect of double volleys at short intervals is abolished by curare in doses ineffective with respect to transmission of the conditioning nerve impulse. After a short period of tetanic stimulation, in the course of which transmission block is attained, the effect of single volleys in inducing repetitive activity is increased for several minutes (WERNER 1960a).

From the time course of augmentation and diminution of postactivation repetition by a conditioning volley, WERNER (1960a) inferred that motor nerve terminals are capable of sustaining, under appropriate conditions and after invasion by a nerve volley, negative and positive afterpotentials of a time course similar to that of nerve fibres with slow conduction velocity. Accordingly, the terminals would act with respect to contiguous axon segments initially as the current sink (i.e., the generator event for antidromic activity), and subsequently as a more prolonged current source. It was also suggested that the phasic interrelation between transmission and repetitiveness may be viewed as a result of these phasic membrane potential changes of motor nerve terminals (WERNER 1960a), and that they may

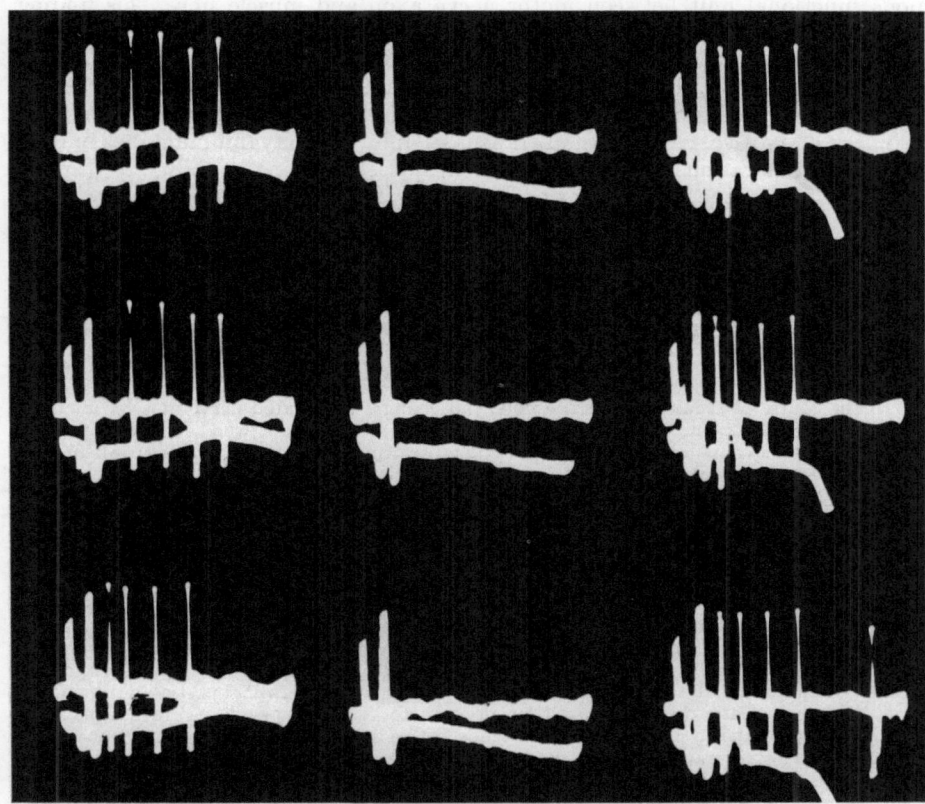

Fig. 19. Depression of repetitive motor-nerve activity by d-tubocurarine, and antagonism of curare-block by tetanic conditioning; motor unit of *gastrocnemius* muscle; chloralose anesthesia (80 mg/kg, i.v.). The record in the upper trace of each pair was obtained from the severed distal end of an L 7 ventral root filament. A square wave pulse (0.1 msec duration) was applied every 7 seconds to the same ventral root filament as used for recording. Muscle activity appears in the lower trace of each pair, and was recorded from a motor unit activated from the ventral root filament. The negative variation in both nerve and muscle is upward. Left column: repetitive nerve activity after intra-arterial injection of 50 µg/kg 3-hydroxy-phenyldiethylmethylammonium. Middle column: absence of repetitive nerve activity after intra- arterial injection of 50 µg/kg 3-hydroxy-phenyldiethylmethyl-ammonium, following intra-arterial injection of 5.0 µ/kg d-tubocurarine. Right column: 2 min after record of middle column was taken, the ventral root filament was stimulated for 10 sec at a frequency of 200/sec. Subsequently, single stimuli were applied (as before the tetanic conditioning, at a rate of one every seven seconds). (From: WERNER, unpublished record)

be identified with the oscillatory potential changes which constitute the "nerve reaction" of polarizable nerve membranes (LORENTE DE NÓ 1947).

That the existence of such a terminal focus for drug action must be considered in the interpretation of studies, physiological or pharmacological, on neuromuscular transmission is also apparent from the fact that d-tubocurarine and gallamine triethiodide suppress drug-induced repetitive activity in nerve and muscle; this effect manifests itself in doses below those which block transmission

(WERNER 1959). It is, therefore, possible to demonstrate in preparations pretreated with hydroxyanilinium ions that subparalytic doses of d-tubocurarine,
concomitantly with abolishing the repetitive activity, restore transmission for
subsequent nerve volleys. This action of curare is obviously a corollary to its
restoring effect on tetanic excitability depressed by physostigmine or neostigmine
(BRISCOE 1938). In accordance with the evidence for the existence of an autonomous functional unit between motor nerve axon and muscle fibre, this finding
indicates that curare has also a presynaptic site of action. The suppressive action
of curare on repetitive nerve and muscle activity is remarkably persistent; it is
not antagonized by physostigmine or hydroxyanilinium ions in doses exceeding
those which restore transmission in fully curarized neuromuscular junctions (see
also page 620). Also, restoration of transmission by hydroxyanilinium ions in fully
curarized preparations is not accompanied by recovery of the ability to respond
repetitively to single nerve volleys. The anticurare action of these agents is, thus,
limited to transmission and does not extend to repetition. However, short tetanic
conditioning is capable of restoring the repetitive reactivity of curarized nerve
and muscle (Fig. 19).

B. Responses of individual units. Amphibian and mammalian muscle

I. Neurally-evoked activity

In the course of studies on electric potential changes at isolated nerve-muscle junctions
in the frog, KUFFLER made several significant observations which were decisive for interpretation of the events associated with junctional transmission (cf. KUFFLER 1948). In particular, KUFFLER (1943) showed that the endplate region is about 1000 times more sensitive
to depolarization by locally applied ACh than other areas of the muscle fibre. Evidence was
obtained also that the junctional potential gives rise to the muscle spike by spreading electrotonically, and thereby critically depolarizing the region adjacent to the endplate (KUFFLER
1942c; KUFFLER 1942a). However, KATZ (1948) pointed out that the suggestion of a brief
transmitter action and prolonged passive decay applies to curare-treated muscle but not
necessarily to the eserinized muscle in which the active period is prolonged. In frog sartorius
muscle, a maximal cathodal shock applied to the terminal portion of the motor axon leads
to the initial rise of the endplate potential after a delay of 1.0 msec. This time was thought
to consist of conduction time in the terminal motor fibre, a "setting-up" time, and a true delay
period; assuming that the nature of electrotonic spread over the terminal portion of the motor
nerve is not essentially different from that along motor axons, KUFFLER (1948) estimated a
true delay time of 0.5 to 0.8 msec. The existence of this delay, not to be accounted for within
the theory of electric transmission in the form held at that time by ECCLES (1946), was highly
suggestive of the presence of a humoral transmitter agent. The humoral theory was further
greatly strengthened by the absence of trans-synaptic spread of subthreshold cathodic pulses
applied to terminal nerve branches (KUFFLER 1948). This argument may, however, be less
convincing than it appears at first since the effect beyond a block of a subthreshold potential
is also labile in nerve axons and likely to require active local response of the blocked region
(BULLOCK and TURNER 1950).

A comparison of the effect on the junctional region of a test volley after a conditioning
neural impulse with that after a conditioning ("antidromic") muscle impulse revealed that
after neural excitation, the endplate remains refractory for a longer period of time than after
"antidromic" stimulation (KUFFLER 1942b). Physostigmine prolongs the refractoriness for
a neural test volley after neural conditioning, concomitantly with its prolonging effect on the
endplate negativity (see also ECCLES et al. 1942).

Measurements of the transmembrane potential at the junctional region largely confirmed
previous results obtained with external recording techniques; in addition, some essential new
aspects of the transmitter process were revealed. FATT and KATZ (1951) determined that in
curarized nerve-muscle junctions of frogs, a net electric charge of 8×10^{-10} coulomb is transferred upon the arrival of each nerve volley; this corresponds to 8×10^{-15} mol. of univalent
cations. In normal muscle, this quantity is 3 to 4 times larger.

FATT and KATZ (1951) made the significant observation that during normal transmission
the electric response of the endplate differs from that of other parts of the muscle membrane,
in that the neurally evoked junctional potential fails by approximately 15 mV to reach the
level which is attained by a membrane action potential; however, this difference in attained

potential is not seen when the muscle fibre is stimulated directly. This phenomena was explained by assuming that the junctional region contains receptors which, on reaction with ACh, lead to a "short-circuit" of the membrane, and consequently to ionic movements in accordance with concentration gradients; furthermore, it was, necessary to assume that such "chemoreceptors" of the endplate region are not activated by the local currents of propagated muscle impulses. Additional supporting evidence for the "short-circuit" theory was subsequently put forward by demonstrating that transmitter action at the junctional region tends to re-set the active membrane potential and to shift it toward an equilibrium level of about 10 to 20 mV internal negativity; moreover, transmitter action is followed by a large local increase in membrane conductance, greater than that which occurs during the peak of a directly elicited muscle spike (DEL CASTILLO and KATZ 1954d, 1955b). In summary, then, the transmitter elicits at the motor endplate a response distinct from the muscle- or nerve action potential in that it consists of a smaller potential change (without reversal of membrane potential), but a larger change of membrane conductance (per unit area) (FATT and KATZ 1951, cf. OGATA and WRIGHT 1960).

The effects of neostigmine on the amplitude and duration of the endplate potential recorded with intracellular electrodes (FATT and KATZ 1951) are of a magnitude similar to those observed with external electrodes in the whole muscle (ECCLES and MACFARLANE 1949). A striking phenomenon was noticed, however, when neostigmine was added to muscles kept in Na^+-deficient solutions: the local potential was lengthened enormously and, instead of passing through a sharp peak, maintained a plateau for some 30 to 40 msec, from which it declined to one-half in about 100 msec (FATT and KATZ 1951). Under these conditions, a charge equivalent to at least 10^{-12} univalent ions passes through the "endplate sink." FATT (1954) pointed out that the prolongation of transmitter action appears as a constant feature whenever junctional transmission is, by means other than curarization, prevented from setting up propagated impulses in muscle fibres. Accordingly, prolongation of transmitter action was also seen when the junctional response was set up during the refractory period of muscle (KUFFLER 1942b).

When transmission is blocked as a result of the presence in the muscle bath of ACh, nicotine, or succinyldicholine, neurally evoked junctional negativity can be recorded, the time course of which is identical with that of endplate potentials in curarized preparations; in contrast, in the presence of decamethonium junctional negativities are markedly prolonged (THESLEFF 1955a). In concentrations which reduce the ChE activity of frog muscle preparations by 50%, decamethonium causes a considerable prolongation of the endplate potential, whereas neostigmine, at equal degree of ChE inhibition, does not alter the duration of endplate potentials in curarized preparations. Prolongation of junctional negativity by decamethonium is not associated with depression of direct excitability of the muscle fibre (THESLEFF 1955a, b).

Immersion of frog muscles into Ringer solution containing edrophonium (10 μg/l) gives rise to a condition in which a single nerve volley is able to elicit repetitive activity of the muscle fibre. At the same time, it causes a persistent delay in the repolarization of the membrane at the endplate such that the membrane potential may be assumed not to return to its resting level between successive action potentials (NASTUK and ALEXANDER 1954). In the presence of d-tubocurarine in the Ringer solution, edrophonium at a concentration of 10 mg/l causes an increase in the amplitude of the endplate potential to a point where propagated action potentials are initiated (NASTUK and ALEXANDER 1954). Like neostigmine, edrophonium also increases the time required for the junctional potential to reach its increased peak value, and prolongs the time for the local potential to decay to one-half of its peak value; the decay time of the transmembrane potential increases under those conditions about two-to three-fold. Characteristic is the rapid onset of action after exposure of the preparation to the edrophonium-Ringer solution; full development of effect is achieved within some 20 sec. Measurement of the time for decay to the half peak value of the endplate potential reveals a significant fact: at the time of onset of transmission, decay time is 2 to 3 times longer if paralysis by curare is antagonized with edrophonium than it is in the case of restoration of transmission through removal of curare by washing. However, the critical height of the endplate potential for triggering propagated muscle spikes appears to be of the same order of magnitude. A marked prolongation of the junctional potential, exceeding that seen in the curare-Ringer solution by about three times or more, occurs in preparations immersed in Na^+-deficient solutions containing edrophonium at relatively low concentrations (4 μg/l). This effect is comparable to that obtained with neostigmine under identical conditions (FATT and KATZ 1951), i.e., when propagated muscle activity was prevented by lack of Na ions. Only at 50 times higher concentrations does edrophonium lower directly the membrane potential at the junctional region without affecting the transmembrane potential at sites distant from that zone. There is also no evidence that edrophonium might alter the excitability of the membrane at the vicinity of the endplate. In contrast, the m-hydroxy-phenyl-trimethylammonium ion reduces the membrane potential at considerably lower concentrations, and at the same time causes transmission block. NASTUK and ALEXANDER (1954) concluded that the actions of edrophonium on neuromuscular transmission can be explained on the basis of its ChE-inhibiting activity in vitro, since no evidence for a different mechanism of action could be obtained.

II. Spontaneous activity

At the junctional region of muscle fibres, there is usually found in the absence of nerve stimulation a continuous display of randomly recurring pulses, exhibiting the characteristics of neurally evoked junctional activity except that the amplitude of the spontaneous pulses is about 100 times smaller (FATT and KATZ 1952a; for review, see KATZ 1958a, b). Furthermore, it is possible to locate at the fibre surface discrete spots from which spontaneous potentials, occurring in random sequences, can be recorded externally. The discharges so recorded differ in certain essential aspects from the internally recorded "miniature endplate potentials" (FATT and KATZ 1952a): the localization of the external potentials is very critical in that movement of the microelectrode for a few microns results in disappearance of activity in the records; also, shape, polarity, and frequency pattern of internally and externally recorded activity are different. The extracellular field associated with the occurrence of a spontaneous "miniature endplate potential" is extremely localized, whereas the field along the inside of the muscle membrane during a miniature discharge spreads electrotonically over a much greater distance. Consequently, focal extracellular recording does not capture more than 1 to 10% of the internally recorded activity (DEL CASTILLO and KATZ 1956b). The spontaneous activity is not seen in the nerve-free region of muscle fibre nor is it observed in muscles the motor nerve supply to which has been interrupted one or two weeks prior to the experiment.

After transient disappearance on denervation, local spontaneous activity is gradually resumed at the denervated endplates, though at much lower rates than in innervated muscle. Electron microscopy revealed that Schwann cells occupied the place of the nerve endings at the time of resumption of spontaneous discharges. Supersensitivity to ACh develops after some weeks of denervation and when local spontaneous activity has reached its final intensity (BIRKS et al. 1960).

The random sequence in which the miniature responses of innervated muscle occur indicated that the nerve terminals are undergoing random fluctuations in their excitatory state, and that occasionally in the course of these fluctuations a critical level is reached which becomes manifest as a "miniature endplate potential"; the time sequence of these discharges is apparently best described as a time-dependent stochastic process, except at very brief discharge intervals, when some form of interaction occurs (FATT and KATZ 1952a; LILEY 1956a). The outstanding novelty introduced by the discovery of the spontaneous miniature discharges consists in the recognition of a presynaptic apparatus composed of a population of units which may discharge individually at random, or synchronously after arrival of a neural volley (DEL CASTILLO and KATZ 1954a, 1956a). Accordingly, the neurally-evoked endplate potential is viewed as the postsynaptic result of a composite presynaptic event to which can be assigned a certain "quantum content," i.e., a number of individual units of transmitter activity. Several factors were found to alter the probability of any one quantal transmitter unit to respond to a nerve volley; preceding nerve impulses (DEL CASTILLO and KATZ 1954b; BROOKS 1956) lead to "facilitation", which is very conspicuous when the "quantum content" of the neural volleys has been reduced by increase of Mg-ion concentration or by deficiency of Ca-ions. Thus, facilitation (i.e., recruitment of quantal units of transmitter activity) occurs at a very early phase of the sequence of events constituting neuromuscular transmission. Conversely, prolonged nerve stimulation in normal (or slightly curarized) frog muscles causes a progressive depression of response to a test volley; this is interpreted as a sign of reduction of quantum content, while at the same time frequency of random miniature discharges greatly increases (DEL CASTILLO and KATZ 1954b). In the rat diaphragm, the increase of discharge frequency after repetitive indirect stimulation exhibits a time course closely resembling that of post-tetanic potentiation of the endplate potential in curarized muscle (LILEY 1956a).

Some indirect evidence points to a relation between the magnitude of the presynaptic neural response and the quantum content of the transmitted response (DEL CASTILLO and KATZ 1954c, WERNER 1961b). Application of a moderate anelectrotonus to the terminal portion of a motor axon leads presumably to hyperpolarization of its membrane and thereby creates a condition under which activity could result in membrane potential changes of larger magnitude than normal; indeed, anodic polarization of nerve terminals facilitates the junctional negativity in curarized frog nerve-muscle preparations. Anodic currents above a certain threshold strength also initiate prolonged outbursts of miniature potentials (DEL CASTILLO and KATZ 1954c). This effect may be ascribed to an increased intensity of transmitter action, since the anelectrotonic current flow is confined to the nerve structures and does not traverse the synapse (KUFFLER 1948). In mammalian nerve-muscle preparations, polarization of motor nerve terminals leads to different effects: electrotonic hyperpolarization of motor nerve arborizations reduces the frequency of miniature discharges, whereas depolarization augments discharge frequency; LILEY (1956b) demonstrated a linear relationship between the discharge rate and the electrotonic displacement of the terminal membrane potential. Essentially, these observations reveal that postsynaptic events can be modified by local electrotonic changes in presynaptic nerve endings without involving nerve impulses (DEL CASTILLO and KATZ 1954c). Moreover, these observations indicate that electrotonic current flow along motor nerve terminal is possible in spite of their presumably high attenuating resistance (BULLOCK 1951), and that such current flow produces profound alterations in that it increases dramatically the frequency of spontaneous discharges. It is, however, important to note that the activity in preterminal nerve endings cannot be directly compared with propagated spike activity in nerve axons, since the former continues in abnormal ionic environment which abolishes nerve conduction (DEL CASTILLO and KATZ 1955b).

The spontaneous discharges in normal muscle are affected by curare and neostigmine in the same manner as neurally evoked junctional potentials: d-tubocurarine greatly reduces the size of "miniature endplate potentials," whereas neostigmine causes a graded increase of their amplitude and duration (Fig. 20). In frog muscle, neostigmine does not significantly alter the frequency of spontaneous random discharges (FATT and KATZ 1952a; FURUKAWA et al. 1957) nor does locally applied ACh affect the rate of spontaneous firing (DEL CASTILLO and KATZ 1955a); however, in mammalian preparations, neostigmine exerts an influence on the recurrence rate of spontaneous discharges which depends critically on the concentration used. With increasing concentrations, there is transient augmentation of amplitude and duration, and frequency diminishes (BOYD and MARTIN 1956a, b). In general, there exists an optimal concentration at which the frequency of the spontaneous potentials increases. The spontaneous miniature activity which reappears in frog muscle some time after severance of the motor nerve exhibits a pharmacologic reactivity identical with that of normal frog muscle (BIRKS et al. 1960).

Assuming that curare acts only postsynaptically and that neostigmine acts only by virtue of ChE inhibition, FATT and KATZ (1952a) concluded that the spontaneous activity at the junctional region, both internally and externally recorded, could be attributed to the release of ACh. The evidence for quantal transmitter action was related to the existence in motor nerve terminals of sub-microscopic vesicles (ROBERTSON 1956) which were believed to contain ACh; release of the supposed ACh content of such vesicles was suggested to occur as a result of critical collision of the vesicles with the presynaptic membrane (DEL CASTILLO and KATZ 1956a). In denervated muscle, ACh release was ascribed to the Schwann cells (BIRKS et al. 1960). In fact, WHITTAKER (1959) isolated from

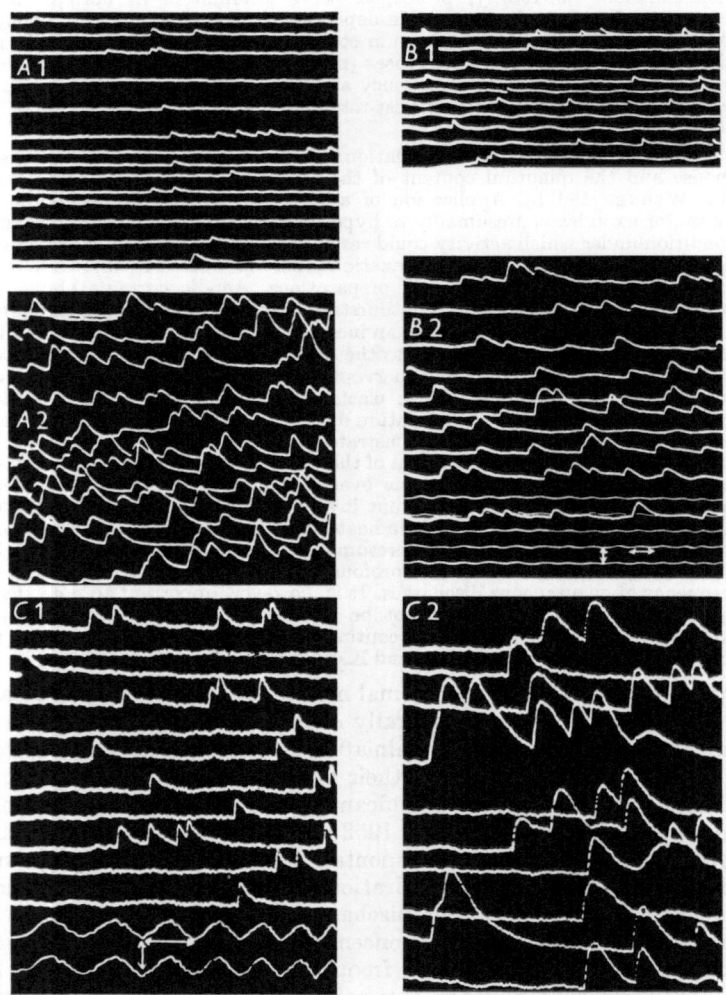

Fig. 20. Effect of neostigmine on size and time course of miniature endplate potentials. A, B and C: three different endplates of frog muscle (A and C from *m. ext. l. digit. IV*; B from *sartorius*). 1: in normal Ringer; 2: after addition of 10^{-6} M neostigmine bromide. (In C 2, potential changes of slow rise can be seen, beside those of the usual rapid rate of rise. This was also observed in several other experiments and is presumably to be explained by electrotonic spread from an accessory endplate of the same fibre.) Arrows indicate 1 mV scale and 20 msec. (From: FATT and KATZ 1952a)

sucrose homogenates of rabbit and guinea pig brain a particle fraction of diameter mostly in the range of 0.02 to 0.08 μ; some of these particles appeared in electron micrographs as vesicles, and most of the particle-bound ACh was contained in this fraction.

The effect of neostigmine to increase the frequency of spontaneous miniature discharges in mammalian muscle suggests an action of this agent on nerve terminals (BOYD and MARTIN 1956a). Apparently, mammalian muscle is also highly susceptible to depression of amplitude and duration of spontaneous discharges by neostigmine. The question arises whether, and under what conditions, such activity in nerve terminals as that revealed by postsynaptic miniature potentials leads to a backfiring into the main motor axon and, by axon reflex, to activity in the entire motor unit. In mammalian muscle, retrograde motor nerve activity can be set up by neostigmine (MASLAND and WIGTON 1940). In frog muscle, however, the level of spontaneous activity remains usually subthreshold for either nerve or muscle, and fibrillatory activity in the presence of neostigmine is only occasionally seen (FATT and KATZ 1952a).

Ammonium ions, on the other hand, elicit increased discharge of miniature endplate potentials accompanied by marked fibrillation; this effect of ammonium ions is suppressed by curare, and is not observed in denervated preparations (FURUKAWA et al. 1957). Also, in the presence of guanidine, spontaneous miniature endplate potentials reach a magnitude sufficient for eliciting propagated muscle action potentials. Concomitantly, guanidine increases the amplitude of the neurally evoked endplate potential in curarized muscle without changing the sensitivity of the endplate to ACh (OTSUKA and ENDO 1960a).

An interesting discrepancy arises when the effects of neostigmine are examined in low Na^+ media: the mean size of the spontaneous internally recorded potentials decreases to about 1/2 to 1/3 of the control amplitude obtained in solutions with normal Na^+ content (FATT and KATZ 1952b). However, the neurally evoked endplate potential was previously shown to be enormously exaggerated under identical conditions (FATT and KATZ 1951). Similarly, edrophonium augments and prolongs considerably the neurally evoked endplate potential in low Na^+ muscles (NASTUK and ALEXANDER 1954). Thus, neostigmine seems to be much less effective in augmenting, in Na^+-poor preparations, the "spontaneous" rather than the "responsive" junctional negativity.

One may have to consider the possibility that neostigmine and edrophonium act with respect to the "responsive" junctional negativity as the quaternary ammonium ions, which in Na^+-deprived B and C fibres of frogs cause prolongation of the nerve action potential (LORENTE DE NÓ 1949). Assuming an analogous action on motor nerve terminals, these agents could enable the terminal arborizations to respond in low-Na^+ solutions with prolonged activity to an incoming volley. The prolonging action of certain quaternary ammonium ions on electric activity of excitable tissue in low-Na^+ media is apparently a phenomenon of more general significance; it was observed in crustacean muscle (FATT and KATZ 1953) and nerve fibres (BURKE et al. 1953), and in frog muscle fibres (HAGIWARA and WATANABE 1955). An equivalent effect on terminal motor nerve fibres in the frog would imply a presynaptic action of neostigmine and edrophonium, due to the quaternary ammonium character of these agents, superimposed on whatever effect they may have as ChE inhibitors. The preferential effect of these agents on neurally evoked activity has its counterpart in the fact that Na-ions are not essential for the maintenance of spontaneous miniature discharges (DEL CASTILLO and KATZ 1955b).

III. Drug-receptor interactions at individual junctions

The stimulating action of ACh at individual motor endplates was demonstrated by BUCHTHAL and LINDHARD (1937) and KUFFLER (1943). An initial negativity of the junctional region is readily seen to lead to the origin of the first muscle spike; immediately after the spike, the potential returns to the baseline and the negativity may then be built up again. This sequence can be repeated several times and can result in a train of discharges. With concentrations of ACh near threshold, small monophasic potentials may be recorded. During application of ACh to the endplates, no potentials could be recorded from ventral roots in frogs; in cats, however, MASLAND and WIGTON (1940) observed antidromic activity in ventral roots after injections of ACh. On the other hand, DIAMOND (1959) found regenerating and normal motor nerve fibres of cats to be relatively resistant to excitation by ACh. Exposure of the frog nerve-muscle junction to physostigmine prior to application of ACh augmented the ability of ACh to cause local negative potentials at the junctional region, but this effect was not regularly obtained (KUFFLER 1943).

The receptors which take part in this reaction to ACh are apparently restricted to the external surface of the junctional region, i.e., the side of the muscle membrane which makes contact with the nerve endings (DEL CASTILLO and KATZ 1955a); this conclusion is derived from experiments in which ACh was applied electrophoretically to single endplates by means of micropipettes (NASTUK 1951, 1953, 1954). The inefficacy of intracellular application was observed not only with ACh, but also with its stable analog, carbaminoylcholine (DEL CASTILLO and KATZ 1955a). Exposure of the muscle to neostigmine enhances the depolarizing effect of a slow continuous outflux of ACh from the micropipette, but the sensitivity of the receptive area to "close-range" electrophoretically released pulses of ACh remains largely unaltered, though increase was observed in some instances. Local junctional potentials elicited by electrophoretically released pulses of carbaminoylcholine decay with about half the speed of ACh potentials elicited in the same way. In the presence of neostigmine, the time course of ACh potentials becomes indistinguishable from that of potentials elicited by jets of carbaminoylcholine ions (DEL CASTILLO and KATZ 1957c). Slowness of onset and considerably prolonged decay distinguish the potentials produced by electrophoretic application of decamethonium, nicotine, and succinylcholine from depolarization with ACh (DEL CASTILLO and KATZ 1957d). The depolarization by close-range pulses of ACh also rises to a maximum relatively slowly and reaches its peak in the course of some 13 msec, while the neurally evoked endplate potential or its quantal components reach their peak value in about one msec (DEL CASTILLO and KATZ 1955a). Choline, like neostigmine, potentiates the depolarizing effect of topically applied ACh; decamethonium enhances the effect of ACh after an initial phase of depression (DEL CASTILLO and KATZ 1957d). After prior exposure to neostigmine, this augmenting effect of stable quaternary ammonium ions on depolarization by ACh is converted into depression. Curare abolishes the reactivity of the junctional region to ACh without affecting membrane resting potential, resistance, or capacity (DEL CASTILLO and KATZ 1957a). The inhibitory action of curare on local depolarization by ACh is accompanied by reversible reduction of amplitude of spontaneous miniature discharges at the junctional region (DEL CASTILLO and KATZ 1957b).

Two main results emerged from these investigations, both essentially substantiating pharmacologic evidence obtained from observations on drug interactions in the isolated frog rectus muscle preparation: these are, (1) potentiation of response to ACh by stable quaternary ammonium ions, and (2) the ability of certain agents to manifest either depolarizing or curare-like activity, depending on the conditions. The latter observation suggested to DEL CASTILLO and KATZ (1957d) the possibility that such agents might form competitively, as an intermediate step in the reaction that leads to depolarization, an inert drug-receptor compound. This reaction may be represented in the form $S + R \rightleftarrows SR \rightleftarrows SR'$, where SR' is the hypothetical depolarizing compound; according to this concept, whether an agent acts predominantly as a depolarizer or as a competitive blocking agent would depend solely on the rate constants of the two steps of this reaction. A subsequent step in the sequence of reaction appears to result in the formation of refractory receptors, as evidenced by the fact that repeated application of ACh or related agents leads to a transient loss of sensitivity (THESLEFF 1955a, b; 1956; KATZ and THESLEFF 1957b; AXELSSON and THESLEFF 1958). The potentiation of response to ACh by neostigmine was, however, ascribed to ChE inhibiton rather than to an effect analogous to that obtained with choline and other stable quaternary ammonium ions, although electrophoretically applied neostigmine led only to depression of reactivity to ACh. The low rate constant of inhibition of ChE by neostigmine obviously complicates the interpretation of this finding.

This difficulty was avoided by the use of edrophonium, which is known to equilibrate rapidly with ChE *in vitro* (WILSON 1955). In fact, potential changes elicited by single pulses of ACh are enhanced during the period of electrophoretic application of edrophonium. The potentiating effect of edrophonium subsides within less than one second after termination of its iontophoretic application (KATZ and THESLEFF 1957a); assuming that the augmenting effect of edrophonium is due to ChE inhibition, a time constant of 0.1 sec for dissociation of the enzyme-edrophonium complex could be determined. The sensitivity to carbaminoylcholine is not increased by edrophonium, but at higher concentrations of edrophonium, carbaminoylcholine exerts less depolarizing activity. In higher concentrations, edrophonium is evidently capable of interacting with receptors, and one may assume that the edrophonium-receptor complex has less depolarizing "efficacy" than the carbaminoylcholine-receptor compound (KATZ and THESLEFF 1957a). In the presence of neostigmine, edrophonium does not enhance the depolarizing potency of ACh, but depression of reactivity to ACh prevails at higher concentrations of edrophonium; thus, neostigmine essentially converts the manifestations of the ACh-edrophonium interaction into those of the carbachol-edrophonium combination.

KATZ and THESLEFF (1957a) considered these findings in harmony with the general concept that quaternary ammonium ions may act at the neuromuscular junction in either of two ways: i.e., by specific inhibition of ChE or by direct receptor interaction. Neostigmine and edrophonium were viewed as "specific" antiesterases exhibiting a substantial margin between affinities for ChE and for receptor structures; choline and decamethonium, on the other hand, were considered to exemplify agents with about equal affinity for receptor and ChE (DEL CASTILLO and KATZ 1957d). One may, however, raise the question whether this analysis of drug action at the level of individual units has removed the essential arbitrariness of division of agents into a class of primary ChE inhibitors and a class of agents with predominant receptor affinity (see page 626).

Denervation does not result in change of sensitivity of endplate receptors to electrophoretically applied ACh, but it leads to increase of the muscle membrane area responsive to ACh (AXELSSON and THESLEFF 1959; MILEDI 1960a). Enlargement of the chemoreceptive membrane area occurs also in partially denervated muscle fibres, but remains restricted to the neighborhood of the denervated endplate. It has been suggested that the receptor molecules of the muscle fibre are being produced continually at the endplate from which they would "over-flow" and spread along the fibre surface but for the inhibiting influence of the motor nerve (MILEDI 1960a). Nevertheless, extrajunctional ACh receptors were also demonstrated in innervated mammalian muscle, though their density decreases rapidly with distance from the junctional region (MILEDI 1960b; KATZ and MILEDI 1961). Some evidence for a generalized action of ACh, choline, and d-TC along the membrane of frog sartorius muscle fibres was claimed by OCHS and MUKHERJEE (1959). The receptors of denervated mammalian muscle respond not only to ACh but also to carbaminoylcholine with transient depolarization; d-tubocurarine reversibly reduces their sensitivity to ACh. Unlike the potentiating effect on response to ACh in innervated muscle, edrophonium inhibits in denervated muscle the response to ACh and produces some membrane depolarization (AXELSSON and THESLEFF 1959).

C. The relationship between cholinesterase inhibition and drug-induced neuromuscular facilitation

The increase in neurally-evoked contractile response produced by chemical agents has been generally viewed as a signal of ChE inhibition ever since this effect was first observed in mammals with physostigmine (BROWN et al. 1936). Recognition of physostigmine's potent anti-ChE activity, and the supposition that accumulation of ACh at the neuromuscular junction results in twitch potentiation, left little choice but to conclude that physostigmine potentiation was the consequence of ChE inhibition. The concept of a causal relationship between twitch potentiation and ChE inhibition was enforced by the impressive correlation between these two parameters in a number of carbamate esters (BACQ and BROWN 1937). Anticurare activity was assumed to be another consequence of ChE inhibition; it was therefore reasonable to expect a number of subsequent investigators to determine whether significant correlation existed also between anticurare and anti-ChE activities. This was, in fact, demonstrated by the experiments of BLASCHKO et al. (1949) on mammalian muscle and by SMITH et al. (1952) and HOBBIGER (1952) on frog muscle. Meanwhile, still another action of drugs on neuromuscular transmission was considered as causally related to ChE inhibition, namely, prolongation of the endplate potential (EPP). This relationship was revealed by demonstrating a correlation between anti-ChE activities of a group of carbamate esters and their effectiveness in prolonging the EPP in frog muscle (ECCLES and MACFARLANE 1949). The significance of this finding relates to the fact that drug-induced twitch potentiation and curare antagonism were both shown to be associated with prolongation of the EPP (ECCLES et al. 1941a, 1942); that this effect on the EPP also results from ACh accumulation seemed to be the only assumption compatible with the experimental evidence and the ACh-AChE theory of neuromuscular transmission. More recently, FATT and KATZ (1951) and NASTUK and ALEXANDER (1954) have demonstrated prolongation of the intracellularly recorded EPP by neostigmine and edrophonium, respectively, thus strengthening previous hypotheses regarding the action of these ChE inhibitors.

In the historical development of ideas relating to the mechanism of action of twitch potentiating and anticurare drugs, another important effect of such drugs has been generally ignored, i.e., the action on the motor nerve terminal originally demonstrated by MASLAND and WIGTON (1940) for neostigmine and by FENG and LI (1941) for physostigmine (see page 634). Such an action has now been demonstrated for a variety of hydroxyanilinium ions (RIKER et al. 1957; RIKER et al. 1959a) and phenyltrialkylammonium and tetraalkylammonium ions (KUPERMAN and WERNER 1960). Recognition of the motor nerve terminals as a focus for drug action not only furnishes a basis for further inquiry into the actions of so-called ChE inhibitors on neuromuscular transmission; it also indicates that ChE inhibition is not the only, or perhaps not even the primary cause of the facilitatory actions of these agents. There is, of course, the possibility that these compounds interact with a presynaptically-located site similar or identical to endplate AChE; significant in this regard is the recent discovery that in sympathetic ganglia, the functional AChE is entirely presynaptic (KOELLE and KOELLE 1959). Although this is undoubtedly not the case at the motor nerve terminals, nevertheless it must be determined whether the drug-receptor combination at this site leads directly to facilitation of the transmitter process, or whether it results in accumulation of transmitter substance in the presence of inhibited AChE at the site of transmitter liberation (KOELLE 1961). At any rate, the problem of an essential similarity between cellular receptors and ChE is again brought into focus and appears to be responsible for the difficulty of determining experimentally mechanisms and loci of drug action at the neuromuscular junction. Accordingly, the conclusions reached may depend primarily on the methods used, a situation not unique to the science of pharmacology.

The concept that ChE and cellular receptor sites are essentially similar with respect to drug reactivity was first proposed by ROEPKE (1937), and has been repeatedly restated in various modifications and on different grounds of inferential evidence (WESCOE and RIKER 1951; HARDEGG 1952; ZUPANCIC 1953; NACHMANSOHN and WILSON 1955; ALTAMIRANO et al. 1955a; STERN 1956). In fact, RIKER (1953) pointed out the value of this concept in accounting for the complex relationships between effects of quaternary ammonium ions *in vivo* and their anti-ChE activities *in vitro*. This idea has been supported also by several other investigators, but only a postsynaptic site of drug action has been taken into consideration (ARIENS et al. 1956a, b; COHEN and POSTHUMUS 1956). Indeed, the recognition of a presynaptic site for ChE deposition and drug responses adds a new dimension of complexity to the interpretation of pharmacologic studies of neuromuscular transmission.

From the work of WILSON and BERGMANN (1950) it has become apparent that the protein molecules of ChE *in vitro* can be conceived to possess at least two reactive groups: the "anionic site" reacting by coulombic forces with ions of opposite charge, and an "esteratic site" capable of reacting with carbonyl groups and alkylphosphates (WILSON 1951; BURGEN and HOBBIGER 1951). Possibly, the "esteratic site" also provides for interaction with phenolic groups (WILSON and QUAN 1958). In AChE, two anionic sites may exist in close proximity to each other (BERGMANN and SEGAL 1954).

NACHMANSOHN and WILSON (1955) and ALTAMIRANO et al. (1955a) pointed out that the number of conceivable interactions between a small molecule like ACh and proteins is limited. Consequently, for significant interaction to take place, summation of several weak contributions is required; this results in severe restriction of the number of molecular configurations capable of reacting with a given protein. Accordingly, all proteins which interact strongly with ACh must be similarly constituted at the binding site; AChE and receptor cannot significantly differ, and the former serves as model for the latter.

The reactivity of junctional receptors with simple tetraalkylammonium ions is well-established from the investigations of ING and WRIGHT (1933), RAVENTOS (1937a) and ALLES and KNOEFEL (1939). Therefore, the question arises whether junctional receptors possess, in addition to the reactivity with cations, the property of interacting directly with carbonyl or equivalent groups, and organophosphates. On theoretical grounds, PFEIFFER (1948) suggested that in ACh and related compounds, the keto and carbonyl oxygen atoms of the ester linkage might take part in the reaction with cellular receptors. More direct evidence was obtained by WELSH and TAUB (1951): inclusion of a keto group at position 4 of the alkyl chain considerably enhanced the nicotinic activity of the unsubstituted amyltrimethylammonium ion. In a series of nuclear-substituted phenylethers of choline, HEY (1952) obtained supportive evidence for the concept that nicotinic activity is inversely related to the electron density of the ether oxygen. These results comprise circumstantial evidence favoring the proposition that the chemical reactivity of ChE's *in vitro* and cellular receptors *in vivo* are essentially similar.

On the other hand, JACOB and TAZIEFF-DEPIERRE (1957) summarized evidence which points to a divergence between anti-ChE activity and muscle depressant potency within homologous series of agents: in the case of the *bis-(m-*trialcoylammonium phenoxy) alcanes, ChE inhibition and muscle depression attain optimal degrees with agents of different chain-lengths between functional groups; quaternary ammonium ions with single functional groups are powerful muscle depressants and weak anti-ChE agents, whereas single inhibitors of the tertiary diamine series lack muscle depressant action. For these, and a number of other reasons (cf., BOVET et al. 1949; DEPIERRE and FUNKE 1952; JACOB 1955), JACOB and TAZIEFF-DEPIERRE assumed that the active groups responsible for ChE inhibition did not determine muscle depressant activity. Accordingly, muscle depression would be attributed primarily to the cationic group, while enzyme inhibition would be essentially dependent on the presence of suitable groups to react with the "esteratic site."

Many compounds which potentiate the isometric twitch tension and antagonize curariform paralysis in mammalian muscle, possess relatively weak anti-ChE activity; the pKi's for such agents vary from 10^{-2} to 10^{-5} M, in contrast to the range of 10^{-6} to 10^{-8} M and even less for hydroxyanilinium, carbamyl, and organophosphorus ChE inhibitors. The problem remains to define the mechanism of facilitatory action of these agents, and it is in this connection that the decision to ascribe the facilitation to ChE inhibition or to some other mechanism often appears arbitrary. The facilitatory compounds in this category of weak ChE inhibitors are characterized chemically as quaternary ammonium ions of either methonium or ethonium type; primary, secondary, and tertiary amines; and amidines. This chemical characterization is based on the nitrogen atom because this atom is apparently the common structural requisite for neuromuscular facilitation; quaternization and the presence of a second functional group in the molecule apparently serve only to (1) increase facilitatory potency, (2) raise the ceiling response and (3) increase anti-ChE activity.

The methonium ions in this category are decamethonium (C_{10}), duodecamethonium (C_{12}), tetramethylammonium (ZAIMIS 1951), phenyltrimethylammonium ion (WESCOE and RIKER 1951), choline (HUTTER 1952a), and a variety of ortho-substituted phenyltrimethylammonium ions (KUPERMAN et al. 1961a). Facilitatory actions of these agents have been observed in mammalian nerve-muscle preparations *in situ*; in the isolated rat phrenic nerve-diaphragm preparation, twitch potentiation by cyclopentyl- and cyclohexyltrimethylammonium ions has been reported (STANDAERT and FRIESS 1960). The capacity of all these depolarizing ions to depress transmission necessitates a judicious choice of dosage in order to demonstrate twitch potentiation; significantly, such an effect is obtainable only with the smaller doses and is more easily achieved with intravenous, or distant intra-arterial, rather than close intra-arterial administration.

In addition to methonium ions, a group of stable non-depolarizing ethonium ions and tertiary amines have been found to act as facilitatory agents at the neuromuscular junction; these also possess insignificant anti-ChE activity when measured *in vitro*. One of the earliest recognized ions in this category is tetraethylammonium (NEt_4). The striking ability of NEt_4 to cause repetitive nerve discharge in response to single shocks in frog nerve (COWAN and WALTER 1937) and squid axon (TASAKI and HAGIWARA 1957) has a counterpart in the effect of NEt_4 at the frog neuromuscular junction; ING and WRIGHT (1931) first showed the NEt_4 potentiation of frog sartorius to nerve stimulation, an effect probably achieved by prolongation of the negative afterpotential in the fine intramuscular nerve terminations, and consequently, the conversion of a single nerve shock into muscle repetition (KOKETSU 1958). The prominent anticurare action of NEt_4 was revealed in the rat and kitten phrenic nerve-diaphragm preparations and in the cat gastrocnemius (KENSLER 1949; SULLIVAN and KENSLER 1950; KENSLER 1950). The kitten diaphragm *in vitro*, like the frog *sartorius in vivo*, responds to single nerve shocks with twitch augmentation in the presence of NEt_4 (SULLIVAN and KENSLER 1950). Surprisingly, the demonstration of this effect in the adult cat *gastrocnemius* preparation was found to require neostigmine pretreatment (KENSLER 1950). It is now known, however, that NEt_4 potentiation can be achieved in this muscle without prior neostigmine administration, provided stimulus parameters are used which do not evoke repetitive orthodromic nerve firing (KUPERMAN et al. 1960a).

The isolated rat phrenic-diaphragm preparation responds with twitch augmentation to the polymethylene *bis*-triethylammonium salts, the methylene bridges of which range in number from 2 to 10 (BARLOW and ING 1948); facilitation was obtained most consistently with the C_2 congener. Gallamine triethiodide, generally considered as a curare-like neuromuscular depressant, augments slightly the twitch response of cat *tibialis* muscle to nerve stimulation (RIKER and WESCOE 1951). This interesting observation has been confirmed repeatedly in the cat gastrocnemius, and such potentiation can even be enhanced by pretreatment with a subthreshold dose of physostigmine (KUPERMAN, unpublished observations). In addition, $PNEt_3$ augments isometric twitch tension in cat muscle and is considerably more potent in this respect than its non-aromatic congener, NEt_4 (KUPERMAN et al. 1960a). It is apparent then that a variety of *mono-*, *bis-*, and *tris*-triethylammonium ions have a weak but definite facilitatory action on neuromuscular transmission.

The augmentative actions of the ethonium ions can be revealed only within a certain dosage range; as with the methonium ions, pure depression appears with higher doses. The biphasic action of facilitatory drugs is, therefore, not entirely dependent on "receptor inactivation" (KATZ and THESLEFF 1957b; NASTUK and ALVING 1958) or depolarization depression (RIKER 1957). The depressant effect appears to be universally associated with molecular configurations suitable for effecting neuromuscular facilitation.

Another category of agents which potentiate the transmitter process despite exceedingly weak anti-ChE activity includes catechol and its tertiary amine derivatives (see page 609). Catechol itself is an effective anticurare agent in the rat diaphragm preparation (MOGEY and YOUNG 1949). The capacity of epinephrine and many of its primary and tertiary amine analogues to augment isometric twitch tension in mammalian muscle is a well recognized phenomenon, but one which has never been adequately explained (BÜLBRING and BURN 1942; BURN and HUTCHEON 1949; HUIDOBRO et al. 1952). However, KRNJEVIC and MILEDI (1958b) have now shown that epinephrine increases the frequency of spontaneous miniature discharges in mammalian muscle, an effect which can be attributed to a direct action on presynaptic terminals. Again, the catecholamines are no exception to the fact that structural requisites for facilitation and depression exist within a single molecular configuration, and that the attainment of one response or the other is dependent largely upon proper selection of dosage. Indeed, the augmentative actions of the catechols are not especially obvious excepting after prior administration of subthreshold doses of neostigmine.

The anticurare action of guanidine was originally investigated by FENG (1940), who found that the amplitude of the endplate potential in curarized frog muscle is increased by it. This effect of guanidine has been recently confirmed by OTSUKA and ENDO (1960a), using intracellular recording technique. FENG also demonstrated in both amphibian (1938) and mammalian endplate (1941b) that guanidine has an effect on the presynaptic terminals in the same concentrations as those which antagonize curare. The twitch potentiating action of guanidine has been demonstrated in the isolated kitten phrenic nerve-diaphragm preparation (CONDOURIS and GHAZAL 1957) and in the cat nerve-muscle preparation *in situ* (KUPERMAN et al. 1961b). Again, as is the case with all other facilitatory drugs tested thus far, the dose of guanidine necessary to demonstrate twitch potentiation must be carefully selected to avoid depressant effects.

The first analysis of the mechanism of facilitatory action by a compound not generally viewed as a ChE inhibitor was achieved by ZAIMIS (1951) with the drug C_{10}. It had been shown previously that C_{10} in small intravenous doses produces a prominent increase in twitch tension (PATON and ZAIMIS 1949). The notion of a cause and effect relationship between this action and ChE inhibition led to a comparison between C_{10} and the closely related C_{12} with respect to anti-AChE and twitch potentiating potencies. Any previous assumption of a correlation between these two parameters was negated for this series by the finding that C_{12}, although a considerably weaker facilitatory agent than C_{10}, possesses a ten-fold more potent anti-AChE activity. In the extension of this work by ZAIMIS (1951), a marked and immediate twitch potentiation was obtained after intra-arterial administration of C_{10}. Significantly, this action was greatly enhanced by the prior injection of doses of physostigmine or neostigmine too low to be effective alone; the C_{12} potentiation was also augmented in this manner. It was shown further that appropriate doses of the simple mono-quaternary ion, tetramethylammonium (NMe_4), enhance isometric twitch tension, and that this can also be potentiated by neostigmine pretreatment; NMe_4 has no significant anti-ChE action *in vitro* (BARLOW and ING 1948).

ZAIMIS (1951) reasoned that the capacity of methonium ions to convert a single twitch response into an incomplete tetanus was the result of a direct action on the endplate membrane. The supposition that depolarization of the postsynaptic membrane is capable of producing a repetitive response in single muscle fibres cannot be questioned; but that such repetition in individual units can account completely for enhancement of twitch tension of the whole muscle is open to debate. Furthermore, the interaction of the drug-induced depolarization with nerve stimulation must be considered. With those facilitatory agents postulated to act only through ChE inhibition, the nerve impulse is supposedly required to permit accumulation of transmitter substance at the junctional foci; but in the presence of a stable methonium ion, acting *per se* to reduce the resting potential of the postsynaptic membrane, the application of the nerve shock should only add to the intensity of this effect, thereby increasing the likelihood of transmission block. The occurrence of C_{10} fasciculation in whole motor units of human muscle (CHURCHILL-DAVIDSON and RICHARDSON 1952) also leads one to question a randomized depolarization of endplates as the basis for neuromuscular facilitation.

Perhaps a clue to the nature of C_{10} neuromuscular facilitation is the pronounced enhancement of this effect by physostigmine or neostigmine (ZAIMIS 1951). ZAIMIS assumed that subthreshold doses of physostigmine produce a non-specific increase in the excitability of muscle. This assumption, although never actually experimentally verified, has been accepted in most instances wherein physostigmine or neostigmine was used to reveal or enhance drug-induced facilitation. The essential problem was succinctly stated by BROWN (1937c): "So specific is the effect of eserine that a powerful potentiation by it of the effect of a nerve excitation can be taken as strong presumptive evidence that the effect is transmitted by ACh. Nevertheless, caution must be used, if the deduction is based on this only, since eserine undoubtedly has the property of causing some rise of cellular excitability by an apparently non-specific action. The degree of this non-specific effect can usually be determined by assessing the degree of potentiation by eserine of the action of stable choline esters, choline itself, the quaternary ammonium bases, or a more general cellular stimulant such as $K^+ \ldots$"

One may wonder whether the designation of this action as "non-specific" is justified in view of the fact that only about 1/10 of the threshold potentiating dose of physostigmine is required for its demonstration. Furthermore, measurements of the contractile response to intra-arterial injection of methonium ions, or of the effect of such ions upon the fibrillary discharge frequency in chronically denervated muscle, revealed that physostigmine does not sensitize the preparations for the excitatory actions of these ions (WERNER and KUPERMAN, unpublished observations).

STOVNER (1958a) has adopted the alternative view that the action of DFP to augment NEt_4 potentiation is the consequence of a partial inhibition of AChE; accordingly, a background of instability is created in which changes in transmission can be easily detected. Presumably, this argument would hold for the similar effects of other cholinesterase inhibitors and indeed, this has been put forward by HUTTER (1952a) for the enhancement by physostigmine of choline-induced potentiation.

Where then is the site of the "non-specific" effect of physostigmine and other anti-ChE agents? Intra-arterially administered doses of physostigmine potentiate frequency and duration of the antidromic nerve repetition produced subsequent to a nerve impulse upon injection of hydroxyanilinium ions; the doses of physostigmine used are about 1/10 of those needed to produce postactivation nerve repetition by themselves. Such drug-induced post-activation repetitive discharge has been shown to originate from the motor nerve terminals (see page 635). Also significant is the ability of these low concentrations of physostigmine to convert a preparation which does not respond with antidromic discharge to any dose of certain hydroxyanilinium ions to one which does (WERNER 1960a). Further evidence for the presynaptic action of physostigmine derives from the work of FENG and LI (1941a) in which it was shown that subthreshold doses augment post-tetanic potentiation of the neurally evoked twitch response.

The highly specific action of physostigmine on the motor nerve endings, and the recognition of these endings as a focus for neuromuscular facilitation induced by hydroxyanilinium ions, neostigmine, physostigmine, and DFP (see page 635) points to the same locus for the facilitatory effects of C_{10}. Indeed, postactivation nerve repetition by close intra-arterial injection of C_{10} has now been demonstrated by WERNER (unpublished observations), and the suppression of C_{10} twitch augmentation by ether (PATON and ZAIMIS 1951) and pentobarbital (HUIDOBRO et al. 1952) finds explanation in the depressant actions of these agents on presynaptic terminals (RIKER et al. 1959b). The same evidence and conclusions with regard to the focus for facilitatory action can probably be applied to ACh (BROWN 1937a; HUNT 1947), NMe_4 and C_{12} (ZAIMIS 1951), and epinephrine and other catecholamines (HUIDOBRO et al. 1952). A presynaptic locus for facilitatory action has already been postulated for choline (HUTTER 1952a), NEt_4 (STOVNER 1958; KOKETSU 1958), epinephrine (KRNJEVIC and MILEDI 1958b), and guanidine (OTSUKA and ENDO 1960a). These actions have been viewed within the context of the ACh theory of transmission, i.e., a drug-induced increase in the amounts of transmitter liberated by the motor nerve endings per nerve volley.

The hypothesis of increased transmitter release by facilitatory drugs is compatible with the effect of these agents to increase the amplitude of the curarized endplate potential with no simultaneous prolongation of time course. Actually, NEt_4 increases slightly the duration of this local potential in the amphibian (KOKETSU 1958); NEt_4 also augments intensity and duration of the active transmitter phase at small motor nerve junctions (OOMURA and TOMITA 1960). In the presence of curare, even a potent anti-ChE agent like neostigmine is severely limited in its capacity to prolong the endplate potential (FATT and KATZ 1953). Accordingly, if an agent does not modify greatly the time course of the endplate potential in the absence of curare, such modification could be entirely abolished in its presence. Therefore, it is an open question, according to this kind of evidence, whether the effect of NEt_4 and similar agents on the local potential differs qualitatively from that of the powerful anti-ChE agents. The work of TAKEUCHI and TAKEUCHI (1959) suggests that the endplate current at amphibian neuromuscular junctions is determined primarily by the time course of the transmitter event originating from nerve terminals, and is only to a smaller extent modified by transmitter removal.

On the premise that drug action at a presynaptic site modifies the transmitter process, potentiating agents may be postulated to act by altering the time course and magnitude of a stimulus-bound excitatory state in the motor nerve terminals which, in turn, controls the graded release of transmitter. KOKETSU (1958) has recorded the increase of negative afterpotential in the intramuscular neuronal branches of the frog under the influence of NEt_4. Such an effect may be analogous to the prolongation of negative afterpotential in squid axon by intracellularly administered NEt_4 (TASAKI and HAGIWARA 1957), and also to the NEt_4 augmentation of the falling phase of crustacean and frog muscle action potential in media low in sodium (BURKE et al. 1953; HAGIWARA and WATANABE 1955). The motor axon terminals in various species of crustacea are particularly sensitive to chemical excitation with a variety of agents, including tetraalkylammonium ions, physostigmine, DDT, and a host of hydrocarbons (WELSH and GORDON 1947; BURKE et al. 1953; WIERSMA 1953; REUBEN et al. 1959; for review see HOYLE 1957). In low sodium medium, BURKE et al. (1953) detected not only the NEt_4-induced post-activation repetitive nerve discharge originating from crustacean nerve endings, but also a concurrent marked augmentation of contractile response. It was concluded that the presynaptic effect is attributable to prolongation of the negative afterpotential and its concomitant supernormal phase of excitability.

Such a conclusion was based on the premise that terminal portions of nerve fibres are, in general, considerably more prone to develop afterpotentials than the axon (KATZ 1950). From the time course for summation and refractoriness of retrograde motor nerve activity in cats, WERNER (1960a) inferred that invasion of nerve terminals by impulses in the presence of physostigmine, 3-OH-PNEt₃, and other agents, leads to negative and positive afterpotentials of a time course similar to that of nerve fibres with slow conduction velocity.

There appeared to be no hesitancy in adopting the viewpoint of a presynaptic and direct mechanism in drug-induced facilitation of crustacean neuromuscular transmission, perhaps because of the absence of evidence for chemical transmission at this junction. Indeed, KATZ (1936) had once suggested that excitation at the crustacean neuromuscular junction is more likely due to a physico-chemical event than a specific chemical transmitter. Evidence has now been produced, however, which indicates the chemical nature of the transmitter process at the excitatory junctional foci (VAN DER KLOOT 1960). Accordingly, the nature of drug-induced facilitation of crustacean muscle awaits reevaluation on this basis. Some other points of relevance to a pharmacological study of neuromuscular facilitation in crustacea have been discussed by EASTON (1957): muscle potentiation by repetitive nerve stimuli was interpreted in terms of penetration of impulses, during the negative afterpotential, into partially blocked nerve terminals; inhibition was interpreted partly in terms of the interaction of impulses in presynaptic terminals. The work of DUN (1956) had previously suggested that the safety factor of conduction in the terminal arborizations of a neuron is very low, due to the large core resistance and the sudden increase in total area to be depolarized.

The supposition that drug-induced neuromuscular facilitation is related to the exaggeration of afterpotentials in the unmyelinated terminals of motor nerve can be supported along two lines of circumstantial evidence: (1) the effects of such agents on ion transport; (2) direct effects on polarizability of nerve membranes.

In principle, it is not difficult to account for the generation of afterpotentials by drug effects on ionic transport mechanisms: RITCHIE and STRAUB (1957) and GREENGARD and STRAUB (1958) obtained evidence that negative afterpotentials in mammalian C fibres are associated with a transient increase of K^+ concentration in the vicinity of the excitable membrane (see also: SHANES 1951; FRANKEN-HAEUSER and HODGKIN 1956); the positive afterpotential was ascribed to an increase of Na^+ extrusion after activity, accompanied by faster K^+ absorption and consequent decrease of K^+ concentration in the vicinity of the membrane. RIKER (1953) suggested that the physostigmine-induced prolongation of endplate potential may be due partly to the presence of this agent per se, and not to accumulated ACh: it was postulated that the attachment of physostigmine, certain related tertiary amines, quaternary amines, or phosphonium ions to membrane receptor sites alters recovery processes by modifying permeability to K^+ and/or Na^+ directly. There is now an abundance of data relating to effects of anti-ChE agents on ion transport. (See also Chapters 6 and 11.)

In squid axon (ROTHENBERG 1950), frog skin (KIRSCHNER 1953, 1955; KOBLICK 1958), erythrocytes (HOLLAND and GREIG 1950), Chironomus anal papillae (KOCH 1954a), Eriocheir gills (KOCH 1954a, b), and frog muscle (VAN DER KLOOT 1958), the active transport of Na^+ is blocked by anti-ChE drugs. Significantly, a parallelism between intracellular ChE inhibition and decrease of Na^+ efflux has been demonstrated by VAN DER KLOOT (1956, 1958). Binding of physostigmine by cell components of erythrocytes leads to the loss of equivalent amounts of intracellular K ions (CHRISTENSEN and RIGGS 1951; TAYLOR and WELLER 1950). Conversely, ACh displaces bound physostigmine from red blood cells (HOLLAND and AUDITORE 1956). STRICKLAND and THOMPSON (1955) showed that the rate of exit of K^+ from chicken brain slices increased sharply in the presence of high concentrations of anti-ChE agents; inhibition of the intracellular enzyme was almost complete at lower inhibitor concentrations.

In an important study, FATT and GINSBORG (1958) suggested that the prolongation of crustacean muscle action potential by NEt_4 is related to an increased permeability of the muscle fibre membrane to Ca^{++}. It was inferred from the data of HODGKIN and KEYNES (1957) for squid axon that depolarization of the crustacean muscle fibre increases Ca^{++} conductance; in the presence of NEt_4 this effect would then be permitted to continue for a longer period. KOKETSU et al. (1959a, b) showed that NEt_4 and other quaternary ammonium ions can maintain excitability of frog spinal ganglion cells in Na⁺-free medium, but only if Ca-ions are present. The action potentials produced by the quaternary ammonium ion in the absence of Na⁺ again revealed the characteristic prolongation of time course. KOKETSU et al. (1959b) concluded that Ca^{++} plays an important role in the excitatory process even under normal conditions, but neither Ca^{++} nor quaternary ammonium ions appear to act as charge carriers for the production of action potentials. The recognition of the role of Ca-ions in the excitatory processes of the membrane lends new perspective to the viewpoint which attempts to account for some actions of quaternary ammonium ions in terms of their effects on ionic transfer mechanisms.

In the isolated guinea pig auricle, a suggestive correlation between the rate of hydrolysis of ACh and exchange of K⁺ and Na⁺ has been established: inhibition of hydrolysis of ACh by physostigmine was paralleled by a decrease in ionic exchange. HOLLAND et al. (1952) assumed on the basis of these findings that the process of substrate hydrolysis by AChE is intimately linked with ionic permeability. However, addition of physostigmine to the perfusion fluid of skeletal muscles of cats increases the K⁺release by intra-arterially injected single doses of ACh (KRAUPP et al. 1955b); in fact, with low doses of ACh, K⁺ is liberated from innervated eserinized muscle at a rate approximating that of its release from non-eserinized, chronically denervated muscle; but at higher doses of ACh, a progressive decrease of K⁺ liberation occurs, so that the dose-response line joins that of non-eserinized normal muscle (Fig. 21). This led KRAUPP et al. (1955b) to the conclusion that physostigmine alters the sensitivity of skeletal muscle to the K⁺-liberating action of ACh in a way that is not entirely explicable on the basis of ChE inhibition. Characteristically, physostigmine does not lower the threshold dose of ACh in chronically denervated muscle, although its total cholinesterase activity remains essentially unaltered (BROOKS and MYERS 1952). Physostigmine by itself, in concentrations of 10^{-7} to 5×10^{-6} M, does not cause any liberation of K⁺ from innervated or denervated mammalian skeletal muscles (KRAUPP et al. 1955b). Lowering of the extracellular Na⁺ concentra-

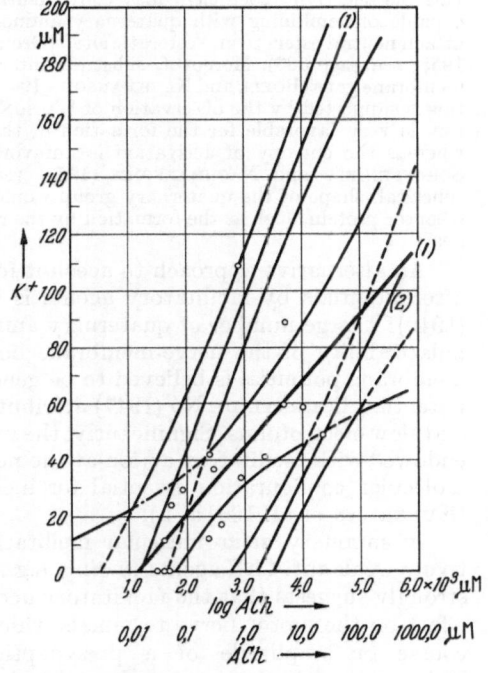

Fig. 21. Dose-response lines (and confidence limits) of K⁺ liberation from perfused cat hind limb skeletal muscle. Line 1: chronically denervated muscle. Line 2: innervated normal muscle. Line I: innervated muscle, in presence of physostigmine (10^{-7} M) in the perfusion fluid. ACh was injected in single doses, plotted logarithmically on the abscissa; the quantity of liberated K⁺ (in μM) is plotted linearly on the ordinate. (From KRAUPP et al. 1955b)

tion, or addition of d-tubocurarine to the perfusion fluid, suppresses the output of ⁺K after injection of single doses of ACh into the circulation (KRAUPP 1956). On the other hand, tetramethylammonium, injected intra-arterially in single doses into the normal perfusion fluid, releases more K⁺, and for markedly longer periods of time, than maximally effective doses of ACh liberate from eserinized muscle (WERNER et al. 1955).

The interpretation of actions on ionic transfer in terms of uncomplicated permutite-like cation-exchange processes (ZIPF 1927) ignores the absence of ionic equivalency between the dose of quaternary ammonium cation and release of intracellular K⁺, the latter by far exceeding the former (see Fig. 21). On the other hand, there is suggestive evidence that the molecules of ChE may interact with substrates or inhibitors in a way that can be described quantitatively as an ion-exchange reaction (ZIFF et al. 1938). Indeed, fixation of ACh by homogenates of brain tissue (CORTEGGIANI 1937; MANN et al. 1939; HOBBIGER and WERNER 1949) was demonstrated, and the same may be true for any quaternary ion. BERGMAN and SHIMONI (1953) greatly refined this model concept by giving special consideration to the selectivity coefficient (K_D) of ion exchangers:

$$K_D = \left(\frac{n_1}{n_2}\right)_{exchanger} \cdot \left(\frac{n_2}{n_1}\right)_{solute} \quad (n_1, n_2 = \text{molar concentrations of two ion species}).$$

More specifically, BERGMAN and SHIMONI (1953) proposed that K_D could vary with current flow or other factors which alter the degree of cross-linking within the matrix of the exchanger; different ionic equilibria would result from changes of K_D. The enzyme catalyzed reaction:

$$ACh + H_2O \rightarrow acetic\ acid + choline$$

was thought to represent a buffer system for K_D insofar as it quickly reversed any local changes of free hydrogen ion concentrations that might result from current flow. The proposal of a variable selectivity coefficient may conveniently be extended to include any receptor that is capable of combining with quaternary ammonium ions through coulombic forces, and to attach neutral esters to an "esteratic site" (Group A and B receptors of COHEN and POSTHUMUS 1955; see page 583). Moreover, substrate interaction with active centers of ChE located in membrane gaps (BOELL and NACHMANSOHN 1940) could result in changes of their configuration; this is supported by the observation of WILSON and CABIB (1956) that the entropy of activation is very favorable for the formation of the acetyl enzyme when ACh is the substrate, whereas the entropy of activation is unfavorable for the tertiary analogue. Accordingly, SCHOFFENIELS and NACHMANSOHN (1957) reasoned that the tetrahedral, approximately spherical, shape of the quaternary group would also facilitate a configurational change of a receptor protein, such as the formation by the receptor of an envelope around the quaternary head.

An alternative approach to account for the postulated augmentation of nerve afterpotentials by facilitatory agents is based on the work of LORENTE DE NÓ (1949): a large number of quaternary ammonium ions were found to increase the polarizability of the nerve-membrane boundary at which the L-fraction of the membrane potential is believed to be generated; to this component of membrane potential, LORENTE DE NÓ (1947) attributed negative and positive afterpotentials and slow electrotonus. Significantly, the minimal structural requirements of agents endowed with facilitatory action at the neuromuscular junction are similar to the molecular configuration essential for increase of nerve-membrane polarizability (KUPERMAN et al. 1961a, b).

In summary, neuromuscular facilitation produced by drugs which are relatively weak anti-ChE agents *in vitro*, e.g., NEt_4, has been discussed. The evidence strongly suggests that the facilitatory actions of these agents are produced by an effect on the motor nerve terminals which consists in the alteration of the time course or amplitude of a presynaptic stimulus-bound excitatory process. This process, in turn, must be related to the graded release of transmitter. Structure-activity considerations reveal that modification of presynaptic events is a fundamental property of the quaternary ammonium ion and, to a lesser extent, of the tricovalent N-atom. Also, the N-atom is the minimal structural requisite for neuromuscular facilitation and for affinity to ChE (except in the organophosphorus compounds). The potent *in vitro* ChE inhibitors which contain the tetra- or tricovalent N-atom also produce a presynaptic action, probably of the same type as that caused by the weak anti-ChE facilitatory compounds. Thus, the essential problem to be resolved in this area of investigation is apparently not whether a facilitatory agent can or cannot be classed as a ChE inhibitor. Rather, the problem is this: to describe, in quantitative terms, how much of the facilitatory action of a chemical agent, be it a potent or weak ChE inhibitor *in vitro*, can be attributed to direct presynaptic actions on the one hand or to inhibition of junctional ChE on the other.

D. Junctional transmission in electric organs

The study of the transmitter process in electric fishes, and its susceptibility to modification by chemical agents, appears of relevance in the context of this review since it has been established for all electric fishes (except *Malapterurus*) that the electric organ is derived from skeletal muscle; in *Malapterurus*, this organ is believed to originate from glandular tissue (cf. KEYNES 1957). The evolutionary aspects and biologic significance of electric organs were recently carefully examined by LISSMANN (1958); their anatomy was exhaustively described by ROSENBERG (1928) and BALLOWITZ (1938). In spite of the seemingly homologous origin of electric tissue in most species, considerable difference exists in the structural organization of synaptic regions (FESSARD 1952). In elasmobranchs, like *Torpedo* and *Raia*, terminal nerve branches form a nerve net of anastomoses of extraordinary density to the extent that the appearance of a "nerve membrane" is created (KÖLLIKER 1856). In teleosts, like *Mormyrus* and *Gymnotus*, the nerve terminals form basket-like endings with the nerve branches sparsely distributed. In the electroplates of *Electrophorus electricus*, there are some 50,000 to 100,000 individual synaptic contact points separated from each other by distances of 5 to 30 μ (cf. SCHOFFENIELS and NACHMANSOHN 1957; LUFT 1958). The genera *Malopterurus* and *Gymnarchus*, of the telost-group, possess synaptic formations in the form of deeply planted end knobs of restricted localization at the electroplate.

The arrangement of electroplates in series, parallel, or both, depends in general on the natural habitat of the species, so that the internal resistance of the combination of units is matched to the resistance of the external circuit through which discharge takes place (COX et al. 1946). One of the most striking histological characteristics of most electroplates is the considerable folding and convolution of one or both surfaces. As a rule, the face on which the nerve terminates is smooth compared with the opposite, non-nervous face which is often covered with large papillae. Through the latter surface large currents flow during discharge at the innervated surface without causing an appreciable potential drop (KEYNES and MARTINS-FERREIRA 1953). Accordingly, conductance must be very high at this membrane. The presence of a system of canaliculi and vesicles at the non-innervated surface suggests the operation of a vesicular ion transport mechanism of high efficiency (LUFT 1958).

The morphologically recognizable species differences of synaptic organization appear correlated with differences in synaptic excitability and the nature of electric discharge (FESSARD 1952). It is, therefore, appropriate to discuss the transmission process in elasmobranchs and teleosts separately.

1. Elasmobranchs: Raia, Torpedines

In 1937, MARNAY discovered a remarkably high cholinesterase activity in electric organs of *Torpedo marmorata*: 1 g of electric organ is capable of hydrolyzing 2 to 3 g ACh per hour (cf. NACHMANSOHN 1955). Subsequently, FELDBERG and FESSARD (1942) determined that the electric organ of *Torpedo marmorata* contains 40 to 100 μg ACh per gram fresh tissue, and that on stimulation of the nerve in the presence of physostigmine, significant amounts of ACh appear in the perfusion fluid. Furthermore, on intra-arterial injection, ACh exerted an electrogenic effect in that it elicited electric discharges; the addition of physostigmine to the perfusion fluid led to a prolongation of the descending phase of single nervous discharges, associated with rapid fatigue on repetitive stimulation.

The electroplate of *Raia* responds only to stimulation of its nerve; presumably, each electroplate is innervated by several nerve fibres with different thresholds, and each fibre supplies a variable number of presynaptic endings on any particular electroplate. Earlier work of AUGER and FESSARD (1939) and FESSARD (1947) resulted in the demonstration of a synaptic delay of several msec duration. In *Torpedo*, the electric organ becomes totally inexcitable after curarization or degeneration of the nerve supply (FESSARD 1946). For these reasons, it appeared likely that the electroplates resemble only the endplate formation of skeletal muscle rather than the muscle fibre proper. This contention received confirmation from measurements of transmembrane potentials in single electroplates: the potential change on activation does not usually exceed the level of depolarization, while overshoot, if present at all, does not amount to more than a few millivolts (BROCK and ECCLES 1958). The minimal synaptic delay in these experiments was found to be 1.5 msec; *d*-tubocurarine suppressed the electric response to nervous stimulation, and neostigmine prolonged the declining phase.

The electric characteristics of response at electroplates of *Raia* are such that they fulfill the defining criteria of a postsynaptic potential (GRUNDFEST 1957a). These electroplates appear to exemplify with particular sharpness the fundamental differentiation of post-junctional excitable membrane from non-junctional excitable membrane, the former being inexcitable by electric current or local circuit depolarization, but responsive to synaptic action only (GRUNDFEST 1957b). This, in itself, does not necessarily imply that agents which modify the electric response of electroplates act at a postsynaptic site; however, the evidence regarding humoral transmission of excitation from nerve to electroplate appears to favor the view that neostigmine prolongs the postsynaptic potential by virtue of its ChE inhibiting activity.

2. Telosts: Electrophorus, Gymnarchus, Gymnotus

Electric organs of *Electrophorus electricus* also possess an extraordinarily high concentration of AChE; NACHMANSOHN et al. (1942, 1946) found a direct proportionality between concentrations of AChE and the voltage (per cm) of discharges. This correlation is contrasted by the absence of any parallelism between electric parameters and distribution of respiratory and glycolytic enzymes, or phosphorylated compounds (like ATP) (cf. NACHMANSOHN 1952). Electroplates contain also an abundance of an additional esterase which is capable of hydrolyzing ethylmonochloracetate but seems to lack the anionic group of AChE. Accordingly, it does not hydrolyze ACh (SCHLEYER 1955). The ethylmonochloracetate-hydrolyzing enzyme requires for its inhibition considerably larger concentrations of physostigmine or neostigmine than AChE. Accordingly, SCHLEYER (1955) demonstrated that physostigmine freely penetrates to the assayable enzyme in intact electroplates; neostigmine reaches the site of the assayable enzyme only when its concentration gradient is about ten-times steeper than that required for the penetration of physostigmine. Interestingly, neither ACh, its tertiary amine analogue (dimethylaminoethylacetate), nor, neostigmine can, in measurable amounts, gain access to more than a small fraction of the total AChE present in intact electroplates (ALTAMIRANO et al. 1955a).

Unlike *Torpedo*, the electric organ of *Electrophorus* is not discharged by the injection of ACh (ALTAMIRANO et al. 1955b). However, it was suggested that the high concentration of ChE at the innervated side of the electroplates (COUCEIRO et al. 1955), and the concomitant occurence of exhaustion of ACh stores and fatigue of the neurally evoked discharge (CHAGAS et al. 1953) point to a cholinergic transmitter mechanism. In accordance with this view, the ACh content of the main organ of *Electrophorus electricus* does not change on direct stimulation (CHAGAS 1952). Under the influence of physostigmine, homosynaptic facilitation of discharge is augmented and prolonged (HARRIS and MIRANDA 1955; ALBE-FESSARD and CHAGAS 1954).

In contrast to *Torpedo*, the innervated electroplate of *Electrophorus* is responsive to direct as well as to neural stimulation (ALTAMIRANO et al. 1953; ALBE-FESSARD and CHAGAS 1955a, b). The extracellularly recorded electrical response to stimulation of one nerve with single pulses is followed by an initial graded response of about 3 msec duration and a maximal amplitude of one-third of the spike height.

In a single-layered preparation of electroplates, each nerve supplies some 5 to 7 cells. A single maximal nerve volley produces a spike discharge in some electroplates, while in others only a graded postsynaptic potential appears. Spike discharges can be elicited in these cells by firing a second nerve volley within a facilitation interval of about 10 to 80 msec. Neostigmine and physostigmine lead to a considerable increase in amplitude of the spike height elicited by conditioning and test stimuli, but the time course of facilitation and duration of the postsynaptic potential are not greatly affected (ALTAMIRANO et al. 1955b).

The accumulated evidence points to the presence, at the innervated face of electroplates of *Electrophorus electricus*, of two different types of responsive membranes (KEYNES and MARTINS-FERREIRA 1953; ALTAMIRANO et al. 1954; GRUNDFEST 1957a, b). During the absolute refractory period for spike discharges, a graded local response can develop in response to a neural stimulus; the local response is not prevented by inactivation of the spike discharge with de- or hyperpolarizing currents. Contrariwise, the prefatory graded potential is not obtained on direct stimulation. The two electrical events are believed to be generated in the same membrane which is visualized to be of composite nature, some "patches" giving rise to the spikes while others generate (on neural activation only) a postsynaptic potential (GRUND-FEST 1957a). Transfer of excitation from the neurally activated postsynaptic membrane component to the spike generating membrane patches appears to take place through initiation, by local circuit action, of a local response in the electrically excitable membrane patches. This local response, although normally fused with the postsynaptic potential, is subject to refractoriness; consequently, the "pure" postsynaptic potential may be demonstrated only during absolute refractoriness of the electrically excitable membrane component (ALTAMIRANO et al. 1954).

With the recognition in the electroplate membrane of a differentiation in postsynaptic and in electrically excitable ("nonsynaptic") areas, it became pertinent to inquire into the differential reactivities to chemical agents of these distinct membrane components.

In experiments with ACh, ALTAMIRANO et al. (1955b) found that the response to direct stimulation of electroplates is more critically affected than the neurally evoked postsynaptic potential. Interestingly, this selective action of ACh on the action potential of nonsynaptic membrane could be obtained in the absence of any change of the resting transmembrane potential (ALTAMIRANO 1956). With higher concentrations of ACh or related agents, reduction of the transmembrane potential took place, but postsynaptic potentials could be elicited through neural excitation while membrane potentials were as low as 10 to 20 mV (ALTAMIRANO et al. 1955b). The effects of ACh on the electroplate were essentially irreversible after removal of the agent; however, addition of d-tubocurarine or procaine in the presence of ACh restored selectively the reduced membrane potential to normal, whereas inactivation of the spike-discharge mechanism persisted. On the basis of these findings, and assuming that d-tubocurarine acted only postsynaptically, ALTAMIRANO (1956) reasoned that ACh (externally applied) initiates depolarization selectively from an action on the postsynaptic membrane. This, in turn, leads through local circuit action to depolarization of neighboring "nonsynaptic" membrane areas. Against this contention, one may raise the objection that the action of curare may not, at least in its entirety, be postsynaptic (see page 638). In any case, non-depolarizing agents, like procaine and d-tubocurarine, affected the nonsynaptic membrane component in the absence of ACh by converting the directly elicited spike discharge into a graded and decrementally conducted response.

Like ACh, neostigmine, decamethonium, and carbamylcholine also were shown by ALTAMIRANO et al. (1955a, b) to depolarize the electrically excitable membrane component secondarily to local circuit action originating from the postsynaptic membrane (see also: CHAGAS and ALBE-FESSARD 1954). Conversely, potent inhibitors of ChE, like physostigmine or DFP, did not abolish the electrogenic responsiveness of the directly excitable membrane component, although these agents converted the propagated into graded and decrementally conducted responses (GRUNDFEST 1957b).

Taking these observations and their interpretations as starting point for a broad classification of drug actions at synapses, GRUNDFEST (1957a) suggested that agents commonly designated as "depolarizers" have in common the capacity to activate specifically the synaptically excitable membrane component; accordingly, such agents should preferably be named "synapse activating" (GRUNDFEST 1957a). Whatever effects these agents appear to have on "nonsynaptic" membrane components are conceived as secondary, and mediated through electrical, local circuit action. Accordingly, interference with the ACh-AChE system was not considered of primary significance for drug action on electrical excitability (GRUNDFEST 1957b).

Results and conclusions, in some respects different from those of ALTAMIRANO (1956) and GRUNDFEST (1957a, b) were reported by NACHMANSOHN and WILSON (1955) and SCHOFFENIELS and NACHMANSOHN (1957) (see also: ALTAMIRANO et al. 1955a; for review, see NACHMANSOHN 1959). A method was used which permitted the simultaneous evaluation of effects of agents on electrical membrane characteristics and on the activity of AChE in intact electroplates. It was concluded that binding of agents to receptor as well as inhibition of AChE result in block of the propagated spike. With agents like procaine, decamethonium, or carb-aminoylcholine, AChE (assayed by means of ethylchloracetate; see page 656) was only slightly inhibited, while spike propagation was abolished. In contrast, physo-stigmine, DFP, and neostigmine blocked spike propagation only when appreciable inhibition of AChE prevailed. All quaternary compounds tested (except d-tubo-curarine) blocked spike propagation and simultaneously depolarized the electro-plate membrane; the tertiary agents (e.g., the tertiary analogue of neostigmine) with the exception of dimethylaminoethylacetate, blocked propagation of the spike without lowering the membrane potential. The depolarization by carb-aminoylcholine was reversed by the tertiary, non-depolarizing agents. Tertiary (non-depolarizing) and quaternary (depolarizing) compounds were assumed to react with identical receptors. Two principal inferences were drawn from these observations: (1) depending on the nature of the agent, drug-receptor interaction may consist in attachment of agents to receptors only (i.e., non-depolarizing type) or may lead to subsequent changes in the receptor configuration, manifested as depolarization, (2) drug receptor interaction may specifically take place without concomitant inhibition of AChE; consequently, receptor and AChE may be viewed as two different reactive sites.

It is of great interest that depolarization by quaternary ammonium agents is largely irreversible, despite the fact that most of the quaternary ammonium agents used in these experiments act reversibly on AChE *in vitro*. In contrast to the largely irreversible depolarization by neostigmine, spike depression by physo-stigmine is completely reversible after removal of the drug from the bathing solution (SCHOFFENIELS and NACHMANSOHN 1957). This, as well as its structural similarity to agents of the ACh-group, and the speed of onset of action, made it appear likely that neostigmine depolarizes primarily as a result of the reaction with ACh receptors and not by virtue of its ChE inhibitory activity (NACHMANSOHN 1955).

SCHOFFENIELS and NACHMANSOHN (1957) affirmed that block of electrical activity by quaternary ammonium agents cannot be dissociated from their depolarizing activity; they did not corroborate the finding of ALTAMIRANO (1956) that in the presence of d-tubocurarine, ACh blocks the propagated spike without affecting the resting membrane potential. Moreover, an isolated single electroplate preparation permitted exclusive aplication of agents to the innervated, or non-innervated membrane only. Surprisingly, the nonsynaptic membrane patches were not affected by quaternary ammonium ions, even if applied from the inside of the cell. These data furnish evidence that the quaternary ammonium agents, although capable of penetrating the non-innervated membrane, interact exclusively with receptors at postsynaptic membranes. Furthermore, it is implied that the non-synaptic membrane patches are at both their external and internal surface surrounded by a structure impermeable to quaternary ammonium agents (SCHOF-FENIELS and NACHMANSOHN 1957). In accordance with this interpretation, SCHOF-FENIELS et al. (1958) demonstrated that lipid soluble quaternary ammonium derivatives (e.g., β-acetoxy-ethyldimethyl-duodecyl-ammonium iodide and py-ridine methiodide dodeciodide) blocked conduction in relatively low concentrations.

3. General implications

The demonstration in electroplates of *Electrophorus electricus* of specific re-ceptors distinct from AChE reinforces the evidence obtained at the amphibian neuromuscular junction that quaternary ammonium ions may act in either of two ways, i.e., by specific inhibition of ChE, or by direct receptor interaction (cf. KATZ and THESLEFF 1957a). In the case of neostigmine, both actions appear to overlap closely (NACHMANSOHN 1955). Attention is thereby redirected to the statement of WESCOE and RIKER (1951) that, in many cases, division of quaternary ions into those that act through ChE inhibition and into others acting by direct receptor interaction is essentially arbitrary.

In the reasoning that ChE inhibition *per se* results in conduction block at the electroplate membrane, emphasis is placed on three basic assumptions: these are (1) curare acts exclusively at the postsynaptic membrane, (2) tertiary and quaternary ammonium agents act on identical receptors, and (3) tertiary agents (as a rule) occupy receptor sites without changing their configuration, whereas quaternary agents, in consequence of receptor interaction, generally initiate depolarization. Plausible as some of these premises may appear, the possibility of drug action on synaptic transmission at sites other than the postsynaptic membrane, and not recognizable as variation of postsynaptic resting membrane potential, deserves further attention.

Acknowledgments

Although the ideas and observations of several hundred investigators are expressed in this review, the authors would like to acknowledge particularly the thoughtful and inspirational advice of Professor W. F. RIKER, Jr. Also, the efficient and cooperative secretarial assistance of Miss DIANE MUNSON is gratefully acknowledged. The authors' unpublished experiments discussed in this review were supported by USPHS Grants B-1447 and B-2605.

Literature

ABDON, N. O.: Liberation of acetylcholine from the precursor in voluntary muscles without motor-end plates. Acta pharmacol. (Kbh.) 1, 325—335 (1945).

—, and T. BJARKE: The mechanism of acetylcholine liberation in striped muscles. Acta pharmacol. (Kbh.) 1, 1—17 (1945).

—, and S. O. HAMMARSKJOLD: Is any free acetylcholine preformed in resting muscles or in the heart? Acta physiol. scand. 8, 75—96 (1944).

—, and K. LJUNGDALHL-OSTBERG: A method for quantitative determination of acetylcholine precursor and free acetylcholine in tissues. Acta physiol. scand. 8, 103—121 (1944).

ACHESON, G. H.: Physiology of neuro-muscular junctions: Chemical aspects. Fed. Proc. 7, 447—457 (1948).

ADRIAN, E. D., and D. W. BRONK: The discharge of impulses in motor nerve fibres, Part II. The frequency of discharge in reflex and voluntary contractions. J. Physiol. (Lond.) 67, 119—51 (1929).

—, and K. LUCAS: On the summation of propagated disturbances in nerve and muscle. J. Physiol. (Lond.) 44, 68—124 (1912).

AESCHLIMANN, J. A., and M. REINERT: The pharmacological action of some analogues of physostigmine. J. Pharmacol. exp. Ther. 43, 413—444 (1931).

—, and A. STEMPEL: Some analogs of prostigmin. Jubilee Volume Emil Barell 306—313, 1946.

ALBE-FESSARD, D., et C. CHAGAS: Étude de la sommation à la jonction nerf-électroplaque chez le Gymnote (Electrophorus electricus). J. Physiol. Path. gén. 46, 823—834 (1954).

— — Mise en évidence d'un potentiel de jonction par dérivation intra-cellulaire dans une électroplaque de l'organe de Sachs du Gymnote. C. R. Acad. Sci. (Paris) 239, 1682—1684 (1955a).

— — Étude par dérivation intracellulaire des effets sommatifs de deux stimulations nerveuses successives au nivence d'une électroplaque de Gymnote. C. R. Acad. Sci. (Paris) 239, 1857—1859 (1955b).

ALDRIDGE, W. N.: Some properties of specific cholinesterase with particular reference to the mechanism of inhibition by diethyl p-nitrophenyl thiophosphate (E 605) and analogues. Biochem. J. 46, 451—460 (1950).

ALLES, G. A., and P. K. KNOEFEL: Comparative physiological actions of alkyltrimethyl-ammonium and alkali metal salts. Univ. Calif. Publ. Pharmacol. 1, 187—212 (1939).

ALTAMIRANO, M.: Electrical properties of the innervated membrane of the electroplax of electric eel. J. cell. comp. Physiol. 46, 249—277 (1955).
— Effect of acetylcholine in the electroplax of electric eel. Biochim. biophys. Acta 20, 323 to 336 (1956).
— C. W. COATES, H. GRUNDFEST and D. NACHMANSOHN: Mechanisms of bioelectric activity in electric tissue. I. The response to indirect and direct stimulation of electroplaques of electrophorus electricus. J. gen. Physiol. 37, 91—110 (1953).
— — — Mechanisms of direct and neural excitability in electroplaques of electric eel. J. gen. Physiol. 38, 319—360 (1954).
— — — and D. NACHMANSOHN: Electrical activity in electric tissue, III. Modifications of electrical activity by acetylcholine and related compounds. Biochim. biophys. Acta 16, 449—463 (1955b).
— W. L. SCHLEYER, C. W. COATES and D. NACHMANSOHN: Electrical activity in electrical tissue; I. The differences between tertiary and quaternary Nitrogen compounds in relation to their chemical and electrical activities. Biochim. biophys. Acta 16, 268—282 (1955a).
ARIENS, E. J., and W. M. DE GROOT: Affinity and intrinsic-activity in the theory of competitive inhibition, III: Homologous decamethonium derivatives and succinylcholine esters. Arch. int. Pharmacodyn. 99, 193—205 (1951).
— A. M. SIMONIS and W. M. DE GROOT: Affinity and intrinsic-activity in the theory of competitive- and non-competitive inhibition and an analysis of some forms of dualism in action. Arch. int. Pharmacodyn. 100, 298—322 (1955).
— J. M. v. ROSSUM and A. M. SIMONIS: A theoretical basis of molecular pharmacology, II. Interactions of one or two compounds with two interdependent receptor systems. Arzneimittel-Forsch. 6, 611—621 (1956a).
— — — A theoretical basis of molecular pharmacology. Arzneimittel Forsch. 6, 737—746 (1956b).
ARNOLD, A., A. E. SORIA and F. K. KIRCHNER: A new anticholinesterase oxamide. Proc. Soc. exper. Biol. (N. Y.) 87, 393—394 (1954).
AUGER, D., and A. FESSARD: Étude oscillographique des décharges de l'appareil électrique des Raies. Ann. Physiol. Physicochim. biol. 15, 261—270 (1939).
AXELSSON, J., E. GJONE and K. NAESS: The effect of d-tubocurarine on the inhibition of tetanic contractions produced by cholinesterase inhibitors. Acta pharmacol. (Kbh.) 13, 319—336 (1957).
—, and S. THESLEFF: The "desensitizing" effect of acetylcholine on the mammalian motor end-plate. Acta physiol. scand. 43, 15—26 (1958).
— — A study of supersensitivity in denervated mammalian skeletal muscle. J. Physiol. (Lond.) 147, 177—193 (1959).
BACQ, Z. M.: Action du D.F.P. (diisopropylphosphonate) sur le rectus isolé d'Amphibien et l'intestin isolé de mammifère. C. R. Soc. Biol. (Paris) 141, 856—859 (1947).
—, and G. L. BROWN: Pharmacological experiments on mammalian voluntary muscle in relation to the theory of chemical transmission. J. Physiol. (Lond.) 89, 45—60 (1937).
BALLOWITZ, E.: Elektrische Organe, in: Handbuch der vergl. Anatomie 5, 657—683 (1938).
BARLOW, R. B., and H. R. ING: Curare-like action of polymethylene bis-quaternary ammonium salts. Brit. J. Pharmacol. 3, 298—304 (1948).
BARNES, J. M., and J. I. DUFF: The role of cholinesterase at the myoneural junction. Brit. J. Pharmacol. 8, 334—339 (1953).
BARSTAD, J. A. B.: The effect of d-tubocurarine on the neuromuscular blocks caused by diisopropylfluorophosphate and acetylcholine. Arch. int. Pharmacodyn. 107, 4—20 (1956a).
— The effect of di-isopropylfluorophosphate on the neuro-muscular transmission and the importance of cholinesterase for the transmission of single impulses. Arch. int. Pharmacodyn. 107, 21—32 (1956b).
— Cholinesterase inhibition and the effect of anticholinesterases on indirectly evoked single and tetanic muscle contractions in the phrenic nerve-diaphragm preparation from the rat. Arch. int. Pharmacodyn. 128, 143—168 (1960).
BENSON, W. M.: Inhibition of cholinesterase by adrenaline. Proc. Soc. exp. Biol. (N. Y.) 68, 598—601 (1948).
—, and W. J. MEEK: Hydrolysis of choline esters in the presence of adrenalin. Amer. J. Physiol. 158, 327—331 (1949).
BERGMANN, F., and R. SEGAL: The relationship of quaternary ammonium salts to the anionic sites of true and pseudo cholinesterase. Biochem. J. 58, 692—698 (1954).
—, and A. SHIMONI: The changes in the nerve membrane and the role of cholinesterase in the conductive process. Biochem. biophys. Acta 10, 49—54 (1953).
BERNARD, M. C.: Analyse physiologique des propriétés des syotèmes musculaire et nerveux au moyen du curare. C. R. Acad. Sci. (Paris) 43, 825—829 (1856).

BERNHARD, C. G., U. S. v. EULER and C. R. SKOGLUND: Post-tetanic action potentials in mammalian muscle. Acta physiol. scand. 2, 284—288 (1941).

BERRY, W. K., and C. L. EVANS: Cholinesterase and neuromuscular block. J. Physiol. (Lond.) 115, 46P—47P (1951).

BIRKS, R., B. KATZ and R. MILEDI: Physiological and structural changes at the amphibian myoneural junction, in the course of nerve degeneration. J. Physiol. (Lond.) 150, 145—168 (1960).

BISHOP, G. B.: Natural history of the nerve impulse. Physiol. Rev. 36, 376—399 (1956).

BLABER, L. C.: The antagonism of muscle relaxants by ambenonium and methoxyambenonium in the cat. Brit. J. Pharmacol. 15, 476—484 (1960).

—, and W. C. BOWMAN: A comparison between the effects of edrophonium and choline in the skeletal muscles of the cat. Brit. J. Pharmacol. 14, 456—466 (1959).

BLASCHKO, H., E. BÜLBRING and T. C. CHOU: Tubocurarine antagonism and inhibition of cholinesterases. Brit. J. Pharmacol. 4, 29—32 (1949).

BOEHM, R.: Einige Beobachtungen über die Nervenendwirkung des Curarin. Arch. exp. Path. Pharmak. 35, 16—22 (1895).

— Curare und Curarealkaloide. Heffters Handb. exper. Pharmakol. 2, Part 1, 179—248. Berlin: Julius Springer 1920.

BOELL, E. J., and D. NACHMANSOHN: Localization of cholinesterase in nerve fibres. Science 92, 513—514 (1940).

BOVET, D., F. BOVET-NITTI, S. GUARINO, V. G. LONGO et R. FUSCO: Recherches sur les poisons curarisants de synthèse, III. Partie: Succinylcholine et dérivés aliphatiques. Arch. int. Pharmacodyn. 88, 1—50 (1951).

— S. COURVOISIER, R. DUCROT et R. HORCLOIS: Recherches sur les poisons curarisants de synthèse Ire Partie: Bis-quinoloxy-alkanes et Bis-aminophenoxy-alkanes. Arch. int. Pharmacodyn. 80, 137—158 (1949).

BOVET-NITTI, F.: Hydrolysis by cholinesterase of some curarizing agents. Rendiconti Dell'Instituto Superiore di Sanita, 12, Partie 1—11—111, 138—157, 1949 (Italian).

BOWMAN, W. C.: The neuromuscular blocking action of benzoquinonium chloride in the cat and in the hen. Brit. J. Pharmacol. 13, 521—530 (1958).

BOYD, I. A., and A. R. MARTIN: Spontaneous subthreshold activity at mammalian neuro-muscular junctions. J. Physiol. (Lond.) 132, 61—73 (1956a).

— — The endplate potential in mammalian muscle. J. Physiol. 132, 74—91 (1956b).

BRAND, H.: A propos du mode d'action du décaméthonium et de l'amyl-triméthylammonium sur la préparation isolée nerf phrénique-diaphragme du rat. Experientia (Basel) 8/7, 273 (1952).

BRECHT, K., u. H. FENEIS: Über tonische und phasische Reaktionen einzelner quergestreifter Muskelfasern und des Ganzmuskels. Z. Biol. 103, 355—380 (1950).

BREMER, F.: Researches on the contracture of skeletal muscle. J. Physiol. (Lond.) 76, 65—94 (1932).

—, et F. KLEYNTJENS: Nouvelles recherches sur le phénomène de la sommation d'influx nerveux. Arch. int. Physiol. 45, 382—414 (1937).

—, et J. TITECA: Antonie curarique et inhibition de Wedensky. Arch. int. Physiol. 42, 223 à 250 (1935).

BRINGLING, J. C., and C. M. SMITH: A characterization of the stimulation of mammalian muscle spindles by succinylcholine. J. Pharmacol. exp. Ther. 129, 56—60 (1960).

BRINKMAN, R., and M. RUITER: Die humorale Übertragung der neurogenen Skelettmuskel-erregung auf den Darm. Pflügers Arch. ges. Physiol. 204, 766—768 (1924).

— — Die humorale Übertragung der Skelettmuskelreizung eines ersten auf den Darm eines zweiten Frosches. Pflügers Arch. ges. Physiol. 208, 58—62 (1925).

BRISCOE, G.: The antagonism between curarine and prostigmin and its relation to the myasthenia problem. Lancet 1936a I, 469—472.

— The antagonism between curarine and acetylcholine. J. Physiol. (Lond.) 87, 425—428 (1936b).

— The anti-curare action of substance 36. Lancet 1937 I, 621—623.

— Changes in muscle contraction curves produced by drugs of the eserine and curarine groups. J Physiol (Lond.) 93, 194—205 (1938).

BROCK, L. G., and R. M. ECCLES: The membrane potentials during rest and activity of the ray electroplate. J. Physiol. (Lond.) 142, 251—274 (1958).

BROOKS, V. B.: The action of botulinum toxin on motor-nerve filaments. J. Physiol. (Lond.) 123, 501—515 (1954).

— An intracellular study of the action of repetitive nerve volleys and of botulinum toxin on miniature end-plate potentials. J. Physiol. (Lond.) 134, 264—277 (1956).

—, and D. K. MYERS: Cholinesterase content of normal and denervated skeletal muscle in the guinea-pig. J. Physiol. (Lond.) 116, 158—167 (1952).

BROWN, G. L.: Action potentials of normal mammalian muscle. Effects of acetylcholine and eserine. J. Physiol. (Lond.) **89**, 220—237 (1937a).
— The actions of acetylcholine on denervated mammalian and frog's muscle. J. Physiol. (Lond.) **89**, 438—461 (1937b).
— Transmission at nerve endings by acetylcholine. Physiol. Rev. **17**, 485—513 (1937c).
— Effect of small doses of curarine on neuromuscular conduction. J. Physiol. (Lond.) **92**, 23—24P (1938).
— E. BÜLBRING and B. D. BURNS: The action of adrenaline on mammalian skeletal muscle. J. Physiol. (Lond.) **107**, 115—128 (1948).
—, and B. D. BURNS: Fatigue and neuromuscular block in mammalian skeletal muscle. Proc. Roy. Soc. (B) **136**, 182—195 (1949).
— — and W. FELDBERG: The action of diisopropylfluorophosphate on neuromuscular transmission. J. Physiol. (Lond.) **106**, 36P (1947).
— H. H. DALE and W. FELDBERG: Reactions of the normal mammalian muscle to acetylcholine and to eserine. J. Physiol. (Lond.) **87**, 394—424 (1936).
—, and U. S. v. EULER: The after-effects of a tetanus on mammalian muscle. J. Physiol. (Lond.) **93**, 39—60 (1938).
—, and A. M. HARVEY: Neuro-muscular conduction in the fowl. J. Physiol. (Lond.) **93**, 285—300 (1938a).
— — Reactions of avian muscle to acetylcholine and eserine. J. Physiol. (Lond.) **94**, 101—117 (1938b).
— — Neuro-muscular transmission in the extrinsic muscles of the eye. J. Physiol. (Lond.) **99**, 379—399 (1941).
BROWN, M. C., and P. B. C. MATTHEWS: The effect on a muscle twitch of the back response of its motor nerve fibres. J. Physiol. (Lond.) **150**, 332—346 (1960).
BROWN, R. V., A. M. KUNKEL, L. M. SOMERS and J. H. WILLS: Pyridine-2-aldoxime methiodide in the treatment of sarin and tabun poisoning, with notes on its pharmacology. J. Pharmacol. exp. Ther. **120**, 276—284 (1957).
BUCHTHAL, F., C. GULD and P. ROSENFALCK: Multielectrode study of the territory of a motor unit. Acta physiol. scand. **39**, 83—104 (1957).
—, and J. LINDHARD: Direct application of acetylcholine to motor endplates of voluntary muscle fibres. J. Physiol. (Lond.) **90**, 82—83P (1937).
— — Transmission of impulses from nerve to muscle fibre. Acta physiol. scand. **4**, 136—148 (1942).
BÜLBRING, E.: Observations on the isolated phrenic nerve diaphragm preparation of the rat. Brit. J. Pharmacol. **1**, 38—61 (1946).
—, and J. H. BURN: The interrelation of prostigmine, adrenaline and ephedrine in skeletal muscle. J. Physiol. (Lond.) **101**, 224—235 (1942).
—, and T. C. CHOU: The relative activity of prostigmine homologues and other substances as antagonists to tubocurarine. Brit. J. Pharmacol. **2**, 8—22 (1947).
BULLOCK, T. H.: Conduction and transmission of nerve impulses. Ann. Rev. Physiol. **13**, 261—280 (1951).
— D. NACHMANSOHN and M. A. ROTHENBERG: Effects of inhibitors of choline esterase on the nerve action potential. J. Neurophysiol. **9**, 9—22 (1946).
—, and R. S. TURNER: Events associated with conduction failure in nerve fibres. J. cell. comp. Physiol. **36**, 59—81 (1950).
BURGEN, A. S. V.: The mechanism of action of anticholinesterase drugs. Brit. J. Pharmacol. **4**, 219—228 (1949).
—, and L. M. CHIPMAN: The location of cholinesterase in the central nervous system. Quart. J. exp. Physiol. **37**, 61—74 (1952).
— F. DICKENS and L. J. ZATMAN: The action of botulinum toxin on the neuro-muscular junction. J. Physiol. (Lond.) **109**, 10—24 (1949a).
—, and F. HOBBIGER: The inhibition of cholinesterases by alkylphosphates and alkylphenolphosphates. Brit. J. Pharmacol. **6**, 593—605 (1951).
— C. A. KEELE and D. SLOME: Pharmacological actions of tetraethylpyrophosphate and hexaethyltetraphosphate. J. Pharmacol. exp. Ther. **96**, 396—409 (1949b).
BURKE, J. C., C. R. LINEGAR, M. W. FRANK and A. R. McINTYRE: Eserine and neostigmine antagonism to d-tubocurarine. Anaesthesiol. **9**, 251—257 (1948).
BURKE, W., B. KATZ and X. MACHNE: The effect of quaternary ammonium ions on crustacean nerve fibres. J. Physiol. (Lond.) **122**, 588—598 (1953).
BURN, J. H.: The relation of adrenaline to acetylcholine in the nervous system. Physiol. Rev. **25**, 377—394 (1945).
—, and D. E. HUTCHEON: The action of noradrenaline. Brit. J. Pharmacol. **4**, 373—380 (1949).
BURNS, B. D., G. B. FRANK and G. SALMOIRAGHI: The mechanism of after-discharges caused by veratrine in frog's skeletal muscles. Brit. J. Pharmacol. **10**, 363—370 (1955).

BURNS, B. D. and W. D. M PATON: Depolarization of the motor end-plate by decamethonium and acetylcholine J. Physiol. (Lond.) 115, 41—73 (1951).

BUTTLE, G. A. H., and E. J. ZAIMIS: The action of decamethonium iodide in birds. J. Pharm. (Lond.) 1, 991—992 (1949).

CANDOLE, DE, C. A., W. W. DOUGLAS, C. L. EVANS, R. HOLMES, K. E. V. SPENCER, R. W. TERRANCE and K. M. WILSON: The failure of respiration in death by anticholinesterase poisoning. Brit. J. Pharmacol. 8, 466—475 (1953).

CANNON, W. B., and A. ROSENBLUETH: Some conditions affecting the late stages of neuromuscular transmission. Amer. J. Physiol. 130, 219—229 (1940).

CASTILLO, J. C., and E. J. DE BEER: The neuromuscular blocking action of succinylcholine (Diacetylcholine). J. Pharmacol. exp. Ther. 99, 458—464 (1950).

CASTILLO, J. DEL, and B. KATZ: Quantal components of the end-plate potential. J. Physiol. (Lond.) 124, 560—573 (1954a).

— — Statistical factors involved in neuromuscular facilitation and depression. J. Physiol. (Lond.) 124, 574—585 (1954b).

— — Changes in end-plate activity produced by presynaptic polarization. J. Physiol. (Lond.) 124, 586—604 (1954c).

— — The membrane change produced by the neuromuscular transmitter. J. Physiol. (Lond.) 125, 546—565 (1954d).

— — On the localization of acetylcholine receptors. J. Physiol. (Lond.) 128, 157—181 (1955a).

— — Local activity at a depolarized nerve-muscle junction. J. Physiol. (Lond.) 128, 396—411 (1955b).

— — Biophysical aspects of neuro-muscular transmission. Progr. Biophys. Biophysic.-Chem. 6, 122—170 (1956a).

— — Localization of active spots within the neuromuscular junction of the frog. J. Physiol. (Lond.) 132, 630—649 (1956b).

— — A study of curare action with an electrical micromethod. Proc. roy. Soc. (B) 146, 339—356 (1957a).

— — The identity of 'intrinsic' and 'extrinsic' acetylcholine receptors in the motor end-plate. Proc. roy. Soc. (B) 146, 357—361 (1957b).

— — A comparison of acetylcholine and stable depolarizing agents. Proc. roy. Soc. (B) 146, 362—368 (1957c).

— — Interaction at end-plate receptors between different choline derivatives. Proc. roy. Soc. (B) 146, 369—381 (1957d).

CHAGAS, C.: Utilisation de l'acetylcholine pendant la décharge chez electrophorus electricus. L. C. R. Acad. Sci. (Paris) 234, 663—665 (1952).

—, and D. ALBE-FESSARD: Action de divers curarisants sur l'organe électrique de l'Electrophorus electricus (Linnaeus) Acta physiol. lat.-amer. 4, 50—60 (1954).

— L. SOLLERO, H. MARTINS-FERREIRA and H. C. PARREIRA: On the utilization of acetylcholine during the electric discharge of Electrophorus electricus (Linnaeus). II. An. Acad. Bras. Cien. 25, 327—329 (1953).

CHANG, H. C., and J. H. GADDUM: Choline esters in tissue extracts. J. Physiol. (Lond.) 79, 255—285 (1933).

CHENNELLS, M., W. F. FLOYD and S. WRIGHT: Action of condensed alkyl phosphates on the nerve-muscle preparation and the central nervous system of the cat. J. Physiol. (Lond.) 108, 375—397 (1949).

CHEYMOL, J., R. DELABY, P. CHABRIER, H. NAJER et F. BOURILLET: Activité Acétylcholinomimétique de quelques Dérivés de la carbaminoylcholine. Arch. int. Pharmacodyn. 98, 161—182 (1954).

CHRISTENSEN, H. N., and R. T. RIGGS: Physostigmine uptake by cells and its effect on potassium exchange. J. biol. Chem. 193, 621—626 (1951).

CHURCHILL-DAVIDSON, H. C., and A. T. RICHARDSON: Decamethonum Iodide (C_{10}): Some observations on its action using electromyography. Proc. Roy. Soc. Med. 45, 179—185 (1952). (Section of Anesthetics, pp. 13—19.)

COHEN, J. A., and C. H. POSTHUMUS: The mechanism of action of anti-cholinesterases. Acta physiol. pharmacol. neerl. 4, 17—36 (1955).

— — The mechanism of action of anti-cholinesterases. III. The action of anti-cholinesterases on the phrenic nerve diaphragm preparation of the rat. Acta physiol. pharmacol. neerl. 5, 385—397 (1957).

— M. G. P. J. WARRINGA and I. INDORF: Relationship between the pharmacological action of neuromuscular drugs and their capacity to inhibit esterases. Acta physiol. pharmacol. neerl. 4, 187—200 (1955).

CONDOURIS, G. A., and A. GHAZAL: Evaluation of the interaction of the guanidinium ion with several neuromuscular blocking agents on a mammalian neuromuscular preparation. Fed. Proc. 16, 289 (1957).

COPPÉE, G.: La transmission neuro-musculaire: Curarisation, décurarisation et renforcement à la jonction myo-neurale. Arch. int. Physiol. **53**, 327—507 (1943).

CORTEGGIANI, E.: Recherches sur l'acetylcholine libre et combiné dans le cerveau. C. R. Soc. Biol. (Paris) **124**, 1197—1198 (1937).

COUCEIRO, A., D. F. DE ALMEIDA and M. MIRANDA: The presence of cholinesterase in the electric tissue of *Electrophorus electricus* by the myristoylcholine method of Gomori. An. Acad. Bras. Cien. **27**, 49—56 (1955).

COUTEAUX, R.: Morphological and cytochemical observations on the post-synaptic membrane at motor end-plates and ganglionic synapses. Exp. Cell. Res. Suppl. **5**, 294—322 (1958).

COWAN, S. L.: The effect of certain substances on the transmission of excitation from motor nerve to voluntary muscle. J. Physiol. (Lond.) **86**, 61P—62P (1936a).

— The effects of drugs on transmission from nerve to voluntary muscle and "accomodation" to different rates of destruction of the chemical transmitter. J. Physiol. (Lond.) **87**, 43P (1936b).

— The initiation of all-or-none responses in muscle by acetylcholine. J. Physiol. (Lond.) **88**, 3P—5P (1936c).

— The action of eserine-like and curare-like substances on the responses of frog's nerve-muscle preparations to repetitive stimulation. J. Physiol. (Lond.) **93**, 215—262 (1938).

— The actions of eserine-like compounds upon frog's nerve-muscle preparations, and conditions in which a single shock can evoke an augmented muscular response. Proc. roy. Soc. (B) **129**, 356—391 (1940a).

— The actions of eserine-like compounds upon frog's nerve-muscle preparations, and the blocking of neuromuscular conduction. Proc. roy. Soc. (B) **129**, 392—411 (1940b).

—, and W. G. WALTER: The effects of tetraethylammonium iodide on the electrical response and the accomodation of nerve. J. Physiol. (Lond.) **91**, 101—126 (1937).

COX, R. T., C. W. COATES and M. V. BROWN: Electrical characteristics of electric tissue. Ann. N. Y. Acad. Sci. **47**, 487—500 (1946).

CREESE, R., D. B. TAYLOR and B. TILTON: Rate of antagonism of *d*-tubocurarine by potassium ions. Brit. J. Pharmacol. **17**, 101—106 (1961).

CREVIER, M., et L. F. BELANGER: Étude quantitative de l'activité cholinesterasique de la plaque motrice par voie d'histophotométrie. Canad J Biochem. **34**, 869—881 (1956).

DALE, H. H.: Pharmacology and nerve-endings. Proc. roy. Soc. Med. **28**, 319—322 (1934).

—, and W. FELDBERG: Chemical transmission at motor nerve endings in voluntary muscle. J. Physiol. (Lond.) **81**, 39P—40P (1934).

— — and M. VOGT: Release of acetylcholine at voluntary motor nerve-endings. J. Physiol. (Lond.) **86**, 353—380 (1936).

—, and J. H. GADDUM: Reactions of *denervated* voluntary muscle and their bearing on the mode of action of parasympathetic and related nerves J. Physiol (Lond.) **70**, 109—144 (1930)

DALLEMAGNE, M., J., J.-M.GERNAY et E. PHILIPPOT: Antagonisme réciproque du tubocurare et d'un dérive de l'ammonium quaternarie curarimimetique (1). Arch. int. Physiol. **59**, 26—39 (1951).

DAVISON, A. N.: Return of cholinesterase activity in the rat after inhibition by Organophosphorus compounds, I. Diethyl p-nitrophenyl phosphate (E_{600}, Paraoxon). Biochem. J. **54**, 583—590 (1953).

— Return of cholinesterase activity in the rat after inhibition by organophosphorus compounds, 2. A comparative study of true and pseudo cholinesterase. Biochem. J. **60**, 339 to 346 (1955).

DE BEER, E. J., J. C. CASTILLO, A. P. PHILLIPS, R. V. FANELLI, A. L. WNUCK and S. NORTON: Synthetic drugs influencing neuromuscular activity. Ann. N. Y. Acad. Sci. **54**, Art. 3, 362—371 (1951).

DENZ, F. A.: On the histochemistry of the myoneural junction. Brit. J. exp. Path. **34**, 329 to 339 (1953).

DEPIERRE, F., et A. FUNKE: Action de l'iodure de tétraméthylammonium et des iodures d'hydroxyphényltriméthylammonium sur la transmission neuro-musculaire. C. R. Acad. Sci. (Paris) **230**, 2242—2243 (1950).

— — Relations entre la structure des dihalogénométhylates de bis-(aminophenoxy) alcanes et arylalcanes et leur action sur la transmission neuromusculaire. C. R. Acad. Sci. (Paris) **235**, 267—269 (1952).

DIAMOND, J.: The effects of injecting acetylcholine into normal and regenerating nerves. J. Physiol. (Lond.) **145**, 611—629 (1959).

DOUGLAS, W. W., and P. B. C. MATTHEWS: Acute tetraethylpyrophosphate poisoning in cats with its modification by atropine or hyoscine. J. Physiol. (Lond.) **116**, 202—218 (1952).

—, and W. D. M. PATON: The mechanisms of motor end-plate depolarization due to a cholinesterase-inhibiting drug. J. Physiol. (Lond.) **124**, 325—344 (1954).

DUN, F. T.: The attenuation of electrotonic potential in the motor terminal arborization. J. Physiol. (Lond.) **133**, 42P—43P (1956).

—, and T. P. FENG: Studies on the neuromuscular junction. XIX. Retrograde discharges from motor nerve endings in veratrinized muscle. Chin. J. Physiol. **15**, 405—432 (1940a).

— — Studies on the neuromuscular junction. XX. The site of origin of the junctional after-discharge in muscles treated with guanidine, barium or eserine. Chin. J. Physiol. **15**, 433—444 (1940b).

EASTON, D. M.: Facilitation in crustacean neuromuscular system. Fed. Proc. **11**, 39 (1952).

— Facilitation and inhibition in crustacean neuromuscular system. Physiol. comp. ('s-Grav.) **4**, 415—428 (1957).

ECCLES, J. C.: An electrical hypothesis of synaptic and neuro-muscular transmission. I. Present theoretical position. Ann. N. Y. Acad. Sci. **47**, 429—455 (1946).

— B. KATZ and S. W. KUFFLER: Electric potential changes accompanying neuromuscular transmission. Biol. Symp. **3**, 349—370 (1941a).

— — — Nature of the "endplate potential" in curarized muscle. J. Neurophysiol. **4**, 362 to 387 (1941b).

— — — Effect of eserine on neuromuscular transmission. J. Neurophysiol. **5**, 211—230 (1942).

—, and W. V. MACFARLANE: Actions of anti-cholinesterases on endplate potential of frog muscle. J. Neurophysiol. **12**, 59—80 (1949).

—, and W. J. O'CONNOR: Action potentials evoked by indirect stimulation of curarized muscle. J. Physiol. (Lond.) **94**, 9—11P (1938).

— — Responses which nerve impulses evoke in mammalian striated muscles. J. Physiol. (Lond.) **97**, 44—102 (1939).

ELLIS, S., O. KRAYER and F. L. PLACHTE: Studies on physostigmine and related substances. III. Breakdown products of physostigmine; their inhibitory effect on cholinesterase and their pharmacological action. J. Pharmacol. exp. Ther. **79**, 309—319 (1943).

EMMELIN, N.: The action of some indifferent narcotics on the acetylcholine sensitivity of the rectus muscle of the frog. Skand. Arch. Physiol. **83**, 69—76 (1940).

— Evipan and the parasympathetic nervous system. Acta physiol. scand. **2**, 289—310 (1941).

ENGBAEK, L.: Investigations on the course and localization of magnesium anesthesia. A comparison with ether anesthesia. Acta pharmacal. (Kbh.) **4**, Suppl. 1, 1—189 (1948).

ENGELHART, E., u. O. LOEWI: Fermentative Acetylcholinspaltung im Blut und ihre Hemmung durch Physostigmin. Naunyn-Schmideberg's Arch. exp. Path. Pharmak. **150**, 1—13 (1930).

EVANS, C. LOWATT: Neuromuscular block by anticholinesterases. J. Physiol. (Lond.) **114**, 6P (1951).

EYZAGUIRRE, C.: The electrical activity of mammalian intrafusal fibres. J. Physiol. (Lond.) **150**, 169—185 (1960).

FATT, P.: The electromotive action of acetylcholine at the motor end-plate. J. Physiol. (Lond.) **111**, 408—422 (1950).

— Biophysics of junctional transmission. Physiol. Rev. **34**, 674—710 (1954).

—, and B. L. GINSBORG: The ionic requirements for the production of action potentials in crustacean muscles fibres. J. Physiol (Lond.) **142**, 516—543 (1958).

—, and B. KATZ: An analysis of the end-plate potential recorded with an intracellular electrode. J. Physiol. (Lond.) **115**, 320—370 (1951).

— — Spontaneous subthreshold activity at motor nerve endings. J. Physiol. (Lond.) **117**, 109—128 (1952a).

— — The effect of sodium ions on neuromuscular transmission. J. Physiol. (Lond.) **118**, 73—87 (1952b).

— — The electrical properties of crustacean muscle fibres. J. Physiol. (Lond.) **120**, 171—204 (1953).

FELDBERG, W., and A. FESSARD: The cholinergic nature of the nerves to the electric organ of the Torpedo (Torpedo Marmorata). J. Physiol. (Lond.) **101**, 200—216 (1942).

FENG, T. P.: Studies on the neuromuscular junction, I. The inhibition at the neuromuscular junction. Chin. J. Physiol. **10**, 417—434 (1936).

— Studies on the neuromuscular junction. IV. The nature of junctional inhibition. Chin. J. Physiol. **11**, 437—450 (1937a).

— Studies on the neuromuscular junction. V. The succession of inhibitory and facilitatory effects of prolonged high frequency stimulation on neuromuscular transmission. Chin. J. Physiol. **11**, 451—470 (1937b).

— Studies on the Neuromuscular junction. VI. Potentiation by eserine of response to single indirect stimulus in amphibian nerve-muscle preparations. Chin. J. Physiol. **12**, 51—58 (1937c).

— Studies on the neuromuscular junction. X. The effects of guanidine. Chin. J. Physiol. **13**, 119—140 (1938).

— Studies on the neuromuscular junction. XVIII. The local potentials around N-M junctions induced by single and multiple volleys. Chin. J. Physiol. **15**, 367—404 (1940).

FENG, T. P. The local activity around the skeletal N-M junctions produced by nerve impulses. Biol. Symp. **3**, 121—152 (1941).
— L. Y. LEE, C. W. MENG and S. C. WANG: Studies on the neuromuscular junction. IX. The after effects of tetanization on N-M transmission in cat. Chin. J. Physiol. **13**, 79—108(1938).
—, and T. H. LI: Studies on the neuromuscular junction. XXIII. A new aspect of the phenomena of eserine potentiation and post-tetanic facilitation in mammalian muscles. Chin. J. Physiol. **16**, 37—56 (1941a).
— — Studies on the neuromuscular junction. XXIV. The repetitive discharges of mammalian motor nerve endings after treatment with veratrine, barium and guanidine. Chin. J. Physiol. **16**, 143—156 (1941b).
— — Studies on the neuromuscular junction. XXV. Eserine-like actions of aliphatic alcohols and ketones. Chin. J. Physiol. **16**, 317—340 (1941c).
— — and Y. C. TING: Studies on the neuromuscular junction. XII. Repetitive discharges and inhibitory after-effect in post-tetanically facilitated responses of cat muscles to single nerve volleys. Chin. J. Physiol. **14**, 55—80 (1939a).
— — — Studies on the neuromuscular junction. XV. The inhibition following eserine-potentiated and post-tetanically facilitated responses of mammalian muscles. Chin. J. Physiol. **14**, 337—356 (1939b).
—, and S. C. SHEN: Studies on the neuro-muscular junction. III. The contracture in eserinized muscle produced by nerve stimulation. Chin. J. Physiol. **11**, 51—70 (1937).
FESSARD, A.: Some basic aspects of the activity of electric plates. Ann. N. Y. Acad. Sci. **47**, 501—514 (1946).
— Recherches sur le fonctionnement des organes électriques. I. Analyse des formes de décharge obtenues par divers procédés d'excitation. Arch. int. Physiol. **55**, 1—26 (1947).
— Diversity of transmission processes as exemplified by specific synapses in electric organs. Proc. Roy. Soc. (Lond.) (B) **140**, 186—191 (1952).
FILLENZ, M., and M. HANAFIN: Acetylcholine and neuromuscular transmission. J. Neurophysiol. **10**, 189—195 (1947).
FINERTY, J. C.: Effects of di*iso*propylfluorophosphate (DFP) on acetylcholine stimulation of the frog rectus abdominis muscle. Amer. J. Physiol. **151**, 107—109 (1947).
FLECKENSTEIN, A., H. HILLE u. W. E. ADAM: Aufhebung der Kontraktur-Wirkung depolarisierender Katelektrotonica durch Repolarisation im Anelektrotonus. Pflügers Arch. ges. Physiol. **253**, 264—282 (1951).
FRANKENHAEUSER, B., and A. L. HODGKIN: The after effects of impulses in the giant axon of Loligo. J. Physiol. (Lond.) **131**, 341—376 (1956).
FRASER, P. J.: Hydrolysis of succinylcholine salts. Brit. J. Pharmacol. **9**, 429—436 (1954).
FREDRIKSSON, T.: Pharmacological properties of methyl-fluoro-phosphorylcholines. Two synthetic cholinergic drugs. Arch. int. Pharmacodyn. **113**, 101—113 (1957).
— Further studies on fluoro-phosphorylcholines. Pharmacological properties of two new analogues. Arch. int. Pharmacodyn. **115**, 474—482 (1958).
FUNKE, A., et F. DEPIERRE: Propriétés anti-curarisantes de quelques sels d'ammonium quaternaire dérivés d'aminophenols. C. R. Acad. Sci. (Paris) **230**, 245—247 (1950).
— — et M. W. KRUCKER: Exaltation de l'activité anticholinestérasique de sels d'ammonium quaternaires des phenoxyalcanes par l'introduction de groupements uréthanés. C. R. Acad. Sci. (Paris) **234**, 762—764 (1952).
— J. JACOB et K. DANIKEN: Propriétés analgésiques et anticholinestérasiques des dichlorhydrate et du diiodomethylate de la bis-(pipéridinomethyl-coumaranyl-5) cétone. C. R. Acad. Sci. (Paris) **236**, 149—151 (1953).
FURUKAWA, T.: Properties of the procaine endplate potential. Jap. J. Physiol. **7**, 199—212 (1957).
— A. FURUKAWA and T. TAKAGI: Fibrillation of muscle fibres produced by ammonium ions and its relation to spontaneous activity at the neuromuscular junction. Jap. J. Physiol. **7**, 252—263 (1957).
GASSER, H. S.: Contractures of skeletal muscle. Physiol Rev. **10**, 35—109 (1930).
—, and H. H. DALE: The pharmacology of denervated mammalian muscle. II. Some phenomena of antagonism, and the formation of lactic acid in chemical contracture. J. Pharmacol. exp. Ther. **2**, 287—315 (1926).
GIACOBINI, E.: The distribution and localization of cholinesterase in nerve cells. Acta physiol. scand. **45**, Suppl. 156, 1—45 (1959).
GINSBORG, B. L.: Spontaneous activity in muscle fibres of the chick. J. Physiol. (Lond.) **150**, 707—717 (1960).
GINZEL, K. H., H. KLUPP u. G. WERNER: Zur Pharmakologie von α-ω-bis-quaternären Ammoniumverbindungen. I. Mitteilung: Neuromuskuläre und ganglionäre Wirkungen des Adipinsäure-bis-Cholinesters. Arch. int. Pharmacodyn. **86**, 385—406 (1951a).

GINZEL, K. H., H. KLUPP u. G. WERNER: Zur Pharmakologie von α-ω-bis-quarternären Ammoniumverbindungen. III. Mitteilung: Die fermentative Spaltung einiger aliphatischer Dicarbonsäureester und die Steigerung ihrer Wirksamkeit durch Eserin. Arch. int. Pharmacodyn. 87, 351—365 (1951 b).

— — — Die Wirkung einiger aliphatischer α-ω-bis-quaternären Ammonium-Verbindungen auf die Skeletmuskulatur. Naunyn-Schmiedeberg's Arch. exp. Path. Pharmak. 213, 453 bis 466 (1951 c).

— — — Zur Pharmakologie von α-ω-bis-quaternären Ammonium-Verbindungen. II. Mitteilung: Arch. int. Pharmacodyn. 87, 79—98 (1951 d).

— — — Die Wirkungsweise einiger α-ω-bis-quaternären Ammonium-Verbindungen an der Skeletmuskulatur. Naunyn-Schmiedeberg's Arch. exp. Path. Pharmak. 215, 103—118 (1952).

GJONE, E.: The effect of decamethonium and succinylcholine on muscle contractions evoked by direct stimulation. Acta pharmacol. (Kbh.) 11, 377—387 (1955).

GOFFART, M.: Recherches relatives à l'action de l'adrenaline sur le muscle strié de mammifère. I. Potentiation par l'adrenaline de la contraction maximale du muscle non fatigué. Arch. int. Physiol. 60, 318—349 (1952).

—, and J. M. RITCHIE: The effect of adrenaline on the contraction of mammalian skeletal muscle. J. Physiol. (Lond.) 116, 357—371 (1952).

GOLDSTEIN, A.: The mechanism of enzyme-inhibitor substrate reactions. J. gen. Physiol. 27, 529—580 (1944).

GOPFERT, H., u. H. SCHAEFER: Über den direkt und indirekt erregten Aktionsstrom und die Funktion der motorischen Endplatte. Pflügers Arch. ges. Physiol. 239, 597—619 (1937).

GOUTIER, R.: Sensibilisation aux ions potassium par les methylanthines (1). Arch. int. Physiol. 57, 154—172 (1949a).

— Action des methylxanthines sur la transmission neuro-musculaire (1). Arch. int. Physiol. 57, 185—200 (1949b).

GREENGARD, P., and R. W. STRAUB: Afterpotentials in mammalian nonmyelinated nerve fibres. J. Physiol. (Lond.) 144, 442—462 (1958).

GROB, D.: The anticholinesterase activity in vitro of the insecticide Parathion (p-nitrophenyl-diethyl Thionophosphate). Johns Hopk. Hosp. Bull. 87, 95—105 (1950).

—, and A. M. HARVEY: Observations on the effects of tetraethyl pyrophosphate (TEPP) in man, and on its use in the treatment of myasthenia gravis. Johns Hopk. Hosp. Bull. 84, 532—567 (1949).

GROBLEWSKI, G. E., B. P. MCNAMARA and J. H. WILLS: Stimulation of denervated muscle by DFP and related compounds. J. Pharmacol. exp. Ther. 118, 116—122 (1956).

GRUNDFEST, H.: Excitation triggers in post-junctional cells. In: Physiological Triggers, edit. T.-H. Bullock, Amer. Physiol. Soc., Washington, D. C., 1957a.

— The mechanisms of discharge of the electric organs in relation to general and comparative electrophysiology. Progress in Biophysics and Biophysical Chemistry; edit. I. A. V. BUTLER and B. KATZ 7, 1—85 (1957b).

GUNTHER, P. G.: Die Morphologischen Grundlagen der Bewegungs- und Halteleistung (Tetanus und Tonus) des Zwerchfells. Acta anat. (Basel) 14, 54—64 (1952).

GUTTMAN, S. A., R. G. MORTON and D. T. WILBER: Enhancement of muscle contraction after tetanus. Amer. J. Physiol. 119, 463—473 (1937).

HAGIWARA, S., and A. WATANABE: The effect of tetraethylammonium chloride on the muscle membrane examined with an intracellular microelectrode. J. Physiol. (Lond.) 129, 513 to 527 (1955).

HALL, R. A., and M. W. PARKES: The effect of drugs upon neuromuscular transmission in the guinea-pig. J. Physiol. (Lond.) 122, 274—281 (1953).

HARDEGG, W. H.: Zur Kinetik der Cholinesterasen-Hemmung durch Prostigmin. Naunyn-Schmiedeberg's exp. Path. Pharmak. 214, 540—555 (1952).

HARRIS, E. J., and M. MIRANDA: The prolongation of facilitation in the electric eel by anti-cholinesterase. J. Physiol. (Lond.) 130, 24 P, (1955).

HARVEY, A. M.: The action of procaine on neuromuscular transmission. Johns Hopk. Hosp. Bull. 65, 223—238 (1939a).

— The action of quinine on skeletal muscle. J. Physiol. (Lond.) 95, 45—67 (1939b).

— B. F. JONES, S. TALBOT and D. GROB: The effect of Diisopropyl fluorophosphate (DFP) on neuromuscular transmission in normal individuals and in patients with myasthenia gravis. Fed. Proc. 5, 182 (1946).

HAWKINS, R. D., and B. MENDEL: True cholinesterases with pronounced resistance to eserine. J. cell. comp. Physiol. 27, 69—85 (1946).

HEINBECKER, P., and S. W. BARTLEY: Action of ether and nembutal on the nervous system. J. Neurophysiol. 3, 219—236 (1940).

HEY, P.: On relationships between structure and nicotine-like stimulant activity in choline esters and ethers. Brit. J. Pharmacol. 7, 117—129 (1952).

HILL, A. V.: Excitation and accomodation in nerve. Proc. Roy. Soc. (B) 119, 305—355 (1936).

HOBBIGER, F.: The action of carbamic esters and tetraethylpyrophosphate on normal and curarized frog rectus muscle. Brit. J. Pharmacol. 5, 37—48 (1950).

— Inhibition of cholinesterases by irreversible inhibitors *in vitro* and *in vivo*. Brit. J. Pharmacol. 6, 21—30 (1951).

— The mechanism of anticurare action of certain neostigmine analogues. Brit. J. Pharmacol. 7, 223—236 (1952).

—, u. G. WERNER: Über das chemische Gleichgewicht von Acetylcholin im Zentralnervensystem. Z. Vitaminforsch. 2, 234—250 (1949).

HODGKIN, A. L., and R. D. KEYNES: Movements of labelled calcium in squid giant axon. J. Physiol. (Lond.) 138, 253—281 (1957).

HOLLAND, W. C., and G. V. AUDITORE: Effect of acetylcholine on rate of uptake and equilibrium distribution of physostigmine in human erythrocytes. J. appl. Physiol. 9, 147—152 (1956).

— C. E. DUNN and M. E. GREIG: Studies on permeability. VII. Effect of several substrates and inhibitors of acetyl cholinesterase on permeability of isolated auricles to Na and K. Amer. J. Physiol. 168, 546—556 (1952).

—, and M. E. GREIG: Studies on permeability. II. The effect of acetylcholine and physostigmine on the permeability to potassium of dog erythrocytes. Arch. Biochem. 26, 151 to 155 (1950).

HOLMES, P. E. B., D. J. JENDEN and D. B. TAYLOR: The analysis of the mode of action of curare on neuromuscular transmission; the effect of temperature changes. J. Pharmacol. exp. Ther. 103, 382—402 (1951).

HOLMES, R., and E. L. ROBINS: The reversal by oximes of neuromuscular block produced by anticholinesterases. Brit. J. Pharmacol. 10, 490—495 (1955).

HOLMSTEDT, B.: Synthesis and pharmacology of dimethylamido-ethoxy-phosphoryl cyanide (Tabun) together with a description of some allied anticholinesterase compounds containing the N-P bond. Acta physiol. scand. 25, Suppl. 90, 1—120 (1951).

HOLTON, P., and H. R. ING: The specificity of the trimethylammonium group in acetylcholine. Brit. J. Pharmacol. 4, 190—196 (1949).

HOPPE, J. O.: A new series of synthetic curare-like compounds. Ann. N. Y. Acad. Sci. 54, 395—406 (1951).

HOYLE, G.: Comparative physiology of the nervous control of muscular contraction. Cambridge Monographs in Experimental Biology, Cambridge Univ. Press 8, 1957.

HUIDOBRO, F., L. CUBILLOS and C. EYZAGUIRRE: On certain effects of decamethonium (C_{10}) on the mammalian neuromuscular preparation. Acta physiol. lat.-amer. 3, 169—182 (1952).

HUNT, C. C.: The effect of di-isopropyl fluorophosphate on neuromuscular transmission. J. pharmacol. exp. Ther. 91, 77—83 (1947).

— Drug effects on mammalian muscle spindles. Fed. Proc. 11, 75 (1952).

—, and S. W. KUFFLER: Pharmacology of the neuromuscular junction. Pharmacol. Rev. 2, 96—120 (1950).

—, and W. F. RIKER, jr.: The effect of chronic poisoning with di-isopropyl fluorophosphate on neuromuscular function in the cat. J. Pharmacol. exp. Ther. 91, 298—305 (1947).

HUTTER, O. F.: Effect of choline on neuromuscular transmission in the cat. J. Physiol. 117, 241—250 (1952a).

— Post-tetanic restoration of neuromuscular transmission blocked by d-tubocurarine. J. Physiol. (Lond.) 118, 216—227 (1952b).

—, and W. R. LOEWENSTEIN: Nature of neuromuscular facilitation by sympathetic stimulation in the frog. J. Physiol. (Lond.) 130, 559—571 (1955).

—, and W. TRAUTWEIN: Neuromuscular facilitation by stretch of motor nerve-endings. J. Physiol. (Lond.) 133, 610—625 (1956).

ING, H. R.: The curariform action of onium salts. Physiol. Rev. (Lond.) 16, 527—544 (1936).

—, and W. M. WRIGHT: The curareform action of quaternary ammonium salts. Proc. roy. Soc. (B) 109, 337—353 (1931).

— — Further studies on the pharmacological properties of onium salts. Proc. roy. Soc. (B) 114, 48—63 (1933).

JACO, N. T., and D. R. WOOD: The interaction between procaine, cocaine, adrenaline and prostigmine on skeletal muscle. J. pharmacol. (Kbh.) 82, 63—73 (1944).

JACOB, J.: Actions d'un inhibiteur sélectif des acétylcholinestérases, le 3318 CT, sur la transmission neuromusculaire du chat. Experientia (Basel) 10, 496 (1954).

— Proprietes antiacétylcholinestérasiques spécifiques du-di-iodométhylate de la Bis-(piperidinomethyl-coumaranyl-5) cétone (3318 CT). I. Relations entre la structure chimique et le pouvoir antiacétylcholinesterasique. Pouvoirs inhibiteurs, *in vitro* et *in vivo*. Arch. int. Pharmacodyn. 101, 446—468 (1955).

JACOB, J., et A. FUNKE: Relations entre la structure chimique et les propriétés anticholinestérasiques d'un groupe d'inhibiteurs sélectifs de l'acétylcholinestérase globulaire du chien. C. R. Acad. Sci. (Paris) 237, 1809—1811 (1953).
—, et M. PECOT-DECHAVASSINE: Actions de la néostigmine, du 3318 CT sur la sensibilité du rectus de grenouille aux esters acétique, propionique et butyrique de la choline. Experientia (Basel) 11/6, 235—236 (1955).
— — Hydrolyse enzymatique de la propionylcholine, de l'acetylthiocholine et de la butyrylthiocholine par le rectus de grenouille. Experientia (Basel) 14/9, 330 (1958).
—, et TAZIEFF-DEPIERRE F.: Actions neuromusculaires des composes anticholinesterasiques. In: Curare and Curare agents, p. 304—318, edit. D. BOVET, F. BOVET-NITTI and G. B. MARINI-BETTOLO. Amsterdam: Elsevier 1957.
JACOBSOHN, D., u. G. KAHLSON: Die Anticurarewirkung einiger Stoffe mit lähmender Wirkung auf die Acetylcholinesterase. Skand. Arch. Physiol. 79, 27—31 (1938).
JENDEN, D. J.: A quantitative interpretation of eserine-acetylcholine interaction in the frog rectus abdominis. J. cell. comp. Physiol. 51, 309—469 (1958).
— K. KAMIJO and D. B. TAYLOR: The action of decamethonium on the isolated rabbit lumbrical muscle. J. Pharmacol. exp. Ther. 111, 229—240 (1954).
KAHLSON, G., u. B. UVNAS: Die Bedeutung der Acetylcholinesterase sowie der spezifischen Rezeptoren für die Acetylcholinempfindlichkeit kontraktiler Substrate. Skand. Arch. Physiol. 78, 40—58 (1938).
KARCZMAR, A. G.: Antagonism between a bis-quaternary oxamide, WIN 8078, and depolarizing and competitive blocking agents. J. Pharmacol. exp. Ther. 119, 39—47 (1957).
—, and S. W. HOWARD: Antagonism of d-tubocurarine and other pharmacologic properties of certain bis-quaternary salts of basically substituted oxamides (WIN 8077 and analogs). J. pharmacol. exp. Ther. 113, 30 (1955).
KATO, G., T. HAYASHI, T. OTA, M. NAKAYAMA, H. TAMURA, M. TAKEUCHI, K. KANAI and S. MATSUYAMA: Explanation of Wedensky inhibition. Part I. Amer. J. Physiol. 89, 471 to 481 (1929).
KATZ, B.: Neuromuscular transmission in crabs. J. Physiol. (Lond.) 87, 199—221 (1936).
— The "anti-curare" action of a subthreshold catelectrotonus. J. Physiol. (Lond.) 95, 286 to 304 (1939).
— The electrical properties of the muscle fibre membrane. Proc. roy. Soc. (B) 135, 506—534 (1948).
— Action potentials from a sensory nerve ending. J. Physiol. (Lond.) 111, 248—260 (1950).
— Microphysiology of the neuro-muscular junction. A physiological 'quantum of action' at the myoneural junction. Johns Hopk. Hosp. Bull. 102, 275—295 (1958a).
— Microphysiology of the neuro-muscular junction. The chemo-receptor function of the motor end-plate. Johns Hopk. Hosp. Bull. 102, 296—312 (1958b).
—, and R. MILEDI: The localized action of "end-plate drugs" in the twitch fibres of the frog. J. Physiol. (Lond.) 155, 399—415 (1961).
—, and S. THESLEFF: The interaction between endrophonium (Tensilon) and acetylcholine at the motor end-plate. Brit. J. Pharmacol. 12, 260—264 (1957a).
— — A study of the "Densitization" produced by acetylcholine at the motor end-plate. J. Physiol. (Lond.) 138, 63—80 (1957b).
KENSLER, C. J.: The antagonism of curare by congo red and related compounds. J. Pharmacol. exp. Ther. 95, 28—44 (1949).
— The anticurare activity of tetraethylammonium ion in the cat. Brit. J. Pharmacol. 5, 204—209 (1950).
—, and R. W. ELSNER: Tetraethylammonium and cholinesterase activity. J. Pharmacol. exp. Ther. 102, 196—199 (1951).
KEWITZ, H.: A specific antidote against lethal alkyl phosphate intoxication. III. Repair of chemical lesion. Arch. Biochem. 66, 263—270 (1957).
KEYNES, R. D.: Electric organ, in: The Physiology of Fishes, Edit. M. E. BROWN, 2, 323 to 343, New York: Academic Press, Inc. 1957.
—, and H. MARTINS-FERREIRA: Membrane potentials in the electroplates of the electric eel. J. Physiol. (Lond.) 119, 315—351 (1953).
KING, H.: Curare alkaloids; part I: Tubocurarine. J. Chem. Soc. 1935 II, 1381—1389.
KIRSCHNER, L.: Effect of cholinesterase inhibitors and atropine on active sodium transport across frog skin. Nature (Lond.) 172, 348—349 (1953).
— The effect of atropine and the curares on the active transport of sodium by the skin of rana esculenta. J. cell. comp. Physiol. 45, 89—102 (1955).
KIRSCHNER, L. B., and W. E. STONE: Action of inhibitors at the myoneural junction. J. gen. Physiol. 34, 821—834 (1951).
KLUPP, H., O. KRAUPP, H. STORMANN u. CH. STUMPF: Über die Pharmakologischen Eigenschaften einiger Polymethylen-Dicarbaminsäure Bischolinester. Arch. int. Pharmacodyn. 96, 161—182 (1953).

KOBINGER, W., u. O. KRAUPP: Über die Wechselwirkungen von d-Tubocurarin, Eserin und depolarisierenden Substanzen am isolierten Rattenzwerchfell, untersucht am Beispiel des Octamethylen-Biscarbaminoylcholins. Arch. exp. Path. Pharmak. **225**, 237—250 (1955).

KOBLICK, D. C.: An enzymatic ion exchange model for active sodium transport. J. gen. Physiol. **42**, 635—645 (1958).

KOCH, H. J.: Cholinesterase and active transport of sodium chloride through the isolated gills of the crab Eriocheir sinesis (M. Edw.) in: Recent Developments in Cell Physiology, ed. by J. A. KITCHING, p. 15—27. London: Butterworths Scientific Publications 1954a.

— L'intervention de cholinestérases dans l'absorption et le transport actif de matieres minerales par les branchies du Crabe "Eriocheir sinesis M. E.". Arch. int. Physiol. **62**, 136 (1954b).

KOELLE, G. B.: Protection of cholinesterase against irreversible inactivation by di-isopropyl fluorophosphate *in vitro*. J. Pharmacol. exp. Ther. **88**, 232—237 (1946).

— The histochemical differentiation of types of cholinesterases and their localizations in tissues of the cat. J. Pharmacol. exp. Ther. **100**, 158—179 (1950).

— Histochemical demonstration of reversible anticholinesterase action at selective cellular sites *in vivo*. J. Pharmacol. exp. Ther. **120**, 488—503 (1957a).

— Histochemical demonstration of reactivation of acetylcholinesterase *in vivo*. Science **125**, 1195—1196 (1957b).

— Neurohumoral agents as a mechanism of nervous integration, in: Evolution of nervous control; edit. A. D. BASS. Amer. Ass. Adv. sci., Publ. No. **52**, 87—114 (1959).

— A proposed dual neurohumoral role of Acetylcholine: its function at the pre- and post-synaptic sites. Nature (Lond.) **190**, 208—211 (1961).

—, and A. GILMAN: The chronic toxicity of di-isopropyl fluorophosphate (DFP) in dogs, monkeys and rats. J. Pharmacol. exp. Ther. **87**, 435—448 (1946).

— — Anticholinesterase drugs. Pharmacol. Rev. **1**, 166—216 (1949).

—, and E. C. STEINER: The cerebral distributions of a tertiary and a quaternary anticholinesterase agent following intravenous and intraventricular injection. J. Pharmacol. exp. Ther. **118**, 420—434 (1956).

KOELLE, W. A., and G. B. KOELLE: The localization of external or functional acetylcholinesterase at the synapses of autonomic ganglia. J. Pharmacol. exp. Ther. **126**, 1—8 (1959).

KOKETSU, K.: Action of tetraethylammonium chloride on neuromuscular transmission in frogs. Amer. J. Physiol. **193**, 213—218 (1958).

— J. A. CERF and S. NISHI: Effect of quaternary ammonium ions on electrical activity of spinal ganglion cells in frogs. J. Neurophysiol. **22**, 177—194 (1959a).

— — — Further observations on electrical activity of frog spinal ganglion cells in sodium-free solutions. J. Neurophysiol. **22**, 693—703 (1959b).

KÖLLIKER, M.: Sur la terminaison des nerfs dans l'organe électrique de la Torpille. C. R. Acad Sci. (Paris) **43**, 792—794 (1856).

KOPPANYI, T., and A. E. VIVIANO: Prevention and treatment of d-tubocurarine poisoning. Science **100**, 474—475 (1944).

KOSTER, R.: Synergisms and antagonisms between physostigmine and di-isopropyl fluorophosphate in cats. J. Pharmacol. exp. Ther. **88**, 39—46 (1946).

KOSTYUK, P. G.: Intracellular recording of muscle fibre potentials using repeated stimulation. Biofizika **3**, No. 3, 274—285 (1958).

KRAATZ, C. P., M. I. GLUCKMAN and H. L. SHIELDS: The effects of thiopental and pentobarbital on voluntary muscle. J. Pharmacol. exp. Ther. **107**, 437—458 (1953).

KRAUPP, O.: Elektrolytverschiebungen in der innervierten und denervierten Skeletmuskulatur durch Acetylcholin bei Durchströmung mit natriumchloridarmer Blut-Tyrode-Lösung. Arch. exp. Path. Pharmak. **228**, 271—287 (1956).

— H. KLUPP, H. STORMANN and CH. STUMPF: Cholinesterasehemmwirkung und neuromuskuläre Wirksamkeit von Bischolin-Polymethylendicarbaminsäure estern. Naunyn-Schmiedeberg's Arch. exp. Path. Pharmak. **222**, 180—182 (1954).

— W. KOBINGER, H. STORMANN u. G. WERNER: Über den Einfluß von Eserin und d-Tubocurarin auf die Freisetzung von Kaliumionen aus der Skeletmuskulatur durch Acetylcholin. Naunyn-Schmiedeberg's Arch. exp. Path. Pharmak. **226**, 403—416 (1955b).

— CH. STUMPF, E. HERZFELD u. B. PILLAT: Pharmakologische Eigenschaften einiger langwirksamer Cholinesterase-Hemmkörper aus der Reihe der Polymethylen-Bis-(Carbaminoyl-m-Trimethylammoniumphenole). Arch. int. Pharmacodyn. **102**, 281—303 (1955a).

KRAYER, O., A. GOLDSTEIN and F. L. PLACHTE: Studies on physostigmine and related substances. I. Quantitative relation between dosage of physostigmine and inhibition of cholinesterase activity in the blood serum of dogs. J. Pharmacol exp. Ther. **80**, 8—30(1944).

KREITMAIR, H.: Eine neue Klasse Cholinester. Naunyn-Schmiedeberg's Arch. exp. Path. Pharmak. **164**, 346—356 (1932).

KRNJEVIĆ, K., and R. MILEDI: Failure of neuromuscular propagation in rats. J. Physiol. (Lond.) **140**, 440—461 (1958a).
— — Some effects produced by adrenaline upon neuromuscular propagation in rats. J. Physiol. (Lond.) **141**, 291—304 (1958b).
— — Presynaptic failure of neuromuscular propagation in rats. J. Physiol. (Lond.) **149**, 1—22 (1959).
—, and J. F. MITCHELL: Release of acetylcholine in rat diaphragm. Nature (Lond.) **186**, 241 (1960).
— — The release of acetylcholine in the isolated rat diaphragm. J. Physiol. (Lond.) **155**, 246—262 (1961).
KRÜGER, P.: Die Grundlagen des Tetanus und Tonus der quergestreiften Skeletmuskelfasern der Wirbeltiere. Experientia (Basel) **6/2**, 75 (1950).
KRÜGER, R., u. P. G. GUNTHER: Innervation und pharmakologisches Verhalten des M. Gastrocnemius und M. Pectoralis Maior der Vögel. Acta anat. (Basel) **33**, 325—338 (1958).
KRUTA, V.: L'acétylcholine produite à l'extrémité des nerfs moteurs est-elle pratiquement efficace pour la contraction musculaire? Arch. int. Physiol. **41**, 187—200 (1935).
KUFFLER, S. W.: Electric potential changes at an isolated nerve-muscle junction. J. Neurophysiol. **5**, 18—26 (1942a).
— Responses during refractory period at myoneural junction in isolated nerve-muscle fibre preparation. J. Neurophysiol. **5**, 199—209 (1942b).
— Further study on transmission in an isolated nerve-muscle fibre preparation. J. Neurophysiol. **5**, 302—322 (1942c).
— Specific excitability of the endplate region in normal and denervated muscle. J. Neurophysiol. **6**, 99—110 (1943).
— Electric excitability of nerve muscle fibre preparations. J. Neurophysiol. **8**, 75—86 (1945).
— Physiology of neuro-muscular junctions: Electrical aspects. Fed. Proc. **7**, 437—446 (1948).
— Incomplete neuromuscular transmission in twitch system of frog's skeletal muscles. Fed. Proc. **11**, 87 (1952).
—, and R. W. GERARD: The small-nerve motor system to skeletal muscle. J. Neurophysiol. **10**, 383—394 (1947).
—, and E. M. VAUGHAN-WILLIAMS: Small-nerve junctional potentials. The distribution of small motor nerves to frog skeletal muscle, and the membrane characteristics of the fibres they innervate. J. Physiol. (Lond.) **121**, 289—317 (1953a).
— — Properties of the slow skeletal muscle fibres of the frog. J. Physiol. (Lond.) **121**, 318 to 340 (1953b).
KUNKEL, A. M., J. H. WILLS and J. S. MONIER: Antagonists to neuromuscular block produced by sarin. Proc. Soc. exp. Biol. (N. Y.) **92**, 529—532 (1956).
KUPERMAN, A. S.: Depression of mammalian neuromuscular transmission. Fed. Proc. **19**, 173 (1960).
— The molecular requirements of neuromuscular facilitation in mammals. J. Pharmacol. exp. Ther. (In preparation, 1961b).
— E. GILL and W. F. RIKER jr.: The relationship between cholinesterase inhibition and drug-induced facilitation of mammalian neuromuscular transmission. J. Pharmacol. exp. Ther. **132**, 65—73 (1961a).
—, and G. WERNER: Interaction between repetitive nerve stimulation and twitch-potentiating agents at the neuromuscular junction. Nature (Lond.) **188**, 1032—1033 (1960).
LANDS, A. M., A. G. KARCZMAR, J. W. HOWARD and A. ARNOLD: An evaluation of the pharmacologic actions of some bis-quaternary salts of basically substituted oxamides (WIN 8077 and analogs). J. Pharmacol. exp. Ther. **115**, 185—198 (1955).
LANGLEY, J. N.: On the reaction of cells and of nerve endings to certain poisons, chiefly as regards the reaction of striated muscle to nicotine and curare. J. Physiol. (Lond.) **33**, 374—413 (1905).
— On the contraction of muscle, chiefly in relation to the presence of receptive substances. J. Physiol. (Lond.) **36**, 346—384 (1907).
—, and T. KATO: The physiological action of physostigmine and its action on denervated skelltal muscle. J. Physiol. (Lond.) **49**, 410—431 (1915).
LAPORTE, Y., and R. LORENTE DE NÓ: Potential changes evoked in a curarized sympathetic ganglion by presynaptic volleys of impulses. J. cell. comp. Physiol. **35**, 61—106 (1950).
LARRABEE, M. G., and J. M. POSTERNAK: Selective action of anesthetics on synapses and axons in mammalian sympathetic ganglia. J. Neurophysiol. **15**, 91—114 (1952).
LAURENT, L. P. E.: Clinical observations on the use of prostigmin in the treatment of myasthenia gravis. Brit. med. J. **1**, 463—467 (1935).
LEHMANN, G.: The "curare-like" action of inhibitors of cholinesterase. Jubilee Volume Emil Barell, 314—326, 1946.

LEVIN, A. P., and B. J. JANDORF: Inactivation of cholinesterase by compounds related to neostigmine. J. Pharmacol. exp. Ther. **113**, 206—211 (1955).

LI, T. H., and Y. C. TING: Studies on the neuromuscular junction. XXI. Responses of cat muscles to acetylcholine during Wedensky inhibition and post-tetanic facilitation. Chin. J. Physiol. **16**, 1—8 (1941).

LILEY, A. W.: An investigation of spontaneous activity at neuromuscular junction of the rat. J. Physiol. (Lond.) **132**, 650—666 (1956a).

— The effects of presynaptic polarization on the spontaneous activity at the mammalian neuromuscular junction. J. Physiol. (Lond.) **134**, 427—443 (1956b).

—, and K. A. K. NORTH: An electrical investigation of effects of repetitive stimulation on mammalian neuromuscular junction. J. Neurophysiol. **16**, 509—527 (1953).

LILLEHEIL, G., and K. NAESS: A presynaptic effect of d-tubocurarine in the neuromuscular junction. Acta physiol. scand. **52**, 120—136 (1961).

LISSMANN, H. W.: On the function and evolution of electric organs in fish. J. exp. Biol. **35**, 156—191 (1958).

LLOYD, D. P. C.: Stimulation of peripheral nerve terminations by active muscle. J. Neurophysiol. **5**, 153—165 (1942).

LOCKE, S.: Fractionation of the motor unit during repetitive response to prostigmine. Nature (Lond.) **190**, 452—453 (1961).

—, and E. HENNEMAN: Fractionation of motor units by curare. Exper. Neurology **2**, 638—651 (1960).

LOEWI, O., u. E. NAVRATIL: Über humorale Übertragbarkeit der Herznervenwirkung. X. Mitteilung. Über das Schicksal des Vagusstoffs. Pflügers Arch. ges. Physiol. **214**, 678—688 (1926).

LORENTE DE NÓ, R.: Publications from the Rockefeller Institute of Medical Research. Vols. 131 and 132, 1947.

— On the effect of certain quaternary ammonium ions upon the frog nerve. J. cell. comp. Physiol. **33**, Suppl. I and II, 1—231 (1949).

LOW, H., and L.-E. TAMMELIN: On succinylcholine, a neuromuscular blocking drug, and its synergism with TEPP. Acta physiol. scand. **23**, 78—84 (1951).

LUFT, J. H.: The fine structure of electric tissue. Exp. Cell. Res. Suppl. **5**, 168—182 (1958).

LÜLLMANN, H., u. W. FÖRSTER: Über die Wirkungen neuromuskulär blockierender Substanzen auf den Rückenmuskel des Blutegels und den M. rectus abd. des Frosches. Naunyn-Schmiedeberg's Arch. exp. Path. Pharmak. **217**, 217—224 (1953).

LUNDBERG, A., and H. QUILISCH: Presynaptic potentiation and depression of neuromuscular transmission in frog and rat. Acta physiol. scand. **30**, 111—120 (1953).

MAANEN, E. F. v.: Antagonism of d-tubocurarine by neostigmine methylsulfate. Fed. Proc. **9**, 323 (1950a).

— The antagonism between acetylcholine and the curare alkaloids, d-tubocurarine, c-curarine-I, c-toxiferine-II and B-erythroidine in the rectus abdominis of the frog. J. Pharmacol. exp. Ther. **89**, 255—264 (1950b).

MAASKE, C. A., T. E. BOYD and J. J. BROSNAN: Inhibition and impulse summation at the mammalian neuromuscular junction. J. Neurophysiol. **1**, 332—341 (1938).

MACFARLANE, D. W., E. W. PELIKAN and K. R. UNNA: Evaluation of curarizing drugs in man. V. Antagonism to curarizing effects of d-tubocurarine by neostigmine, m-hydroxy phenyltrimethylammonium and m-hydroxy phenylethyldimethylammonium. J. pharmacol. (Kbh.) **100**, 382—392 (1950).

MANN, I. P. G., M. TENNENBAUM and I. H. QUASTEL: Acetylcholine metabolism in central nervous system; the effects of potassium and other cations on acetylcholine liberation. Biochem. J. **33**, 822—835 (1939).

MARNAY, A.: Cholinestérase dans l'organe électrique de la torpille. C. R. Soc. Biol. (Paris) **126**, 573—574 (1937).

—, and D. NACHMANSOHN: Choline esterase in voluntary muscle. J. Physiol. (Lond.) **92**, 37 to 47 (1938).

MASLAND, R. L., and R. S. WIGTON: Nerve activity accompanying fasciculation produced by prostigmin. J. Neurophysiol. **3**, 269—275 (1940).

MATTHEWS, P. B. C., and G. RUSHWORTH: The relative sensitivity of muscle nerve fibres to procaine. J. Physiol. (Lond.) **135**, 263—269 (1957).

McDOWALL, R. J. S., and R. WATSON: The inhibitory action of acetylcholine with special reference to small doses. J. Physiol. (Lond.) **114**, 515—520 (1951)

McISAAC, R. J., and G. B. KOELLE: Comparison of the effects of inhibition of external, internal and total acetylcholinesterase upon ganglionic transmission. J. Pharmacol. exp. Ther. **126**, 9—20 (1959).

McNAMARA, B. P., E. F. MURTHA, A. D. BERGNER, E. M. ROBINSON, C. W. BENDER and J. H. WILLS: Studies on the mechanism of action of DFP and TEPP. J. Pharmacol. exp. Ther. **110**, 232—240 (1954).

MEETER, E.: The relation between end-plate depolarization and the repetitive response elicited in the isolated rat phrenic nerve-diaphragm preparation by DFP. J. Physiol. (Lond.) 144, 38—51 (1958).

MENG, C.-W.: The role of cholinesterase in the sensitization of the muscle to acetylcholine. Chin. J. Physiol. 15, 143—150 (1940).

MERTON, P. A.: Interaction between muscle fibres in a twitch. J. Physiol. (Lond.) 124, 311 to 324 (1954).

— Problems of muscular fatigue. Brit. med. Bull. 12, 219—221 (1956).

MILEDI, R.: The acetylcholine sensitivity of frog muscle fibres after complete or partial denervation. J. Physiol. (Lond.) 151, 1—23 (1960a).

— Junctional and extrajunctional acetylcholine receptors in skeletal muscle fibres. J. Physiol. (Lond.) 151, 24—30 (1960b).

MIQUEL, O.: The action of physostigmine, di-isopropyl fluorophosphate and other parasympathomimetic drugs on the rectus muscle of the frog. J. Pharmacol. exp. Ther. 88, 67—71 (1946).

MODELL, W., S. KROP, P. HITCHCOCK and W. F. RIKER jr.: General systemic actions of diisopropyl fluorophosphate (DFP) in cats. J. Pharmacol. exp. Ther. 87, 400—413 (1946).

MOGEY, G A., and J. W. TREVAN: Response of the phrenic nerve of the rat to rectangular pulses of direct current. J. Physiol. (Lond.) 107, 28P (1948).

—, and P. A. YOUNG: The antagonism of curarizing activity by phenolic substances. Brit. J. Pharmacol. 4, 359—365 (1949).

MONTAGU, K. A.: On the mechanism of action of adrenaline in skeletal nerve-muscle. J. Physiol. (Lond.) 128, 619—628 (1955).

MURTHA, E. F., B. P. MCNAMARA, L. J. EDBERG, A. D. BERGNER and J. H. WILLS: Studies on the pharmacology of tetraethylpyrophosphate. J. Pharmacol. exp. Ther. 115, 291—299 (1955).

MUSCHOLL, E.: Elektrophysiologische Untersuchung der einzelnen Faseranteile des isolierten Rattenzwerchfelles. Pflügers Arch. ges. Physiol. 264, 467—483 (1957).

NACHMANSOHN, D.: Chemical mechanisms of nerve activity, in: Modern Trends in Physiology and Biochemistry; edit. E. S. Guzman Barron; p. 229—276, 1952.

— Die Rolle des Acetylcholins in den Elementarvorgängen der Nervenleitung. Ergebn. Physiol. 48, 575—683 (1955).

— Chemical and molecular basis of nerve activity. Academic Press, 1959.

— C. W. COATES and M. A. ROTHENBERG: Studies on cholinesterase. II. Enzyme activity and voltage of the action potential in electric tissue. J. biol. Chem. 163, 39—48 (1946).

— R. T. COX, C. W. COATES and A. L. MACHADO: Action potential in the electric organ of electrophorus electricus (Linnaeus). I. Choline esterase and respiration. J. Neurophysiol. 5, 499—515 (1942).

—, and I. B. WILSON: The enzymic hydrolysis and synthesis of acetylcholine. Advanc. Enzymol. 12, 259—334 (1951).

— — Molecular basis for generation of bioelectric potentials, in: Electrochemistry in Biology and Medicine, edit. T. Shedlovsky, p. 167—186, 1955.

NAESS, K.: A comparison of the effect of ether and curare on the neuro-muscular transmission, investigated by means of prostigmine. Acta physiol. scand. 20, 117—124 (1950).

— The peripheral effects of magnesium and curare. Acta pharmacol. (Kbh.) 8, 137—148 (1952a).

— The mechanism of action of curare. Acta pharmacol. (Kbh.) 8, 149—163 (1952b).

— Effects of brief and protracted curarization. Acta pharmacol. (Kbh.) 8, 400—408 (1952c).

— The specificity of diisopropyl-fluorophosphate (DFP). Acta pharmacol. (Kbh.) 12, 154—163 (1956).

—, and E. SÖGNEN: Combined action of diisopropylfluorophosphate (DFP) and botulinum toxin on the rat diaphragm preparation. Acta pharmacol. (Kbh.) 14, 333—340 (1958).

NASTUK, W. L.: Membrane potential changes at a single muscle endplate produced by acetylcholine. Fed. Proc. 10, 96 (1951).

— Membrane potential changes at a single muscle end-plate produced by transitory application of acetylcholine with an electrically controlled microjet. Fed. Proc. 12, 102 (1953).

— Relation between extracellular Na$^+$ and the depolarizing action of acetylcholine on the end-plate membrane. Fed. Proc. 13, 104 (1954).

—, and J. T. ALEXANDER: The action of 3-hydroxyphenyldimethylethylammonium (Tensilon) on neuromuscular transmission in the frog. J. Pharmacol. exp. Ther. 111, 302—328 (1954).

—, and B. O. ALVING: Further study of 3-hydroxy phenyldimethylethylammonium (Edrophonium) and its closely related analogues with respect to activity at the neuromuscular junction. Biochem. Pharmacol. 1, 307—322 (1958).

OCHS, S., and A. K. MUKHERJEE: Action of acetylcholine, choline and d-tubocurarine on the membrane of frog sartorius muscle fibres. Amer. J. Physiol. 196, 1191—1196 (1959).

OESTER, Y. T., and C. A. MAASKE: Quinine: Effects on normal and denervated skeletal muscle, and on the acetylcholine and physostigmine actions on skeletal muscle. J. Pharmacol. exp. Ther. 66, 133—145 (1939).

OGATA, M., and E. B. WRIGHT: Intracellular recording of neuromuscular junction action potential in single isolated nerve-muscle fiber. J. Neurophysiol. 23, 647—658 (1960).

OOMURA, Y., and T. TOMITA: Analysis of the junction potential of a small nerve. Nature (Lond.) 188, 416—417 (1960).

ORD, M. G., and R. H. S. THOMPSON: The distribution of cholinesterase types in mammalian tissues. Biochem. J. 46, 346—352 (1950).

OTSUKA, M., and M. ENDO: The effect of guanidine on neuromuscular transmission. J. Pharmacol. exp. Ther. 128, 273—281 (1960a).

— — Presynaptic nature of neuromuscular depression in the frog. Nature (Lond.) 188, 501—502 (1960b).

PAL, J.: Physostigmin, ein Gegengift des Curare. Zbl. Physiol. 14, 255—258 (1900).

PATON, W. D. M.: A theory of drug action based on the rate of drug-receptor combination. Proc. Roy. Soc. (B) 154, 21—69 (1961).

—, and E. J. ZAIMIS: The pharmacological actions of polymethylene bis-trimethylammonium salts. Brit. J. Pharmacol. 4, 381—400 (1949).

— — The action of d-tubocurarine and of decamethonium on respiratory and other muscles in the cat. J. Physiol. (Lond.) 112, 311—331 (1951).

— — The methonium compounds. Pharmacol. Rev. 4, 219—253 (1952).

PELIKAN, W. W., C. M. SMITH and K. R. UNNA: Mode of action of antagonists to curare. II. Anti-curare action of hydroxyphenyltrialkylammonium compounds in avian muscle. J. Pharmacol. exp. Ther. 111, 30—42 (1954).

PFEIFFER, C.: Nature and spatial relationships of the prosthetic chemical groups required for maximal muscarinic action. Science 107, 94—96 (1948).

PHILIPPOT, E.: Action de quelques dérives lauryles de l'ammonium quaternaire sur la transmission neuro-musculaire ches le rat. Arch. int. Pharmacodyn. 107, 123—125 (1956).

—, et J. SCHLAG: L'action des Sels D'alkyltriméthylammonium et d'alkyltriéthylammonium sur le potentiel de démarcation du muscle strié. Arch. int. Pharmacodyn. 106, 260—274 (1956).

PICK, E. P., and G. V. RICHARDS: The syergism of anesthetics and hypnotics with curare and curare-like alkaloids. J. Pharmacol. exp. Ther. 90, 1—13 (1947).

PILLAT, B., P. H. CLODI, O. KRAUPP u. G. WERNER: Die Wirkung von Biscarbaminoylcholinestern auf das Endplattenpotential, untersucht am Musculus gracilis der Katze. Naunyn-Schmiedeberg's Arch. exp. Path. Pharmak. 226, 563—569 (1955).

PIRQUET, A. F. v.: Zur Frage der posttetanischen Verstärkung indirekt durch Einzelreize ausgelöster Muskelreaktionen. Pflügers Arch. ges. Physiol. 240, 763—768 (1938).

PRESTON, J. B., and E. F. v. MAANEN: Effects of frequency of stimulation on the paralyzing dose of neuromuscular blocking agents. J. Pharmacol. exp. Ther. 107, 165—171 (1953).

PRITCHARD, E., and E. A. BLACK: Wedensky inhibition in myasthenia gravis. J. Physiol. (Lond.) 78, 3P (1933).

QUILLIAM, J. P., and F. G. STRONG: Some observations upon the pharmacological activity of di-isopropyl fluorophosphonate. Brit. J. Pharmacol. 4, 168—176 (1949).

—, and D. B. TAYLOR: Antagonism between curare and the potassium ion. Nature (Lond.) 160, 603 (1947).

RAJAPURKAR, M. V., and G. B. KOELLE: Reactivation of DFP-inactivated acetylcholinesterase by monoisonitroso-acetone (MINA) and diacetyl mono oxime (DAM) in vivo. J. Pharmacol exp. Ther. 123, 247—253 (1958).

RANDALL, L. O.: Anticurare action of phenolic quaternary salts. J. Pharmacol. exp. Ther. 100, 83—93 (1950).

— Synthetic curare-like agents and their antagonists. Ann. N. Y. Acad. Sci. 54, Art. 3, 460 to 474 (1951).

—, and G. LEHMANN: Pharmacological properties of some neostigmine analogs. J. Pharmacol. exp. Ther. 99, 16—32 (1950).

RAVENTOS, J.: Pharmacological actions of quaternary ammonium salts. Quart. J. exp. Physiol. 26, 361—374 (1937a).

— The effects of arterial injections of drugs on the frog's gastrocnemius. J. Physiol. (Lond.) 90, 8P—9P (1937b).

RAVIN, A.: Effects of quinine on mammalian skeletal muscle. Amer. J. Physiol. 131, 228—239 (1940).

REUBEN, J. P., F. BERGMANN and H. GRUNDFEST: Chemical excitation of presynaptic terminals at the lobster neuromuscular junctions. Biol. Bull. 117, 424 (1959).

RIESSER, O.: Untersuchungen an überlebenden roten und weißen Kaninchenmuskeln. Pflügers Arch. ges. Physiol. 190, 137—157 (1921).

RIKER, W. F., jr.: Excitatory and anti-curare properties of acetylcholine and related quaternary ammonium compounds at the neuromuscular junction. Pharmacol. Rev. 5, 1—86 (1953).
— Neuromuscular transmission. A. Analysis of the mechanism of quaternary ammonium action at the neuromuscular junction. Tokyo J. Med. Sci. 65, 107—115 (1957).
— J. ROBERTS, J. REILLY and B. B. ROY: Effect of onium charge attenuation on activity of quaternary amines on mammalian neuromuscular junction. Fed. Proc. 13, No. 1, 1304 (1954).
— — F. G. STANDAERT and H. FUJIMORI: The motor nerve terminal as the primary focus for drug-induced facilitation of neuromuscular transmission. J. Pharmacol. exp. Ther. 121, 286—312 (1957).
— G. WERNER, J. ROBERTS and A. S. KUPERMAN: The presynaptic element in neuromuscular transmission. Ann. N. Y. Acad. Sci. 81, 328—344 (1959a).
— — — Pharmacologic evidence for the existence of a presynaptic event in neuromuscular transmission. J. Pharmacol. exp. Ther. 125, 150—158 (1959b).
—, and W. C. WESCOE: The direct action of prostigmine on skeletal muscle; its relationship to the choline esters. J. Pharmacol. exp. Ther. 88, 58—66 (1946).
— — Studies on the inter-relationship of certain cholinergic compounds. V. The significance of the actions of the 3-hydroxy phenyltrimethylammonium ion on neuromuscular function. J. Pharmacol. exp. Ther. 100, 454—464 (1950).
— — The pharmacology of flaxedil with observations on certain analogues. Ann. N. Y. Acad. Sci. 54, 373—394 (1951).
— — and M. J. BROTHERS: Studies on the inter-relationship of certain cholinergic compounds. II. The effects of 3-acetoxy phenyltrimethylammonium methylsulfate on neuromuscular function. J. Pharmacol. exp. Ther. 97, 208—221 (1949).
RITCHIE, J. M., and R. W. STRAUB: The hyperpolarization which follows activity in mammalian nonmedulated fibres. J. Physiol. (Lond.) 136, 80—97 (1957).
ROBERTSON, J. D.: The ultrastructure of a reptilian myoneural junction. J. biophys. biochem. Cytol. 2, 381—393 (1956).
ROEPKE, M. H.: A study of choline esterase. J. Pharmacol. exp. Ther. 59, 264—276 (1937).
ROSENBERG, H.: Die elektrischen Organe; in: Handb. norm. pathol. Physiol. 8/2, 876—925 (1928).
ROSENBLUETH, A.: The transmission of nerve impulses at neuroeffector junctions and peripheral synapses. John Wiley & Sons, Inc. 1950.
—, and W. B. CANNON: Some features of the early stages of neuromuscular transmission. Amer. J. Physiol. 130, 205—218 (1940).
— D. B. LINDSLEY and R. S. MORISON: A study of some decurarizing substances. Amer. J. Physiol. 115, 53—68 (1936).
—, and J. V. LUCO: A study of denervated mammalian skeletal muscle. Amer. J. Physiol. 120, 781—797 (1937).
—, and R. S. MORISON: Curarization, fatigue and Wedensky inhibition. Amer. J. Physiol. 119, 236—256 (1937).
ROTHBERGER, J. C.: Über die gegenseitigen Beziehungen zwischen Curare und Physostigmin. Pflügers Arch. ges. Physiol. 87, 117—169 (1901).
ROTHENBERG, M. A.: Studies on permeability in relation to nerve function. II. Ionic movements across axonal membranes. Biochim. biophys. Acta 4, 96—114 (1950).
RUMMEL, W., u. R. SCHULZ: Gegenüberstellung von blockierenden und deblockierenden Substanzen am Zwerchfellphrenicuspräparat der Ratte. Naunyn-Schmiedeberg's Arch. exp. Path. Pharmak. 222, 533—539 (1954).
SAMOJLOFF, A.: Aktionsströme bei summierten Muskelzuckungen. Arch. Anat. Physiol. Lpz. 1—22, 1908.
SCHAEFER, H.: Über einen lokalen Erregungsstrom an der motirischen Endplatte. Pflügers Arch. ges. Physiol. 242, 364—381 (1939).
SCHLEYER, W. L.: Electrical activity in electric tissue. II. Evaluation of esterase activity in intact electroplax. Biochim. biophys. Acta 16, 396—403 (1955).
SCHOFFENIELS, E., and D. NACHMANSOHN: An isolated single electroplax preparation. I. New data on the effect of acetylcholine and related compounds. Biochim. biophys. Acta 26, 1—15 (1957).
— I. B. WILSON and D. NACHMANSOHN: Overshoot and block of conduction by lipid soluble acetylcholine analogues. Biochim. biophys, Acta 27, 629—633 (1958).
SECHER, O.: The peripheral action of ether estimated on isolated nerve muscle preparation. III. Antagonistic and synergistic actions of ether and neostigmine. Acta pharmacol. (Kbh.) 7, 103—118 (1951).
SHANES, A. M.: Potassium movement in relation to nerve activity. J. gen. Physiol. 34, 795 to 807 (1951).

676   Literature

SIRNES, T. B.: Some effects of barbituric acid derivatives on the function of the mammalian skeletal muscle. Acta pharmacol. (Kbh.) 10, Suppl. 1, 1—170 (1954).
SMITH, C. M., H. L. COHEN, E. W. PELIKAN and K. R. UNNA: Mode of action of antagonists to curare. J. Pharmacol. exp. Ther. 105, 391—399 (1952).
— J. C. MEAD and K. R. UNNA: Antagonism of tubocurarine. III. Time course of action of pyridostigmin, neostigmine and edrophonium in vivo and in vitro. J. Pharmacol. exp. Ther. 120, 215—228 (1957).
SOMERS, G. F.: Studies on the pharmacology of succinylcholine. Brit. J. Pharmacol. 8, 19—21 (1953).
SOMMERKAMP, H.: Das Substrat der Dauerverkürzung am Froschmuskel. Naunyn-Schmiedeberg's Arch. exp. Path. Pharmak. 128, 99—115 (1928).
STANDAERT, F. G.: Effect of pH on twitch facilitating potency of 3-hydroxyphenyltriethylammonium ion. Proc. Soc. exp. Biol. (N. Y.) 102, 138—139 (1959).
— The action of d-tubocurarine on the motor nerve terminal. Fed. Proc. 20, 304 (1961).
—, and S. L. FRIESS: Steric configuration and the activity at the mammalian neuromuscular junction of cyclic aminoalcohol derivatives. J. Pharmacol. exp. Ther. 128, 55—64 (1960).
STEDMAN, E.: XCIV. Studies on the relationship between chemical constitution and physiologic action. Part I. Position isomerism in relation to the miotic activity of some synthetic urethanes. Biochem. J. 20, 719—734 (1926).
— III. Studies on the relationship between chemical constitution and physiological action. Part II. The miotic activity of urethanes derived from the isomeric hydroxy-benzyl-dimethylamines. Biochem. J. 23, 17—24 (1929).
—, and G. BARGER: Physostigmine. (Eserine); part III. J. chem. Soc. 127, 247—258 (1925).
—, and E. STEDMAN: The methyl urethanes of the isomeric-hydroxyphenyl-ethyldimethyl-amines and their miotic activity. J. chem. Soc. 131, 609—617 (1929).
— — CCCV. The purification of choline-esterase. Biochem. J. 29, 2563—2567 (1935).
— — and L. H. EASSON: Cholinesterase. An enzyme present in the blood serum of the horse. Biochem. J. 26, 2056—2066 (1932).
STERN, P.: Straubs Theorie im Lichte der heutigen Auffassung der neuromuskulären Transmission. Acta neuroveget. 13, 209—216 (1956).
STEWART, W. C.: The effects of sarin and atropine on the respiratory center and neuromuscular junctions of the rat. Canad. J. Biochem. 37, 651—660 (1959).
STOVNER, J.: The effect of tetraethylammonium (TEA) and temperature on the neuromuscular block produced by magnesium. Acta physiol. scand. 41, 370—383 (1957).
— The interaction of tetraethylammonium (TEA) and diisopropylfluorophosphate (DFP) on myoneural junction. Acta pharmacol. (Kbh.) 15, 55—69 (1958a).
— The anticurare activity of tetraethylammonium (TEA). Acta pharmacol. (Kbh.) 14, 317—332 (1958b).
— The release of Acetylcholine from mammalian motor nerve endings. Brit. J. Pharmacol. 15, 417—424 (1961a).
STRAUGHAN, D. W.: The action of procaine at the neuromuscular junction. J. Pharm. Pharmacol. 13, 49—52 (1961b).
STRAUS, O. H., and A. GOLDSTEIN: Zone behavior of enzymes. J. gen. Physiol. 26, 559—585 (1943).
STRICKLAND, K. P., and R. H. S. THOMPSON: On the mechanism of potassium loss from brain slices induced by cholinesterase inhibitors. Biochem. J. 60, 468—475 (1955).
SULLIVAN, W. J., and C. J. KENSLER: Action of tetraethylammonium bromide and acetylcholine in the kitten phrenic nerve diaphragm preparation. Fed. Proc. 9, 319 (1950).
TAKEUCHI, A., and N. TAKEUCHI: Active phase of frog's end-plate potential. J. Neurophysiol. 22, 395—411 (1959).
TASAKI, I., and S. HAGIWARA: Demonstration of two stable potential states in the squid giant axon under tetraethylammonium chloride. J. gen. Physiol. 40, 859—885 (1957).
—, and K. MIZUTANI: Comparative studies on the activities of the muscle evoked by two kinds of motor nerve fibres. Jap. J. med. Sci. 10, 237—244 (1944).
—, and M. TSUKAGOSHI: Comparative studies on the activities of the muscle evoked by two kinds of motor nerve fibres. Part II. Jap. J. med. Sci. 10, 245—251 (1944).
TAUGNER, R., and A. FLECKENSTEIN: Versuche am doppelten Zwerchfellphrenikuspräparat der Ratte. Naunyn-Schmiedeberg's Arch. exp. Path. Pharmak. 209, 286—306 (1950).
TAYLOR, I. M., and J. M. WELLER: Studies on the permeability of human erythrocytes to potassium. Biol. Bull. 99, 311 (1950).
THESLEFF, S.: The mode of neuromuscular block caused by acetylcholine, nicotine, decamethonium and succinylcholine. Acta physiol. scand. 34, 218—231 (1955a).
— The effects of acetylcholine, decamethonium and succinylcholine on neuromuscular transmission in the rat. Acta physiol. scand. 34, 386—392 (1955b).

THESLEFF S. A further analysis of the neuromuscular block caused by acetylcholine. Acta physiol. scand. **37**, 330—334 (1956).
— Motor endplate 'desensitization' by repetitive nerve stimuli. J. Physiol. (Lond.) **148**, 659 to 664 (1959).
— Supersensitivity of skeletal muscle produced by botulinum toxin. J. Physiol. (Lond.) **151**, 598—607 (1960).
—, and K. R. UNNA: Differences in mode of neuromuscular blockade in a series of symmetric bis-quaternary ammonium salts. J. Pharmacol. exp. Ther. **111**, 99—113 (1954).
THIES, R. E.: Electrophysiological studies of acetylcholine release during repetitive neuromuscular transmission. Thesis, The Rockefeller Institute, New York (1960).
TODRICK, A.: The inhibition of cholinesterases by antagonists of acetylcholine and histamine. Brit. J. Pharmacol. **9**, 76—83 (1954).
TOMAN, J. E. P.: The neuropharmacology of anti-epileptics. EEC Clin. Neurophysiol. **1**, 33 to 44 (1949).
TREVAN, J. W.: Bertram Louis Abraham Lecture, Royal College of Physicians, 1948 (quoted from: Mogey, G. A. and P. A. Young). Brit. J. Pharmacol. **4**, 359—365 (1949).
VAHLQUIST, B.: On the esterase activity of human blood plasma. Skand. arch. Physiol. **72**, 133—160 (1935).
VAN DER KLOOT, W. G.: Cholinesterase and sodium transport by frog muscle. Nature (Lond.) **178**, 366—367 (1956).
— The effect of enzyme inhibition on the resting potential and on the ion distribution of the sartorius muscle of the frog. J. gen. Physiol. **41**, 879—900 (1958).
— Factor S-A substance which excites crustacean muscle. J. Neurochem. **5**, 245—252 (1960).
VAN DER MEER, C., and E. MEETER: The mechanism of action of anticholinesterases. II. The effect of diisopropylfluorophosphonate (DFP) on the isolated rat phrenic nerve-diaphragm preparation. A. Irreversible effects. Acta physiol. pharmacol. neerl. **4**, 454—571 (1956a).
— — The mechanism of action of anticholinesterases. II. The effect of diisopropylfluorophosphonate (DFP) in the isolated rat phrenic nerve-diaphragm preparation. B. Reversible effects. Acta physiol. pharmacol. neerl. **4**, 472—481 (1956b).
WACHHOLDER, K., and F. NOTHMANN: Jahreszeitliches Schwanken zwischen „tonischem" und „nicht tonischem" Verhalten von Wirbeltiermuskeln. Pflügers Arch. ges. Physiol. **229**, 120—132 (1932).
—, and J. VON LEDEBUR: Untersuchungen über „tonische" und „nicht tonische" Wirbeltiermuskeln. Pflügers Arch. ges. Physiol. **225**, 627—642 (1930).
— — Die Erregbarkeit der „tonischen" und „nicht tonischen" Fasern eines Muskels bei direkter und indirekter Reizung. Ein kritischer Beitrag zur Frage des Isochronismus von Nerv und Muskel. Pflügers Arch. ges. Physiol. **228**, 183—197 (1931).
WALKER, M. B.: Treatment of myasthenia gravis with physostigmine. Lancet **1934 I**, 1200 to 1201.
WELSH, J. H., and H. T. GORDON: The mode of action of certain insecticides on the arthropod nerve axon. J. cell. comp. Physiol. **30**, 147—171 (1947).
—, and R. TAUB: The significance of the carbonyl group and ether oxygen in the reaction of acetylcholine with receptor substance. J. Pharmacol. exp. Ther. **103**, 62—73 (1951).
WERNER, G.: The presynaptic action of d-tubocurarine and flaxedil at the neuromuscular junction. Fed. Proc. **18**, 458 (1959).
— Neuromuscular facilitation and antidromic discharges in motor nerves; their relation to activity in motor nerve terminals. J. Neurophysiol. **23**, 171—187 (1960a).
— Generation of antidromic activity in motor nerves. J. Neurophysiol. **23**, 453—461 (1960b).
— Antidromic activity in motor nerves and its relation to a generator event in nerve terminals. J. Neurophysiol. **24**, 401—413 (1961a).
— Spontaneous miniature activity and gradation of transmission at the neuromuscular function. Experientia (Basel) **17**, 95—96 (1961b).
— O. KRAUPP, W. KOBINGER u. H. STORMANN: Freisetzung von Kaliumionen aus innervierter und denervierter Skeletmuskulatur durch Tetramethylammoniumbromid. Naunyn-Schmiedeberg's Arch. exp. Path. Pharmak. **227**, 1—11 (1955).
— W. F. RIKER, J. ROBERTS and A. S. KUPERMAN: A new approach to the study of neuromuscular transmission. Army Chemical Center., Symp. IX: Vol. 1, 33—45 (1959).
WESCOE, W. C., and W. F. RIKER jr.: The pharmacology of anti-curare agents. Ann. N. Y. Acad. Sci. **54**, 438—455 (1951).
— —, and V. L. BEACH: Studies on the inter-relationship of certain cholinergic compounds. III. The reactions between 3-acetoxy phenyltrimethylammonium methylsulfate, 3-hydroxy phenyltrimethylammonium bromide and cholinesterases. J. Pharmacol. exp. Ther. **99**, 265—276 (1950).
— —, and M. J. BROTHERS: Studies of the inter-relationship of certain cholinergic compounds. I. The pharmacology of 3-acetoxy phenyltrimethylammonium methylsulfate. J. Pharmacol. exp. Ther. **97**, 190—207 (1949).

WHITE, A. C., and E. STEDMAN: On the physostigmine-like action of certain synthetic urethanes. J. Pharmacol. exp. Ther. 41, 259—288 (1931).

WHITTAKER, V. P.: Hydrolysis of succinylcholine by cholinesterase: simultaneous utilization of paper chromatography and Warburg technique. Experientia (Basel) 7/6, 217—218 (1951) (Italian).

— The isolation and characterization of acetylcholine containing particles from brain. Biochem. J. 72, 694—706 (1959).

WIERSMA, C. A. G.: The efferent innervation of muscle. Biol. Symp. 3, 259—289 (1941).

WILLS, J. H., A. M. KUNKEL, R. V. BROWN and G. E. GROBLEWSKI: Pyridine-2-aldoxime methiodide and poisoning by anticholinesterases. Science 125, 743—744 (1957).

WILSON, A. T., and S. WRIGHT: Anti-curare action of potassium and other substances. Quart. J. exp. Physiol. 26, 127—139 (1936).

WILSON, I. B.: Mechanism of hydrolysis: New evidence for an acylated enzyme as intermediate. Biochim. biophys. Acta 7, 520—525 (1951).

— Acetylcholinesterase: XII: Further studies on binding forces. J. biol. Chem. 197, 215—225 (1952).

— The interaction of tensilon and neostigmine with acetylcholinesterase (1). Arch. int. Pharmacodyn. 104, 204—213 (1955).

—, and F. BERGMANN: Studies on cholinesterase. VII. the active surface of acetylcholine esterase derived from effects of pH on inhibitors. J. biol. Chem. 185, 479—489 (1950).

—, and E. CABIB: Acetylcholinesterase: Enthalpies and Entropies of activation. J. Amer. chem. Soc. 78, 202—207 (1956).

—, and C. QUAN: Acetylcholinesterase studies on molecular complementariness. Arch. Biochem. 73, 131—143 (1958).

ZAIMIS, E. J.: The action of decamethonium on normal and denervated mammalian muscle. J. Physiol. (Lond.) 112, 176—190 (1951).

ZIFF, M., F. P. JAHN and R. R. RENSHAW: The acetylcholine-cholinesterase system. J. Amer. chem. Soc. 60, 179—182 (1938).

ZIPF, K.: Die Austauschbindung als Grundlage der Aufnahme basischer und saurer Fremdsubstanzen in die Zelle. Teil I und II. Naunyn-Schmiedeberg's Arch. exp. Path. Pharmak. 124, 259—325 (1927).

ZUPANCIC, A. O.: The mode of action of acetylcholine. A theory extended to a hypothesis on the mode of action of other biologically active substances. Acta physiol. scand. 29, 63—71 (1953).

Chapter 14

Actions at the Central Nervous System

By

Xenia Machne and Klaus R. W. Unna*

Contents

Introduction

A number of comprehensive reviews has been devoted to the function of acetylcholine (ACh) in the central nervous system (C.N.S.) (FELDBERG 1945, 1950,
Symposium on Neurohumoral Transmission 1954, PERRY 1956). The reviews
mustered the evidence regarding cholinergic mechanisms in the C.N.S. Frequently,
results obtained with anticholinesterase (anti-ChE) agents are included in these
reviews as supportive of cholinergic transmission. The same applies to numerous
original contributions dealing with cholinergic transmission of impulses in the
brain; few investigations have been devoted exclusively to study of the effects of
anti-ChE agents on the C.N.S. The only complete review of the pharmacology of

---

* The authors express their gratitude to Miss PEGGY J. DAVIS for her assistance in the
literature search.

anti-ChE agents presently available is the excellent one by HOLMSTEDT (1959) which, however, does not include cholinesterase (ChE) inhibitors other than organophosphorus compounds.

Knowledge of the role of ACh is fragmentary, most observations having been limited to a particular site within the C.N.S. The data on anti-ChE agents follow the scatter of experimentation with ACh; thus they are biased. Many of these investigations employing anti-ChE agents and interpreting their effects as supportive of a cholinergic mechanism in the brain are open to criticism and reinvestigation for a variety of reasons. The effect of anti-ChE agents has rarely been correlated with their primary mode of action, namely, inhibition of specific enzymes. In many studies, single and arbitrarily large doses of anti-ChE agents have been employed without considering the possibility that large doses may have effects opposite to those of small doses which are expected to facilitate the action of ACh in transmitting impulses across neuronal synapses. A critical survey of present evidence reveals the lack of pertinent data regarding the effects of different doses of anti-ChE agents on the same test object, and the correlation of these effects with the spectrum of action of a wide dose range of ACh. Very few attempts have been successful in obtaining information on a correlation between a dose effect on a certain function of the brain and an enzyme effect. Crucial evidence is not at hand to link the functional effect of any anti-ChE agent in the brain to inhibition of a specific enzyme at a specific cellular site. Difficulties and baffling frustrations in experimenting on central neurons (as compared to the dissectable peripheral ones) and possibly the ever present temptations to operate in analogies have so far prevented the experimenters from reaching these specific objectives. At present, it appears to the reviewers that the wealth of observations made by so many contributors in this field can not be explained by a unit concept of mode of action. Advances in methodology and further arduous experimentation are expected to provide indisputable facts regarding sites and modes of action of anti-ChE agents in the C.N.S.; such knowledge will be essential for an advance in our understanding of interneuronal communication and brain function.

This chapter will consist mainly of observations on the effects of anti-ChE agents on particular sites of the C.N.S.; it will follow the few established paths of methodology. Present experimental methods measure effects of anti-ChE agents indirectly by responses to electrical stimulation of nerves or neuronal aggregates within the brain, by responses to ACh or anoxia, or by the antagonistic action of cholinergic blocking agents. Thus, anatomical site does not necessarily mean site of drug action, but is rather understood as the site where drug effects have been measured.

Only the results of experiments in which the central origin of drug effects was established will be considered. Data on ChE levels in the brain have been included only where such information has contributed to the interpretation of the effects of anti-ChE agents on brain function.

The scarcity of data does not permit a differentiation of ChE inhibitors according to their duration of action and reversibility, their action on true ChE (specific ChE, acetylcholinesterase, AChE) and pseudo-cholinesterase (nonspecific ChE, BuChE), or their ability to penetrate the blood-brain barrier. In the absence of information on dose-response relations, no emphasis has been placed on relative potencies.

The presentation will progress in anatomical fashion, starting from the cortex. The headings serve to group observations on anti-ChE effects made in a certain functional area without implying site of action.

A. Cerebral cortex, hippocampus, and midbrain reticular formation

I. Isolated cerebral cortex

Topical application of ACh (0.2 to 1%) preceded by local application of physostigmine (eserine) (1%) to cat's cortex enhanced the low amplitude electrical activity which may be recorded from isolated cortical areas (KRISTIANSEN and COURTOIS 1949) and produced a convulsive type of activity in the silent slab (INFANTELLINA 1955). On the other hand, topical application of ACh or eserine alone depressed the cortical response to electrical stimulation. Intracarotid injection of ACh in doses from 0.2 to 0.4 μg restored electrical activity, while larger doses were ineffective (INFANTELLINA 1955). The author suggested the possibility that ACh may have a stimulant effect on deep layers of the cortex and an inhibitory action on superficial elements. However, the contrasting results may have depended entirely on drug concentration at different cortical levels.

II. Topical application

Application of eserine (1%) to the cortex of cats or rabbits caused reduction in amplitude of electrocortical activity (MILLER et al. 1940). Comparable effects were elicited by ACh (0.001 to 1%). Acetylcholine (0.2 to 1%) applied to the previously eserinized cortex evoked characteristic spikes in the electroencephalogram (EEG). CHATFIELD and DEMPSEY (1942) noted that 1% neostigmine (Prostigmine) produced a transient depression of spontaneous electrical activity of the cortex of the cat, while ACh (1%) was ineffective. However, ACh applied after neostigmine increased the spontaneous activity. The "primary" cortical response to stimulation of a peripheral nerve with single shocks was either unchanged or slightly reduced after treatment. The repetitive response which under nembutal anesthesia sometimes follows the primary sensory potential was instead greatly increased in magnitude and duration. BECKETT and GELLHORN (1948) found that application of eserine sulfate (1%) followed by ACh (10%) to cortical suppressor areas caused a temporary suppression or diminution of electrocortical activity and elimination of the responsiveness of the motor cortex to electrical stimulation in cats and monkeys. The responsiveness to afferent stimuli, on the other hand, was enhanced. The authors inferred from these observations that ACh has a stimulant action on suppressor neurones as well as on other cortical neurones. CHATFIELD and PURPURA (1954) reported that neostigmine (2%) and ACh (2%) topically applied to the sensory cortex of the cat depressed evoked primary potentials and simultaneously elicited spontaneous spiking in the EEG. To explain their results, the authors postulated the existence of two cholinergic mechanisms, one of which would be inhibitory of the other. The inhibitory mechanism cannot be presently identified with any known cerebral system. CHATFIELD and LORD (1955) examined the effects of atropine (2%) on evoked cortical potentials in the cat. Atropine increased the amplitude of the potentials and facilitated transmission of impulses in transcortical pathways. Even after maximal effects had been reached, neostigmine and ACh could subsequently cause a further augmentation of the atropine effects. The authors concluded that atropine probably acts in deeper cortical layers by blocking a presumably cholinergic cortical inhibitory system, while ACh may be involved in transmission within specific afferent and other systems in the cerebral cortex. BONNET (1957, 1958) examined the effects of eserine on the sustained negative cortical potential or dendritic response elicited by repetitive stimulation of the surface of the cortex, of non-specific thalamic nuclei, of the mesencephalic reticular formation, and of specific thalamic nuclei in *encéphale isolé* preparations of cats.

Eserine sulfate (1 to 5%), applied locally to the recording site, augmented the amplitude and the duration of the dendritic response. This result was taken to support the view that cholinergic transmission may occur at axo-dendritic synapses, although neither atropine nor dihydro-β-erythroidine exhibited antagonistic action.

Topical application of ACh (0.01 to 1%) decreased or abolished the activity of single units in the cerebellar cortex of the cat (CREPAX et al. 1957). Eserine (1%) was usually ineffective; sometimes it produced a slight decrease in activity. Acetylcholine after eserine increased the frequency of firing, and burst-like discharges appeared.

The difficulty in drawing any conclusions from these data is apparent. The variety of methods employed to evaluate drug effects, the great range of doses in which the drugs were used, and the fact that the experiments were performed on different species and preparations exclude the possibility of a direct comparison of the results obtained by different authors. There is general agreement with regard to the results obtained when ACh was applied after eserine or neostigmine, in that the changes observed indicate a stimulant action. Contrasting results were obtained when anti-ChE agents alone were applied to the cortex. The discrepancies suggest that not all their effects are attributable to ChE inhibition.

III. Effects on the electrical activity of the cortex and of the hippocampus induced by intracarotid or systemic administration

1. Physostigmine and neostigmine

Intracarotid injection of physostigmine or neostigmine (0.1 to 0.5 mg/kg) in cats with a high spinal section produced electrocortical arousal (BREMER and CHATONNET 1949). The primary response to brief auditory stimuli was occluded. Atropine (0.5 mg/kg i.v.) abolished the effects. BRADLEY and ELKES (1953, 1957) examined the effects of physostigmine and neostigmine in the conscious cat. Physostigmine (0.05 to 0.1 mg/kg i.p.) produced fast, low amplitude activity without concomitant behavioral alertness. It abolished the slow activity produced by atropine, and it also abolished, in acute preparations, the sleep patterns produced by high spinal or midbrain sections. Neostigmine (0.2 to 0.4 mg/kg) caused an effect on the electrical activity of the brain only in doses which produced marked peripheral effects.

Several authors studied the action of eserine (0.05 to 0.25 mg/kg i.v.) on the electrical activity of rabbit brain. LONGO and SILVESTRINI (1957) observed a widespread desynchronization of the EEG waves and blockade of the cortical recruiting response obtained by stimulation of the anteromedial nuclei of the thalamus. BRÜCKE and STUMPF (1957) obtained typical electrical arousal patterns in the hippocampus, and SAILER and STUMPF (1957) noted that physostigmine produced electrical patterns of arousal both in the neocortex and in the hippocampus which were comparable to those obtained by stimulation of the reticular formation. However, after septal lesions, eserine produced in the hippocampus high frequency activity similar to neocortical arousal (MAYER and STUMPF 1958). Thus, the pattern of arousal elicited by physostigmine in the hippocampus when the brain is intact may be only the result of the effects on the reticular formation, which in turn drives the hippocampal rhythm. According to BROWN and GANGLOFF (1959), EEG arousal induced by eserine was not accompanied by behavioral changes in rabbits. Physostigmine (0.1 to 0.3 mg/kg i.v.) produced electrocortical activation in rabbits in which the brain had been transected at the ponto-mesencephalic junction, but was ineffective in animals in which the midbrain had been transected (WHITE and DAIGNEAULT 1959).

No change in the electrical activity was obtained by MAC LEAN (1957a) after injecting physostigmine into the cat's hippocampus through implanted needles; on the other hand, ACh (50 μg) in conjunction with physostigmine induced in the hippocampus rhythmic potentials at about 20/second followed by high-voltage spikes.

BREMER and STOUPEL (1959) re-examined the action of eserine (0.2 mg/kg i.v.) in *encéphale isolé* preparations of cats. Eserine was found to prolong the facilitation of cortical evoked potentials which is normally produced by a preceding conditioning shock to the reticular formation. The effect was abolished by 2 mg/kg of atropine. These findings support the hypothesis of a cholinergic relay in reticulo-cortical paths.

2. Other anticholinesterase agents

On repeated administration of di*iso*propyl phosphorofluoridate (DFP) to man, EEG changes consisting in an increase in amplitude and frequency were reported by GROB et al. (1947). These effects were abolished by atropine.

WESCOE et al. (1948) injected DFP (3 mg i.v.) into cats and monkeys. The drug produced consistently an increase in frequency and decrease in voltage in electrocortical potentials. The action of DFP could be prevented by atropine (3 mg i.v.). FREEDMAN et al. (1949), ESSIG et al. (1950), and HAMPSON et al. (1950) described grand mal like EEG patterns in rabbits after intracarotid injection of DFP (0.1 to 1 mg/kg). Intracarotid injection of DFP in cats augmented the potentials evoked in the optic cortex by stimulation of the optic tract (MARAZZI and HART 1950). Intravenous injection of DFP in doses up to 3 to 4 mg/kg abolished the spindle activity in cats with high spinal or midbrain sections (BRADLEY et al. 1953). In the animals anesthetized with pentobarbital, DFP replaced the barbiturate spindles by a 4 to 6/second rhythm, which could be abolished by midbrain section. RINALDI and HIMWICH (1955) described long lasting patterns of alertness in rabbits after intracarotid injection of DFP (0.3 to 1.1 mg/kg). The effects could be abolished by atropine (0.5 to 1 mg/kg i.v.). DESMEDT and LA GRUTTA (1955a, 1955b, 1957) attempted to find out whether pharmacological arousal elicited by anti-ChE drugs could be attributed to differential inactivation of either the AChE or the pseudo-ChE of the brain. For this purpose they chose a number of compounds which are known to inhibit selectively either type of ChE, including DFP, Ro-2-0683 (Nu 683, the dimethylcarbamate of [2-hydroxy-5-phenylbenzyl]-trimethylammonium Br), BW 284C51e (1,5-*bis*[4-allyldimethylammoniumphenyl] pentan-3-one dibromide), and Ro-2-1250 (Nu 1250, the N-*p*-chlorophenyl-N-methylcarbamate of *m*-hydroxyphenyltrimethylammonium Br). Since the selectivity varies from one species to another, they first assessed the degree of selectivity of the inhibitors on homogenates of cat's brain; DFP and Ro-2-0683 inactivated pseudo-ChE at much lower concentrations than AChE; conversely, Ro-2-1250 and BW 284C51e were more efficient against AChE. In addition, the inhibitors were standardized *in vivo* by examining their potentiating action on the indirect twitch of the cat's tibialis muscle; the inhibitors selective for AChE potentiated the twitch more effectively than the inhibitors selective for pseudo-ChE. Intracarotid injection of all four anti-ChE agents accelerated and desynchronized the spontaneous cerebral rythm and produced occlusion of the surface-positive evoked potentials in sensory areas in *encéphale isolé* preparations of cats. However, the inhibitors selective for pseudo-ChE were much more effective in producing arousal than those selective for AChE (mean threshold doses: 5 μg Ro-2-0683 or 12 μg DFP vs.

70 μg Ro-2-1250 or 225 μg BW 284C51e). Similar results were also obtained in the preparation "*cerveau sans reticulée*", and upon intraarterial injection in preparations in which, by means of various ligatures, the drug was forced into the internal maxillary or the ascending pharyngeal artery. Thus, the authors concluded that the pharmacological arousal produced in the cat's brain by small doses of anti-ChE agents results from inhibition of the pseudo-ChE and not of the AChE.

DESMEDT and FRANKEN (1957) were able to produce EEG arousal by injecting 100 μg of eserine i.v. into cats after transection of the brain at the level of the mammillary bodies. On the other hand, the same dose of eserine had no effect on the behavior of cats which had been decorticated several days prior to the tests. These findings indicate that EEG activation induced by anti-ChE agents depends on drug effects which occur at the cortical level rather than within the reticular formation.

IV. Effects on the midbrain reticular formation and the diffuse thalamic projection system

Intracarotid injection of eserine (10 to 50 μg) produced an increase in the frequency of firing of single reticular units in the mesencephalic tegmentum of the cat (DESMEDT and SCHLAG 1957). The cortical recruiting response obtained in rabbits by stimulation of the antero-medial nuclei of the thalamus was reduced after i.v. injection of eserine (0.025 to 0.1 mg/kg) (LONGO and SILVESTRINI 1957, SAILER and STUMPF 1957). Physostigmine (0.020 to 0.035 mg/kg i.v.) lowered the threshold of electrical stimulation of the reticular formation for EEG arousal, while the threshold for behavioral arousal was unaltered (BRADLEY and KEY 1958). According to BROWN and GANGLOFF (1959), eserine (100 μg/kg i.v.) had no effect on the arousal induced by stimulation of the reticular formation in rabbits.

There is general agreement that intracarotid or systemic administration of ChE inhibitors in appropriate doses elicits electrocortical patterns of arousal. Although anti-ChE agents appear to enhance the activity of the reticular formation, experimental evidence indicates that EEG activation obtained with various anti-ChE agents depends at least in part on drug effects which occur at the cortical level.

On the assumption that a cholinergic mechanism may exist at some level of the reticulo-cortical paths involved in producing electrocortical "arousal", RIEHL and UNNA (1960) investigated the action of muscarine and arecoline on the EEG. Both muscarine and arecoline produced patterns of EEG activation in small doses (0.01 to 0.5 μg/kg, and 0.5 to 1.0 μg/kg, respectively). Methylatropine antagonized completely the effects of muscarine. Those of large doses of arecoline (50 μg/kg) were not abolished by methylatropine. Thus, besides "muscarinic" synapses, atropine-resistant or "nicotinic" synapses may be involved in the EEG activation response.

Although a considerable amount of evidence has been brought forward to support the existence of a cholinergic mechanism along these pathways, none of the present data contributes much to the knowledge of the site at which this cholinergic mechanism is located: cholinergic synapses may be found in both, the cortex and the reticular formation.

V. Action on convulsive activity

WILLIAMS and RUSSELL (1941) observed that subcutaneous injection of eserine salicylate in doses not large enough to cause peripheral autonomic effects (1 to 2 mg) reduced petit mal activity in the EEG induced by overbreathing and also spontaneous epileptic discharges, while larger doses increased epileptic activity. Neostigmine (0.6 to 2 mg, subcutaneously) invariably caused an increase in the petit mal activity. In patients with histories suggesting idiopathic epilepsy but with normal EEG patterns, eserine (0.15 to 0.35 mg) may evoke in the EEG episodes characteristic of petit mal activity (LESNÝ and VOJTA 1960).

KEITH and STAVRAKI (1935) were unable to modify convulsions induced by thujone in cats and rabbits by i.v. administration of 1 mg/kg of eserine. Local application of ACh (0.2%) or eserine (0.2 to 1%) enhanced strychnine spikes in the cerebral cortex of rabbits (SJÖSTRAND 1937). SCHWEITZER and WRIGHT (1937a) examined the anti-strychnine action of neostigmine (0.5 to 1 mg/kg), Stedman's "meta" compound (the methylcarbamic ester of m-hydroxyphenyltrimethyl ammonium I) (0.1 to 0.2 mg/kg), and eserine injected i.v. in chloralosed cats. Eserine did not influence the convulsions, while the other two drugs diminished, abolished, or delayed the onset of strychnine (0.1 to 1 mg/kg) convulsions. DARROW et al. (1944) reported that physostigmine (0.27 to 0.67 mg i.v.) prevented the effects of hyperventilation on the EEG in cats. Eserine administered i.v. (0.1 mg/kg) or applied directly (0.1 to 1%) to the exposed cortex of cats has been reported to facilitate the convulsive response to a series of widely different chemical substances (strychnine, picrotoxin, pentylenetetrazol, mescaline) by HYDE et al. (1949). Neostigmine (0.025 to 0.1 mg/kg i.v.), like eserine, exerted a facilitating effect on convulsive activity in doses which were without significant effect on blood pressure or heart rate. Diisopropyl phosphorofluoridate was without effect whether administered i.v. (0.02 to 1 mg/kg) or applied directly (0.002 to 10%) to the cortex. Spiking produced by topical application of curare or penicillin in cats was inhibited by i.v. injection of eserine (0.25 mg/kg); i.v. injection of neostigmine (0.1 mg/kg) had no effect (FUNDERBURK and CASE 1951).

The contradictory results do not permit one to draw any conclusions about the mechanism by which anti-ChE agents may enhance convulsive activity; present data do not support a facilitating action on cholinergic transmission. This conclusion is in keeping with the results obtained in investigations of the possible role of ACh in epilepsy. Many authors have assumed that the convulsant effects of ACh (observed both in man and in experimental animals) simulate conditions which occur in other experimental types of epilepsy as well as in human epilepsy. However, no satisfactory evidence has been brought forward to support this view. An investigation by ARDUINI and MACHNE (1948) on the Jacksonian epilepsy produced in rabbits by application of ACh in minimum concentrations of 4 to 10% to the masticatory cortex showed that the convulsant effects of ACh were potentiated by local eserine and prevented by i.v. injection of atropine. However, atropine never abolished or decreased faradic, spontaneous, or reflex epilepsy. These observations and the fact that the convulsant doses of ACh are so excessive that they could hardly be compared with the physiological concentrations of the transmitter, led the authors to conclude that their results had only a pharmacological meaning and did not favor the possibility that epilepsy might be due to accumulation of the transmitter at a synaptic level. Furthermore, it should be noted that while small doses of ACh (0.2 μg) injected into the carotid artery have a stimulant action on the cortex, larger doses depress the cortex and may even abolish epileptic discharges elicited by topical application of strychnine and by afferent sensory stimulation (MORUZZI 1946). Thus, the significance of the presence of ACh in the cerebrospinal fluid of epileptic patients and of the concomitant changes in cerebrospinal fluid cholinesterase fraction patterns reported by TOWER and McEACHERN (1949a, b) awaits further elucidation.

VI. In amphibians

Studies on the isolated frog brain by BROOKS et al. (1949) included measurements of the effects of a great number of agents on electrical activity, on ChE activity, and on O_2 consumption. With the exception of eserine, ChE inhibitors (DFP, tetraethyl pyrophosphate [TEPP], eserine) added to the fluid surrounding the brain decreased oxygen consumption at concentrations which did not inhibit ChE activity. The anti-ChE agents did not produce the same electrical pattern. Di*iso*prophyl phosphofluoridate depressed the amplitude of the waves, while TEPP and eserine increased it; eserine and DFP, but not TEPP, markedly slowed the rhythm. The authors concluded that the changes in electrical activity were related to decreased O_2 consumption since similar effects were obtained with fluoroacetates. The effects of DFP and TEPP on electrical patterns were independent of ChE inhibition; eserine antagonized the effects of DFP on metabolism and function as measured by electrical potentials.

B. Effects of anticholinesterase drugs on behavior

CHUTE et al. (1940) noted that the addition of eserine (0.00,000,25 to 0.00,000,3%) to the perfusion fluid increased reflex excitability in the isolated cat's brain, with spontaneous movements followed by depression.

SCHIFF et al. (1950), APRISON et al. (1954), HARWOOD (1954), DIAMANT (1954), and DIAMANT and HEILBRONN (1957) examined the vestibular syndrome (compulsive circling) caused by intracarotid injection of ChE inhibitors (DFP, 0.1 to 2 mg/kg; Tabun (ethyl-N,N-dimethyl phosphoramidocyanidate), 0.03 mg/kg; TEPP (tetraethyl pyrophosphate), 0.2 to 0.3 mg/kg; Paraoxon (diethyl 4-nitrophenyl phosphate, Mintacol, E 600), 0.5 to 1 mg/kg; eserine, 0.1 to 0.4 mg/kg) in rabbits, cats, and guinea pigs. The results indicate that the syndrome was probably induced by central excitation, since it could not be obtained after destruction of the vestibular nuclei in the brain stem. Although an asymmetric depletion of ChE in the two hemispheres could be demonstrated, it was not established that the enzyme-inhibiting action of anti-ChE agents was responsible for the occurrence of the syndrome. In guinea pigs, ACh elicited the syndrome only in exceptional cases, while methacholine (Mecholyl) was effective in approximately one third of the cases. Dimenhydrinate and diphenhydramine corrected the abnormal behavior in rabbits. Microinjection of DFP into the caudate nucleus also produced forced circus movements (WHITE 1956) which could be prevented by atropine; the ChE activity in the caudate nucleus was greatly decreased with respect to normal.

Intrathecal injections of eserine (10 μg to 1 mg), neostigmine (50 μg to 1 mg), Sarin (*iso*propyl methylphosphonofluoridate) (1 to 10 μg/kg), and DFP (10 μg to 2 mg) produced in different species (cats, dogs, sheep, and rats) abnormal movements, alteration of awareness, electrographic changes, and neuro-vegetative effects (EMMELIN and JACOBSOHN 1945, MUIRHEAD-COOKE et al. 1952, COOKE and SHERWOOD 1954, FELDBERG and SHERWOOD 1954, HEYMANS et al. 1956, HORNYKIEWICZ and KOBINGER 1956, PALMER 1959, BROWN 1959, 1960). Similar effects had been observed also in man (HENDERSON and WILSON 1936).

EGLIN (1953) injected ACh in conjunction with eserine into the lateral and posterior groups of nuclei of the hypothalamus of cats. The animals showed angry behavior but were submissive to petting between growls. Application of physostigmine with ACh to the posterior cingulate gyrus in cats elicited changes of sexual behavior (MAC LEAN 1955). When the same drugs were applied to the hippocampus in unrestrained cats, the animals exhibited pseudocatatonic manifestations associated with hippocampal seizure discharges (MAC LEAN 1954, 1957b).

PICKFORD (1947), DUKE et al. (1950), and ABRAHAMS and PICKFORD (1956) described the effects of injections of eserine salicylate (7 μg) and DFP (120 μg) into the supraoptic nucleus of choralose-anesthetized dogs. The administration of eserine resulted in an inhibition of the rate of urine flow. The immediate effect of DFP was a profound inhibition of urine flow, while its delayed effects consisted in a marked polyuria, lasting up to 19 days. GROSSMAN (1960) reported that chemical stimulation of the hypothalamus with ACh plus physostigmine caused an increase of water intake in rats.

Eserine restored normal maze-traversing in rats, the performance of which had been impaired by atropine administration (MIKHEL'SON et al. 1954). KRECH et al. (1956) determined the level of ChE activity in the visual and somesthetic areas of the cerebral cortex of rats previously tested in the KRECH hypothesis apparatus under the progressively solvable training procedure. The results suggested that a high ChE level was associated with an ability to maintain a probabilistic response pattern, while a low ChE level was associated with a more thorough commitment to the dominant stimulus. CHOW and JOHN (1958) injected physostigmine and DFP (doses up to 7 μg) either into the lateral ventricle or into the cerebral cortex of rats and observed that the drugs did not alter the behavioral performance in running a maze. The results were taken to indicate that "hypotheses behavior" does not depend on cortical levels of ACh.

The only study of the effects of an anti-ChE agent on perception reported that inhalation of Sarin increased significantly the absolute visual (scotopic) threshold in man (RUBIN and GOLDBERG 1958).

C. Respiratory and cardiovascular effects due to central action

SCHWEITZER and WRIGHT (1938a) studied the effects of neostigmine and eserine on the respiration of cats under chloralose anesthesia. Small doses of neostigmine (0.25 mg i.v.) acted as a stimulant, while larger doses (over 0.5 mg i.v.) had an inhibitory effect, either preceded or followed by periods of respiratory stimulation. The initial stimulation could be abolished by elimination of the vaso-sensory nerves. The inhibition and secondary stimulation were at least in part attributable to drug action on the central nervous system. Eserine (2 mg or more, i.v.) depressed the respiration, but was less potent than neostigmine in this respect. GESELL and HANSEN (1943) observed that i.a. or i.v. injections of eserine (0.7 to 3 mg) produced in the dog a reinforcement of thoracic expiratory contractions and a temporary irregularity of torsal inspiratory contractions associated with subnormal pulmonary ventilation. The effects occurred also after chemoreceptor denervation. Respiration could be restored by injection of atropine, 1 mg i.v. HEYMANS et al. (1946) were unable to demonstrate any central action of neostigmine (0.75 to 2 mg i.v.) or of DFP (0.1 to 4 mg/kg i.v.) in cross-circulation experiments in the dog, even when the injected doses apparently inhibited ChE activity completely. SISKEL FREY and GESELL (1948) compared the effects of several anti-ChE agents (physostigmine, neostigmine, DFP) and concluded that moderate doses produced coordinated hyperpnoea, while larger doses produced uncoordinated hyperpnoeic activity with total ventilation diminished rather than increased. All these effects were attributed to central potentiation of nervous activity. MILLER (1949) noted that eserine (0.15 mg/kg i.v.) induced in decerebrate cats increased respiration and tongue retractions which were enhanced by topical application of ACh to the floor of the fourth ventricle. Injection of eserine and of DFP into the vertebral artery was found to augment the temporal summation of repetitive stimuli applied to the carotid nerve and studied by recording the reflex response of breathing in the dog (GESELL and SISKEL FREY 1950).

ERDMANN et al. (1955) observed that i.v. injection of Parathion (0,0-diethyl 0-[4-nitrophenyl] phosphorothioate, E 605) (1 to 3 mg/kg) and of eserine (0.5 to

2 mg/kg) produced in dogs and cats an increase in the frequency of respiration and the minute volume, and facilitation of the vagal influence on respiration. The effects were abolished by atropine (1 mg/kg i.v.). Larger doses of Parathion (10 to 20 mg/kg) or eserine (4 mg/kg) produced respiratory paralysis. Injection into the internal carotid artery of Parathion (0.1 to 0.5 mg/kg) produced the same results. Neostigmine (0.1 to 0.5 mg/kg) was ineffective when injected i.v.; i.a., only very large doses (0.25 mg/kg) had a slight stimulant action.

The effects of eserine, neostigmine, DFP, TEPP, OMPA (octamethyl pyrophosphortetramide), and Parathion on the frequency of respiration, pulmonary ventilation, and central excitability (CO_2 test, threshold for apnoea by centripetal excitation of the vagus) were studied in dogs by PAULET (1956). Intravenous injection of the six agents in small doses ($\leq 1/3$ LD_{50}) produced acceleration of the respiratory frequency and hyperventilation. The organophosphorus compounds increased central excitability to CO_2, while eserine and neostigmine decreased it. All depressed the ability of the vagus to produce apnoea. Larger doses ($\geq 1/2$ LD_{50}) had a depressant action. The alterations in frequency and changes in ventilation could be attributed to drug action on bulbar centers, since they could be obtained after elimination of sino-carotid chemoreceptors. On the contrary, the changes in central excitability disappeared after section of the nerve of Hering and both vagi. The intensity of the reaction varied with the injected agent, and the six ChE inhibitors could be classified in order of decreasing activity as follows: eserine > neostigmine=OMPA > DFP=TEPP=Parathion. Atropine reduced partially the effects of eserine, DFP and OMPA, but had no effect on the changes induced by neostigmine, Parathion, or TEPP. Measurements of the degree of inhibition of ChE induced in the bulbar region showed that there was absolutely no relation between ChE activity and respiratory function. Thus, the author concluded that anti-ChE agents have a double action on respiratory activity: a direct central action which is independent of ChE inhibition, and a reflex action initiated by the chemoreceptors. The data were not considered to be supportive of a cholinergic synaptic mechanism at the level of the central respiratory neurones.

SCHAUMANN and JOB (1958) examined the effects of Phospholine (2-diethoxy-phosphinylthioethyl-trimethylammonium I, echothiophate, 217-MI) and its tertiary analogue, Compound 217-AO, on the central control of respiration in experiments on rats. The action potentials of the left cut phrenic nerve were recorded as well as the contraction of the innervated right diaphragm. The drugs were injected into the jugular vein. Phospholine, which does not penetrate the blood-brain barrier (KOELLE and STEINER 1956), was ineffective in doses as large as 2 mg/kg. On the other hand, 217-AO (0.1 to 0.3 mg/kg) inhibited the respiration without visibly impairing neuromuscular transmission. The effect could be prevented by atropine (5 mg/kg).

Respiratory failure following large doses of ChE inhibitors (DFP, Sarin, TEPP, Paraoxon) appears to be caused by depression of the respiratory center as well as by paralysis of the respiratory muscles, bronchorrhea, and bronchoconstriction (KRIVOY and MARAZZI 1951, DOUGLAS and MATTHEWS 1952, DE CANDOLE et al. 1953, WRIGHT 1954, SAKI et al. 1958, SCHAUMANN 1959).

Although there are some discrepancies with regard to the doses, the majority of authors agree about the effects of eserine and neostigmine in that both stimulation and respiratory depression were observed, the latter with relatively larger doses. With respect to other anti-ChE agents, and particularly to the organophosphorus compounds, it should be pointed out that the majority of authors examined only the mechanisms involved in respiratory depression induced by these agents, while little information is available about the effects of relatively small doses.

Although direct central stimulation was noted with small doses of Parathion, DFP, TEPP, and OMPA, constrasting results were obtained with centripetal stimulation of the vagus, and cannot presently be explained.

Cardiovascular effects elicited by anti-ChE agents have been reported by many authors. While large doses were reported unanimously to produce bradycardia and hypotension, the results obtained with relatively small doses were variable. No effect, hypertension, or hypotension, was noted with different agents and sometimes for the same agent, depending on the route of administration and the species on which the experiments were performed. Only few detailed investigations about the mechanisms involved in these actions have been carried out. The pressor response elicited by centripetal stimulation of the vagus of the perfused isolated head of the dog was enhanced by administration of eserine (1 mg/kg i.v.) to the donor (CHANG et al. 1937). HEYMANS et al. (1946) and HEYMANS and JACOB (1947) reported a direct central excitatory action on the vagal nucleus with eserine, but the injection of neostigmine or of DFP (up to 6 mg/kg i.v. to the donor) into the perfused isolated head of dogs did not increase either the direct or the reflex excitability (carotid sinus or aortic pressoreceptor stimulation) of the cardio-inhibitory and vasomotor centers; very large doses had a depressant action. No change in either central transmission or direct excitability of the cardio-inhibitory center was obtained in the dog after Nu-683 (CALDEYRO and GARCIA AUSTT 1949). Tetraethyl pyrophosphate (0.07 to 0.2 mg/kg i.v.) facilitated central transmission and augmented central excitability in the dog (PAULET 1954). Cardiovascular effects on rats have been attributed, at least in part, to an action of these drugs on the central nervous system (DIRNHUBER and CULLUMBINE 1955, HORNYKIEWICZ and KOBINGER 1956). However, no correlation has been established between ChE inhibition and the cardiovascular changes of central origin.

Blood-brain barrier

KOELLE and STEINER (1956) examined the permeability of the blood-brain barrier to the anti-ChE agent 217-AO (2-diethoxyphosphinylthioethyldimethyl-amine acid oxalate) and its quaternary methiodide derivative, 217-MI (echothiophate, Phospholine), in the rabbit. Following i.v. injection, the tertiary compound produced 90% inactivation of the total brain AChE, whereas the quaternary derivative caused no measurable inhibition; a slight inhibition of brain AChE was noted when 217-MI was injected into the carotid artery. Marked inactivation of the AChE of the whole brain followed instead injection of 217-MI into the lateral ventricle, thus showing that the blood-brain barrier limits the passage of the quaternary agent from the circulation to the cerebral AChE. PAULET et al. (1957) investigated the changes in permeability of the blood-brain barrier induced by anti-ChE agents in the rat; as a test substance they used sulfanilamide. Neostigmine, Parathion and octamethylpyrophosphoramide (OMPA) increased the permeability of the blood-brain barrier; the effect appeared to be entirely independent of the anti-ChE activity of these agents.

D. Spinal cord

I. Reflexes

1. In mammals

SCHWEITZER and WRIGHT (1937b, 1937c, 1938b) and SCHWEITZER et al. (1939) studied the action of a large number of anti-ChE agents on the reflex activity of the spinal cord of cats under chloralose anesthesia. Experiments were performed in which a hindlimb was separately perfused or its circulation was temporarily occluded so as to detect direct actions on the spinal cord. Eserine (0.03 to 0.2 mg/kg i.v.) markedly increased the knee jerk, while larger doses (up to 0.75 mg/kg i.v.) produced an increase in tone and convulsive movements. These effects were mostly due to a direct action on the central nervous system and more precisely on the low spinal somatic centers, since they could be obtained also after midthoracic spinal transection. Occasionally initial inhibition preceded excitation. Atropine (0.5 to 2 mg/kg i.v.) did not antagonize to any marked extent the excitatory action of eserine on reflex activity. Neostigmine (0.2 to 1 mg i.v.) depressed or abolished the knee jerk, partly by a central action, which was unaffected by atropine (1 mg/kg i.v.).

These authors also made a comprehensive study of hordenine and its derivates. The dimethylcarbamic ester of hordenine hydrochloride or sulphate (5 to 30 mg/kg i.v.) increased the knee jerk and produced convulsions. Sometimes initial depression was observed. Atropine (1 mg/kg i.v.) had only a slightly antagonistic action. The dimethylcarbamic ester of hordenine methiodide or methylsulphate (5 to 10 mg/kg i.v.) and the dimethylcarbamic ester of methyl hordenine methylsulphate (5 to 30 mg/kg i.v.) depressed the knee jerk. Previous administration of atropine did not alter the results. All the observed effects were of central origin. Hordenine hydrochloride or sulphate and hordenine methiodide or methylsulphate, which do not exhibit anti-ChE action *in vitro*, depressed the knee jerk.

Finally, the action of various anti-ChE agents and their phenolic bases, after removal of the urethane grouping, was examined. Eseroline HCl (0.5 to 20 mg i.v.) produced a slight increase in reflex activity, which was followed by depression. Eserine methiodide (2 mg i.v.), the dimethyl carbamic ester of *m*-hydroxyphenyl diethyl methyl ammonium iodide (0,2 mg i.v.), and miotine methiodide (1 to 10 mg i.v.) depressed the knee jerk by a central action which was not antagonized by atropine. The methyl carbamic ester of *m*-hydroxyphenyl dimethyl ammonium HCl (10 to 15 mg i.v., after atropine) and the dimethyl carbamic ester of *m*-hydroxyphenyl dimethylamine HCl (0.1 g i.v.) increased the knee jerk by a central action. Miotine HCl (10 to 30 mg i.v.) depressed the knee jerk but produced simultaneously convulsive movements, thus indicating both inhibitory and excitatory actions on the central nervous system. These results led the authors to conclude that all quaternary compounds had an inhibitory action, while tertiary compounds had an excitatory action, with the partial exception of miotine HCl. The suggestion was made that anti-ChE agents capable of penetrating into the cells will act as convulsants, while those which do not will act as depressants. With regard to the mode of action, the authors believed that their findings supported the possibility that the excitatory action of tertiary anti-ChE agents may depend on their anti-ChE activity.

MERLIS and LAWSON (1939) studied the effects of eserine on the knee jerk, tibialis anticus reflex, and the crossed quadriceps reflex in chloralosed and barbitalized dogs. Eserine salicylate perfused through the lumbar subarachnoid space in the intact or spinal animal (cord transected at T_{10}) depressed the knee jerk and augmented the flexion reflex. The crossed extensor reflex was augmented in the extremity in which the knee jerk was depressed. The same effects were obtained on intravenous injection (0.01 to 2 mg/kg).

McKAIL et al. (1941) confirmed that eserine (0.1 to 0.5 mg i.v.) enhanced both excitatory and inhibitory reflex responses in lightly anesthetized cats. On the other hand, they noted that the motor response to cortical stimulation, as well as that to pyramidal tract stimulation, was depressed.

BÜLBRING and BURN (1941) examined the effects of eserine and neostigmine in dogs in which the spinal cord was sectioned in the lower thoracic region. They devised a system in which there were two circulations of perfusing blood, the one supplying the spinal cord, and the other the muscles. Both eserine sulphate (0.2 to 0.5 mg) and neostigmine methylsulphate (0.5 to 1 mg) depressed the knee jerk, while larger doses (1 to 5 mg and 2 to 5 mg, respectively) abolished it. The flexor reflex was augmented by both drugs, although the response to neostigmine was less consistent. Atropine (1 to 2 mg) antagonized all effects.

CALMA and WRIGHT (1944, 1947) and CALMA (1949) found that intravenous injection of eserine (up to 4 mg) increased the tension of the quadriceps muscle in decerebrate cats. Intrathecal injection of eserine (0.2 to 0.6 mg) or neostigmine (0.2 to 0.5 mg) in chloralosed cats increased the knee jerk and the crossed extensor reflex, while it had a variable effect on the flexor reflex. Intra-aortic injection of eserine (0.1 to 0.2 mg/kg) in cats was reported to increase the monosynaptic extensor and polysynaptic flexor reflexes, while the monosynaptic flexor reflex was decreased (TAVERNER 1954). KISSEL and DOMINO (1959) reexamined the effects of physostigmine (25, 50, and 100 μg/kg i.v.) and of neostigmine (25 and 50 μg/kg i.v.) in cats after stabilizing the arterial blood pressure. Both agents produced an increase in the patellar reflex and in crossed extension, while ipsilateral inhibition remained unchanged.

Diisopropyl phosphorofluoridate, HETP (hexaethyltetraphosphate, a mixture of organophosphorus compounds of which TEPP is the major active component), and TEPP potentiated in cats both extensor and flexor reflexes on intravenous as well as on intrathecal injection (CHENNELS and WRIGHT 1947. CHENNELS et al. 1949, 1951). McNAMARA et al. (1954) investigated the mechanism of action of DFP (3 to 25 mg/kg i.m.) and of TEPP (0.5 to 2 mg/kg i.m.) in cats. The former abolished spinal cord and respiratory reflexes (ipsilateral flexor reflex of anterior tibialis muscle, knee jerk, Hering-Breuer reflex) after a brief period of potentiation. No correlation with ChE levels could be established. Tetraethylpyrophosphate abolished the same reflexes at dose levels which produced only moderate decrease of ChE activity and which altered only slightly peripheral neuromuscular function. Parathion (1 to 6 mg i.v.) depressed the contralateral extensor reflex and the ipsilateral flexor reflex; the patellar reflex was enhanced (ERDMANN and SCHAEFER 1954).

Neostigmine reduced the facilitatory and the inhibitory actions of the reticular formation on spinal reflexes (BROOKS et al. 1956).

2. In man

KREMER et al. (1937) showed that the introduction of 1 mg neostigmine into the cerebro-spinal fluid by means of lumbar puncture in patients with hemiplegia decreased or abolished tendon reflexes and muscle tone in the legs and sometimes in the arms also, without change in sensation. KREMER (1942) compared the effects of intrathecal injection of neostigmine (0.1 to 1.5 mg) and eserine sulphate (0.25 to 1 mg) in patients with evidence of pyramidal tract involvement and subjects with a normal central nervous system. Neostigmine produced depression of muscle tone and spinal reflexes. The distal part of the cord was involved first, and the depression gradually ascended. Nausea, vomiting, and drowsiness commonly occurred with large doses. Circulatory and respiratory changes were small and inconsistent. Bladder emptying was temporarily abolished. The same results were obtained in three subjects with normal spinal cords. Eserine produced a transient depression of spinal reflexes followed by a rapid return to a level exceeding that

44*

noted prior to the injection. Drug injection below the level of a spinal block produced effects which were strictly limited to the cord region distal to the block.
Unlike neostigmine, eserine produced subjective sensory disturbances (warmth
and tingling sensation in the legs) and hypersensitivity to touch, which resulted
in pain.

II. Ventral root potentials

1. In mammals

WIKLER (1945) examined the effects of eserine salicylate (0.25 mg/kg i.v.) on
the reflex discharges recorded from ventral roots (L_7 and L_8) upon peripheral nerve
or dorsal root stimulation in spinal cats. The two-neurone arc reflex discharges
were enhanced, while the multineurone arc discharges were little affected by
eserine. Eserine (0.01%) had no effect on single or repetitive synaptic potentials
recorded from ventral roots of the cat's spinal cord (ECCLES 1946). FELDBERG
et al. (1953) examined the effects of close arterial injection of ACh and eserine on
the activity of the cervical cord of the cat. The second cervical nerve was stimulated
and reflex discharges or root potentials were recorded from the first and second
cervical nerve or ventral roots, respectively. Both ACh and eserine increased the
amplitude and decreased the latency of the ventral root potentials.

The action of Tabun on spinal cord reflexes and on spinal cord potentials was
studied by SKOGLUND (1952) and HOLMSTEDT and SKOGLUND (1953), and by BERN-
HARD and SKOGLUND (1953), respectively. Low spinal, decapitate, decerebrate, or
Dial (diallyl barbituric acid)-anesthetized cats, which were artificially respired, were
used. The drug was injected either intravenously or intraarterially. Intraarterial
injection into the lumbar cord was performed through a catheter placed in the
aorta above the lumbar arteries, all other branches being tied with the exception
of the iliac arteries, which were temporarily clamped during injection. Afferent
nerves or dorsal roots were stimulated and recordings were made from ventral
root filaments and from the spinal cord. The minimum doses which influenced
transmission following i.v. injection varied from 50 to 200 μg, while 5 to 10 μg
was effective intraarterially. Both mono- and multisynaptic flexor reflexes showed
initial facilitation, and depression with larger doses. Maximal facilitation was
obtained with 30 μg i.a., and depression appeared after 40 to 50 μg i.a. The monosynaptic extensor reflex was always decreased independently of the dose. Fifteen
μg i.a. depressed the positive cord dorsum potential elicited by stimulation of
low threshold cutaneous fibers, indicating an effect on the membrane potential of
propriospinal neurones. HAASE et al. (1957) studied several anti-ChE agents in
low spinal cats. They stimulated peripheral nerves or dorsal roots and recorded
reflex discharges from ventral roots (L_7, S_1, and S_2). All drugs produced ,upon i.v.
injection, increase of the monosynaptic stretch reflex discharge. Only Tabun depressed the monosynaptic flexor reflex, while the effects of other agents were
inconsistent. Sarin produced a brief initial depression of all reflexes. (Upon i.a.
injection Tabun gave variable results and it was shown that the discrepancies
were probably due to uneven distribution of the drug.) Atropine antagonized both
the excitatory and the depressant actions observed in these experiments.

2. In amphibians

· Injection of eserine (50 to 200 μg) into the right aortic arch increased the
afterdischarge of spinal reflexes (BONNET and BREMER 1937). BREMER and
KLEYNTJENS (1937) studied central summation in spinal frogs. Eserine sulphate
(0.1 to 0.6 mg/25 g injected into the abdominal vein) increased the amplitude of

the reflex contraction but did not modify the summation curve of the homo-lateral flexion reflex. In toads, both contralateral and homolateral extensor re-flexes were abolished by neostigmine in high concentrations (TORDA 1940). Neo-stigmine (0.0003 to 0.0006 M) had no detectable effect on the synaptic potentials set up in the anesthetized spinal cord of the frog by dorsal root volleys, even when they were rapidly repetitive (ECCLES 1947). KOLMODIN and SKOGLUND (1953) found that Paraoxon caused typical changes in isolated spinal cord segments of the frog. The slow negative potentials which may be recorded from the dorsal and ventral horn regions increased in amplitude and in duration, and the postsynaptic cell discharges were increased with low doses (1 to 10 μg per ml) and depressed by high doses.

TAKAGI (1954) tested several anti-ChE agents on dorsal column-root prepara-tions of the Japanese toad. The amplitude of slow potentials was increased by low doses (DFP 0.01 to 0.001%, TEPP 0.1 to 0.001%) and decreased by high con-centrations (DFP 0.05%, TEPP 1 to 0.1%). The author suggested that the effects might be explained by a physicochemical mechanism rather than by a 'pharma-cological' action. ERDMANN and SCHAEFER (1954) reported a decrease of the contralateral extensor reflex in decerebrate frogs after intraaortic injection (0.1 mg) or topical application (in concentrations of 0.0001%) of Parathion.

III. Single neurone activity

ECCLES et al. (1953, 1954, 1956) reported data strongly supporting the view that a group of interneurones lying in the ventral horn of the lumbar segment of the spinal cord of the cat are normally discharged by the release of ACh from the terminals of motor axon collaterals. These interneurones, the functional pro-perties of which were first described by RENSHAW (1941, 1946), would in turn inhibit adjacent motoneurones. The characterization of the synapse between motor axon collaterals and Renshaw cells was based on the observation that Renshaw cells were stimulated by i.v. or i.a. injection of ACh, nicotine, and several anti-ChE agents, including eserine, NU 2126 (the dimethylcarbamate of 3-hydroxy-2-dimethylaminomethyl pyridine dihydrochloride), TEPP, and DFP, and de-pressed by dihydro-β-erythroidine. However, neostigmine and several cholinomi-metic agents (methacholine, succinylcholine, arecoline) had no significant effect when given either i.v. or i.a. Furthermore, atropine depressed the activity only slightly; tubocurarine and decamethonium were ineffective.

The anomalous behavior of these cells when tested with certain drugs spe-cifically acting on other cholinergic synapses suggested that they are surrounded by at least two diffusional barriers, the blood-brain barrier and a second barrier more intimately related to the synaptic terminals on the cells. To overcome some of these problems, the pharmacological properties of the Renshaw cells were reexamined by applying drugs electrophoretically in the immediate vicinity of the cells (CURTIS and ECCLES 1958a, b, CURTIS and PHILLIS 1960). Drugs such as neostigmine and some cholinomimetic agents which were relatively ineffective when administered over other routes, became quite effective when applied near the cells. However, among the tested blocking agents, only dihydro-β-erythroidine had a considerable effect on transynaptically evoked discharges and abolished the activity elicited by ACh or nicotine. Atropine had a more powerful depressant action when applied electrophoretically than upon i.v. administration; however, in addition to its blocking action on cholinergic synapses, it appeared to have also a direct action on the postsynaptic membrane. Locally applied tubocurarine was only slightly effective, especially when the interneurones were activated transynaptically. Decamethonium, which on the neuromuscular junction exhibits anti-ChE action besides a depolarizing action (DEL CASTILLO and KATZ 1957a, b), had no significant effect on the activity evoked transynaptically; it enhanced the discharge elicited by ACh and decreased the discharge elicited by nicotine.

The evidence obtained with the method of electrophoretic application of drugs may be taken to confirm the cholinergic nature of transmission between motor axon collaterals and Renshaw cells. The results obtained with blocking agents are not necessarily in contrast with this view and may be attributed to specific properties of the synapse as well as to the presence of the diffusional barrier postulated by the authors.

The effects of physostigmine (i.v.) on the frequency of spike activity of the Renshaw cells in cats were also examined by LONGO et al. (1960). Although the drug was found to prolong the duration of the Renshaw burst, the results were inconsistent with the hypothesis that the duration of the burst is determined solely by the rate of hydrolysis of ACh.

KOLMODIN and SKOGLUND (1954) reported that Paraoxon elicited burst discharges and decreased the membrane resting potential of interneurones in the ventral horn of the lumbar cord of decapitated cats.

Effects on spinal cord activity have been measured by changes in muscle reflexes and by changes in ventral root potentials. Although in the earlier experiments muscle contraction was the endpoint of the observed reflex, most authors have carefully excluded effects on the muscle itself and on the neuromuscular junction. The data obtained by investigating ventral root potentials definitely show that the changes in reflex activity induced by anti-ChE agents were of central origin. The data agree in that polysynaptic reflexes were enhanced by low doses and depressed by large doses of all anti-ChE agents examined. No such consistency was found with respect to the monosynaptic extensor reflex. In cats, low doses usually produced enhancement, while in dogs and in man the reflex was consistently depressed. Differences in anesthesia, in the reflex preparation, and in species may account for this discrepancy.

With regard to the mechanism of action, the majority of experimenters found that the spinal effects of anti-ChE agents were atropine-resistant. The only available data on concomitant ChE levels did not show correlation with functional changes in the spinal cord.

The cholinergic nature of transmission between motor axon collaterals and Renshaw cells seems to be established beyond any reasonable doubt. With the direct micro-injection technique it has been possible to show that all anti-ChE agents tested enhanced the rate of firing of Renshaw cells; however, the time course of the effects of anti-ChE agents apparently does not support the view that the effects were directly related to anti-ChE activity.

Literature

ABRAHAMS, V. C., and M. PICKFORD: The effect of anticholinesterases injected into the supraoptic nuclei of chloralosed dogs on the release of the oxytoxic factor of the posterior pituitary. J. Physiol. (Lond.) **133**, 330—333 (1956).
APRISON, M. H., P. NATHAN and H. E. HIMWICH: Brain acetylcholinesterase activities in rabbits exhibiting three behavioral patterns following the intracarotid injection of di-*iso*-propyl fluorophosphate. Amer. J. Physiol. **177**, 175—178 (1954).
ARDUINI, A., e X. MACHNE: Sul meccanismo e sul significato dell'azione convulsivante della acetilcolina. Arch. Fisiol. **48**, 152—161 (1948).
BECKETT, S., and E. GELLHORN: Role of acetylcholine in the activity of sensorimotor and suppressor areas of the cortex. Amer. J. Physiol. **153**, 113—120 (1948).

BERNHARD, C. G., and C. R. SKOGLUND: Potential changes in spinal cord following intra-arterial administration of adrenaline and noradrenaline as compared with acetylcholine effects. Acta physiol. scand. **29**, Supp. 106, 435—454 (1953).

BONNET, V.: La transmission synaptic d'influx au niveau des dentrites superficiels de l'écorce cérébrale. Arch. int. Physiol. **65**, 506—511 (1957).

— Mécanisme des réactions des dendrites superficiels de l'écorce cérébrale à différentes stimulations. J. Physiol. (Paris) **50**, 163—166 (1958).

—, and F. BREMER: A study of the after-discharge of spinal reflexes of the frog and toad. J. Physiol. (Lond.) **90**, 45—47P (1937).

BRADLEY, P. B., S. CERQUIGLINI and J. ELKES: Some effects of di-isopropylfluorophosphate on the electrical activity of the brain of the cat. J. Physiol. (Lond.) **121**, 51—52P (1953).

—, and J. ELKES: The effect of atropine, hyoscyamine, physostigmine and neostigmine on the electrical activity of the brain of the conscious cat. J. Physiol. (Lond.) **120**, 14—15P (1953).

— — The effects of some drugs on the electrical activity of the brain. Brain **80**, 77—117 (1957).

—, and B. J. KEY: The effect of drugs on arousal responses produced by electrical stimulation of the reticular formation of the brain. Electroenceph. clin. Neurophysiol. **10**, 97—110 (1958).

BREMER, F., et J. CHATONNET: Acétylcholine et cortex cérébrale. Arch. int. Physiol. **57**, 106—109 (1949).

—, et F. KLEYNTJENS: Nouvelles recherches sur le phénomène de la sommation d'influx nerveux. Arch. int. Physiol. **45**, 382—414 (1937).

—, et N. STOUPEL: Étude pharmacologique de la facilitation des réponses corticales dans l'éveil réticulaire. Arch. int. Pharmacodyn. **122**, 234—248 (1959).

BROOKS, C. McC., K. KOIZUMI and A. A. SIEBENS: Inhibitory action of bulbar and suprabulbar reticular formation on the spinal reflex pathway. Amer. J. Physiol. **184**, 497—504 (1956).

BROOKS, V. B., R. E. RANSMEIER and R. W. GERARD: Action of anticholinesterases, drugs and intermediates on respiration and electrical activity of the isolated frog brain. Amer. J. Physiol. **157**, 299—316 (1949).

BROWN, B. B., and H. GANGLOFF: Effects of deanol, d-amphetamine and eserine on evoked brain activity in rabbits. Proc. West. Pharm. Soc. (San Francisco) **2**, 58—64 (1959).

BROWN, R. V.: The central effects of atropine and P2S in dogs poisoned by intrathecal sarin. J. Physiol. (Lond.) **149**, 49—50P (1959).

— The effects of intracisternal Sarin and pyridine-2-aldoxime methyl methanesulphonate in anaesthetized dogs. Brit. J. Pharmacol. **15**, 170—174 (1960).

BRÜCKE, F. TH., and CH. STUMPF: The pharmacology of "arousal reactions". In: S. GARATTINI and V. GHETTI, Eds., Psychotropic Drugs-Int. Symp. on Psychotropic Drugs, 319 to 324. Milan, Italy. Amsterdam-London-New York-Princeton: Elsevier Publishers 1957.

BÜLBRING, G., and J. H. BURN: Observations bearing on synaptic transmission by acetylcholine in the spinal cord. J. Physiol. (Lond.) **100**, 337—368 (1941).

CALDEYRO, R., et E. GARCIA AUSTT: Sur la pharmacologie du diméthylcarbamate d'hydroxyphényl-benzyl-triméthylammonium (Nu 683). Arch. int. Pharmacodyn. **79**, 454—460 (1949).

CALMA, I.: Observations on the action of prostigmine on the spinal cord of the cat. J. Physiol. (Lond.) **108**, 282—291 (1949).

—, and S. WRIGHT: Action of acetylcholine, atropine and eserine on the central nervous system of the decerebrate cat. J. Physiol. (Lond.) **103**, 93—102 (1944).

— — Action of intrathecally injected eserine on the spinal cord of the cat. J. Physiol. (Lond.) **106**, 80—94 (1947).

CHANG, H. C., K. F. CHIA, C. H. HSU and R. K. S. LIM: Humoral transmission of nerve impulses at central synapses. I. Sinus and vagus afferent nerves. Chin. J. Physiol. **12**, 1—36 (1937).

CHATFIELD, P. O., and E. W. DEMPSEY: Some effects of prostigmine and acetylcholine on cortical potentials. Amer. J. Physiol. **135**, 633—640 (1942).

—, and J. T. LORD: Effects of atropine, prostigmine and acetylcholine on evoked cortical potentials. Electroenceph. clin. Neurophysiol. **7**, 553—556 (1955).

—, and D. P. PURPURA: Augmentation of evoked cortical potentials by topical application of prostigmine and acetylcholine after atropinization of cortex. Electroenceph. clin. Neurophysiol. **6**, 287—298 (1954).

CHENNELLS, M., W. F. FLOYD and S. WRIGHT: Action of condensed alkyl phosphates on the nerve-muscle preparation and the central nervous system of the cat. J. Physiol. (Lond.) **108**, 375—397 (1949).

— — — The action of di-isopropylfluorophosphonate on the central nervous system of the cat. J. Physiol. (Lond.) **114**, 107—118 (1951).

—, and S. WRIGHT: Central excitant action of di-isopropylfluorophosphonate (DFP). Nature (Lond.) **160**, 503 (1947).

CHOW, K. L., and E. R. JOHN: Effects of intracerebral injection of anti-cholinesterase drugs on behavior of rats. Science 128, 781—782 (1958).

CHUTE, A. L., W. FELDBERG and D. H. SMYTH: Liberation of acetylcholine from the perfused cat's brain. Quart. J. exp. Physiol. 30, 65—72 (1940).

COOKE, P. M., and S. L. SHERWOOD: The effect of introduction of some drugs into the cerebral ventricles on the electrical activity of the brain of cats. Electroenceph. clin. Neurophysiol. 6, 425—431 (1954).

CREPAX, P., A. NIGRO e P. L. PARMEGGIANI: Fattori che regolano l'attività unitaria cortico-cerebellare e modificazioni dell'attività medesima per effetto di stimoli chimici. Arch. Sci. Biol. 41, 163—190 (1957).

CURTIS, D. R., and R. M. ECCLES: The excitation of Renshaw cells by pharmacological agents applied electrophoretically. J. Physiol. (Lond.) 141, 435—445 (1958a).

— — The effect of diffusional barriers upon the pharmacology of cells within the central nervous system. J. Physiol. (Lond.) 141, 446—463 (1958b).

—, and J. W. PHILLIS: The action of procaine and atropine on spinal neurones. J. Physiol. (Lond.) 153, 17—34 (1960).

DARROW, W., J. R. GREEN, E. W. DAVIS and H. W. GAROL: Parasympathetic regulation of high potential in the electroencephalogram. J. Neurophysiol. 7, 217—226 (1944).

DE CANDOLE, C. A., W. W. DOUGLAS, G. LOVATT EVANS, R. HOLMES, K. E. V. SPENCER, R. W. TORRANCE and K. M. WILSON: The failure of respiration in death by anticholinesterase poisoning. Brit. J. Pharmacol. 8, 466—475 (1953).

DEL CASTILLO, J., and B. KATZ: A comparison of acetylcholine and stable depolarizing agents. Proc. roy. Soc. B, 146, 362—368 (1957a).

— — Interaction at end-plate receptors between different choline derivatives. Proc. roy. Soc. B, 146, 369—381 (1957b).

DESMEDT, J. E., et L. FRANKEN: Mecanismes neuro-humoraux et synergie reticulocorticale. Fourth Internat. Congress of Electroencephalography and Clinical Neurophysiology. Brussels, 1957. Electroenceph. clin. Neurophysiol. Supp. 7, pp. 356—360.

—, and G. LA GRUTTA: Control of brain potentials by pseudocholinesterase. J. Physiol. (Lond.) 129, 46—47P (1955a).

— — Un Preparato che permette lo studio dell'attività spontanea ed evocata della corteccia cerebrale di gatto dopo esclusione della formazione reticolare meso-diencefalica: il "cerveau sans réticulée". Boll. Soc. ital. Biol. sper. 312, 913—915 (1955b).

— — The effect of selective inhibition of pseudocholinesterase on the spontaneous and evoked activity of the cat's cerebral cortex. J. Physiol. (Lond.) 136, 20—40 (1957).

—, et J. SCHLAG: Mise en évidence d'éléments cholinergiques dans la formation réticulée mesencephalique. J. Physiol. (Paris) 49, 136—138 (1957).

DIAMANT, H.: Cholinesterase inhibitors and vestibular function. A study of a vestibular syndrome in guinea pigs caused by intracarotid centripetal injection of cholinesterase inhibitors and cholinesters. Acta otolaryng. (Stockh.) Supp. 111, 5—84 (1954).

—, and E. HEILBRONN: The effect of intracarotid centripetal injection of cholinesterase inhibitors on the nuclear region of the vestibular nerve. Acta physiol. scand. 39, 209—215 (1957).

DIRNHURBER, P., and H. CULLUMBINE: The effect of anticholinesterase agents on the rat's blood pressure. Brit. J. Pharmacol. 10, 12—15 (1955).

DOUGLAS, W. W., and P. B. C. MATTHEWS: Acute tetraethylpyrophosphate poisoning in cats and its modification by atropine or hyoscine. J. Physiol. (Lond.) 116, 202—218 (1952).

DUKE, H. N., M. PICKFORD and J. A. WATT: The immediate and delayed effects of di-isopropylfluorophosphate injected into the supraoptic nuclei of dogs. J. Physiol. (Lond.) 111, 81—88 (1950).

ECCLES, J. C.: Synaptic potentials of motoneurones. J. Neurophysiol. 9, 87—120 (1946).

— Acetylcholine and synaptic transmission in the spinal cord. J. Neurophysiol. 10, 197—204 (1947).

— R. M. ECCLES and P. FATT: Pharmacological investigations on a central synapse operated by acetylcholine. J. Physiol. (Lond.) 131, 154—169 (1956).

—, P. FATT and K. KOKETSU: Cholinergic and inhibitory synapses in a central nervous pathway. Aust. J. biol. Sci. 16, 50—54 (1953).

— — — Cholinergic and inhibitory synapses in a pathway from motor-axon collaterals to motoneurones. J. Physiol. (Lond.) 126, 524—562 (1954).

EGLIN, J. M.: A study of behavioral effects following intra-hypothalamic injection of acetylcholine with eserine in the waking animal. Unpublished thesis for degree of Doctor of Medicine, Yale U. School of Med., 1953. Quoted by MacLean 1955.

EMMELIN, N., and D. JACOBSOHN: Some effects of acetylcholine, eserine and prostigmine when injected into the hypothalamus. Acta physiol. scand. 9, 97—111 (1945).

ERDMANN, W. D., H. D. KEMPE u. W. LÜHNING: Über die Wirkung von Esteraseblockern (E 605, Eserine und Prostigmin) auf das Atemzentrum von Katze und Hund. Naunyn-Schmiedeberg's Arch. exp. Path. Pharmak. 225, 359—368 (1955).

—, u. K. P. SCHAEFER: Über die Wirkung von Diäthyl-p-nitrophenylthiophosphat (E 605) auf Rückenmarksreflexe an der Katze. Naunyn-Schmiedeberg's Arch. exp. Path. Pharmak. 223, 517—532 (1954).

ESSIG, C. F., J. L. HAMPSON, P. D. BALES, A. WILLIS and H. E. HIMWICH: Effect of Panparnit on brain wave changes induced by DFP. Science 111, 38—39 (1950).

FELDBERG, W.: Present views on the mode of action of acetylcholine in the central nervous system. Physiol. Rev. 25, 596—642 (1945).

— The role of acetylcholine in the central nervous system. Brit. med. Bull. 6, 312—321 (1950).

— J. A. B. GRAY and W. L. M. PERRY: Effects of close arterial injections of acetylcholine on the activity of the cervical spinal cord of the cat. J. Physiol. (Lond.) 119, 428—438 (1953).

—, and S. L. SHERWOOD: Behavior of cats after intraventricular injections of eserine and DFP. J. Physiol. (Lond.) 125, 488—500 (1954).

FREEDMAN, A. M., P. D. BALES, A. WILLIS and H. E. HIMWICH: Experimental production of electrical major convulsive patterns. Amer. J. Physiol. 156, 117—123 (1949).

FUNDERBURK, W. H., and T. J. CASE: The effect of atropine on cortical potentials. Electroenceph. clin. Neurophysiol. 3, 213—223 (1951).

GESELL, R., and E. T. HANSEN: Eserine, acetylcholine, atropine and nervous integration. Amer. J. Physiol. 139, 371—385 (1943).

—, and J. SISKEL FREY: Temporal summation of stimuli studied with the aid of anticholinesterases. Amer. J. Physiol. 160, 375—384 (1950).

GROB, D., A. M. HARVEY, O. R. LANGWORTHY and J. L. LILIENTHAL, jr.: The administration of di-isopropyl fluorophosphate (DFP) to man. III. Effect on the central nervous system with special reference to the electrical activity of the brain. Johns Hopk. Hosp. Bull. 81, 257—266 (1947).

GROSSMAN, S. P.: Eating or drinking elicited by direct adrenergic or cholinergic stimulation of hypothalamus. Science 132, 301—302 (1960).

HAASE, J., D. LÜCKE, F. SCHELER, R. SCHÜTZ, B. MÜHLBERG u. W. KOLL: Die Wirkung von Cholinesterasegiften auf Reflexsysteme der tiefspinalen Katze. Naunyn-Schmiedeberg's Arch. exp. Path. Pharmak. 232, 274—276 (1957).

HAMPSON, J. L., C. F. ESSIG, A. McCAULEY and H. E. HIMWICH: Effects of di-isopropyl fluorophosphate (DFP) on electroencephalogram and cholinesterase activity. Electroenceph. clin. Neurophysiol. 2, 41—48 (1950).

HARWOOD, C. T.: Cholinesterase activity and electroencephalograms during circling induced by the intracarotid injection of di-isopropyl fluorophosphate (DFP). Amer. J. Physiol. 177, 171—174 (1954).

HENDERSON, W. R., and W. C. WILSON: Intraventricular injection of acetylcholine and eserine in man. Quart. J. exp. Physiol. 26, 83—95 (1936).

HEYMANS, C., et J. JACOB: Sur la pharmacologie du di-isopropyl fluorophosphonate (DFP) et le rôle des cholinestérases. Arch. int. Pharmacodyn. 74, 233—252 (1947).

— R. PANNIER et R. VERBEKE: Influence des anticholinéstérases prostigmine, éserine et di-isopropylfluorophosphate, et de l'atropine sur la transmission centrale et périphérique des excitations nerveuses. Arch. int. Pharmacodyn. 72, 405—429 (1946).

— A. POCHET et H. VAN HOUTTE: Contributions à la pharmacologie du Sarin et du Tabun. Arch. int. Pharmacodyn. 104, 293—332 (1956).

HOLMSTEDT, B.: Pharmacology of organophosphorus cholinesterase inhibitors. Pharmacol. Rev. 11, 567—688 (1959).

—, and C. R. SKOGLUND: The action on spinal reflexes of dimethyl-amido-ethoxy-phosphoryl cyanide, "Tabun", a cholinesterase inhibitor. Acta physiol. scand. Supp. 106, 29, 410—427 (1953).

HORNYKIEWICZ, O., u. W. KOBINGER: Über den Einfluß von Eserine, Tetraäthylpyrophosphat (TEPP), und Neostigmin auf den Blutdruck und die pressorischen Carotissinusreflexe der Ratte. Naunyn-Schmiedeberg's Arch. exp. Path. Pharmak. 228, 493—500 (1956).

HYDE, J., S. BECKETT and E. GELLHORN: Acetylcholine and convulsive activity. J. Neurophysiol. 12, 17—27 (1949).

INFANTELLINA, F.: Azione dell'acetilcolina, dell'eserina e dell'atropina sul lembo isolato di corteccia cerebrale di gatto. Arch. Sci. biol. (Bologna) 39, 209—232 (1955).

KEITH, H. M., and G. W. STAVRAKY: Experimental convulsions induced by administration of Thujone. Arch. Neurol. Psychiat. 34, 1022—1040 (1935).

KISSEL, J. W., and E. F. DOMINO: The effects of some possible neurohumoral agents on spinal cord reflexes. J. Pharmacol. exp. Ther. 125, 168—177 (1959).

698   Literature

KOELLE, G. B., and E. C. STEINER: The cerebral distributions of a tertiary and a quaternary
    anticholinesterase agent following intravenous and intraventricular injection. J. Pharmacol.
    exp. Ther. 118, 420—434 (1956).
KOLMODIN, G. M., and C. R. SKOGLUND: Potentials within isolated segments of the frog's
    spinal cord during reflex activation and changes induced by cholinesterase inhibitors and
    temperature variations. Acta physiol. scand. Supp. 106, 29, 503—529 (1953).
— — Properties and functional differentiation of interneurons in the ventral horn of the cat's
    lumbar cord as revealed by intracellular recording. Experientia (Basel) 10, 505—506 (1954).
KRECH, D., M. R. ROSENZWEIG and E. L. BENNETT: Dimensions of discrimination and level of
    cholinesterase activity in the cerebral cortex of the rat. J. comp. physiol. Psychol. 49,
    261—268 (1956).
KREMER, M.: Action of intrathecally injected prostimine, acetylcholine and eserine on the
    central nervous system in man. Quart. J. exp. Physiol. 31, 337—357 (1942).
— H. E. S. PEARSON and S. WRIGHT: Action of prostigmine on spinal cord in man. J. Physiol.
    (Lond.) 89, 21—23P (1937).
KRISTIANSEN, K., and G. COURTOIS: Rhythmic electrical activity from isolated cerebral cortex.
    Electroenceph. clin. Neurophysiol. 1, 265—272 (1949).
KRIVOY, W. A., and S. MARRAZZI: Evaluation of the central action of anticholinesterases in
    producing respiratory paralysis. Fed. Proc. 10, 316 (1951).
LESNÝ, I., and V. VOJTA: Eserine activation of the electroencephalogram in children. Elec-
    troenceph. clin. Neurophysiol. 12, 742—743 (1960).
LONGO, V. G., W. R. MARTIN and K. R. UNNA: A pharmacological study on the Renshaw cell.
    J. Pharmacol. exp. Ther. 129, 61—68 (1960).
—, and B. SILVESTRINI: Action of eserine and amphetamine on the electrical activity of the
    rabbit brain. J. Pharmacol. exp. Ther. 120, 160—170 (1957).
MacLEAN, P. D.: The limbic system and its hippocampal formation. Studies in animals and
    their possible application to man. J. Neurosurg. 11, 29—44 (1954).
— The limbic system ("Visceral Brain") in relation to central grey and reticulum of the brain
    stem. Evidence of interdependence in emotional processes. Psychosom. Med. 17, 355—366
    (1955).
— Chemical and electrical stimulation of hippocampus in unrestrained animals. I. Methods
    and electroencephalgraphic findings. A.M.A. Arch. Neurol. Psychiat. 78, 113—127 (1957a).
— Chemical and electrical stimulation of hippocampus in unrestrained animals. II. Behavioral
    findings. A.M.A. Arch. Neurol. Psychiat. 78, 128—142 (1957b).
MARRAZZI, S., and E. R. HART: Cholinergic sensitivity in an afferent cerebral system. Fed.
    Proc. 9, 85 (1950).
MAYER, C., u. CH. STUMPF: Die Physostigminwirkung auf die Hippocampus-Tätigkeit nach
    Septumläsionen. Naunyn-Schmiedeberg's Arch. exp. Path. Pharmak. 234, 490—500
    (1958).
McKAIL, R. A., S. OBRADOR and W. C. WILSON: The action of acetylcholine, eserine and other
    substances on some motor responses of the central nervous system. J. Physiol. (Lond.) 99,
    312—328 (1941).
McNAMARA, B. P., E. F. MURTHA, A. D. BERGNER, E. M. ROBINSON, C. W. BENDER and J. H.
    WILLS: Studies on the mechanism of action of DFP and TEPP. J. Pharmacol. exp. Ther.
    110, 232—240 (1954).
MERLIS, J. K., and H. LAWSON: The effect of eserine on spinal reflexes in the dog. J. Neuro-
    physiol. 2, 566—572 (1939).
MIKHEL'SON, M. LA., E. K. ROZHKOVA, E. K. and N. V. SAVATEEV: Antagonistic action of
    cholinolytic and anticholinesterase substances (translated from Russian). Bjull eksp. Biol.
    Med. 37, 7—12 (1954).
MILLER, F. R.: Effects of eserine and acetylcholine on the respiratory centers and hypoglossal
    nuclei. Canad. J. Res. 27, E, 374—386 (1949).
— G. W. STAVRAKY and G. A. WOONTON: Effects of eserine, acetylcholine and atropine on the
    electrocorticogram. J. Neurophysiol. 3, 131—138 (1940).
MORUZZI, G.: L'epilessia sperimentale. N. Zanichelli Ed., Bologna 1946.
MUIRHEAD-COOKE, P., E. RIDLEY and S. L. SHERWOOD: The effect of some drugs, injected
    into the cerebral ventricles, on the EEG. Electroenceph. clin. Neurophysiol. 4, 253 (1952).
PALMER, A. C.: Injection of drugs into the cerebral ventricle of sheep. J. Physiol. (Lond.) 149,
    209—214 (1959).
PAULET, G.: Nouvelle contribution à l'étude de l'action pharmacologique du tétraéthylpyro-
    phosphate (TEPP). Arch. int. Pharmacodyn. 97, 157—185 (1954).
— Activité cholinéstérasique et fonctionnement des centres respiratoires. J. Physiol. (Paris)
    48, 915—936 (1956).
— H. MARSOL et H. COQ: Cholinéstérase et perméabilité de la barrière hématoencéphalique.
    J. Physiol. (Paris) 49, 342—345 (1957).

PERRY, W. L. M.: Central and synaptic transmission (Pharmacological aspects). Ann. Rev. Physiol. **18**, 279—308 (1956).

PICKFORD, M.: The action of acetylcholine in the supraoptic nucleus of the chloralosed dog. J. Physiol. (Lond.) **106**, 264—270 (1947).

RENSHAW, B.: Influence of discharge of motoneurones upon excitation of neighboring motoneurones. J. Neurophysiol. **4**, 167—183 (1941).

— Central effects of centripetal impulses in axons of spinal ventral roots. J. Neurophysiol. **9**, 191—204 (1946).

RIEHL, J.-L., and K. R. UNNA: Effects of muscarine on the central nervous system. Recent Advances in Biol. Psychiatry. Chapter 25, 345—362 (1960).

RINALDI, F., and H. E. HIMWICH: Alerting responses and actions of atropine and cholinergic drugs. Arch. Neurol. Psychiat. (Chicago) **73**, 387—395 (1955).

RUBIN, L. S., and M. N. GOLDBERG: Effect of tertiary and quaternary atropine salts on absolute scotopic threshold changes produced by an anticholinesterase (Sarin). J. appl. Physiol. **12**, 305—310 (1958).

SAILER, S., u. CH. STUMPF: Weitere Hinweise auf den Cholinergen Mechanismus der "arousal reaction". Naunyn-Schmiederberg's Arch. exp. Path. Pharmak. **232**, 277—278 (1957).

SAKAI, F., J. DAL RI, W. D. ERDMANN und G. SCHMIDT: Über die Atemlähmung durch Parathion oder Paraoxon und ihre antagonistische Beeinflußbarkeit. Naunyn-Schmiedeberg's Arch. exp. Path. Pharmak. **234**, 210—219 (1958).

SCHAUMANN, W.: Über den Einfluß von Atropin auf die zentrale Hemmung der Atmung durch Anticholinesterasen. Naunyn-Schmiedeberg's Arch. exp. Path. Pharmak. **236**, 415—420 (1959).

—, and C. JOB: Differential effects of a quaternary cholinesterase inhibitor, phospholine and its tertiary analogue, compound 217-AO, on central control of respiration and on neuromuscular transmission. The antagonism by 217-AO of the respiratory arrest caused by morphine. J. Pharmacol. exp. Ther. **123**, 114—120 (1958).

SCHIFF, M., W. G. ESMOND and H. E. HIMWICH: Forced circling movements (adversive syndrome). Correction with dimenhydrinate (Dramamine). Arch. Otolaryng. (Chicago) **51**, 672—677 (1950).

SCHWEITZER, A., E. STEDMAN and S. WRIGHT: Central action of anticholinesterases. J. Physiol. (Lond.) **96**, 302—336 (1939).

—, and S. WRIGHT: The anti-strychnine action of acetylcholine, prostigmine and related substances, and of central vagus stimulation. J. Physiol. (Lond.) **90**, 310—329 (1937a).

— — The action of eserine and related compounds and of acetylcholine on the central nervous system. J. Physiol. (Lond.) **89**, 165—197 (1937b).

— — Further observations on the action of acetylcholine, prostigmine and related substances on the knee jerk. J. Physiol. (Lond.) **89**, 384—402 (1937c).

— — Action of prostigmine and acetylcholine on respiration. Quart. J. exp. Physiol. **28**, 33—47 (1938a).

— — Action of hordenine compounds on the central nervous system. J. Physiol. (Lond.) **92**, 422—438 (1938b).

SISKEL FREY, J., and R. GESELL: A comparative study of the effects of several anticholinesterases on central nervous integration. Fed. Proc. **7**, 37 (1948).

SJÖSTRAND, T.: Potential changes in the cerebral cortex of the rabbit arising from cellular activity and the transmission of impulses in the white matter. J. Physiol. (Lond.) **90**, 41—43P (1937).

SKOGLUND, C. R.: Factors that modify transmission through the spinal cord. Cold Spr. Harb. Symp. quant. Biol. **17**, 233—244 (1952).

Symposium on Neurohumoral Transmission. Physiol. Soc. of Philadelphia, September 11—12, 1953. Pharmacol. Rev. **6**, 2—131 (1954).

TAKAGI, S. F.: The slow potential observed in the dorsal column-root preparations II. The concentration effects of drugs on the slow potential. Jap. J. Physiol. **4**, 91—101 (1954).

TAVERNER, D.: The action of eserine sulphate on the spinal cord of the cat. Brit. J. Pharmacol. **9**, 84—90 (1954).

TORDA, C.: Effect of acetylcholine, prostigmine, potassium, and fatigue on the crossed extensor reflex and on its reflex inhibition in the toad. J. Physiol. (Lond.) **97**, 357—362 (1940).

TOWER, D. B., and D. McEACHERN: Actylcholine and neuronal activity. I. Cholinesterase patterns and acetylcholine in the cerebrospinal fluids of patients with craniocerebral trauma. Canad. J. Res., E, **27**, 105—119 (1949a).

— — Acetylcholine and neuronal activity. II. Acetylcholine and cholinesterase activity in the cerebrospinal fluids of patients with epilepsy. Canad. J. Res., E, **27**, 120—131 (1949b).

WESCOE, W. C., R. E. GREEN, B. P. McNAMARA and S. KROP: The influence of atropine and scopolamine on the central effects of DFP. J. Pharmacol. exp Ther. **92**, 63—72 (1948).

WHITE, R. P.: Relationship between behavioral changes and brain cholinesterase activity following graded intracerebral injections of DFP. Proc. Soc. exp. Biol. (N. Y.) **93**, 113—116 (1956).

—, and E. A. DAIGNEAULT: The antagonism of atropine to the EEG effects of adrenergic drugs. J. Pharmacol. exp. Ther. **125**, 339—346 (1959).

WIKLER, A.: Effects of morphine, nembutal, ether and eserine on two-neuron and multineuron reflexes in the cat. Proc. Soc. exp. Biol. (N. Y.) **58**, 193—196 (1945).

WILLIAMS, D., and W. R. RUSSELL: Action of eserine and prostigmine on epileptic cerebral discharges. Lancet **240**, 476—479 (1941).

WRIGHT, P. G.: An analysis of the central and peripheral components of respiratory failure produced by anticholinesterase poisoning in the rabbit. J. Physiol. (Lond.) **126**, 52—70 (1954).

HANDBUCH
DER EXPERIMENTELLEN
PHARMAKOLOGIE

BEGRÜNDET VON A. HEFFTER
FORTGEFÜHRT VON W. HEUBNER

ERGÄNZUNGSWERK

HERAUSGEGEBEN VON

O. EICHLER   UND   A. FARAH

PROFESSOR DER PHARMAKOLOGIE
AN DER UNIVERSITÄT HEIDELBERG

PROFESSOR DER PHARMAKOLOGIE
AN DER STATE UNIVERSITY OF NEW YORK

FÜNFZEHNTER BAND

CHOLINESTERASES AND
ANTICHOLINESTERASE AGENTS

SUB-EDITOR
GEORGE B. KOELLE

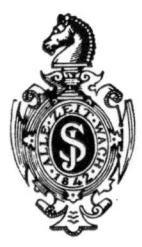

Springer-Verlag Berlin Heidelberg GmbH

1963

CHOLINESTERASES AND ANTICHOLINESTERASE AGENTS

CONTRIBUTORS

K. B. AUGUSTINSSON · L. E. CHADWICK · J. A. COHEN · H. CULLUMBINE · D. R. DAVIES · K. P. DuBOIS · D. GROB · C. O. HEBB · F. HOBBIGER · BO HOLMSTEDT · A. G. KARCZMAR · G. B. KOELLE · N. KRISHNA · A. S. KUPERMAN · I. H. LEOPOLD · J. P. LONG · X. MACHNE · L. A. MOUNTER · D. NACHMANSOHN · R. A. OOSTERBAAN · K. R. W. UNNA · G. WERNER · V. P. WHITTAKER · J. H. WILLS · E. ZAIMIS

SUB-EDITOR

GEORGE B. KOELLE

WITH 176 FIGURES

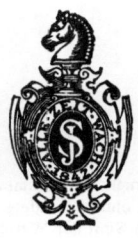

Springer-Verlag Berlin Heidelberg GmbH

1963

ISBN 978-3-642-99877-5   ISBN 978-3-642-99875-1 (eBook)
DOI 10. 1007/978-3-642-99875-1

Ursprünglich erschienen bei Springer-Verlag oHG. Berlin · Göttingen · Heidelberg 1963

Softcover reprint of the hardcover 1st edition 1963
Library of Congress Catalog Card Number Agr 25 — 699

Preface

Although the anticholinesterase (anti-ChE) agents have only limited applications in therapy, and from the viewpoint of practical significance they are more appropriately classified as toxic compounds or insecticides than as drugs, in their capacity of pharmacological tools they have few equals. The concept of neurohumoral transmission was originally established largely from experiments in which physostigmine, or eserine, was employed to protect acetylcholine (ACh), the transmitter of the cholinergic nerves, from rapid hydrolytic destruction by acetylcholinesterase (AChE) and other cholinesterases (ChE's). Since then, a great number of additional reversible and irreversible anti-ChE agents also have been indispensable in studies of synaptic and neuroeffector transmission, and of other physiological processes. At the same time, there is practically no other class of compounds for which a mechanism of pharmacological action can be described in such concrete biochemical and physiological terms. Consequently, it is not surprising that a huge literature has developed on these several closely interdependent topics. The assembling and proper correlation of this material for the present volume has taken the collaborative efforts of over two dozen investigators. It is believed that their contributions to this end will prove invaluable to future investigators in providing a ready, inclusive source of established information, in defining areas where further studies are indicated, and in preventing unnecessary duplication of past work. How well these aims have been accomplished will be for time and the reader to judge.

The volume is divided into four major sections. The first (I, Chapters 1 to 6) presents the biochemical and physiological background which is essential to an understanding of the primary mechanism of action of the anti-ChE agents. This includes the identification and distribution of ACh and other naturally occurring choline esters (Chapter 1), the known facts about the enzyme choline acetylase (ChAc), which catalyzes the final step in the synthesis of ACh (Chapter 2), and the current knowledge and hypotheses concerning the formation, storage, and liberation of ACh *in vivo* (Chapter 3). Chapter 4 presents a classification of the cholinesterases (ChE's) and the methods employed for their determination. The nomenclature and abbreviations used here are with few exceptions followed in the other chapters of the volume. The embryonic appearance and development of ChE's in various phyla are considered in relation to function in Chapter 5. Chapter 6 describes the cytological localizations of AChE and other ChE's throughout the body, and considers the possible functions of the enzymes and their known substrate, ACh, on the basis of these observations and pertinent data from physiological studies.

Section II is devoted to the chemistry of the anti-ChE agents. This includes the biochemical problems of the nature of the reactions between the various types of inhibitors and the enzymes (Chapter 7), and the pathways of metabolic degradation of the organophosphorus anti-ChE agents (Chapter 10), as well as the chemical classifications and relationships between structure and pharmacological actions of the reversible (Chapter 8) and organophosphorus (Chapter 9) anti-ChE agents.

The systematic pharmacology of the anti-ChE agents is covered in Section III. Here, the authors have attempted to distinguish as well as possible between effects due to inhibition or inactivation of ChE's and those which are more reasonably attributable to other mechanisms. The first four Chapters (11 to 14) of this Section discuss actions at sites where it is generally acknowledged that cholinergic transmission occurs, *i.e.*, at autonomic effector sites (11), autonomic ganglia (12), the neuromuscular junction of skeletal muscle (13), and certain regions of the central nervous system (14). The hypothesis that ACh and AChE are involved directly in the propagation of conducted axonal impulses is presented in Chapter 15; evidence to the contrary is considered in Chapter 6. The remaining two chapters here deal with the actions of anti-ChE agents on insects and other invertebrates (16), and on growth and development (17).

The final section (IV) treats the toxicological and therapeutic aspects of the anti-ChE agents. The general toxicological evaluation and the specific neurotoxic actions of the organophosphorus anti-ChE agents are presented in Chapters 18 and 19, respectively. Chapter 20 describes the pharmacology of the various types of antagonists of anti-ChE agents, with the exception of the compounds which reactivate alkylphosphorylated AChE; the latter are discussed in Chapter 21. The current clinical application of these findings to the treatment of intoxication with anti-ChE agents is presented in Chapter 22. Finally, the therapeutic uses of anti-ChE agents in myasthenia gravis (Chapter 23) and glaucoma (Chapter 24) are considered.

The Editor takes great pleasure in expressing to his collaborators in the preparation of this volume his deepest appreciation of their contributions and of their cooperative spirit and forbearance in bringing them into final form. He is most grateful for the invaluable editorial and secretarial help he has received from Miss CORNELIA GEESEY, Mrs. ZAROUG KABAKIAN, and Mrs. MARIAN SULLIVAN. For the accomplishment of this own investigative work, much of which is included in Chapter 6, he is deeply indebted to the stimulating participation of his past and present colleagues whose work is cited and acknowledged there. It is particularly appropriate to note the inspiration which he received from his early mentor, the late Dr. JONAS S. FRIEDENWALD, whose enthusiasm, genius, and kindly guidance first interested him in the application of histochemistry to pharmacological problems.

Finally, it is obviously not an Editor's prerogative to offer personal dedication of the work produced by his collaborators. However, his own efforts in assembling, contributing to, and editing this volume are dedicated with deepest affection to WIN, and to PETER, BILLY, and JONATHAN, who provided both constant inspiration and generous relinquishment of their rightful claims to the hours taken for its compilation.

Philadelphia. September, 1961   G. B. K.

List of Contributors

KLAS-BERTIL AUGUSTINSSON, Ph.D., Associate Professor, Institute of Organic Chemistry and Biochemistry, University of Stockholm, Stockholm 6, Sweden.

L. E. CHADWICK, Ph.D., Head, Department of Entomology, University of Illinois, Urbana, Ill., U.S.A.

J. A. COHEN, Ph.D., Professor of Applied Enzymology and Radiobiology, University of Leyden, and Director of the Medical Biological Laboratory, RVO-TNO, Rijswijk, Z.H., The Netherlands.

HARRY CULLUMBINE, M.D., Visiting Lecturer, Department of Pharmacology, Graduate School of Medicine, University of Pennsylvania, Philadelphia 4, Pa., U.S.A.

D. R. DAVIES, Senior Principal Scientific Officer, The Chemical Defence Experimental Establishment, Porton Down, Salisbury, England.

KENNETH P. DuBOIS, Ph.D., Professor of Pharmacology, University of Chicago, Chicago 37, Ill., U.S.A.

DAVID GROB, M.D., Professor of Medicine, State University of New York College of Medicine, and Director of Medical Services, Maimonides Hospital of Brooklyn, Brooklyn 19, N. Y., U.S.A.

CATHERINE O. HEBB, Ph.D., Head, Subdepartment of Chemical Physiology, Agricultural Research Council, Institute of Animal Physiology, Babraham, Cambridge, England.

F. HOBBIGER, M.D., D.Sc., Ph.D., Reader in Pharmacology, Middlesex Hospital Medical School, London, W. 1, England.

BO HOLMSTEDT, M.D., Associate Professor, Department of Pharmacology, Karolinska Institutet, Stockholm 60, Sweden.

ALEXANDER G. KARCZMAR, Ph.D., Professor and Chairman, Department of Pharmacology and Therapeutics, Stritch School of Medicine, University of Loyola, Chicago 12, Ill., U.S.A.

GEORGE B. KOELLE, Ph.D., M.D., Professor and Chairman, Department of Pharmacology, Schools of Medicine, University of Pennsylvania, Philadelphia 4, Pa., U.S.A.

NARENDRA KRISHNA, M.B.B.S., D.Sc. (Med.), Instructor in Ophthalmology, Graduate School of Medicine, University of Pennsylvania, and Research Associate, Wills Eye Hospital, Philadelphia 30, Pa., U.S.A.

ALBERT S. KUPERMAN, Ph.D., Assistant Professor of Pharmacology, Cornell University Medical College, New York 21, N. Y., U.S.A.

IRVING H. LEOPOLD, M.D., D.Sc. (Med.), Professor and Chairman, Department of Ophthalmology, Graduate School of Medicine, University of Pennsylvania, and Medical and Research Director, Wills Eye Hospital, Philadelphia 30, Pa., U.S.A.

J. P. LONG, Ph.D., Associate Professor, Department of Pharmacology, College of Medicine, State University of Iowa, Iowa City, Ia., U.S.A.

XENIA MACHNE, M.D., Assistant Professor of Pharmacology, University of Illinois College of Medicine, Chicago 12, Ill., U.S.A.

L. A. MOUNTER, Ph.D., Associate Professor, Department of Biophysics, Medical College of Virginia, Richmond 19, Va., U.S.A.

DAVID NACHMANSOHN, M.D., Professor of Biochemistry, College of Physicians and Surgeons, Columbia University, New York 32, N. Y., U.S.A.

R. A. OOSTERBAAN, Ph.D., Head of the Biochemical Department of the Medical Biological Laboratory, RVO-TNO, Rijswijk, Z.H., The Netherlands.

KLAUS R. W. UNNA, M.D., Professor and Head, Department of Pharmacology, University of Illinois College of Medicine, Chicago 12, Ill., U.S.A.

GERHARD WERNER, M.D., Associate Professor of Pharmacology, Cornell University Medical College, New York 21, N. Y., U.S.A.

V. P. WHITTAKER, D.Phil. (Oxon.), Member of the Scientific Staff, Biochemistry Department, Agricultural Research Council, Institute of Animal Physiology, Babraham, Cambridge, England.

J. H. WILLS, Ph.D., Chief, Physiology Division, Directorate of Medical Research, U.S. Army Chemical Research and Development Laboratories, Army Chemical Center, Maryland, U.S.A.

ELEANOR ZAIMIS, M.D., Professor of Pharmacology, University of London, Royal Free Hospital School of Medicine, London, W.C. 1, England.

Contents

I. Components of Cholinergic Systems: Acetylcholine (ACh), Choline Acetylase (ChAc), and Acetylcholinesterase (AChE)

II. Chemical Classification and Biochemical Reactions of the Anticholinesterase (Anti-ChE) Agents

III. Systematic Pharmacology of the Anticholinesterase (Anti-ChE) Agents

IV. Toxicology and Therapeutic Applications of the Anticholinesterase (Anti-ChE) Agents

Chapter 15

Actions on Axons, and Evidence for the Role of Acetylcholine in Axonal Conduction*

By

DAVID NACHMANSOHN

With 16 Figures

Contents

    * This work was supported in part by the National Science Foundation, Grants No. G-4331
and 12901, by the Division of Research Grants and Fellowships, National Institutes of Health,
Grant No. B-400, U.S. Public Health Service, and by a gift from the Muscular Dystrophy
Association of America, Inc.

A. Events during activity recorded by physical methods

I. Ion movements

A characteristic feature of living cells is the unequal distribution of ions between the interior and the outer environment. K-ions are present in high concentrations inside cells, usually 10 to 20 times as high as in the surrounding fluid; the reverse is true for the Na-ion concentration. Conducting cells are endowed with the special ability to use these ionic concentration gradients for generating electric currents. In a fluid medium ions must be the carriers of these currents.

The "membrane theory" (BERNSTEIN 1902) assumed that nerve fibers are surrounded by a semipermeable membrane, selectively permeable to K^+. The membrane is charged positively on the outside and negatively on the inside. On stimulation the active region of the membrane becomes permeable to all ions and is thereby depolarized. Currents are generated and stimulate the adjacent points; the same process takes place there. In this way successive parts of the membrane are activated and the impulse is propagated along the axon. Measurements carried out with electrodes inserted into squid giant axon revealed, however, that at the activated point there is not merely a depolarization, but a reversal of polarity (CURTIS and COLE 1942, HODGKIN and HUXLEY 1945). By this "overshoot" the potential of the action current becomes about twice as great as the resting potential. During activity the membrane resistance is greatly decreased; in the squid giant axon it drops from 1000 to 40 Ohms cm² (COLE and CURTIS 1939).

The availability of radioactive ions after the Second World War made it possible to measure ion movements in rest and during activity. ROTHENBERG (1949, 1950), using the squid giant axon, found that 4 $\mu\mu$moles of Na^+ per cm² surface per impulse enter the interior. The figure was confirmed by HODGKIN and his associates (HODGKIN 1951). An equivalent amount of K^+ moves to the outside, since the cell must maintain electrical neutrality (KEYNES and LEWIS 1951 a, b). The analysis of ion movements during activity has been extended by the Cambridge group by the use of the so-called "voltage clamp" method, worked out by COLE (1949, 1955). Their investigations have shown that at first there is a strong and rapid, but transitory increase of Na-conductance, coinciding with the rising phase of the action current. Subsequently, there is a smaller increase of K-conductance; K^+ moves to the outside during the falling phase (HODGKIN 1957).

During the last few years SCHOFFENIELS has developed a single isolated electroplax preparation which permits the study of ion flux across the innervated and non-innervated membranes (SCHOFFENIELS and NACHMANSOHN 1957, SCHOFFENIELS 1959 a). Using this preparation, WHITTAM and GUINNEBAULT (1960) found an efflux of 5 to 8 $\mu\mu$moles K^+ per cm² per impulse. This figure is very close to that obtained with the squid giant axon. The results suggest that the ion movements underlying electric currents, which had been demonstrated on special types of invertebrate axons, may be a process similar in all excitable membranes.

We may then consider as reasonably well established that during activity ions move across the conducting membrane, and that the membrane conductance changes in a specific way during activity. This immediately raises the question as to the mechanism which is responsible for these changes and which controls these special ion movements across conducting membranes. What is the nature of the transitory changes taking place in the membrane, of the forces by which Na-conductance suddenly increases so markedly, followed by a much smaller increase of K-conductance ? Some special events must take place in the conducting membrane by which the ionic concentration gradients, the potential source of EMF which is inactive in the resting state, are suddenly used for the generation of electric currents. Understanding of nerve activity is impossible without a knowledge of these events.

In reviewing the ionic movements underlying electrical activity, HODGKIN (1951) attributed the initial heat production, measured some 30 years ago by A. V. HILL and his associates, to the mixing of Na^+ and K^+. This interpretation attributes the heat released to purely physical processes and thus implies that no chemical reaction takes place in the elementary processes of generating the currents, since a chemical reaction would contribute to the heat produced. In discussing the nature of the permeability change in his Ferrier lecture, HODGKIN (1957) did not consider the possibility of a chemical reaction's being responsible for this process. In contrast, the chemical forces controlling the ion movements during nerve activity and the molecular events in the elementary processes of conduction have been in the center of the studies of the author of this review (NACHMANSOHN 1955a, b, 1959).

II. Heat production

The view of purely physical processes as the source of the initial heat is contradicted by the recent measurements of A. V. HILL and his associates on the initial heat production. In the early measurements of A. V. HILL and his associates the initial heat production was found to be rather small, 2×10^{-6} cal/g/impulse. Recently, however, HILL and his associates (ABBOTT et al. 1958b, HILL 1960, ABBOTT 1960) took up these measurements with still faster recording equipment than that which was previously available. Using *Maja* nerve at 0°C, they found that the initial heat production takes place in two successive phases: a positive heat, averaging in a single impulse about 9×10^{-6} cal/g nerve. This phase is very rapid and coincides roughly with activity. The positive heat is followed by a negative heat produced within 100 to 300 milliseconds, averaging about -7×10^{-6} cal/g nerve. With the previous method only the difference between the two processes, the "net heat" (2×10^{-6} cal/g nerve/impulse) was recorded. Making some necessary corrections the authors arrived at values of 14×10^{-6} cal and -12×10^{-6} cal/g nerve/impulse at 0°C. The ions are assumed to move across a membrane of about 50 Å thickness; the observed permeability change must take place in this layer; so should chemical events associated with this change. The surface in 1 g *Maja* nerve is estimated to be 10^4 cm². Referring the heat to 1 g active material instead of to 1 g nerve, HILL and his associates arrived at the remarkably high amount of 2.8×10^{-3} cal/g/impulse, which is the same order of magnitude as the heat produced per gram in a muscle during a single twitch.

The observations on heat production in *Maja* nerve are supported by measurements on the heat released by the discharge of the electric organ of *Torpedo marmorata* (ABBOTT et al. 1958a). Three successive phases of heat associated with the discharge were observed: the first phase was always a positive heat, produced most likely simultaneously with the discharge; this positive phase is closely followed by a negative one in which heat is absorbed, but which is usually masked by a prolonged phase in which heat is again produced. The results are in contradiction with those of BERNSTEIN and TSCHERMAK (1906) who thought they had observed a negative heat associated with the discharge of the fish. They assumed that the energy of the discharge is provided by the diffusion of ions in the direction of their concentration gradients. The recent observation carried out with greatly improved recording instruments are incompatible with the simple explanation offered by BERNSTEIN and TSCHERMAK and the fundamentally similar views of HODGKIN (1951).

III. Temperature coefficient

Another type of physical recording pertinent for the problem is the temperature coefficient. There are relatively few data reported in the world literature about the Q_{10} of bioelectric currents. HODGKIN and KATZ (1950) did find high temperature coefficients, but this finding was not considered as relevant to the problem of the nature of the conducting process.

Recently, SCHOFFENIELS (1958, 1959b) has evaluated the Q_{10} and the energy of activation of bioelectric potentials over a wide range of temperature, using the isolated single electroplax of the electric organ of *Electrophorus electricus*. The duration of the action potential, of the postsynaptic potential, and of the latency period of synaptic transmission decrease with rise of temperature, whereas the height of the spike and of the postsynaptic potential remain unchanged. Since during the action potential there is a marked transitory change of permeability, the duration of the spike is a good measure of this change and pertinent for the question whether or not chemical reactions are required for this process. A straight line was obtained when the logarithm of the reciprocal of the half width of the spike was plotted against the reciprocal of the absolute temperature according to the principle of Arrhenius. The Q_{10} of the action potential determined by SCHOFFENIELS is about 3.6, and the energy of activation 21,000 cal/mole.

IV. Necessity of biochemical studies

Once it is recognized that there is the necessity of a chemical reaction which is responsible for the Na-conductance, the question arises: what is the specific chemical system with which conducting cells are endowed? Such a system must obviously have quite a few very special features enabling it to fulfill the function postulated. Moreover, once it has been shown that the system has the necessary properties, it must be demonstrated also that it functions in the living cell in the way proposed. The chemical analysis of every biological process is complex and full of inherent difficulties, especially when it takes place in one thousandth of a second or less and on such a small scale that its detection offers great obstacles even for physical methods. However, the rapid advances of dynamic biochemistry, especially the spectacular progress in enzyme and protein chemistry, have provided the biologist with extremely powerful tools for analyzing cellular function.

For several decades physiologists have been interested in the role of acetyl-choline (ACh), an ester which appears to be specifically linked with nerve activity. The compound has been assumed to be a "neurohumoral transmitter", i.e., that ACh is secreted from nerve endings, crosses the intercellular space and acts as a mediator of nerve impulses from the nerve ending to the effector cell, nerve, or muscle (DALE 1937). This hypothesis, resulting to a large extent from essentially pharmacological observations, is discussed in its various aspects in Chapters 3, 6, 11, 12, 13, and 14 of the present volume. However, it was considered by many neurophysiologists to be unsatisfactory in many respects and in contradiction with other conclusions based on electrophysiological results. They have found it particularly difficult to accept the assumption of a basic difference between the physicochemical mechanism of synaptic transmission and axonal conduction (see, e.g., ERLANGER 1939, FULTON 1938, LORENTE DE NÓ 1938). Not the facts observed were questioned but their interpretation.

In this impasse it appeared necessary to analyze the process underlying nerve activity with chemical methods. Chemical analysis seemed to offer the greatest promise that it would become possible to explain (eventually) the pharmacological observations and to find an interpretation of the role of ACh which would reconcile the opposing views and integrate the facts reported.

A new approach was initiated by the author about twenty-five years ago, based on biochemical methods and on notions and principles similar to those used in the analysis of the biochemical basis of other cellular function, notably of muscular contraction. The sequence of energy transformations associated with nerve activity has been established. The enzymes responsible for the hydrolysis and formation of ACh have been studied and these reactions have been integrated into the metabolic pathways of the nerve cell; the enzymes and proteins of the system have been isolated and purified and their reaction mechanisms have been analyzed. Many relationships have been established between chemical reactions and molecular forces in proteins, studied *in vitro*, and the physical and electrical events occurring in intact cells (NACHMANSOHN 1952, 1955a, b; 1957, 1959, NACHMANSOHN and WILSON 1951, 1956).

The results of these investigations very early necessitated a modification of the original hypothesis of neurohumoral transmission. According to the author's concept which emerged, the release and the action of ACh are not *inter*cellular, but *intra*cellular, or rather intramembranous processes which take place within the axonal and synaptic membranes and which control ion movements. The ACh system provides the mechanism with which the conducting fibers of the animal kingdom are endowed and which enables them to use the ionic concentration gradients, the potential source of electromotive force, for their special function. The reaction of the ester with a receptor protein is essential for the permeability changes taking place during activity, i.e., for the generation of bioelectric currents propagating nerve impulses across synapses as well as along axons. A detailed presentation of the unified concept and of its development, and the various experimental and theoretical aspects of the problem may be found in a recent Monograph (NACHMANSOHN 1959). The opposite viewpoint, that ACh is not involved in axonal conduction, is presented in several chapters of this book (*vide* Chapter 6, pp. 268—273). The controversial questions have been fully discussed in the monograph and a repetition is considered to be unnecessary. Therefore, this chapter summarizes and emphasizes only those aspects which support the assumption of the essential role of ACh in the elementary process generating bioelectric currents. It includes pertinent recent evidence obtained since the publication of the monograph.

B. Evidence for the essentiality of acetylcholinesterase (AChE) in conduction

I. Physiologically significant features of the enzyme

A study of the enzymes catalyzing the hydrolysis and the formation of ACh offers many interesting biochemical aspects. Many features, however, such as occurrence, concentration, localization, speed of reaction, and others, are pertinent for the understanding of the biological role of the ester. Certain prerequisites are required for the postulate that the action of ACh changes Na-conductance during activity, and that the inactivation of ACh by enzymatic hydrolysis reverses the effect and permits the rapid return of Na-conductance to its normal value. Thus, knowledge of the enzyme hydrolyzing the ester is, in addition to its biochemical interest, of paramount importance for interpreting the function of the esterase and consequently of its substrate in nerve activity.

Many types of esterases are present in the animal body. However, there is a special type of esterase which has several features different from other esterases, although some modifications may occasionally be encountered. This enzyme has a relatively high affinity to ACh and has been referred to as acetylcholinesterase (AChE) (AUGUSTINSSON and NACHMANSOHN 1949), a term which has been generally accepted. The enzyme has been reported in greatly varying concentrations in conducting tissue throughout the animal kingdom. It has been found by the author in all types of nerves: motor and sensory fibers, sympathetic and parasympathetic (so-called "cholinergic" and "adrenergic"), peripheral and central, vertebrate and invertebrate, and in various types of muscle. While there have been claims to the contrary for certain neurons (GIACOBINI 1957, HOLMSTEDT and SJOQVIST 1959), these may be attributable to the limited sensitivity of the methods employed. Its occurrence has been demonstrated in monocellular organisms provided with cilia for their movements, such as *Tetrahymena geleii S* (SEAMAN and HOULIHAN 1951). It is essentially absent from certain non-conducting tissue such as liver and kidney.

The concentration of AChE in nerve fibers is remarkably high; on the average, 5 to 50 mg ACh may be split per gram nerve fiber (fresh weight) per hour (NACHMANSOHN 1955b, 1959). These figures, however, do not indicate the actual concentration. The enzyme is localized predominantly in or near the surface membranes. This has been demonstrated in experiments with squid giant axons where no enzyme was detected in the axoplasm, whereas all the enzyme was found in the envelope in which the active membrane must be localized (BOELL and NACHMANSOHN 1940, NACHMANSOHN and MEYERHOF 1941). Observations from other laboratories support this observation. The actual concentration per gram active material must then be several orders of magnitude higher than the figures obtained per gram whole tissue. The apparently low values found in some conducting tissues may be a reflection of the large fraction of inactive material in the samples tested compared with the fraction of active material.

The enzyme concentration in nerve and muscle fibers increases in the region of myoneural and synaptic junctions on the average by a factor of 3 to 6. This result has been obtained with a great variety of tissues. This difference of activity between axonal and synaptic membranes appears to be rather small and may be due, either partly or entirely, to the increased surface area of the membranes at junctions. In a recent paper, GIACOBINI and HOLMSTEDT (1960) reported values of motor endplate AChE which differed by a factor ranging from 3-fold to 100-fold from the values for muscle fibers. However, their procedure was entirely different, and the apparent discrepancy may not be real. This aspect will be discussed more fully in a later section (p. 732).

Quite recently, DETTBARN (1962) found AChE in *Nitella*, an aquatic plant capable of propagating impulses by electric currents in a way similar to that of conducting fibers of animal cells, only the speed of propagation is markedly smaller. The enzyme activity amounts to 6 to 8 μmoles of ACh split per gram tissue per hour, as compared with 40 to 60 μmoles per gram squid giant axon. The enzyme appears to be of the specific type (AChE). This finding suggests the possibility of a mechanism of propagation by electric currents in the plant similar to that used in animal cells. If this assumption should be confirmed by further studies, the observations would add a new example of the biochemical unity of life.

An outstanding feature of the enzyme is the high rate of the hydrolytic process. The enzyme is one of the fastest acting enzymes known. It has a very high turnover number. Early investigations suggested the high value of twenty million (ROTHENBERG and NACHMANSOHN 1946). According to recent still unpublished data of Dr. CLAIRE LAWLER, the figure is about three times higher. In its pure form the enzyme appears to be a polymer containing about 100 active sites. One active site splits one molecule of ester within less than one-tenth of a millisecond. The turnover time is at most 40 to 60 microseconds, but may be even smaller (LAWLER 1961). The high speed of action and the high concentrations in conducting tissues are particularly pertinent for the evaluation of the biological function of the substrate. A chemical reaction which plays an essential role in the generation of bioelectric potentials must take place with the speed comparable to that of the electrical process. If the action of ACh on a protein is responsible for the increased Na-conductance, and the hydrolysis of the ester for the return to the resting state, theory requires the hydrolytic process to have a speed comparable to that of the physical events. The increase of Na-conductance reaches its peak in about 1/10 of a millisecond and then decreases. The speed of the enzymatic action thus satisfies a pertinent prerequisite, since it permits one to attribute to AChE the function of inactivating ACh, thereby enabling the return of Na-conductance to the resting value within the required time limits.

II. Inseparability of electrical and enzyme activity

The occurrence of the enzyme in all animal cells able to generate bioelectric currents and to conduct impulses, the predominant and peculiar localization in the region where the conducting membrane is located, and the high rate of the hydrolytic action are physiologically significant features, pertinent prerequisites for the assumption that the action of ACh and its hydrolysis by AChE play an essential role in the Na-conductance change which generates bioelectric currents. However, the fact alone that the enzyme has the extraordinary features for the proposed special role is, although suggestive, not yet conclusive. A crucial test requires the demonstration of a direct correlation between electrical and enzyme activity. If the proposed concept is correct, it should be impossible to separate electrical and enzyme activity.

Extensive investigation with different types of highly specific and potent inhibitors, such as physostigmine (eserine), applied to a great number of different nerve fibers under a variety of conditions and with different procedures, indicates that such a separation is impossible.

Eserine, a potent and specific inhibitor of ChE, blocks conduction. This block is readily reversible, as would be expected from the reversible nature of the inhibitory process (BULLOCK et al. 1946). In contrast to eserine, neostigmine, an equally potent competitive inhibitor of AChE, does not block conduction, even if applied in very high concentrations for prolonged periods of time. It could be shown, however, as one might have suspected, that structural barriers do not permit the compound to enter the cell interior. When squid giant axons were exposed to neostigmine in 10^{-2} M concentrations for several hours, not a trace of the compound was found in the axoplasm, in contrast to analogous experiments with eserine. Neostigmine would have been detectable in 10^{-8} M concentration.

During World War II a group of organophosphorus compounds became known which are highly potent irreversible inhibitors of AChE and esterases in general. These compounds were used originally as insecticides, but some of them, due to their volatile character, are extremely potent "nerve gases", potential chemical warface agents [e.g., Sarin, Tabun, diisopropyl-phosphorofluoridate (DFP); see Chapters 9 and 19]. Because of the irreversible nature of this inhibition, these compounds are for several reasons extremely useful tools for studying the relationship of enzyme and electrical activity, and for the analysis of the mechanism of hydrolytic action. The latter aspect will be discussed in a later section. There are, however, many pitfalls in such analysis, described on previous occasions (NACHMANSOHN 1959). In some early studies, when many of the pitfalls were not yet known, it seemed possible to inactivate the enzyme completely while conduction was still unimpaired. Subsequent investigations using these compounds have shown that it is impossible under any condition to separate electrical and enzyme activity. A striking parallelism was established between irreversible block of conduction and decrease of enzyme activity as a function of time and of temperature. Measurements in the author's laboratory indicate that electrical activity in axons ceases when the enzyme activity falls to about 20% of the initial concentration; the excess of this enzyme above the functional minimum required seems to be about 5-fold in most axons studied (NACHMANSOHN 1959). This is within the usual range of excess of many enzyme concentrations. The inseparability of electrical and chemical activity was shown with a great many types of nerve fibers, motor and sensory, sympathetic and parasympathetic, central and peripheral, vertebrate and invertebrate, as well as with muscles (NACHMANSOHN 1955, 1959). Thus, the generality of the relationship appears to be firmly established.

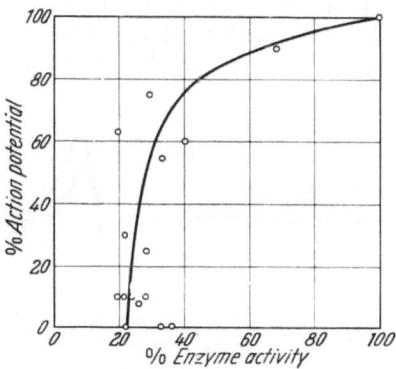

The inseparability of enzyme and electrical activity was demonstrated on intact nerve fibers of crab (Fig. 1). In these observations evidence was offered that different factors such as the concentration of the inhibitor, its chemical structure, and other properties affect the speed with which the 20% level is obtained, but not the level itself (WILSON and COHEN 1953). The demonstration of the functional interdependence of electrical and enzyme activity eliminated the objection that the concentrations of inhibitor required are high, much higher than those required to inhibit enzyme activity *in vitro* or to block synaptic activity. It would seem that the outside concentration is completely irrelevant since it is possible to demonstrate that as long as there is electrical activity the enzyme activity is not decreased below a certain critical level. It is only the concentration of the inhibitor at the site of action which is pertinent. The existence of structural barriers prohibiting many compounds from entering the

Fig. 1. Inseparability of electrical and esterase activity in axons. Crab nerve fibers were exposed to DFP (0.02 to 0.04 M). Enzyme activity was determined on intact fibers. No electrical activity can be evoked when enzyme activity falls to about 20% of the initial value

cell has been well known for a long time. For the specific problem under discussion, the experiments with neostigmine mentioned before are pertinent evidence. An analogous experiment was carried out with DFP, which in contrast to neostigmine is highly lipid soluble.

Nevertheless, when squid giant axons were exposed to 1 mg of DFP/ml, it was found that at the time when conduction was blocked, the concentration in the interior was less than 1 μg per g axoplasm; this is less than one thousandth of the outside concentration. Although we do not know what the concentration at the active site may be, the experiments demonstrate the existence of a complex structural barrier and the difficulty in attempting to correlate the outside concentration for the relationship between enzyme and functional activity.

An interesting new confirmation in this respect was provided by the recent experiments of DETTBARN (1960a) on Ranvier nodes of a single frog sciatic nerve fiber, in which he used the technique worked out by STAEM-

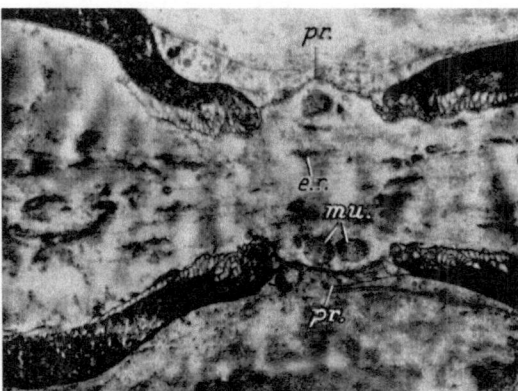

Fig. 2. Longitudinal section of a node fixed in permanganate. The unmyelinated nodal region is characterized by a collar of minute processes (pr.) of the two Schwann cells meeting at the node. Magnification: × 16,000 (from J. D. ROBERTSON 1960)

PFLI (1956). Electron microscope studies of ROBERTSON (1960) have revealed that the conducting membrane at the node of Ranier is covered only by a very thin and apparently "porous" structure (Fig. 2). On exposure of the node to 200 to 300 μg eserine/ml, DETTBARN found conduction blocked in about 30 seconds (Fig. 3). Applied to the intact frog sciatic nerve eserine, at a concentration of 5 mg/ml, blocks in 30 minutes. By removing inactive extraneous material (fat, connective tissue, etc.), the dose required to block electrical activity in the conducting membrane of a myelinated nerve fiber was decreased by a factor of 1000. With 30 to 60 μg of eserine/ml, block of conduction in a Ranvier node was achieved within minutes.

If the action of ACh increases Na-conductance and the return to the resting state is due to hydrolysis of the ester, a decrease in the rate of removal should increase the spike height and amplitude before blocking conduction. As was first

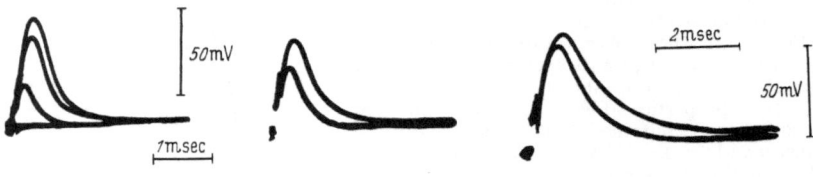

Fig. 3   Fig. 4

Fig. 3. Effect of eserine (300 μg/ml) on the mononodal action potential of a single nerve fiber preparation of the frog sciatic nerve. Electrical activity was blocked in 30 sec. After the return to Ringer's solution, conduction was restored within 40 sec. The spike reached its original height after 10 min. pH 7.7. t = 23°C' (DETTBARN 1960a)

Fig. 4. An increased spike height and a prolongation of the descending phase produced at a node of Ranvier of a single frog nerve fiber by 10^{-6} M eserine (3 μg/ml) (DETTBARN 1960a)

pointed out by ECCLES in a discussion in 1946 at a meeting of the New York Academy of Sciences, such an effect of inhibitors of cholinesterase on the spike should be expected from theory (see Chapter 6, p. 270). There are several factors,

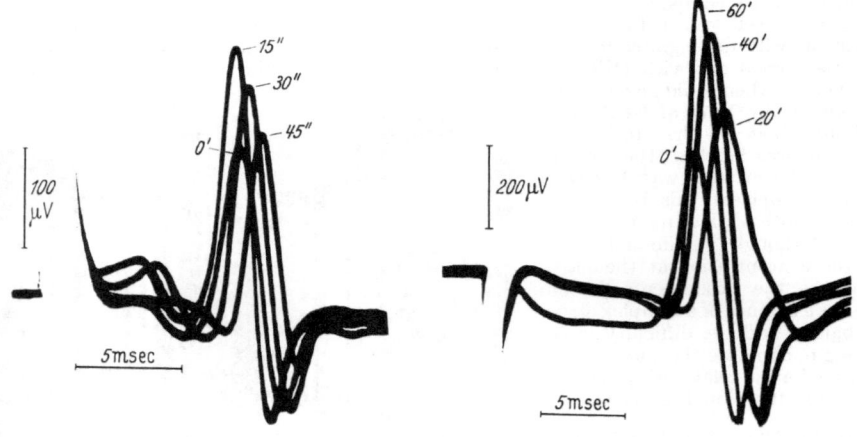

Fig. 5   Fig. 6

Fig. 5. Increase of spike height in a frog sartorius muscle on exposure to Paraoxon (1.5 mg/ml). Records shown (superimposed) were taken at 0 time and 15, 30, and 45 sec after exposure

Fig. 6. Increase of spike height in a frog sartorius muscle during recovery after the muscle had been exposed to Paraoxon (1 mg/ml) for 10 min. Records shown were taken at 0 time and 20, 40, and 60 min after the start of the experiment

however, which may complicate the picture. The effect postulated will take place only at a very definite level of enzyme activity. Below the minimum compatible with electric activity, conduction fails. As long as an excess of enzyme is present, no change of the spike potential would be expected. The appropriate range of the level of enzyme activity may be extremely narrow and the period of time during which this level is maintained may be extremely short. In multifiber preparations such as the frog sciatic nerve, where the spike is the resultant of the electrical activity of several thousand fibers, the effect may be masked. Some inhibitors of the enzyme, as will be seen later, also have a high affinity to the receptor protein and this factor may modify the picture. However, by applying 1.5 to 10 μg eserine/ml to Ranvier nodes of single frog sciatic fibers, DETTBARN (1960a) did indeed observe an increase of spike height and amplitude (Fig. 4). Diethyl 4-nitrophenyl phosphate (Paraoxon) produced similar and sometimes even stronger effects.

An increased spike height and amplitude was recently observed in strips of frog sartorius muscle on exposure to either eserine or Paraoxon (Fig. 5) (HINTER-BUCHNER and NACHMANSOHN 1960). Under conditions in which the latter had not yet produced irreversible block, the increase of the spike potential was sometimes very pronounced in the recovery period, which is usually much longer than that during which the electrical activity disappears; diffusion of the inhibitor from the outside to the inside is faster than the reverse (higher concentration gradient) (Fig. 6). The period during which the appropriate level of enzyme activity prevails may therefore be longer.

III. Electrical activity produced by a specific chemical reaction

Recently, a new type of evidence has been obtained for the essentiality of AChE in electrical activity. If the irreversible inhibition of the enzyme by organophosphorus compounds is responsible for the irreversible block of electrical activity in

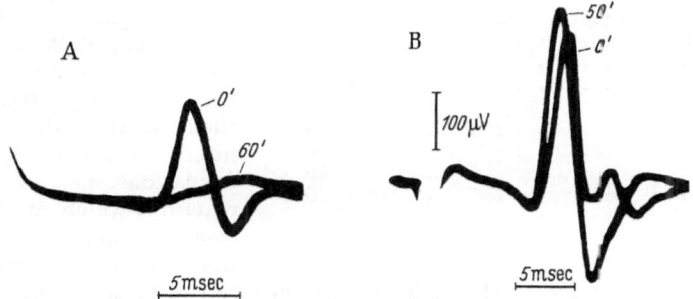

Fig. 7. Reappearance of electrical activity by the action of benzoylpyridine oxime methiodide in a muscle exposed to Paraoxon until irreversible block was achieved. Two strips dissected from a frog sartorius muscle were exposed to 1.5 mg/ml of Paraoxon for 8 min. A, control. Action potential was abolished within 3.5 min. The strip was washed 3 times with and then kept in Ringer solution. Records shown were taken at 0 and 60 min. B, second strip was washed 3 times with Ringer's solution and then kept in 10^{-2} M benzoyl-pyridine oxime methiodide from the 9th to the 45th min after the start of the experiment. Records were taken at 0 and 50 min

conducting membranes, as proposed by the author in 1946, then electrical activity should reappear if the enzyme activity could be restored by a chemical reaction. An extremely potent and highly specific compound has been developed, pyridine-2-aldoxime methiodide (P-2-AM), which reactivates specifically AChE inhibited by certain organophosphorus compounds by displacing the phosphoryl group from the enzyme (see section D and Chapter 21). Pyridine-2-aldoxime methiodide is a quaternary ammonium compound, and lipid-insoluble. It will therefore not reach the conducting membrane, as will be discussed later. However, benzoyl-pyridine oxime methiodide is somewhat lipid soluble and nearly as potent as P-2-AM.

Strips of frog sartorius muscle were exposed to Paraoxon until irreversible block was achieved. When the strips were bathed in the benzoyl derivative, a restoration of electrical activity was obtained (Fig. 7) (HINTERBUCHNER and NACHMANSOHN 1960). However, these experiments were in some respects not fully satisfactory. The multifiber preparation selected offered some special problems, the organophosphorus compound some others. But the essential principle was established: electrical activity of a conducting membrane, abolished by specific inhibitors of AChE which phosphorylate the enzyme, was restored by a compound which specifically reactivates phosphorylated AChE.

C. Sequence of energy transformations. Integration of acetylcholine (ACh) into metabolic pathways

I. Acetylcholinesterase (AChE) in electric organs

Early in this century OTTO MEYERHOF (1913) postulated that knowledge of the sequence of energy transformations is essential for the understanding of the biochemistry of cellular function. The transformation of chemical into mechanical energy in muscle takes place on a scale which is much more readily accessible to biochemical measurements than the chemical reactions controlling ion movements across conducting membranes during activity. However, nature has provided biologists with an invaluable tool for studying chemical mechanisms underlying electrical activity: the electric organs of fish. These organs are the most powerful bioelectric generators created by nature. Moreover, they are highly specialized in their function. Here the magnitude of the energy transformations, i.e., of chemical reactions which are linked to electrical activity, is in the range of measurement. The electrical characteristics of the cellular unit, the electroplax, are similar to those in nerve and muscle cells; it is only the arrangement of the units in series by which the discharge becomes so powerful. Among the various species *Electrophorus electricus*, the so-called "electric eel", has the most powerful organ. It has 5000 to 6000 electroplax in series, the discharge is about 600 volts. For various reasons it is a most suitable material for many studies. The electroplax of this species has both synaptic and conducting membranes which can be readily distinguished functionally (see Chapter 13). The use of these fish for the study of biochemical processes underlying the generation of bioelectricity, which was initiated by the writer in 1937, proved to be of decisive value for further developments in this field.

Table 1. *Acetylcholinesterase concentration in the main electric organ of Electrophorus electricus compared with some other tissues*

Tissue	Acetylcholine hydrolyzed (mg/gm/hr)
Mammalian (guinea pig) at 37°C	
Muscle fibers	8— 15
Nerve fibers	10— 15
Brain	80—100
Frog at 23°C	
Muscle fibers	3— 6
Nerve fibers	5—10
Brain	40—80
Electric organ, *E. electricus*, at 23°C. .	2000—4000
Mammalian kidney	0
Mammalian liver	0

The strong electric organs of *Torpedo* and *Electrophorus* contain a strikingly high concentration of AChE: as the very first measurements revealed, the electric organs of these two species are capable of hydrolyzing 2 to 4 g of ACh per g tissue (fresh weight) per hour. This is high even compared to other conducting tissue (see Table 1), and particularly remarkable in view of the high water and low protein content of the tissue, 93 and 2%, respectively. The actual concentration per gram active membrane is actually several orders of magnitude higher, since once again the enzyme is localized in an extremely small fraction of the tissue. Such an extraordinary concentration of a specific enzyme in an organ which is highly specialized for generating electric currents at once suggests the possibility of a direct relationship with the primary function. The electric organ of *Electrophorus* has unique structural features which permit the correlation of function (electrical activity) with enzyme activity (NACHMANSOHN 1959). A direct proportionality was found to exist in this organ between voltage per cm and enzyme concentration (NACHMANSOHN et al. 1941; NACHMANSOHN et al. 1946).

The organs offer an exceptionally favorable material for preparing enzyme solutions (NACHMANSOHN and LEDERER 1939). Highly active and purified enzyme preparations were obtained (ROTHENBERG and NACHMANSOHN 1947; LAWLER 1959). This made possible the study of many pertinent properties of the enzyme and has permitted the analysis of the molecular forces in the active site, as will be described in the sections to follow.

II. Discovery of choline acetylase (ChAc)

The release of energy by the breakdown of phosphocreatine during the discharge of *Electrophorus* is more than adequate to account for the total electrical energy released (NACHMANSOHN, COX, COATES and MACHADO 1943). It was assumed on the basis of analogy with events known to take place in muscular contraction, that ATP hydrolysis would precede that of phosphocreatine. But it appeared unlikely for many reasons that ATP would be directly associated with the elementary process as in muscular contraction. If the action of ACh and its hydrolysis are responsible for the primary event, then the free energy (ΔF) of ATP hydrolysis should be used for the resynthesis of ACh, i.e., for the acetylation of choline. This would, of course, not be the only function of the energy provided by ATP hydrolysis. The restoration of the original ion distribution, i.e., the extrusion of Na^+ and the uptake of K^+ against the concentration gradients, also requires a supply of energy and this must be another function of ATP.

The assumption that ATP hydrolysis may provide the energy for the acetylation of choline proved to be correct. An enzyme, choline acetylase (ChAc), was extracted in 1943 from brain and electric tissue which, in the presence of ATP, was capable of synthesizing ACh in solution (NACHMANSOHN and MACHADO 1943). This was the first enzymatic acetylation achieved in solution and the first demonstration that the energy of ATP hydrolysis may be used for acylation reactions; it suggested that the energy of ATP, until then linked only with glycolysis, may be used for biosynthetic reactions in general. It was also found in the same year that the system requires a coenzyme, since it became rapidly inactivated during dialysis (NACHMANSOHN, JOHN and WAELSCH 1943). These observations opened the way for the study of acetylating mechanisms in general, and during the following decade the investigation of this reaction mechanism became one of the most active fields in biochemistry.

Choline acetylase has been found to be present in a great variety of conducting tissues: in motor and sensory axons, in invertebrate and vertebrate, in central and peripheral nerve tissue, and in muscle. Choline acetylase is absent from non-conducting tissue such as liver and kidney. Thus, it is apparent that the system forming and hydrolyzing ACh is a specific feature of tissues capable of generating electric currents.

A more detailed discussion of various aspects of choline acetylase may be found in Chapters 2 and 3.

III. Depolarizing action of acetylcholine (ACh)

The significance of the discovery of ChAc for understanding the chemical basis of nerve activity was the evidence that in the sequence of energy transformations ACh hydrolysis and synthesis precede the other chemical reactions. Thereby, the integration of the metabolism of ACh in the intermediary cellular pathways was achieved. It could be argued that theoretically another chemical reaction may precede that of ACh. Such an assumption is contradicted by the fact that ACh has a depolarizing action. This was first proposed by MONNIER and DUBUISSON (1934) and COWAN (1936) and experimentally demonstrated on *Torpedo* (Fig. 8) (FELDBERG et al. 1940). This depolarizing (electrogenic) action makes it difficult to speculate that the ester may have an entirely different function which takes place in some mysterious way during recovery. There are, of course, other compounds and substances which may mimic this action, but only the ACh system has the prerequisites to be associated with the permeability changes which occur in a conducting membrane during activity.

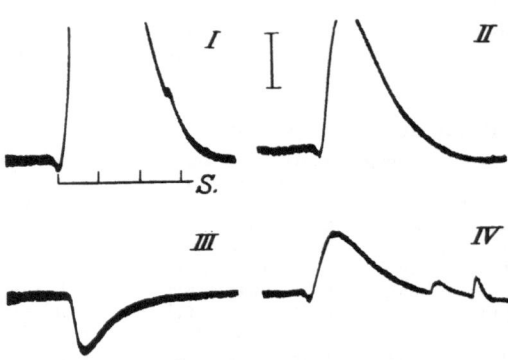

Fig. 8. Depolarizing action of ACh. The potential changes are produced by intra-arterial injection of ACh into the electric organ of *Torpedo marmorata*, in the presence of eserine. I, II and IV present the effects of 10, 5, and 2.5 μg of ACh; at III only perfusion fluid was injected. 0.5 Millivolt indicated at II. Time in seconds

IV. Sensory receptors

Both AChE and ChAc are present in sensory fibers; inhibitors of ChE block conduction in dorsal roots and other sensory fibers in the same way as in motor fibers. This action supports the assumption of the functional necessity of the enzyme for conduction in both types of fibers (BULLOCK et al. 1947, COHEN 1956). Acetylcholine and analogous compounds activate sensory receptor endings as well as effector cells at synaptic junctions (SKOUBY 1951, ZOTTERMAN 1953, BUCHTHAL 1954). Recently, LOEWENSTEIN and MOLINS (1958) determined the ChE distribution in Pacinian corpuscles obtained from the mesentery and pancreas of the cat. The various parts of the corpuscle were separated by dissection and the enzyme activity was determined in the different structures. By far the largest fraction of the enzyme was found to be localized in the axon, nerve ending, and in the thin hull of core structure which surrounds the ending. The ChE or ChE's present in the structures around the nerve ending, precisely where the generation of electrical activity of this receptor organ has been shown to take place, are able to hydrolyze 0.7×10^9 molecules of ACh/millisecond. This activity is remarkably close to the figure obtained for the AChE in a single motor endplate of frog sartorius muscle, which is 1.6×10^9 molecules/millisecond (NACHMANSOHN 1939). The data provide further support for the view that the ACh system has the same physiological role in the generation of bioelectric potentials in sensory receptors as in motor endplates. In the former there is, however, no synaptic junction which makes it difficult to picture the release and action of the ester other than intracellular.

V. The elementary process

The picture of the role of the ACh system in the elementary process of conduction which has emerged from the data accumulated may be described as follows (Fig. 9): In the resting condition, ACh (o-) is in a bound and inactive form. It may be tentatively called the storage form (S). Excitation of the membrane, by current or any other stimulus, leads to a dissociation of the complex, and ACh is released. The free ester acts upon a receptor protein (R), and this action upon the receptor is essential for the change of ionic permeability, i.e., for the increased Na-conductance and thus the generation of bioelectric potentials. Some facts to be discussed later suggest that ACh may act by changing the configuration of the receptor protein.

The complex between ACh and the receptor is in a dynamic equilibrium with the free ester and the receptor. The free ester is susceptible to attack by AChE (E). The enzymatic hydrolysis of ACh will permit the receptor to return to its resting condition. Sodium-conductance returns to its original level. Thus the action of the enzyme leads to immediate recovery and ends the cycle of the elementary process. It is the speed of this inactivation process which makes rapid restoration of the membrane possible and permits the nerve to respond to the next stimulus within a millesecond or less. All these events, which control the ion movements during activity, must take place within the structure which functions as a barrier for these ions in rest. Structural organization of the components within a membrane of 100 Å or less may greatly contribute to the speed, precision, and efficiency of the reactions. The further recovery leads to the resynthesis of ACh in its bound form by ChAc and the other components of the acetylating system. At this point, the cyclic processes known for other cells enter the picture.

The evidence summarized so far is considered to have established a solid basis for the view that ACh is the "specific operative substance" in the elementary process of conduction of nerve impulses in the sense applied by MEYERHOF to the role

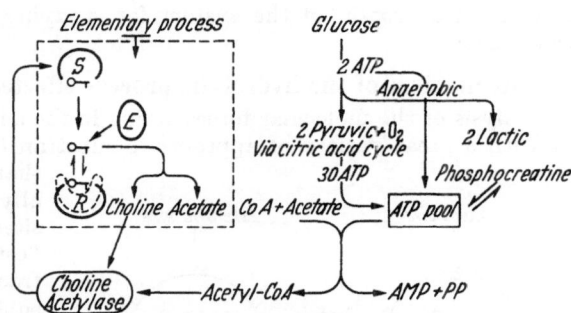

Fig. 9. Schematic presentation of the elementary process and of the sequence of energy transformations associated with conduction and integration of the ACh system into the metabolic pathways. For details see text

of ATP in muscular contraction. Just as the latter is inseparably associated with motility, ACh is considered essential for the primary events generating bioelectricity in conducting membranes throughout the animal kingdom. Although the action of the ester appears essential for the ionic conductance changes taking place during activity, an analysis of the detailed mechanism is still in the initial stage. This will be discussed more fully in connection with the molecular forces acting in the proteins of the ACh system. Obviously, many additional factors and membrane constituents must be important, about which virtually nothing is known at present. Suggestions as to the precise mechanism of action must, therefore, clearly be only tentative. This, of course, cannot be construed as an argument against the essential role proposed.

D. Molecular forces in the proteins of the acetylcholine system and their relation to function

During the last decade much pertinent information has been obtained by the analysis of the molecular forces acting in the proteins of the ACh system. In several instances it was possible to establish relationships between the reactions of the proteins in solution and the function of the intact cell. In some cases such relationships were found to parallel those of specific electrical events.

Four proteins, as we have seen, are directly tied to the function of ACh. Two of them, the two enzymes, have been isolated and are available for analysis in purified form in solution. The existence of a receptor as a distinct cell constituent was first demonstrated on intact cells only (ALTAMIRANO et al. 1955, NACHMAN-SOHN 1955b), but recently EHRENPREIS has isolated the putative receptor protein from electric tissue of *Electrophorus* (EHRENPREIS 1959, 1961). The storage form has not been isolated, and nothing definite is known about its properties and characteristics (see Chapter 3). A molecule such as ACh has only a limited number of possibilities of reacting with a protein; the molecular forces acting between the small molecule and the macromolecules of the system must, therefore, be similar. Relatively small modifications in the surface of the protein may lead to important changes in function. Information obtained by the analysis of molecular forces in one protein will, therefore, provide valuable information for an understanding of the reactions with other proteins. Acetylcholinesterase is for many reasons the most suitable protein of the system for studying the molecular forces in the active surface.

I. Mechanism of the hydrolytic process effected by acetylcholinesterase

Analysis of the molecular forces acting in the active surface of AChE, carried out with a great variety of appropriate substrates and inhibitors, has revealed that the surface has two functionally and spatially separated subsites: an "anionic" site and an "esteratic" site. The former attracts the cationic group of the substrate by COULOMBIC and VAN DER WAALS' forces. The esteratic site has an acidic and a basic or nucleophilic group, symbolized by H and G. The nucleophilic group forms a covalent bond with the electrophilic carbon of the carbonyl group (Fig. 10) (BERGMANN et al. 1950).

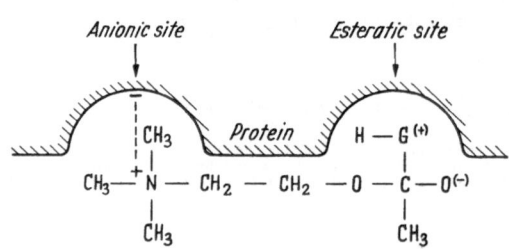

Fig. 10. Schematic presentation of the interaction of the active groups in the surface of AChE and the substrate; the Michaelis-Menten complex

The following mechanism has been proposed for the hydrolytic process (WILSON et al. 1950).

$$H-\overset{\cdot\cdot}{G} + R-\overset{\overset{O}{\parallel}}{C}-OR' \rightleftarrows R'\overset{H-G}{\underset{R}{\overset{\cdot\cdot}{O}}}\overset{\parallel}{C}-O^{(-)} \rightleftarrows \overset{G^{(+)}}{\underset{R}{\overset{\parallel}{C}}}-O^{(-)} + R'OH$$

$$(A) \qquad (B)$$

$$H-\overset{\cdot\cdot}{O}: + \overset{G^{(+)}}{\underset{R}{\overset{\parallel}{C}}}-O^{(-)} \rightleftarrows \overset{H-G^{(+)}}{\underset{R}{HO-C}}-O^{(-)} \rightleftarrows H-\overset{\cdot\cdot}{G} + R-\overset{\overset{O}{\parallel}}{C}-OH$$

$$(B) \qquad (C)$$

The alcohol is eliminated from the enzyme substrate complex by an electronic shift and as a result of the first phase an acetylated enzyme is formed. This reacts with H_2O to form acetate, thus regenerating the enzyme. Experimental evidence in support of this mechanism has been offered in many ways. A detailed discussion may be found in several reviews (NACHMANSOHN 1955b, NACHMANSOHN 1959, NACHMANSOHN and WILSON 1951, WILSON 1954). A full account of the information concerning the active centers of the enzyme will be found in Chapters 7 and 21.

II. Mechanism of "nerve gas" action and development of a powerful antidote

Knowledge of the molecular forces in the active sites of the enzyme has greatly helped the understanding of various aspects of nerve function. An illustration is the analysis of the mechanism of the action of organophosphorus compounds, to which belong the widely used insecticides and the "nerve gases". The information led to the development of an extremely potent antidote. All esterases are irreversibly inhibited by the action of these compounds. Their lethal action, however, is due to the inhibition of AChE, i.e., to a specific chemical lesion (NACHMANSOHN and FELD 1947).

Even before the mechanism of the hydrolytic process had been analyzed, BURGEN (1949) proposed that the action of alkylphosphates must be due to a phosphorylation of the enzyme by a process in which the acidic group is eliminated and the phosphoryl radical is transferred to some polar group on the enzyme. The analysis of the molecular forces in the active site and the explanation of the hydrolytic process fully support the mechanism of alkylphosphate action suggested by BURGEN. The nucleophilic group in the esteratic site of the enzyme attacks the phosphorus atom in an S_N2 reaction (WILSON and BERGMANN 1950). Instead of an acylated enzyme, the physiological intermediary, a phosphorylated enzyme is formed. But whereas the acylated form reacts extremely fast, within a fraction of a millisecond, with water to form acetate and restored enzyme, the phosphorylated enzyme does not react with water at all or does so extremely slowly, requiring days or weeks. The enzyme is inactivated, and because of the loss of its vital function death ensues.

Once the mechanism of alkylphosphate poisoning was recognized, it seemed possible to reverse the inhibition of the enzyme by a nucleophilic group which would attack the phosphorus atom and remove the phosphoryl group from the enzyme in a displacement reaction; thereby the enzymatic activity would be restored. Hydroxylamine is a nucleophilic agent which had been shown to attack the carbon of the carbonyl group of the acetylated enzyme (HESTRIN 1949, 1950). When this compound was applied to the phosphorylated enzyme, it was found that it is indeed capable of reactivating the enzyme. In 0.7 M concentration, about 50% of the enzyme activity inhibited by tetraethyl pyrophosphate was restored in about 5 hours (WILSON 1951).

Wilson reasoned that by attaching the active nucleophilic group to a cationic quaternary nitrogen group at a proper atomic distance, the attack on the phosphorus atom should be greatly promoted. The cationic group of the molecule would be attracted to the anionic site and the nucleophilic atom would thus be directed towards the P atom. This would be analogous to the fact that ACh is a greatly superior substrate for AChE compared to ethyl acetate, since the presence of the cationic group increases the force of binding by more than 1000-fold and helps the compound to be attracted and oriented on the protein surface. Among a series of compounds synthesized the most potent reactivator turned out to be pyridine-2-aldoxime methiodide (P-2-AM). When this compound was tested, its ability to reactivate alkylphosphate -inhibited AChE *in vitro* was found to be about 1 million times as high as that of hydroxylamine (WILSON and GINSBURG 1955). The active molecule has the following structure (the *anti*-form):

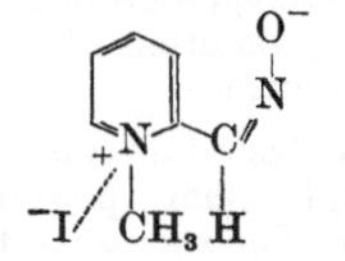

It may be mentioned that shortly after the description of P-2-AM by WILSON and GINS-BURG (1955) in this laboratory, CHILDS et al. (1955) described a series of oximes which they had synthesized independently, in view of WILSON's earlier studies with hydroxamic acids. One of them was P-2-AM.

When P-2-AM was applied by KEWITZ to animals, it proved to be an extremely potent antidote (KEWITZ and WILSON 1955). In combination with atropine, which protects the receptor protein, animals survived 10- to 20-fold lethal doses of nerve gas (KEWITZ et al. 1956).

An outstanding early toxic effect is paralysis of the diaphragm. It appeared, therefore, logical to test the AChE activity in the diaphragm of P-2-AM treated animals. A marked reactivation of the AChE in this tissue has been demonstrated in animals exposed to alkylphosphate and treated with P-2-AM (KEWITZ 1957). In brain the first experiments on the reactivation of AChE by P-2-AM were inconclusive (KEWITZ and NACHMANSOHN 1957). Studies on the effect of P-2-AM on the electroencephalogram of rabbits exposed to Sarin suggested, however, some action on the brain (LONGO et al. 1960). Recently, ROSENBERG (1960) using chloroform extraction procedures in which some earlier inadequacies were eliminated, found a significant reactivation of AChE by P-2-AM in various brain centers of the rabbit. Reactivation was not equally strong in all parts but seemed most marked in the pons, the region of area postrema, and the remainder of the medulla. The observations support the view that the principal action of P-2-AM is due to the reactivation of the enzyme activity, the repair of the chemical lesion. It is true that direct reaction with some of the alkylphosphates does also occur and this factor may in some cases also contribute to the antidotal action. However, this reaction is very slow, especially with some of the alkylphosphates tested such as Paraoxon, and therefore inefficient so that this cannot be the principal factor of the antidotal power of P-2-AM.

The ability of P-2-AM to reactivate the enzyme attacking the phosphoryl group naturally depends on the structure and properties of the latter. Some will be readily detached by P-2-AM, others only poorly, and some not at all. The phosphorylated enzyme formed after the reaction with Tabun or octamethylpyrophosphoramide (OMPA) (when the latter has been transformed in the organism into an active form) is not reactivated by P-2-AM at all. Consequently, it should be expected, if the theory proposed is correct, that in those cases P-2-AM is not an antidote. This is indeed the case. Pyridine-2-aldoxime methiodide has only a very small protective effect after poisoning by Tabun and none against OMPA. The slight protection against Tabun must be attributed to a direct reaction in the blood between drug and P-2-AM, since this reaction is relatively fast, in any case faster than with some other alkylphosphates tested. These negative results are further evidence for the view that the antidotal properties of P-2-AM must be attributed to the repair of the specific chemical lesion, i.e., to the reactivation of the phosphorylated enzyme and not to a direct reaction with alkylphosphate; it is a really efficient antidote against only those compounds which form a phosphorylated enzyme that can be readily reactivated by P-2-AM in vitro (KEWITZ 1957).

In order to explain the extraordinary power of P-2-AM to reactivate alkylphosphate -inhibited enzyme, Wilson and his associates undertook a systematic study of the "geometry" of the enzyme. They prepared a series of derivatives of phenyltrimethylammonium ions to obtain information about the degree of binding in terms of the respective positions of various atoms of the inhibitor and of the enzyme. It turned out that P-2-AM has a perfect complementary conformation to the phosphorylated enzyme (WILSON and QUAN 1958, WILSON et al. 1958, WILSON 1959). When the quaternary nitrogen is attached, through Coulombic forces, to the anionic site of the enzyme, the nucleophilic oxygen atom of the oxime is exactly one bond length away from the P atom. If the oxime group is in the 4-position, the compound is still a very good reactivator, although about 40 times poorer, but in the 3-position, it is virtually inactive. Both results are in agreement with theory derived from these studies.

In view of the molecular complementariness of P-2-AM to the phosphorylated AChE, it is to be expected that this compound exerts the extraordinary power of reactivation only in the case of this particular enzyme. The reactivation of phosphorylated serum esterase by P-2-AM proved indeed to be much less efficient. For phosphorylated chymotrypsin, P-2-AM is a very poor reactivator. Moreover, there is no difference between P-2-, P-3, and P-4-AM. These facts provide additional evidence that the reactivating power of P-2-AM is not due to an especially high intrinsic power of the oxygen atom to attack the P atom, but to molecular complementariness and to the special promotion of the reaction by the cationic nitrogen located in the most favorable atomic distance.

Pyridine-2-aldoxime methiodide was tested on a large scale by NAMBA and HIRAKI (1958) on humans suffering from acute alkylphosphate poisoning in Japan where insecticides are widely used and are of vital importance. The success of the treatment was striking and many lives were saved. Other dramatic recoveries in severe poisoning of humans have been described elsewhere (e.g., ERDMANN et al. 1958).

The theoretical explanation of the mechanism of action of organophosphorus compounds and the preparation of a powerful antidote as developed in the reviewer's laboratory, have been described in more detail in a recent monograph (NACHMANSOHN 1959). The correctness of these views has been generally recognized and the implications have been widely accepted. They formed the basis of much subsequent work in many laboratories during the last few years (see Chapters 7 and 21).

The analysis of the molecular forces of the active site, the mechanism of the hydrolytic process, and the design of a compound capable of reactivating AChE inhibited by organophosphates have been discussed, although only very briefly, as an illustration of the basic approach of the author to the problem of nerve function. The principle used has been the investigation of the properties of enzymes and proteins in solution and the use of the information obtained *in vitro* for the understanding of their action in the intact cell. One example, described in a preceding section, is the restoration of electrical activity in a conducting membrane after its apparently irreversible block by organophosphate, achieved by the reactivation of the enzyme with the aid of a compound removing specifically the phosphoryl group from the esteratic site. The systematic development of a powerful antidote against organophosphate poisoning acting not only on the intact cell but even in the whole animals is another example.

E. The acetylcholine receptor

I. Studies on the intact electroplax

Another illustration of how the analysis of the molecular forces acting in the proteins of the ACh system has been helpful in the interpretation of problems of conduction is the information obtained about the interaction between ACh and the receptor.

During the analysis of the role of VAN DER WAALS' forces acting in the enzyme substrate complex formation, a remarkable fact was observed: if one substitutes the protons of an ammonium ion by methyl groups, each of the first three methyl groups increase the *binding* by a factor of about 7. The fourth methyl group is without effect. Similar results were obtained with hydroxyethyl ammonium ion: the fourth alkyl (third methyl) group does not increase the binding (WILSON 1952).

In striking contrast the difference in *enzymatic activity* is extremely marked between tertiary and quaternary nitrogen derivatives; the rate of formation of acetyl enzyme by AChE was found to be about 10 times as high with ACh as substrate as with its tertiary analogue, dimethylaminoethyl acetate. A similar difference was observed in the activity of ChAc towards choline and its tertiary analogue, dimethylethanolamine. The latter compound is acetylated at a rate only 8% of that of the former (BERMAN et al. 1953, BERMAN-REISBERG 1957).

The question arises as to the significance of these striking differences of enzyme activity due to the presence of one extra methyl group. The binding forces, as we have seen, are not increased. The quaternary nitrogen is a saturated group and is less reactive than a tertiary nitrogen because at neutral pH the latter is in equilibrium with a small concentration of conjugated base which has a free pair of electrons. Chemical reactivity then cannot be the answer and another explanation must be found. A clue may be the tetrahedral structure of the quaternary nitrogen group. Such a structure is more or less spherical. If a molecule like this is attracted to a protein surface, the fourth alkyl will not have direct contact since it is oriented in a direction away from the protein. One way in which the protein could be simultaneously in contact with all the methyl groups would be by enveloping the molecule. This implies a change of configuration of the protein during its active state in the enzymatic process.

This possibility has found some experimental support in studies on the enthalpies and entropies of activation, ΔH^* and ΔS^*, of the esters of ethanolamine and its methylated derivatives (WILSON and CABIB 1956). Substitution of the first two protons by methyl groups did not greatly change the activation energies. But the third additional methyl group has a very pronounced effect. The enthalpy of activation, ΔH^*, of the hydrolysis of ACh is about —14,000 cal/mole as compared with about —8000 cal of that of the tertiary analogue. The high ΔH^* indicates that conditions for the hydrolysis of the quaternary ester are less favorable. But the entropy of activation, ΔS^*, is extremely favorable for the quaternary compared to that of the tertiary compound. The value for the tertiary is —7 to —9 entropy units (e.u.), whereas it is strongly positive with the quaternary, about + 15 to + 30 e.u. This extraordinary difference of the entropy of activation produced by the presence of the extra methyl group can be explained in terms of rearrangement of the protein molecule, i.e., a change in configuration. A rearrangement of acidic and basic groups due to a change of configuration of proteins was proposed by KURT H. MEYER (1937) as a possible basis for the change of permeability to ions during conduction. Does ACh produce such an effect when reacting with the receptor ?

A receptor was postulated 50 years ago by LANGLEY (1907). Its existence as a cell constituent distinct from AChE has been experimentally demonstrated by a combination of two methods, which permitted a distinction to be made between compounds acting predominantly on the receptor, those acting on the enzyme, or on both (ALTAMIRANO et al. 1955, NACHMANSOHN 1955b).

Segments of electric tissue containing one to three rows of electroplax were isolated. The effects upon the electrical activity of compounds acting on the ACh system were measured with microelectrodes inserted into the interior of the cell. At the same time the AChE activity was determined on the row of intact cells. In this way it has been demonstrated that some compounds, such as ACh, carbamylcholine, procaine, and tubocurarine, block conduction without affecting the esterase. In the presence of these compounds, the enzyme activity remains at a high level, even at a 200 fold concentration above that producing block. Consequently, the blocking action cannot be attributed to the effect on the esterase but to that upon a different but similar cell constituent, the long postulated receptor. With other compounds the enzyme activity is at quite a low level when electrical activity stops. In these cases the blocking action on conduction may be attributed, either partly or entirely, to the decrease of enzyme activity to a level incompatible with electrical activity.

The compounds acting on the receptor may be divided into two distinctly different types according to the way in which they affect electrical activity. One type blocks conduction without depolarization, the other blocks and simultaneously depolarizes the membrane. In one case the barrier to ion movements evidently remains unchanged when activity stops; in the other case, it is removed, similarly to the situation prevailing during activity. Quaternary compounds, such as ACh, carbamylcholine, decamethonium, and others, usually belong to the latter category. Most tertiary analogues, as for example procaine and tetracaine, block but do not depolarize. An interesting example of how the presence of the extra methyl group profoundly changes the effect on electrical activity is the striking difference between the effect of neostigmine and that of its tertiary analogue: the quaternary compound blocks with depolarization, while the same molecular structure without the extra methyl group blocks but does not depolarize (Figs. 11 and 12).

If one associates the transient change of permeability on conducting tissues with the reaction between ACh and the receptor, one must assume that ACh not only combines with the receptor but produces a simultaneous change. This was postulated by CLARK (1937) some twenty years ago. We have, therefore, introduced the distinction between receptor activators which effect this change, and receptor inhibitors which combine with the receptor but do not produce a change. The latter apparently block the access of ACh to the active site. These two different types of interaction are analogous to those in enzyme chemistry where it is possible to distinguish between enzyme substrates and inhibitors.

If one accepts the idea that the molecular forces acting between ACh and the proteins associated with its function are more or less similar, one may visualize that the receptor in the active state undergoes a change in configuration comparable to that suggested to occur in the enzyme during activity. Such an action may well be associated with the change of permeability taking place in the active membrane. One possible picture would be that positively charged amino groups may form an obstacle for the rapid passage of Na^+. A small, even very limited change in a long protein chain may remove a strategically located positive charge by a few Å, thereby greatly increasing the rate of flow. Folding or unfolding of a small section of a helical or nonhelical portion of a protein may be enough for such a process and thus act as a trigger. According to the most recent data (unpublished experiments of W. D. DETTBARN), 1 g of squid giant axon may on the average hydrolyze about 80 μmole of ACh per hour. This value is several times as high as the figure obtained previously. Assuming an average diameter of 400 μ and a surface area of 80 cm^2 per g of squid giant axon, 30×10^{-14} mole of ACh may be split per cm^2 per msec. However, we know that only 20% of this activity, i.e., enough AChE for hydrolyzing 6×10^{-14} mole of ACh, is required for

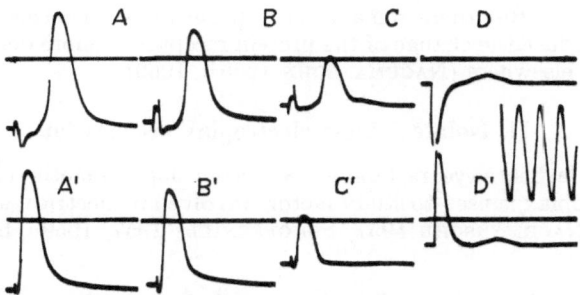

Fig. 11. Effect of neostigmine on the response of the electroplax of *Electrophorus* to stimulation. Experimenta arrangement in this and next figure: the tip of one microelectrode is fixed on the outside of the electroplax close to the innervated membrane; the other electrode is inserted through the non-innervated face and fixed just opposite the first electrode. The upper horizontal line appearing in the cathode ray oscilloscope corresponds to the potential difference between the two electrodes. As long as both are outside the cell, the difference is 0. When the second electrode is inserted, the lower line appears. The distance between the two lines indicates the potential difference in rest between the inside and outside, usually about 80 mV. A—D neural, A'—D' direct stimulation. A, A' control, A, B' 1 min, C, C' 2 min, D, D' 9 min after addition of 8 μmol/ml of neostigmine. The propagated spike is blocked and at the same time the potential difference is decreased. Stimulation: 25/sec. Calibration: 1000 cycles and 100 mV.

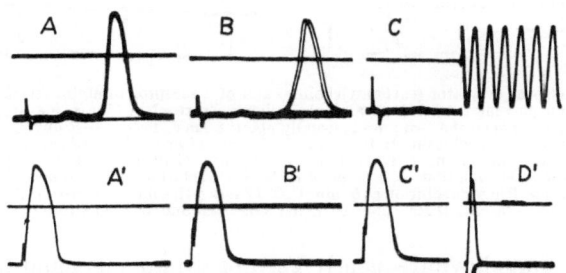

Fig. 12. Effect of the tertiary analog of neostigmine on the resting potential and the action current of an electroplax. A—C: neural, A'—D': direct stimulation. A, A': Control. B, B': 2 min. after addition of 3 μmol/ml of the compound to the Ringer's solution. C, C': 7$^1/_2$ min afterward. The propagated spike was blocked after 15 min. D': after 176 min. Resting potential same as in the control, in spite of the addition of 10 μg/ml of carbamylcholine 124 min before the recording of D'.

maintaining electrical activity. This is a figure which is 80 times smaller than the amount of ions entering the interior per cm^2 per impulse. We do not know the actual period of time during which the removal takes place; this period may be slightly less or slightly more than 1 millisecond. But the difference between the number of Na ions entering per cm^2 surface per impulse and the number of molecules of ACh metabolized per cm^2 per msec appears consistent with the assumption of a trigger action of ACh.

Since the receptor inhibitor must react with the same receptor site as a receptor activator, it follows that if an inhibitor is applied first at the proper concentration it should prevent the activation of the receptor by the subsequent addition of an activator. It has been found that depolarization by the receptor activator carbamylcholine is antagonized by procaine, *d*-tubocurarine, or the tertiary analogue of neostigmine. Since the receptor inhibitors and activators are competitive, the effect of one should be overcome by increased concentrations of the other, and this indeed proved to be the case (SCHOFFENIELS and NACHMANSOHN 1957).

The features required for a molecule to be a receptor activator are still poorly understood. This is analogous to the situation with enzyme inhibitors and substrates. A great variety of compounds may be inhibitors, but only a few have the specifications for being a substrate. The cationic nitrogen group seems to be an important factor in promoting activation, and the carbonyl group another although less essential one. But there remain many problems with respect to the factors required to produce the change of the protein receptor. A more detailed discussion may be found elsewhere (NACHMANSOHN 1955b, 1959).

II. Isolated single electroplax preparation

During the last three years, SCHOFFENIELS developed a method in which a single isolated electroplax is used to study factors involved in electrical activity (SCHOFFENIELS and NACHMANSOHN 1957, SCHOFFENIELS 1957, 1959a, b). Preparations

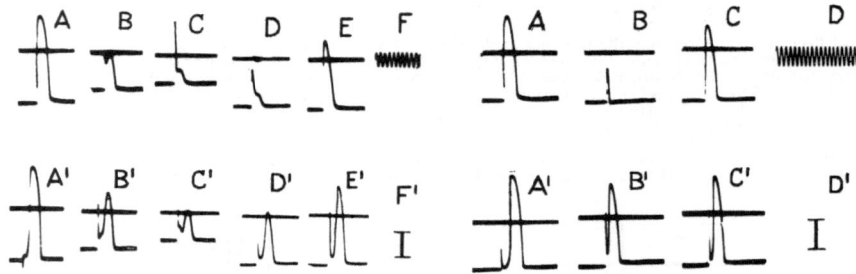

Fig. 13. Effects of a receptor activator (carbamylcholine) and of a receptor inhibitor (tetracaine) on the resting potential and the action current recorded on a single isolated electroplax. The value of the resting potential measured by the distance between the two lines is usually about 85 mV. Left: A—E direct, A'—E' indirect stimulation. A, A' control in Ringer's solution. B, B' 1 min, C, C' 4 min after addition of carbamylcholine, 5×10^{-5} M Return to Ringer's solution at 5 min; D, D' 12 min; E, E' 20 min. Calibration: F 1000 cps; F' 50 mV. Right: A—C direct, A'—C' indirect stimulation. A, A' control in Ringer's solution. B, B' $5\frac{1}{2}$ min after addition of tetracaine, 5×10^{-5} M. Return to Ringer's solution at 6 min; C, C' 17 min (stimulus strength: A' 30 V, B' 100 V, C' 60V). Calibration: D 1000 cps; D' 50 mV (HIGMAN and BARTELS 1961)

of single cellular units have frequently been of paramount importance in studies aimed at the understanding of cellular function. The new method has contributed greatly to resolving previous difficulties; it is a promising tool for further studies.

A single electroplax is dissected and kept between a nylon sheet with a window adjusted to the dimensions of the cell and another nylon sheet with a grid consisting of nylon threads. The cell is placed between two chambers in such a way that it separates two pools of fluid. The innervated membrane of the electroplax has a more or less rectangular shape and is, therefore, uniquely suitable for the study of ion movements between the two chambers across membranes. One face is innervated and has also a conducting membrane, while the other is not innervated. It is possible, with radioactive material and appropriate arrangements, to follow the rates of flux across the two types of membranes separately. The preparation is by far superior to those previously used. It eliminates many disturbing factors, especially various structural barriers which were an obstacle to the study of physical and chemical effects on electrical manifestations. The isolated single electroplax and the isolated single frog sciatic fiber offer two extremely sensitive tools for correlating reactions with proteins and enzymes, observed *in vitro*, to cellular function.

With the new preparation the effects with ACh and related compounds were obtained at much lower concentrations and were reversible for the first time (SCHOFFENIELS and NACHMANSOHN 1957, ROSENBERG et al. 1960, ROSENBERG and

HIGMAN 1960). In the latest observations, ACh acts, rapidly and reversibly, in concentrations of less than 0.5 μg/ml, decamethonium in about the same concentration, and carbamylcholine in about 3 to 5 μg/ml. The difference between the effects of a receptor activator and a receptor inhibitor, recorded on this monocellular preparation with intracellular electrodes, is shown in Fig. 13. In this preparation curare blocks even the directly evoked electrical activity, although the concentration required, about 1 mg/ml, is very much higher than that required to block the neurally evoked response. This question will be discussed in the following section.

Investigations have been initiated on the flux rates of Na- and K-ions under different conditions across innervated and non-innervated membranes (WHITTAM and GUINNEBAULT 1960). One important result has been mentioned in the first section. Merely as an illustration, the data of measurements of K⁺ efflux from an electroplax are shown in Fig. 14. In this experiment, the effect of various frequencies of stimulation on the efflux of potassium is seen after a steady state had been reached.

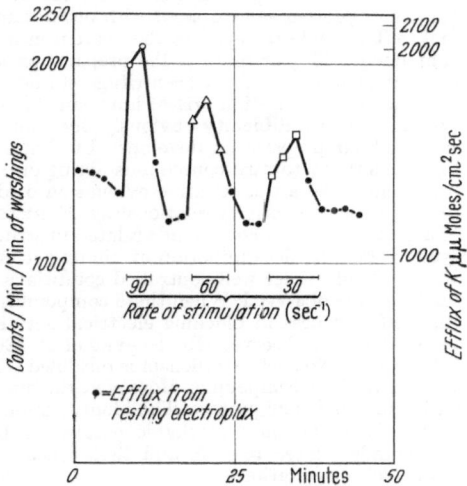

Fig. 14. The effect of direct stimulation of an electroplax on the efflux of potassium

III. Isolation and identification of the acetylcholine receptor protein

Once the experimental evidence for the existence of a receptor as a distinct cell constituent was obtained, the problem of the isolation of this protein arose. CHAGAS and his co-workers were the first to attempt the isolation (CHAGAS et al. 1958, CHAGAS 1959a, b). Using a radioactively labelled curare-like substance, the triethiodide of gallamine (TRIEG), they found that, following its introduction *in vivo* or *in vitro*, this compound was bound to a component or components present in extracts of electric tissue of *Electrophorus* when these extracts were dialyzed against distilled water. However, complex formation was markedly reduced even by very dilute salt solutions (0.02 M). This and various other facts raised the question of whether the macromolecule which was responsible for binding was indeed the receptor. Since TRIEG has three cationic nitrogen atoms, it is possible that unspecific Coulombic and van der Waals' forces led to complex formation with a number of macromolecules which might be unspecific components of the extract and not identical with the receptor. Such a possibility is indeed suggested by the report that the component responsible for a considerable amount of the binding is an acidic polysaccharide.

The problem has been investigated by EHRENPREIS (1959, 1960) with a procedure which differs from that used by CHAGAS and his associates. Tissue extracts of electric organ have been subjected to ammonium sulfate fractionation. The resulting protein fractions have been examined by equilibrium dialysis for their ability to bind curare and other related substances known to react with the ACh system, and more specifically with the receptor. This procedure eliminated other components which were found by EHRENPREIS to react with curare, such as nucleic acids and acidic polysaccharides (EHRENPREIS and FISHMAN 1960).

When d-tubocurarine is added to the fraction obtained with ammonium sulfate at 30% saturation, part of the protein is precipitated. But whereas most other proteins and macromolecules which form complexes with curare go easily into solution at high ionic strength, the precipitate of this fraction is solubilized only partly by dialysis at pH 7.5 and an ionic strength of 0.1 μ. The remaining precipitate, however, is solubilized at pH 9 (EHRENPREIS 1960). d-Tubocurarine has in addition to two quaternary nitrogen atoms two phenolic hydroxy groups which possibly form hydrogen bonds with this particular protein. At pH 9 they are dissociated and the protein goes into solution. This striking difference in the behavior of this particular protein as compared with other macromolecules and proteins is fortunate, since it makes it possible to separate the protein in a relatively simple way and more or less as one component: 90% or more of the preparation is formed by this particular protein, according to electrophoretic and ultracentrifuge studies.

The crucial question arises: how can this protein be identified with be the ACh receptor protein? Such a difficulty obviously does not arise in enzyme purification. At this point the monocellular preparation developed by SCHOFFENIELS (l.c.) became instrumental due to its high sensitivity toward compounds acting on the ACh receptor. The preparation readily permits, therefore, a quantitative evaluation of differences in potency and is most suitable for testing structure-activity relationships. EHRENPREIS tested the binding strength to this protein of a great variety of compounds related in structure to ACh and known to react with the ACh system. For the determination of binding strength he used equilibrium dialysis according to KLOTZ (1946) under well controlled conditions of pH and ionic strength. Great differences in binding were observed. When these compounds were tested by ROSENBERG and HIGMAN as to their effectiveness in blocking electrical activity of the monocellular electroplax, a striking parallelism was observed (ROSENBERG et al. 1960, ROSENBERG and HIGMAN 1960, and unpublished data). No such parallelism is obtained with other proteins although some of them show binding to these compounds. Moreover, the binding is usually much weaker than that obtained with this particular protein. The identification of this protein with the ACh receptor protein is thus based on the remarkable parallelism between binding in vitro of a great variety of compounds related to ACh and their effectiveness in affecting electrical activity of the intact cell preparation.

It may be noted that there seems to exist a difference between receptor activators and receptor inhibitors as far as binding is concerned. Acetylcholine and other activators are bound to the receptor protein, but in this case the binding seems to be poorer than that of receptor inhibitors when related to their effectiveness on the electroplax. A similar phenomenon is, of course, encountered in enzyme chemistry. Inhibitors are frequently much more strongly bound than substrates. The dissociation constant of neostigmine-or physostigmine-AChE complex is 10^{-7}, that of ACh-AChE 10^{-4}. Even in the case of substrates, strength of binding by no means parallels their reaction rate with the enzyme. Acetylcholine, for instance, is much more poorly bound to AChE than butyrylcholine, but it is a 150 times better substrate. The explanation may be that for a compound to produce rapidly and efficiently the reversible action required, a strong binding may be unfavorable. Much further investigation of the ACh receptor protein is required for a proper characterization of its various properties; extensive studies are now in progress.

IV. Effect of local anesthetics. Essentiality of the acetylcholine receptor protein for electrical activity

Of particular interest are the results obtained with local anesthetics in the course of these studies. Procaine and many other local anesthetics are analogous

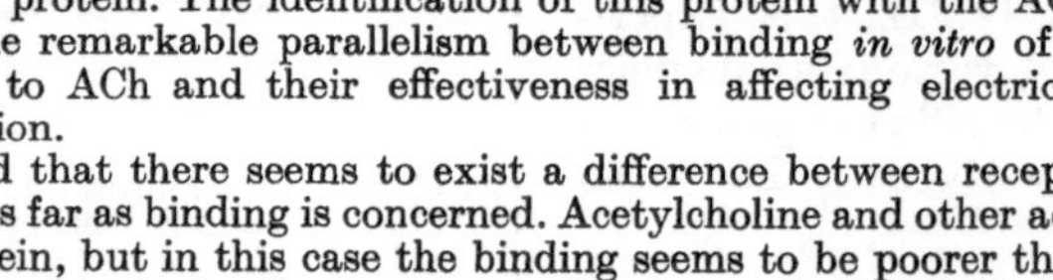

Acetylcholine   Procaine

Fig. 15. Analogy of the structure of a local anesthetic (procaine) to that of ACh

in structure to ACh (Fig. 15). The substitution of a methyl group on the nitrogen atom by a proton makes this compound lipid soluble since at neutral pH part of the molecules are in uncharged form. Lipid solubility is still further enhanced by the substitution of the methyl group on the carbon of the carbonyl by an aniline ring. In tetracaine, one hydrogen on the nitrogen of the aniline is substituted by a butyl group. It has long been maintained by the author that these local anesthetics block electrical activity by competitive action as typical "antimetabolites" of ACh, and support for this view was obtained in studies on the electroplax (ALTAMIRANO et al. 1955, SCHOFFENIELS and NACHMANSOHN 1957). These analogues apparently combine with the active site of the receptor thereby preventing the action of acetylcholine released intracellularly. However, lacking the quaternary group and being receptor inhibitors, they do not produce the change of the protein required for increased permeability. They block electrical activity without depolarization.

Recently, ROSENBERG and HIGMAN (1960) compared procaine, tetracaine, and dibucaine as to their ability to affect electrical activity of the monocellular electroplax preparation. Tetracaine proved to be about 15 times as effective as procaine, and dibucaine was twice as effective as tetracaine. In view of these strong differences, EHRENPREIS and KELLOCK (1960) tested the binding strength of these three local anesthetics to the ACh receptor protein in solution. Again, as with other series of tertiary, and mono- and *bis*-quaternary nitrogen derivatives, a striking parallelism was obtained between binding in solution and the potency on the intact cell. With tetracaine, which was studied in more detail, the specificity of the binding is quite pronounced. The binding is strong in low concentrations. A number of proteins and other macromolecules show some binding, but only in rather high concentration of the drug, and even then the binding is very much weaker than that to the receptor protein. The experiments support the assumption of the competitive nature of the action of local anesthetics.

A still further extension of the evidence for this mode of action of local anesthetics is offered by the experiments of HIGMAN and BARTELS (1961). It is postulated that local anesthetics, being receptor inhibitors, block electrical activity by reacting with the active site of the ACh receptor protein, thereby preventing the change produced by ACh or other receptor activators. If this is the case, a cell exposed to ACh and depolarized should be repolarized by tetracaine in concentrations adequate to displace ACh from the active site and thereby restore the receptor protein to its resting condition. Increasing concentrations of ACh should again be able to displace tetracaine and to depolarize again the cell in the presence of tetracaine. This result predicted from theory has been obtained by the two authors. They exposed a monocellular preparation of the electroplax to 2.5×10^{-6} M ACh in the presence of 5×10^{-5} M physostigmine, and tested the electrical characteristics with intracellular electrodes. Electrical activity was rapidly blocked, within 2 to 3 min, after the addition of ACh; simultaneously the cell was depolarized. On removal of ACh and physostigmine, electrical activity was rapidly restored and the cell was repolarized. If, however, tetracaine, 5×10^{-5} M, was added to the depolarized cell after block of electrical activity by ACh and physostigmine and in their presence, the cell became repolarized, although the activity did, of course, not recur, as expected by theory: the receptor inhibitor displaces the receptor activator from the receptor protein. It has been possible to overcome the effect of the inhibitor by higher concentrations of activators (carbamylcholine) and to depolarize the cell again.

The competitive nature of these actions becomes even more apparent by contrast with a compound which blocks activity in a noncompetitive way, namely the marine toxin obtained from pufferfish. This compound blocks electrical activity at 7×10^{-8} M without depolarization. It has no affinity to AChE or to ACh receptor protein in solution. The effect must be attributed to the reaction with another cell constituent (DETTBARN et al. 1960). If this toxin is applied to the electroplax in a concentration 10 times as high as that required to block electrical activity and the cell is then exposed to ACh and physostigmine in the usual minimal concentrations, in the presence of the high concentration of toxin, rapid depolarization takes place in the same way as in the absence of the toxin.

These developments are of interest in two respects. They provide an explanation of the mode of action of local anesthetics on axonal conduction in that their effects must be attributed to a specific chemical reaction with a specific cell constituent rather than to some unknown general effect. Secondly, they offer additional strong evidence for the proposed role of ACh in conduction. In view of the well known generality of the local anesthetics which block electrical activity in all types of nerves, motor and sensory, adrenergic and cholinergic, and in view of the specificity of the reaction of tetracaine with the ACh receptor protein, it is difficult to envisage an alternative explanation. The data provide evidence for the essentiality of the ACh receptor protein, thereby supplementing the evidence for the essentiality of AChE in conduction.

Since the local anesthetics are tertiary nitrogen derivatives, the charge of the nitrogen group is pH-dependent. In the reaction between AChE and tertiary nitrogen derivatives, the neutral forms are poorer inhibitors and substrates than the charged ones, due to the absence of Coulombic forces. A similar pH effect is obtained in the reaction between a local anesthetic such as tetracaine and the ACh receptor protein *in vitro*. The effect on the electrical activity of the electroplax shows a parallel dependence: the lower the pH, the stronger and faster the action. The responses to neural and direct stimulation in the presence of procaine or tetracaine or dibucaine are equally affected by the changes of pH: the rate of block changes in a parallel way in both types of response with the change of pH. The strength of action of the three compounds on the two types of response also shows the same ratio (BARTELS et al. 1960). Thus, the structure — activity relationship obtained with these compounds is the same for both conducting and synaptic membranes and has the same pH-dependence. The observations suggest a similar chemical reaction at both sites and thus support the unified concept of the chemical events in the membrane in axonal conduction and synaptic transmission.

F. Effects of quaternary ammonium ions on conduction

I. Structural barriers for lipid-insoluble quaternary ammonium ions

The powerful action of ACh on synaptic junctions was one of two essential observations on which the theory of neurohumoral transmission was based. Applied to axons, ACh has no effect even in very high concentrations. This failure of ACh to affect electrical activity in axons has been for many years one of the main objections to the theory of an essential role of the ester in conduction.

However, as mentioned before, axons are surrounded by complex structural barriers which apparently protect the conducting membrane against the action of many compounds. Acetylcholine is a methylated quaternary ammonium salt. This type of compound is poorly lipid-soluble; for such, the barrier seems to be particularly impervious. The experimental demonstration of the inability of neostigmine to enter the axon has been mentioned before. In contrast to neostigmine, its tertiary analogue — although a hundred times weaker as an inhibitor of ChE than the quaternary form — blocks electrical and enzyme activity as was shown on intact axons (WILSON and COHEN 1953). The inability of ACh to enter the interior of the axon was demonstrated in the following way: squid giant axons were exposed to a solution containing ACh labeled with N^{15}, in a concentration of 0.1 M; the isotopic nitrogen was not found in the interior of the axon (ROTHENBERG et al. 1948) whereas a labeled tertiary nitrogen compound entered readily.

II. Action of lipid-soluble quaternary ammonium ions

Recently, a series of lipid-soluble quaternary ammonium ions has been prepared by substituting a dodecyl group for a methyl on the nitrogen. The analogue of acetylcholine, β-acetoxyethyldimethyl dodecyl ammonium iodide, has been referred to as noracetylcholine 12 (nor-ACh-12). Other compounds prepared were pyridinium dodeciodide (PDI) and a lipid-soluble analogue of P-2-AM, pyridine aldoxime dodeciodide (PAD). All these lipid-soluble quaternary ammonium ions block axonal conduction of crab and lobster nerve in relatively low concentrations (about 10^{-4} M). They depolarize the conducting membrane of the electroplax of *Electrophorus electricus* even after complete block of the synaptic junctions by *d*-tubocurarine; this indicates that the compounds affect the conducting membrane directly (SCHOFFENIELS et al. 1958, ROSENBERG and HIGMAN 1961). They produce muscular contraction of both frog rectus abdominis and sartorius muscle. As in the electroplax, the action is not blocked by curare in contrast to that of the lipid insoluble nitrogen derivatives. The effects of nor-ACh-12 on the rectus abdominis are reversible and may be repeated many times. The effects on the muscle emphasize the significance of the action of these quaternary ammonium ions, lipid-soluble analogues of ACh, because they are able to reproduce the biological action postulated for the physiological role of the ester (HINTERBUCHNER et al. 1958, HINTERBUCHNER and WILSON 1959a, b).

Using the Ranvier node of single frog sciatic fibers, STAEMPFLI (1958) obtained an increase in amplitude and duration of the spike potential with nor-ACh-12 in 3×10^{-5} M. With higher concentrations depolarization was observed. The effects take place within seconds; this is a rather high speed, only slightly less than that observed with high K^+ concentrations. The actions in low concentrations are readily reversible. Even more potent effects were obtained by DETTBARN (1960a) with PAD: electrical activity was affected in 10^{-7} M (equivalent to 0.02 $\mu g/ml$ of ACh); depolarization occurred with 10^{-6} M.

In higher concentrations the lipid-soluble quaternary ammonium ions may have an unspecific "detergent" action. They will interact with a variety of macromolecules by Coulombic and van der Waals' forces. The relatively low concentrations used and the various biological effects described suggest, however, a more specific type of action on the ACh system.

For the interpretation of the effects of these compounds as well as for determining the specificity of their action, it has been tested whether or not they react with the ACh system. Evidence in this direction has been obtained by tests for the competitive action with eserine (DETTBARN et al. 1958, DETTBARN 1959). This compound inhibits the enzyme and is also a receptor inhibitor. When eserine is added to the desheathed frog tibialis nerve, subsequent addition of PAD in otherwise effective concentration has absolutely no effect. Higher concentrations of PAD do overcome the protective action of eserine. The antagonism between the two compounds is typical for a competitive action.

Another question pertinent for the significance of the action of the lipid-soluble quaternary ammonium ions is whether their effect on permeability is specific or indiscriminate. Do they change permeability to Na^+ in a way which differs from that of the change in permeability to K^+? This problem was tested by DETTBARN (1959b, 1960a) with desheathed frog tibialis nerve. The preparation was exposed to PDI, nor-ACh-12, and PAD with appropriate modifications of the Ringer's solution. The permeability to Na^+ was increased; that to K^+, at the concentration used, showed a slight but definite decrease. Thus, the depolarization observed with these quaternary ammonium ions appears to be effected by a marked specific increase of permeability to Na^+ which is difficult to reconcile with an unspecific detergent action.

Whether the compounds act primarily on the receptor, on the esterase, or on the storage protein apparently depends on their structural features and on the concentrations used, and will, therefore, differ according to experimental conditions, type of compound and preparation, etc. At present, insufficient information is available as to this particular aspect. But this distinction has little bearing on the main question. The pertinent result is the evidence that lipid-soluble analogues of ACh, in low concentrations and apparently by a specific reaction, may produce the same effects in conducting membranes as those postulated to take place intracellularly by the release of ACh, whereas these effects are not reproducible with lipid-insoluble compounds from the outside due to structural barriers surrounding the axon.

III. The action of curare

The classical observations of CLAUDE BERNARD that curare acts on the neuromuscular junction only and does not affect nerve and muscle fibers was a factor of great importance in the development of the concepts of a special mechanism of synaptic transmission, including the hypothesis of neurohumoral transmission. It has been suspected for a long time and has now been shown *in vitro* that curare forms a complex with the ACh receptor protein isolated by EHRENPREIS (1959, 1960). The two cationic groups react with two apparently correspondingly located negative groups, one of them being the anionic site of the active surface. In addition, binding is enhanced by van der Waals' forces. Hydrogen bonding of the phenolic hydroxy groups may be an additional factor, but this has still to be ascertained. Because curare is bound to the receptor, it prevents the action of the ester released during activity. In spite of its two quaternary nitrogen atoms, it is a receptor inhibitor, apparently being unable to produce the folding in the receptor because of its large size [classified by BOVET (1951) as "pachycurare"].

It has been emphasized repeatedly that quaternary nitrogen derivatives are unable to penetrate the structural barriers. This has been offered as explanation for the limitation of curare action to the junction. However, during the last 3 years it has been possible to obtain rapid and reversible block of electrical activity of axons with curare or ACh or with both. Either preparations were used where the conducting membrane of the axon seems to be poorly protected, or the structural barriers were reduced by chemical treatment. At Ranvier nodes the conducting membrane is poorly covered, as mentioned before, and we have seen that there eserine acts rapidly and in low concentrations. Therefore, DETTBARN (1960b) applied, d-tubocurarine to Ranvier nodes of single frog sciatic fibers; a rapid and completely reversible block of electrical activity was obtained. Within a few minutes the spike had disappeared (Fig. 16). The concentration required was usually 10^{-3} M, although in 30% of the cases 5×10^{-3} M was used. Neostigmine blocks in about the same concentration, which is about 10 times higher than that required for eserine. Evidently charged molecules penetrate poorly compared to uncharged ones. Quaternary compounds such as curare and neostigmine, classically known to act exclusively on the neuromuscular junction, have been unequivocally shown to act on the axonal membrane.

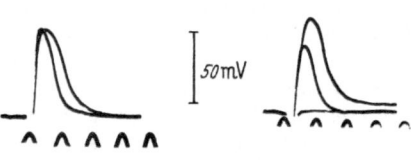

Fig. 16. Block of electrical activity at the node of Ranvier of a single frog nerve fiber preparation exposed to d-tubocurarine chloride (10^{-3} M). a: before and 40 sec after exposure, increased duration of spike. b: after 100 sec complete block of conduction. Four min after return to Ringer's solution height of spike has returned to normal. t = 24°C, time: 1000 cycles/sec (DETTBARN 1960b)

An action of ACh on the unmyelinated C fibers of desheathed rabbit vagus was recently observed by ARMETT and RITCHIE (1960). The ester depolarizes the axons, reduces the spike height, and slows conduction. The greater the concentration of ACh, the stronger the action. The effects are reversible. Although the observations require considerable amplification for the interpretation of certain aspects, they demonstrate that ACh is able to affect reversibly the electrical activity of axons (see also Chapter 6). A direct action of ACh on somatic nerve fibers without removal of the sheath or any other treatment has been recently obtained by DETTBARN and DAVIS (1962) on bundles of the walking leg of lobsters. Acetylcholine rapidly and reversibly blocked electrical activity. It depolarized the membrane within seconds after its application; the effect took place only in the presence of sodium ions, but the question whether and how far the observed increase of conductance is specific for Na$^+$ still requires further studies. But apparently, the axons of this preparation are surrounded by barriers sufficiently strong to prevent ACh from reaching the conducting membrane. This direct action of ACh appears particularly pertinent in the light of the previously discussed demonstration of the inseparable association of electrical activity with the ACh system when lipid soluble inhibitors of either AChE or of the ACh receptor protein are used.

WALSH and DEAL (1959) attempted to remove the barriers for lipid soluble quaternary ammonium ions. They found indeed that after pretreatment with the cationic detergent cetyltrimethylammonium bromide, conduction in frog sciatic nerve bundles was reversibly affected by curare, ACh, and neostigmine.

Still more recently, ROSENBERG and EHRENPREIS (1961 a,b) applied a series of enzymes to squid giant axons to test whether the structural barriers could be reduced to a degree that compounds not acting on the intact fiber would produce effects. Several enzymes tested did not change the response. But when cobra venom (10 μg/ml) was applied, particularly in combination with cetyltrimethyl-ammonium chloride (10 μg/ml), the effect was striking: curare (d-tubocurarine chloride), completely inactive in the highest concentrations tested before the treatment, blocked electrical activity rapidly and reversibly. The concentrations of curare required were about 10^{-3} M, and in some cases 5×10^{-4} M. Acetylcholine, however, had even in very high concentrations only a slight effect. This and other facts suggested that the reduction of the barriers was still quite incomplete. ROSENBERG and PODLESKI (1962) tested, therefore, some other venoms. With cottonmouth moccasin venom, they obtained much stronger effects: curare reversibly blocked conduction in concentrations which were lower than those effective after treatment with cobra venom. The treatment with the cottonmouth moccasin venom rendered ACh effective. The breakdown of barriers by this venom was also shown by P. ROSENBERG and F. C. G. HOSKIN with the aid of radioactively labelled ACh and dimethyl curarine: following the treatment the compounds readily penetrated into the axoplasm of the giant axon of squid (unpublished observations).

The startling evidence for the action of curare and ACh on the conducting membrane of axons removes one of the major factors upon which the assumption of a special mechanism of transmission across the neuromuscular junction was based. The limitation of the effect of curare to the junction has profoundly influenced the thinking of physiologists since the classical experiments of CLAUDE BERNARD. Clearly, these observations were correct, but the interpretation must be modified. It is not the difference of the mechanism which limits to the junction the actions of curare and ACh in a nerve-muscle preparation, but the inaccessibility of the conducting membrane in the fibers. What has long been apparent on the basis of biochemical and physicochemical data, has now been clearly and unequivocally demonstrated on the intact cell, by a type of experiment which furnishes "direct" evidence according to the physiological way of thinking.

In contrast to the failure of lipid insoluble compounds to block conduction of untreated squid giant axons, exposure to tertiary nitrogen derivatives readily affects their electrical activity. This was shown by BULLOCK et al. (1946) with physostigmine and strychnine. ROSENBERG and EHRENPREIS (1961 b) applied a number of tertiary nitrogen derivatives such as atropine, methantheline, diphenhydramine, local anesthetics, etc., to the untreated isolated squid giant axons. The stronger their binding strength to the ACh receptor protein was found to be *in vitro*, the greater was their ability to affect electrical activity of the axons. Moreover, when the concentrations required for these effects are compared to those previously reported by ROSENBERG and HIGMAN (1960) as being effective at the synaptic junction of the mono-cellular electroplax preparation, they are surprisingly similar although the two types of preparation are so different. The greatest differences in concentrations found were tenfold.

G. Summary of the basic evidence which indicates the essential role of acetylcholine in the generation of bioelectric currents

1. The conducting membrane is endowed with the unique and specific ability to use the ionic concentration gradients, existing between the interior of living cells and their outer environment, for generating bioelectric currents which propagate impulses. A rapid transitory change of Na-conductance permits the flow of ions. Thus, a specific mechanism present in conducting membranes must be postulated for the process.

2. The strong initial heat coinciding with electrical activity, the high energy of activation, and the high temperature coefficient show that the electrical activity requires a chemical reaction. Since the Na-conductance change is the specific event responsible for electrical activity, the chemical reaction must be linked to this specific process.

The following facts are evidence that the action of ACh is essential for the rapid transitory change of conductance.

3. The enzymes forming and hydrolyzing ACh, i.e., ChAc and AChE, respectively, occur in the conducting tissues of the animal kingdom and in the various types of fibers; they are not present in significant concentrations in non-conducting tissues, such as liver and kidney. This fact suggests a specific role of the ACh system in conducting tissue.

4. If the action of ACh increases Na-conductance, its rapid return to the initial value should be made possible by the rapid removal of ACh by AChE. The high speed of the enzyme activity satisfies this crucial prerequisite. The enzyme is one of the fastest acting enzymes known, the turnover time being around 40 to 60 microseconds.

5. The concentration of AChE is very high in nerve fibers. The average activities, referred to g tissue (fresh weight), are about 0.01 to 0.06 g ester split per hour in fibers, and 0.1 to 0.3 g in brain or ganglia. The enzyme is, however, not evenly distributed, but localized in the region of the conducting membrane. In some muscle fibers the enzyme appears to be relatively low. The discrepancy between the weight of active material and total tissue weight is of course usually greater in muscle than in nerve tissue; this may account for the apparently low values in some muscle tissue. Per g active material the concentration must be extremely high, permitting the inactivation of significant amounts of ACh per millisecond.

6. Electric organs of *Electrophorus* and *Torpedo*, the most powerful bioelectric generators created by nature and tissues highly specialized in their function, are capable of hydrolyzing two to four g of ACh per g fresh tissue per hour, in spite of the fact that these tissues contain 93% water and only 2% protein. The activity per g active material must be several orders of magnitude higher.

These features are physiologically significant, and prerequisites for attributing to the ACh system this specific property of conducting membranes, namely to change Na-conductance and to generate electricity. The following direct evidence has been obtained:

7. It has not been possible to separate electrical and AChE activity. With potent and specific reversible inhibitors electrical activity of axons is blocked reversibly, and with irreversible inhibitors, under certain conditions, irreversibly. The author has found that about 20% of the initial enzyme activity is required for unimpaired conduction. The functional interdependence of enzyme and electrical activity has been demonstrated with a variety of procedures and under a variety of conditions. It has been tested on a great variety of types of conducting fibers, motor and sensory fibers, "cholinergic" and "adrenergic", central and peripheral, vertebrate and invertebrate, and on muscle fibers. The interdependence of electrical and enzyme activity has been demonstrated on intact axons.

8. Electrical activity, irreversibly blocked by an organophosphate anti-ChE agent, can be restored by a specific chemical reaction, namely by the reactivation of the enzyme by benzoyl pyridine oxime methiodide, a compound displacing the phosphoryl group specifically from AChE.

9. According to theory, electrical activity if produced by the action of ACh on the ACh receptor protein. This receptor protein, tentatively isolated as a single component in solution, has been shown to react specifically with local anesthetics, known to block electrical activity. The stronger the binding of local anesthetics to the protein in solution, the stronger is the effect on electrical activity in the intact cell. The competitive nature between the action of local anesthetics and that of ACh has been demonstrated on the intact cell. The evidence for the essentiality of the ACh receptor protein for generating bioelectricity thus supplements that for the essentiality of AChE.

10. The failure of ACh to act on axons has been considered to be strong evidence against a possible role in conduction. The same reasoning has been applied to the action of curare, known for more than a century to be limited to the junction and generally assumed to react with the ACh receptor. However, it has been shown that this failure must be attributed to the existence of structural barriers preventing lipid-insoluble quaternary nitrogen derivatives from entering the axon. After a long exposure to very high concentration of neostigmine (0.01 M) and ACh (0.1 M), the compounds are not found in the axoplasm, in contrast to tertiary nitrogen derivatives which do enter.

11. Recently, rapid and reversible block of electrical activity of axons has been obtained with curare and with ACh. This effect was obtained on special preparations, where the structural barriers surrounding the axon are apparently not sufficiently strong for preventing the compounds from reaching the membrane. Curare was found to act on Ranvier nodes of single myelinated fibers, ACh on somatic fibers of the walking leg of lobster, and on fibers of the desheathed vagus nerve of rabbit. An alternative procedure to demonstrate the intrinsic ability of ACh and curare to affect axonal conduction, almost certainly by reacting with the ACh receptor protein, has been a chemical pretreatment aimed at reducing the barriers, such as a detergent or venoms. The cottonmouth moccasin venom was found to be particularly efficient: after treatment with this venom, curare and ACh rapidly and reversibly blocked

conduction of the giant axon of squid, while they were even in highest concentrations inactive before the exposure to the venom.

12. In the sequence of energy transformations, ACh hydrolysis precedes that of ATP. It is capable of a depolarizing (electrogenic) action, thereby excluding a role in recovery. Other compounds have a depolarizing action but none of them satisfies the prerequisites to have the physiological function attributed to ACh.

It has thus been shown that the ester has the properties required for the specific operative substance in the elementary process of nerve activity in the sense defined by MEYERHOF for ATP in the elementary process of muscular activity.

H. Neuromuscular and synaptic transmission

We have discussed so far the evidence for the concept that the release and the action of ACh are intracellular (intramembranous) processes inseparably associated with the permeability changes in axonal membranes during the generation of bio-electric currents. The question naturally occurs of whether it is still justified, in view of the new information, to maintain the hypothesis of neurohumoral transmission in its original form. Do the experimental facts support an *inter*cellular role of ACh at synaptic junctions in contrast to the *intra*cellular one in the axon ? This viewpoint has been presented in several other chapters of this volume (see Chapter 6). The reader interested in the views of the author concerning this special problem is referred to the recent monograph of the author (1959). Here only a few pertinent aspects may be briefly discussed.

I. The basis of the original hypothesis

The original hypothesis of neurohumoral transmission was based essentially on two facts: 1. ACh has a powerful action on synaptic junctions. It does not affect, even in high concentration, axonal conduction. 2. When nerves are stimulated, ACh appears in the perfusion fluid of synaptic junctions, although only in the presence of eserine. These two observations, and several ancillary findings (see Chapters 3, 6, 11, 12, 13, 14), were taken as evidence that the physiological function of ACh is limited to the synaptic junction and that the ester, released from the nerve terminal, acts on the effector cell.

The failure of ACh and other quaternary ammonium ions to affect conduction when applied externally has found an experimentally supported explanation in the existence of structural barriers, discussed before. As to the appearance of ACh in the perfusion fluid, this observation does not reveal its mode of action. As was emphatically and repeatedly stressed by DALE (1937) and his collaborators, ACh appears only if eserine is present in the perfusion fluid. Obviously, if one interferes with the rapid physiological removal of ACh by the esterase, ACh when released, would be expected to diffuse from the pre- and postsynaptic membranes into the surrounding medium. In physiological conditions, i.e. in the absence of eserine, only the hydrolytic products would be expected to leak out following stimulation. This is exactly what has been observed by EMMELIN and MacINTOSH (1956). Leakage of either the ester or its hydrolytic products would occur only at synaptic junctions where, as we have seen, no structural barrier exists for ACh. No such leakage would be expected from the intact fiber. If, however, the nerve fiber is cut and stimulated, ACh is released from the cut surface where the protecting barrier is no longer an obstacle, as was shown more than twenty years ago (CALABRO 1933, BERGAMI et al. 1936) and has since then been confirmed by many investigators.

It is accepted as an established fact that ACh is released exclusively from the nerve ending. In many decades of research on the role of ACh in synaptic transmission, there exists only one experimental observation in support of this view: when the nerve fiber is cut and the ending has degenerated, no ACh is detectable in the perfusion fluid after direct stimulation of the muscle fiber (DALE et al. 1936). However, this observation has not been confirmed. McINTYRE et al. (1950), McINTYRE (1959) has challenged this finding by his demonstration that ACh is released from muscle even after complete degeneration of the nerve endings. He has offered a reasonable explanation for the apparently negative results of the previous experiments.

The original observations had stimulated much interesting research, but they do not permit an interpretation of the precise mode of action of ACh on a cellular and subcellular level.

II. More recent data on synaptic transmission

During the last 20 years, much new information has accumulated with respect to the various aspects of neuromuscular and synaptic transmission.

Structure. Investigations with the light and electron microscopes on the structure of the neuromuscular junction have shown that the nerve terminals lie in troughs and are surrounded by complex branching and anastomosing folds (COUTEAUX 1955, ROBERTSON 1956). A compound membrane about 500 A thick, referred to by ROBERTSON as the "synaptic membrane complex", separates axoplasm from sarcoplasm. It consists of 5 distinct layers. Whether the middle layer is the continuation of the outer membranes covering axonal and muscle fibers, or whether it is an artifact, is still an open question. It appears quite obvious that such an extraordinarily complex morphological structure must greatly influence the electrical fields generated during activity as well as the responses to these currents. One would assume *a priori* that certain properties and electrical events should present marked deviations when compared to those in a simple cylinder, such as the axon. ECCLES (1946) has stressed the importance of "geometry" for the response even in such simple structures as axons. The effect of geometry must be incomparably greater and more complex in a structure such as the neuromuscular junction. However, no direct information exists at present in this respect.

In electron microscope pictures, DE ROBERTIS and BENNETT (1955) observed the presence of vesicles near the nerve terminals . They suggested that these vesicles may be associated with ACh release, in line with the hypothesis of neurohumoral transmission. Later, a considerable amount of speculation developed about these vesicles (DEL CASTILLO and KATZ 1956). They were considered to be little carrier corpuscles, "packages" of ACh, and the number of ACh molecules per vesicle was calculated (see Chapter 3). Some further developments are in condradiction with these speculations. Vesicles have been found in many different places in the nervous systems, at postsynaptic sites as well as in the presynaptic areas (see EDWARDS et al. 1958). There is no evidence that these vesicles are in any way associated with the action of ACh.

Electrical signs. The endplate potential. The discovery of a special endplate potential (GÖPFERT and SCHAEFER 1938) and the study of its characteristics with microelectrodes inserted in the close vicinity of the endplate have revealed many interesting facts (see Chapter 13). It is generally agreed today that the endplate potentials are produced by ACh through its depolarizing action there. But the question still remains, where does the ACh generating the endplate potential come from ? Since, as discussed above, the question can be raised as to whether it is actually secreted from the nerve terminals, the alternative explanation appears to the author more likely, viz., that the ester is released within the postsynaptic membrane by ion movements initiated by the depolarization of the nerve terminal.

For several years the observation of "miniature" endplate potentials during resting conditions has been used as evidence for "quantal" release of ACh from nerve terminals (FATT and KATZ 1952). Without considering alternative interpretations, the assumed ability of nerve endings to secrete ACh was presented as evidence for neurohumoral transmission. However, the miniature endplate potentials persist after degeneration of the nerve terminals (KATZ and MILEDI 1959). Thus, the interpretation proposed now appears untenable.

If the ionic concentration gradients are the local source of energy for the small currents in the axon, and this potential source of energy is made available at excited points by the action of ACh, currents in the terminals might be generated in a similar way. A propagated disturbance, reaching the postsynaptic membrane, may mobilize ACh in order to produce the postsynaptic potential. Action currents of a fiber are able to stimulate adjacent fibers under appropriate conditions, i.e., under suitable composition of the outer milieu. Such favorable conditions may well prevail at the junctions where the membranes are so close to each other and not separated by insulating material. Although there is at present no satisfactory information based on direct measurements about the precise nature of the transmitting processes across junctions, there is in the view of the author no adequate evidence for the assumption of a role of ACh at junctions basically different from that in axonal membranes requiring the idea of ACh being released in one cell and acting on the membrane of a second cell. The available data are considered most readily compatible with the view that ACh plays an essential role within the pre- and postsynaptic membranes during activity without actually crossing the gap.

Inhibitory synaptic activity has long been known. Synaptic potentials recorded with intracellular electrodes in some cases revealed a transient increase of the membrane potential, i.e., a hyperpolarization (ECCLES 1957).

It is certainly good reasoning to attribute hyperpolarization to a chemical reaction. It would be difficult to explain it in purely physical terms. But this applies equally to depolarization. Both phenomena must involve conductance changes and, therefore, chemical reactions in the membrane, whether the latter is synaptic or axonal. Inhibition and excitation are more or less mirror images. Acetylcholine is known to be capable of producing both events. This is not surprising or extraordinary. It is known that ATP is required for muscular relaxation as well as contraction, depending on ancillary regulatory factors such as the relaxing factor which in turn depends on ions, etc. Even in a membrane of 80 Å thickness in which the action of ACh is postulated to take place, there may be a variety of factors controlling and regulating the system, and additional chemical factors may be provided from the environment. All these factors may easily determine the effect of ACh: they may increase or antagonize the action and they may lead to hyper- or to depolarization. The currents coming from the nerve endings are too weak to produce activation of the membrane (ECCLES 1957). There can hardly be any disagreement with this view. But the question is, how is the necessary chemical energy mobilized? This is the real problem and the answer cannot be decided only on the basis of electrical manifestations or pharmacological effects.

III. The concentration of acetylcholinesterase at synaptic junctions

Of particular interest is the problem of the concentration of AChE at synaptic junctions in relation to that in fibers. A considerable amount of confusion exists about this problem. The author admits to share the responsibility for this situation. Some clarification appears necessary.

The theory of neurohumoral transmission requires the removal of ACh by AChE within the brief period of one or a few milliseconds (depending on the type of preparation). In 1937, Miss ANETTE MARNAY and the author determined the concentration and distribution of ChE in frog sartorius muscle. They found that in the part containing motor endplates the concentration of the enzyme was about three to four times as high as in the pelvic end which is free of motor endplates (MARNAY and NACHMANSOHN 1937, 1938). Knowing the number of endplates in the muscle, it was possible to calculate that per motor endplate about 1.6×10^9 molecules of ACh may be split per millesecond, an amount which indeed permits the assumption of an active role of ACh in the process of synaptic transmission, although obviously it does not indicate what this role may be (NACHMANSOHN 1939).

However, at that time, the author assumed that AChE is evenly distributed in nerve and muscle fibers outside the endplate and only more concentrated at the junction. If one refers the concentrations in the fibers and at the endplates to the corresponding volumes, the data seem to indicate that the actual concentration at the motor endplates is several thousand times higher than in the fibers, since the endplates form an extremely small fraction of the volume of the fiber, probably less than one-thousandth.

Later, however, it was found that the enzyme is not evenly distributed in fibers, but localized in the region of the surface membrane. This was first suggested in experiments on the superior cervical ganglion of cat. The enzyme activity of this tissue amounts to about 600 mg of ester split per gram per hour, whereas in the preganglionic fibers only 50 mg are split per gram per hour. After section of the fibers, the activity falls within a week to 240 mg/g per hour and then remains constant. If this decrease is due to the degeneration of the terminals, as is suggested by the temporal coincidence of the two processes, how can the decrease of concentration be so great? There seemed to be a higher enzyme concentration in the fibers inside the ganglion than at the outside. The nerve terminals branch many times in the ganglion and form an extremely extensive end-arborization. One possibility to explain this increased concentration inside the ganglion would be a high concentration of the enzyme near the surface membrane. The large increase in surface area due to the end-arborization would then explain the high concentration in the fibers inside the ganglion and the strong decrease of enzyme activity within the ganglia when the terminals degenerate (COUTEAUX and NACHMANSOHN 1940). It was this observation which led the author to test the distribution of ChE between axoplasm and sheath of the squid giant axon (BOELL and NACHMANSOHN 1940, NACHMANSOHN and MEYERHOF 1941). As mentioned before, the result was the demonstration of the absence of detectable ChE from the axoplasm and, therefore, presumably its exclusive localization in the sheath. The experiments on the superior cervical ganglion suggested, moreover, that the enzyme must be present in high concentrations in pre- and postsynaptic membranes. These observations on the peculiar localization of ChE were one of the results which, in connection with many others, suggested to the author the unified concept of the role of ACh in conduction and transmission of impulses rather than one limited to the junction.

In the experiments of COUTEAUX and NACHMANSOHN (1940) no distinction was made between AChE and other nonspecific esterases. The superior cervical ganglion contains both types (SAWYER and HOLLINSHEAD 1945, KOELLE 1951). The values for the total esterase activity found by SAWYER and HOLLINSHEAD are lower than those reported previously. However, the enzyme activity was determined after glycerine extraction. This may involve some losses which may account for the differences, since the extraction may have been incomplete. In the preganglionic fibers the enzyme was essentially AChE, whereas in the ganglion a considerable fraction was another type of esterase. After section of the preganglionic fibers AChE in the ganglion fell during the first 8 to 10 days to about 20% of the initial value and remained at this level for several weeks, indicating that even after the disappearance of the preganglionic fibers part of this specific enzyme is still present in the ganglion. The data are thus essentially in agreement with those reported previously (see also Chapter 6).

Following the observations of MARNAY and NACHMANSOHN on frog sartorius muscle, COUTEAUX and NACHMANSOHN (1940) (COUTEAUX 1942) investigated the concentration and distribution of ChE in mammalian muscle. In the guinea pig gastrocnemius, the nerve fibers with all their branches including the motor endplates are localized in a well defined zone. When sections of the frozen muscle are prepared with the microtome in an appropriate way, most sections are virtually free of motor endplates; only a few are extremely rich in nerve fibers and endplates. In the latter sections the concentration of ChE is 3 to 5 times higher than in the sections free of nerve fibers and endplates. What is the interpretation of this difference?

As mentioned before, electron microscope studies have revealed that the nerve terminals lie in gutters. These gutters are formed by complex folds of the muscular membrane whereby the surface area is greatly increased. An estimation of this increase of surface area is not available at present. But it is apparent that an increase of three- to five-fold of enzyme concentration in the part of the muscle containing the junctions may be due at least to a large extent to the increase of surface area. Although it is possible that per unit surface area the enzyme concentration is higher at the junction, the difference might be only minor.

The results reported by GIACOBINI and HOLMSTEDT (1960) using microgasometric techniques fail to clarify the situation. Their individual values for the same type of nerve tissue (motor and sensory fibers) show very large variations: the differences range from 500 to 1000% or more. These variations are in striking contrast to the very narrow range of variations encountered in experiments with standard chemical techniques when the same type of tissue is used. The largeness of the variations may be a reflection that use of so extremely small fractions of tissue, of the order of 0.1 to 0.01 μg, may involve much greater variations of active membranes present in each sample than when larger amounts are utilized giving average values. The absolute values of AChE concentrations are much higher than any figure reported so far in the literature. In thick motor fibers innervating the rectus abdominus muscle of rats, the AChE activity, expressed in the customary way, amounts to 1 to 20 g ACh split per gram tissue per hour. In sensory fibers the concentrations are lower by a factor of about 10, but still extremely high. Per motor endplate the amounts split are about 1 to 5 g ACh/g/hour; these high values may be due to the presence of more active material obtained by microdissection techniques than that used in earlier determinations in which the activity was determined in whole fibers containing much connective tissue and fat. They support the view of the author concerning the high concentration of AChE in axons. In muscle fibers free of nerve elements the values are of the order of only one tenth to one hundredth of those in nerve fibers or endplates, but the activity still amounts to about 20 to 100 mg ACh split per g/hour, which is higher than the values obtained by COUTEAUX and NACHMANSOHN (1940) in muscle fibers of guinea-pigs free of nerve elements, although in this case the difference is relatively small. The reason for the much smaller discrepancy may be that the authors had to use much more tissue even with their micro techniques and that the amount of active surface material in relation to inactive material was much smaller than in the case of axons or endplates. In spite of the application of microgasometric techniques the results do not permit, as the authors themselves acknowledge, an estimation of enzyme activity per unit of surface area or volume. Basically these studies do not change the picture obtained twenty years ago by the author and his associates.

In summary, although the early data about the concentration of ChE in muscle and the absolute values for the activity per motor endplate are correct, the interpretation assuming an unusually high concentration at motor endplates in contrast to the low concentration in fibers must be modified. The enzyme is localized in the surface region and the increase of activity at junctions may be attributed — either entirely or to a large extent — to the remarkable increase in surface area. Thus, the author believes there is no justification, on the basis of enzyme activity, to attribute to the substrate a role at the junction which differs from that in the fiber.

Let us now consider in the light of these chemical data the results obtained with histochemical staining techniques.

When KOELLE and FRIEDENWALD (1949) introduced their well known technique, they noticed at once the strong staining of motor endplates in contrast to the rest of the muscle fiber. This seemed to support the original interpretation of an extraordinary concentration of the enzyme at the junction. However, in the following decade KOELLE (1951, 1955) himself, as other investigators in the field, pointed out the many pitfalls inherent in this as in many other staining techniques for localizing enzyme activity in the cell. The great value of the method and its many potentialities are not questioned and much interesting information has been obtained. But it is necessary to recognize the limitations and to avoid the pitfalls. The method can supplement chemical data and provide additional information which the chemical methods cannot do. But it cannot possibly contradict unequivocal results of chemical determinations. When chemical measurements have established the presence of the enzyme, the failure of the staining technique to reveal its activity cannot be used as evidence against the chemical data. Pictures of muscle treated with KOELLE's method show a strong coloration of motor endplates in contrast to the faint coloration in the fibers. Recently, in still unpublished experiments, Dr. WOLFGANG ZENKER found in human vocal muscles with KOELLE's histochemical staining technique a strong coloration of the surface of the muscle fibers in parts completely free of nerve elements (personal communication). However, histochemical staining techniques do not permit precise quantitative evaluation as do chemical methods. Their value lies in different directions (see Chapter 6).

IV. Presence of the ACh system on the two sides of the junction

For the understanding of the precise role of ACh at the junction it is of interest to know exactly where the various proteins of the ACh system are located. If the action of ACh is intracellular or intramembraneous, then they should be present on both sides of the junction, i.e., in the pre- and postsynaptic membranes. If this is the case it would seem inconsistent with the theory of neurohumoral transmission.

The early experiments on the superior cervical ganglion of cat discussed before indicated that high concentrations of ChE's are present in nerve terminals as well as in the effector cell. Chemical determinations with other biological preparations have shown similarly the presence of ChE's on both sides (FENG and TING 1938, NACHMANSOHN and HOFF 1944, STOERK and MORPETH 1944). Attempts at precise localization with histochemical staining methods at first encountered considerable technical difficulties. Recently, however, KOELLE and KOELLE (1959) found additional definite evidence for the localization of AChE in axon terminals of various ganglia of the cat by applying new procedures in which staining techniques were used in combination with reversible and irreversible enzyme inhibitors (KOELLE 1957), and by comparing the ganglia before and after denervation. At some postsynaptic sites the enzyme appeared to be absent. However, once again it appears questionable whether failure of histochemical techniques to find the enzyme can be used as evidence for its absence, unless experiments would be devised confirming this absence by chemical methods. It appears to the author most significant that, by designing experiments in which a resourceful combination of methods has been applied, the demonstration of the presence of ChE in nerve terminals has been achieved, at least in some of them, although only a few years earlier this problem seemed to have encountered nearly insurmountable technical difficulties (see, e.g., COUTEAUX 1955). This subject is discussed in detail in Chapter 6.

Choline acetylase is present in nerve and muscle fibers and, as discussed before, ACh appears in the perfusion fluid of active muscle after complete degeneration of nerve terminals. This indicates that ACh may be formed on both sides of the junction, or in adjacent cellular elements.

Acetylcholine receptors are also present on both sides, i.e., in the terminal as well as in the postsynaptic membrane. For many years it was assumed that ACh applied externally acts only on the synaptic membrane. However, 20 years ago,

MASLAND and WIGTON (1940) reported that neostigmine, following injection, produced rapid bursts of electrical activity in the motor roots in addition to its action upon the electrical activity on the muscle fiber. Curare blocked both muscle and nerve response. The authors concluded that their observations provide evidence that ACh and neostigmine stimulate the motor nerve terminal as well as the muscle; the concept of a specific local effect of ACh on the muscle at the myoneural junction was, in the view of the authors, unable to explain the findings. MASLAND and WIGTON's observations were borne out by findings of other investigators. Recently, RIKER and his associates (1959) fully confirmed these results and concluded that ACh receptors must be present in nerve terminals. In this connection the response to ACh demonstrated with several sensory nerve terminals may also be recalled.

V. Present state

There is general agreement that ACh plays an essential role in neuromuscular transmission. The difference of opinion in this instance concerns the precise mechanism of action, the question of whether ACh acts in both pre- and post-synaptic membranes to generate ion movements, or whether it acts as a "chemical mediator" between two cells. The events in the synaptic junctions differ in many respects from those in the axon: these differences may be due to the striking differences in structure and organization which must affect electrical fields, time relations, response to chemical agents, etc. But, in accordance with the author's hypothesis, the ACh system specifically concerned with the control of ion movements across membranes does not differ fundamentally in its function at the synapse from that in the axon.

Certain general principles resulting from advances in dynamic biochemistry make it *a priori* difficult, from a biochemical point of view, to accept the mode of action proposed by the hypothesis of neurohumoral transmission. Many biochemical reactions are highly organized structurally, as has been shown in studies of electron microscopy in conjunction with enzyme chemistry. A process such as oxidation, e.g., was found to be localized in the cristae of mitochondria; electron transfer proceeds here in a well organized pattern. It appears difficult to assume that the fastest and most precise function developed by nature, the propagation of nerve impulses, includes chemical processes at certain points which are structurally not organized; that they are not even intracellular, but intercellular and therefore random; that a substance produced in one cell acts upon a specific protein in another cell. All reactions taking place in a living cell are chemically and energetically coupled by complex enzymatic systems. This coupling of enzyme catalyzed reactions is one of the most distinctive biochemical attributes of living matter. Is it reasonable to believe that a sort of uncoupling takes place in the ACh system, so that one part of the reaction, namely the formation and the release of the ester, is localized in one cell, while the reaction with the receptor and the hydrolysis by the esterase take place in another cell? The presence of the complete system at both sides of the gap makes the assumption of an unorganized and split system unlikely. Anything is possible, but to put the hypothesis of neurohumoral transmission on a firmer basis much more and better evidence is necessary than that existing at present.

It is of interest that DALE (1954), in quoting from a lecture he had given in New York in 1937, envisaged the possibility of a much wider role of ACh than was considered at that time: "If the liberation of a chemical mediator at a nerve ending should prove to be not a process peculiar and limited to that ending but merely a local intensification, to ensure transmission to a contiguous cell, of a process which actually figures in the propagation of the impulse along the nerve fiber, we should have to make yet a further revision of our existing conceptions. Some minds have undoubtedly felt difficulty in postulating a complete breach in the nature of the processes concerned in transmission, where the excitation passes from nerve ending to effector cell. This particular difficulty would then disappear but only at the cost of a more fundamental change of conception concerning the nature of the propagated wave of excitation than any which has yet been seriously considered". This statement is all the more remarkable since at that time there was no experimental basis for such an assumption. It appears to the author even more significant that DALE, one of the great pioneers of the theory of neurohumoral transmission, recalled in 1953 his statement of 1937 and warned the audience not to consider the theory of neurohumoral transmission as being the final answer (DALE 1954).

DALE is reluctant to accept the unified theory; he considers it as a simplification which might lead us astray in biology. Methods of approach greatly influence our thinking. The remarkable unity of biochemical principles and systems throughout the great diversity of living cells must influence the reasoning of the investigator attacking the problem primarily by chemical analysis. Physiology and pharmacology study manifestations of intact cells characterized by a nearly infinite variety of organization and structure. Eventually an integration of the various aspects must be achieved on a molecular level.

Literature

ABBOTT, B. C.: Heat production in nerve and electric organ. J. gen. Physiol. **43**, Suppl., 119 to 127 (1960).
— X. AUBERT and A. FESSARD: La production de chaleur associée à la décharge du tissue électrique de la Torpille. J. Physiol (Paris) **50**, 99—102 (1958a).
— A. V. HILL and J. V. HOWARTH: The positive and negative heat production associated with a nerve impulse. Proc. Roy. Soc. B. **148**, 149—187 (1958b).
ALTAMIRANO, M., W. L. SCHLEYER, C. W. COATES and D. NACHMANSOHN: Electrical activity in electric tissue. I. The difference between tertiary and quaternary nitrogen compounds in relation to their chemical and electrical activities. Biochim. biophys. Acta **16**, 268—282 (1955).
ARMETT, CH. J., and J. M. RITCHIE: The action of acetylcholine on conduction in mammalian non-myelinated fibres and its prevention by anticholinesterase. J. Physiol. (Lond.) **152**, 141—158 (1960).
AUGUSTINSSON, K. B., and D. NACHMANSOHN: Distinction between acetylcholine esterase and other choline ester splitting enzymes. Science **110**, 98—99 (1949).
BARTELS, E., W. D. DETTBARN, H. HIGMAN and P. ROSENBERG: Acetylcholine receptor protein and nerve activity. II. Cationic group in local anesthetics and electrical response. Biochem. Biophys. Res. Comm. **2**, 316—319 (1960b).
BERGAMI, G., G. CANTONI e T. GUALTIEROTTI: Sulla liberazione di sostanze biologicamento attive dalla superficie di taglio di nervi durante l'eccitamento fisiologico o provocato. I. La loro azione sul preparato di muscolo dorsale di sanguisuga. Arch. Ist. biochim. ital. **8**, 267—298 (1936).
BERGMANN, F., I. B. WILSON and D. NACHMANSOHN: Acetylcholinesterase. IX. Structural features determining the inhibition by amino acids and related compounds. J. biol. Chem. **186**, 693—703 (1950).
BERMAN-REISBERG, R.: Properties and biological significance of choline acetylase. Yale J. Biol. Med. **29**, 403—435 (1957).
BERMAN, R., I. B. WILSON and D. NACHMANSOHN: Choline acetylase specificity in relation to biological function. Biochim. biophys. Acta **12**, 315—324 (1953).
BERNSTEIN, J.: Untersuchungen zur Thermodynamik der bioelektrischen Ströme. Pflügers Arch. ges. Physiol. **92**, 521—562 (1902).
—, and A. TSCHERMAK: Untersuchungen zur Thermodynamik der bioelektrischen Ströme. Pflügers Arch. ges. Physiol. **112**, 439—531 (1906).
BOELL, E. J., and D. NACHMANSOHN: Localization of choline esterase in nerve fibers. Science **92**, 513—514 (1940).

736   Literature

BOVET, D.: Some aspects of the relationship between chemical constitution and curare-like
    activity. Ann. N. Y. Acad. Sci. 54, 407—437 (1951).
BUCHTHAL, F.: The effect of acetylcholine-like substances on sensory receptors. Pharmacol.
    Rev. 6, 97—98 (1954).
BULLOCK, T. H., H. GRUNDFEST, D. NACHMANSOHN and M. A. ROTHENBERG: Generality of
    the role of acetylcholine in nerve and muscle conduction. J. Neurophysiol. 10, 11—21 (1947).
— D. NACHMANSOHN and M. A. ROTHENBERG: Effects of inhibitors of choline esterase on
    the nerve action potential. J. Neurophysiol. 9, 9—22 (1946).
BURGEN, A. S. V.: The mechanism of action of anticholinesterase drugs. Brit. J. Pharmacol.
    4, 219—288 (1949).
CALABRO, Q.: Sulla regolazione neuro-umorale cardiaca. Riv. biol. 15, 299—320 (1933).
CHAGAS, C.: Studies on the mechanism of curarization. Ann. N. Y. Acad. Sci. 81, 345—357
    (1959a).
— Studies on the mechanism of curare fixation by cells. In: D. BOVET, F. BOVET-NITTI and
    G. B. MARINI-BETTOLO, Eds., Curare and Curare-Like Agents, 327—345. Amsterdam:
    Elsevier 1959b.
— E. PENNA-FRANCA, K. NISHIE and E. J. GARCIA: A study of the specificity of the complex
    formed by galamine triethiodide with a macromolecular constituent of the electric organ.
    Arch. Biochem. 75, 251—259 (1958).
CHILDS, A. F., D. R. DAVIES, A. L. GREEN and J. P. RUTLAND: The reactivation by oximes
    and hydroxamic acids of cholinesterase inhibited by organophosphorus compounds. Brit.
    J. Pharmacol. 10, 462—465 (1955).
CLARK, A. J.: General pharmacology. In: W. HEUBNER and J. SCHUELLER, Eds., Handb.
    Experiment. Pharmacol., IV. Berlin: Springer 1937.
COHEN, M.: Concentration of choline acetylase in conducting tissue. Arch. Biochem. 60,
    284—296 (1956).
COLE, K. S.: Dynamic electrical characteristics of the squid axon membrane. Arch. Sci.
    physiol. 3, 253—258 (1949).
—   Ions, potentials and the nerve impulse. In: T. SHEDLOVSKY, Ed., Electrochemistry in
    Biology and Medicine, 121—140. New York: John Wiley and Sons 1955.
—, and H. J. CURTIS: Electric impedance of the squid giant axon during activity. J. gen.
    Physiol 22, 649—670 (1939).
COUTEAUX, R.: La cholinestérase des plaques motrices après section du nerf moteur. Bull.
    biol. France Belg. 76, 14—57 (1942).
— Localization of cholinesterases at neuromuscular junctions. Intern. Rev. Cytol. 4, 335—375
    (1955).
—, and D. NACHMANSOHN: Changes of cholinesterase at end plates of voluntary muscle
    following section of sciatic nerve. Proc. Soc. exp. Biol. (N. Y.) 43, 177—181 (1940).
COWAN, S. L.: The initiation of all-or-none responses in muscle by acetylcholine. J. Physiol.
    (Lond.) 88, 4P (1936).
CURTIS, H. J., and K. S. COLE: Membrane resting and action potentials from the squid giant
    axon. J. cell. comp. Physiol. 19, 135—144 (1942).
DALE, H. H.: Transmission of nervous effects by acetylcholine. In: Harvey Lectures, vol. 32,
    229—245. Springfield: Charles C. Thomas 1937.
— The beginnings and the prospects of neurohumoral transmission. Pharmacol. Rev. 6,
    7—13 (1954).
— W. FELDBERG and M. VOGT: Release of acetylcholine at voluntary motor nerve endings.
    J. Physiol. (Lond.) 86, 353—380 (1936).
DEL CASTILLO, J., and B. KATZ: Biophysical aspects of neuro-muscular transmission. In:
    J. A. V. BUTLER, Ed., Progress in Biophysics, 6, 121—170. London and New York:
    Pergamon Press 1956.
DE ROBERTIS, E., and H. S. BENNETT: Some features of the submicroscopic morphology of
    synapses in frog and earth worm. J. biophys. biochem. Cytol. 1, 47—58 (1955).
DETTBARN, W. D.: Action of lipid soluble quaternary ammonium ions on the resting potential
    of myelinated nerve fibers of the frog. Biochim. Biophys. Acta 32, 381—386 (1959a).
— Distinction between sodium and potassium in change in permeability effected by lipid-
    soluble analogues of acetylcholine. Nature (Lond.) 183, 465—466 (1959b).
— New evidence for the role of acetylcholine in conduction. Biochim. Biophys. Acta 41,
    377—386 (1960a).
— Effect of curare on conduction in myelinated, isolated nerve fibres of the frog. Nature
    (Lond.) 186, 891—892 (1960b).
— Acetylcholinesterase activity in Nitella. Nature 194, 1175—6, 1962.
—, and F. A. DAVIS: Effect of acetylcholine on the electrical activity of somatic nerves of the
    lobster. Science, 132, 716—717, 1962.

DETTBARN, W. D., H. HIGMAN, P. ROSENBERG and D. NACHMANSOHN: Rapid and reversible block of electrical activity by powerful marine biotoxins. Science **132**, 300—301 (1960).
— I. B. WILSON and D. NACHMANSOHN: Action of lipid soluble quaternary ammonium ions on conducting membranes. Science **128**, 1275—1276 (1958).
ECCLES, J. C.: An electrical hypothesis of synaptic and neuromuscular transmission. Ann. N. Y. Acad. Sci. **47**, 429—455 (1946).
— The Physiology of Nerve Cells. Baltimore: The Johns Hopkins Press, 1957.
EDWARDS, G. A., H. RUSKA and E. DE HARVEN: Electron Microscopy of peripheral nerves and neuromuscular junctions in the wasp leg. J. biophys. biochem. Cytol. **4**, 107—113 (1958).
EMMELIN, N., and F. C. MACINTOSH: The release of acetylcholine from perfused sympathetic ganglia and skeletal muscles. J. Physiol. (Lond.) **131**, 477—496 (1956).
EHRENPREIS, S.: Interaction of curare and related substances with acetylcholine receptor-like protein. Science **129**, 1613—1614 (1959).
— Isolation and identification of the acetylcholine receptor protein from electric tissue. Biochim. biophys. Acta **44**, 561—577 (1960).
—, and M. M. FISHMAN: The interaction of quaternary ammonium compounds with chondroitin sulfate. Biochim. biophys. Acta **44**, 577—585 (1960).
—, and M. G. KELLOCK: Acetylcholine receptor protein and nerve activity. I. Specific reaction of local anesthetics with the protein. Biochem. Biophys. Res. Comm. **2**, 311—315 (1960).
ERDMANN, W. D., F. SAKAI and F. SCHELER: Erfahrungen bei der spezifischen Behandlung einer E 605-Vergiftung mit Atropin und dem Esterasereactivator PAM. Dtsch. med. Wschr. **83**, 1359—1362 (1958).
ERLANGER, J.: The initiation of impulses in axons. J. Neurophysiol. **2**, 370—379 (1939).
FATT, P., and B. KATZ: Spontaneous subthreshold activity at motor nerve endings. J. Physiol. (Lond.) **117**, 109—128 (1952).
FELDBERG, W., A. FESSARD and D. NACHMANSOHN: The cholinergic nature of the nervous supply to the electrical organ of the *Torpedo (Torpedo marmorata)*. J. Physiol. (Lond.) **97**, 3P—5P (1940).
FENG, T. P., and V. C. TING: Studies on the neuromuscular junction. XI. A note on the local concentration of cholinesterase at motor nerve endings. Chin. J. Physiol. **13**, 141—144 (1938).
FULTON, J. F.: Physiology of the Nervous System. New York: Oxford University Press 1938, 1943, 1949.
GIACOBINI, E.: Quantitative determination of cholinesterase in individual sympathetic cells. J. Neurochem. **1**, 234—244 (1957).
—, and B. HOLMSTEDT: Cholinesterase in muscles: a histochemical and microgasometric study. Acta pharmacol. (Kbh.) **17**, 94—105 (1960).
HESTRIN, S.: Acylation reactions mediated by purified acetylcholine esterase. J. biol. Chem. **180**, 879—881 (1949).
— Acylation reactions mediated by purified acetylcholine esterase. Biochim. biophys. Acta **4**, 310—321 (1950).
HIGMAN, H. B., and E. BARTELS: The competitive nature of the action of acetylcholine and local anesthetics. Biochim. biophys. Acta **54**, 543—554 (1961).
HILL, A. V.: The heat production of muscle. In: D. NACHMANSOHN, Ed., Molecular Biology. Elementary Processes of Nerve Conduction and Muscle Contraction, 17—24. New York: Academic Press 1960.
HINTERBUCHNER, L. P., and D. NACHMANSOHN: Electrical activity evoked by a specific chemical reaction. Biochim. biophys. Acta **44**, 554—560 (1960).
—, and I. B. WILSON: Muscle response to long chain quaternary ammonium ions. I. Biochim. biophys. Acta **31**, 323—327 (1959a).
— — Muscle response to long chain quaternary ammonium ions. II. Biochim. biophys. Acta **32**, 375—380 (1959b).
— — and E. SCHOFFENIELS: Effect of lipid soluble analogues of acetylcholine on muscle. Fed. Proc. **17**, 71 (1958).
HODGKIN, A. L.: The ionic basis of electrical activity in nerve and muscle. Biol. Rev. **26**, 338—409 (1951).
— Ionic movements and electrical activity in giant nerve fibers. Proc. Roy. Soc. B., **148**, 1—37 (1957).
HOLMSTEDT, B., and F. SJOQVIST: Distribution of acetylcholinesterase in the ganglion cells of various sympathetic ganglia. Acta physiol. scand. **47**, 284—296 (1959).
KATZ, B., and R. MILEDI: Spontaneous subthreshold activity at denervated amphibian end plates. J. Physiol. (Lond.) **146**, 44P—45P (1959).
KEWITZ, H.: A specific antidote against lethal alkyl phosphate intoxication. III. Repair of chemical lesion. Arch. Biochem. **66**, 263—270 (1957).

KEWITZ, H., and D. NACHMANSOHN: A specific antidote against lethal alkylphosphate intoxication.IV. Effects in brain. Arch. Biochem. **66**, 271—283 (1957).

—, and I. B. WILSON: A specific antidote against lethal alkylphosphate intoxication. Arch. Biochem. **60**, 261—263 (1956).

— — and D. NACHMANSOHN: A specific antidote against lethal alkyl phosphate intoxication. II. Antidotal properties. Arch. Biochem. **64**, 456—465 (1956).

KEYNES, R. D., and P. R. LEWIS: The leakage of radioactive potassium from stimulated nerve. J. Physiol. (Lond.) **113**, 99—114 (1951a).

— — The sodium and potassium content of cephalopod nerve fibers. J. Physiol. (Lond.) **114**, 151—182 (1951b).

KLOTZ, I. M., F. M. WALKER and R. B. PIVAN: The binding by organic ions by proteins. J. Amer. chem. Soc. **68**, 1486—1490 (1946).

KOELLE, G. B.: The elimination of enzymatic diffusion artifacts in the histochemical localization of cholinesterases, and a survey of their cellular distributions. J. Pharmacol. exp. Ther. **103**, 153—171 (1951).

— The histochemical identification of acetylcholinesterase in cholinergic, adrenergic, and sensory neurons. J. Pharmacol. exp. Ther. **114**, 167—184 (1955).

— Histochemical demonstration of reversible cholinesterase action at selective cellular sites *in vivo*. J. Pharmacol. exp. Ther. **120**, 488—503 (1957).

—, and J. S. FRIEDENWALD: A histochemical method for localizing cholinesterase activity. Proc. Soc. exp. Biol. (N. Y.) **70**, 617—622 (1949).

KOELLE, W. A., and G. B. KOELLE: Correlation of cytological localization and function of nervonal acetylcholinesterase; external or functional AChE. Fed. Proc. **17**, 384 (1958).

LANGLEY, T. N.: On the contraction of muscle, chiefly in relation to the presence of receptive substances. Par. I. J. Physiol. (Lond.) **36**, 347—389 (1907).

LAWLER, H. C.: A simplified procedure for the partial purification of acetylcholinesterase from electric tissue. J. biol. Chem. **234**, 799—801 (1959).

— Turnovertime of acetylcholinesterase. J. biol. Chem. **236**, 2296—2301 (1961).

LOEWENSTEIN, W. R., and D. MOLINS: Cholinesterase in a receptor. Science **128**, 1284 (1958).

LONGO, V. G., D. NACHMANSOHN and D. BOVET: Aspects électroencéphalographiques de l'antagonisme entre le iodométhylate de 2-pyridine aldoxime (PAM) et le méthylfluorophosphate d'isopropyle (Sarin). Arch. int. Pharmacodyn. **123**, 282—290 (1960).

LORENTE DE NÓ, R.: Liberation of acetylcholine by the superior cervical sympathetic ganglion and the nodosum ganglion of the vagus. Amer. J. Physiol. **121**, 331—349 (1938).

MARNAY, A., and D. NACHMANSOHN: Sur la répartition de la cholinestérase dans le muscle couturier de la grenouille. C. R. Soc. Biol. (Paris) **125**, 41—43 (1937).

— —Cholinesterase in voluntary muscle. J. Physiol. (Lond.) **92**, 37—47 (1938).

MASLAND, R. L., and R. S. WIGTON: Nerve activity accompanying fasciculation produced by Prostigmine. J. Neurophysiol. **3**, 269—275 (1940).

McINTYRE, A. R.: Neuromuscular transmission and normal and denervated muscle-sensitivity to curare and acetylcholine. In: D. BOVET, F. BOVET-NITTI, and G. B. MARINI-BETTOLO, Eds., Curare and Curare-Like Agents, 211—218, Amsterdam: Elsevier 1959.

— F. M. DOWNING, A. L. BENNETT and A. L. DUNN: Acetylcholine content of tyrode solution perfused through muscles as affected by calcium and procaine hydrochloride. Proc. Soc. exp. Biol. (N. Y.) **74**, 180—185 (1950).

MEYER, K. H.: La perméabilité des membranes. V. Sur l'origine des courants bioélectriques. Helv. chim. Acta **20**, 634—644 (1937).

MEYERHOF, O.: Zur Energetik der Zellvorgänge. Göttingen: Vandenhoek und Ruprecht 1913.

MONNIER, A. M., and M. DUBUISSON: L'action des nerfs extrinsèques du coeur considérée comme phénomène de subordination. Arch. int. Physiol. **38**, 180—222 (1934).

NACHMANSOHN, D.: Cholinesterase in voluntary muscle. J. Physiol. (Lond.) **95**, 29—35 (1939).

— Chemical mechanisms of nerve activity. In: E. S. G. BARRON, Ed., Modern Trends of Physiology and Biochemistry, 229—276. New York: Academic Press 1952.

— Metabolism and function of the nerve cell. In: Harvey Lectures 1953/1954, 57—99. New York: Academic Press 1955a.

— Die Rolle des Azetylcholins in den Elementarvorgängen der Nervenleitung. Asher-Spiro: Ergebn. Physiol. **48**, 575—683 (1955b).

— Chemical and Molecular Basis of Nerve Activity. New York: Academic Press 1959.

— Chemical factors controlling nerve activity. Science **134**, 1962—1968 (1961).

— C. W. COATES and R. T. COX: Electric potential and activity of choline esterase in the electric organ of *Electrophorus electricus* (Linnaeus). J. gen. Physiol. **25**, 75—88 (1941).

— — and M. A. ROTHENBERG: Studies on cholinesterase. II. Enzyme activity and voltage of the action potential in electric tissue. J. biol. Chem. **163**, 39—48 (1946).

NACHMANSOHN, D., R. T. COX, C. W. COATES and A. L. MACHADO: Action potential and enzyme activity in the electric organ of Electrophorus electricus (Linnaeus). II. Phosphocreatine as energy source of the action potential. J. Neurophysiol. 6, 383—396 (1943).
—, and E. A. FELD: Studies on cholinesterase. IV. On the mechanism of diisopropyl fluorophosphate (DFP) action in vivo. J. biol. Chem. 171, 715—724 (1947).
—, and E. C. HOFF: Effects of doral root section on cholinesterase concentration in spinal cord of cats. J. Neurophysiol. 7, 27—36 (1944).
— H. M. JOHN and H. WAELSCH: Effect of glutamic acid on the formation of acetylcholine. J. biol. Chem. 150, 485—486 (1943).
—, and E. LEDERER: Sur la biochimie de la cholinesterase. Bull. Soc. Chim. biol. (Paris) 21, 797—808 (1939).
—, and A. L. MACHADO: The formation of acetylcholine. A new enzyme 'choline acetylase". J. Neurophysiol. 6, 397—404 (1943).
—, and B. MEYERHOF: Relation between electrical changes during nerve activity and concentration of cholinesterase. J. Neurophysiol. 4, 348—361 (1941).
—, and I. B. WILSON: The enzymic hydrolysis and synthesis of acetylcholine. In: F. F. NORD, Ed. Advanc. Enzymol. 12, 259—339 (1951).
— — Trends in the biochemistry of nerve activity. In: D. E. GREEN, Ed. Currents in Biochemical Research, 628—652. New York: Interscience 1956.
NAMBA, T., and K. HIRAKI: PAM (Pyridine-2-aldoxime methiodide) therapy for alkylphosphate poisoning. J. Amer. med. Ass. 166, 1834—1839 (1958).
RIKER, W. F. jr., G. WERNER, J. ROBERS and A. KUPERMAN: The presynaptic element in neuromuscular transmission. Ann. N. Y. Acad. Sci. 81, 328—344 (1959).
ROBERTSON, J. D.: The ultrastructure of a reptilian myoneural junction. J. biophys. biochem. Cytol. 2, 381—394 (1956).
— The molecular biology of cell membranes. In: D. NACHMANSOHN, Ed. Molecular Biology. Elementary Processes of Nerve Conduction and Muscle Contraction, 87—151. New York: Academic Press 1960.
ROSENBERG, P.: In vivo reactivation by PAM of brain cholinesterase inhibited by paraoxon. Biochem. Pharmacol. 3, 212—219 (1960).
—, and S. EHRENPREIS: Reversible block of axonal conduction by curare after treatment with cobra venom and a detergent. Nature (Lond.) 190, 728—729 (1961a).
—, — Reversible block of axonal conduction by curare after treatment withcobra venom. Biochem. Pharmacol. 8, 192—206 (1961b).
—, and T. R. PODLESKI: Block of axonal conduction by acetylcholine and t-Tubocurarine after treatment with cottonmouth moccasin venom. J. Pharmacol. Exp. Ther. in press.
—, and H. HIGMAN: An improved isolated single electroplax preparation. II. Compounds acting on the conducting membrane. Biochim. biophys. Acta 45, 348—354 (1960).
— — and D. NACHMANSOHN: An improved isolated single electroplax preparation. I. Effect of compounds acting primarily at the synapses. Biochim. biophys. Acta 44, 151—160 (1960).
ROTHENBERG, M. A.: Studies on the permeability of nerve membranes to ions. Trans. Amer. neurol. Ass., 230 (1949).
— studies on permeability in relation to nerve function. II. Ionic movements across axonal membranes. Biochim. biophys. Acta 4, 96—114 (1950).
—, and NACHMANSOHN: Studies on cholinesterase. III. Purification of the enzyme from electric tissue by fractional ammonium sulfate precipitation. J. biol. Chem. 168, 223—231 (1947).
— D. B. SPRINSON and D. NACHMANSOHN: Site of action of acetylcholine. J. Neurophysiol. 11, 111—116 (1948).
SAWYER, C. H., and W. H. HOLLINSHEAD: Cholinesterase in sympathetic fibers and ganglia. J. Neurophysiol. 8, 137—153 (1945).
SCHOFFENIELS, E.: Electrical activity of isolated single electroplax of electric eel as affected by temperature. Science 127, 1117—1118 (1958).
— Ion movements studied with single isolated electroplax. Ann. N. Y. Acad. Sci. 81, 285—306 (1959a).
— Les bases physiques et chimiques des potentiels bioélectriques chez Electrophorus electricus L. Thèse d'agrégation, Université de Liège, Liège 1959b.
—, and D. NACHMANSOHN: An isolated single electroplax preparation. I. New data on the effect of acetylcholine and related compounds. Biochim. biophys. Acta 26, 1—15 (1957).
— I. B. WILSON and D. NACHMANSOHN: Overshoot and block of conduction by lipid soluble acetylcholine analogues. Biochim. biophys. Acta 27, 629—633 (1958).
SEAMAN, G. R., and R. K. HOULIHAN: Enzyme systems in Tetrahymena geleii S. II. Acetylcholinesterase activity. Its relation to motility of the organism and to coordinated ciliary action in general. J. cell. comp. Physiol. 37, 309—321 (1951).
SKOUBY, A. P.: Sensitization of pain receptors by cholinergic substances. Acta physiol. scand. 24, 174—191 (1951).

STAEMPFLI, R.: Nouvelle méthode pour enrégistrer le potentiel d'action d'un seul étranglement de Ranvier et sa modification par un brusque changement de la concentration du milieu extérieur. J. Physiol. (Paris) **48**, 710—714 (1956).
— Die Wirkung von Nor-Acetylcholin 12 auf die erregbare Membran des Ranvierschen Schnürrings. Helv. physiol. pharmacol. Acta **16**, C32—C33 (1958).
STOERK, H. C., and E. MORPETH: Choline esterase activity of skeletal muscle in various conditions. Proc. Soc. exp. Biol. (N. Y.) **57**, 154—159 (1944).
WALSH, R. R., and S. E. DEAL: Reversible conduction block produced by lipid insoluble quaternary ammonium ions in acetyltrimethylammonium bromide treated nerves. Amer. J. Physiol. **197**, 547—550 (1959).
WHITTAM, R., and M. GUINNEBAULT: The efflux of potassium from electroplax of electric eels. J. gen. Physiol. **43**, 1171—1191 (1960).
WILSON, I. B.: Acetylcholinesterase. XI. Reversibility of tetraethyl pyrophosphate inhibition. J. biol. Chem. **190**, 111—117 (1951).
— Acetylcholinesterase. XII. Further studies of binding forces. J. biol. Chem. **197**, 215—225 (1952).
— The mechanism of enzyme hydrolyses studied with acetylcholinesterase. In: W. D. McELROY and B. GLASS, Eds. The Mechanism of Enzyme Action, 642—657. Baltimore: The Johns Hopkins Press 1954.
— Promotion of acetylcholinesterase activity by the anionic site. Faraday Soc. Disc. **20**, 119—125 (1955).
— Molecular complementarity in antidotes for nerve gases. Ann. N. Y. Acad. Sci. **81**, 307—316 (1959).
—, and F. BERGMANN: Studies on cholinesterase. VII. J. biol. Chem. **185**, 479—489 (1950).
— — and D. NACHMANSOHN: Acetylcholinesterase. X. Mechanism of the catalysis of acylation reaction. J. biol. Chem. **186**, 781—790 (1950).
—, and E. CABIB: Acetylcholinesterase: Enthalpies and entropies of activation. J. Amer. chem. Soc. **78**, 202—207 (1956).
—, and M. COHEN: The essentiality of acetylcholinesterase in conduction. Biochim. biophys. Acta **11**, 147—156 (1953).
— — A powerful reactivator of alkylphosphate-inhibited acetylcholinesterase. Biochim. biophys. Acta **18**, 168—170 (1955).
— S. GINSBURG and C. QUAN: Molecular complementariness as basis of reactivation of alkylphosphate inhibited enzyme. Arch. Biochem. **77**, 286—296 (1958).
—, and C. QUAN: Acetylcholinesterase studies on molecular complementariness. Arch. Biochem. **73**, 131—143 (1958).
ZOTTERMAN, Y.: Sensory Receptors. In: D. NACHMANSOHN, Ed. Transact. of the 4th Conference on "Nerve Impulse". 140—206. New York: Josiah Macy, Jr. Foundation 1953.

Chapter 16

Actions on Insects and Other Invertebrates

By

L. E. Chadwick

Contents

Introduction

Reports in the late 1940's of work done earlier with various synthetic organo-phosphorus chemicals as potential insecticides (SCHRADER 1947) have stimulated enormous industrial activity in this field. By way of illustration, MOOREFIELD and LANHAM (1959) estimated that over 50,000 such compounds had already been made and tested against insects. Thirty-six of these were said to be in commercial production: 33 dialkyl phosphates, 2 aminophosphates, and 1 phosphonate. FUKUTO et al. (1959, p. 1121) found the number in use to be "30 or more", of which 2 were esters of phosphonic acid.

Such unprecedented developments have naturally brought with them some increase in basic studies concerned with the mode of action of agents of this sort on insects and mammals, although the growing amount of investigation devoted to fundamentals still must be reckoned very slight in comparison with the intense effort that obviously has gone into synthesis and screening (O'BRIEN 1959b).

Expanded production of anti-cholinesterase (anti-ChE) agents for insect control has been due not merely to repeated demonstrations that many of these chemicals are highly effective killers of insects and to the commercial urge to "get on the boat". Two other factors have had considerable influence. The first of these is the widespread assumption that the essentials of the mode of action of these toxicants are rather thoroughly understood. This feeling, be it right or wrong, has given the developer of insecticides some degree of confidence that he is able to meet on a rational rather than on a hit-or-miss basis certain of the many problems he must face in synthesizing, manufacturing, formulating, distributing, and using these materials, so that he has tended to risk operations on a broader scale. It is of interest that in spite of the existence of such a set of guiding principles, out of over 50,000 organophosphorus compounds recently prepared with entomological purposes in mind, only approximately thirty are currently in the insecticide market.

A second phenomenon that has lent impetus to the development of anti-ChE agents as insecticides is the growing prevalence, in an appreciable number of medically and agriculturally important insect species, of resistance toward other classes of chemicals. In several instances, extensive use of chemical control measures has led, through selection pressure, to the emergence of insect populations so tolerant of the toxicants previously employed against them that continued use of these agents is no longer economical. Examples of such resistance first became of noteworthy practical concern shortly after the awakening of general interest in the anti-ChE insecticides. Although some similar resistance to organophosphorus compounds has since occurred and more is to be expected, both with them and with the carbamates, it has generally been slower to appear and of lesser extent, so that the anti-ChE insecticides have enjoyed at least a temporary advantage in this area. Interest in this class of control agents has been particularly strong because resistance toward chemicals is regarded by many as the principal obstacle that confronts the practicing entomologist today.

Several excellent reviews that examine the chemical, toxicological, and physiological aspects of the anti-ChE insecticides have appeared in the entomological literature, e.g., METCALF 1955, 1959; KEARNS 1956; MARTIN 1956, 1959; SPENCER and O'BRIEN 1957; WINTERINGHAM and LEWIS 1959; FUKUTO 1961; and the series of papers devoted to these topics in the *Symposium on Metabolism of Insecticides* in the 1959 issue of the Canadian Journal of Biochemistry and Physiology. Many of these articles are referred to individually in other parts of this chapter. At least one extensive and extremely useful volume concerning these matters has been published (O'BRIEN 1960). O'BRIEN's book includes detailed consideration of the enzymic and other processes of activation and degradation of anti-ChE agents in the insect body, subjects that are not reviewed in this chapter. Problems involved in the resistance of insects to organophosphorus compounds also receive only cursory consideration here. The interested reader is directed to these earlier summaries for fuller orientation.

One must recognize in any event that the rate at which agents are being added in this field is such that no present compendium can be expected to stay fully up to date for long. Attention at this time will therefore be focussed mainly on an examination of the premises that are held concerning the mode of action of these agents, and on relating the newer experimental data to these concepts. Ideally, such a discussion should be able to draw heavily on knowledge developed with all phyla and classes of invertebrates. It is unfortunate, however, that the unparalleled burgeoning of the anti-ChE agents as insecticides has done little to promote the study of their *mechanism of action* in other invertebrates. Even with the mites (class *Arachnida*, order *Acarina*), although these are economically troublesome and although organophosphorus agents are used extensively in their control, few such studies have been made (CASIDA 1955; VOSS 1959; McENROE 1960; SMISSAERT 1960; MEHROTRA 1961a, 1961c). Except for the occasional application of one or another organophosphorus compound as a convenient enzyme inhibitor with some invertebrate other than an insect or a mite, or the equally rare use of another invertebrate as a test organism for bioassay of some of these poisons (v., for example, CALLAWAY, DIRNHUBER and WILSON 1952: *Gammarus*; SEUME 1957:

Daphnia), little attention has been paid in recent years to their effects on animals other than insects or mammals.

A few of these chemicals have been used somewhat more freely in connection with general studies of nervous function. Data on the structure and physiology of the nervous systems of insects and crustaceans, many of which are pertinent to our problem, have been reviewed thoroughly by such authors as WELSH and SCHALLEK (1946), PROSSER (1946, 1950, 1954 a), ROEDER (1958), the contributors to WATERMAN (1960, 1961), and others.

The effect of the anti-ChE agents most generally recognized in insects is implicit in the name: that is, these compounds are inhibitors of enzymes that hydrolyze acetylcholine (ACh).

The most frequently adopted theory of their action on insects and other invertebrates is well presented by SMALLMAN (1959), and is approximately as follows:

1. Cholinesterase is regarded as vital to nervous function, probably by removing ACh, which is considered as the normal nervous transmitter, but which blocks transmission when it is allowed to accumulate to excess.

2. Anti-ChE agents inhibit the enzyme(s) responsible for the rapid destruction of ACh released during normal nervous activity; hence, in the poisoned animal ACh accumulates, nervous function is wholly blocked or at least greatly impaired, and death ensues as a logical sequel.

Cholinesterases (ChE's) in invertebrates

A. Nature and distribution

I. Classification

Insects and other invertebrates contain numerous enzymes that catalyze the hydrolysis of various esters, and many of these enzymes are inactivated by anti-ChE compounds. Several proposals have been made, analogous to those put forward for the comparable vertebrate enzymes, for classifying these esterases, largely on the basis of their activity toward types of substrates or inhibitors or both; but it seems that no simple arrangement can represent adequately the diversity met with in practice.

Speaking only of those enzymes the primary activity of which seems to be the hydrolysis of ACh, CASIDA (1954, p. 20P) has said: "The insect acetylcholinesterases appear to be a group of related enzymes with widely divergent properties. These organo-phosphate sensitive esterases differ greatly in their substrate specificity, susceptibility to inhibitors and activity on mixed substrates. Insects considered to be quite similar taxonomically bear little similarity in the properties of their acetylesterases (i.e., *Homoptera* — leafhoppers, aphids, white flies and scales); yet distantly related forms may be quite similar (leafhoppers and honeybee; mites and scale insects). Esterases from different organ systems of the same insect hydrolysing the same substrate may be completely different in properties. The balance and properties of the esterases may shift markedly during development (housefly and wax moth) (v. Chapter 17). Sex differences may be quite distinct. Properties resembling those of specific cholinesterase appeared in whole leafhoppers, heads of adult wax moths and flies, and in the ventral nerve cord of roaches; nonspecific characteristics were evident in pea aphids, mites and carpet beetle larvae. Enzymes of many intermediate types were also observed. No consistent classification of these esterases appears possible at this time." CASIDA (1955) has given the detailed basis of these judgments; evidence of such complications has also been reported by METCALF et al. (1955), and by various others.

In spite of the well-authenticated complexities of the situation, it is necessary in order to limit our discussion to treat the several enzymes as representative of only a few classes. Realizing that no such simplification can depict adequately the continuous spectrum of properties with which we are to deal, the system proposed by MOUNTER and WHITTAKER (1953) seems most suitable. It distinguishes the *cholinesterases* (ChE's), inhibited both by organophosphates and by carbamates; *aliesterases* (AliE's), inhibited by organophosphates but not by carbamates; and *aryl esterases* (ArE's), inhibited by neither.

It is more or less implicit in the names of these classes that each utilizes a particular type of substrate. Though such a generalization has multiple exceptions, it is often helpful to keep in mind certain trends of this nature. Thus, several of the choline esters, though not all of them, may be looked on as preferred substrates of the ChE's. Acetylcholine is of particular interest in this respect, although it is not always the substrate most rapidly hydrolyzed, even at its optimal concentration. As a greater variety of substrates is tested, it is found that certain esterases which meet other criteria of ChE's will utilize various other alkyl esters and even aryl esters also (v., e.g., WOLFE and THORN 1958). Ordinarily, excess concentrations of substrate inhibit these ChE's; an optimal substrate concentration results, usually of the order of 10^{-3} to 10^{-2} M. Activity toward benzoylcholine is slight.

Aliesterases hydrolyze preferentially various alkyl esters other than the choline esters, though some of them as here defined attack choline esters also. Generally AliE's are not inhibited by excess substrate, but in one instance an optimal concentration of ethyl butyrate has been reported (STEGWEE 1959). The same author (1960) has found that one insect AliE, or group of AliE's, is differentially susceptible to inhibition by tri-*ortho*-cresyl phosphate (TOCP), which is relatively ineffective against ChE's.

As their name suggests, ArE's are most active against aryl esters, of which o-nitrophenyl acetate has been most used experimentally, but they may hydrolyze other types of esters also. Since, by our adopted definition, they are not inhibited by anti-ChE agents, their first interest to us here is that they may be responsible in part for the hydrolysis of compounds that are regarded as the normal substrates of ChE's; thus, the presence of ArE's may obscure the interpretation of the activity of ChE inhibitors. Some ArE's utilize also organophosphorus compounds as substrates and thus detoxify them (METCALF et al. 1956); this is probably their most significant role in relation to the effect of anti-ChE agents.

From the foregoing discussion, it is evident that the terms "acetylcholinesterase" (AChE) and "butyrocholinesterase" (BuChE), as defined in Chapter 4 for mammalian species, are not always appropriate for insects. In many of the reports cited in the present chapter, the methods used do not permit distinction of the particular ChE, or mixtures of ChE's, studied. For these reasons, in the sections which follow, the terminology of the original authors is used in many cases. In general, the terms "specific ChE" and "true ChE" are equivalent to "AChE", and "non-specific ChE" and "pseudo-ChE" to "BuChE".

So far as is now known, the general similarity of the various ester-splitting enzymes in insects and mammals is more striking than their differences, although further differences will probably be discovered. In the sections that follow, the distinctions will be stressed.

II. Distribution in invertebrates

1. General

Cholinesterase in insects was first reported by GAUTRELET (1938), who found a high titre of ChE and ACh in the head of bees. CORTEGGIANI and SERFATY (1939) extended these observations to a number of other orders of insects and arachnids. Cholinesterase has since been demonstrated in numerous hexapods, and it probably occurs in all of them and in other arthropods as well, although experimental proofs of its presence naturally are few relative to the number of species extant. Several reports attest the prevalence of ChE in decapod crustaceans, for example, WALOP and BOOT (1950), WALOP (1951), in various tissues of *Carcinus (= Carcinides)*; WILSON and COHEN (1953) in nerves of a walking leg of *Libinia*; H. J. KOCH (1954a, 1954b) and KOCH et al. (1954a, 1954b) in blood and gill tissue of *Eriocheir*; and MAYNARD and MAYNARD (1960) in muscle receptor organs of *Homarus*. KOCH's finding of ChE in *Eriocheir* blood is unusual; like many other students of the *Crustacea*, R. I. SMITH (1939) found little or no ChE in the blood of *Cambarus*. The distribution of ChE in crustaceans has been reviewed by WELSH (1961).

From all other groups of *Metazoa*, down to ctenophores and coelenterates, ChE has been reported also, though not from all species studied (PROSSER 1946). According to AUGUSTINSSON (1948, 1950), ChE had been demonstrated in some hydrozoans and anthozoans, although such an enzyme had not been recorded from scyphozoans, ctenophores, or sponges, or from *Protozoa*. However, BAYER and WENSE (1936) had already reported ChE in *Paramecium*, while SEAMAN and HOULIHAN (1951) later added the ciliate *Tetrahymena* to the list of microorganisms possessing an AChE.

2. Adult insects

The titre of ChE found in the non-nervous tissue of insects is usually very low or even zero. Thus, in the fat body, muscle, and testis of the cockroach, ChE activity of only about 1% or 2% of that in the nerve cord was found (CHAMBERLAIN and HOSKINS 1951). STEGWEE (1952), in endeavoring to assess the ChE activity of peripheral nerve in *Periplaneta*, found that whole leg muscle, including the nerve branches and endings, has about 8% of the ChE activity of the central nervous system (CNS). He had previously (1951) observed with *Hydrophilus* that leg muscle has about 7% of the activity of CNS, wing muscles ca. 2%, and intestine ca. 3%; there was no activity in blood.

The most frequent observations similarly have indicated the absence of ChE from insect hemolymph [earlier data reviewed by BACQ (1947) and since corroborated by many others]. A few contrary reports in the literature have not been well substantiated.

In *Periplaneta*, COLHOUN (1959b) could not demonstrate ChE activity in coxal muscle, and only a questionable activity in what he designated as "flight muscle"; in denervated muscle he was unable to find any indications of ChE. One infers that the positive results others have sometimes obtained with insect muscle may reflect either the presence in the tissues of a small proportion of nervous elements or the ACh-splitting activity of "non-specific" esterases; in any case, the values observed have been minor compared to those ordinarily found with portions of the CNS, in which much at least of the activity may properly be attributed to "specific" ChE's.

By way of contrast with the figures for other tissues, the titre of ChE in the brain of a housefly, which is by no means atypical among insects in this respect, is nearly equivalent on a weight basis to that in the electric organ of *Electrophorus* or *Torpedo*; homogenates of these fly heads split 11 to 13 mmol ACh/g tissue/hr at 37° (METCALF 1955).

3. Embryonic and postembryonic development of insect ChE

Cholinesterase often is absent even from nervous tissue in the very young insect embryo (subject reviewed by SMITH and WAGENKNECHT 1959, and in Chapter 5). Changes in various esterases in the egg of *Oncopeltus* have been demonstrated by SALKELD (1960, 1961).

The time of appearance of ChE in fertile insect eggs varies with different species. Generally, ChE can first be detected about at the mid-point of embryonic development. Sometimes it is found before the appearance of ACh; in other cases both have been reported to arise simultaneously. Perhaps most often ChE appears shortly after ACh. In several instances, ChE activity in the developing organism was not measurable until the nervous system became functional and coordinated movements began, but in others the initial occurrence and subsequent increase of ChE could be followed even before blastokinesis. Generally ChE has not been recorded before neuroblast formation, with which its appearance often seems to coincide (however, v. Chapter 5).

Again, during diapause of the *Cecropia* silkworm pupa, ChE and ACh vanished from the brain, which at the same time became electrically quiescent (VAN DER KLOOT 1955). Interestingly, there was no correlation between these events and the titre of choline acetylase (ChAc) in the brain, and no change during diapause in the (normal) concentration of ACh in the *ventral* ganglia, although VAN DER KLOOT observed that in the brain the concentration of ACh increased gradually during exposure of the diapausing pupae to cold.

Like several other biochemical constituents of the body, ChE usually has not reached its final level at the time of emergence of the adult. In the honey bee, ChE activity of the whole brain increased significantly during the first week of adult life, continuing undiminished thereafter until old age (ROCKSTEIN 1950). Throughout this time there was a decrease in the average number of nerve cells, amounting ultimately to some 35 % of the initial count, so that the ratio *enzyme : cell* increased; however, the exact location of the enzyme in relation to the cells is not known in this insect. The titre of ChE in the head of the housefly also rises appreciably during the first day or two following emergence, and then remains constant throughout the rest of life. During this time, the ChE level in females was somewhat lower than in males of equal age (BABERS and PRATT 1950; CHADWICK and LOVELL unpublished). CHAMBERLAIN and HOSKINS (1951) found that breis of female cockroach cords had only about 60 % of the ChE activity of cords from males.

The ontogenesis of ChE's in insects and other species is treated in detail in Chapter 5.

4. Insect nervous system

Cholinesterase is widely distributed in the adult insect nervous system, and also occurs here in mites (McENROE 1960).

In the ventral ganglia of the cockroach, ACh-splitting activity was approximately twice as great as in the pooled fibrous connectives and the basal portions of the peripheral nerve trunks (RICHARDS and CUTKOMP 1945), while the abdominal portion of these cords (including ganglia) was about 57 % as active as the (larger) thoracic portion (CHAMBERLAIN and HOSKINS 1951). In all parts of the cockroach nervous system that he examined, COLHOUN (1959c) measured considerable ChE activity. He gave a tabulation in which the ChE values he obtained were compared with those of ACh and ChAc in the same tissues. COLHOUN's measurements (*ibid.*, Table 1) revealed that ChE activity was highest in the thoracic ganglia, in the 6th abdominal ganglion, and in the ventral nerve cord. The titre of ChE in the supra- and sub-oesophageal ganglia, in the cercal nerves (predominantly sensory), and in the 5th leg nerves (predominantly motor) was only about half that of the thoracic ganglia. A rather similar distribution of ChE activity in the roach was reported by IYATOMI and KANEHISA (1958), except that they found the greatest amount of enzyme in the brain.

About two-thirds of the measurable ChE of houseflies was in the head, one-third in the thorax, which contains the composite thoracico-abdominal nerve mass, and none in the abdomen (CHADWICK and LOVELL unpublished). Rather similarly, VAN ASPEREN (1959a) measured the following distribution of a "specific" ChE in houseflies: head, 68%; thorax, 27%; abdomen, 5%; STEGWEE (1960) found corresponding values of 64%, 23%, and 13%. MENGLE and CASIDA (1960) stated that 75% of the ChE activity of their housefly preparations was due to the heads, and 25% to thoraces plus abdomens. In the *Musca* thorax, 91% of the ChE was located in the ganglionic tissue (STEGWEE 1960).

The figures of MEANS (1942), determined with the Cartesian diver for ChE in the grass-hopper *Melanoplus*, are quite low compared to those of more recent studies with this and other insects. TAHMISIAN (1943) has reported ChE in the egg of this species.

Apparently the distribution of ChE in certain insects may be obscured by the presence of endogenous inhibitory compounds. LORD and POTTER (1953), for instance, found ACh-hydrolyzing activity in the heads and thoraces of *Tribolium*, but not in extracts prepared from whole insects. Further analysis indicated the presence in the abdomen of this insect of a water-soluble, dialysable, stable, reversible inhibitor. Nothing more is known of its chemical nature. An endogenous inhibitor was present also in extracts of whole *Dysdercus*.

Histochemical experiments with thiocholine esters and several organophosphate inhibitors have indicated the presence of ChE's in the cockroach along the surface of the neuronal material both in ganglionic and interganglionic regions (WINTON et al. 1958), but these and several of the grosser studies mentioned above are not necessarily conclusive as to the specificity or exact histological location of the enzyme(s) involved. Although it is probable that many of the investigators cited here were dealing largely with "specific" ChE's, as was certainly the case in the work of VAN ASPEREN (1959), others, for example METCALF et al. (1956), have shown that the cockroach CNS contains a significant fraction of choline ester-splitting AliE; one cannot then always judge the extent to which AliE's and ArE's may have contributed to some of the observations hitherto reported relative to ChE activity.

In a more detailed histochemical study with the blood-sucking bug, *Rhodnius*, WIGGLESWORTH (1958) found a "specific" ChE that was limited to the neuropile, the nerve roots, and the larger nerves in the brain and in the thoracico-abdominal nerve mass. The enzyme was absent from the axons; it was confined to the inter-neuronal cytoplasm, a product of the glial cells, and was most concentrated in the synaptic regions. A "nonspecific" ChE, *not* equivalent to the "pseudo-ChE" of mammals, was also present. It occurred in traces in the nerve cells of the ganglia, there was more of it in the glial layer between the cells, and it was plentiful in the cells of the perineurium. Many other tissues contained "nonspecific"esterases which did not hydrolyze acetylthiocholine; these included salivary glands, alimentary canal, pericardial cells, hemocytes, oenocytes, dermal glands, epidermal cells, germ cells, and fat body. No esterase of any kind was detected at muscle endplates. Further details in regard to the location of these esterases in *Rhodnius* are given by WIGGLESWORTH (1959a, 1959b).

From the available findings, which obviously require completion, one can conclude with certainty that the great bulk of "specific" ChE in insects is located in the CNS, and that its principal function is to be sought there. It is not clear whether its distribution within this organ system varies in different insects. With insects other than the hemipteron studied by WIGGLESWORTH, one can only surmise that the "specific" enzyme(s) may be spread along the tissue both in the fibrous interganglionic regions and over the ganglia, though decisive information on this question would be welcome. Except for such data as are summarized here and a few observations cited below (p. 769, 771, 772) in the sections on AliE's and ArE's, little is known about the distribution in insects of choline ester-splitting enzymes other than ChE's. There is considerable likelihood that esterases other than ChE's are responsible for at least part of the ACh-hydrolyzing activity that has been found, for example, in the longitudinal connectives; however, the data that attest the presence of ChE in peripheral axons also render it likely that ChE's do occur in appreciable titre in the fibrous as well as in the cellular portions of the CNS. It has been suggested that inhibition of AliE's may have more to do with the poisoning of insects by organophosphates than the inhibition of ChE itself. We shall return to this problem later.

The location in the CNS of ChE in relation to ACh (v. p. 754—756) is also by no means certain. Although the available data are not sufficiently refined to indicate more than that there is considerable overlap in the distribution of the two materials, it is obvious that much of the neuronal substrate must normally be kept from contact with the enzyme or the ACh would be undetectable. One possibility is that ACh within the tissues, although close to the enzyme, is held there in a bound form that is not readily hydrolyzable. Or again, the ACh may be separated from the ChE by structural barriers. Certain observations suggest that at least a portion of the ChE is relatively free to move. Thus, MIKALONIS and BROWN (1941) found that ChE diffused from isolated cockroach cords into the Ringer's solution surrounding them, while CHADWICK and HILL (1947) measured with excised whole cords about half the ACh-splitting activity of cord homogenates. In these instances it is possible, though undemonstrated, that enzyme diffused from the cords, or substrate into them, via the cut ends of the peripheral nerves or of the connectives.

It is generally held that ACh, because of its ionized condition, is unable to penetrate the intact cord (KOLBEZEN et al. 1954, O'BRIEN 1957b, 1959a, 1959b, O'BRIEN and FISHER 1958), although some of these authors have themselves called attention to exceptions that are not reconciled easily with the basic thesis. Apart from difficulties of this nature, there is the demonstration of BOCCACCI et al. (1960) that iodoacetic acid enters the nervous tissue of the intact cockroach without apparent difficulty. Nevertheless, the general rule that ionization or strong polarity of compounds does not favor their entry into insect nervous tissue is well supported. TWAROG and ROEDER (1956, 1957) showed that the nerve sheath of *Periplaneta* helps to bar exogenous ACh from the synapses of the 6th abdominal ganglion, when they succeeded in demonstrating a synaptic action of ACh only with desheathed cords (cf. YAMASAKI and NARAHASHI 1958b, 1960). TWAROG and ROEDER found that even after desheathing, ACh concentrations of 10^{-4} M to 10^{-3} M were required; since many synapses in vertebrates are much more sensitive to applied ACh, some students have inferred that the cockroach nerve cord contains yet other barriers to ACh, though no such barriers have been visible. WALOP (1951) too had concluded that crustacean synapses and axons are protected from the penetration of ACh by a sheath, a view espoused by WELSH (1961). The alternative is to regard these arthropod synapses as relatively refractory to ACh, which raises the otherwise unsupported possibility that some other substance is the normal mediator. If so, this unknown transmitter cannot be an ester of choline, inasmuch as several investigators have found that ACh is the only detectable choline ester in insect nervous tissue (v. p. 754 below).

B. Properties of insect ChE

I. Subcellular fractions

The ChE of insects exists in homogenates both in soluble and insoluble forms, which are interconvertible and the activity of which toward ACh is apparently unaffected by the shift (SMALLMAN and WOLFE 1956). The same investigators found that if fly head homogenates were suspended in 0.25 M sucrose, some 40%

of the ChE activity was precipitated by centrifuging at 500 g, another 20 % between 500 g and 5,000 g, and a further 20 % between 15,000 g and 26,000 g. The remaining activity could not be removed from the supernatant by centrifuging at 50,000 g for 1 hr. SMALLMAN and WOLFE decided that most of the particulate form of the enzyme was associated under these conditions with large cell fragments and nuclei, and another portion with a microsomal fraction, while a final 20 % was actually in solution. Essentially comparable results with *Musca* ChE were obtained by METCALF et al. (1956), who at the same time investigated the solubilities of ChE and ArE from whole bee brei.

SMALLMAN and WOLFE found that the distribution of fly head ChE between the particulate and soluble fractions was influenced by the concentration of salt present. Addition of salts increased the proportion of enzyme in the gross particulate form, and this reached an equilibrium value of about 70% between 0.05 N and 0.1 N KCl, with no further change up to 0.5 N KCl. Similar results were obtained with bee heads and brains, and with roach nerve cords. The form of the precipitation curves suggests that salt promotes adsorption of the enzyme to particulate matter present in the homogenates.

The level of the equilibrium between the two enzyme fractions depends also on pH. In aqueous suspensions, SMALLMAN and WOLFE (1956) found all the ChE activity in the particulate form at pH 4.0. As the pH was raised, activity in the soluble fraction increased until it reached levels of 90 % or more at pH 8.0 and higher, while the particulate activity showed a reciprocal decrease. The authors demonstrated that such pH differences account for the apparently different solubilities of ChE's from bee and fly heads, such as were noted by BABERS and PRATT (1951).

II. Effects of salt and pH on activity

Salt concentrations and pH affect not only the solubility of insect ChE, but also the hydrolytic activity.

The rate at which ACh was broken down by fly head homogenates was progressively increased, up to 2 or 3 times the values observed in aqueous suspensions, by the addition of NaCl, KCl, MgCl$_2$, CaCl$_2$, or NaNO$_3$ at concentrations up to 0.5 N (CHADWICK et al. 1953). In spite of small but definite differences between the effects of some of the salts, there was evidently no requirement for any specific cation. At still higher salt concentrations, ChE activity was reversibly depressed. Corroboratory data were produced by SMALLMAN and WOLFE (1954, 1956), who also found that activity was reduced by bicarbonate, fluoride, and hydrogen phosphate ions, while it was increased by chloride, bromide, iodide, nitrate, sulfite, oxalate, and citrate. In addition, they demonstrated with erythrocyte ChE that the optimal substrate concentration was increased as the concentration of NaCl was raised. Maximum activation by NaCl occurred between pS 3 and pS 2. A similar shift in pS optimum and an increase in K$_s$(ACh) were observed by WOLFE and SMALLMAN (1956) with fly head homogenates when the concentration of NaCl was raised progressively from zero to 0.5 N. VAN ASPEREN (1959a) too found that ChE activity in houseflies was favored by 0.5 N NaCl. In the absence of salt, the rate of hydrolysis of ACh was depressed 14%/mole of added glycerol and 31%/mole by sucrose (CHADWICK et al. 1953).

The pH optimum for fly head ChE (at 25°; ACh, 0.015 M; NaCl, 0.5 N; 1 head/ml) was found to be at least as high as 8.0 and probably as high as 9.0 (CHADWICK et al. 1954). In the absence of added salt, the activity-pH curve reached a flat maximum between pH 8.0 and 9.0 (WOLFE and SMALLMAN 1956). The latter writers stated that neither they nor CHADWICK et al. found any shift in the pH optimum on changing the substrate concentration, but they reported also a regular variation in optimal pS and in Ks with a change in pH. From the relationship between pK$_s$ and pH, they computed a pK of 7.6 for the enzyme, which is close to the pK of 7.7 found by HASE (1952) with horse serum ChE; therefore, the two enzymes possess anionic sites of similar ionization constant.

Like nearly all ChE's, fly head ChE has a pH optimum on the alkaline side of neutrality. The value of pH 5.75 reported by BABERS and PRATT (1950) is aberrant, although the reasons for their finding are not evident. STEGWEE (1951) measured an optimum of pH 7.4 for the ChE's of the CNS of both the cockroach *Periplaneta* and the beetle *Hydrophilus*. The pH optimum of ChE from roach intestinal extracts was determined to be 6.5 to 7.0 in bicarbonate solution by KOOISTRA (1950).

The reduction in ChE activity that occurs when fly head suspensions at 25° are held at pH values other than 8.0 is not entirely reversible, but the permanent loss does not exceed 25 % during exposures of 30 min until one passes below pH 5.0 or above pH 10.5 (CHADWICK et al. 1954). At pH 3.5 or less, nearly all activity is destroyed under these conditions. As became evident at pH 4.0, the course of inactivation follows two successive first order reactions. During the initial 35 min of exposure at pH 4.0, about 65 % of the original activity was lost; a slower reaction that occurred thereafter led to a total decrement of about 80 % at the end of 2 hr. Housefly ChE was entirely precipitated from such suspensions at pH 5.0 to 5.1; though it was not so rapidly inactivated at this pH level, still it could not be reconverted to the soluble form.

III. Temperature characteristics and heat denaturation

The temperature dependence of insect ChE has been measured, with ACh as substrate, in the developing eggs of the grasshopper (TAHMISIAN 1943), in the oriental fruit fly (ROAN and MAEDA 1953), in housefly heads (WOLFE and SMALLMAN 1956, CHADWICK 1957, CHADWICK and LOVELL 1958), in blowfly heads (LEWIS and SMALLMAN 1956), and in the cockroach nerve cord (RICHARDS 1958). The data of TAHMISIAN do not define the relationship for grasshopper eggs below 35°, but L. D. CARLSON (1941) had studied the ability of the same preparation to hydrolyze methyl butyrate over a wider temperature range. Presumably AliE activity, if present, was included in CARLSON's determinations.

The only other invertebrate for which we have found comparable measurements is the lobster (BULLOCK et al. 1947).

With nearly all these preparations, as is true also with most preparations of vertebrate ChE's, activity is directly proportional to temperature over the entire range of temperatures at which heat inactivation occurs; furthermore, as demonstrated for fly head ChE by CHADWICK and LOVELL (1958), the activity of that portion of the enzyme which has not been denatured by heat may continue to show this proportionality even at higher temperatures. At whatever temperature the Q_{10} is determined, it is low, generally not more than 1.3 to 1.5, with extreme values of 1.7 or 1.8. Data in which log rate is proportional to the reciprocal of absolute temperature are exceptional. RICHARDS (1958) plotted his results with the cockroach on such ordinates for the sake of comparing them with the temperature relationships of other processes, but remarked that the ChE curve is unsatisfactory. One is forced to conclude either that the kinetics of the reaction between ChE and ACh are influenced in most cases by unknown complicating factors, or else that the reaction is limited by some physical process that has not been identified.

However, an instance where the observations with insect ChE do appear to conform to the van't Hoff-Arrhenius formulation is found in the study of LEWIS and SMALLMAN (1956), who measured between 5° and 25° the ChE activity of *Calliphora* heads that had been frozen previously in nitrogen. Their results, plotted as log rate against $1/T_{abs.}$, gave a straight line between 10° and 25° from which one can calculate an apparent energy of activation (ΔE^*) of about 8,000 cal/mole/degree. The rate they measured at 5° is only about 10% too low to fit the line defined by the other data. In one of the few experiments where observations equally suitable for such a calculation were made with a vertebrate ChE, ORMEROD (1953), studying the hydrolysis of 8 derivatives of benzoylcholine by horse serum ChE, found apparent energies of activation ranging, with the different substrates, from 5,000 to 13,000 cal/mole/degree. DAVIES (1955) determined a constant ΔE^* of 4,200 to 4,600 cal/mole/degree for hydrolysis of ACh by a partly purified preparation of this same enzyme, but could not obtain data adequate for this purpose with whole or diluted horse serum. Such measurements of the apparent energy of activation give estimates of the overall energy requirement for the hydrolysis of substrate by ChE, but of course do not permit one to assign exact values for the true changes in free energy and entropy associated with each of the several steps in the reaction, which as yet could not be analyzed independently. Some comparable determinations for the reactions of vertebrate ChE's with various inhibitors have been made by several investigators (reviewed by CHADWICK 1957, p. 55ff.), and ALDRIDGE (1954) has reported that reversal of the phosphorylation by Paraoxon (E 600, 0,0-dimethyl 0-p-nitrophenyl phosphate) of erythrocyte AChE has a ΔE^* of about 14 kcal/mole per degree.

At present, nothing that is known about the activity-temperature relationships seems to offer any prospect of permitting one to distinguish on this basis between vertebrate and invertebrate ChE's.

To those who would like to be able to signal such differences, it is perhaps more encouraging that although ChE's from both sources are inactivated rapidly at temperatures of 55° and above, there do appear distinctions between vertebrate and invertebrate enzymes in regard to their denaturation by heat. A review of this information concerning vertebrate ChE's has been given by CHADWICK (1957). For invertebrates such data have been obtained only with fly head ChE (WOLFE and SMALLMAN 1956, METCALF et al. 1956, CHADWICK 1957, CHADWICK and LOVELL 1958). The most extensive observations have been reported by WOLFE and SMALLMAN, who treated separately the responses of the particulate and soluble enzyme fractions. They found ΔE^*'s for the denaturation reactions of 79,000 cal/mole per degree and 37,000 cal/mole per degree for the soluble and particulate forms of ChE, respectively. CHADWICK and LOVELL calculated a value of 44,500 ± 4,667 cal/mole per degree for their preparation, in which at pH 8.0 the enzyme presumably was mostly in the soluble state. Less heat lability than they found would perhaps have been expected, especially since the preparation contained 0.5 N NaCl, which WOLFE and SMALLMAN showed exerts a protective effect on the soluble form of the enzyme. However, as SMALLMAN (in lit.) pointed out, we do not have such information with respect to the rates of denaturation of mixtures in known proportions of the soluble and particulate forms of the enzyme, so we cannot judge what interactions might be expected.

Despite a moderate degree of similarity between the determinations of ΔE^* by the two groups of workers, there is no explanation of why what seems to be the same enzyme should in other respects exhibit such wide differences in stability to heating as have been found by the various investigators. By comparing the values of k (the rate constants for the reaction) measured in the various experiments, one sees that the enzyme, in bicarbonate buffer under apparently similar conditions, was inactivated 50 times *less* rapidly at 50° in the tests made by METCALF et al. (1956) than in those of WOLFE and SMALLMAN (1956). When, on the other hand, one compares the data of WOLFE and SMALLMAN for the soluble enzyme in 0.5 N NaCl at 50° with those of CHADWICK and LOVELL (1958) for homogenates of whole fly heads, one finds that inactivation was about 20 times *more* rapid in the latter case. Thus it appears that the stability difference for fly head ChE in the experiments of METCALF et al. and those of CHADWICK and LOVELL was of the order of 1000-fold. Such apparent discrepancies remain to be explained. Accounting for these disagreements should throw more light on the denaturation process and on the nature of the protection afforded by adjuvants in solution.

IV. Stability and the effects of some organic solvents

In some contrast with several types of enzymes other than ChE's, the ChE's of insects, like those of many other animals, are relatively stable, at least in the impure state.

Thus, the ChE activity of whole homogenates of houseflies in bicarbonate Ringer (NaCl, 0.5 N; NaHCO₃, 0.025 M) decreased only 1% in 2 hr at 37°, and only 4% in 24 hr at 20° (VAN ASPEREN 1959a). Breis of fly heads or of cockroach nervous tissue may be stored without change in ChE activity at 2° to 3° for weeks or months if the pH is kept slightly above neutrality. The activity of a solution of ChE from the crab, *Carcinus*, decreased 50% in a week at 2° to 4° (WALOP and BOOT 1955). Normal enzyme in whole fly heads or in their homogenates remains apparently unaltered for at least 3 months when frozen and held at −20°; however such enzyme, after inhibition with DFP (di*iso*propyl phosphorofluoridate), regained a considerable fraction of its activity in this time (CHADWICK and LOVELL unpublished).

Heat denaturation of fly head ChE (v. above) begins to be measurable at temperatures of 30° to 35° (CHADWICK and LOVELL 1958), whereas in the mammalian ChE's that have been tested such irreversible denaturation is slight at 50° and below. Mammalian enzymes, however, show some *reversible* inactivation between 40° and 50°; nothing of this sort has been seen in insect material.

WINTON et al. (1958) found that the ChE of roach nerve cords, dried at 37° for 15 min, was still capable of hydrolyzing acetylthiocholine. Similar activity in *Rhodnius* ChE was seen by WIGGLESWORTH (1958) after whole organs or their frozen sections had been incubated for 24 hr in cold formaldehyde solution.

On the other hand, addition of small percentages of ethanol to fly head homogenates at room temperature resulted in a complete loss of enzymic activity (CHADWICK and LOVELL unpublished). The ChE of *Tenebrio* larvae and *Tribolium* adults was completely inhibited by 33.3% ethanol (LORD and POTTER 1950, 1951; O'BRIEN 1953). Apparently some fly head ChE is more sensitive to ethanol than hemipteran ChE, for which O'BRIEN (1956a) found nearly direct proportionality between degree of inhibition and the concentration of ethanol. In O'BRIEN's experiments, 18% ethanol gave 45% inhibition; but ethanol, methanol, and propylene glycol also protected the enzyme to some extent against inhibition by organophosphates. METCALF et al. (1956) observed that 3.3% and 10% ethanol caused no depression of ACh hydrolysis by fly head brei, while 20% ethanol inhibited the enzyme 72%. Phenyl acetate hydrolysis by the same brei was inhibited 0%, 8%, and 90% by these same ethanol concentrations, respectively. On the other hand, with bee head brei both 3.3% and 10% ethanol caused marked *activation* of the hydrolyzing enzyme with both substrates. When bee head brei was kept overnight in the refrigerator with addition of 15% ethanol, 39% of the ACh-hydrolyzing activity and 50% of the phenyl acetate-hydrolyzing activity were precipitated. Similar treatment with 30% ethanol largely destroyed enzymic activity against these substrates, both in the precipitate and in the supernatant.

According to VAN ASPEREN (1960 unpublished; cf. DAUTERMAN et al. 1962), 2% *n*-butanol strongly increased the activity of fly head ChE, whereas ethanol and acetone up to about 10% concentration had little effect on it. All these solvents distinctly decreased the inhibition by organophosphates. Cholinesterase activation by *n*-butanol was also observed with purified bovine erythrocyte ChE and with a purified soluble preparation of fly head ChE. In contrast, AliE activity (substrate, methyl butyrate) was markedly inhibited by low concentrations of *n*-butanol, but only by higher concentrations of ethanol or acetone. The organic solvents did not alter the inhibition of AliE by Diazoxon (0,0-diethyl 0-(2-*iso*propyl-4-methyl-6-pyrimidil) phosphorothioate).

The attempt to obtain a concentrate of insect ChE in the form of an acetone powder has frequently been unsuccessful. Thus, LORD and POTTER (1945a) found that extracts of acetone powders of *Dysdercus fasciatus*, *Tenebrio molitor*, and *Tribolium castaneum* did not hydrolyze ACh, although a similar preparation from *Blattella germanica* did. DAUTERMAN et al. (1962) have obtained 157-fold purification of fly head ChE by means of ammonium sulfate fractionation and calcium phosphate gel adsorption.

Acetylcholine (ACh) in invertebrates

A. Identification and general occurrence

Acetylcholine is distributed extensively throughout the animal kingdom above coelenterates (v. PROSSER 1946, 1950 for tabulations) and ACh has also been found in the protozoans, *Paramecium* (BAYER and WENSE 1936) and *Trypanosoma*

(BÜLBRING et al. 1949). The latter authors could not detect any ACh in the erythrocytic stages of *Plasmodium*. Many but not all of the claims, though they may be correct, are founded only on circumstantial evidence from pharmacological investigations, rather than on direct chemical identification.

Such was long the case with insects, where the presence of ACh-like materials has been known since the work of BACQ (1935a). It was not until the report of AUGUSTINSSON and GRAHN (1954) that ACh in insects was identified unequivocally, in extracts from bee heads. LEWIS (1953), using chromatographic methods, had already shown that a substance synthesized rapidly in extracts from blowflies was in all probability ACh. Acetylcholine was soon identified by chemical as well as by other means in the work of CHEFURKA and SMALLMAN (1955, 1956) and of WINTERINGHAM and HARRISON (1956) with extracts of housefly heads, and by CHANG and KEARNS (1955) in nervous tissue of the cockroach. In these instances, ACh appeared to be the only choline ester present, as was also found in later experiments with extracts of the eggs of the housefly and milkweed bug by MEHROTRA (1960a). MEHROTRA (1961a) has also identified ACh as the sole choline ester in mites.

Most recent workers who have assayed ACh in insect extracts have returned to the less exacting but likewise less specific pharmacological tests. In general, these investigators have employed the eserinized frog's *rectus abdominis* muscle and corrected for the possible presence of sensitizing substances by means of the method of FELDBERG (1945, 1950). A full account of the methods available for the assay and identification of ACh and other choline esters is given in Chapter 1.

Like ChE, ACh in invertebrate tissues has been found predominantly in the nervous system (v. PROSSER 1946, 1950, WELSH 1961). Very little or none normally occurs in the blood (CORTEGGIANI and SERFATY 1939, COLHOUN 1958a, 1959b), though R. I. SMITH (1939) found appreciable amounts in *Cambarus* hemolymph. Most other non-nervous tissues are also low in ACh (BACQ 1935a, 1935b; COLHOUN 1959b). In various tissues of molluscs, annelids, and echinoderms, only slight amounts generally have been reported, but exceptions are known. VINCENT and JULLIEN (1938) stated that the hearts of lamellibranchs and of cephalopods were poor in ACh, but that relatively large amounts occurred in the hearts of *Pulmonata*. The *Murex* heart was said to be especially rich in ACh. BACQ (1935a), who found no ACh in octopus blood, or in the whole bodies of ascidians, coelenterates, or *Porifera*, measured the large amount of 77 μg ACh/g in the cerebral ganglia of the octopus, a value that compares favorably with those found in vertebrate nervous tissue.

The numerous measurements of the quantities of ACh in insects are reviewed below.

B. Ontogenesis in insects

Acetylcholine, like ChE, first appears in insect eggs about at the midpoint of embryonic development, but in some species it occurs here at somewhat different times as regards both the stage of growth and the time of appearance of ChE (v. review by E. H. SMITH and WAGENKNECHT 1959). Although ACh was found before ChE in some instances studied, there are species in which the two appeared simultaneously, and others in which ChE was detectable first. The level of ACh recoverable from insect eggs seemed, in certain examples, to depend in some degree on the level of activity that had been attained by the ChE system (CHINO 1957). This suggests that at least part of the ACh within these particular intact eggs must have had access to the enzyme. The ontogenesis of ACh is discussed more fully in Chapter 5.

C. The state of ACh in vivo

In insect nerve, ACh apparently exists in two forms, as is seen when one attempts to extract endogenous ACh for assay. What is usually called "free ACh" is ordinarily released simply by homogenizing the tissue in Ringer's solution eserinized to prevent hydrolysis of the ACh by the ChE simultaneously mobilized. Roach nerve tissue differs from mammalian nerve tissue in that a large proportion of its ACh may be released merely by immersion of the cords in hypertonic solutions or by mechanical disruption, or by the two procedures in conjunction (COLHOUN 1958b). These observations suggest that much of the ACh in insects is not held in chemical combination, but instead occupies a "structural compartment." More drastic procedures must be used to liberate "bound ACh," which is evidently held more firmly to some tissue constituent. Acid treatment (pH 3 to 4) and higher temperatures are often combined for this purpose. At present we have no certain knowledge of the respective physiological rôles, locations within the tissues, or relative proportions of these two forms of ACh, or of how they may be related to one another. The terms "free ACh" and "bound ACh" are not used in the same sense by all authors. For example, COLHOUN (1958d) considered as "bound" any ACh within the tissue that was not free to reach by diffusion the ChE present. Under this definition, ACh that appeared in the blood during certain conditions of intoxication was considered by the author to have been "free," although one really knows nothing of its previous history. A discussion of "free" and "bound" ACh in crustaceans is given by WELSH (1961).

In relation to this general question, CAVANAUGH and TOBIAS (1949) presented evidence from rat brain preparations that is compatible with the notion that bound ACh is held loosely, by adsorption, in precursor form. Thermal liberation of free ACh from bound precursor in these preparations was rather rapid, even at relatively low temperatures. These workers showed also that ACh could be protected from active ChE by adsorption on charcoal. Possibilities of this nature seem not to have been investigated in insects, nor, for that matter, to have been followed up in studies with vertebrates. This subject is discussed fully in Chapter 3.

Although CORTEGGIANI and SERFATY (1939) had reported that all ACh extractible from the CNS of insects and arachnids is free, later investigators have forced a revision of this estimate. Thus, in the nerve cord of the cockroach thorax, TOBIAS et al. (1946) found that normally about one-fourth of the ACh is in the bound form.

D. Distribution and concentration of ACh in insects and mites

TOBIAS et al. (1946) reported an average total ACh concentration of 46 μg/g for cockroach thoracic nerve cords, but ROEDER (1948) found only 32 to 38 μg ACh/g wet weight in this tissue. The difference between the foregoing values, though not great, exemplifies the rather numerous discrepancies in the ACh levels for various insect tissues published by different workers. Some resolution of such disagreements was attempted by LEWIS (1953), who called attention to the extremely active ACh synthesizing system in homogenates of the blowflies *Calliphora* and *Lucilia*. LEWIS suggested that the higher values found for ACh in insects, such as those observed by TOBIAS et al., were in part the result of synthesis of new ACh during the extraction procedures. This suggestion was reiterated by LEWIS and SMALLMAN (1956). They showed that in order to obtain valid estimates of ACh in insect material, both the ChE and choline acetylase (ChAc), which are present in very high titre, must be fully inactivated before the tissue is homogenized. With many sources of ACh, the concentrations of these enzymes are not such as to necessitate precautions of this nature. Having compared various methods for extracting ACh from the nervous tissues of insects, LEWIS and SMALLMAN recommended boiling the heads or other parts in Ringer's solution for

1.5 min immediately after they are taken from the animal, and following this with extraction in 1% trichloroacetic acid (TCA). By these means they obtained an average value of 36.7 μg ACh/g for the isolated thoracic nerve cord of the cockroach, and 50 μg/g when ventral strips of integument and muscle were included. In view of the low levels of ACh ordinarily reported for other than nervous tissues, the source of this difference in their observations is not clear. FOWLER and LEWIS (1958) got slightly but significantly higher yields of ACh from blowfly heads than had been found previously by homogenizing them at $-70°$ in alcoholic or ethereal TCA. The alcohol or ether served merely as a vehicle to ensure rapid penetration of the TCA at the low temperature, and was evaporated completely before the residue was extracted with an aqueous medium.

COLHOUN (1958c, 1959a, 1959c) measured somewhat higher levels of ACh in normal cockroach nerve tissue than were found by earlier workers, although he adopted the procedure of LEWIS and SMALLMAN with only minor alterations. COLHOUN's values were reported in terms of the chloride (1958c, 1958d, 1959c) or bromide (1958a), those of LEWIS and SMALLMAN and of FOWLER and LEWIS as ACh-ion. Presumably the figures of TOBIAS et al. and of ROEDER are for ACh-ion or the free ester. Adjusting COLHOUN's results accordingly, one finds that he measured on the average about 63 μg ACh ester/g thoracic nerve cord in the normal cockroach (COLHOUN 1958c, 1959c Table 1). He gave also determinations for other parts of the CNS. In the brain he found about 80% more ACh than in the thoracic cord. The thoracic connectives had only about 25 μg ACh ester/g, and the thoracic ganglia about 76 μg. Measurable amounts of ACh were recovered also from the cercal nerves and the 5th leg nerve. Muscle, heart, and blood lacked ACh. The definite finding of ACh in the peripheral nerves is a significant addition to our knowledge of the distribution of this substance. COLHOUN (1958c) noted that in *Periplaneta* ACh seemed to be confined to nervous tissue, and that he had been unable to find any in denervated muscle of this insect.

Although COLHOUN's (1959c) values for roach brains (ca. 115 μg ACh ester/g) seem rather high, they are apparently paralleled in other insects. By using estimates of LOWNE (1893—1895) and of METCALF and MARCH (1950) for the approximate weight of the nervous tissue in fly heads, LEWIS and SMALLMAN (1956) calculated the probable tissue concentrations of ACh in whole fly heads as being between 170 and 500 μg ACh/g. COLHOUN employed a perhaps more realistic ratio (1.8 : 1) of total head weight to brain weight in flies, and so computed a considerably lower concentration of ACh in fly brain tissue (80.2 μg/g). Consequently he concluded that the roach brain contains more ACh on a weight basis.

In further evaluation of methods for estimating ACh, COLHOUN and GILLEBERG (1961) pointed out that traces of TCA in the extraction medium may have a depressant effect on contraction of the frequently used frog's *rectus abdominis*. Therefore, they advised avoiding the use of TCA for extracting ACh from cockroach nervous tissue.

According to LEWIS and FOWLER (1956), the whole blowfly (*Calliphora*) contains about 0.15 μg ACh-ion. Two-thirds is in the head, one-third in the thorax, and none (less than 0.005 μg) in the abdomen, a distribution that agrees strikingly with that for ChE in the body of the housefly (v. above, p. 748).

Large amounts of ACh occur in honey and in the food elaborated by nurse bees (v. GOLDSCHMIDT and BURKERT 1955, HENSCHLER 1956 for data and an introduction to the literature). Apparently the ester is produced by the salivary glands and hence much of the ACh of the bee head, which usually is attributed to the brain, may be present in the glands instead.

MEHROTRA (1961a) found about 25 μg ACh/g in the mite, *Tetranychus*.

Changes in the ACh content of insects

A. Treatment with anti-ChE agents and other chemicals

I. General

Changes in the content and distribution of ACh in insects have been measured under various experimental conditions, and attempts have been made to extract from the data indications of the underlying mechanisms. Where intoxication by anti-ChE agents has been involved, the usual expectation has been that, if an ACh-ChE system of nervous transmission is present, inhibition of the enzyme should result in a significant accumulation of the ester.

In passing, we may note that, although some fairly large increases in ACh have been seen following the use of various drugs or other treatments, there have been no reports of a comparably large decrease, under any conditions, in the normal content of ACh. After the administration of tri-*ortho*-cresyl phosphate (TOCP) to houseflies, STEGWEE (1960) found a relatively slight drop in ACh. Lowering the temperature from 25° to 15° also caused a small decrease in ACh (COLHOUN 1958c).

II. Biphasic nature of the usual increase in ACh

TOBIAS et al. (1946) recorded increases of some 200% in the free ACh of the nervous tissue of cockroaches prostrate for some hours following dosage with DDT (1,1-*bis*-(*p*-chlorophenyl)-2,2,2-trichloroethane) and Gammexane (γ-hexachlorocyclohexane), neither of which causes any measurable inhibition of ChE.

The general failure of chlorinated hydrocarbon insecticides to inhibit ChE *in vitro* has been demonstrated many times, and normal ChE activity ordinarily has been found also in preparations from insects treated with these agents. STEGWEE's (1952) observation of reduced ChE activity in the DDT-treated cockroach has not been repeatable, and seems to have been due to some unknown contaminant in the DDT-formulation he tested. Moreover, MOOREFIELD and TEFFT (1958) showed that inhibition *in vitro* of ChE by carbamates was not interfered with in any way by DDT, BHC[1], Toxaphene[2], Dieldrin[3], or Aldrin[4], nor by rotenone[5] or pyrethrins[6]. A reversible inhibition of ChE by these insecticides *in vivo*, which might be postulated as passing undetected in assay, is unlikely. An indication that DDT may nevertheless affect ChE in some unknown manner *in vivo* is seen in the report of STERNBURG et al. (1959), that DDT-prostrate cockroaches are protected against tetramethyl pyrophosphate; apparently there is here some interference with access of the inhibitor to the enzyme.

In the experiments of TOBIAS et al., increases in ACh comparable to those found after treatment with DDT or Gammexane were produced also by poisoning with eserine or barbital, which were found to be inhibitors of ChE, as well as by cyclopropane anesthesia. However, CO_2-prostration of similar duration did not affect ACh content. With the shrimp, *Gammarus*, these workers found that

---

[1] A technical mixture of hexachlorocyclohexanes.

[2] Octachlorocamphene, empirical formula $C_{10}H_{10}Cl_8$, constituents unknown.

[3] 1,2,3,4,10,10-hexachloro-6,7-epoxy-1,4,4a,5,6,7,8,8a-octahydro-1,4-*endo*, *exo*-5,8-dimethanonaphthalene.

[4] 1,2,3,4,10,10-hexachloro-1,4,4a,5,8,8a-hexahydro-1,4-*endo*,*exo*-5,8-dimethanonaphthalene.

[5] One of several rotenoids, active principles of resins extracted from a number of leguminous plants.

[6] A mixture of several insecticidally active ingredients (pyrethroids) extracted from plants of the genus *Chrysanthemum*, family *Compositae*.

prostration with DDT or Gammexane evoked only smaller rises in ACh (ca. 35 %), while none occurred in the frog or rat. The increases in ACh in the nerve cords of the roach and shrimp were entirely in the connectives.

Similar changes in the ACh extractible from cockroach nerve cords 24 hr after lethal doses of the anti-ChE agent tetraethyl pyrophosphate (TEPP) were obtained by COLHOUN (1958a, 1958c), but he could find no shift in the relative proportions of ACh in various parts of the nervous system. However, during the first half-hour after TEPP-poisoning, COLHOUN noticed a smaller, transient increase in ACh; this had not been remarked in the experiments of TOBIAS et al. nor in COLHOUN's own work with DDT.

WINTERINGHAM and HARRISON (1956), after poisoning houseflies with 10 μg DFP, also found a transient rise of ACh in the thorax (Table 1).

Table 1. μg ACh/Musca thorax at intervals after DFP-treatment
(from WINTERINGHAM and HARRISON 1956)

	0.5 hr	2 hr
untreated	0.007	0.007
DFP, topical	0.025	0.009

Both phases of ACh increase were seen by SMALLMAN and FISHER (1958) in houseflies dosed with four organophosphorus compounds (TEPP, Parathion (0,0-diethyl 0-(4-nitrophenyl) phosphorothioate), Malathion (0,0-dimethyl S-(1,2-dicarboethoxyethyl) phosphorodithioate), or DFP). These investigators observed a slight initial rise and fall in ACh, which reached a peak only approximately 20 % above normal in 0.5 hr, approximately at the time when complete inhibition of ChE appreared to have been attained. Later, except with DFP, there was a much larger increase in ACh; with Parathion, which produced irreversible inactivation of the enzyme, the late rise continued until the end of the experiment (18 hr). In the studies with TEPP and Malathion there was some renewal of ChE activity after the maximal depression had occurred, and more or less simultaneously there was a decrease in the previously augmented concentration of ACh. SMALLMAN and FISHER found these results in agreement with the expectation that the level of ACh should vary reciprocally with that of the enzymic removal system. Absence of the anticipated late increase in ACh when DFP was the toxicant had also been noted by WINTERINGHAM and HARRISON (1956).

III. Effects of P-2-AM and TOCP

Further complications arise from data obtained by COLHOUN (1959c). In cockroaches pretreated with P-2-AM (pyridine-2-aldoxime methiodide) before being dosed with TEPP, no *early* change in ACh content occurred, but a later rise took place as usual. Pyridine-2-aldoxime methiodide is thought to promote regeneration of active ChE from the phosphorylated, inhibited enzyme. Whether the P-2-AM penetrated to the cockroach ChE *in vivo* is in some doubt, but that it had a delaying effect on the expected course of TEPP-poisoning is certain; however, in spite of its presumably alleviating action, the treated roaches died. Pyridine-2-aldoxime methiodide failed also to save DFP-poisoned houseflies (WINTERINGHAM and HARRISON 1956, WINTERINGHAM et al. 1957, WINTERINGHAM 1957, WINTERINGHAM and LEWIS 1959).

Equally confusing are the results of STEGWEE (1960), who showed that the normal level of ACh in houseflies was reduced approximately 10 % by treatment with 100 μg of TOCP (tri-*ortho*-cresyl phosphate), which seemed to have no effect on their ChE or on their well-being; furthermore, following subsequent dosage with 0.2 μg TEPP, the ACh content of the flies increased, though it rose less rapidly than in flies exposed to TEPP alone. The possibility that TOCP might have affected the ACh-synthesizing system was mentioned, though there was no other supporting evidence. Of the flies that had received the combined treatment with TOCP and TEPP, only 77 % died, whereas 96 % of the flies succumbed when they had received only TEPP. Thus, the pretreatment with TOCP might be regarded as having given some protection; but, since the level of ACh in the flies dosed with both compounds rose only until it equalled that of normal flies that had received no treatment whatever, there was evidently no simple relationship between the degree of toxicity and the average level of ACh.

IV. "Substrate protection"

Yet other uncertainties have been uncovered by VAN ASPEREN (1958a). The research of this investigator indicates that spuriously high values for the degree of inhibition of ChE after treatment *in vivo* with anti-ChE agents may be found in analyses of insect homogenates, because some of the yet unreacted anti-ChE agent may be held in the nervous tissue and may not reach the enzyme until the samples are prepared for assay. For this reason, as recognized by SMALLMAN (1959) some of the apparent correlations reported earlier between degree of ChE inhibition and ACh content may be suspect. VAN ASPEREN's findings led him to recommend the technique, since widely adopted, of "substrate protection," in which substrate solutions of adequate strength rather than the usual media are used for homogenizing the tissue, with the object of preventing any further inhibition of ChE during preparation. Although both earlier and later workers have shown that this precaution is not essential in *all* cases, at present it is not always clear which of the previously published observations may have given an erroneous picture of the true course and ultimate degree of ChE inhibition *in vivo*. Until such problems have been reinvestigated, some of the ostensible correlations between symptom-matology and degree of inhibition of ChE have to be accepted with reservations. In direct relation to our present problem, STEGWEE (1960) showed, by means of the method of "substrate protection," that inhibition of ChE in houseflies poisoned with TEPP occurs less rapidly than was thought by SMALLMAN and FISHER (1953), so that the actual relationship between ACh content and level of ChE inhibition is not exactly as it appeared to be from the measurements these workers made. In particular, it seems that the late rise in concentration of ACh probably began before maximal (average) inhibition of ChE had been attained.

In relation to the question of "substrate protection" it should be pointed out that the technique cannot guarantee *no* migration whatever of unreacted anti-ChE to as yet unhibited enzyme. The presence of substrate will protect, but the protection it offers is competitive. If an anti-ChE is held in the tissue, some, when released by grinding, will reach the ChE before substrate can do so and, in the case of some organophosphorus agents, will cause inhibition the nature of which will probably be permanent. The amount of inhibition that may thus occur will be of significance in relation to some problems.

V. ACh changes in eggs

Further data that bear on the relationship between the effects of anti-ChE agents and ChE content have been obtained with insect eggs. Poisoning of housefly eggs with Parathion resulted in complete inhibition of ChE and in a subsequent increase of about 50 % in ACh content (MEHROTRA and SMALLMAN 1957, MEHROTRA 1960b). The studies of CHINO (1957), in which eserine was used mainly in connection with the extraction of ACh from silkworm eggs at various

ages, do not seem pertinent to this point, although they have been cited in relation
to it in the literature; however, DAVID (1959) found that eggs of *Pieris* showed
lower ChE values and a higher than normal ACh content either when they were
exposed directly to Paraoxon or were taken from plants that had been treated
with this agent. This topic is considered in detail in Chapter 17.

VI. Distributional shifts in ACh

An interesting movement of ACh in the insect body after anti-ChE poisoning
was called attention to by LEWIS and FOWLER (1956). In their experiments, they
used DFP at the high dosage of 10 μg/blowfly, or about 250 to 300 mg/kg. This
caused paralysis in about 3 min. After 0.5 hr, the ACh content of the head,
originally some 0.11 μg, began to drop, and at 3.5 hr it had fallen to 25% of the
original level. The ACh content of the thorax (0.035 μg at the start) doubled in
the first hour and remained at this new value. The same quantity (0.07 μg) was
reached at 3.5 hr in the abdomen, which was lacking in ACh at the beginning.
Thus there appears to have been a transfer of ACh from head to abdomen. These
observations were corroborated by SMALLMAN and FISHER (1958), who also found
indications of a similar shift in ACh after intoxication of flies with other anti-ChE
agents, though they could not prove a redistribution of ACh in the latter instances
because of the large overall increases in ACh that took place.

LEWIS and FOWLER noted that the abdominal ACh became concentrated in
the hindgut, and suspected that the ACh had been transported from the head in
the hemolymph, although they were unable to demonstrate that this was the
pathway. SMALLMAN and FISHER also found that ACh became concentrated in
the hindgut of flies poisoned with DFP or with other anti-ChE agents. In support
of the notion of LEWIS and FOWLER that this ACh had been carried in the blood,
SMALLMAN and FISHER pointed to COLHOUN's (1958a) demonstration of ACh in
the blood of TEPP-treated roaches and to their own similar finding in flies poisoned with Paraoxon. However, it is proper to mention in this connection that
COLHOUN himself (1958a, 1958d) was inclined to doubt that the ACh he found
in the blood had been released from the nervous system. Its amount was small,
even at the maximal level 2 hr after treatment, and its quantity fell subsequently,
at a time when the concentration of ACh in the cord was rising to much greater
values than before. One may reason, however, that if the ACh liberated into the
blood were being sequestered rapidly into the hindgut, its concentration in the
blood might remain small at all times, irrespective of the concentrations reached
in the nervous system; hence, COLHOUN's argument for its having originated
elsewhere need not settle the matter.

VII. Summary

Despite the difficulties in their final interpretation, the experiments described
in the foregoing section delineate certain general characteristics of the changes that
may occur in ACh content when insects are subjected to drastic treatments. In
particular, poisoning with anti-ChE agents results initially in a relatively small,
transient increase of ACh in the nervous system (in the absence of P-2-AM).
After the insects have reached a stage of prostration (from which, as a rule, few
of them recover if they have been "knocked down" by irreversible inhibitors,
although some recuperation may be attained, even with these compounds, by
means of a suitable choice of sublethal doses), there begins a prolonged rise in
ACh, and the ester ultimately reaches levels much greater than normal. A quantitatively similar *late* increase in ACh also follows prostration by various chemicals

that are not anti-ChE agents, and may occur likewise after prostration from other, but not from all, causes. LEWIS et al. (1960) have shown that, in general, ACh content rises during stress caused by a variety of means other than insecticides.

Notwithstanding the likelihood first emphasized by LEWIS (1953), that much synthesis of ACh may occur in homogenates of insect nervous tissue unless preventive steps are taken, his own experiments as well as those of several other workers prove that exposing insects to such toxicants as DDT, Gammexane, and various anti-ChE agents activates an ACh-producing mechanism in these animals. Of considerable interest in this connection is the fact that, in spite of large increases of ACh content *in vivo*, which we have seen may occur without the benefit of ChE inhibition, no change in the synthesizing capacity *in vitro* was detected by TOBIAS et al. (1946), WINTERINGHAM and HARRISON (1956), SMALLMAN and FISHER (1958), or COLHOUN (1958c); however, this was not so in the experiments of LEWIS (1953). The numerous negative results raise the suspicion that the ChAc system, as it has been studied in isolation, may not be the sole source of ACh in the living organism.

The as yet sparse observations on insects pretreated with P-2-AM or with TOCP simply do not fit into any of the present theories regarding the genesis of ACh or its physiological rôle in these organisms.

B. Changes induced by other treatment

I. Electrical stimulation

According to the view that ACh is the normal nervous mediator, the quantity of ACh released should be augmented by increased nervous activity. In agreement with this hypothesis, MIKALONIS and BROWN (1941) found a higher than average level of ACh associated with high endogenous electrical activity of excised cockroach nerve cords. COLHOUN (1958a) investigated this situation further. He showed that placing cockroach nerve cords in eserine sulfate, 10^{-4} M, increased their ACh content, which rose still more when the cords were simultaneously stimulated electrically. TOBIAS et al. (1946) had noted earlier an increase in the nerve cord ACh of cockroaches prostrated by injections of eserine or barbital, both of which reduced ChE activity and very likely augmented the nervous discharge. The effect of ACh applied to the desheathed 6th abdominal ganglion of the cockroach was enhanced to some extent by pretreating the preparation with eserine (TWAROG and ROEDER 1957, YAMASAKI and NARAHASHI 1958b, 1960). It is noteworthy that in the experiments of COLHOUN there was little or no diffusion of ACh into the surrounding perfusion fluid, an observation that may indicate the presence in the intact nerve cord of a barrier to outward movement of ACh analogous to, or perhaps even identical with, the obstacle to inward diffusion which is represented in part at least by the nerve sheath.

In summary of this subsection, few attempts have been made to assess the effect of increased nervous activity on the level of ACh in the nervous system. Such data as have been collected do not contradict the hypothesis that an increase in ACh might be expected to result from augmented nervous discharge; but the problem is a complex one, beset with numerous difficulties as regards both theory and technique. Although a definite solution would be most desirable, one can hardly claim that such has been attained, and it seems rather unlikely that one could be.

II. Temperature of holding

The observations outlined above concerning the behavior of ACh all refer to insects that had been under considerable degrees of stress, the rôle of which in causing increases in ACh has been emphasized, as was noted, by Lewis et al. (1960). It is likewise of interest that the level of ACh may shift appreciably as the result of somewhat milder treatment.

Colhoun (1958c) found that holding roaches for 20 hr at different temperatures caused measurable variation in the ACh content of the thoracic nerve cord. Taking as 100% the level of 76.8 μg ACh/g observed at 25°, the average values he found were 127% at 35°, 94% at 15°, and 111% at 9°. In line with the view advanced by Lewis et al., one might suppose that in these experiments some degree of stress was afforded by the prolonged exposure at very high or very low temperatures. The ACh of roaches first kept for 20 hr at 35° and then placed for 2 hr at 15° dropped only part way toward the level characteristic of the lower temperature, but reached this value after the animals had been for 20 hr in the cold.

ACh Synthesis in invertebrates

The relatively large concentrations of ACh and the high titre of ChE in the nervous tissue of insects and other arthropods afford a basis for a hypothesis of cholinergic impulse transmission, even though the mere presence of these substances cannot prove the existence of such a system. Also, whereas essential ACh-synthesizing pathways would seem implicit in the high concentrations of ester that have been found, the demonstration of a mechanism for the rapid synthesis of ACh remains an important element of such an hypothesis. For the present subject, it is equally legitimate to enquire, where such a synthetic system exists, whether and how greatly its activity may be affected by anti-ChE agents.

A. Choline acetylase in invertebrates other than insects

The presence of choline acetylase (ChAc) in the pathogenic flagellate, *Trypanosoma*, was shown by Bülbring et al. (1949).

According to Bueding (1952), Nachmansohn informed him of unpublished evidence that acetone powders of schistosomes contain ChAc.

Bülbring et al. (1953) found that ACh was synthesized by nerve-free gill plates of the mussel, *Mytilus*, while Berman et al. (1953) studied the production of ACh by the head ganglion of the squid.

Synthesis of ACh by homogenates of abdominal ganglia of the crab, *Carcinides*, was reported by Walop (1950, 1951). He found that such preparations would form up to 480 μg ACh/g tissue/hr in the presence of cysteine in a nitrogen atmosphere. The tissue was suspended in a phosphate buffer, with the addition of NaCl, NaF, sodium acetate, and ATP. Easton (1950) also reported a similar ChAC in nervous tissue of *Cambarus* and *Cancer*.

Choline acetylase also occurs in the mite, *Tetranychus*, acetone powders of which are able to synthesize as much as 20 μmol ACh/g powder/hr (Mehrotra, 1961c).

B. Choline acetylase in adult insects

Early evidence of ACh-synthesis by insect nervous tissue was provided by Tobias et al. (1946) and by Lewis (1953). Tobias et al. found that eserinized homogenates of cockroach nerve cord produced 47 μg ACh/g tissue/30 min when incubated anaerobically with choline, ATP, and yeast juice, without an added acetyl donor. Lewis observed that the ACh content of blowfly homogenates increased from 7.5 μg ACh/g to 35 μg/g when incubated for 5 hr with eserine, and that the rate of such synthesis was greater in extracts from insects previously exposed to lethal doses of DDT, although this apparently had not been the case in the experiments of TOBIAS et al.

A more thorough study of the mechanism for ACh-synthesis was carried out by SMALLMAN (1956) with extracts of acetone powders from heads of the blowfly, *Lucilia*. Rates of synthesis as high as 100 μg ACh/g acetone powder/hr were obtained when the powders were incubated with ATP, coenzyme A (CoA), choline, and acetate or citrate. Separate enzyme systems were evidently present for acetylation of CoA from acetate or citrate, respectively; the final rate of acetylation of choline by ChAc was shown to depend on the quantity of acetyl CoA present. As had been found with squid head ganglion by BERMAN et al. (1953), the formation of ACh was more rapid when acetate was the acetyl donor, in which respect vertebrate ChAc systems are said to differ (see Chapter 3). SMALLMAN calculated that on the basis of the weight of nervous tissue, as distinct from the total weight of bodily materials present in his preparations, the blowfly brain has about half the synthesizing activity of the purified preparations from the squid.

SMALLMAN and PAL (1957) demonstrated ChAc activity in homogenates of cockroach nerve cords. The formation of ACh was most rapid when acetyl CoA was supplied, and was reduced in the presence of ATPase, which lowered the rate of production of acetyl CoA. As had been noted with houseflies, the ChAc activity was higher than in mice. The enzyme in roaches differed from mammalian ChAc also in that, after centrifuging, activity was found to be associated with the supernatant rather than with the mitochondria.

FRONTALI (1958) showed that ACh, which she identified chemically as well as pharmacologically, was produced by head extracts from houseflies, both in the presence and absence of added substrate (acetate or citrate, plus choline). With propionate as substrate, propionylcholine was formed, together with a small amount of ACh. Only ACh was found when formate or butyrate was supplied. There was no synthesis with phosphoryl choline.

A housefly ChAc preparation with a 5-fold increase in specific activity was prepared by BOCCACCI et al. (1960). The activity of ChAc in these flies agreed with that determined by SMALLMAN (1956) for *Lucilia*. In the adult housefly, ChAc activity increased about 77% from the time of emergence until the 2nd day of adult life, and then remained at the new level until the 5th day, when a decline set in. By the 8th day, ChAc activity had fallen to about 85% of the initial value, and did not change further; the experiment was carried until the flies were 14 days old.

Significantly, treatment of these houseflies or of cockroaches with 10 $\times$ the LD$_{50}$ of iodoacetic acid (IAA), which reacts strongly with sulfhydryl groups, did not alter the activity of ChAc extracts from the insects, even though inhibition of glyceraldehyde-3-phosphate dehydrogenase in the same nervous tissue showed that the IAA had penetrated, notwithstanding its ionization. That IAA is intrinsically a poor inhibitor of insect ChAc was demonstrated further by the results obtained with it *in vitro*, where even 10^{-1} M IAA caused only 37% reduction in ACh synthesis, while lower concentrations caused none.

Study of the synthesis of ACh by homogenates of housefly heads was carried further by MEHROTRA (1961 b). He was able to concentrate the ChAc 20-fold by means of ammonium sulfate fractionation. The Michaelis-Menten constant, K_m, was determined as 6.6×10^{-4} M with respect to acetyl CoA as a substrate. The K_m with respect to choline was 4.4×10^{-4} M when chemically produced CoA was used, but was only 3.3×10^{-4} M when the CoA was produced enzymically. The V_{max}-was about 3 times greater with enzymically than with chemically produced CoA.

COLHOUN (1958a, 1958c) had already extended our knowledge of the formation of ACh by homogenates of cockroach nerve tissue and muscle. He incubated the eserinized preparations with CoA, acetyl phosphate, transacetylase, choline, salts, and buffer at 30°, which he found to be the optimum temperature here and with the housefly. Exact proportions of the medium were given by MEHROTRA (1961 b). The greatest synthetic activity obtained by COLHOUN was from the ganglia of the brain (ca. 50 μg ACh/g roach tissue/hr) and ventral nerve cord, with lesser amounts produced by tissues containing only nerve fibers (2 μg ACh/g leg nerve/hr). No activity was found in coxal or flight muscles.

C. Choline acetylase in insect eggs

The ability of the eggs of various *Lepidoptera* to synthesize ACh was investigated by YUSHIMA (1957) and by CHINO (1957). They found that ChAc was absent initially, but that it appeared rather early in development, preceding the appearance of ChE, rose presently to a maximum, and then declined to a slight extent before emergence. Acetylcholine was first detectable in these eggs about at the same time that the synthesizing system appeared.

The order in which these several constituents were detected in the developing eggs of the housefly and milkweed bug, *Oncopeltus*, was: ChAc, ChE, ACh (MEHROTRA 1960a). MEHROTRA likewise observed a slight decline in the level of ChAc shortly before emergence, at which time both ChE and ACh continued to rise. As in other examples where both ChE and ACh have been detected in the same general locus, it is evident here that not all the ACh in the living system can have had access to the enzyme or it would not have been detected. Equally, since we have no way of knowing what proportion of the ACh initially produced may have been destroyed in this way, we are unable to gauge the actual rate of ACh-synthesis *in vivo* in such a situation; our present unrefined methods of analysis show only that ChE was also present.

MEHROTRA found that 25° was optimal for ChAc activity in preparations of eggs from either species, which is lower than the value of 30° recorded by COLHOUN for ChAc from adult insects. The best temperature for synthesis of ACh by vertebrate extracts is considerably higher (v. Chapter 2).

D. Effects of anti-ChE agents on insect choline acetylase

According to WINTERINGHAM and colleagues (WINTERINGHAM and HARRISON 1956, WINTERINGHAM et al. 1957, WINTERINGHAM 1957, WINTERINGHAM and LEWIS 1959), DFP not only inhibits ChE in houseflies but also may interfere *in vivo* with their synthesis of ACh, although addition of DFP to housefly homogenates was without effect on the ChAc system *in vitro*. The latter observation has been confirmed (SMALLMAN and FISHER 1958). WINTERINGHAM et al. suggested that the synthesis of ACh *in vivo* may be regulated by the demand, which would be expected to fall off after nervous discharge had been greatly reduced by nearly complete inhibition of ChE; in this way they attempted to rationalize a lack of increase in the ACh accumulated by flies dosed with moderate amounts of DFP. But, in view of the often large increases in ACh seen in flies after inhibition of their ChE by other organophosphorus compounds, it does not seem that this explanation can be generally valid.

As noted previously, the ChAc system was not found to be more (or less) active than normal in measurements *in vitro* with preparations from TEPP-poisoned cockroaches (COLHOUN 1959c).

E. Comment

In summary, there appears to be widely distributed among insects a ChAc system for the synthesis of ACh, and similar systems have been found in several other arthropods as well as in a few invertebrates from other phyla. Like ACh and ChE, the ChAc of arthropods is concentrated in the nervous tissue, where it is present in high titre. Nothing is known about its precise histological location. Choline acetylase comes into being rather early in the developing insect embryo, apparently before ChE.

The properties of insect ChAc's resemble those of vertebrate ChAc, though they differ in several details, notably in the lower temperature optima, in the absence of important reactive sulfhydryl groupings, in the fact that acetate seems to be the preferred acetyl donor in insects, and in the lack of association with mitochondria. According to BETTINI and BOCCACCI (1958), IAA and other sulfhydryl inhibitors have been shown to inactivate squid ChAc, so that a simple contrast of the vertebrate and invertebrate enzymes from this viewpoint is evidently not possible.

In spite of the high activity of the ChAc mechanisms of insects, there is room to doubt that all of the large amounts of ACh observed under certain conditions have been derived from these sources, since sizeable increases in ACh frequently have been recorded following procedures that neither inhibited ChE nor caused any demonstrable activation of the ChAc system.

Other effects of anti-ChE agents on insects, etc.

A. On enzymes

I. Cholinesterases

As in other animals, in insects ChE-inhibition is ordinarily the most conspicuous effect of the anti-ChE agents. The chemical nature of these reactions appears fully comparable to that which has been investigated intensively with other organisms (cf. Chapter 7). For general discussions of the subject as it relates particularly to insecticidal materials, reference may be made to the works of METCALF (1955, 1959) and O'BRIEN (1960).

Among the various chemical classes of known ChE-inhibitors only the organophosphorus compounds and the carbamates have been studied to any great extent with insects. Reports of inhibition by other kinds of agents are few, and in some cases questionable.

The organophosphorus compounds are believed to react with insect ChE's, and with AliE's also, to form highly stable phosphorylated complexes. The reactions are competitive with hydrolysis of substrate. *In vitro*, the complexes may be dephosphorylated slowly, depending on the particular alkylphosphate group, with ultimate regeneration of active enzyme (but not of inhibitor); agents such as P-2-AM apparently accelerate the process with insect enzyme (COLHOUN 1959c), although they have not been shown to exert any protective effect against the lethal action of anti-ChE agents *in vivo*. However, insects that survive near-lethal exposures to organophosphorus agents may spontaneously recover considerable ACh-hydrolyzing ability within only a few hours of a large degree of ChE-inhibition (CHAMBERLAIN and HOSKINS 1951, O'BRIEN 1956b, MENGLE and CASIDA 1958, HOPF and TAYLOR 1958, SMALLMAN and FISHER 1958, STEGWEE 1960, MENGLE and O'BRIEN 1960). In some of these instances regeneration of ChE has been thought to be hastened by other enzymes in the body. The nature of such postulated enzymes or other "highly labile reactivating factors" is unknown.

By using P-2-AM, MENGLE and O'BRIEN (1960) were able to show that fly head ChE *in vitro*, like ChE from vertebrate sources, passed from an initial stage of inhibition, during which P-2-AM was effective, into a condition in which regeneration by these means was no longer possible. The rate of "ageing" of the inhibited ChE was dependent on the nature of the alkoxy substituents of the inactivating agents, in the descending order: methyl-, ethyl-, *iso*-propyl-.

Inhibition of insect ChE's by carbamates is also competitive, but is usually readily reversible (v. CASIDA et al. 1960). According to the classification of esterases used in this chapter, AliE's are relatively insensitive to carbamates; ArE's are insensitive both to them and to organophosphorus compounds. Phenyl carbamates are said to cause initially a considerable increase in the titre of ChE measurable in the nervous system of cockroaches exposed to these agents (WALOP et al. 1956, MELTZER 1958). After a lapse of time, this activation turns into inhibition. These authors theorized that the carbamates act first by being adsorbed to protein and consequently expelling bound ChE, but there is no proof that this is the mechanism involved.

The rates of reaction of a given inhibitor with ChE's from different sources ordinarily differ to some extent, though there are many anti-ChE agents for which the rates of combination with various ChE's are quite similar. The general impression gained from the entomological literature is that insect enzymes on the whole are somewhat more susceptible to inhibitors than are the mammalian ChE's. This impression is perhaps biased by the fact that there has been a vigorous effort to produce anti-ChE agents with a toxicity differential favoring their use as insecticides, so that compounds that do not show such a differential tend to be dropped rather quickly from further investigation. That there are differences in sensitivity among various ChE's is clear, but the nature and degrees of these differences are not at present predictable. Certain striking distinctions of this sort among the ChE's of different insects have been noted, for example by METCALF and MARCH (1950), though they have been questioned by other workers (v. O'BRIEN 1960, for discussion). Comparative studies based on leads of this kind may well be fruitful in the development of insecticides for specific purposes, as well as in explaining the characteristics of the various enzymes and of the nature of the binding that takes place between enzyme and inhibitor.

1. Toxicity in relation to degree of inhibition

Many entomologists have taken for granted that a high degree of inhibition of ChE must be produced by an anti-ChE agent if the compound is to be effective in killing insects. This impression is *not* invariably correct. Observations by CHADWICK and HILL (1947), ROEDER (1948), METCALF and MARCH (1949), CHAMBERLAIN and HOSKINS (1951), CASIDA (1955), and by BENJAMINI et al. (1959), among others, have contributed to this viewpoint, even though many of these reports have included indications that there are important exceptions to such a generalization.

The fact that appreciably lower levels of ChE inhibition may be observed during the early symptoms of poisoning, and sometimes even at death, has been documented abundantly (HOPF 1952, O'BRIEN 1956b, HOPF and TAYLOR 1958, VAN ASPEREN 1958a, 1959b, 1959c, 1960a, 1960b, COLHOUN 1959a, STEGWEE 1959, 1960, POTTER 1960, MENGLE and O'BRIEN 1960, EDDY et al. 1960, PLAPP and BIGLEY 1961), so that one is compelled to recognize, whatever the inter-

pretation, that there is not any *essential* relationship between the average percentage of ChE-inhibition produced *in vivo* by anti-ChE agents and their insecticidal potency. Evidently differences in this respect exist between agents as well
as between insect species.

Moreover, as various students have realized, the available data are not
adequate for either the acceptance or definitive rejection of the basic hypothesis.
O'BRIEN (1956 b, p. 489) pinpointed the difficulty: "However, it is total ChE that
is being studied, and it is not impossible that a localized and important site of the
enzyme is following a different pattern of inhibition and recovery." This outlook
is strengthened by histochemical findings such as those of MOLLOY, summarized
by POTTER (1960), that ChE inhibition of Diazinon-poisoned flies occurred predominantly in the thoracico-abdominal nerve mass rather than in the cerebral
ganglia, as some might have anticipated. Similar conclusions had already been
reached on other grounds, for insects by VAN ASPEREN (1958a, 1959b, 1960) and
for mammalian tissues by KOELLE (1957; see Chapter 6).

We should emphasize that it is a *possibility* rather than a *certainty* to which
O'BRIEN (1956 b) and these other workers have directed our attention, and that
the essential guidance offered by the often conflicting and yet equally well-
authenticated observations is that the student of the mechanism of action of the
anti-ChE agents needs to look beyond the superficially apparent for the true and
fundamentally significant relationships.

In connection with this question as to how the level of ChE inhibition may
be connected with lethal effectiveness, one must reject the *general* validity of a
logically correct deduction made by MENGLE and O'BRIEN (1960) with regard to
Malathion (0,0-dimethyl S-(1,2-dicarbethoxyethyl) phosphorodithioate).

MENGLE and O'BRIEN observed that houseflies treated with an LD_{50} of Malathion soon experienced average ChE inhibition of 95% to 100%. But 24 hr later
the average inhibition of the entire population (dead and alive) was only 50%,
by which time the survivors were known (MENGLE and CASIDA 1958) to have
achieved essentially complete reactivation of ChE. Therefore, one reasons with
MENGLE and O'BRIEN, inhibition in the dead must have remained total; in other
words, the flies originally doomed to die had suffered complete inhibition and had
subsequently shown no recovery of enzymic ChE activity. One has difficulty in
finding a flaw in this argument; however, it cannot explain observations such as
those of VAN ASPEREN (1960a), that "knockdown" of flies with five other organophosphorus compounds occurred at times when the average ChE inhibition ranged
only from 27% to 51%, a type of result that has been obtained by numerous
other workers. Again we may only conclude that there is no readily apparent
overall correlation between the average degree of ChE inhibition, as we are able
to measure it, and the symptomatology seen in various insect species after treatment with different anti-ChE agents.

II. Aliesterases (AliE's) and aryl esterases (ArE's)

1. General

Accepting the well-established potency of anti-ChE agents as inhibitors of the
ACh-hydrolyzing enzymes of insects, we should next review the data that concern
the presence of AliE's and ArE's in these animals. The insect CNS evidently
contains esterases other than ChE's. Some of these enzymes, as well as similar
ones elsewhere in the body, are affected strongly by anti-ChE agents, and hence
might be of significance in the mode of intoxication. In support of this possibility,
attention has been called to the sometimes relatively poorer correlation between

the degree of inhibition of ChE's and the toxic effects; to the occurrence of toxicity at periods when ChE's are totally absent while certain of these other esterases are present; to the detoxication by ArE's of organophosphorus compounds, which may be treated by some ArE's as substrates; and to competition between AliE's, ArE's, and ChE's for the limited supply of an applied inhibitor.

Observations regarding AliE's and ArE's of insects, though numerous, are fragmentary; there exist no more than surmises as to their possible natural functions in these animals. Such esterases have been found in all insects in which they have been looked for, i.e., two or three dozen species, and apparantly occur in all developmental stages from the early embryo onwards. Evidently a fuller analysis of their normal rôles, and of their impact on the effects of anti-ChE agents, will require much further investigation. Furthermore, in the studies that have been made, distinctions between AliE's and ArE's often were not drawn or were based on criteria other than those arbitrarily adopted for this report. We shall not make an attempt here to review the part played by esterases in insect digestion, a topic which has been considered by Day and Waterhouse (1953) and by Gilmour (1961). For these several reasons, our account of AliE's and ArE's must remain incomplete; we shall indicate only something of the nature of such enzymes, and mention the sources of information that concern them, particularly in their presumed or actual relations to the poisoning of insects by anti-ChE agents.

Extracts that hydrolyzed ethyl butyrate and o-nitrophenyl acetate, but not ACh, and which were inhibited by TEPP, were prepared from eggs, larvae, or adults of 7 species of insects by Lord and Potter (1950, 1951). The enzyme(s) that hydrolyzed o-nitrophenyl acetate occurred in eggs of Diataraxia and Ephestia less than 24 hr old, as well as in older eggs; TEPP or Parathion killed these young eggs before the nervous system had differentiated and also inhibited the AliE's at a time when no ChE was present. That inhibition of these AliE's might constitute a significant feature of poisoning by anti-ChE agents was suggested.

The same authors (1953) extended their observations to 4 additional species of insect, all of which were found to contain a TEPP-inhibitable AliE. It was shown that all preparations of these various species that would hydrolyze ACh would also hydrolyze o-nitrophenyl acetate (1954a); but extracts could be made from them that would hydrolyze only the aryl compound.

The presence here of at least two enzymes was thus apparent. These were designated as a ChE and a "general esterase." In comparative tests with 4 insect species and 4 organophosphorus inhibitors, Lord and Potter (1954b) found that their "general esterase" was inhibited at lower concentrations of the anti-ChE agent in 10 cases, while ChE was the more readily inhibited only in 4. In 2 cases, both enzymes were about equally susceptible. The "general esterase" occurred in eggs of Diataraxia throughout their development, whereas ChE appeared only after 5.5 days of incubation.

According to Hopf (1952), enzymes in the nerve cord of Locusta hydrolyzed o-nitrophenyl acetate and ACh, and the hydrolysis of both substrates was inhibited about equally by TEPP. Four other non-polar organophosphorus compounds were tested, with similar results. There was little if any hydrolysis of ethyl butyrate by these enzymes. Correlation between toxicity and inhibition of ChE by the agents was poor. This fact suggested to Hopf that some other toxic effect was involved in their insecticidal action.

Another phenyl esterase was identified in Locusta ganglia by Hopf and Taylor (1958). This enzyme was poorly inhibited by ethoxy ethylphosphophenylthioethyl triethylammonium iodide, an effective inhibitor of ChE, and perhaps should be designated an ArE. The behavior of some locusts, the CNS ChE of which, but not this ArE, was completely inhibited after they were treated with this anti-ChE agent, appeared to remain normal. Though the compound was said to penetrate the nerve sheath with difficulty, some was found to do so, and to inactivate the ChE entirely, both in locusts that became prostrated and in others that seemed un-affected. Precautions taken by the investigators indicate that during the prep-aration of samples for analysis there was no transfer of excess inhibitor to previously uninhibited ChE. The implication of these observations, which is at variance with the usual concept of the mode of action of organophosphorus com-pounds, is then that normal behavior in insects is possible in the face of complete inhibition of the ChE of the CNS.

CASIDA (1955) studied the hydrolytic action of acetylesterases from a variety of species and stages of insects with various substrates, substrate mixtures, and several inhibitors. As indicated in the quotation from CASIDA (1954) on p. 744, these important results do not fall into a simple pattern, but it seems certain that among the enzymes CASIDA investigated were some that would be classified here as AliE's.

2. Aryl esterases (ArE's)

Although somewhat less study has been devoted to ArE's than to AliE's in insects, METCALF et al. (1956) made a thorough investigation of an aryl esterase found in large amounts in bees; this ArE, which was not inhibited by Paraoxon or neostigmine at 10^{-3} M, hydrolyzed approximately 20 aromatic esters at rela-tively rapid rates. With phenyl acetate as substrate, K_s was determined as 4.36×10^{-3} and V_{max} as 1.39. The titre of this ArE was highest in the bee abdomen, and lowest in the head, in which ChE and AliE predominated. METCALF et al. also found that fly heads and cockroach nerve cords contained largely ChE, some AliE, and no ArE. These results were corroborated histochemically by WINTON et al. (1958). The ArE of bees obviously is not of importance as a target of organo-phosphorus compounds, but was considered to have some significance in their detoxication.

O'BRIEN (1957b) concluded that the cockroach nerve cord *in situ* contained a phenyl acetate-hydrolyzing esterase that was inhibited only 50% by TEPP, 10^{-4} M. Since METCALF et al. (1956) had already shown that this tissue contains only a ChE and an AliE, both of which were organophosphorus sensitive, it is probable that the locus of O'BRIEN's TEPP-insensitive enzyme was actually in the body, outside the nerve cord, and that the TEPP-inhibited hydrolysis he observed was due to the ChE and AliE that were present in the cord. If so, it would not then follow, as O'BRIEN believed, that the ArE had been inhibited 50% by the TEPP; possibly it was not inhibited by TEPP at all at the concentra-tion tested, and hence was even less likely to have played a part in TEPP-intoxica-tion than O'BRIEN decided.

It is possible that some of the esterases found in *Rhodnius* by WIGGLESWORTH (1958, 1959a, 1959b), that did not hydrolyze acetylthiocholine, were ArE's.

3. Distribution and development in insect eggs

SMITH and WAGENKNECHT (1956) noted the presence of a Parathion-resistant esterase in the eggs of *Lepidoptera*. Although they did not test this enzyme with carbamate inhibitors, it is conceivable that it was insensitive to them also and hence should be classified as an ArE. However, doubt is cast on this conjecture by later analyses by SALKELD (1960, 1961) of the development and distribution of esterases in eggs of *Oncopeltus*. Of the various organophosphate-insensitive esterases she found in these embryos, one is concentrated in the neuropile and appears to be the forerunner of the ChE of the nymphs, although it is not inhibited by such agents as DFP or *iso*-octamethylpyrophosphoramide until after hatching.

With *Pieris*, POTTER et al. (1957) found that all stages of the eggs of this cabbage-butterfly would hydrolyze *o*-nitrophenyl acetate, but that there was no ability to hydrolyze ACh until the eggs were 5 or more days old. Nevertheless, high doses of TEPP applied at early stages stopped development promptly. With lower doses, development proceeded to completion, yet many of the embryos failed to hatch.

Earlier findings of POTTER and coworkers with respect to esterases in insect eggs have been mentioned in the passages above.

From more recent work of SOLLY, POTTER (1960) has reported evidence for the presence of at least 3 esterases in eggs of *Pieris* aged 0 to 12 hr, while results with purified breis of 5-day-old eggs were best explained by assuming there are in them no less than 5 distinct esterases. These conclusions are based on the rates of hydrolysis, after electrophoretic fractionation of purified bries, of the phenyl esters of acetic, propionic, butyric, and caproic acids, and on the differing degrees of their inhibition by Paraoxon and by eserine. The experiments were facilitated by an improved procedure for removing a naturally occurring inhibitor from the breis, which could then be freeze-dried without loss of esteratic activity.

A portion of the enzyme from the younger eggs that hydrolyzed phenyl acetate (PhAc) does not fit into the classification of esterases employed here, because it was inhibited by eserine, 10^{-4} M, but was insensitive to Paraoxon, 10^{-4} M. The rest of the hydrolysis of PhAc was interfered with by both types of inhibitor, so that the enzyme concerned in it could be designated a ChE except for the earlier report (POTTER et al. 1957) that there was almost no hydrolysis of ACh by *Pieris* eggs at this stage. Possibly the previous results had been affected by the presence of an endogenous inhibitor, while in the later experiments ACh apparently was not tested. Or, we may be confronted with complications such as those mentioned above in the accounts of the work of SMITH and WAGNEKNECHT and of SALKELD. At any rate, this portion of SOLLY's data indicates the presence of at least two enzymes.

Additionally, not less than two other enzymes from these eggs seem to have been involved in the studies with phenyl propionate (PhPr), since here Paraoxon gave only partial inhibition of hydrolysis. Inasmuch as neither of these enzymes was sensitive to eserine, one of them may have been an AliE and the other an ArE; but neither could be identical with either of the PhAc-hydrolyzing enzymes, both of which were eserine-sensitive.

With these breis, the entire hydrolysis of phenyl butyrate and phenyl caproate was sensitive to Paraoxon and insensitive to eserine, so that on such a basis this activity could be ascribed to the same AliE that split PhPr.

Summarizing the present analysis of these observations, a minimum of 4 esterases must have been present in *Pieris* eggs at the 0 to 12 hr stage, rather than only the 3 reported by POTTER (1960). His progress report does not give similarly detailed information about the 5-day-old eggs. Our recapitulation of the results of these experiments of limited scope illustrates the manifold complications attendant on any effort to analyze and classify the types of esteratic activity met with in insect material.

4. Houseflies

Considerable study has been made of esterases other than ChE in houseflies; a fair proportion of this work, to which we shall presently give separate attention, is concerned also with the problem of organophosphorus resistance in these insects.

An AliE in *Musca* was investigated by VAN ASPEREN (1957, 1958a). It was present mainly in the thorax. This enzyme, for which methyl butyrate was used as substrate, was inhibited by DDVP (0,0-dimethyl 0—2,2-dichloro-vinyl phosphate), DFP, Parathion, or Paraoxon. The presence of methyl butyrate protected the enzyme against inhibition by DDVP. At the time when the flies were first knocked down by DDVP-poisoning, ChE was inhibited only 27% to 46%, but their AliE was inhibited 83%. More extensive data in support of this observation were accumlated later (VAN ASPEREN 1959c, 1960a, 1960b). The I_{50} (DDVP) for housefly head ChE was 1.5×10^{-7} M (VAN ASPEREN 1958b). VAN ASPEREN judged that some effect of the anti-ChE agent other than ChE inhibition was important in intoxication; possibly, he suggested, this was inhibition of AliE.

VAN ASPEREN and OPPENOORTH (1959) then showed that the AliE of houseflies was not inhibited by eserine, 10^{-5} M, although housefly ChE was. Unlike the ChE, this AliE was extremely sensitive to heating in slightly alkaline media, and was inactivated as much as 85% in 1 hr at 37°, pH 8.3. The temperature coefficient of inactivation was large, suggesting a denaturation. Cholinesterase in the housefly was characterized by the ability to split esters of choline and of acetic acid; in contrast, the AliE hydrolyzed esters of acetic and butyric acids, but not choline esters (VAN ASPEREN 1959a).

Comparative tests with Paraoxon led to the conclusion that at least 2 separate AliE's were present, one Paraoxon-sensitive and the other inhibited only by high concentrations of this substance. On the basis of substrate activities also, there appeared to be 2 or more AliE's. VAN ASPEREN and OPPENOORTH emphasized that the enzymes that could be differentiated thus by their substrate specificity should not automatically be regarded as identical with those distinguished by their relative sensitivity to Paraoxon; they suspected that there may be several distinct AliE's in these insects. Under the criteria adopted for this discussion, the Paraoxon-insensitive esterase found by VAN ASPEREN and OPPENOORTH is not an AliE, but can be considered an ArE.

In a further study, VAN ASPEREN (1959a) concluded that *Musca* contains a ChE, an AliE (probably actually more than one such enzyme), and likely an ArE. Thirteen substrates and three inhibitors were used in the attempt to characterize these enzymes. The ChE, with 68% of its activity in the head, 27% in the thorax, and 5% in the abdomen, was evidently associated for the most part with the nervous tissue. In contrast, the head had only about 21% of the activity of the combined AliE and ArE fractions, the thorax 39%, and the abdomen 40%; clearly, a considerable part of these enzymes was elsewhere than in the nervous system.

Work of STEGWEE (1959, 1960) on the housefly is especially useful for comparison with the results obtained by others with the same species. STEGWEE found in *Musca* a ChE, an AliE which he considered identical with VAN ASPEREN's (Paraoxon-sensitive) AliE, and an ArE. The AliE was not inhibited *in vitro* by eserine, 10^{-5} M, but both it and housefly ChE were inhibited by TEPP, 10^{-6} M. Acetylcholine was hydrolyzed by the ChE only, and ethyl butyrate only by the AliE; both utilized phenyl acetate and tributyrin. The substrate optimum for ethyl butyrate with the AliE was 1.7×10^{-2} M. Substrate optima have not been reported previously for such esterases. The AliE split also methyl butyrate and triacetin. STEGWEE's AliE, like VAN ASPEREN's, is evidently situated largely outside the CNS, for although 91% of the thoracic ChE was found in the ganglion, only 4% of the AliE was there. Also present was a TEPP-insensitive esterase (an ArE), which would hydrolyze triacetin or phenyl acetate. Its general distribution was similar to that of the AliE.

The partition of these three enzymes in the main regions of the body was as given in Table 2.

This relative distribution of the enzymes makes it very unlikely that inhibition of AliE's has a direct part in the nervous dysfunction associated with intoxication by anti-ChE agents. One may note that BIGLEY and PLAPP (1960) found only ChE in housefly heads, but AliE in the remainder of the body.

Decisive as to possible further rôles of AliE's in the poisoning of *Musca* by anti-ChE agents is STEGWEE's (1960) additional evidence that housefly AliE could be inhibited completely by topical applications of 100 μg of tri-*ortho*-cresyl-phosphate (TOCP), without affecting their ChE and also without causing any toxic signs. Nevertheless, the ChE of these flies could still be inhibited in the usual manner by later dosage with TEPP. The flies so treated became paralyzed more slowly, however, than those that received only TEPP; furthermore, unexplained changes in their ACh content took place. After treatment with TOCP, the amount of ACh recoverable from them was reduced to 90% of the value normal for untreated flies, and then rose only to the normal level when the usually lethal dose of TEPP was given. Only 77% of these flies died, as against 96% of those that received TEPP alone.

Table 2. *Per cent of esteratic activity in the body regions of the housefly* (after STEGWEE 1960)

Enzyme type	Head	Thorax	Abdomen
ChE	64	23	13
AliE	16	33	51
ArE	20	32	48

These observations demonstrate clearly that inhibition of AliE alone cannot be a significant feature of organophosphorus poisoning in adult flies; this means that those who are not satisfied that inhibition of ChE is the primary step in such intoxication must search for yet another possible mechanism. Moreover, STEGWEE's data contain a suggestion that accumulation of ACh may be important in such poisoning, although it is hard to interpret the fact the rise in ACh in doubly-treated flies brought this ester only to the level normal for wholly untreated specimens. As O'BRIEN (1956 b) had done, STEGWEE took refuge in the surmise that overall measurements of ChE and ACh, which are all that could be made, may not reflect the true concentrations of these materials at significant loci, and properly proposed to attempt observations of greater refinement. This statement, of course, is more an excuse than an explanation.

5. Resistance to organophosphorus compounds

The basis of insect resistance to organophosphorus chemicals is a burning question, with which many investigators continue to concern themselves. The problem has been most prominent in, although not confined exclusively to, houseflies.

The possible rôle of "general esterase" (LORD and POTTER) in organophosphate resistance in houseflies was examined by LORD and SOLLY (1956), with results that, like those of less detailed experiments with the same strain reported by CHADWICK (1954), failed to provide any explanation of the physiological nature of the resistance. LORD and SOLLY found that ACh, triacetin, and tributyrin, respectively, were hydrolyzed by resistant flies at the same rates as by normally susceptible flies. Although the resistant flies were about twice as tolerant of Paraoxon as normals (and more tolerant of some other anti-ChE's; CHADWICK 1954), extracts of heads, thoraces, and abdomens, presumably containing the A-esterase of ALDRIDGE (1953), caused no breakdown of Paraoxon *in vitro*. *In vivo*, the concentration of Paraoxon dropped rapidly and to an equal extent in both strains, which evidently possessed efficient mechanisms of detoxication or excretion or both.

Unfortunately, a thorough analysis of the physiological basis of organophosphorus resistance in different strains of *Drosophila* by RASMUSON and HOLMSTEDT (1958) also did not uncover a definite cause for the phenomenon. Additional data on this problem, and a discussion of it, have been added by MENGLE and CASIDA (1960), and many other authors have suggested factors that might be concerned, but, speaking physiologically, the subject is still a mystery. Perspective may nevertheless be gained by a brief review of some of the data.

A most interesting observation is that of VAN ASPEREN and OPPENOORTH (1959). These workers found that AliE activity was 2 to 6 times lower in 5 organophosphorus-resistant strains of houseflies than in 6 normally susceptible strains, with either tributyrin, phenyl acetate, phenyl propionate, ethyl butyrate, or methyl butyrate as substrate. With amyl acetate or triacetin, AliE activity was about equal in both types of flies, and so was their ChE activity. The decreased hydrolysis of methyl butyrate by resistant flies did not depend on any change in the affinity of their AliE for the substrate, nor was there any evidence for the presence of either enhancing or inhibitory materials in either type of strain. Evidently the resistant flies simply had less than the usual quota of AliE, as others (e.g., BIGLEY and PLAPP 1960, PLAPP and BIGLEY 1961) have in part confirmed.

VAN ASPEREN and OPPENOORTH (1959) found that an ArE accounted for 34% of the hydrolysis of methyl butyrate in organophosphorus-resistant flies, but for only 4% in susceptible flies. Since the total activity of AliE plus ArE in the resistant flies was only about one-fifth of that in the susceptible strains, it follows that a considerable reduction in Paraoxon-sensitive AliE was associated with the resistance.

EDDY et al. (1960) reported that resistant and susceptible houseflies resembled one another at all stages of post-embryonic growth with respect to the changing levels of ChE content, but that AliE activity was lower in larvae and pupae of resistant flies as well as in adults. Highest AliE activity was reached in 3-day-old larvae and early in the pupal stage. Although larvae and adults of a Parathion-resistant strain were from 3 to 13 times less susceptible than normals, resistant pupae were at least 100 times less susceptible.

A plausible explanation of the low AliE activity of resistant housefly strains has been put forward (OPPENOORTH 1959b, VAN ASPEREN and OPPENOORTH 1960, OPPENOORTH and VAN ASPEREN 1960), and bolstered with experimental data. The presumption adopted is that, via a series of mutants of a single gene which is responsible for the elaboration of the AliE in normal flies, a related group of "phosphatases" is produced instead. These "phosphatases" differ only by a slight change in the constitution of their protein from the normal AliE, which they replace; but unlike it they are active in the degradation of organophosphorus compounds, and thereby confer a degree of resistance on their possessors. This proposal fits with the genetic data of OPPENOORTH (1959b) and of NGUY and BUSVINE (1960), according to which a single series of alleles is primarily responsible for resistance in most organophosphate-resistant strains of houseflies.

This theory evidently agrees with the conclusion reached as a result of the studies of STEGWEE (1959, 1960), that inhibition of AliE is not *per se* a significant feature of organophosphorus poisoning; but some investigators question whether the mechanism of resistance postulated by OPPENOORTH and VAN ASPEREN is as yet sufficiently supported, and whether it is adequate to account for the varying degrees and, in some instances, large amounts of organophosphorus-resistance displayed by certain strains of houseflies. The situation has been evaluated by MENGLE and CASIDA (1960) (see also PLAPP and BIGLEY 1961). In reference to it, one may note that OPPENOORTH (1959b) and OPPENOORTH and VAN ASPEREN (1960) have themselves called attention to at least one resistant strain of housefly in which additional physiological factors apparently are involved. A valuable discussion of enzymic changes in relation to insecticide susceptibility is given by GORDON (1961).

6. General comment on AliE's and ArE's

Insects clearly contain numerous esterases other than ChE's. Those enzymes that are readily inhibited by organophosphorus compounds but not by carbamates we have designated here as AliE's, and those insensitive to either type of inhibitor, as ArE's. In general, these enzymes are inactive toward ACh and other choline esters, although exceptions have been reported. The normal functions of AliE's and ArE's are unknown; actually the same is true even of insect ChE's, the natural substrate of which, on quite reasonable but yet still circumstantial evidence, has widely been assumed rather than proven to be ACh.

Aliesterases and ArE's, unlike ChE, are distributed in the insect body largely outside the nervous system. Although AliE's are readily inhibited by organophosphorus insecticides, apparently they are not involved directly in the lethal action of these materials, at least not in post-embryonic stages. AliE's are present in insect embryos before the advent of ChE; the latter enzyme, therefore, cannot be held responsible for the lethality of anti-ChE agents to such early developmental stages; but, although the AliE's may then be inhibited, there is no other indication that they in turn may be responsible for the toxic effects. Complete inhibition of AliE's in adult houseflies does not seem to produce abnormal behavior.

Being equally or more sensitive than ChE to many organophosphorus agents, the AliE's may to some extent afford competitive protection against these anti-ChE agents. In many strains of resistant houseflies, AliE's apparently are replaced in part by ArE's. Inasmuch as organophosphorus compounds may serve as substrates for some ArE's, the latter may then reduce the concentrations of the anti-ChE agents by degrading them more rapidly than normal, but the quantitative aspects of this situation do not at present account satisfactorily for the degrees of resistance that have been found. Nor has any other adequate explanation of organophosphorus resistance been brought forward, although intensive investigation has ruled out several other theoretical possibilities.

B. Miscellaneous effects

In evaluating the mode of action of anti-ChE agents, all their known physiological effects must be considered if the issue is not to be prejudged in favor of those mechanisms that happen to be the most conspicuous or which, for various reasons, may have been investigated most intensively. A number of the observations now to be reviewed seem more or less random and may prove to be unrelated to our main topic, but nevertheless deserve attention at this stage of our incomplete understanding of the subject. A separate section is reserved for discussion of the more numerous data that have to do with the actions of these agents on nervous function.

I. Reactions during embryonic development

When insect eggs are poisoned with moderate doses of organophosphorus compounds, embryonic development proceeds normally, irrespective of the stage at treatment, until the usual time for hatching (SCHWARZ 1950, SPEYER 1950, SMITH and AVENS 1954, SMITH and WAGENKNECHT 1956, POTTER et al. 1957, MEHROTRA and SMALLMAN 1957, MEHROTRA 1960b). Many of the apparently fully developed embryos then fail to emerge, or succumb during the process, and many of those that succeed in hatching die soon afterwards. Evidence has been obtained in support of the interpretation that these effects result from a delayed inhibition of ChE, which at the time of treatment is not yet vitally concerned with function or may even be absent (SMITH and WAGENKNECHT 1959). Death is not due merely to retention of anti-ChE agent by the chorion and embryonic membranes, which are ingested by the hatching larva (MOLLOY, in POTTER 1960).

In eggs thus poisoned with Parathion, oxygen-uptake follows the ordinary pattern of increase until a day or two before hatching. Thereupon an abnormal decline sets in and progresses, in the case of unhatched eggs, until death; this follows a few days after the usual time for emergence (STAUDENMAYER 1953, SMITH 1955). The respiratory decrease can be ascribed to a reduction in body activity, consequent upon inhibition of nervous system ChE, although there is no proof that this is the causal connection. With Paraoxon, however, a somewhat different pattern has been seen (STAUDENMAYER 1955). Here the decline in O_2-consumption begins, with *Bombyx*, 7 days before hatching; i.e., 2 days before any ChE activity is detectable. From these observations it is logical to conclude, with STAUDENMAYER, that Paraoxon has been shown to have toxic effects beyond those associated with the inhibition of ChE. It is not clear why there should be a difference of this kind noted in the mode of action of Parathion and Paraoxon, since Parathion is thought to act via its conversion to the actively inhibitory Paraoxon (METCALF and MARCH 1953).

Actions of some of the anti-ChE agents other than ChE-inhibition are likewise obvious in other instances. Thus, in certain of the experiments of HOLZ (1949), embryonic development appears to have been halted early by Parathion, probably before the appearance of ChE; this was so in eggs of silkworms, aphids, and psyllids, and sometimes with eggs of red spider mites, though not with walking-stick insects or with a geometrid moth.

Incidentally, BABERS (1958) stated that he and PRATT, in unpublished experiments, had been unable to demonstrate any ChE in either Parathion-resistant or -susceptible *Tetranychus bimaculatus* Harvey. However, CASIDA (1954, 1955) had already reported the presence of "nonspecific" esterases in *Acarus siro* L.; VOSS (1959) has since found ChE in *Tetranychus urticae* Koch, and McENROE (1960) has documented the occurrence of ChE in the nervous system of *Tetranychus telarius* L., while MEHROTRA (1961a, 1961c) has also shown the presence of ACh and ChAc in this last species, so that there is no basis here for denying to the acarinids generally a possible rôle of ChE-inhibition in the mode of action of anti-ChE agents on them.

In experiments of MEHROTRA (1960b) with Parathion-treatment of developing eggs of *Musca* and *Oncopeltus*, the ChE was inhibited and the accumulation of ACh was greater than in controls, findings consistent with the hypothesis that excess ACh, resulting from a failure of the normal process of destruction, was the actual lethal agent. However, it must be emphasized that such data, indicative though they may be, cannot suffice to prove this hypothesis beyond doubt; they are not even pertinent to some of the actions that have been reported for anti-ChE agents.

Thus, for instance, SCHWARZ (1950) found that doses of Parathion somewhat in excess of those required to kill the eggs interfered with development in *Leptinotarsa*, or even stopped it altogether; SPEYER (1950) likewise noted a delay in the embryogenesis of *Agelastica*. Parathion or TEPP killed eggs of *Diataraxia* or *Ephestia* at an early stage when no ChE was present (LORD and POTTER 1951). The eggs of *Pieris* reacted similarly to high doses of TEPP applied early, but proceeded to the point of hatching when lower doses were used (POTTER et al.

1957). The significance of such observations has sometimes been questioned on the ground that relatively large doses of the toxicant may have been required to produce effects that seemed unrelated to ChE-inhibition. However, granting that a lethal result of smaller doses may have more practical interest in some circumstances, we are still too uncertain of the toxic mechanism of action of the anti-ChE agents in any situation to overlook any physiological effect of which they may be capable. Moreover, whatever the mechanism of interest, the concentration of the poison at the site of toxic action is unknown. In fact, the differing sensitivity of the eggs of different insect species toward anti-ChE agents appears to be a complicated matter that is far from having been fully explained (O'BRIEN and SMITH 1961).

The actions of anti-ChE agents during embryological development in insects and other species are discussed in Chapter 17.

II. Respiration of adult insects

Increases in the respiratory exchange of adult insects treated with anti-ChE agents have been noted by several investigators. LORD (1950) showed that dusts containing Parathion or HETP (so-called "hexaethyltetraphosphate," the active ingredient of which is TEPP) increased the O_2-consumption of *Tenebrio* markedly, while HARVEY and BROWN (1951) found that injections of Parathion or TEPP stimulated respiration in *Blattella*. With TEPP, the effect on this cockroach was immediate, but that with Parathion was delayed, possibly while this compound was being converted *in vivo* to Paraoxon. Respiratory increases of this sort are a logical consequence of heightened bodily activity induced by the neurotoxic action of the anti-ChE agents, although the fact that respiration often remains abnormally high long after prostration and apparent quiescence, as noted for example by WINTERINGHAM and HARRISON (1956) with DFP-poisoned houseflies, is harder to account for on such a basis. Also a respiratory increase does not invariably occur in organophosphorus poisoning; O'BRIEN (1956b) reported no enhancement of respiration in the Malathion-poisoned cockroach. GOSTICK (1961) found that after dosage with Malathion, there was increased oxygen uptake in the mealworm beetle, *Alphitobius*, only in individuals that were prostrated, and that these always died.

The further possibility, that organophosphates might have some more specific effect on the respiratory enzymic chain, was examined in *Periplaneta* by MORRISON and BROWN (1954). They found that TEPP, Parathion, Schradan (OMPA, octamethyl-pyrophosphortetramide), and Malathion all increased the activity of the cytochrome oxidase system *in vitro* at 10^{-5} M, the effect being most marked with TEPP and Malathion, and transitory with Parathion. At 10^{-3} M, TEPP was significantly activating and Schradan slightly so, while Parathion and Malathion caused complete inhibition at 20 and 40 min, respectively. The authors offered no explanation of these results, nor is the reviewer prepared to do so except to say that their bearing on the significant mode of toxic action of the agents is doubtful. When BROWN and BROWN (1956) investigated this matter in the living cockroach, they found that the effect on the level of cytochrome oxidase of injected Parathion or Malathion was very slight. O'BRIEN (1956b, 1957a) similarly showed that Malathion is not a potent inhibitor of the enzymes of carbohydrate metabolism in the cockroach and housefly, and that the toxic effect of Malathion on these insects cannot be ascribed to its interference with the tricarboxylic acid cycle. McALLAN and BROWN (1960) found no depression of glutamate-aspartate transamination in homogenates of the fat body from cockroaches killed with Malathion.

WINTERINGHAM and associates (WINTERINGHAM and HARRISON 1956, WIN-
TERINGHAM et al. 1957, WINTERINGHAM 1957, 1958, WINTERINGHAM and LEWIS
1959) observed that exposures of houseflies to lethal doses of DFP produced not
only increased respiration but also a delayed though sustained accumulation of
glutamine, which they regarded as suggestive of interference with amino acid
metabolism, if it were not merely a consequence of the more active respiration.
To the reviewer it seems that there are so many possible sources of an increase
in glutamine that this observation, though of interest, can give little indication
of what biochemical systems have been deranged. The authors cited observed no
significant effect of DFP on the phosphorus metabolism of the insect; that is to
say, no changes were measurable in the quantities of the phosphorus-containing
ingredients in their extracts. On the basis of these various findings, taken together
with the inefficacy of P-2-AM and atropine in therapy with this species, the
workers concluded that DFP might possibly be causing other fatal biochemical
lesions in addition to ChE inhibition. Their suggestion that inhibition of ChE by
DFP may depress ACh synthesis *in vivo* has already been mentioned (p. 764).

According to WIESMANN and KOCHER (1951), treatment of houseflies with the
carbamate, Pyrolan (1-phenyl-3-methyl-pyrazolyl-(5)-dimethyl carbamate), had
several actions in addition to the inhibition of ChE. They observed increases both
in respiratory rate and in rate of water loss. Carbon dioxide-production rose about
400% in 5 min. In *Periplaneta* the pH of the blood fell from about 6.9—7.0 to 6.3,
and that of muscle from about 6.7—6.8 to 6.1. WIESMANN and KOCHER attributed
these changes in acidity to excess production of lactic acid, as a consequence of
the muscle spasms induced by the poison. Although a general explanation in terms
of the release of acid metabolites may be correct, there is some question as to
whether lactic acid *per se* is formed in sufficient amounts by insect muscle to
produce acidosis (v. BOETTIGER 1960). In any event, it seems possible that most
of the effects cited by WIESMANN and KOCHER were secondary to ChE inhibition.

III. Heart and blood

Acetylcholine and anti-ChE agents have often been found to affect the functioning of the heart in various invertebrates. In addition to earlier reviews, there
have been those of KRIJGSMAN (1952) on arthropods, of KRIJGSMAN and DIVARIS
(1955) on molluscs, of BEARD (1953) and of JONES (1956) on insects, and of
MAYNARD (1960) on *Crustacea*.

Many of the studies with insects have produced results similar to those of
DAVENPORT (1949), who showed that ACh accelerated the rate of heartbeat of
the orthopteron, *Stenopelmatus*, and caused transitory tetany at high concentrations. Thus, KRIJGSMAN and KRIJGSMAN (1950) found that ACh and anti-ChE
agents are accelerators of the isolated heart of *Periplaneta*; but ORSER and BROWN
(1951) succeeded with injected Parathion in causing only a very small change in
the rate of heartbeat of this species. The effects of ACh on the heart of *Stenopelmatus* that had been reported by DAVENPORT were corroborated, however, by
METCALF et al. (1955). Also, they observed similar phenomena in *Periplaneta*,
and found that pretreatment with eserine or TEPP sensitized the preparations
to ACh.

Such observations as those cited are for the most part consistent with the view
that the hearts in question are under a cholinergic system of control.

Nevertheless, one fact that emerges from a consideration of all the observations
on the hearts of invertebrates is that to speak simply of "the invertebrate heart"
in comparison or contrast with the vertebrate heart is an oversimplification. In

the reviews of KRIJGSMAN (1952) and of KRIJGSMAN and DIVARIS (1955) the conclusions reached, stated in the simplest terms, were that the arthropod heart is neurogenic and the molluscan heart, myogenic; yet a more recent analysis of the structure, physiology, and pharmacology of the insect heart alone by JONES (1956) indicates that functionally there are at least three types of heart in this one class: neurogenic, innervated myogenic, and non-innervated myogenic. With the crustacean, *Daphnia*, BEKKER and KRIJGSMAN (1951) had already obtained evidence that this animal has a myogenic heart, while BEARD (1953) concluded from his extensive survey of the data on insect hearts that there was at that date no agreement as to the neurogenic or myogenic origin of the heartbeat in this group. NEEDHAM (1954) is sometimes cited as authority for the presence of a cholinergic mechanism in the heart of the crustacean, *Asellus*, but his statement (p. 272) is: "Acetylcholine accelerated in relatively high concentration. Adrenalin had no consistent effect." MAYNARD (1955) found that ACh excited the cardiac ganglion of *Homarus* and *Panulirus*; in his review (1960) he concluded that cladoceran and anostracan hearts are probably myogenic, and the hearts of all other crustaceans examined probably neurogenic.

Apparently, the hearts of molluscs also encompass a wide range of responses to cholinomimetic agents. PILGRIM (1954), in an experimental survey of about 10 species of lamellibranchs, found that seeming discrepancies in the results of earlier workers actually represented points obtained with different species in a graded series of reactions. PILGRIM decided that the evidence available to him was not sufficient to permit postulating cholinergic transmission at the ventricle of these animals; certain observations suggested an action of ACh primarily on the contractile elements themselves, though the pacemaker might also be affected. Of especial interest here is the fact that the heart of *Venus*, a well-known object for the estimation of low concentrations of ACh, is very insensitive to such anti-ChE agents as physostigmine, neostigmine, and DFP (TOWER and McEACHERN 1948).

The central point in the various complexities that have come to light is not that cholinergic mechanisms of cardiac regulation do not exist among some of these species, for they do, but rather that among the invertebrates there are hearts that physiologically and pharmacologically are of several different kinds. Some invertebrate hearts are not obviously subject to ACh or to ChE inhibitors, while with others we do not know enough as yet about these matters to predict with confidence the nature, in any one group, of the reactions to anti-ChE agents of any hitherto uninvestigated species. Studies with such materials constitute one of our strongest weapons in the effort to understand the varied physiology of the different invertebrate hearts, but until we have attained a fuller comprehension of the subject we must avoid the temptation to overgeneralize.

There is at present little indication that insects are dependent for continued life on the integrity of the heart and circulation, so that if these functions are disrupted by anti-ChE agents (and there is evidence that they sometimes may be), such interference seems unlikely to be of first-line importance in the lethal effects of these chemicals.

IV. Body wall and intestine

Apparently, the excitatory system of the *anterior retractor byssus* muscle of the lamellibranch mollusc, *Mytilus*, is cholinergic (TWAROG 1954). This muscle contains both ACh and ChE, as well as 5-hydroxytryptamine. Acetylcholine at concentrations of 10^{-6} M or more caused depolarization and tonic contraction; the effects were potentiated by eserine and blocked by certain agents antagonistic to ACh. Relaxation of the tonic contractions that were produced by ACh or by electrical or mechanical stimulation was prevented by 5-hydroxytryptamine at concentrations of 10^{-9} M and above. Acetylcholine, 10^{-7} or greater, caused contraction of this muscle, plus the electrical activity characteristic of excitation (HOYLE and LOWY 1956).

Rather similar observations have been made with annelids. NICHOL (1952), working with the sabellid worm, *Branchiomma*, found that eserine or DFP augmented the previously known effect of ACh in causing contraction of the body wall. Likewise, the muscle response of the sipunculid, *Phascolosoma*, was enhanced by physostigmine, and PROSSER and MELTON (1954) concluded therefore that not only the nerves that elicit graded all-or-none muscle potentials but also those that elicit end-plate potentials were probably cholinergic.

In the sea-cucumber, *Thyone*, also, PROSSER (1954b) felt that the innervation may be cholinergic, since the response to electric shocks was much greater after the muscle had been soaked in 10^{-7} M to 10^{-8} M eserine, while responsiveness was lost with concentrations of 10^{-6} M or higher.

In complete contrast with such data from other invertebrate phyla, it has been noticed often that ACh and anti-ChE agents are usually without effect on the somatic muscles of insects (e.g., HARLOW 1958), but apparently observations of this nature do not extend to the intestinal musculature of these animals. Here, for instance, KOOISTRA (1950) showed that ACh and acetyl-β-methyl choline (methacholine) at concentrations of the order of 10^{-6} M improved weak intestinal contractions of *Periplaneta*, and that contraction was increased by eserine, 3.5×10^{-5} M. With HETP, optimal contraction was obtained at 10^{-7} M; higher doses caused paralysis. Similar results were obtained with Parathion.

More pronounced effects of this nature had been observed by MOONEY and OBRESHKOVE (1948) with another arthropod, the cladoceran, *Simocephalus*. In this crustacean, vigorous intestinal contractions were produced by neostigmine, ACh, carbaminoylcholine, and acetyl-β-methylcholine. Atropine blocked the action of these agents, but neostigmine was synergistic with the effect of ACh.

The somatic muscles of crustaceans, like those of insects, have ordinarily been reported as refractory to cholinomimetic materials (v. WIERSMA 1961a). It is therefore of particular interest that MAYNARD and MAYNARD (1960) found ChE in the muscle receptor organs of *Homarus*. The enzyme, identified histochemically, occurred in the sensory neurones and in motor and accessory fibers, but was most concentrated in the semitendinous region of the fast-adapting muscle receptor organs. Somewhat less ChE was found in those receptors that had been shown physiologically to be slow-adapting. Since muscle receptors, apparently of the same general kind, have been demonstrated in insects by FINLAYSON and LOWENSTEIN (1955, 1958), the possibility that they may have a similar pharmacology, if a somewhat unexpected one, should be considered.

In spite of the general insensitivity of crustacean muscle to ACh, injections of this ester or of anti-ChE agents into certain crabs reduced the frequency of autotomy of legs (WELSH and HASKIN 1939). Also, effects similar to those caused by ACh followed injection into various crabs of extracts from coelenterate tentacles (WELSH 1955).

A histological study of changes in the gut epithelium of the beetle, *Leptinotarsa*, after ingestion of various materials was made by H. A. KOCH (1960). Neither physostigmine nor atropine produced noticeable changes, except at high concentrations. An insecticidal preparation of esters of thiophosphoric acid resulted in excessive secretion by the midgut, with the formation of a vacuole in the greatly swollen nucleus of many cells. However, these observations resembled those made with DDT, and were ascribed to a similar interference with cellular metabolism which was regarded as characteristic of lipophilic contact insecticides generally. In summary, no effects definitely peculiar to the anti-ChE agents were identified.

V. Excretion

The Malpighian tubules are generally regarded as the excretory organs of insects, and at present there appears to be no evidence that their excretory function is affected in any way by anti-ChE agents. The rate of clearance of indigo carmine from the blood was not altered significantly by pretreating *Periplaneta* with 0.12 μg of Parathion (PATTON et al. 1959).

From other experiments with anti-ChE agents there have come, however, suggestions of other excretory routes, the significance of which has not as yet been explored. Thus, both LEWIS and FOWLER (1956) and SMALLMAN and FISHER (1958) noted that ACh became concentrated in the hindgut of flies that had been poisoned with organophosphorus compounds. The source of this abnormal ACh was thought to be the CNS, although COLHOUN (1958a, 1958d) was inclined to seek its origin elsewhere; in any case it was presumably transported by the blood, even though the experimental data do not suffice to show whether the ACh entered the hindgut directly or was simply accumulated there after having made its way into the lumen via the Malpighian tubes or at some more anterior level. By means of parabiosis, BALL and BECK (1951) proved the transport of a toxicant in the blood of *Periplaneta* after the injection of Parathion, which was collected from the foregut tissue of the specimen that had only a blood connection with the treated insect.

Perhaps even less expected was the discovery of ROAN et al. (1950), that four injected organophosphorus[32] agents or their P[32]-containing degradation products were removed rapidly from the blood into the lumen of the foregut of *Periplaneta*.

JOCHUM (1953) gave much consideration to the movement of body fluids in Parathion-poisoned insects. He called attention to the observation of ROAN et al. (1950), that blood failed to flow from the clipped appendages of insects prostrate from organophosphorus agents, which CHAMBERLAIN and HOSKINS (1951), like SCHRADER (1952), had also noticed. According to JOCHUM, the cause of this "dryness" is that the body fluid has shifted almost completely into the gut lumen, via the accessory glands of the foregut and the midgut epithelium. In *Bombyx* larvae, he stated, this loss of fluid could be delayed greatly by ligaturing immediately behind the head, a procedure that prevented the fluid from passing into the gut via the accessory glands; death was thereby delayed. JOCHUM envisaged the metabolic disorder consequent upon the removal of much water from the tissues, rather than the inhibition of ChE in the nervous system, as being primarily responsible for the fatal effects of the organophosphorus agents. Though many students would regard this interpretation as overdrawn, there remains the fact of significant water loss to the gut in many instances of organophosphorus poisoning; it is obvious that such an event could have drastic metabolic consequences. The rôle of such processes in the mode of lethal action of the anti-ChE agents therefore deserves additional study, which conceivably might serve to account for some of the anomalies with which we are confronted at present.

Apparently there has been no attempt made to discern the way in which organophosphorus compounds may produce such changes, although the fact that such poisoning may result in gross movements of water is well established, at least in some instances.

Evidently, the main route of excretion of the organophosphorus agents is not always the foregut. CASIDA (1955) found that, although some agents followed this pathway, others did not; for instance, most of the compound dimethyl 1-carbo-methoxy-1-propen-2-yl phosphate accumulated in the hindgut, with fairly large amounts in the nervous tissue. See ARTHUR and CASIDA (1957).

VI. Ion transport

Evidence for the importance of a cholinergic system in the active transport of ions across cellular membranes in arthropods has been accumulated chiefly by H. J. KOCH and coworkers (KOCH 1954a, 1954b, KOCH et al. 1954a, 1954b). Apparently the gills of the crab, *Eriocheir*, contain an AChE, blockage of which by physostigmine, DFP, quaternary ammonium salts, basic dyes, or *d*-tubocurarine reversibly inhibits the active transport of NaCl. Inhibition of the process by TEPP was not reversible by simple washing, but could be reversed by choline. Active transport of Na^+ by the anal papillae of the larval gnat, *Chironomus*, has similar characteristics (as also had been reported earlier for ion transport across frog skin), and the presence of ChE in the papillae was inferred from the transport-blocking effects of anti-ChE agents. In this connection, it should be mentioned that frogs, which can effect considerable ionregulatory and respiratory exchange through the skin, are able to survive huge doses of DFP (CRESCITELLI et al. 1946). See also Chapters 6 (p. 275), 11 (p. 519), and 12 (p. 562).

VII. Molting and metamorphosis

Variations of ACh and ChE in the brain during metamorphosis of certain silkworms (VAN DER KLOOT 1955) have been considered elsewhere in this volume (v. p. 747 and Chapter 5).

Perhaps highly significant in relation to this subject is the discovery of MONRO (1958), that diapause in the pupa of some *Lepidoptera* was prolonged, apparently without harming the insects in other ways, by injections of eserine. MONRO surmised that inhibition of ChE in some manner prevents release of the brain hormone that is essential for the reinitiation of development. Before this suggestion can be accepted, it would seem desirable to investigate the effect of many other anti-ChE agents.

In further reference to this unsolved but most intriguing problem, a few additional observations should be considered, although their pertinence to the subject is no more than conjectural. SCHREIBER (1957), for instance, found that regular ingestion of small amounts of atropine or of some of its derivatives, while apparently innocuous to *Leptinotarsa* in the early larval instars, resulted in greatly increased mortality during the 4th larval stage and in interference with metamorphosis. With *Trialeurodes*, MCMULLEN (1959) somewhat similarly noticed that the insecticidal effects of ethylene-*bis*-dithiocarbamates differed from those of Perthane (2,2-*bis*-(*p*-ethylphenyl)-1,1-dichloroethane) or of Malathion in that they caused a very slow death. The treated whiteflies survived for an unusually long time, during which they apparently fed, but although they became bloated molting did not occur and eventually they died.

Are such incidents perhaps additional examples of interference with an essential rôle of ACh or ChE in regulating the periodic activity of the brain hormone in the molting cycle?

VIII. Spawning of Hydractinia

Observations of YOSHIDA (1959) suggest the possibility that a cholinergic system is involved in the spawning of the coelenterate, *Hydractinia*. This process, which normally is governed by the proportion between light and dark periods in the daily exposure, was inhibited by ACh, 5×10^{-4}, or by eserine, 10^{-4}, and by higher concentrations of these agents. According to AUGUSTINSSON (1948), *Tubularia* was the only hydrozoan for which ChE had been reported; perhaps this substance is distributed more widely than has been thought.

IX. Luminescence

Anti-ChE agents apparently affect at least some types of biological luminescence, as has been studied with slime from the annelid, *Chaetopterus* (JOHNSON 1959), and with various bacteria (JOHNSON and PLOUGH 1959). Though the latter organisms are not invertebrate animals, observations made on them help to clarify information gathered with luminescent material of invertebrate origin and may also be significant in relation to the mode of action of anti-ChE agents generally.

With the slime of *Chaetopterus*, the luminescence of which decayed gradually after isolation, the addition of DFP, 1.7×10^{-4} M to 2×10^{-3} M, caused a sudden inhibition of from 28% to 71% in light production. This effect was reversible on dilution. The further addition of atropine, 3×10^{-3} M, in the one experiment for which this was graphed, resulted in an immediate slight decrease in luminescence beyond that which had already been caused by DFP. When plotted on a log-log scale, the decrease in luminescence relative to the concentration of DFP could be described by a straight line of slope 0.8, about the same relationship as was obtained for the effect of this agent on bacterial luminescence at the optimum temperature.

The luminescence of three species of bacteria was affected rather similarly by DFP, Sarin (*iso*propyl-methylphosphonofluoridate), and eserine. JOHNSON and PLOUGH (1959) were able to distinguish three components in the response. First, there was a rapid inhibition that was reversible on dilution and on raising the temperature from a colder level toward the bacterial optimum. In the second place, with low drug concentrations, a gradual recovery from inhibition was seen; this was most prominent at low temperature. Finally, there ensued a progressive increase in irreversible inhibition of luminescence, which took place when high concentrations of agent were used. This process had a large temperature coefficient and was ascribed to the denaturation of some protein essential to the light-producing reaction. The authors felt that this last process might have parallels with the better-known progressive and essentially permanent inactivation of ChE by such compounds as DFP or Sarin.

As had been the case in the studies with *Chaetopterus*, atropine at concentrations 10 or more times greater than that of DFP did not counteract the initial decrease in bacterial luminescence, to which in fact atropine contributed to a slight extent.

In considering the possible significance of such studies with bacteria in relation to our general problem, it is pertinent to recall that there has not been unanimous agreement on the existence of cholinergic mechanisms in these organisms. VINCENT and DE PRAT (1945) succeeded in documenting indications of only slight ChE activity in some 10 bacterial species they examined. In order to achieve measurable values for the hydrolysis of ACh by these bacteria, VINCENT and DE PRAT were forced to continue their determinations for a week, and then obtained rates only some 0.01% to 0.03% of those they found with serum; in spite of carefully planned and executed controls, the possibility remained that not all the bacterial activity they recorded was due to esteratic hydrolysis.

SCHALLER (1942) reported evidence of ChE activity in suspensions of both entire and autolyzed Type I *Pneumococcus*, but BERNOUILLI and BLOCH (1944) found no hydrolysis of ACh by 10 pneumococcal strains.

STEPHENSON and ROWATT (1947) demonstrated the presence of an ACh-producing system in *Lactobacillus plantarium* from sauerkraut. Though, in further studies, they could find no ACh in 20 streptococcal strains, they listed several earlier investigations of others that showed production of ACh during fermentation of plant juices by lactic acid bacteria. No ChE has been reported in the latter, and the physiological rôle of ACh in these organisms is unknown. An adaptively produced ChE, the properties of which were not identical with those of either of the main types of animal ChE's, was found in cutures of *Pseudomonas* from fermenting cucumber by GOLDSTEIN and GOLDSTEIN (1953), and was studied further by FITCH (1961).

One may conclude that in general there is little indication that cholinergic mechanisms are important in bacteria; no claim for the operation of such a mechanism in their experiments was made by JOHNSON and PLOUGH (1959).

In fireflies, the induction of "pseudoflashes" by means of the return of hypoxic animals to air, occurs more rapidly in decapitated animals if these have received an injection of 10^{-3} M eserine (A. D. CARLSON 1959). This observation has been taken as indicating neural involvement in the "pseudoflash". The central nature of this involvement is also indicated by the fact that in lanterns with central connections but not in denervated ones, eserine induces asynchronous unit activity which may go through regular cycles of block and recovery (CASE and BUCK 1959).

C. Nervous function

Three aspects of nervous activity in insects have been studied most extensively: *axonal conduction*, in peripheral sensory and motor nerves as well as in internuncial and motor fibers within the CNS, *synaptic transmission*, and *spontaneous discharge*.

The arthropod CNS, when isolated from sensory input, normally exhibits a considerable amount of axonal discharge, the source of which appears to be in neuronal cell bodies in the ganglia (PROSSER 1934, 1943; ROEDER 1955, 1958; STERNBURG 1960). Internuncial activity of this type is referred to as "spontaneous." Besides, many sensory nerves are constantly carrying impulses from the receptors they serve, even when these receptors are receiving no evident stimulation. Ordinary sensory input then modulates the already existing pattern of afferent activity, which also is designated as "spontaneous."

Information regarding the neural effects of anti-ChE agents has been developed mainly with preparations in which these three aspects of nervous function may be followed readily. Also available for study are various cellular membrane potentials, synaptic potentials, etc. (e.g., BOISTEL and CORABOEUF 1954, HAGIWARA and WATANABE 1954, TWAROG and ROEDER 1956, McCANN et al. 1958, YAMASAKI and NARAHASHI 1957, 1958a, NARAHASHI 1960), but these potentials have not been investigated extensively in relation to the action of anti-ChE agents. Some observations of the effect of anti-ChE agents on postsynaptic excitatory potentials in insects have been recorded by YAMASAKI and NARAHASHI (1958b, 1959, 1960) and by NARAHASHI and YAMASAKI (1960).

I. Neuromyal junctions

Anti-cholinesterase agents are without demonstrable effect on transmission at the neuromyal junctions of insects and crustaceans; in fact the general dearth of chemicals that will divorce arthropod muscles from nervous control has deterred physiological investigation at these sites (v. WIERSMA 1961a). The supposition has been expressed that the lack of effect here is due simply to the failure to penetrate. There is evidence, indeed, that compounds such as ACh, atropine, and various highly ionized or highly polar organic agents do not gain access readily to the CNS of insects (v. p. 749 above). Hence, there is reason for surmising that chemicals of this nature may be hindered similarly in reaching the neuromyal junctions, even though there is no direct evidence that this is the case. But it is obvious that many of the non-ionized anti-ChE agents penetrate all other parts of the nervous system rapidly, so that, except for their failure to interfere with nervous stimulation of the muscles, there is no demonstrated cause to assume that they too are excluded from the motor endplates (STERNBURG 1960).

Thus, there are no positive indications that ACh serves as a neuromyal transmitter in insects, or in crustaceans (WIERSMA 1961a). Possibly it is pertinent to this question of the possible release of ACh at the motor nerve endings on muscle, that continuing injections of ACh into denervated *Telea* pupae failed to stimulate muscle differentiation; the inference from this work is that, although motor innervation is known to be essential for the process, apparently it is not ACh set free at the motor endings that is the controlling factor (NÜESCH 1957). There are several objections that legitimately may be raised against the inclusion of this datum in the present context, and perhaps it is best regarded simply as one more among several negative observations. Rather more decisive is the fact that the best histochemical studies (v. p. 748) indicate strongly that there is no ChE at these sites in insects.

For all these reasons, it is incumbent upon those who would maintain that a cholinergic system of neuromyal transmission operates in arthropods to produce some positive proof of its existence. The evidence available is all to the contrary.

Even at the vertebrate neuromyal junction, where ChE has been abundantly demonstrated, reason has been found to question whether the esterase is invariably essential for transmission (e.g., BROOKS and FUORTES 1952, BARNES and DUFF 1953, McNAMARA et al. 1954, BARSTAD 1956).

II. Axons

There is likewise little effect of anti-ChE agents on axonal conduction in arthropods, and such alterations as have been seen are for the most part clearly unrelated to inhibition of ChE. After treatment with anti-ChE agents, a moderate increase in the threshold of the afferent nerves of insects to electrical stimulation was noted regularly (ROEDER et al. 1947, ROEDER 1948), but axonal conduction throughout the remainder of the nervous system was not affected until the agents had been applied in concentrations very much greater (10 to 1,000 times) than those that inhibit ChE completely. With TEPP, such high concentrations halted axonal conduction reversibly; this action was shown to be the result of acid liberated by hydrolysis of the inhibitor (ROEDER 1948). Axonal conduction was similarly inhibited by high concentrations of DFP, but in this instance neutralization of the solutions did not restore normal function; the mechanism of the effect remained unexplained, although the block was nevertheless removed rapidly by washing. Possibly, the fluoride ion set free by hydrolysis of the agent was responsible. Even such axonic effects have not been demonstrable with all anti-ChE agents. Comparable block was obtained with high concentrations of only three out of seven other extremely active organophosphorus compounds (ROEDER and KENNEDY 1955).

The reversibility of the effect, when it did occur, proves that it cannot have been due to inactivation of ChE, since inhibition caused by chemicals of this sort persisted during washing; the occurrence of a block does show that either the anti-ChE agents or derivatives of them had penetrated the tissues to the point of interfering with normal axonic function. That the unchanged compounds, or their possible degradation products, had entered the tissue was attested to also by the fact that the axonal ChE, which is evidently present in considerable titre (v. p. 747), had been inhibited. Hence the return of axonal conduction is conclusive in demonstrating that ChE is not essential for this function in insects.

There is, however, no explanation as to how the anti-ChE agents raised the threshold for electrical stimulation in sensory axons, an observation that has been corroborated in various laboratories. Conceivably, this effect might be linked with the inhibition of ChE, although the mechanism of such a connection is not apparent.

III. Synapses

Synaptic transmission in insects is particularly easily disrupted by anti-ChE agents, as is seen clearly, for example, in studies with the 6th abdominal ganglion of the cockroach. Here the ascending sensory fibers from the cercus impinge upon the giant internuncial neurones of the ventral cord. The normal situation in these relatively stable synapses is that each adequate impulse in the cercal nerve evokes a single propagated potential in the postsynaptic giant fiber. In generalizing from results obtained with this preparation, one must keep in mind that the insect CNS contains a variety of synapses which differ somewhat in their response to drugs and other types of treatment, and that little investigation has been made of the effects of anti-ChE agents at other sites.

The fullest picture of synaptic reactions to anti-ChE agents in insects has been developed by Roeder and associates (Roeder et al. 1947, Roeder 1948, Roeder and Kennedy 1955, Twarog and Roeder 1957). Corroboratory data and further details have been added by other workers. For purposes of discussion it is useful to consider the observed events in the following somewhat schematized sequence, which adheres approximately to the order of their occurrence with time after treatment, or with rising concentrations of agent. It should be understood that the effects elicited are not invariably identical from one preparation to another or with all the inhibitors investigated, and that they have been described from excised nerve cords rather than from the intact CNS.

1. After-discharge

A conspicuous early effect of anti-ChE agents is a prolonged after-discharge in the postsynaptic fibers, following each adequate presynaptic stimulus. Instead of the usual single propagated impulse in the giant fibers, there is a train of high frequency potentials which may last for as long as 15 to 30 sec. Such an after-discharge is often followed by complete synaptic block, recovery from which occurs spontaneously (usually within a few minutes) to be succeeded by alternating periods of facilitation and block for long periods of time. Washing the preparation with saline solution does *not* reverse this condition. The concentrations of inhibitors that produce it (Roeder 1948) are similar to those that had been found by Chadwick and Hill (1947) to cause 90 to 95% inhibition of the ChE in the cockroach nervous system.

Yamasaki and Narahashi (1958b, 1959, 1960) pointed out that after application of anti-ChE agents, there was a marked increase in and prolongation of the excitatory postsynaptic potentials, with a superimposed long after-discharge. Eventually there was produced a persistent ganglionic depolarization which was associated with synaptic block. Repolarization and recovery of synaptic transmission occurred after some time, following which alternate depolarization and repolarization sometimes took place without presynaptic stimulation.

Twarog and Roeder (1957) called attention to the additional fact that even before the occurrence of conspicuous after-discharge in the giant fibers, there was an after-discharge of smaller magnitude, which they referred to as the "delayed response," in other ascending fibers emanating from the ganglion. This "delayed response" appeared while the activity of the giant fibers was still synchronized with the presynaptic stimulation. The synapses or cells that mediated the "delayed reponse" were evidently even more sensitive to the action of anti-ChE agents and other neuroactive materials than were those which are associated with the giant fibers.

By surgically desheathing parts of the nerve cord, these same authors, unlike earlier workers, were able to show a reproducible effect of ACh at 10^{-3} M on cockroach synapses. Pretreatment with eserine reduced the required concentration of ACh 10-fold (results corroborated by YAMASAKI and NARAHASHI 1958b, 1960). In crustaceans, although ACh was without effect on the lateral synapses or on spontaneous activity (WIERSMA 1961b), eserine blocked the synapses and enhanced spontaneous activity, despite its failure to bring to light any effect of ACh.

2. Synchronized synaptic response

In insects, with several anti-ChE agents, increasing the concentration beyond that required to produce a condition of after-discharge and alternating block in the giant fibers resulted in the return of a superficially normal response to presynaptic stimulation (ROEDER and KENNEDY 1955). Each stimulus in the cercal nerve then called forth a single giant fiber spike, of the same magnitude as in the untreated preparation. Transmission became fatigued more rapidly than normally, and washing the preparation restored it only to the condition of after-discharge and block, which apparently was irreversible.

The synchronized synaptic response, following the stage of facilitation, was not seen after treatment with DFP or TEPP [in the form of "hexaethyl tetraphosphate" (HETP)]. STERNBURG et al. (1959) and STERNBURG (1960) observed, however, that after the initial bout of after-discharge caused by 10^{-3} M TEPP or its methyl homolog (a concentration much higher than is needed to produce facilitation), continued treatment of the preparation with fresh batches of the same strength of inhibitor restored the ganglion, apparently permanently, to a condition of seemingly normal spontaneous activity and (except for greater susceptibility to fatigue) synaptic transmission.

3. Continous block

Although synaptic block of relatively short duration, alternating with periods of after-discharge, appeared after treatment with low doses of anti-ChE agents, the use of concentrations still higher than those which then resulted in the return of a synchronized synaptic response produced a continuing inability to transmit, which lasted as long as the high concentration of agent was maintained (ROEDER and KENNEDY 1955). The effect could be reversed by washing with saline solution, although this might take as long as 2 or 3 hr. On washing, the block usually was replaced first by a period of synchronized response which led in turn to the after-discharge state. In some cases, washing led directly to after-discharges. The block was thus of a different nature from that produced initially by lower concentrations of agent, and, because of its reversible character, cannot have been the result of inhibition of ChE. Concomitantly, one sees that some degree of synaptic transmission, often of near normal quality, was possible in the presence of completely inhibited ChE. Owing to the absence of the intervening state of synchronized responses, it was not possible for ROEDER and KENNEDY to distinguish two types of block in the actions of DFP, TEPP (HETP), and physostigmine, although they observed both with several other anti-ChE agents.

4. Comment on synaptic effects

The reversible nature of the synaptic effects in insects, other than those of the initial after-discharge and block, indicates that the conditions designated as "synchronized synaptic response" and "continuous block" cannot be consequences of "irreversible" inhibition of ChE by the organophosphorus agents employed. With reversible inhibitors, such as physostigmine, washing restores the preparation to a completely normal condition, except that there is a tendency for it to be refractory to further doses of the agent (v. KRUPP et al. 1952). Such restoration to wholly normal transmission is not possible with organophosphorus compounds. It is logical, therefore, to ascribe the irreversible condition of after-discharge and block to ChE-inhibition, without, however, attempting at this point to define how inhibition operates to produce the observed result. But the other phenomena must then be attributed to some other effect or effects of the agents.

On the assumption that the inhibition of ChE will result in the accumulation of excess mediator, which is in turn responsible for the initial condition of alternating after-discharge and block, ROEDER and KENNEDY (1955) suggested that the additional effects observed with still higher concentrations of anti-ChE agents might reflect a competition between them and the (presumed) mediator for postsynaptic receptor sites, i.e., a replacement of natural mediator by the anti-ChE agents at these sites. ROEDER and KENNEDY mentioned that in order to be competitive inhibitors of the enzyme, these anti-ChE agents must in this sense be similar structurally to the natural substrate, and that it is conceivable therefore that they should also be able to replace it at other loci. This possibility was noted purely as a hypothetical means of explaining the observations, with awareness that it would not account satisfactorily for all of the phenomena witnessed; what is certain is that these anti-ChE agents have synaptic (and other) actions beyond those attributable to inhibition of ChE's.

IV. Spontaneous activity

Apart from the fact that changes in spontaneous activity take place under the influence of anti-ChE agents, little is known about how these compounds affect it. This is hardly surprising, since the genesis and nature of spontaneous activity in normal circumstances is poorly understood. For the sake of bringing this portion of our analysis as nearly up-to-date as possible, much of the following description of observations on spontaneous activity is based on as yet unpublished experiments by STERNBURG and his associates (v. also STERNBURG 1960).

When anti-ChE agents are applied to the excised cockroach nerve cord there is, at the time when synaptic facilitation and after-discharge in the giant fibers are appearing, a great increase in the number of spontaneous impulses recorded in the abdominal connectives. Coincident with synaptic block, there comes a period of complete electrical quiescence. Presently spontaneous activity reappears, usually before transmission across the synapse can again be accomplished, and while the synapse is in the state of alternating after-discharge and block, spontaneous activity cycles simultaneously. In thoroughly poisoned preparations, in which all detectable ChE has been inhibited, spontaneous activity may then continue at a seemingly normal level for many hours, even though the synapses may remain refractory to afferent stimulation, as they sometimes do. If the early changes in spontaneous activity are to be regarded as the result of inhibition of ChE, it is unlikely that the subsequent re-establishment of spontaneous activity and its prolonged continuation in the presence of high concentrations of organophosphorus compounds are dependent on the activity of the enzyme.

Discussion

The foregoing information shows decisively that there can be no single mechanism of action of the anti-ChE agents on insects; it seems of primary importance that this fact be more generally recognized.

As one obvious but perhaps not overwhelmingly important illustration, effects of anti-ChE agents that take place when ChE is not present cannot properly be attributed to its inhibition. This is certainly the case with some of the instances of interference with embryonic development in insects.

Nevertheless, apart from a few comparable examples, the correlations between inhibition of ChE's and toxic manifestations, though subject to multiple exceptions, some of which we have been at pains to delineate, are both numerous and impressive; consequently most students will agree with this reviewer, that the phenomena of ChE-inhibition, disruption of nervous function, and toxicity, are in many instances clearly linked in insects.

This statement should not be construed, however, to mean that the existence of a cholinergic system has been demonstrated definitely in insects, for it has not. Though many entomologists have adhered somewhat uncritically to such a scheme, which superficially accords well with many of the most conspicuous data, this view has sometimes been taken without full realization that even in better studied groups of animals, cholinergic transmission has been proven conclusively for only a limited number of pathways. An enormous amount of investigation has been required to establish the importance of cholinergic transmission at such few loci as the vertebrate nerve-muscle junction and some sympathetic synapses, but even here not to the full satisfaction of many vertebrate neurophysiologists. Most authorities have meanwhile become convinced that quite different mechanisms regulate nervous activity at many other sites.

Since various phases of nervous performance in insects have been studied relatively little, knowledge of the mechanisms in operation here is much less complete. Moreover, it is doubtful *a priori* that nervous processes in insects should be identical in all details with those in vertebrates, while diversity among the hexapods should be no less. Consequently, one is not surprised to find that some of the facts developed in studies on insects with the anti-ChE agents do not fit snugly into a cholinergic theory of nervous function.

Our principal conclusions from the voluminous data set forth above are then:

1. Correlation between the capacity of anti-ChE agents to produce inhibition of ChE and the toxic effects of the agents on insects is in general so strong that in many instances the inhibition of ChE seems to be causally concerned.

2. Nevertheless, there is reason to suspect that this toxicity is rarely exercised through what is ordinarily understood as a cholinergic mechanism.

Without attempting to rehearse here the multiple observations, already detailed from a variety of sources, that contribute to this second conclusion, we may summarize the evidence in the statement that, if a cholinergic system is anywhere of vital importance in the neurotoxic action of anti-ChE agents on insects, this can be only at very limited loci (certain synapses in the nervous system). Several other nervous functions in insects have been shown not to involve the operation of such a system, while still others have not been sufficiently studied to permit a decision; with them, information either for or against such a hypothesis has not been produced.

The presence of much ACh, ChE, and ChAc throughout the nervous system of insects is usually looked on as a strong point in favor of the existence of a cholinergic system, and it is true that such a system would be unimaginable in the absence of these materials; yet, actually their occurrence in high concentration throughout the nervous tissue, extending even to regions the function of which is surely not dependent on the operation of a cholinergic mechanism, weakens the case for the general significance of such a system.

Difficulties are also encountered in the attempt to invoke a cholinergic theory of transmission, even at those few synapses for which some evidence has been obtained that such a system might be operative. In the first place, it is not clear why blockage at these particular synapses alone should prove fatal; this fact suggests some additional toxic action of the anti-ChE compounds. Conceivably, these agents could be acting through interference with a cholinergic mechanism at other wholly hypothetical sites; if so, evidence for the existence of such sites, and of their dependence on a cholinergic mechanism, is needed. Again, one may wonder why a fatal outcome should follow temporary disruption of certain synapses and spontaneous nervous activity, when normal or nearly normal performance often is soon regained by them in the face of continuing or augmented inhibition of ChE. The latter observation, which is well authenticated, shows that a cholinergic mechanism cannot be indispensable for these functions, even if one chooses to interpret the initial abnormality as due to the derangement of a system of the kind postulated.

The actual cause of death is of course in no way understood in insects, whether the train of events leading to it has been set in motion by interference with a cholinergic mechanism or in some other manner.

The realistic view is then that the observations that have so far been collected in regard to the mode of action of anti-ChE agents on insects and other invertebrate animals emphasize the need for much more information about the process, in all its various aspects. In particular, the data already available warn us against the too facile assumption that all the toxic actions of these materials can be explained satisfactorily by postulating any one relatively simple and ubiquitous physiological mechanism.

Acknowledgment. Completion of this review was supported in part by PHS Research Grant RG-7891 from the Division of General Medical Sciences, U.S. Public Health Service.

Literature

ALDRIDGE, W. N.: Serum esterases. 2. An enzyme hydrolysing diethyl *p*-nitrophenyl phosphate (E 600) and its identity with the A-esterase of mammalian sera. Biochem. J. **53**, 117—124 (1953).
— Anticholinesterases. Inhibition of cholinesterase by organophosphorus compounds and reversal of this reaction: mechanisms involved. Chem. and Ind. **1954**, (17), 473—476.
ARTHUR, B. W., and J. E. CASIDA: Metabolism and selectivity of 0,0-dimethyl 2,2,2-trichloro-1-hydroxyethyl phosphonate and its acetyl and vinyl derivatives. J. agric. Food. Chem. **5**, 186—192 (1957).
ASPEREN, K. VAN: Werking en specificiteit van DDVP. Meded. Landbouwhogeschool Gent **22**, 447—456 (1957).
— Mode of action of organophosphorus insecticides. Nature (Lond.) **181**, 355—356 (1958a).
— The mode of action of an organophosphorus insecticide (DDVP). Some experiments and a theoretical discussion. Entom. Exptl. et Appl. **1**, 130—137 (1958b).
— Distribution and substrate specificity of esterases in the housefly, *Musca domestica* L. J. Insect Physiol. **3**, 306—322 (1959a).
— De meting van de door fosforinsekticiden veroorzakte cholinesteraseremming *in vivo* bij zoogdieren en insekten. Meded. Landbouwhogeschool Gent **24**, 925—932 (1959b).
— Esterase inhibition in the housefly (Musca domestica L.) by organophosphorus compounds. Rec. Trav. chim. Pays-Bas **78**, 872—873 (1959c).
— Mode of action and metabolism of some organic phosphorus insecticides in houseflies. Proc. Fourth int. Congr. Crop Prot., Hamburg 1957, **2**, 1173—1176 (1960a).

ASPEREN, K. VAN: Toxic action of organophosphorus compounds and esterase inhibition in houseflies. Biochem. Pharmacol. **3**, 136—146 (1960b).
— Properties and purification of housefly cholinesterase (personal communication) (1960c).
—, and F. J. OPPENOORTH: Organophosphate resistance and esterase activity in houseflies. Entom. Exptl. et Appl. **2**, 48—57 (1959).
— — The interaction between organophosphorus insecticides and esterases in homogenates of organophosphate susceptible and resistant houseflies. Entom. Exptl. et Appl. **3**, 68—83 (1960).
AUGUSTINSSON, K.-B.: Cholinesterases: a study in comparative enzymology. Acta physiol. scand. **15** (Suppl. 52), x + 182 pp. (1948).
— Acetylcholine esterase and cholinesterases. In: J. B. SUMNER and K. MYRBÄCK, Eds. The Enzymes, 443—472. New York: Academic Press 1950.
—, and M. GRAHN: The occurrence of choline esters in the honey-bee. Arch. physiol. scand. **32**, 174—190 (1954).
BABERS, F. H.: Biochemistry and physiology of resistance of insects to insecticides. Indian J. Malar. **12**, 517—529 (1958).
—, and J. J. PRATT jr.: Studies on the resistance of insects to insecticides. I. Cholinesterase in house flies (*Musca domestica* L.) resistant to DDT. Physiol. Zool. **23**, 58—63 (1950).
— — A comparison of the cholinesterase in the heads of the house fly, the cockroach, and the honey bee. Physiol. Zool. **24**, 127—131 (1951).
BACQ, Z. M.: Recherches sur la physiologie et la pharmacologie du système nerveux autonome. XVII. — Les esters de la choline dans les extraits de tissus des invertébrés. Arch. int. Physiol. **42**, 24—42 (1935a).
— Recherches sur la physiologie et la pharmacologie du système nerveux autonome. XIX. — La choline-estérase chez les invertébrés. L'insensibilité des Crustacés à l'acétylcholine. Arch. int. Physiol. **42**, 47—60 (1935b).
— L'acétylcholine et l'adrénaline chez les invertébrés. Biol. Rev. **22**, 73—91 (1947).
BALL, H. J., and S. D. BECK: The role of the circulatory and nervous systems in the toxic action of Parathion. J. econ. Entom. **44**, 558—564 (1951).
BARNES, J. M., and J. I. DUFF: The role of cholinesterase at the myoneural junction. Brit. J. Pharmacol. **8**, 334—339 (1953).
BARSTAD, J. A. B.: The effect of diisopropylfluorophosphate on the neuromuscular transmission and the importance of cholinesterase for the transmission of single impulses. Arch. int. Pharmacodyn. **107**, 21—32 (1956).
BAYER, G., and T. WENSE: Über einen Nachweis von Hormonen in einzelligen Tieren. I. Mitteilung. Cholin und Acetylcholin im Paramecium. Pflügers Arch. ges. Physiol. **237**, 417—422 (1936).
BEARD, R. L.: Circulation. In: K. D. ROEDER, Ed. Insect Physiology, 232—272. New York: John Wiley and Sons, Inc. 1953.
BEKKER, J. M., and B. J. KRIJGSMAN: Physiological investigations into the heart function of *Daphnia*. J. Physiol. (Lond.) **115**, 249—257 (1951).
BENJAMINI, E., R. L. METCALF and T. R. FUKUTO: The chemistry and mode of action of the insecticide, 0,0-diethyl 0-*p*-methylsulfinylphenyl phosphorothionate and its analogues. J. econ. Entom. **52**, 94—98 (1959).
BERMAN, R., I. B. WILSON and D. NACHMANSOHN: Choline acetylase activity in relation to biological function. Biochim. biophys. Acta **12**, 315—324 (1953).
BERNOUILLI, P., and H. BLOCH: Über den Esterase-Gehalt verschiedener Pneumokokken-Typen. Helv. chim. Acta **27**, 362—366 (1944).
BETTINI, S., and M. BOCCACCI: In: Discussion of F. P. W. WINTERINGHAM (1958). Fourth int. Congr. Biochem. **12**, 211—213 (1958).
BIGLEY, W. S., and F. W. PLAPP jr.: Cholinesterase and ali-esterase activity in organo-phosphorus-susceptible and -resistant house flies. Ann. entom. Soc. Amer. **53**, 360—364 (1960).
BOCCACCI, M., G. NATALIZI and S. BETTINI: Research on the mode of action of halogen containing alkylating agents on insects. J. Insect Physiol. **4**, 20—26 (1960).
BOETTIGER, E.: Insect flight muscles and their basic physiology. Ann. Rev. Entom. **5**, 1—16 (1960).
BOISTEL, J., and E. CORABOEUF: Potentiel de membrane et potentiels d'action de nerf d'insecte recueullis à l'aide de microélectrodes intracellulaires. C. R. Acad. Sci. (Paris) **238**, 2116—2118 (1954).
BROOKS, C. Mc., and M. G. F. FUORTES: Excitation, conduction and synaptic transmission in the nervous system. Ann. Rev. Physiol. **14**, 363—390 (1952).
BROWN, B. E., and A. W. A. BROWN: The effects of insecticidal poisoning on the level of cytochrome oxidase in the American cockroach. J. econ. Entom. **49**, 675—679 (1956).

BUEDING, E.: Acetylcholinesterase activity of *Schistosoma mansoni*. Brit. J. Pharmacol. **7**, 563—566 (1952).

BÜLBRING, E., E. M. LOWRIE and A. U. PARDOE: The presence of acetylcholine in *Trypanosoma rhodesiense* and its absence from *Plasmodium gallinaceum*. Brit. J. Pharmacol **4**, 290—294 (1949).

— J. H. BURN and H. J. SHELLEY: Acetylcholine and ciliary movement in the gill plates of *Mytilus edulis*. Proc. roy. Soc. B **141**, 445—466 (1953).

BULLOCK, T. H., H. GRUNDFEST, D. NACHMANSOHN and M. S. ROTHENBERG: Effect of di-isopropyl fluorophosphate (DFP) on action potential and cholinesterase of nerve. II. J. Neurophysiol. **10**, 53—78 (1947).

CALLAWAY, S., P. DIRNHUBER and K. M. WILSON: A new method for the bioassay of cholinesterase inhibitors. Nature (Lond.) **170**, 843 (1952).

CARLSON, A. D.: Neural involvement in the firefly pseudoflash. Biol. Bull. Wood's Hole **117**, 407 (1959).

CARLSON, L. D.: Enzymes in ontogenesis (Orthoptera). XVII. Esterases in the grasshopper egg. Biol. Bull. Wood's Hole **81**, 375—387 (1941).

CASE, J. F., and J. B. BUCK: Central nervous aspects of firefly excitation. Biol. Bull. Wood's Hole **117**, 393 (1959).

CASIDA, J. E.: Comparative enzymology of certain insect acetylesterases in relation to poisoning by organophosphate insecticides. J. Physiol. (Lond.) **127**, 20P—21P (1954).

— Comparative enzymology of certain insect acetylesterases in relation to poisoning by organophosphorus insecticides. Biochem. J. **60**, 487—496 (1955).

— K.-B. AUGUSTINSSON and G. JONSSON: Solubility, toxicity and reaction mechanism with esterases of certain carbamate insecticides. J. econ. Entom. **53**, 205—212 (1960).

CAVANAUGH, D. J., and J. M. TOBIAS: Studies on bound acetylcholine. Fed. Proc. **8**, 22—23 (1949).

CHADWICK, L. E.: Recent advances in basic studies on insect physiology in relation to mechanisms of resistance to insecticides. R. C. Ist. sup. Sanità (Suppl.), First int. Symposium Control Vectors Disease, 219—234 (1954).

— Temperature dependence of cholinesterase activity. In: F. H. JOHNSON, Ed. The Influence of Temperature on Biological Systems, 49—59. Baltimore: Waverley Press 1957.

—, and D. L. HILL: Inhibition of cholinesterase by di-isopropylfluorophosphate, physostigmine and hexaethyltetraphosphate in the roach. J. Neurophysiol. **10**, 235—246 (1947).

—, and J. B. LOVELL: The effect of temperature on the activity of fly head cholinesterase. Proc. Tenth int. Congr. Entom. **2**, 19—27 (1958).

— — (unpublished data).

— — and V. E. EGNER: The effect of various suspension media on the activity of cholinesterase from flies. Biol. Bull., Wood's Hole **104**, 323—333 (1953).

— — — The relationship between pH and the activity of cholinesterase from flies. Biol. Bull., Wood's Hole **106**, 139—148 (1954).

CHAMBERLAIN, W. F., and W. M. HOSKINS: The inhibition of cholinesterase in the American roach by organic insecticides and related phosphorus-containing compounds. J. econ. Entom. **44**, 177—191 (1951).

CHANG, S. C., and C. W. KEARNS: The occurrence of acetylcholine in the nerve tissue of American cockroaches. Program Third Annual Meeting entom. Soc. Amer. 30—31 (1955).

CHEFURKA, W., and B. N. SMALLMAN: Identity of the acetylcholine-like substance in the housefly. Nature (Lond.) **175**, 946 (1955).

— The occurrence of acetylcholine in the housefly, Musca domestica L. Canad. J. Biochem. **34**, 731—742 (1956).

CHINO, H.: Enzymatic synthesis and hydrolysis of acetylcholine in the eggs of the silkworm, *Bombyx mori*. Annot. zool. jap. **30**, 106—113 (1957).

COLHOUN, E. H.: Tetraethyl pyrophosphate and acetylcholine in Periplaneta americana. Science **127**, 25 (1958a).

— Physical release of acetylcholine from the thoracic nerve cord of *Periplaneta americana* L. Nature (Lond.) **181**, 490 (1958b).

— Acetylcholine in *Periplaneta americana* L. — I. Acetylcholine levels in nervous tissue. J. Insect Physiol. **2**, 108—116 (1958c).

— Acetylcholine in *Periplaneta americana* L. — II. Actylcholine and nervous activity. J. Insect Physiol. **2**, 117—127 (1958d).

— Acetylcholine in Periplaneta americana L. III. Acetylcholine in roaches treated with tetraethyl pyrophosphate and 2,2-bis (p-chlorophenyl)-1,1,1-trichloroethane. Canad. J. Biochem. **37**, 259—272 (1959a).

— Some physiological and pharmacological effects of chlorinated hydrocarbon and organophosphorus poisoning. Proc. N. Cent. Branch entom. Soc. Amer. **14**, 35—37 (1959b).

COLHOUN, E. H.: Physiological events in organophosphorus poisoning. Canad. J. Biochem. **37**, 1127—1134 (1959c).
—, and J. GILLEBERG: The estimation and extraction of acetylcholine from nervous tissue of the American cockroach. Ann. entom. Soc. Amer. **34**, 140—141 (1961).
CORTEGGIANI, E. et A. SERFATY: Acétylcholine et cholinestérase chez les insectes et les arachnides. C. R. Soc. Biol. (Paris) **131**, 1124—1126 (1939).
CRESCITELLI, F., G. B. KOELLE and A. GILMAN: Transmission of impulses in peripheral nerves treated with di-isopropyl fluorophosphate (DFP). J. Neurophysiol. **9**, 241—252 (1946).
DAUTERMAN, W. C., A. TALENS and K. VAN ASPEREN: Partial purification and properties of flyhead cholinesterase. J. Insect Physiol. **8**, 1—14 (1962).
DAVENPORT, D.: Studies in the pharmacology of the heart of the orthopteron, Stenopelmatus. Physiol. Zool. **22**, 35—44 (1949).
DAVID, W. A. L.: The systemic insecticidal action of Paraoxon on the eggs of *Pieris brassicae* (L.). J. Insect Physiol. **3**, 14—27 (1959).
DAVIES, J. H.: The Kinetics of Butyrocholine Esterase. Ph. D. Thesis, Univ. Bristol, 1—169. Bristol England 1955.
DAY, M. F., and D. F. WATERHOUSE: The mechanism of digestion. In: K. D. ROEDER, Ed. Insect Physiology 311—330. New York: John Wiley & Sons, Inc. 1953.
EASTON, D. M.: Synthesis of acetylcholine in crustacean nerve and nerve extract. J. biol. Chem. **185**, 813—816 (1950).
EDDY, G. W., F. W. PLAPP, W. S. BIGLEY and D. I. DARROW: 1. Studies on Malathion-resistance in *Culex tarsalis*. 2. *In vitro* studies on house fly cholinesterase and aliesterase. 3. *In vivo* inhibition of cholinesterase and aliesterase. 4. Substrate protection in measuring cholinesterase and aliesterase inhibition. 5. Measurements of ChE and AliE throughout the life cycle of susceptible and resistant flies (personal communication) (1960).
FELDBERG, W.: Synthesis of acetylcholine by tissue of the central nervous system. J. Physiol. (Lond.) **105**, 367—402 (1945).
— Synthesis of acetylcholine (Choline acetylase). Meth. med. Res. **3**, 95—106 (1950).
FINLAYSON, L. H., and O. LOWENSTEIN: A proprioceptor in the body musculature of Lepidoptera. Nature (Lond.) **176**, 1031 (1955).
— The structure and function of abdominal stretch receptors in insects. Proc. roy. Soc. B **148**, 433—449 (1958).
FITCH, W. M.: An unusual cholinesterase. Fed. Proc. **20** (1), Part I, 219 (1961).
FOWLER, K. S., and S. E. LEWIS: The extraction of acetylcholine from frozen insect tissue. J. Physiol. (Lond.) **142**, 165—172 (1958).
FRONTALI, N.: Acetylcholine synthesis in the house fly head. J. Insect Physiol. **1**, 319—326 (1958).
FUKUTO, T. R.: The chemistry of organic insecticides. Ann. Rev. Entom. **6**, 313—332 (1961).
— R. L. METCALF and M. WINTON: Alkyl phosphonic acid esters as insecticides. J. econ. Entom. **52**, 1121—1127 (1959).
GAUTRELET, J.: Existence d'un complexe d'acétylcholine dans le cerveau et divers organes. Ses caractères, sa répartition. Bull. Acad. Méd. (Paris) **120**, 285—291 (1938).
GILMOUR, D.: Biochemistry of Insects. New York: Academic Press 1961.
GOLDSCHMIDT, S., and H. BURKERT: Die Hydrolyse des cholinergischen Honigwirkstoffes und anderer Cholinester mittels Cholinesterasen und deren Hemmung im Honig. Hoppe-Seylers Z. physiol. Chem. **301**, 78—89 (1955).
GOLDSTEIN, D. B., and A. GOLDSTEIN: An adaptive bacterial cholinesterase from a Pseudomonas species. J. gen. Microbiol. **8**, 8—17 (1953).
GORDON, H. T.: Nutritional factors in insect resistance to chemicals. Ann. Rev. Entom. **6**, 27—54 (1961).
GOSTICK, K. G.: The relationships between increased oxygen uptake and locomotor ataxy or death in insecticide-poisoned *Alphitobius laevigatus* F. Ann. appl. Biol. **49**, 46—54 (1961).
HAGIWARA, S., and A. WATANABE: Action potential of insect muscle examined with intracellular electrode. Jap. J. Physiol. **4**, 65—78 (1954).
HARLOW, P. A.: The action of drugs on the nervous system of the locust (*Locusta migratoria*). Ann. appl. Biol. **46**, 55—73 (1958).
HARVEY, G. T., and A. W. A. BROWN: The effect of insecticides on the rate of oxygen consumption of *Blattella*. Canad. J. Zool. **29**, 42—53 (1951).
HASE, E.: Studies on the mechanism of action of cholinesterase. I. Kinetic studies on the action of hydrogen ions upon cholinesterase. J. Biochem. (Tokyo) **39**, 259—266 (1952).
HENSCHLER, D.: Zur Identifizierung von Cholinestern im biologischen Material, insbesondere von Acetylcholin in Bienenfuttersäften. Hoppe-Seylers Z. physiol. Chem. **305**, 34—41 (1956).
HOLZ, W.: Wirkung von E 605-f auf Eier verschiedener Insekten. Anz. Schädlingsk. **22**, 134—138 (1949).

HOPF, H.: Studies on the mode of action of insecticides. I. Injection experiments on the role of cholinesterase inhibition. Ann. appl. Biol. **39**, 193—202 (1952).

—, and R. T. TAYLOR: Role of cholinesterase in insecticidal action. Nature (Lond.) **182**, 1381—1382 (1958).

HOYLE, G., and J. LOWY: The paradox of *Mytilus* muscle. A new interpretation. J. exp. Biol. **33**, 295—311 (1956).

IYATOMI, K., and K. KANEHISA: Localization of cholinesterases in the American cockroach. Jap. J. appl. Entom. Zool. **2**, 1—10 (1958).

JOCHUM, F.: Der Wasserhaushalt bei durch diäthyl-p-nitrophenylthiophosphat (E 605) erkrankten Insekten. Z. Pflanzenkr. **60**, 354—356 (1953).

JOHNSON, F. H.: Kinetics of luminescence in Chaetopterus slime, and the influence of certain factors thereon. J. cell. comp. Physiol. **53**, 259—277 (1959).

—, and B. PLOUGH: The action of DFP and related drugs on bacterial luminescence. J. cell. comp. Physiol. **53**, 279—305 (1959).

JONES, J. C.: Effects of drugs on Anopheles heart rates. J. exp. Zool. **133**, 573—588 (1956).

KEARNS, C. W.: The mode of action of insecticides. Ann. Rev. Entom. **1**, 123—148 (1956).

KOCH, H. A.: Untersuchungen über die Wirkung von Insektiziden und von Pflanzenalkaloiden auf den Darmtraktus des Kartoffelkäfers und seiner Larven. Entom. Exptl. et Appl. **3**, 103—113 (1960).

KOCH, H. J.: L'intervention de cholinestérases dans l'absorption et le transport actif de matières par les branchies du crabe "Eriocheir sinensis M. E.". Arch. int. Physiol. **62**, 136 (1954a).

— Cholinesterase and active transport of sodium chloride through the isolated gills of the crab (*Eriocheir sinensis* (M. Edw.)). In: J. A. KITCHING, Ed. Recent developments in cell physiology, 15—31 (1954b).

— J. EVANS and E. SCHICKS: The active absorption of ions by the isolated gills of the crab Eriocheir sinensis. Meded. Vlaamse Acad. Wet. (1954a).

— — — The importance of cholinesterase for the active absorption of ions by *Eriocheir sinensis* and *Chironomus plumosus*. Meded. Vlaamse Acad. Wet. (1954b).

KOELLE, G. B.: Histochemical demonstration of reversible anticholinesterase action at selective cellular sites *in vivo*. J. Pharmacol. exp. Ther. **120**, 488—503 (1957).

KOLBEZEN, M. J., R. L. METCALF and T. R. FUKUTO: Insecticidal activity of carbamate cholinesterase inhibitors. J. agric. Food. Chem. **2**, 864—870 (1954).

KOOISTRA, G.: Action of acetyl choline in intestine of *Periplaneta americana* L. Physiol. comp. 's-Grav. **2**, 75—79 (1950).

KRIJGSMAN, B. J.: Contractile and pacemaker mechanisms in the heart of arthropods. Biol. Rev. **27**, 320—346 (1952).

—, and G. A. DIVARIS: Contractile and pacemaker mechanisms of the heart of molluscs. Biol. Rev. **30**, 1—39 (1955).

—, and N. E. KRIJGSMAN: Heart mechanism of arthropods. Nature (Lond.) **165**, 936—937 (1950).

KRUPP, H., L. LENDLE and K. STAPENHORST: Pharmakologische Wirkungen am isolierten Ganglien-Muskelpräparat des Gelbrandkäfers. (Zur vergleichenden Pharmakologie des Nerv-Muskelsystems.) Naunyn-Schmiedeberg's Arch. exp. Path. Pharmak. **215**, 443—459 (1952).

LEWIS, S. E.: Acetylcholine in blowflies. Nature (Lond.) **172**, 1004—1005 (1953).

—, and K. S. FOWLER: Effect of diisopropylphosphorofluoridate on the acetylcholine content of flies. Nature (Lond.) **178**, 919—920 (1956).

—, and B. N. SMALLMAN: The estimation of acetylcholine in insects. J. Physiol. (Lond.) **134**, 241—256 (1956).

— J. B. WALLER and K. S. FOWLER: The effect of DDT and physically induced prostration on acetylcholine levels in the cockroach. J. Insect Physiol. **4**, 128—137 (1960).

LORD, K. A.: The effect of insecticides on respiration. II. The effects of a number of insecticides on the oxygen uptake of adult *Tribolium castaneum* Herbst. at 25° C. Ann. appl. Biol. **37**, 105—122 (1950).

—, and C. POTTER: Mechanism of action of organo-phosphorus compounds as insecticides. Nature (Lond.) **166**, 893—894 (1950).

— — Studies on the mechanism of insecticidal action of organo-phosphorus compounds with particular reference to their anti-esterase activity. Ann. appl. Biol. **38**, 495—507 (1951).

— — Hydrolysis of esters by extracts of insects. Nature (Lond.) **172**, 679 (1953).

— — Differences in esterases from insect species: toxicity of organo-phosphorus compounds and *in vitro* anti-esterase activity. J. Sci. Food Agric. **1954** (10), 490—498 (1954a).

— — Organo-phosphorus insecticides. Insecticidal and anti-esterase activity of organo-phosphorus compounds. Chem. and Ind. (Rev.) **1954**, 1214—1217 (1954b).

LORD, K. A., and S. R. B. SOLLY: The rate of disappearance of para-oxon from two strains of houseflies. Chem. and Ind. (Rev.) **1956**, 1352—1353 (1956).

LOWNE, B. T.: The Anatomy, Physiology, Morphology and Development of the Blow-fly, vol. **2**, 450. London: R. H. Porter 1893—1895.

MARTIN, H.: The chemistry of insecticides. Ann. Rev. Entom. **1**, 149—166 (1956).

— The Scientific Principles of Crop Protection. Ed. 4, 216—231. London: Edward Arnold Ltd. (1959).

MAYNARD, D. M.: Activity in a crustacean ganglion. II. Pattern and interaction in burst formation. Biol. Bull., Wood's Hole **109**, 420—436 (1955).

— Circulation and heart function. In: T. H. WATERMAN, Ed. The Physiology of Crustacea **1**, 161—226. New York: Academic Press, Inc. 1960.

MAYNARD, E. A., and D. M. MAYNARD: Cholinesterase in the crustacean muscle receptor organ. J. Histochem. Cytochem. **8**, 376—379 (1960).

McALLAN, J. W., and A. W. A. BROWN: The effect of insecticides on transamination in the American cockroach. J. econ. Entom. **53**, 166—167 (1960).

McCANN, F. V., R. WERMAN and H. GRUNDFEST: Graded or all-or-none electrical activity in insect muscle fibers. Biol. Bull., Wood's Hole **115**, 356—357 (1958).

McENROE, W. D.: Cholinesterase in the two-spotted spider mite. Bull. entom. Soc. Amer. **6**, 150 (1960).

McMULLEN, R. D.: Insecticidal action of ethylene *bis*dithiocarbamates. Nature (Lond.) **184**, 1338 (1959).

McNAMARA, B. P., E. F. MURTHA, A. D. BERGNER, E. M. ROBINSON, C. W. BENDER and J. H. WILLS: Studies on the mechanism of action of DFP and TEPP. J. Pharmacol. exp. Ther. **110**, 232—240 (1954).

MEANS, O. W., jr.: Cholinesterase activity of tissues of adult *Melanoplus differentialis* (Orthoptera, Acrididae). J. cell. comp. Physiol. **20**, 319—324 (1942).

MEHROTRA, K. N.: Development of the cholinergic system in insect eggs. J. Insect Physiol. **5**, 128—142 (1960a).

— Effect of an anticholinesterase on the cholinergic system in insect eggs. Canad. J. Biochem. **38**, 1045—1052 (1960b).

— The occurrence of acetylcholine in the two-spotted mite, *Tetranychus telarius* L. J. Insect Physiol. **6**, 180—184 (1961a).

— Properties of choline acetylase from the house fly, *Musca domestica* L. J. Insect Physiol. **6**, 215—221 (1961b).

— (personal communication) (1961c).

—, and B. N. SMALLMAN: Ovicidal action of organo-phosphorus insecticides. Nature (Lond.) **180**, 97—98 (1957).

MELTZER, J. Unspecific resistance mechanisms in the house-fly, *Musca domestica* L. Indian J. Malar. **12**, 579—588 (1958).

MENGLE, D. C., and J. E. CASIDA: Inhibition and recovery of brain cholinesterase activity in house flies poisoned with organophosphate and carbamate compounds. J. econ. Entom. **51**, 750—755 (1958).

— — Biochemical factors in the acquired resistance of house flies to organophosphate insecticide. J. agric. Food Chem. **8**, 431—437 (1960).

—, and R. D. O'BRIEN: The spontaneous and induced recovery of fly-brain cholinesterase after inhibition by organophosphates. Biochem. J. **75**, 201—207 (1960).

METCALF, R. L.: Organic Insecticides, their Chemistry and Mode of Action. New York: Interscience Publishers 1955.

— The impact of the development of organophosphorus insecticides upon basic and applied science. Bull. entom. Soc. Amer. **5**, 3—15 (1959).

—, and R. B. MARCH: Studies of the mode of action of Parathion and its derivatives and their toxicity to insects. J. econ. Entom. **42**, 721—728 (1949).

— — Properties of acetylcholinesterases from the bee, the fly and the mouse and their relation to insecticide action. J. econ. Entom. **43**, 670—677 (1950).

— — Further studies on the mode of action of organic thionophosphate insecticides. Ann. entom. Soc. Amer. **46**, 63—74 (1953).

— — and M. G. MAXON: Substrate preferences of insect cholinesterases. Ann. entom. Soc. Amer. **48**, 222—228 (1955).

— M. MAXON, T. R. FUKUTO and R. B. MARCH: Aromatic esterase in insects. Ann. entom. Soc. Amer. **49**, 274—279 (1956).

MIKALONIS, S. J., and R. H. BROWN: Acetylcholine and cholinesterase in the insect central nervous system. J. cell. comp. Physiol. **18**, 401—403 (1941).

MOLLOY, F. M.: In: C. POTTER (1960) (q. v.).

MONRO, J.: Cholinesterase and the secretion of the brain hormone in insects. Aust. J. biol. Sci. **11**, 399—406 (1958).

MOONEY, R., and V. OBRESHKOVE: Action of prostigmine, carbaminoyl-choline (Doryl) and acetyl-B-methyl-choline (Mecholyl) on the intestine of a cladoceran. Proc. Soc. exp. Biol. (N. Y.) 68, 42—46 (1948).

MOOREFIELD, H. H., and W. M. LANHAM: A new class of cyclic phosphate insecticides. Oral presentation at First Joint Meeting entom. Soc. Ont., entom. Soc. Canad., entom. Soc. Amer. Detroit, Michigan (1959).

—, and E. R. TEFFT: Application of cholinesterase assay to residue analyses of 1-naphthyl N-methylcarbamate (Sevin). Contr. Boyce Thompson Inst. 19, 295—301 (1958).

MORRISON, P. E., and A. W. A. BROWN: The effect of insecticides on cytochrome oxidase obtained from the American cockroach. J. econ. Entom. 47, 723—730 (1954).

MOUNTER, L. A., and V. P. WHITTAKER: The hydrolysis of esters of phenol by cholinesterases and other esterases. Biochem. J. 54, 551—559 (1953).

NARAHASHI, T.: Excitation and electrical properties of giant axon of cockroaches. In: Electrical Activity of Single Cells, 119—131 (1960).

—, and T. YAMASAKI: Nervous and cholinesterase activities in the cockroach as affected by Demeton and Methyldemeton. Jap. J. appl. Entom. Zool. 1, 64—69 (1960).

NEEDHAM, A. E.: Physiology of the heart of Asellus aquaticus L. Nature (Lond.) 173, 272 (1954).

NGUY, V. D., and J. R. BUSVINE: Studies of the genetics of resistance to Parathion and Malathion in the housefly. Bull. World Hlth. Org. 22, 531—542 (1960).

NICOL, J. A. C.: Muscle activity and drug action in the body wall of the sabellid worm Branchiomma vesiculosum (Montagu). Physiol. comp. 's-Grav. 2, 339—345 (1952).

NÜESCH, H.: Über die Bedeutung des Nervensystems für die Entwicklung anderer Organe. Verh. naturf. Ges. Basel 68, 194—216 (1957).

O'BRIEN, R. D.: Occurrence of cholinesterase in Tenebrio and Tribolium. Nature (Lond.) 172, 162 (1953).

— Protection of cholinesterase by ethanol against inhibition by organophosphates in vitro. J. biol. Chem. 219, 927—931 (1956a).

— The inhibition of cholinesterase and succinoxidase by Malathion and its isomer. J. econ. Entom. 49, 484—490 (1956b).

— The effect of Malathion and its isomer on carbohydrate metabolism of the mouse, cockroach and house fly. J. econ. Entom. 50, 79—84 (1957a).

— Esterases in the semi-intact cockroach. Ann. entom. Soc. Amer. 50, 223—229 (1957b).

— Effect of ionization upon penetration of organophosphates to the nerve cord of the cockroach. J. econ. Entom. 52, 812—816 (1959a).

— Comparative toxicology of some organophosporus compounds in insects and mammals. Canad. J. Biochem. 37, 1113—1122 (1959b).

— Toxic Phosphorus Esters. New York: Academic Press, Inc. 1960.

—, and R. W. FISHER: The relation between ionization and toxicity to insects for some neuropharmacological compounds. J. econ. Entom. 51, 169—175 (1958).

—, and E. H. SMITH: The uptake and metabolism of Parathion by insect eggs. J. econ. Entom. 54, 187—191 (1961).

OPPENOORTH, F. J.: Genetics of resistance to organophosphorus compounds and low aliesterase activity in the housefly. Entom. Exptl. et Appl. 2, 304—319 (1959).

—, and K. VAN ASPEREN: Allelic genes in the housefly producing modified enzymes that cause organophosphate resistance. Science 132, 298—299 (1960).

ORMEROD, W. E.: Hydrolysis of benzoyl choline derivatives by cholinesterase in serum. Biochem. J. 54, 701—704 (1953).

ORSER, W. B., and A. W. A. BROWN: The effect of insecticides on the heartbeat of Periplaneta. Canad. J. Zool. 29, 54—64 (1951).

PATTON, R. L., J. GARDNER and A. D. ANDERSON: The excretory efficiency of the American cockroach, Periplaneta americana L. J. Insect Physiol. 3, 256—261 (1959).

PILGRIM, R. C.: The action of acetylcholine on the hearts of lamellibranch molluscs. J. Physiol. (Lond.) 125, 208—214 (1954).

PLAPP, F. W. jr., and W. S. BIGLEY: Inhibition of house fly ali-esterase and cholinesterase under in vivo conditions by Parathion and Malathion. J. econ. Entom. 54, 103—108 (1961).

POTTER, C.: Insecticides and fungicides department. Rep. Rothamst. exp. Sta. for 1959, 117—131, 267—270 (1960).

— K. A. LORD, J. KENTEN, E. H. SALKELD and D. V. HOLBROOK: Embryonic development and esterase activity of eggs of Pieris brassicae in relation to TEPP poisoning. Ann. appl. Biol. 45, 361—375 (1957).

PROSSER, C. L.: Action potentials in the nervous system of the crayfish. I. Spontaneous impulses. J. cell. comp. Physiol. 4, 185—209 (1934).

— An analysis of the action of salts upon abdominal ganglia of crayfish. J. cell. comp. Physiol. 22, 131—145 (1943).

PROSSER, C. L.: The physiology of nervous systems of invertebrate animals. Physiol. Rev. 26, 337—382 (1946).
— Comparative Animal Physiology. C. L. PROSSER, Ed. Philadelphia: W. B. Saunders Co. 1950.
— Comparative physiology of nervous systems and sense organs. Ann. Rev. Physiol. 16, 103—124 (1954a).
— Activation of a non-propagating muscle in Thyone. J. cell. comp. Physiol. 44, 247—253 (1954b).
—, and C. E. MELTON jr.: Nervous conduction in smooth muscle of Phascolosoma proboscis retractors. J. cell. comp. Physiol. 44, 255—275 (1954).
RASMUSON, B., and B. HOLMSTEDT: Resistance to cholinesterase inhibitors of the organophosphorus group in different strains of Drosophila melanogaster. Genetical and enzyme studies. Kgl. Lantbruks-Högskol. Ann. 24, 89—100 (1958).
RICHARDS, A. G.: Temperature in relation to the activity of single and multiple physiological systems in insects. Proc. Tenth int. Congr. Entom. 2, 67—72 (1958).
—, and L. K. CUTKOMP: The cholinesterase of insect nerve. J. cell. comp. Physiol. 26, 57—61 (1945).
ROAN, C. C., H. E. FERNANDO and C. W. KEARNS: A radiobiological study of four organic phosphates. J. econ. Entom. 43, 319—325 (1950).
—, and S. MAEDA: The cholinesterase of the Oriental fruit fly and its in vitro reactions with various insecticidal compounds. J. econ. Entom. 46, 775—779 (1953).
ROCKSTEIN, M.: The relation of cholinesterase activity to change in cell number with age in the brain of the adult worker honeybee. J. cell. comp. Physiol. 35, 11—24 (1950).
ROEDER, K. D.: V. The effect of anticholinesterases and related substances on nervous activity in the cockroach. Johns Hopk. Hosp. Bull. 83, 587—599 (1948).
— Spontaneous activity and behavior. Sci. Mon. (N. Y.) 80, 362—370 (1955).
— The nervous system. Ann. Rev. Entom. 3, 1—18 (1958).
—, and N. K. KENNEDY: The effect of certain trisubstituted phosphine oxides on synaptic conduction in the roach. J. Pharmacol. exp. Ther. 114, 211—220 (1955).
— — and E. A. SAMPSON: Synaptic conduction to giant fibers of the cockroach and the action of anticholinesterases. J. Neurophysiol. 10, 1—10 (1947).
SALKELD, E. H.: Histochemical studies on the identification and localization of esterases in insect eggs. Bull. entom. Soc. Amer. 6, 150 (1960).
— Histochemical studies on the identification and localization of esterases (personal communication) (1961).
SCHALLER, K.: Über die Spaltung von Acetylcholin durch Pneumokokken. Z. physikal. Chem. 276, 271—274 (1942).
SCHRADER, G.: The development of new insecticides. In: B. I. O. S. Final Rep. No. 714, Item 8. 1947.
— Die Entwicklung neuer Insektizide auf Grundlage organischer Fluor- and Phosphor-Verbindungen. 2. erw. Aufl. Weinheim. Bergstr.
SCHREIBER, K.: Natürliche pflanzliche Resistenzstoffe gegen den Kartoffelkäfer und ihr möglicher Wirkungsmechanismus. Züchter 27, 289—299 (1957).
SCHWARZ, E.: Wirkung von E605-f auf Eier des Kartoffelkäfers. Anz. Schädlingskunde 23, 87 (1950).
SEAMAN, G. R., and R. K. HOULIHAN: Enzyme systems in Tetrahymena geleii S. II. Acetylcholinesterase activity. Its relation to motility of the organism and to coordinated ciliary action in general. J. cell. comp. Physiol. 37, 309—321 (1951).
SEUME, F. W.: Ein Beitrag zur Zucht von Daphnia magna Straus. Anz. Schädlingskunde 30, 25—27 (1957).
SMALLMAN, B. N.: Mechanisms of acetylcholine synthesis in the blowfly. J. Physiol. (Lond.) 132, 343—357 (1956).
— Enzyme relationships in the action of organophosphorus insecticides. Canad. J. Biochem. 37, 1123—1126 (1959).
—, and R. W. FISHER: Effect of anticholinesterases on acetyl choline levels in insects. Canad. J. Biochem. 36, 575—586 (1958).
—, and R. PAL: The activity and intra-cellular distribution of choline acetylase in insect nervous tissue. Bull. entom. Soc. Amer. 3, 25 (1957).
—, and L. S. WOLFE: The effect of salts on the estimation of cholinesterase activity. Enzymologia 17, 133—144 (1954).
— — Soluble and particulate cholinesterase in insects. J. cell. comp. Physiol. 48, 197—214 (1956).
SMISSAERT, H. R.: Preliminary investigations on the physiology of organophosphorus resistance in spider mites. (Personal communication) (1960).
SMITH, E. H.: Further studies on the ovicidal action of Parathion to eggs of the peach tree borer. J. econ. Entom. 48, 727—731 (1955).

SMITH, E. H., and A. W. AVENS: The ovicidal action of Parathion to eggs of the peach tree borer. J. econ. Entom. **47**, 912—917 (1954).
—, and A. C. WAGENKNECHT: The occurrence of cholinesterase in eggs of the peach tree borer and large milkweed bug and its relation to the ovicidal action of Parathion. J. econ. Entom. **49**, 777—783 (1956).
—, — The ovicidal action of organophosphate insecticides. Canad. J. Biochem. **37**, 1135—1144 (1959).
SMITH, R. I.: Acetylcholine in the nervous tissue and blood of crayfish. J. cell. comp. Physiol. **13**, 335—344 (1939).
SPENCER, E. Y., and R. D. O'BRIEN: Chemistry and mode of action of organophosphorus insecticides. Ann. Rev. Entom. **2**, 261—278 (1957).
SPEYER, W.: Haben die modernen Kontaktgifte eine ovicide Wirkung? Nachrbl. dtsch. Pflanzenschutzdienst (Berlin) **2**, 2—3 (1950).
STAUDENMAYER, T.: The influence of "E 605" on the respiration of silkworm eggs. Höfchenbr. Wiss. **6**, 158—166 (English edition) (1953).
— Die Cholinesterase während der Eientwicklung von *Bombyx mori* und die ovizide Wirkung von Phosphorsäureester (E 600 u. E 605). Z. vergl. Physiol. **37**, 416—423 (1955).
STEGWEE, D.: Studies on cholinesterase in insects. Physiol. comp. ('s-Grav.) **2**, 241—247 (1951).
— The effect of Parathion and DDT on cholinesterase activity in the roach. Biochim. biophys. Acta **8**, 187—193 (1952).
— Esterase inhibition and organophosphorus poisoning in the housefly *Musca domestica*. Nature (Lond.) **184**, 1253—1254 (1959).
— The role of esterase inhibition in tetraethyl pyrophosphate poisoning in the house-fly, *Musca domestica* L. Canad. J. Biochem. **38**, 1417—1430 (1960).
STEPHENSON, M., and E. ROWATT: The production of acetylcholine by a strain of *Lactobacillus plantarum*. J. gen. Microbiol. **1**, 279—298 (1947).
STERNBURG, J.: Effect of insecticides on neurophysiological activity in insects. J. agric. Food Chem. **8**, 257—261 (1960).
— S. C. CHANG and C. W. KEARNS: The release of a neuroactive agent by the American cockroach after exposure to DDT or electrical stimulation J. econ. Entom. **52**, 1070—1076 (1959).
TAHMISIAN, T. N.: Enzymes in ontogenesis: choline-esterase in developing *Melanoplus differentialis eggs*. J. exp. Zool. **92**, 199—213 (1943).
TOBIAS, J. M., J. J. KOLLROS and J. SAVIT: Acetylcholine and related substances in the cockroach, fly and crayfish and the effect of DDT. J. cell. comp. Physiol. **28**, 159—182 (1946).
TOWER, D. B., and D. McEACHERN: Experiences with the "Venus" heart method for determining acetylcholine. Canad. J. Res., Sec. E **26**, 183—187 (1948).
TWAROG, B. M.: Responses of a molluscan smooth muscle to acetylcholine and 5-hydroxytryptamine. J. cell. comp. Physiol. **44**, 141—163 (1954).
—, and K. D. ROEDER: Properties of the connective tissue sheath of the cockroach abdominal nerve cord. Biol. Bull., Wood's Hole **111**, 278—286 (1956).
— — Pharmacological observations on the desheathed last abdominal ganglion of the cockroach. Ann. entom. Soc. Amer. **50**, 231—237 (1957).
VAN DER KLOOT, W. G.: The control of neurosecretion and diapause by physiological changes in the brain of the cecropia silkworm. Biol. Bull., Wood's Hole **109**, 276—294 (1955).
VINCENT, D., and A. JULLIEN: L'activité cholinestérasique des extraits myocardiques chez les mollusques. C. R. Soc. Biol. (Paris) **127**, 631—632 (1938).
—, and J. DE PRAT: Essai de recherche de la cholinestérase chez quelques bactéries. C. R. Soc. Biol. (Paris) **139** (2), 1148—1150 (1945).
VOSS, G.: Esterasen bei der Spinnmilbe *Tetranychus urticae* Koch (Acari, Trombidiformes, Tetranychidae). Naturwissenschaften **46**, 652 (1959).
WALOP, J. N.: Acetyl choline formation in the central nervous system of *Carcinus maenas*. Acta physiol. pharmacol. néerl. **1**, 333—335 (1950).
— Studies on acetylcholine in the crustacean central nervous system. Arch. int. Physiol. **59**, 145—156 (1951).
—, and L. M. BOOT: Studies on cholinesterase in *Carcinus maenas*. Biochim. biophys. Acta **4**, 566—571 (1950).
— J. MELTZER and E. JAEGER-DRAAFSEL: Activation of cholinesterase in insects. Proc. XXth physiol. Congr. Brussels **1956**, 562 (1956).
WATERMAN, T. H.: The Physiology of Crustacea, volume 1. T. H. WATERMAN, Ed. New York: Academic Press, Inc. 1960.
— The Physiology of Crustacea, volume 2. T. H. WATERMAN, Ed. New York: Academic Press, Inc. 1961.
WELSH, J. H.: On the nature and action of coelenterate toxins. Rep. Mar. Biol. Oceanogr., Deep-Sea Res. **3** (Suppl.), 287—297 (1955).

WELSH, J. H.: Neurohormones and neurosecretion. In: T. H. WATERMAN, Ed. The Physiology of Crustacea 2, 281—311. New York: Academic Press, Inc. 1961.
—, and H. H. HASKIN: Chemical mediation in crustaceans. III. Acetylcholine and autotomy in Petrolisthes armatus (Gibbes). Biol. Bull., Wood's Hole 76, 405—415 (1939).
—, and W. SCHALLEK: Arthropod nervous systems: a review of their structure and function. Physiol. Rev. 26, 447—478 (1946).
WIERSMA, C. A. G.: The neuromuscular system. In: T. H. WATERMAN, Ed. The Physiology of Crustacea 2, 141—240. New York: Academic Press, Inc. 1961a.
— Reflexes and the central nervous system. In: T. H. WATERMAN, Ed. The Physiology of Crustacea 2, 241—279. New York: Academic Press, Inc. 1961b.
WIESMANN, R., and C. KOCHER: Untersuchungen über ein neues, gegen resistente Musca domestica L. wirksame Insektizid. Z. angew. Entom. 33, 297—321 (1951).
WIGGLESWORTH, V. B.: The distribution of esterase in the nervous system and other tissues of the insect Rhodnius prolixus. Quart. J. micr. Sci. 99, 441—450 (1958).
— The histology of the nervous system of an insect, Rhodnius prolixus (Hemiptera). I. The peripheral nervous system. Quart. J. micr. Sci. 100, 285—298 (1959a).
— The histology of the nervous system of an insect, Rhodnius prolixus (Hemiptera). II.The central ganglia. Quart. J. micr. Sci. 100, 299—313 (1959b).
WILSON, I. B., and M. COHEN: The essentiality of cholinesterase in conduction. Biochim. biophys. Acta 11, 147—156 (1953).
WINTERINGHAM, F. P. W.: Comparative biochemical aspects of insecticidal action. Chem. and Ind. (Rev.) 1957, 1195—1202.
— Comparative aspects of insect biochemistry with particular reference to insecticidal action. Fourth int. Congr. Biochem. 12, 201—210 (discussion, 211—215) (1958).
—, and A. HARRISON: Study of anticholinesterase action in insects by a labelled pool technique. Nature (Lond.) 178, 81—83 (1956).
— — M. A. MCKAY and A. WEATHERLEY: Biochemistry of diisopropylphosphorofluoridate poisoning in the adult housefly. Biochem. J. 65, 49P (1957).
—, and S. E. LEWIS: On the mode of action of insecticides. Ann. Rev. Entom. 4, 303—318 (1959).
WINTON, M. Y., R. L. METCALF and T. R. FUKUTO: The use of acetyl thiocholine in the histochemical study of organophosphorus insecticides. Ann. entom. Soc. Amer. 51, 436—441 (1958).
WOLFE, L. S., and B. N. SMALLMAN: The properties of cholinesterase from insects. J. cell. comp. Physiol. 48, 215—236 (1956).
—, and G. D. THORN: The hydrolysis of p-acetoxyphenylethylamines by insect cholinesterase. Canad. J. Biochem. 36, 145—152 (1958).
YAMASAKI, T., and T. NARAHASHI: Studies on the mechanism of action of insecticides (XIV). Intracellular microelectrode recordings of resting and action potentials from the insect axon and the effects of DDT on the action potential. Botyu-Kagaku 22, 305—313 (1957).
— — Effects of potassium and sodium ions on the resting and action potentials of the giant axon of the cockroach. Nature (Lond.) 182, 1805—1806 (1958a).
— — Synaptic transmission in the cockroach. Nature (Lond.) 182, 1806 (1958b).
— — Electrical properties of the cockroach giant axon. J. Insect Physiol. 3, 230—242 (1959).
— — Synaptic transmission in the last abdominal ganglion of the cockroach. J. Insect Physiol. 4, 1—13 (1960).
YOSHIDA, M.: Effect of acetylcholine and eserine on the spawning of Hydractinia echinata. Nature (Lond.) 184, 1151 (1959).
YUSHIMA, T.: Changes in rate of synthesis of acetylcholine in vitro in eggs of the Asiatic rice borer, Chilo suppressalis (Wlk.) and cabbage armyworm Mamestra brassicae (L.) during embryonic development. J. econ. Entom. 50, 440—443 (1957).

Chapter 17

Ontogenetic Effects

By

Alexander G. Karczmar

With 1 Figure

Contents

Introduction

I. Purpose of employment of anticholinesterase (anti-ChE) agents in studies of phylogenesis and ontogenesis

Cholinesterases (ChE's), enzymes intimately concerned with synaptic transmission as well as with motor activity ("overt behavior"), teleologically should appear in phylogenesis and in ontogenesis at the first occurrence of transmission and of behavioral events. Pertinent results were described and discussed in Chapter 5; while they bear out the general importance of ChE's and particularly of acetylcholinesterase (AChE) for rapidly occurring functions, their coupling with specific phylo- or ontogenetic steps could not be successfully pinpointed in many cases; moreover, it was found expedient to suggest that these enzymes may also play a part in processes other than transmission.

It was pointed out further that if ChE's are involved at crucial evolutionary and ontogenetic stages, anticholinesterase (anti-ChE) agents should become effective at the same stages. While this is a mere transposition to evolution or ontogenesis of one of the well known criteria for acceptance of a transmitter mechanism, namely that the inhibition of the destruction of the transmitter by an enzyme functionally coupled with the pertinent transmission should lead to malfunction (FELDBERG 1957, GIARMAN 1959), it was hoped (SAWYER 1943a, BOELL 1948) that the application of anti-ChE agents in phylogenesis or ontogenesis should clarify the functional significance of ChE's more dramatically than their more orthodox employment.

Somewhat similar hopes were held for the ontogenetic and phylogenetic appearance of ChE's. In Chapter 5, the *phylogenesis* of ChE's was discussed to indicate technical and interpretative problems encountered in philosophically related studies of ChE's in *ontogenesis*; to continue this approach in this Chapter, certain effects of anti-ChE agents in phylogenesis will be first briefly discussed.

II. Effects of anti-ChE agents on unicellular organisms

When it was proposed that in evolution ChE's may appear not only at the time of the emergence of the nervous system and higher function (BULLOCK and NACHMANSOHN 1942) but at the moment of the appearance of ciliary motility and of its fibrillar coordination system (Chapter 5), SEAMAN and HOULIHAN (1951) demonstrated that the protozoan *Tetrahymena gelii* possesses an AChE, and that its ciliary activity can be inhibited by eserine and di*iso*propyl phosphorofluoridate (DFP). Yet, before this is accepted as final evidence of the significance of phylogenetic appearance of AChE, certain methodological aspects of the experiments of SEAMAN and HOULIHAN (o.c.) must be considered.

Firstly, eserine and DFP in concentrations of 4×10^{-7} M inhibited completely the activity of AChE of *Tetrahymena*; yet, inhibition of motility occurred only with concentrations about 10,000 times higher. Enzymic inhibition, while measured in homogenates, should not differ significantly from that which actually obtained *in vivo*, since the lipid soluble compounds eserine and DFP should easily penetrate to the strategic sites of the intact *Tetrahymena*; in fact, much lower concentrations of eserine and DFP could penetrate through the intact skin of aquatic vertebrates and effectively inhibited ChE's (SAWYER 1943a, KOPPANYI and KARCZMAR 1947). Secondly, not only the effects of inhibition by eserine but also by DFP, 10^{-3} M, could be reversed by dilution. The first phase of inhibition by DFP has been claimed to be reversible; however, the irreversible phase was stated to set in a few minutes after exposure to strong concentrations of DFP (NACHMANSOHN et al. 1947). Thus, complete restoration of motility upon dilution 14.4 minutes after exposure to DFP (SEAMAN and HOULIHAN o.c., p. 314) is surprising. Data as to whether or not enzyme activity also returned to normal unfortunately are lacking. It is noteworthy that similar restoration of function in the absence of return of enzymic activity was recorded in higher forms (KARCZMAR and KOPPANYI 1953; cf. p. 819).

All in all, the two points adduced introduced a certain degree of doubt as to whether or not the effects of DFP and eserine on *Tetrahymena* were due to their anti-ChE action. Certain other experiments are of interest in this context.

Effects on seeds, cancer cells, and microorganisms. Diethyl p-nitrophenyl phosphate (Para-oxon), diethyl p-nitrophenyl thiophosphate (Parathion), and DFP inhibited, at concentrations varying from 1.8×10^{-6} to 3.4×10^{-5} M, germination and growth of seeds as well as the growth of human tubercle bacilli, and the proliferation of the lymphoblasts of the mouse sarcoma (MENDEL et al. 1953). The growth inhibition was parallel to that of aliesterases; the growth of certain non-malignant fibroblasts and lymphoblasts was not affected.

Some of the studies on ChE's of unicellular organisms suggested a correlation between these enzymes on the one hand and motility or transmission on the other; some of the data, however, indicated that ChE's may play an entirely different role (Chapter 5). It appears now that the studies with anti-ChE agents do not provide the evidence for function-ChE correlation; in fact, they suggest non-cholinesterasic actions of these agents. Finally, the investigations of SEAMAN and HOULIHAN (o.c.) are an illustration of the caution necessary in interpreting effects of anti-ChE agents. All these aspects of *phylogenetic* studies with anti-ChE agents will be frequently encountered in the case of the investigations of *ontogenetic* effects of these agents.

Morphogenetic, toxic, and melanophore effects of anti-ChE agents during ontogenesis

A. Effects of anti-ChE agents on growth and morphogenesis

Action of anti-ChE agents on growth is not confined to unicellular organisms. Also, in the case of multicellular organisms anti-ChE agents exhibit effects on morphogenesis and growth which sometimes occur prior to neurogenesis and development of motility. Antigrowth and morphogenetic effects of anti-ChE agents were studied on the chick, urodele, and insect embryos; cholinomimetic agents were studied on echinoderms, and their actions are of inherent as well as historical interest.

I. Effects of cholinomimetic agents on echinoderm morphogenesis

Immediately after LANGLEY and HEIDENHAIN proposed at the turn of the century that substances such as atropine and pilocarpine act at the autonomic nerve endings, and thus laid the foundation for the theory of cholinergic transmission (DALE 1937), MATHEWS (1902) argued that these substances act directly on the effector cell. This he tried to demonstrate by the effect of these substances on echinoderm development prior to neurogenesis. Pilocarpine (1:25,000 to 1:50,000) considerably speeded and increased the growth of the echinoderm, *Asterias forbesii*, during blastulation and gastrulation. Atropine (1:100,000) had an opposite effect and caused arrest of development and death at the bipinnaria stage. It is of interest that the concentrations used (from 1.5 to 3.2×10^{-7} M) were of the magnitude of those producing effects on isolated mammalian smooth muscle. Subsequently SOLLMAN, in one of his early publications (1904), not only confirmed the findings of MATHEWS (o.c.) but also demonstrated atropine-pilocarpine antagonism during early sea urchin development; even in concentrations not producing growth retardation, atropine prevented growth stimulation by pilocarpine. On the other hand, atropine depression of growth was less easily antagonized by pilocarpine. This then resembles the situation at the parasympathetic mammalian neuroeffectors where pilocarpine cannot easily break through atropine blockade, while atropine readily prevents effects of large doses of pilocarpine. It should be added that SINGER et al. (1960; cf. Chapter 5) demonstrated that high concentrations of atropine inhibit regenerative growth in *Amblystoma*.

Cholinesterases of the developing sea urchin appear first in the blastula; their concentration rises slowly during a lengthy developmental period prior to the onset of a rapid increase, at which moment they have been associated with the ontogenesis of ciliary motility and of intestinal function (Chapter 5). If anti-ChE agents have a pilocarpine-like, stimulant effect on echinoderm development, and if this effect is mediated by ChE's, this would suggest that these enzymes are coupled in these forms not only with function but also with growth. This is, however, entirely speculative, particularly since anti-ChE agents cause in other forms growth inhibition rather than growth stimulation (cf. infra).

II. Effects of eserine and cholinomimetic agents on chick morphogenesis

In the chick embryo, ANCEL (1945, 1950), LANDAUER (1949, 1953a, b, 1954), KARNOFSKY (1955), and BUEKER and PLATNER (1956) established morphogenetic effects of certain cholinomimetic agents and compared their effects with those of eserine and of other anti-ChE agents. These effects can be obtained both prior to and after the beginning of neurogenesis and function. In fact, eserine and pilocarpine could produce death in 24-hr (LANDAUER o.c., ANCEL o.c.) or in 3 to 4-day old (LEVI-MONTALCINI and VISINTIAI 1938) chick embryos.

LEVI-MONTALCINI and VISINTIAI suggested that mortality at 3 to 4 days is due to the cardiac effect of eserine. However, chick heart has probably no ChE at that stage (cf. Chapter 5). Lethality at 24 hrs, i.e., preceding organ formation, cannot be easily explained. Embryos surviving the treatment exhibit after 72 hrs of development absence of caudal vertebrae and of associated soft parts ("rumplessness"); an intermediate condition characterized by imperfectly formed or fused tail vertebrae has also been noticed. As will be seen, these and related malformations occur also when the treatment is applied later.

The question of doses used in these experiments is of importance, as it has a bearing on the specificity of the lethality of the compounds in question. The drugs were injected into the yolk sac, at 24 hrs of incubation or later (KARNOFSKY o.c.). The lowest doses of pilocarpine and of physostigmine employed were 3 and 5 mg, respectively. If the weight of the 24 hrs old chick embryo, inclusive of the membranes, is estimated at 300 mg, these doses would correspond to about 10 g/kg. The frequency of fatilities ranged between 40 and 70%. In the case of the experiments of LEVI-MONTALCINI and VISINTIAI (o.c.), eserine (1:2,000 to 1:40,000) was applied directly to the embryo after removal of the amniotic fluid. These are then very large doses. In the case of other classes of agents, antimetabolites produce lethality of the chick embryo at hundredths or thousandths of a mg per egg (KARNOFSKY o.c.); even in the case of anti-ChE agents, early *Amblystoma* embryos can be killed by many times weaker concentrations of DFP or of neostigmine (cf. infra, p. 805).

Yet, it should not be lightly concluded that these results represent non-specific toxicity or toxicity related to other than cholinomimetic actions of pilocarpine and physostigmine. What militates against this view is that these and certain other cholinomimetic agents cause specific morphogenetic actions which differ from those produced by other teratogens. Moreover, imidazole (LANDAUER 1953a) and presumably many other agents (KARNOFSKY o.c.) proved innocuous at doses similar to that which produced death in the case of pilocarpine and physostigmine. Finally, a clear-cut relationship between the dose and the extent and frequency of morphogenetic action could be established (LANDAUER 1954). It should be stated, however, that acetylcholine (ACh) and atropine (BUEKER and PLATNER o.c.) proved ineffective.

ANCEL (1945, 1950) was the first to notice the characteristic effects of eserine when this agent is injected at later stages, particularly after 4 days of incubation. He described particularly bone defects affecting the beak, the long bones of the lower extremities and, sometimes, the lower vertebrae ("rumplessness"). LANDAUER (1953a and b, 1954) described this condition in more detail and compared it with that produced by pilocarpine. These studies were pursued further by KARNOFSKY (1955) and BUEKER and PLATNER (1956), and extended to neostigmine and to certain quaternary neostigmine analogs (KARNOFSKY et al. 1954). While on the whole the effects of all these agents were similar and included weak anti-growth action, "rumplessness," and related bone effects, interesting differences between the compounds were also noticed.

Table 1. *Teratogenic effects of cholinomimetic agents and other substances on chick embryo development. Agents injected into the yolk sac on the 4th day of incubation*
Data from LANDAUER (1954), KARNOFSKY (1955), and BUEKER and PLATNER (1956).

Teratogenic substance	Facial skeleton	Long bones of leg	Toes	Other defects (usually with relatively low incidence)
Sulfanil-amide	Parrot beak	Micromelia (bending of tibiotarsus)	Syndactylism	Clubbed down
Physo-stigmine	Parrot beak	Micromelia (bending of tibiotarsus)	Syndactylism (relatively rare)	Clubbed down; "wry neck" and "rumplessness"
Insulin	Short upper or parrot beak, rarely facial coloboma	Micromelia (maximal shortness and bending of tibiotarsus)	Syndactylism (low incidence)	Microphthalmia, buphthalmia, coloboma of upper lid
Boric acid	Short lower beak, facial coloboma, cleft palate	Micromelia (maximal shortness and bending of tarsometatarsus)	Syndactylism (shortening or lack of toes, preferentially of 4th toe)	Curled toe, paralysis
Pilocarpine	Depending on dose: short upper and parrot beak or short lower beak, facial coloboma, and cleft palate	Micromelia (maximal shortness and bending of tarsometatarsus)	Syndactylism (shortening or lack of 1st toe)	Clubbed down, microphthalmia, coloboma of upper lid; never "wry neck" or "rumplessness"
Thallium	Parrot beak	Micromelia (bending of femur and tibiotarsus)	—	Microphthalmia
Quaternary ammonium compds. (TMA, neo-stigmine)	—	Slight micromelia	—	"Wry neck" and "rumplessness"

Eserine produced "parrot beak" (shortening of the mandible and downward curvature of the upper beak). Outside of the facial region, it caused frequently long-bones malformations (micromelia) and rarely syndactylism. At low doses (0.5 mg/egg) it caused also slight thoracic and lumbar kyphosis and retarded formation of eyelids; high doses (1 to 15 mg/egg) induced defects and fissures in the external auditory meatus, shortening of cervical ("wry neck", KARNOFSKY 1955) and thoracic vertebrae ("rumplessness"), bends in the vertebral column, ankylosis, fusion, and defects of the vertebrae. Among rarer effects of physostigmine were atrophic changes in central and autonomic neurones (BUEKER and PLATNER, o.c.) and clubbed down (LANDAUER 1954). Anterior horn cells were hypoplastic or atrophied, the spinal cord was missing in sacral and coccygeal regions, and the brain and brainstem reduced in size. Spinal and sympathetic ganglia were well differentiated but fused.

Neostigmine produced effects resembling those of physostigmine with regard to kyphosis, ankylosis, "wry neck" and "rumplessness," defects in the external auditory meatus, and to malformation of the eyelids; it also mimicked physostigmine in some of the rarer effects of the latter, such as some atrophy of the autonomic and central nervous systems. However, it never produced appendicular or beak changes (KARNOFSKY o.c.). Somewhat similar effects were produced by methyl nicotinium bromide, trimethyl vinyl ammonium chloride, as well as 8 other quaternary compounds; they caused "wry neck" and, in higher doses, growth inhibition, skeletal abnormalities such as micromelia, and edema (KARNOFSKY et al. 1954). Some thirty other quaternary compounds were not effective. Unfortunately, their structures and anti-ChE potencies were not given. It is likely that at least the two neostigmine analogs, methyl nicotinium and trimethyl vinyl ammonium, produced ChE inhibition at the dose of 1 to 10 mg/egg (presumably but not explicitly used).

Finally, *pilocarpine* (0.5 to 12 mg per embryo weighing 5 to 7 g, inclusive of membranes) resembled physostigmine in that it produced beak changes, micromelia, and sometimes clubbed down; however, micromelia was produced only by larger doses, and differed somewhat from that produced by physostigmine; the "parrot beak," so characteristic for physostigmine, occurred relatively rarely with pilocarpine. Shortening of the lower beak occurred usually in the absence of upper beak changes. Vertebral fusion and "wry neck" never occurred with pilocarpine. On the other hand, pilocarpine caused microphthalmia, cleft palate, and triangular coloboma of the upper lip, never caused by physostigmine, as well as syndactylism, only rarely produced by the latter. Finally, while physostigmine and pilocarpine produced sometimes clubbed down, pilocarpine caused a change of pigmentation in certain chick strains. It was not stated clearly whether the pigmentation effect was obtained only with pilocarpine or also with other cholinomimetic agents used (LANDAUER 1953b and 1954). Syndactilism occurred more frequently with pilocarpine than with eserine; it is of interest that pilocarpine, particularly in the case of the lower dose of 3 mg/egg, produced syndactylism independently from, and in absence of, micromelia. Bending of the tibiotarsus was more frequent with pilocarpine, and of the tarsometatarsus with eserine. However, the tarsometatarsus was affected by large doses of pilocarpine. Finally, pilocarpine shortened the first toe and produced syndactylism with regard to the 3rd and 4th toe; physostigmine syndactylism while rare, was less restricted.

An interesting finding with pilocarpine was the induction of white pigmentation in Black Minorca embryos (LANDAUER 1953b and 1954); non-pigmented feathers persisted through the first and disappeared in subsequent plumage. The extents of the skeletal and pigment abnormalities were related; moreover, treatment during developmental periods when skeletal abnormalities could not be invoked (cf. below) did not produce pigment abnormalities. This may have a significance with reference to the mechanism of the morphogenetic action of the cholinomimetic agents (cf. infra).

III. Comment

Are pilocarpine and physostigmine teratologies due to their cholinomimetic action? Cholinesterase is present within the first day of development of the chick embryo which is the time when pilocarpine and physostigmine can be lethal; "rumplessness" and other teratologies cannot be produced before 72 hours of development, which is the time of appearance of ACh (Chapter 5). In fact, BUEKER and PLATNER (1956) suggested that teratologies may be due to muscle contraction; these teratologies would resemble then the "bent" body produced in *Amblystoma* by physostigmine (SAWYER 1943a; vide infra). However, the "bent" could be alleviated by surgery of the muscles and caused no spinal abnormalities; altogether, it seems unlikely that the teratologies in the chick are due to effects of drugs on cholinergic neuromyal transmission. On the other hand, cholinomimetic agents could cause teratologies by affecting the hypothetical relationship between the cholinergic system and growth and morphogenesis.

However, a cholinergic effect should not require concentrations which were necessary to produce teratologies. Also, the teratologies produced by cholinomimetic agents resembled those produced by boric acid, insulin, sulfanilamide, and thallium (Table 1), which militates against the specificity of teratologic action of pilocarpine and physostigmine and against the likelihood that this action is mediated cholinergically. On the other hand, LANDAUER (1954) suggested "physiological relatedness" between these two groups of agents and postulated that they interfere with carbohydrate metabolism. In support of this he cited the fact that agents capable of affecting carbohydrate metabolism can antagonize these malformations, that curled-toe paralysis induced by boric acid resembles the defect due to a flavin-deficient diet of the mothers, that the liver of malformed chicks was found grossly deficient in riboflavin, and finally, that insulin malformations were coincidental with inhibition of glycogenolysis (ZWILLING 1951). Unfortunately, there is no available evidence of the possible effect on carbohydrate metabolism of pilocarpine, physostigmine, or of the quaternary ammonium compounds. Also, malformations similar to these due to insulin can be brought about by sulfanil-amide in the absence of hypoglycemia (LANDAUER 1954).

It should be borne in mind also that while general similarity exists between malformations induced by neostigmine, pilocarpine, eserine, thallium, insulin, sulfanilamide, and boric acid, they also differ from each other in detail (Table 1), and with regard to the developmental period at which they were most effective; finally, the effectiveness of biochemical antagonists differed with regard to various agents enumerated.

It can be speculated therefore, that the compounds in question differ and that they affect specific sequential steps of morphogenesis, which is also the mechanism of developmental action of genes and gene "modifiers".

LANDAUER (1954) suggested that genes, gene "modifiers", and teratogens behave similarly; for instance, sensitivities to teratogens and to genic influences exhibit sharp peaks at certain characteristic development periods. Phenocopies obtained by interaction of genes and gene "modifiers" can be mimicked by various teratogens, including eserine and pilocarpine, or by combining genic factors with teratogens.

IV. Toxic actions of anti-ChE agents on Fundulus and Amblystoma embryos

Early toxic actions of anti-ChE agents similar to those noticed in the chick were observed in the urodeles *Amblystoma punctatum* or *opacum* and in *Fundulus*. In the case of *Amblystoma*, a small percentage of blastulae (HARRISON's stage 8) exo-gastrulated in a 10^{-10} M solution of di*iso*propyl phosphorofluoridate (DFP), while stronger solutions caused death at a rate depending on the concentration (KARCZMAR and KOPPANYI 1953). Similar effects were reported with physostigmine and neostigmine (SAWYER 1947).

It is of interest that some of the concentrations of DFP employed were probably too weak to cause significant enzymic inhibition. However, concentrations of eserine and of neostigmine (0.01 and 0.03%, respectively) which affected somewhat growth and morphogenesis, partic-ularly at earlier stages, should have inhibited ChE's. At 0.1%, neostigmine completely in-hibited growth at the premotile stage 30, although this concentration was well tolerated after stage 40. Resistance to DFP may also increase during development; particularly, embryos of stages 8 to 26 may be less resistant to DFP than motile larvae of stage 34 or older (KARCZMAR and KOPPANYI 1953, KARCZMAR 1955). Similarly in *Fundulus*, eserine (2.5×10^{-4} M) applied at the blastula stage killed the embryos within a week, that is, after somatic movements had developed but prior to the onset of swimming (SAWYER 1944; see also Chapter 5). If eserine was applied at later stages, death occurred more rapidly; this may indicate not so much lower resistances of older *Fundulus* embryos, which would be the reverse of what occurs in *Amblystoma*, but that early, prolonged treatment induces some degree of adaptation (SAWYER o.c.).

In *Amblystoma* larvae of stage 60, death latency also depended upon the con-centration of DFP (KARCZMAR and KOPPANYI 1953).

Larvae could remain alive for weeks in weaker (10^{-7} to 10^{-9} M) concentrations of DFP, exhibiting alternately convulsions and tonic contractures, or for hours or days in stronger (10^{-5} to 10^{-6} M) solutions, exhibiting, after initial convulsions and contracture, flaccid pa-ralysis. In the latter case, viability could be determined only by observation of cardiac func-tion and of gill circulation. KARCZMAR and KOPPANYI (o.c.) claimed that complete inhibition of larval ChE's occurred within the 10^{-5} to 10^{-7} M range of DFP concentration, and that the survival time was a function of DFP concentration rather than of enzyme inhibition. Since, moreover, atropine prolonged life but did not affect DFP convulsions and did not delay their onset, it was concluded that DFP toxicity in the *Amblystoma* larvae was not entirely cholin-ergic in nature, and could not depend solely upon inhibition of ChE's. However, it must be stressed that difference of opinion exists as to the concentration of DFP capable of inhibiting completely larval ChE's (cf. infra, p. 817).

It should be pointed out that earliest morphogenetic and toxic actions of anti-ChE's occur prior to ontogenesis of organ systems and of cardiovascular or nervous function. The enzyme is present at these stages in the case of all Amphibia investigated; it may be present only in trace or small amounts during early development of *Fundulus* (cf. Chapter 5). Altogether, the early morphogenetic and toxic actions of anti-ChE agents may be not cholinergically mediated, and can be related to their teratologic actions on the chick embryo.

V. Morphogenetic effects of anti-ChE agents on urodele embryos and larvae

Anti-ChE agents caused certain morphogenetic effects when applied relatively late in development to premotile (stage 25) or motile (stage 46) *Amblystoma* larvae.

Free-swimming larvae were reared in half-strength Holtfreter solution or in pond water in which the drugs were dissolved. SAWYER (1943a and 1947) used neostigmine and physostigmine at concentrations ranging from 0.0001 to 0.1%. Generally, physostigmine was used at 0.01% (1.5×10^{-4} M) and neostigmine at 0.03% (10^{-3} M); these concentrations are a hundred to a thousand times stronger than those sufficient to inhibit AChE and non-specific ChE *in vitro*. KOPPANYI and KARCZMAR (1947) and KARCZMAR and KOPPANYI (1953) used neostigmine and eserine at 10^{-5} to 10^{-7} M; fresh DFP solutions (10^{-5} to 10^{-9} M) were prepared daily.

Treatment with physostigmine and neostigmine applied at premotile stages caused considerable shortening and a "bent" trunk by stage 37 or 38 (SAWYER 1943a and 1947, KOPPANYI and KARCZMAR 1947, KARCZMAR and KOPPANYI 1953). The larvae remained for a long time in opistho-or pleurothotonos, which superficially resembled the "wry neck" and "rumplessness" described for similarly treated chick embryos. This, however, was not due to a permanent morphogenetic effect on the vertebral column, since the bend (and presumably the shortening) of the trunk could be alleviated by cutting the contracted muscles of the concave side (SAWYER 1943a).

More permanent changes, noticed at stage 41, occurred after treatment with physostigmine or DFP. These agents, as well as ACh, methacholine (Mecholyl, MeCh), and carbaminoylcholine (0.01 to 0.05%, SAWYER 1943a) produced shortening, slight broadening, and decrease in the size of the head ("heterogony," KOPPANYI and KARCZMAR 1947). Physostigmine produced also shrinking of the dorsal fin and considerable reduction of the size of gills. Neostigmine-treated larvae exhibited just the opposite effect; their gills became somewhat longer and the caudal fin higher than those of the controls (SAWYER o.c.).

Since SAWYER (o.c.) observed also with cholinomimetic stimulants pigment changes which normally remain under pituitary control, he applied these agents to hypophysectomized larvae (cf. p. 807) for detailed description); again, physostigmine was effective while neostigmine was either inactive or stimulated gill and tail growth. He concluded therefore that the effect of physostigmine was not mediated centrally or via the pituitary but that it was due to direct peripheral action. He ascribed physostigmine-produced gill atrophy to visually observed constriction of peripheral capillaries in the gill filaments; the additional evidence for this was that epinephrine, which in *Amblystoma* gill produces capillary vasodilation, caused in contradistinction to eserine, an increase in the length of the filaments. However, epinephrine, just as eserine, caused reduction of the height of the caudal fin, and SAWYER concluded that both these agents must cause vasoconstriction of the fin capillaries. It is not clear, however, why the effects of neostigmine on the gill and the tail were opposite to those of eserine; the limiting effect of the quaternary nitrogen atom of neostigmine on the penetration of this compound might account for this difference, even though the actions in question are probably peripheral. Finally, atropine could not reverse either eserine or neostigmine effects on the fin and gills.

It must be pointed out that the effects of physostigmine and DFP other than those on the gills and the fin (for instance anti-ChE "heterogony") are not likely to have been also due to circulatory changes. It may be then that the heterogonic, gill, and fin effects of anti-ChE agents in *Amblystoma* constitute genuine morphogenetic actions. They may be then related to anti-growth and teratologic effects of anti-ChE agents on the early chick, *Fundulus*, and *Amblystoma* embryo. The speculations on the mechanism of these actions were already presented (cf. supra, pp. 804 and 805), and the doubt as to its cholinergic nature expressed. Similarly, the morphogenetic action of anti-ChE agents in *Amblystoma* larvae may be not related to the cholinergic system at all. This may be indicated by the difference between morphogenetic effects in *Amblystoma* of physostigmine, on the one hand, and neostigmine on the other, as well as by the ineffectiveness of atropine in reversing the effects of physostigmine.

B. Melanophore effects of anti-ChE agents during larval development of Amblystoma

I. Pituitary versus nervous control of amphibian color system

Amphibian and fish melanophore systems are sensitive to cholinominetic agents (for review, cf. PARKER 1943, PROSSER 1950, and BROWN 1950). While studying the functional effects of anti-ChE agents in the course of *Amblystoma* development, SAWYER (1943a and b) noticed that these agents affect also the melanophores. His subsequent publication (1947) deals with this problem in detail. To understand better the significance of his experiments, a brief review of color changes in amphibians and fishes is indicated.

Color changes in fishes and amphibians depend on a combination of physiological and morphological factors; the former involve concentration and dispersion[1] of the pigment, and the latter its accumulation and chemical production (cf. BROWN 1950). While tactile, environmental, and psychic (cf. KLEINHOLZ 1938) factors affect chromatophores, the ratio of light striking the animal or its eye directly to the light reflected from the background is by far the most important single environmental factor. This ratio is large when a black background is illuminated and small when the background is white; the animals become dark and pale, respectively, in these two situations, independently of the intensity of total illumination. General illumination is a less important factor; the pigment disperses in light, and concentrates in darkness. These changes can be primary, and due to responses of skin or chromatophores, or they can be secondary and produced via the eyes. During development the primary phase naturally predominates till functionalization of the eyes.

The amphibian color system is thought to depend on pituitary rather than on nervous control. First of all, direct innervation of amphibian melanophores has never been demonstrated. Secondly, the extirpation of the pars tuberalis causes maximal dispersion of melanophores and cessation of response to the background; finally, the removal of the posterior or intermediate lobe produces maximal pallor, while the removal of the anterior lobe of the pituitary does not affect melanophore response. It was accordingly postulated (HOGBEN and WINTON 1923, HOGBEN and SLOME 1931) that a lightening substance (W) is secreted by the pars tuberalis, while a darkening substance B (probably intermedin) is released by the intermediate lobe; the state of pigmentation depends upon the interplay between these antagonistic substances.

Fishes, to the contrary, can exhibit either nervous or hormonal control of chromatophores, or both, depending on species. Hormonal control may be phylogenetically older and it predominates in elasmobranchs. As in *Amphibia*, the hormonal factors are located in the fishes in the pituitary, intermedin (substance B) being released from the posterior lobe; the body-blanching principle (substance W) is also usually present. Chromatophore innervation can be either double with separate dispersing and concentrating fibers, or single concerned only with concentrating the pigment. The dispersing and concentrating fibers release presumably ACh and adrenalin, respectively (PARKER 1940); the evidence for the release of either substance from pertinent fibers and for their role in the control of melanophores is strictly "pharmacologic" (cf. PARKER 1943).

II. Cholinergic control of Amblystoma melanophores

In his experiments SAWYER (1947) used *Amblystoma punctatum* and *Triturus torosus* larvae of pre-motile (stage 25), free-swimming (stage 46), and finally early feeding stages. The secondary visual melanophore response replaces in these forms the primary or pre-pituitary response at stages 37 to 40. Hypophysectomies were performed during stages 28 to 31; they included removal of not only the buccal rudiment but also the floor of the third ventricle. Larvae were kept against northern exposure with a light (tan paper) background, observations always being made between 2 and 4 p.m. While the experiments were carried out over several years and seasonal change of light might have occurred, the epidermis of the control animals shown in SAWYER's (o.c.) figures had a uniform, moderately light coloration. The melanophore concentration or dispersion of the drug-treated animals was qualitatively compared with the skin color of the control larvae, and this was expressed in terms of lightness or darkness. Occasionally, the melanophore index is said to have been used (cf. HOGBEN and SLOME, o.c.). Photography was performed under chloretone (1 : 3,000) anesthesia, which is said to cause

---

[1] Pigment "dispersion," synonymous with "expansion," leads to darkening, and pigment "contraction" or "concentration" leads to lightening of the color of the epidermis and dermis.

melanophore expansion only after a delay. The melanophore-expanding hormone (substance B) was prepared from desiccated mammalian posterior pituitary as a "potentiated" (by the method of CHEN and GEILING 1943) extract (U.S.P. XII); one "unit" consisted of 3.75 cc of the potentiated U.S.P. extract diluted to 15 cc.

In *Amblystoma*, melanophores appear first at stage 34, the pituitary develops during stages 37 to 40, while hormone B (intermedin) was reported present at stage 39. Larvae treated from stage 25 on with 0.01% eserine or 0.03% neostigmine showed dispersion of the pigment (darkening) beginning at stage 37; between stages 41 and 46 the effect of eserine was greater. Sixty percent of animals treated by DFP (0.001%, or 5.4×10^{-5} M) at stage 33 became dark from stage 41 on; dispersion was never as marked as that due to eserine and neostigmine. The action of drugs was faster when they were applied after the appearance of melanophores; when used at stages 45 or 46, eserine was effective in 10 minutes.

Somewhat similar results were obtained with ACh and MeCh (0.05%), and carboaminoylcholine (Doryl, 0.01%). Acetylcholine was particularly effective at stages 37 to 40; the results were variable later; the effects of eserine-ACh or eserine-MeCh combinations resembled essentially those obtained with eserine alone. The effects of ACh or MeCh were blocked by atropine (0.025%) at stages 37 to 41, particularly when atropine was applied early; atropine alone produced some blanching during these stages. Later, however, atropine alone produced darkening of the larvae, and neither then nor at any other stage could it antagonize eserine or neostigmine-produced melanophore dispersion. Finally, the dispersion of melanophores by cholinomimetic agents was only partially antagonized by transferring the animals into darkness, although treated larvae were darker in light than in darkness.

The first blanching of hypophysectomized (stages 28 to 31) non-treated larvae was noticed at stage 41. These larvae were darkened by stages 38 to 40 by eserine, ACh, and neostigmine as much as intact, treated larvae. Later, the effect of cholinomimetic agents decreased till after stage 45 hypophysectomized larvae treated with neostigmine or ACh were as light as hypophysectomized, non-treated larvae; eserine retained some effect through stage 46; this effect again was not counteracted by atropine. Finally, intermedin did not synergise with eserine or neostigmine at stages 43 to 45, at which intermedin could darken the hypophysectomized larvae.

Whenever cholinomimetic and anti-ChE agents produced darkening, both dermal and epidermal melanophores were dispersed and the number of free pigment granules in the epidermal cells augmented; thus, both physiological and morphological changes (vide supra) were involved.

It is of interest that epinephrine produced darkening during pre-pituitary and pituitary phases of development in both intact and hypophysectomized animals; the response declined later in development. Essentially, the mechanism of action of epinephrine is then peripheral, and it becomes unoperative at later stages. In the adult frog and in the case of dually innervated melanophores of adult fish, epinephrine seems to contract the melanophores. Unfortunately, no work has been done on larval or embryonic forms of these animals. Finally, whether in intact or hypophysectomised larvae, nicotine did not affect melanophores at concentrations short of toxic (0.00,001%).

III. Comment

SAWYER suggested that these findings indicate two developmental phases of the cholinergic effect upon melanophores. During the *pre-pituitary phase* of drug responsiveness (stages 37 to 40), cholinomimetic agents stimulate melanophores directly; this is indicated by equipotent action of the quaternary and tertiary ChE inhibitors, and by atropine blockade of melanophore dispersion during this phase. During the *pituitary phase* of drug responsiveness (stages 41 to 46) cholinomimetic agents stimulate some central cholinergic mechanism leading to secretion of intermedin. This is suggested by the ineffectiveness of cholinomimetic agents, and by their lack of synergism with exogenous intermedin, in *hypophysectomized* larvae of stage 45 or 46, as well as by the fact that eserinized or neostigmine-treated intact larvae morphologically resemble BLOUNT's (1932) triple pituitary animals (cf. pp. 806).

Since the pituitary develops in *Amblystoma* during stages 37 to 40, and since in hypophysectomized larvae ACh and neostigmine cause dispersion till stage 45 and eserine even longer, some overlapping between the periods of central and peripheral control may occur.

SAWYER speculated further that the central action of cholinomimetic agents is directed actually not at the pituitary but at the hypothalamus. Indeed, in *Amblystoma*, electric or mechanical stimulation of the hypothalamus causes melanophore dispersion (SHEN 1939); the hypothalamus can in turn activate hypothalamico-hypophysial fibers which, as HERRICK (1939, 1942) has shown, enter the pars intermedia in *Amblystoma* larvae of stages 41 to 46. The median eminence, with its portal system to the adenohypophysis (GREEN 1947), may be also involved. Finally, in mammals, anti-ChE and cholinomimetic agents affect the pituitary, presumably by their action upon the hypothalamus (DUKE et al. 1950; v. also Chapter 6).

It is of interest that at the prepituitary stages, non-innervated *Amblystoma* melanophores respond to anti-ChE and cholinomimetic agents similarly to innervated melanophores of the adult fish (PARKER 1943). It may be speculated that the amphibian color system may have evolved from the innervated system of fishes and maintained its responsiveness, at least during a part of its embryonic development, after having lost its innervation.

Altogether, the behavior of *Amblystoma* melanophores as suggested by SAWYER is somewhat puzzling. While their response would be analogous to that of denervated muscle or of embryonic heart prior to its innervation, the melanophore would then be an organ which is ontogenically never innervated, and which possesses a cholinergic receptor early in development and loses it later on. It is also strange that the emergence of central cholinergic control occurs at the time of the loss of the peripheral response rather than at that of the appearance of intermedin (stage 39), and that the quaternary compound neostigmine should exhibit central effects during post-pituitary stages, although neostigmine may cause central actions upon prolonged treatment (KARCZMAR and KOPPANYI 1953, vide infra, p. 816).

It is also difficult to understand how ACh not only escaped hydrolysis in the course of its absorbtion when used without anti-ChE agents, but also crossed the blood-brain barrier to act on the hypothalamus. In the adult frog, ACh and eserine had either no effect in some experiments (STOPPANI 1942, TEAGUE et al. 1939) or caused direct melanophore expansion (SHEN 1939). Finally, SAWYER stated that he used quantitative measurement of melanophore dispersion only occasionally; thus, his observation of the lack of synergism between extrinsic intermedin and cholinomimetic agents which seems to weigh heavily on his conclusions (cf. supra and o.c., p. 163), may be open to revision.

It could be then speculated that DFP, neostigmine, ACh, and other cholinomimetic drugs act peripherally and that their loss of effectiveness at stages 45—46 in hypophysectomized animals may be due to a change of skin or melanophore permeability in the absence of an intact adrenal-pituitary axis; indeed, decrease of sensitivity to epinephrine occurred in older, both hypophysectomized and intact, larvae.

C. Effects of anti-ChE agents on insect development

I. Early and late ovicidal action of anti-ChE agents

Economic interest in the control of pests led to basic findings on the biology of insects and particularly on the mechanism of action of organophosphorus anti-ChE agents as among the best and most popular means of chemical pest control (cf. Chapters 5 and 16). This action can be directed against the adult and also against the egg and the embryo; the ovicidal effect will be reviewed at present in the light of the data on ontogenesis of insect ChE's (Chapter 5).

The methods used for measuring ChE's have already been described (Chapters 4 and 5). The treatment of insect eggs with anti-ChE agents constitutes an art, and the interpretation of data depends on its full understanding. While this point cannot be covered fully here, the differences between commonly used techniques as well as certain precautions sometimes disregarded will be mentioned briefly.

Eggs can be subjected to anti-ChE agents by dipping them for varying lengths of time in anti-ChE preparations; or by exposing them in their natural habitat, e.g., upon oviposition on the leaf, to an anti-ChE spray, vapor, or "residue"; or by exposing them to treated filter paper; or finally, by injecting the eggs with various agents. Each method and anti-ChE preparation has its own pecularities: when eggs are dipped in an anti-ChE solution or emulsion, it has to be ascertained whether they are actually submerged or stay on the surface of the preparation (HOLZ 1949); also, emulsions, solutions, or vapors may have different stabilities and penetrating powers, and the results obtained with different preparations thus may greatly differ (SMITH and AVENS 1954).

With regard to the manner of observing and recording the data, it is particularly important that the eggs are closely watched after treatment. If this is disregarded, an ovicidal effect may be assumed, whereas actually the development proceeded normally and larvae were killed after hatching by coming into contact with insecticide residue or by ingesting it. Finally, it has to be clearly recognized that lack of ovicidal effect may simply mean that the anti-ChE agent was incapable of penetrating into the egg rather than that it could not kill the embryo; this can be obviated theoretically by injecting the agent into the egg, which is difficult and rarely tried.

An early impression was that anti-ChE agents do not affect the eggs, and that their toxic action is directed at the larvae; as the larvae chew their way out of the chorion, they come into contact with the insecticide present as the surface residue or in the chorion (HOLZ 1949, SCHWARZ 1950, SPEYER 1950, SCHUHMANN 1953). SCHUHMANN (o.c.), for instance, concluded that Parathion is dissolved in the egg shell and the larvae are poisoned on attempting to emerge. Some data indicate that at least in certain forms this is not so.

The data of SMITH and AVENS (1954) indicate that field control in the case of the peach tree borer *Sanninoidea exitiosa* (Say) is due largely to the ovicidal action. Peach borer eggs can be killed by a 2-minute immersion in Parathion suspension (425 to 3400 p.p.m.; SMITH 1955); it is true that the susceptibility increases with age and reaches 100% at 7 days of incubation, i.e., $1^1/_2$ days before hatching, but even at 3 days the lowest concentration used killed 59% of eggs. Moreover, when SMITH sandwiched the eggs between filter paper sheets impregnated by Parathion, 0.035%, susceptibility was greatest at the 1st day of development. It is not known why the direction of the change of susceptibility with age should depend upon the mode of exposure. In fact, other workers recorded either limited change of susceptibility (POTTER 1958) or an increase of susceptibility with age (SCHWARTZ 1950, SALKELD and POTTER 1953, POTTER et al. 1957). Another unexplained finding of SMITH (o.c.) was that while the susceptibility decreases with age continually in the case of exposure of eggs to insecticidal residues, there is a sharp break in the ascent of susceptibility with age in the case of direct exposure.

Ovicidal toxicity of organophosphorus compounds was also reported in the case of the housefly (MEHROTRA and SMALLMAN 1957); the flour moth, *Ephestia kuehniella*; the tomato moth, *Diataraxia oleracea* (LORD and POTTER 1951); milkweed bug, *Oncopeltus fasciatus* (SMITH and WAGENKNECHT 1956); the white butterfly, *Pieris brassicae* (POTTER et al. 1957); and certain aphids, psyllids, and red spider mites (HOLZ 1949, SCHWARZ 1950).

While the ovicidal action of organophosphorus compounds seems thus well substantiated, the finding of early ovicidal action has to be particularly analysed; indeed, ovicidal effect recorded very early in embryonic development may indicate that the toxicity is unrelated to ChE's or to the nervous system. Certain data suggest that this indeed may be the case.

LORD and POTTER (1951) found that while a large percentage of eggs of two moths formed highly developed embryos before death in the case of low (0.0391 to 0.1562%, weight per volume) concentrations of TEPP (tetraethylpyrophosphate), a complete cessation of growth occurred with higher concentrations (up to 0.625%). Similarly, the tomato moth egg showed no development whatsoever if treated within 24 hrs of oviposition with 0.0004 cc of "HETP-TEPP" ("hexaethyltetraphosphate", a mixture of compounds of which TEPP is the major active component) mixture or with Parathion. In the case of the white butterfly (*P. brassicae*; POTTER et al. 1957) some eggs did not develop past stages B or C if treated when newly laid with strong concentrations of TEPP, or past stage E when kept in 0.29 to 2.6% solutions (Chapter 5, Fig. 2); even when the TEPP concentration was only 0.02 to 0.03%, about 10% of eggs died relatively undeveloped.

Similarly, low concentrations of organophosphorus anti-ChE agents prevented hatching, while high concentrations interfered with or stopped the development of the potato beetle, *Leptinotarsa decemlineata* (SCHWARTZ 1950). Finally, it may be that developmental block cannot be produced in some forms: using Parathion, HOLZ (1949) could not affect development of walking sticks *(Phasmidae)* or geometrid moths *(Geometridae)*, while he could produce developmental arrest in silkworms, ophids, psyllids, and certain mites. Also, related anti-ChE agents may produce ovicidal actions either early or late in development; when eggs of the silkworm, *Bombyx mori*, were treated with Paraoxon and Parathion after 14 days of incubation, toxicity arose 3 and 8 days later, respectively, i.e., some 7 and 3 days before hatching (STAUDENMAYER 1955, 1957).

It is of interest that when development could be arrested by the anti-ChE agents, it could generally be stopped also by agents such as Selinon (structural designation unavailable) or carbolic acid derivatives, compounds devoid of anti-ChE action (HOLZ o.c.).

On the other hand, at least in some cases early ovicidal treatment caused no or little immediate developmental changes, and death occurred not long before hatching; in some cases fully developed embryos were present at hatching but failed to emerge or finally died soon after hatching.

In the case of the housefly with the incubation time of 12 hours, exposure to Parathion (2%) residue on filter paper did not arrest development; young flies developed fully but failed to emerge (MEHROTRA and SMALLMAN, o.c.). Similarly in the case of the peach tree borer, incubation period $8^{1}/_{2}$ days, treatment at one day did not affect development. In fact, neither the respiratory rate nor its increase in the course of development was blocked for most of the incubation time; one day prior to hatching respiration ceased to increase, and gradually declined (SMITH and WAGENKNECHT 1956). This was by and large true in the case of low (425) and high (3400 p.p.m.) concentrations of Parathion, and also was independent of the time of treatment; there was, however, an indication that earlier treatment or treatment with higher concentrations of Parathion caused earlier cessation of the increase of respiratory rate.

II. Relationship of the ovicidal effect of organophosphorus compounds to enzymic inhibition and neurogenesis

Two viewpoints were advanced with respect to the mechanism of the ovicidal action of organophosphorus compounds in insects.

1. Implication of ChE and nervous system in ovicidal action

SMITH, SMALLMAN and their associates pointed out that extremely high concentrations of anti-ChE agents were necessary to kill the eggs during early embryonic development, stressed the delayed character of ovicidal treatment, related delayed toxicity to the appearance of the nervous system and of ChE's, and generally correlated ovicidal effect with ChE inhibition.

When peach tree borer eggs were treated with Parathion on the first day of incubation, ChE inhibition occurred following its ontogenetic appearance 3 days later (SMITH and WAGEN-KNECHT 1956; cf. Chapters 5 and 16). Moreover, when eggs of Parathion-insensitive milkweed bugs and Parathion-sensitive peach tree borer were treated between the 4th and 7th day of development, inhibition of the enzyme *in vivo* was proportional to the ovicidal action of Parathion in these two species; 85% inhibition and toxicity occurred in the case of borer eggs exposed to 0.035% Parathion, while the enzyme was only slightly inhibited and there was no death in the case of milkweed bug eggs treated with 0.1% Parathion. *In vitro*, the enzymes of the two species exhibited similar, quite high ID_{50} values of 3×10^{-8} M; independently of the concentration used, inhibition was never higher than 90%. The residual ChE activities of the borer eggs were about the same in the case of experiments *in vitro* and *in vivo*. No further inhibition occurred when breis obtained from the eggs treated *in vivo* were further treated *in vitro*; thus, the enzyme remaining active after the treatment *in vivo* must have been identical with the residual enzyme of the experiments *in vitro*. These data were taken to indicate that differential resistance of the milkweed bug and peach tree borer is related to the degree of ChE inhibition *in vivo*, which in turn depends upon extent of absorbtion; in fact, the nymphs of the milkweed bug are susceptible to Parathion. It must be pointed out, however, that *in vivo* Parathion is oxidised to a more potent anti-ChE agent; thus, the similarity of Parathion inhibitory potency *in vitro* against ChE's of the two species may have no bearing on occurrences *in vivo*.

Finally, housefly eggs exposed to Parathion as early as at 1 hour after oviposition showed complete inhibition of the enzyme at 11 hours, as well as increase of ACh concentration (MEHROTRA and SMALLMAN 1957), and silkworm eggs treated with eserine early in development exhibited an increase in ACh after $8^{1}/_{2}$ days of incubation which was 100% greater than that recorded in controls (CHINO 1957). Accumulation of ACh after insecticide treatment is important since it provides a mechanism for toxicity.

SMITH suggested therefore (cf. SMALLMAN and FISHER 1958) that the mechanism of ovicidal action following early treatment with organophosphorus compounds depends on retention of the insecticide in the eggs after treatment till it can act when ChE's and the nervous system are present. It can be quoted in support of this "storage" theory that eggs treated with Parathion can inhibit ChE *in vitro* (SMITH and WAGENKNECHT 1956); SMITH also auggested that such a storage can occur even in the case of the water-unstable TEPP (KARCZMAR and LONG 1958, HOLMSTEDT 1959), provided it is stored in the lipid fraction of the egg. Death would occur then at a rather advanced stage of embryonic development, usually just before hatching, and it would be due to accumulation of ACh.

There are several difficulties in accepting fully this theory. It is based to an extent on data obtained with Parathion. Yet, probably not all ovicidal action of Paraoxon, a compound generally conceived to be the metabolite responsible for the anti-ChE effect of Parathion, is due to ChE inhibition, since oxygen consumption decreased in Paraoxon-treated *Bombyx* eggs 7 days before hatching and two days before the appearance of ChE (STAUDENMAYER 1957; Chapter 16).

There is also some doubt as to the association of ACh accumulation with death. While it occurs also in adult insects (SMALLMAN and FISHER o.c.) as well as in mammals poisoned by anti-ChE agent's (cf. for instance DUBOIS et al. 1949 and MICHAELIS et al. 1954), this can be caused also by other than anti-ChE treatment (cf. Chapter 16). Moreover, although high levels of ACh were found in the heads of *hatched* houseflies treated with DFP, this rise was followed by a fall to normal values within 2 hrs, death ensuing many hours later (WINTERINGHAM and HARRISON 1956).

Generally, ACh does not accumulate in the adult, following anti-ChE treatment, consistently enough (SMALLMAN and FISHER 1958, LEWIS and FOWLER 1956) to account for death (WINTERINGHAM and HARRISON o.c.); in fact, it is not clear whether insects are vulnerable to ACh accumulation in the head or at another site. This is treated more in detail in Chapter 16.

Finally, VAN ASPEREN (1958) suggested that the extent of ChE inhibition which actually occurs *in vivo* may be significantly lower than that indicated by manometric measurement, and thus not be responsible for insecticidal action. He showed that at toxic concentrations (0.1 mg/g) O-O-dimethyl-0-2,2-dichlorovinyl phosphate inhibits only 27 to 46% of ChE of housefly heads, thoraces, or abdomens provided ACh is added prior to homogenization. VAN ASPEREN commented that addition of ACh protected the enzyme from unbound inhibitor present in the tissues and released during homogenization.

2. Non-ChE mechanisms in ovicidal action

Several writers denied the importance of ChE and of neurogenesis in the action of ovicidal agents. STAUDENMAYER (1957) confirmed in his experiments the delayed action of anti-ChE agents, but argued that this action did not coincide with onto-genesis of ChE's or with neurogenesis; other investigators stressed early ovicidal effects preceding neurogenesis and the appearance of ChE's.

STAUDENMAYER (1953, 1957), who took the decrease of embryonic oxygen consumption as evidence of organophosphorus toxicity, showed that Parathion kills the eggs of *Bombyx mori* two days, and Paraoxon seven days before hatching. Thus, in *Bombyx* the appearance and the rapid increase of ChE activity (5 or 6 days before hatching), and the differentiation of the nervous system (4 days before hatching) occur precociously with regard to Parathion toxicity or late with reference to the ovicidal effect of Paraoxon.

It cannot be gainsaid that developmental arrest and toxicity of anti-ChE agents, when they occur prior to the development of neuroblasts, cannot be related to their neurotropic action. Yet, it can still depend on inactivation of ChE's, since in certain insects the enzymes seem present in very early development stages (Chapter 5). Similarly, anti-ChE and cholino-mimetic agents are capable of morphogenetic and anti-growth effects in echinoderms, amphibians, and in the chick, in which ChE's, ACh, or both are also present very early. It may be speculated that in all these forms the ChE-ACh system may be coupled with another metabolic system (cf. supra, p. 804). However, the presence of ChE in the early or unfertilized insect egg seems to be the exception rather than the rule (cf. Chapter 5). Thus, in insects the early ovicidal action of anti-ChE agents may be due to interference with a metabolic system different from, and not coupled with, the cholinergic one; for instance, WINTERINGHAM and HARRISON (1956) reported that in the fly organophosphorus compounds, besides blocking aliesterases, cause also accumulation of glutamine.

Ali- and aryl-esterases could be involved also, as suggested by POTTER et al. (1957) and LORD and POTTER (1951). POTTER et al. (1957) found an arylesterase in newly laid eggs of *Pieris brassicae* and of two moths (Chapter 5).

It should be noted that enzymes capable of splitting *o*-nitrophenyl acetate and ethyl butyrate are present in the adult insect heads (LORD and POTTER 1951 and 1953; cf. Chapters 5 and 16). However, phenylacetate esterase in question may be different from arylesterases; the latter have been defined as insensitive to organophosphorus compounds (Chapter 16), while the ali- and aryl-esterases described by LORD and POTTER were as affected by Paraoxon, DFP, and also eserine as were AChE and other ChE's.

In the case of several adult forms a rough relationship exists between TEPP content of the insect body, estimated chemically, and insecticidal and anti-ChE activities (LORD and POTTER 1951). As already described (cf. p. 810), HETP and TEPP were found capable of arresting early development of certain eggs (LORD and POTTER 1951, POTTER et al. 1957). Unfortunately, inhibition of the arylesterase *in vivo* was not measured in parallel with the tests of developmental inhibition. Also, VAN ASPEREN (o.c.), while estimating that the actual inhibition of ChE's by an organophosphorus agent was no more than 46%, found a marked inhibition of an aliesterase capable of hydrolysing methylbutyrate; 83% average inhibition was obtained even in homogenates protected by addition of ACh (cf. supra, p. 812, and Chapter 16).

POTTER and LORD hypothesized that all effects of high or low concentrations of TEPP arise immediately, and are mediated via ali- or aryl-esterases. They supported this reasoning by a calculation based on hypothetical figures indicating that TEPP may not be stored in the lipid component of the insect egg upon its adminis-tration nor be released later into the aqueous phase to produce toxicity at that time; they suggested that low concentrations have delayed effects partially because of the instability of TEPP, and partially because only a small proportion of "key systems" is inactivated under these circumstances, so that they become a bottle-neck only later in development.

However, POTTER and LORD may have been influenced by finding aryl- but not cholinesterase early in development of several forms, including *Pieris brassicae* (Chapter 5). Yet, as stated by LORD and POTTER (1953) themselves, only preli-minary attempts were made to demonstrate ChE, and the alcoholic extraction method used (LORD and POTTER 1950) may lead to inhibition of ChE's. In fact,

O'BRIEN (1953) demonstrated ChE in larval and pupal forms in which the enzyme was not found by means of the methods employed by LORD and POTTER (o.c.); he did not, however, study early eggs of *Pieris*.

Moreover, *in vitro*, TEPP was found to be about 2.5 times more potent an inhibitor of the arylesterase than Parathion, yet the latter was many times more toxic than the former to eggs, larvae, and adults of several insects, although in certain forms the difference was relatively small. LORD and POTTER (1951) ascribed this to the fact that TEPP is more unstable than Parathion. They showed that high concentrations of TEPP affect the eggs faster than similar concentrations of Parathion; when concentrations are chosen so as to affect the eggs after a delay only, TEPP may be hydrolyzed prior to the appearance of a TEPP-sensitive step of ontogenesis, and Parathion becomes more effective.

Also, only very strong concentrations of TEPP are rapidly ovicidal; development was arrested prior to neuroblast formation only in 6 to 12% solutions of TEPP, while in the case of 0.1 to 3.0% solutions high percentages of eggs died *after* reaching developmental stages D and E (Chapter 5, Fig. 2). Similarly, Paraoxon and Parathion caused delayed at low, and immediate toxicity at high concentrations (SMITH and WAGENKNECHT 1956).

It may be more reasonable to hypothesize that TEPP and probably other anti-ChE agents have an early and a delayed mechanism of action. In fact, various anti-ChE agents may exhibit these two mechanism to a different degree; for instance, the ratio of concentrations blocking development on the one hand and preventing hatching on the other is 100:1 in the case of Paraoxon, and only 20:1 in the case of TEPP (POTTER 1958). Extensive evidence points to the ChE's and neurogenesis as constituting one of the mechanisms in question, even though conflicting data exist with reference to ACh accumulation as a direct cause of toxicity, and to the extent of ChE inhibition. It seems however quite clear that organophosphorus toxicity can occur also prior to neurogenesis. This additionally is borne out by the evidence that anti-ChE agents exert similar toxic and morphogenetic effects in other phyla.

III. Effects of eserine on insect diapause

Electric silence of the brain correlated with the disappearance of brain, but not ganglionic, ChE and ACh characterizes the onset of diapause in the moth *Platysamia cecropia*; the reverse trend appears at the end of diapause (cf. Chapters 5 and 16). Accordingly, it was postulated by VAN DER KLOOT (1955) that ChE is necessary for electric activity of the brain and for brain neurosecretion, which in turn activates the prothoracic glands and causes the release of their growth hormone.

MONRO (1958) showed subsequently that induction of adult development in the non-diapausing pupa of a noctuid, *Phalenoides plexippus*, was significantly delayed (23.4 against 16.2 days) by injection of 0.01 μg of eserine sulfate per pupa. This form has been shown by MONRO to have an active brain in the pupal stage and to pupate for several days before enough brain hormone is released to induce adult development. MONRO therefore postulated that in this form eserine inhibits, till it is metabolised, neurosecretory activity of the brain.

In the case of *Pieris rapae*, which also does not diapause, the pupation was generally not prolonged by a similar dose of eserine, except in isolated cases (from 6 to 38 days). The explanation of this was that this form secretes enough of brain hormone at pupation to ensure completion of adult development within 6 to 8 days; in fact, *Pieris* can develop in the absence of the brain provided the brain is removed at, rather than before, pupation. Thus, eserine was generally given too late, although by chance it may have been applied before sufficient brain hormone was secreted, in which case artificial diapause occurred. Finally, eserine was given to pupae of *Danaus plexippus* which were unaffected similarly to pupae of *Pieris*, although the adults exhibited muscular twitching or paralysis and frequently could not emerge without help. The non-diapausing *Danaus* has a brain which is inactive after pupation, and it develops into an adult because of the presence of the brain hormone carried over the final larval instar.

It is unfortunate that MONRO did not use *Platysamia*, the diapausing form investigated by VAN DER KLOOT, since on the basis of VAN DER KLOOT's hypothesis its diapause should be prolonged by eserine. In fact, in *Platysamia* pilocarpine prevented the adult development of diapausing pupae (WILLIAMS 1951). While WILLIAMS ascribed this to blockade of cytochrome synthesis by pilocarpine, and MONRO (o.c.) to ChE inhibition, pilocarpine may have prolonged diapause by its cholinomimetic action on the brain; the mechanism of action of anti-ChE agents might be similar. Thus, cholinergic stimulation may induce and prolong diapause. This mechanism may underlie also naturally occurring diapause; while the brains of newly *pupated* animals showed little or no ACh or ChE, VAN DER KLOOT (o.c.) did not assay ACh *prior* to pupation. It may, be, then, that ACh accumulates following the disappearance of ChE and induces brain depression which occurs a few days before pupation (VAN DER KLOOT o.c.) and diapause. Subsequent disappearance of ACh may be due to hydrolysis by enzymes other than AChE or other ChE's, and to diffusion.

MONRO mentioned also an interesting form, the codling moth *Cydia pomonella*, which, while diapausing, walks and spins the cocoon. In many insects the movement may depend upon lower ganglia, over which the brain exerts merely an inhibitory control (ROEDER et al. 1960, MILBURN et al. 1960). Thus, *Cydia* diapause may be triggered, like that of *Platysamia*, by the disappearance of brain ChE and by the cessation of brain activity, while function is maintained by the ganglia. However, MONRO thought that in the diapausing *Cydia*, ChE deficiency is localized and confined to the neurosecretory cells. It would be of interest to study this further by histochemical methods as well as by using anti-ChE agents. Generally, anti-ChE agents other than eserine should be used to test MONRO's and VAN DER KLOOT's hypothesis, particularly since eserine has actions independent of its anti-enzymic potency (curaremimetic or membrane stabilizing effects). It should be stated that several substances which are not ChE-inhibitors, such as diphteria toxin and imidazole compounds, also prolong diapause; it was proposed also that diapause can be correlated with an entirely different mechanism, invoking a defect in the cytochrome systems of insects (SHAPPIRIO and WILLIAMS 1957).

Actions of anti-ChE agents on function during development

A. Effects related mainly to the central nervous system

I. Effects in Amblystoma

YOUNGSTROM was the first (1938a) to observe that amphibian larvae exposed to unspecified concentrations of eserine in the early swimming stages developed contracture, gradual paralysis, and loss of irritability. Effects of DFP, eserine and other anti-ChE agents on *Amblystoma* were described more in detail subsequently.

Amblystoma larvae were exposed to eserine, DFP, N,N'-*bis*-(diethylaminoethyl) oxamide *bis* 2-chlorobenzyl choride (ambenonium), and neostigmine, usually prior to the onset of motility (stages 26—32; SAWYER 1943a, KOPPANYI and KARCZMAR 1947, KARCZMAR and KOPPANYI 1953, BLUM et al. 1958, BOELL 1946, 1948). In the case of DFP, which is unstable in water, the solution was changed 4 times daily; other solutions were changed daily (cf. however p. 819). KARCZMAR (1955) recorded muscle effect of several anti-ChE agents by visual observations of fasciculation and "tail flutter"; in the case of the bisquaternary compound, ambenonium, subsequent indication of the peripheral effect was a d-tubocurarine-like flaccidity. The effect of drugs on ChE's was studied by KARCZMAR and his associates by the manometric method of AMMON (1933) and by BOELL by means of the Cartesian micro-diver (cf. Chapters 4 and 5). Both these groups of workers used occasionally MeCh as the specific substrate of AChE. Finally, SAWYER (1943a) employed for the assay of the enzyme the microtitrimetric method already described (cf. Chapters 4 and 5).

The earliest effect observed may have been confined to the muscle. Fasciculation appeared with ambenonium and DFP at stage 34; surprisingly enough, d-tubocurarine produced flaccidity only one stage later. The shape of the relationship between concentration and latency changed between stages 34 and 58 (Fig. 1) in the case of DFP but not in that of ambenonium.

Since the sensitivity to the quaternary compound did not change with age, it is unlikely that the alteration of the shape of the DFP dose-effect relationship was a function of the change in permeability of larval skin or gills (cf. also KARCZMAR 1955, KARCZMAR and KOPPANYI 1948). KARCZMAR (1955) speculated that the data may indicate sequential development of several discrete receptor structures within the endplate.

Subsequent effects of inhibitors on behavior differed in the case of eserine and DFP on the one hand, and of neostigmine on the other (Table 2). The first effect of DFP could be demonstrated at the onset of the coil movement of the larvae (stage 36; cf. Table 2). The drugs slowed the coil motion, thus exhibiting a tetanizing tendency ("bent"; SAWYER 1943a, KARCZMAR and KOPPANYI 1953). It is of interest that neither drug hastened the onset of the first movement; this is in contradistinction to strychnine which was capable of producing coil or flexion prior to ontogenesis of reflex excitability, and S-movement at the time when controls exhibited only coil motion (BLUM et al. 1958). When DFP and eserine treatment was continued, excitatory actions could be observed at stages 37 to 39; upon stimulation, the larvae swam rapidly, progressing by means of a rapid, small-amplitude "flutter". Subsequently, non-progressive quiver replaced swimming

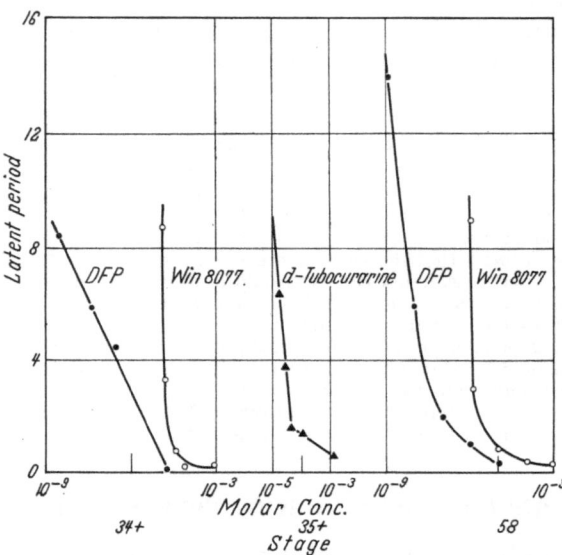

Fig. 1. Relationship between dose and latency of appearance of "overt" effects (cf. Table 2) of neuromyally active agents in *Amblystoma* larvae of various developmental stages. Ordinate: latent period in hours; abscissa: molar concentrations, logarithmic scale: 10^{-3} to 10^{-9} M for DFP and ambenonium (WIN 8077), HARRISON stage 34+; 10^{-3} to 10^{-5} M for *d*-tubocurarine, HARRISON stage 35+; 10^{-3} to 10^{-9} M for DFP and ambenonium, HARRISON stage 58 (from KARCZMAR 1955)

progression; still later, clonic and tonic convulsions resulted (KARCZMAR and KOPPANYI, o.c.; SAWYER, o.c.); after still longer treatment, a few stimulations of the larvae led to reversible paralysis; finally, larvae ceased to respond to stimulation and exhibited permanent paralysis, being at first fixed in pleurothotonos or opisthotonus ("bent") and turning flaccid subsequently (cf. also BOELL 1946).

Neostigmine (3×10^{-4} to 1.5×10^{-3} M) applied for 5 to 6 days caused flutter and, more rarely than eserine, "bent" but never quiver or convulsion (SAWYER 1943a). Essentially similar effects were obtained by KOPPANYI and KARCZMAR (1947) with 2×10^{-7} M solutions of neostigmine during 2 weeks of treatment.

This agrees with data on lack of the effects of neostigmine, given i.v., on electric activity of mammalian brain (e.g., BRADLEY 1958). It seems, however, that in larval *Amblystoma* prolonged treatment with neostigmine may lead to penetration of the drug into the central nervous system, as indicated by development of clonic and tonic convulsions (KOPPANYI and KARCZMAR, o.c.). This may be suggested also by the fact that the thiophosphonate Parathion caused convulsions in the case of larvae of stage 60, while it acted later as a depressant (BLUM et al. 1958). In mammals, Parathion penetrates into the brain less well than several other phosphonates (FRAWLEY et al. 1952). It is possible, then, that the blood-brain barrier is not fully developed in younger *Amblystoma* larvae, which would explain convulsant effects of

Table 2. *Effects of various anticholinesterase agents on behavior and cholinesterase activity of developing Amblystoma*[1]

Stage	Anti-ChE agent	Molar concentration	Cholinesterase inhibition	Effect	Central behavior
34+	DFP	10^{-9} to 10^{-3}	Complete with most concs.	Fasciculation; exaggerated and slow flexure; later paralysis	Early flexure
	Ambenonium	10^{-9} to 10^{-3}	?	As above; paralysis predominates	
36	Physostigmine	1.6×10^{-4}	59%	Slow coil, relaxation delayed	Coil
	Neostigmine[2]	3×10^{-4}	None	None	
37	DFP	10^{-4}	Complete	Rapid flutter	Double coil (S flexure)
38	Physostigmine	1.6×10^{-4}	81%	Tetanic convulsion, non-progressive; quiver, opisthotonus	Early swimming
	Neostigmine	3×10^{-4}	20%	"Flutter swim," little progress; never convulsions	
40	Physostigmine	1.6×10^{-4}	60—70%	Excitement; tetanic convulsion, non-progressive; quiver; opisthotonus; then, paralysis	"Late" swimming
	Neostigmine	3×10^{-4}	47%	"Flutter swim" or little effect; never convulsions	
60	DFP	10^{-9} to 10^{-5}	Complete with most concs.	Excitement, exaggerated swimming; "tail twitch"; myotonic and tetanic convulsions; opisthotonus; then, paralysis	"Late" swimming
	Neostigmine	2×10^{-7} to 10^{-5}	?	Myoclonic and tetanic convulsions after 2 weeks of treatment; then paralysis	
	TEPP	10^{-7}	?	Myotonic and tetanic convulsions; then, paralysis	
	Parathion	?	?	Excitement, clonic and tonic convulsions	
Adult	Parathion	?	?	Depression only	Terrestrial movement

[1] Data from SAWYER 1943a, BOELL 1948, KARCZMAR and KOPPANYI 1953, KARCZMAR 1955, BLUM et al. 1958, cf. also Chapter 5, Table 1.

[2] Molarity calculated for neostigmine methylsulfate from SAWYER's (1943a) Prostigmine (salt not indicated), 0.01%.

Parathion as well as of neostigmine after prolonged treatment; Parathion depression of older larvae may be due to peripheral toxicity of this compound (KARCZMAR 1948).

The difference between the effects of eserine and DFP on the one hand, and of neostigmine on the other can be related to the higher enzymic inhibition obtained with the non-quaternary compounds. For instance, eserine (1.6×10^{-4} to 10^{-5} M, v. Table 2) inhibited ChE's of stage 34 to 36 larvae from 59 to 81%, while neostigmine, even in a concentration of 3×10^{-4} M, never inhibited more than 45% of the enzyme. While the inhibition was measured in whole larvae it is likely that in the case of eserine and DFP central inhibition of ChE was also pronounced.

Certain aspects of these studies differed from one investigator to another. BOELL (1946), who used DFP at the high concentration of 10^{-4} M, did not report toxicity even after several days, contrary to results obtained with similar concentrations by KARCZMAR (1955); death occurred immediately when still stronger concentrations were used (BOELL 1948). If BOELL did not frequently change DFP solutions — he made no statement on this point — his experiments may have been affected by hydrolysis of DFP, phosphonates being very unstable in aqueous solutions (HOLMSTEDT 1959, KARCZMAR and LONG 1958).

While BOELL (1946 and 1948) and SAWYER (1955) obtained with DFP, 5×10^{-7} to 5×10^{-5} M, inhibition ranging from 48 to 90%, KARCZMAR and KOPPANYI (1953) claimed complete inhibition with 10^{-8} to 10^{-7} M DFP solutions. This degree of inhibition may appear high; *in vitro*, the I_{50} value for DFP inhibition of AChE was reported as 6.3×10^{-8} M by DUBOIS and MANGUN (1947), and as 0.75×10^{-5} M by HOLMSTEDT (1959); the LD_{50} of this compound in mice (approximately 2 mg/kg, i.v.) corresponds, on the basis of equidistribution, to a molarity of 0.9×10^{-5}.

More specific correlation between larval behavior and ChE's was attempted by BOELL (1948). BOELL exposed for various periods stage 25 to 27 larvae to 10^{-5} M DFP solution, and returned them to pond water. Enzyme activity reappeared at stage 40 and increased subsequently, till at stage 41 swimming motion of a "primitive" type set on. BOELL suggested that the enzyme present at that time was insufficient to remove endogenous ACh, leading to a behavior comparable to that of controls, stage 37 to 38, enzymic activity of the two larval groups being also similar. YOUNGSTROM (1938b) commented, similarly, that the slow, tetanic character of the coil stage of larvae of stage 34 is due to enzymic insufficiency; all this implies that the enzyme level alone conditions the behavior. While in the presence of the inhibitor the enzyme level may be related to the abnormality of function, it is an oversimplification to suggest that at any stage ChE level alone controls behavior.

If this were so, the bradycardia observed in treated larvae of stage 40 or 41 should also characterise untreated larvae of stage 37, which does not appear to be true. SAWYER (1955) cautioned against the suggestion that the behavior of a larva of an advanced stage with partially inhibited enzyme will be identical with that of a younger larva with similar enzyme activity; rather, any stage of functional development would require a certain amount of enzyme for the function normal for this particular stage.

The same problem of the relationship of enzyme level to function was approached by SAWYER (1955) by taking advantage of the adaptability of larval material to quantitation of functional response.

"Reflex capacity" of larvae, stage 45 or 46, was measured by means of stimulating their back or side once per second for 60 seconds by a fine hair, and scoring positive responses. "On repeated testing, a (control) larva gave a reproducible score varying usually within 2 and 4%" (o.c., p. 563).

Eserine (1.5×10^{-4} M) and DFP (5×10^{-5} M) depressed within 2 hrs of treatment both the "reflex capacity" and enzymic activity by about 60 and 80%, respectively. Even the time course of the enzymic inhibition on the one hand, and of the loss of "reflex capacity" on the other were identical: the 50% points of enzymic and behavioral blockade were recorded at the same time with the coefficient of correlation of 0.93. Neostigmine did not affect either the enzyme or the function.

Considerable impairment of function was found even at the 25% levels of enzymic inhibition. Actually, since SAWYER measured ChE's in the homogenates of whole larvae, the inhibition of the central nervous system and neuroeffector enzyme may have been smaller than indicated. In any event, the data are somewhat surprising since usually 50 to 80% of effector ChE has to be inhibited before any pharmacological, physiological (KOPPANYI and KARCZMAR 1951, KOELLE 1957), or, finally, behavioral (RUSSEL 1958) effects set in. It is also surprising that neostigmine at as a strong concentration as 10^{-3} M produced little if any enzymic inhibition. Larvae of stage 46 exhibit considerable amounts of muscle enzyme, which actually constitutes a marked fraction of the total enzymic activity of the larva (cf. Chapter 5); at least this ChE should be inhibited by neostigmine and this should be revealed even in measurements involving whole larvae.

Recovery from enzymic and functional blockade following eserine and DFP

SAWYER (1943a) kept larvae of stages 36 to 42 in a 0.01% (1.5×10^{-4} M) solution of eserine sulfate for as short as 12 or as long as 135 hrs; enzymic inhibition ranged from 57 to 81%. Subsequent transfer into water led to an apparent average 50% recovery of enzymic activity, whether determined 27 or 51 hrs after termination of treatment, as well as to return toward function characteristic for the larval stage concerned. However, complete normalcy of behavior was not regained within this recovery time; "flutter swim" was exhibited by the treated larvae as compared with the "strong swim" (cf. Chapter 5, Table 1) of the controls. While on the whole these results can be correlated with the reversible character of ChE inhibition by eserine, better enzymic and functional recovery might have been expected 51 hrs after treatment; moreover, abnormal behavior with inhibition as low as 16% (SAWYER o.c.) is somewhat puzzling.

The data obtained with DFP appear even more controversial; parallel recoveries of enzymic and swimming function were found by SAWYER (1955), while KARCZMAR and KOPPANYI (1953) claimed that function can return to normal in the absence of enzymic recovery. Ample evidence (for references, cf. HOLMSTEDT 1959, pp. 614—616) supports the notion that functional adaptation of intact animals and of isolated organs to organophosphorus anti-ChE agents can occur relatively rapidly, probably independently of synthesis of new enzyme. Finally, BOELL (1948) recorded enzymic recovery even in the continued presence of the inhibitor.

BOELL (o.c.) kept premotile, stage 22 larvae in 10^{-4} M DFP solution, which inhibited ChE's completely, and, presumably without removing the inhibitor, recorded the first appearance of the enzyme at stage 40, i.e., after 10 days of DFP treatment. Subsequently, the enzyme activity increased rapidly and BOELL's (o.c.) data indicate that the ratio of enzyme activity of treated and untreated larvae decreased from the initial 1:6 at stage 40 to about 1:3 at stage 45. In other words, treated larvae seemed to compensate for their initial lag in enzyme activity (cf. also SAWYER 1955). Swimming characterized by flutter and early fatigue appeared at stage 40, concomitantly with the appearance of the enzyme. In the case of DFP treatment of motile larvae (stage 34 onward), a much shorter time elapsed prior to both enzymic and functional recovery.

BOELL (o.c.) did not indicate how frequently he prepared fresh DFP solutions in the course of the treatment. It can be assumed then that he used a single DFP solution, and that ChE activity recorded 10 days after treatment (during which time practically all excess DFP would be inactivated by hydrolysis) was that expected to occur in the course of ontogenesis of the enzyme between larval stages 22 and 40 (cf. Chapter 5, Fig. 3). SAWYER (1955) exposed larvae of premotile and early motile stages to DFP, 5×10^{-5} M, causing 90% enzymic inhibition. At stage 45, i.e., after 10 days of treatment, larvae were returned to water. Some recovery of enzyme activity was noticed 1 day later, control levels were reached within 6 days, and swimming ability "improved rapidly". KARCZMAR and KOPPANYI (1953) kept stage 60 larvae in considerably weaker (10^{-7} M) concentrations of DFP for 4 days and noticed, similarly, a rapid recovery of function which occurred within 1 to 2 days of transfer to water. However, the recovery of enzymic activity took at least 6 to 8 days, and thus was much slower than that recorded by SAWYER. Cholinesterase is synthesized faster in stage 36 to 42 larvae, used by SAWYER (1955), than in younger larvae used by BOELL (o.c.; cf. Chapter 5). Thus, the data of SAWYER (o.c.) which indicate rapid functional and enzymic recovery do not disagree essentially with those of BOELL. In the case of the still older larvae (stage 60) used by KARCZMAR and KOPPANYI (o.c.), the synthesis of new enzyme is slow and actually does not keep pace with that of other proteins (cf. Chapter 5). This then agrees with faster recovery of enzymic activity in SAWYER's larvae than in those of KARCZMAR and KOPPANYI; slow recovery of enzyme activity at that stage is, moreover, consistent with in vitro (WILSON 1951) and in vivo (MAZUR and BODANSKY 1946) data on the recovery of organophosphorus-inhibited enzyme.

II. Effects in fishes

Few data on the effects of physostigmine are available in the case of the elasmobranch Scyliorhinus (WHITING 1955) and of the teleost Fundulus (SAWYER 1944). WHITING used physostigmine (concentration not reported), d-tubocurarine, and ACh, 5×10^{-6} g/ml. SAWYER used eserine in concentrations varying from 0.0001 to 0.01%. The solutions were renewed daily. Neither investigator measured ChE activity following physostigmine treatment.

Spontaneous somatic activity of *Fundulus* is myogenic in character, independent of innervation (Chapter 5; COGHILL 1933), and occurs in the presence of only traces of ChE. This is consistent with the finding that eserine did not affect the somatic activity of stage 23—25 of *Fundulus*. However, the reflex reactivity to the compression of the fourth ventricle was affected by eserine at its very onset; the relaxation phase of the response was lengthened, and later in development a stimulus normally causing a single twitch response would initiate a series of twitches and coils in the eserinized embryos. Still later, opisthotonic quiver and tetanic "bent" resembling that described for *Amblystoma* (SAWYER 1943a) was observed in eserinized larvae.

Some resistance to the inhibitor could be developed by initiating the treatment sufficiently early. Paralysis and death did not occur till after a week of treatment with a stronger (0.01%) solution of eserine applied from the blastula stage on; motile embryos of stage 27 died within 12 to 24 hrs after 15 sec treatment with a similar concentration; hatched larvae died within a few hours.

The data obtained in *Scyliorhinus* (WHITING 1955) were interesting. That, similarly to the situation in *Fundulus*, the early somatic activity of the elasmobranch was not affected by eserine could be expected; however, ACh produced at the same stage a marked increase in the frequency of the spontaneous somatic activity. Moreover, physostigmine and d-tubocurarine did not affect the neurogenic and reflexogenic stages of development of *Scyliorhinus*.

III. Comment

In both *Fundulus* and *Amblystoma*, the onset of the rapid increase of ChE occurs after the myogenic phase of behavior (Chapter 5). This may be considered consistent with the fact that anti-ChE agents do not affect function of the myogenic embryo.

The pertinent ChE data are not quite comparable, since they refer to the enzyme of the central nervous system in the case of *Amblystoma* and to that of the whole embryo in that of *Fundulus*. The situation is also obscured by the fact that physostigmine was ineffective in the elasmobranch *Scyliorhinus* both during myogenic and neurogenic phases of development of behavior (WHITING 1955).

First effects of DFP and of a quaternary anti-ChE agent occurred at stage 34 (Fig. 1). Since this is presumably the time of formation of the endplates and of the onset the rapid increase of ChE activity (inasmuch as d-tubocurarine was effective at this stage, while atropine, a weak neuromyal agent, could not block responses to DFP), the early actions of anti-ChE agents in *Amblystoma*, and possibly in *Fundulus*, are probably localized at the myoneural junction and coincide with muscle innervation. On the other hand, cholinomimetic stimulants may affect the skeletal and cardiac muscle before their innervation occurs, at least in the mammal (cf. infra, pp. 823 and 824). This is not unexpected, since cholinergic receptors may appear precociously with regard to innervation and ChE's (cf. infra).

The neuromyal junction may have been involved also in responses to anti-ChE agents of stage 36 *Amblystoma* and of *Fundulus*, stage 23 to 27. Indeed, eserinised spinal or decapitated *Amblystoma* larvae of stage 36 still exhibited "tetanus" or "bent" (SAWYER 1943a). In fact, SAWYER (1943a,1944) favored the motor endplate as the site of action of eserine, both at the onset of the reflex response of *Fundulus* to the compression of the fourth ventricle, and at the flexure stage of *Amblystoma*, and he pointed out that d-tubocurarine blocks the response of *Fundulus* (COGHILL 1933). This, however, does not of course exclude the central nervous system as the site of action of eserine. Atropine prolonged life of DFP treated larvae (KARCZMAR and KOPPANYI 1953), and this protection was probably exerted centrally (KARCZ-MAR and LONG 1958). The repetitive, convulsant effect of eserine on *Fundulus*, stage 27 (SAWYER 1944), suggests a central site of action also in that form. Altogether, in view of the presence of reflex and commissural pathways in both *Fundulus*, stages 23 to 27, and stage 36 *Amblystoma*, and of relatively high levels of ChE's at that developmental stage (Chapter 5, Table 1), anti-ChE agents may have a double site of action at this developmental moment.

Central action is also implicated in the responsiveness of *Amblystoma* to anti-ChE agents later in development. At about stage 40, swimming behavior becomes subservient to the mesencephalon (Chapter 5) and it may be also associated with the peak of ChE activity occurring at this stage prior to its subsequent decrease. This stage is nearly coincidental with the onset of the stimulant effect of anti-ChE agents on swimming motion of *Amblystoma* (cf. p. 816), and on hypothalamic control of the melanophore system (SAWYER 1947; v. supra). Finally, at stages 45 to 46, enzymic inhibition by eserine could be well correlated with quantitated (in terms of "reflex capacity," cf. p. 818) larval behavior. All these indirect indications of the appearance of a cholinergic step in the ontogeny of *Amblystoma* midbrain agree with the suggestion of BRADLEY and ELKES (1957) and of RINALDI and HIMWICH (1955) that in the adult mammal certain mesencephalic systems are cholinergic in nature.

However, discrepancies between enzymic activity and function could be pinpointed also; older *Amblystoma* larvae, which synthesize new enzyme slowly and which as gill-breathers, not subject to death from bronchiolar constriction, are well constituted to survive the first "shock" of anti-ChE treatment, seem to exhibit behavioral adaptation in the absence of reappearance of enzymic activity (KARCZMAR and KOPPANYI 1953); some adaptation seems to be possible also in *Fundulus* (SAWYER 1944). In more general terms, the multineuronal character of the pathways in question, both in *Fundulus* and in *Amblystoma*, makes final analysis of the effects of anti-ChE agents difficult.

In fact, in *Fundulus*, stages 27 and later, anti-ChE agents seemed to cause only convulsions but no excitement (SAWYER 1944). Still another factor should caution against construing the data as implicating causally the cholinergic system in the phenomena described. In *Amblystoma*, depressants such as pentobarbital sodium produce at stages 40 to 42 flutter, coil, multiple flexion, and tetanic and conculsive behavior prior to the onset of anesthesia; this behavior resembles very much that caused by anti-ChE agents applied at this larval stage (BLUM et al. 1958). Thus, depressants "recapitulate in reverse order ... various ontogenetic behavior patterns" (o.c., p. 442). This in turn indicates that *Amblystoma* and probably also *Fundulus* larvae have a limited range of behavioral expression with regard to depression, toxicity, or presumably accumulation of ACh. In other words, many of the changes described in this section may be not specific nor exclusively cholinergic, and thus should be used only with caution for identification of cholinergic synapses.

IV. Effects in mammals

The data on the effects of anti-ChE agents during mammalian development are few, and deal mainly with the postnatal development of the rat. Prenatal development was studied only with regard to ACh sensitivity of the rat muscles (DIAMOND and MILEDI 1959). Thus, in spite of the detailed knowledge of the ontogenesis of ChE's of the mammalian brain (Chapter 5), the limited employment of anti-ChE agents has not as yet shed much additional light on the developmental significance of ChE's in the mammal.

DIAMOND and MILEDI (1959), employing iontophoretic techniques and intracellular electrodes, studied ACh responses of individual fibers of the diaphragm of 19 to 22-day old fetuses, and of young rats up to 14 days of age. In the fetuses as well as just after birth, the whole fiber surface was sensitive to ACh. KHUDOROZHEVA

(1956), working with fetal rabbits (26 days) and cats, obtained ACh contractions by applying it to the gastrocnemius muscle; the exact locus of application was not stated. Spontaneous firing could be recorded also along the whole length of the fibers, although it seemed to originate from the region of the future endplate (DIAMOND and MILEDI o.c.). Subsequently, the ACh-sensitive area began to recede from the tendon ends toward the endplate, and was down to adult dimensions two weeks after birth.

With regard to postnatal development, FREEDMAN and HIMWICH (1948) found that DFP lethality was higher in the newborn than in the adult rat, although the inhibition of total ChE's was, percent-wise, nearly *identical*. ELKES et al. (1955), on the other hand, found that ChE inhibition by DFP *increased* between 4 and 40 days of age; while they, too, seemed to find DFP more toxic to the newborn than to older rats, subtoxic effects of DFP in surviving animals under continuous treatment first decreased and then increased, muscle fasciculation appearing only at 40 days. Finally. DuBois (1961) found no difference in ChE inhibition by equitoxic doses of 0,0-diethyl 0-(4-methylthio-*m*-tolyl) phosphorothioate (DMP) at 23 and 45 days, although a 15-fold decrease in toxicity occurred at puberty (30 to 40 days) in young male (but not female) rats (DuBois and PUCHALA 1961). The decrease in toxicity was explained as due to development, at puberty, of a detoxifying system, present in the liver of the male rat alone.

In view of certain divergence between the results of FREEDMAN and HIMWICH on the one hand and of ELKES et al. on the other, their investigations will be presented in detail. FREED-MAN and HIMWICH (1948) administered DFP i.p. or s.c. in doses of 2 mg/kg. Results were the same with either route. In the s.c. series, 175 rats were divided into 7 groups: new-born controls, treated new-born rats, treated 1 to 3, 6 to 8, 16 to 18 and 32-day old rats, and treated adults. There was a decrease in lethality from 100 to 79% from the day of birth to the 1st to 3rd day of life, a subsequent increase to 87% at 16 to 18 days, and final decrease to 61 and 73% at 32 days and in the adults, respectively. FREEDMAN and HIMWICH did not comment on the dip in viability at 16 to 18 days; in view of the numbers of animals employed it may not have been significant. Inhibition of ChE's was 96 and 97% in newborn and adult rats, respectively.

ELKES et al. (1955) used, in addition to DFP, tetramono*iso*propyl pyrophosphortetramide (*iso*-OMPA) which is a differential but not entirely specific butyrocholinesterase (BuChE) inhibitor, and tricresylphosphate (TCP). Di*iso*propyl phosphorofluoridate, in doses of 2.0 and 2.5 mg/kg, was injected s.c. biweekly from the 6th to 49th day of life and once weekly till the age of 150 days; atropine (0.9 mg/kg) was given prophylactically before each DFP treatment. The other compounds, *iso*-OMPA and TCP, were given s.c. biweekly between the 6th and 24th day of age. The dose of *iso*-OMPA varied from 15 to 40 mg/kg, that of TCP appeared to be 2500 mg/kg. Ten-day old rats showed a 50% inhibition of brain AChE and BuChE, and a 60% inhibition of spinal cord ChE's after having received a total of 5.5 to 6.5 mg/kg of DFP in divided doses. Six out of 7 rats (almost 90%) died by the time they were approximately 2 weeks old after having received a total dose of 7.5 mg/kg DFP in ten days. Twenty-two, 40 and 150-day old rats, which received a total dose of 13.5, 20 to 24.5 and 50 mg/kg of DFP, respectively, showed a 73 to 87% inhibition of brain and spinal cord AChE and BuChE, and a 35% lethality. Thus, both groups of investigators reported somewhat similar lethality in the newborn; in older rats, fewer fatalities were reported by ELKES et al. than by FREEDMAN and HIMWICH.

Coarse tremor, tail spasm, worm-like trunk movements, and marked restlessness charac-terized the rats till the 20th day of age; muscle fasciculation was never present (ELKES et al. o.c.). Between the 25th and 40th day of age rats were relatively free from signs and tolerated DFP better than either before or after this period. After the 40th day, signs of toxicity seemed to increase; muscle fasciculation appeared and hyperreflexia and clonic and tonic convulsions became frequent. Whenever death occurred it was preceded by convulsions, cyanosis, and respiratory failure. Finally, specific inhibition of BuChE with *iso*-OMPA had little effect on the rat at any age studied (ELKES et al., o.c.).

Comment

It is somewhat piquant that both ELKES et al., and FREEDMAN and HIMWICH recurred to postnatal development of ChE to explain their divergent data on ChE inhibition. In the rat, which is born relatively immature, AChE activity increasse immediately after birth (Chapter 5). In view of this, similar percentage enzymic inhibition by DFP in the newborn and adult rat signifies higher absolute activity in the latter which, as suggested by FREEDMAN and HIMWICH, is related to its higher resistance. On the other hand, ELKES et al. (o.c.) explained the increase of enzymic inhibition with age by the falling off at that time of the rate of increase of enzymic activity (cf. Chapter 5). It is not clear why absolute rather than percentage levels of enzyme activity should be decisive for survival, or why the decrease of the rate of enzymic synthesis should lead to the increase of inhibition by DFP.

Also, it might be expected on the basis of the arguments advanced by both groups of investigators that the medulla, which is relatively rich in the enzymes at birth, may be resistant to DFP; the immediate cause of death does not indicate that this is the case.

DESMEDT and LA GRUTTA (1957) were among the few workers to consider brain BuChE as functionally important; in the rat, *bis*-mono*iso*propylamino-fluorophosphine oxide and other specific BuChE inhibitors had little effect (BARNES and DENZ 1953). ELKES et al. (o.c.) found no defect of myelination or pathology of the brain with inhibition of BuChE ranging from 31 to 50% with TCP and *iso*-OMPA, respectively; they suggested that brain BuChE is not related to development of function. Needless to say, these are relatively small changes in enzyme levels.

With regard to the relationship between AChE inhibition and functional disturbance on the one hand, and neurogenesis on the other, the particular vulnerability of the newborn rat reported by FREEDMAN and HIMWICH, or the decrease of this vulnerability between the 25th and 40th day, followed again by sensitization (ELKES et al., o.c.) cannot be elucidated conclusively at present. It should be stressed that ontogenesis of detoxification systems, about which so little is known but which played a part in decrease at puberty toxicity of DMP (DuBOIS and PUCHALA o.c.), could be responsible also for the postnatal decrease of DFP toxicity.

Similarly, the appearance of fasciculation only after the 40th day cannot be easily explained, since the postnatal concentration of the enzyme at the motor endplate, the shift from BuChE to AChE, and the anatomical and functional maturation of the endplate seem completed by the 9th postnatal day (Chapter 5), while the mature sensitivity to ACh is acquired by the 14th day (DIAMOND and MILEDI 1959). This effect of anti-ChE agents can be regarded then as a marker of developmental events not demonstrable at present by biochemical or anatomical approaches; a similar suggestion was made with regard to certain effects of ChE inhibitors at the amphibian neuromyal junction (cf. supra, p. 816).

Finally, it should be pointed out that the results of DIAMOND and MILEDI (1959) and of KHUDOROZHEVA (1956) suggest that the appearance of the cholinergic receptors is precocious with regard to the innervation of the muscle.

B. Cardiac effects of cholinomimetic and anti-ChE agents during ontogenesis

I. Chick and rat hearts

The possibility that the ontogenesis of ChE's of the vertebrate heart is not associated with the establishment of the vagal reflex (Chapter 5, Tables 4 and 5) suggests that during embryogenesis anti-ChE and cholinomimetic agents may have other besides vagomimetic effects. On the other hand, these agents may be expected to produce bradycardia at the time of establishment of cardiac innervation. Only one study of the effects of an anti-ChE on the developing heart (Mc-CARTY et al. 1960) seems available; consequently, the analysis of the relationship of the ontogenesis of cardiac ChE's to cardiac function also will be analysed on the basis of the cardiac effects of other cholinomimetic substances in addition to anti-ChE agents. Finally, this analysis will be extended to the invertebrate heart.

Embryonic hearts were excised and the cardiac beat observed and measured under the binocular microscope in a study carried out on the rat (HALL 1957). In the case of the chick, cardiac function was studied either *in situ* after the chick embryos has been removed from the shell (JONES 1958, FINGL et al. 1952) or in excised hearts (McCARTY et al. 1960). JONES (1958) used a micromanipulator to place the electrodes via incision in the embryonic membranes and measured the heart rates from cathode-ray oscilloscope records. FINGL et al. (1952) used capillary microelectrodes to record after suitable amplification (WOODBURY et al. 1951) the transmembrane potentials of individual heart muscle fibers. Other studies on the hearts *in situ* utilized simple visual observations for estimating cardiac effects of drugs.

An interesting technique was applied to excised chick hearts by McCARTY et al. (1960). The hearts were mounted on a recording apparatus placed in a chamber containing aerated Tyrode's solution at 39°C. The apparatus was an isometric lever constructed from a 0.003 inch wire in the case of 4-day old hearts, and from a 0.006 Nichrome wire in the case of older hearts. The lever was connected with a mirror, and a beam of light was reflected from it to a photocell coupled via a bridge circuit with an oscilloscope. It was shown that the photocell output was directly proportional to the load, and that a contractile force as small as 0.2 mg could be recorded accurately. Contractile amplitude, tone, and heart rate could be measured.

The embryonic *rat* hearts did not respond to ACh (2.5 to 100 mg/l) at $10^{1}/_{2}$ days, but some of them exhibited temporary diastolic arrest (average 60 sec) beginning with the $11^{1}/_{2}$ day of gestation (HALL 1957). Also, ACh slowed the cardiac rate by about 37% whether after or in lieu of the arrest. Both the arrest frequency and degree of bradycardia increased between $11^{1}/_{2}$ and $14^{1}/_{2}$ days of gestation.

Parenthetically, a positive chronotropic effect of epinephrine was first observed at the $11^{1}/_{2}$ day of gestation. It should be stated, however, that epinephrine was always given subsequently to ACh.

Similarly, ACh and epinephrine were effective on the *chick* heart quite early in development. ZINGONI (1956) reported slowing with ACh at 68 hrs; FINGL et al. (1952) and McCARTY et al. (1960) reported slowing, arrest, or both at 3 days, and JONES (1958) at 6 days of development. It is of interest that in the course of much earlier investigations PICKERING (1893, 1895) reported relative insensitivity of the chick heart to muscarine at about 100 hrs.

FINGL et al. (o.c.), JONES (o.c.) and McCARTY et al. (o.c.) used ACh in concentrations of 10^{-5}, 10^{-5} to 10^{-6}, and 10^{-7} to 10^{-8} g/ml, respectively. In the studies of FINGL et al. and JONES, drugs were dripped in 0.5 cc of solution directly upon the heart; in that of McCARTY et al., drugs were added to a 50 ml bath.

Thus, ACh effectiveness antedates the innervation of the chick heart by at least 2 days (cf. however GARREY 1937). Moreover, the reports of the above authors as well as those of TSCHERMAK (1909) and BARRY (1950) agree that the sensitivity of the heart to ACh does not change upon innervation. Even a careful analysis of ACh effects on membrane phenomena of the cardiac cycle failed to reveal any difference due to age or innervation (FINGL et al., o.c.).

FINGL and his associates studied the resting membrane potential, action potential (composed, as described by the authors, of depolarization, repolarization, and an "overshoot"), and temperature coefficient of the various phases of repolarization. Repolarization rates of the atrial and of most phases of the ventricular action potential, the duration of ventricular potential, and finally the temperature coefficients did not change between the 3rd and the 7th day of embryonic age. Acetylcholine reduced resting and action potentials, and decreased the duration of the latter. The authors associated these changes with incomplete depolarization of the excited fiber in the presence of ACh; the enhancement of repolarization was noticed in some experiments. Innervation of the heart had no effect upon ACh response.

Final evidence that cardiac innervation has no effect upon ACh response was provided by JONES (1958). JONES (o.c.) removed the hindbrain to provide an embryo without parasympathetic ganglion cells in the atrial wall of the heart. The embryos preserved nodose, sympathetic, and prevertebral ganglia which do not originate from the hindbrain. The absence of any contribution by these ganglia to the heart was verified histologically; particularly, the innervation of the heart by the distal fibers of the nodose ganglia was not accompanied by formation of parasympathetic neuroblasts (cf. JONES 1942). Even in these hearts ACh caused cardiac slowing or arrest between the 4th and the 9th day of the incubation period; its effects were qualitatively and quantitatively similar to those produced in normally innervated controls.

Physostigmine at 10^{-6} g/ml had no effect upon cardiac rate or amplitude from the 3rd to 9th developmental day (McCARTY et al., o.c.) but it was capable of increasing the cardiac response to ACh. This potentiating action could not be obtained at the time of the first effectiveness of ACh, i.e., in the third day of incubation, but only a day later — some three days before the heart becomes innervated. At this time physostigmine potentiated the cardiac action of ACh in 3 out of 4 hearts tested. Subsequent trials of the drug indicated that the incidence and extent of the potentiating action increased at the time of innervation; thus, physostigmine differed from ACh both in the time of onset of its effectiveness and in that its response was affected by innervation.

Comment

These data for the chick and rat heart, admittedly incomplete insofar as anti-ChE agents are concerned, should be analyzed first of all with regard to ontogenesis of cardiac function and of cardiac ChE's. In the case of the rat heart (Chapter 5, Table 5) the ACh response was recorded barely one day (at $11^1/_2$ days) after the appearance of contractility, AChE, and BuChE, and some 4 days before the vagal innervation penetrated the heart. Somewhat similarly, in the chick ACh became effective perhaps less than one day after the initiation of the cardiac beat, between the 40th and 48th hour of incubation. This is about one day before ChE's can be demonstrated histochemically (ZACKS 1954) and eserine becomes effective (Mc-CARTY et al. 1960), and about 3 days before the heart becomes innervated. Once it had developed, the sensitivity of the chick heart to ACh did not change upon innervation, nor was it affected by prolonging experimentally the period of nervelessness of the developing heart (JONES 1958). It is true that ARMSTRONG (1935) for the fish, and GARREY (1935) for the chick came to different conclusions.

SIPPEL's analysis of ontogenesis of ChE's, particularly insofar as they have a pattern similar to that of enzymes concerned with the energy and "efficiency" of cardiac function, led him (1954 and 1955) to support the speculation of BÜLBRING and her associates (1949, 1954) that cardiac ChE's have to do primarily with cardiac rhythmicity and contractility rather than with vagal function (Chapter 5). It seems at present that not only ChE's but also cardiac response to cholinomimetic agents antedate innervation; moreover, this response may either precede or follow the ontogenetic appearance of ChE's. Since the developmental emergence of response to ACh is clearly concerned with vagomimetic control of the heart, premature ontogeny of ChE's may be by analogy interpreted as related to the same process, particularly since physostigmine potentiation of the ACh response is intensified by innervation. Early ontogeny of ChE's and of ACh could be then construed as an instance of the presence and responsiveness of the cholinergic receptors preceding, or in the absence of, innervation; this certainly obtains at denervated cholinergic or at aneural sites, as was shown very early by LANGLEY (1905) and subsequently by KUSCHINSKY et al. (1954) in the case of the chick amnion (cf. also Chapter 5). Furthermore, precociousness of the cardiac cholinergic system may be analogous with the precocious sensitivity of the mammalian muscle to ACh and development of its ChE prior to the innervation (cf. supra, p. 823). Also, the presence of the cholinergic system may have inductive properties upon prospective innervation of the heart, as was suggested for the central nervous system of *Amblystoma* (Chapter 5).

II. Invertebrate heart

Limited evidence suggests that the precocity or independence of cardiac cholinergic response and of cholinergic sensitivity with regard to innervation may be confined to the vertebrate heart.

The invertebrate heart, studied extensively with reference to cholinomimetic and to a limited extent with regard to anti-ChE agents, presents peculiar cholinergic relationships. Arthropods and molluscs may have innervated myogenic, non-innervated myogenic, or, finally, neurogenic hearts. Neurogenic hearts have a ganglionic, neuronal pacemaker and are accelerated by ACh; innervated myogenic hearts are typically depressed by ACh (JONES 1956b), while non-innervated myogenic hearts are not affected by ACh. Even in the absence of histological evidence, the ACh response may be used to decide whether a heart is myogenic or neurogenic (PROSSER 1942).

Most crustaceans, and *Limulus* have neurogenic hearts both on the basis of their response to ACh and on histologic evidence, although in development they are myogenic at first. The heart of *Limulus* begins contracting on the 21st day of development, while the cardiac ganglion is histologically demonstrable about 9 days later (CARLSON and MEEK 1908). PROSSER (o.c.) did not find any effect of ACh, eserine, or their combinations on the *Limulus* heart rate till the 31st day of development, when the hearts were accelerated by ACh. The *Limulus* heart is then accelerated by ACh at the time of ontogeny of the ganglionic pacemaker.

Insect hearts may be non-innervated and myogenic throughout development, as in the case of *Anopheles*. Accordingly, the *Anopheles* heart does not respond to ACh, MeCh, or eserine in the case of the 4 instars of the larva and the imaginal (adult) stages (JONES 1954, 1956a and b), even though eserine caused convulsions, "quiver" and "fibrillations" in the larvae and adult.

Thus, it seems that the nicotinic or ganglionic effect of ACh on hearts of certain invertebrates is contingent upon the innervation of the heart and, in ontogenesis, it can occur only after the innervation is present. It would be then of interest to know whether or not ontogenesis of ChE and of ACh of the neurogenic crustacean heart is more nearly related to cardiac neurogenesis than that of the vertebrate heart. However, pertinent data are not available; in the adult insect aliesterases rather than ChE predominate outside the brain and abdominal nervous system (cf. Chapter 16). Eserine, TEPP and other anti-ChE agents generally affected cardiac rate and synergized with ACh in the adult insect (KRIJGSMAN and KRIJGSMAN 1950, KRIJGSMAN 1952, METCALF et al. 1955); pharmacological data suggest therefore that ChE's may be localized in the adult insect heart, at least at minute strategic points, and thus escape detection.

The data obtained in *Limulus* which suggest a relationship between the cholinergic system and ontogeny of cardiac innervation strengthen indirectly earlier speculation (vide supra) on the chronotropic role of ontogeny of the cholinergic system, in spite of its precocity, with respect to innervation, in the vertebrate heart.

On the other hand, it might be speculated that if non-innervated myogenic insect hearts possess ChE, the enzyme may be related in this case to contractility, conductivity, and efficiency of cardiac function, as hypothesized for the vertebrate heart (SIPPEL 1955, BÜLL-BRING et al. 1954). Lack of ACh action upon non-innervated myogenic hearts may not be inconsistent with this view. It should be remembered, however, that there are over a million insect species; the study of their cardiac drug responses is barely initiated, and general discussion of the role of the cholinergic system in adult or embryonic insect hearts may be althogether premature (cf. Chapter 16).

Discussion

While the analysis of ontogenesis of ChE's led to a number of conclusions, it brought up as well certain problems (cf. *Introduction* and Chapter 5) which conceivably could be elucidated by results obtained with anti-ChE agents in the course of development.

1. Early and morphogenetic actions of anti-ChE agents

Indubitably, ChE's appear very early in ontogeny, sometimes in the unfertilized egg, and certainly in the blastula of many species (Chapter 5). These precocious ChE's naturally could not be associated with transmission or motility. However, this does not mean necessarily that early ChE's are involved in growth and morphogenesis; they may appear precociously in rudiments of the nervous system and of other tissues. Unfortunately, their fate with regard to, e.g., differentiation of the muscle, was not traced (Chapter 5).

In parallel, anti-ChE agents exhibit anti-growth, toxic, and morphogenetic changes early in development, prior to neurogenesis or emergence of motility; in fact, such effects were obtained even in the case of seeds and cancer cells. However, in spite of the presence of ChE's at the early developmental stages, morphogenetic and related effects of ChE inhibitors do not have to be mediated by ChE's and the cholinergic system. Indeed, high concentrations of anti-ChE agents were generally necessary (cf., however, KARCZMAR and KOPPANYI 1953) to produce such changes; these concentrations may have been sufficient to affect the metabolism of carbohydrates (LANDAUER 1954) or amino-acids (WINTERINGHAM and HARRISON 1956) Incidentally, several ChE inhibitors, particularly organophosphorus compounds, may exhibit non-cholinesterasic actions in the adult (KARCZMAR 1948, KOPPANYI and KARCZMAR 1951).

Altogether, employment of anti-ChE agents did not resolve the problem of the significance of early aneural appearance of ChE's. Of course, the data are still incomplete; systematic investigation of morphogenetic actions of these agents was undertaken mostly in the chick, less so in *Amphibia* and in the insects, and not at all in other species, and only a few anti-ChE agents were utilized.

2. Functional effects of anti-ChE agents

Theoretically, anti-ChE agents could exhibit, during development, functional effects not dependent on neurogenesis, since non-neural roles have been suggested for ChE's (BÜLBRING and BURN 1949). In the case of the heart, the study of ontogenesis of cardiac ChE's suggested that these enzymes may be related to cardiac contractility and rhythmicity (Chapter 5). On the other hand, effects of anti-ChE and cholinomimetic agents during ontogenesis suggested that ChE's are related to the vagal and autonomic control of cardiac function; these studies demonstrated also the emergence of cardiac cholinergic receptors prior to innervation. Parenthetically, the precocious appearance of cholinergic receptors or their presence in denervated and aneural tissues was stressed several times in this Chapter as well as earlier (Chapter 5).

On the whole, a similar relationship between ChE's and neurogenesis emerged from studies with anti-ChE agents. Particularly in the case of *Amblystoma*, these studies indicated the importance of ontogenesis of ChE's with relation to neurogenesis, development of transmission, and of function of the nervous system. Such correlations seem indicated with regard to the neuromyal junction, the so-called "reflex activity," and perhaps to the mesencephalon.

In view of all this, some investigators (YOUNGSTROM 1941, BOELL 1948) felt that amphibian motility and even qualitative patterns of behavior could be related solely to ChE levels. This is an obvious oversimplification. In the first place, the differences in anti-ChE responses at various developmental stages are not sufficiently discrete to warrant their correlation with specific steps in neurogenesis; in an analogous situation, the relatively smooth curves of the phase of rapid increase of ChE's did not lend themselves to concrete hypothesizing (Chapter 5). Moreover, abnormal behavior after aliphatic depressants resembles that induced by anti-ChE agents (BLUM et al. 1958). Finally, adaptability in *Amblystoma* of function to inhibition of ChE's (cf. p. 819) renders the correlation between ChE's and function difficult.

It should be stressed that on theoretical grounds also, ChE's cannot be regarded as the ultimate or only correlate of the development of behavior. It is likely that much of central transmission is not cholinergic in nature (BRADLEY and ELKES 1957). Accordingly, ChE levels and functional effects of anti-ChE agents during ontogeny can be used to identify steps in neurogenesis only if studied with regard to synapses at which ACh has been identified as the transmitter, or which have been analysed pharmacologically as was done in the adult by ECCLES et al. (1956) with regard to the Golgi collaterals to the Renshaw cells. In fact, earlier reliance on the combination of data on ontogenesis of ChE's on the one hand, and on the ontogenetic effects of anti-ChE agents on the other, for the purpose of pinpointing the role of ChE's in stepwise development of transmission and function should be tempered at present by the realization that the effects of the inhibition of ChE's at any ontogenetic moment must depend not only on the ontogenetic presence of ACh, but also on whether or not other transmitter systems are required at any particular developmental moment for the expression of ChE inhibition. It can be easily imagined that if a particular pathway depends on alternating cholinergic and non-cholinergic neurons, the effects of the inhibition of ChE may be apparent only at the ontogenetic completion of the latter step, but not earlier.

Moreover, ontogenesis of transmittive effects of anti-ChE agents cannot be considered solely in terms of its biochemical aspects; structural (KARCZMAR 1955) as well as on other factors particularly important in controlling and modifying drug action also must be considered. Among these factors are the morphogenesis of protective structures such as the blood-brain barrier, changes in their permeability, appearance of detoxification mechanisms, etc. The pertinent data are not as yet available. Altogether, this analysis of actions of anti-ChE agents on both growth and functional ontogenesis reveals, no less than the earlier (Chapter 5) analysis of ontogenesis of ChE's, that ontogenetic functions of ChE's and of the cholinergic system are not as yet fully understood.

References

AMMON, R.: Die fermentative Spaltung des Acetylcholins. Pflügers Arch. ges. Physiol. **233**, 486—491 (1933).
ANCEL, P.: L'achondroplasie. Sa réalisation éxperimentale, sa pathogénie. Ann. Endocr. (Paris) **6**, 1—24 (1945).
— La Chimioteratogenèse chez les vertébrés. Paris. Gaston Doin et Cie 1950.
ARMSTRONG, P. B.: The role of the nerves in the action of acetylcholine on the embryonic heart. J. Physiol. (Lond.) **84**, 20—32 (1935).
BARRY, A.: The effect of epinephrine on the myocardium of the embryonic chick. Circulation **1**, 1362—1368 (1950).
BLOUNT, R. F.: Transplantation and extripation of the pituitary rudiment and the effects upon pigmentation in the urodele embryo. J. exptl. Zool. **63**, 113—141 (1932).
BARNES, J. M., and F. A. DENZ: Experimental demyelination with organophosphorus compounds. J. Path. Bact. **65**, 597—605 (1953).
BLUM, B., T. KOPPANYI, and A. G. KARCZMAR: Drug action on the central nervous system during development of urodele larvae. Arch. int. Pharmacodyn. **115**, 433—451 (1958).
BOELL, E. J.: The effect of di-isopropyl fluorophos on the development of behavior and cholinesterase in Amblystoma punctatum. Anat. Rec. **96**, 500—501 (1946).
— Biochemical differentiation during amphibian development. Ann. N. Y. Acad. Sci. **49**, 773—800 (1948).
BRADLEY, P. B.: The central action of certain drugs in relation to the reticular formation of the brain. In: H. H. JASPER, Ed., Reticular Formation of the Brain, 123—150. Boston: Little, Brown & Co. 1958.
—, and J. ELKES: The distribution of cholinergic and noncholinergic receptors in the brain: electrophysiological evidence. In: D. RICHTER, Ed., Metabolism of the Nervous System, 515—522. New York: Pergamon Press 1957.
BROWN, F. A.: Chromatophores and color change. In: C. LADD PROSSER, Ed., Comparative Animal Physiology, 677—724. Philadelphia: W. B. Saunders Co. 1950.
BUEKER, E. D., and W. S. PLATNER: Effect of cholinergic drugs on development of chick embryo. Proc. Soc. exp. Biol. (N. Y.) **91**, 539—543 (1956).
BÜLBRING, E., and J. H. BURN: Action of acetylcholine on rabbit auricles in relation to acetylcholine synthesis. J. Physiol. (Lond.) **108**, 508—524 (1949).
— S. R. KOTTEGODA and A. SHELLEY: Cholinesterase activity in the auricles of the rabbit's heart and their sensitivity to eserine. J. Physiol. (Lond.) **123**, 204—213 (1954).
BULLOCK, T. H., and D. NACHMANSOHN: Cholinesterase in primitive nervous systems. J. cell. comp. Physiol. **20**, 239—242 (1942).
CARLSON, A. J., and W. J. MEEK: On the mechanism of the embryonic heart rhythm in Limulus. Amer. J. Physiol. **21**, 1—10 (1908).

CHEN, G., and E. M. K. GEILING: Studies on the chemistry and pharmacology of the melano-phore hormone of the pituitary gland. J. Pharmacol. exp. Ther. **78**, 222—237 (1943).

CHINO, H.: Enzymatic synthesis and hydrolysis of acetylcholine in the egg of the silkworm, *Bombyx mori*. Annot. zool. Jap. **30**, 106—113 (1957).

COGHILL, G. E.: Somatic myogenic action in embryos of Fundulus heteroclitus. Proc. Soc. exp. Biol. (N. Y.). **31**, 62—64 (1933).

DALE, H. H.: Transmission of nervous effects by acetylcholine. Harvey Lect. **32**, 229—245 (1937).

DESMEDT, J. E., and G. LA GRUTTA: Effect of selective inhibition of pseudocholinesterase on the spontaneous and evoked activity of the cat's cerebral cortex. J. Physiol. (Lond.) **136**, 20—40 (1957).

DIAMOND, J., and R. MILEDI: The sensitivity of foetal and new-born rat muscle to acetyl-choline. J. Physiol. (Lond.) **149**, 50 P, 1959.

DuBois, K. P.: Personal communication (1961).

—, and E. PUCHALA: Studies on the sex difference in toxicity of a cholinergic phosphorothioate. Proc. Soc. exp. Biol. (N. Y.) **107**, 908—911 (1961).

—, and G. H. MANGUN: Effect of hexaethyl tetraphosphate on choline esterase *in vitro* and *in vivo*. Proc. Soc. exp. Biol. (N. Y.) **64**, 137—139 (1947).

— J. DOULL, P. R. SALERNO and J. M. COON: Studies on the toxicity and mechanism of action of p-nitrophenyl thionophosphate (Parathion). J. Pharmacol. exp. Ther. **95**, 79—91 (1949).

DUKE, H. N., M. PICKFORD and J. A. WATT: The immediate and delayed effects of isopropyl-fluorophosphate injected into supraoptic nuclei of dogs. J. Physiol. (Lond.) **111**, 81—88 (1950).

ECCLES, J. C., R. M. ECCLES and P. FATT: Pharmacological investigations on a central synapse operated by acetylcholine. J. Physiol. (Lond.) **131**, 154—169 (1956).

ELKES, J., J. T. EAYRS and A. TODRICK: In: H. WAELSH, Ed., Biochemistry of the Developing Nervous System, 499—509. New York: Academic Press, Inc. 1955.

FELDBERG, W.: Acetylcholine. In: D. RICHTER, Ed., Metabolism of the Nervous System, 493—510. New York: Pergamon Press, 1957

FINGL, E. L., A. WOODBURY and H. H. HECHT: Effect of innervation and drugs upon direct membrane potentials of embryonic chick myocardium. J. Pharmacol. exp. Ther. **104**, 103—114 (1952).

FRAWLEY, J. P., E. C. HAGAN and O. G. FITZHUGH: A comparative pharmacological and toxicological study of organic phosphate-anticholinesterase compounds. J. Pharmacol. exp. Ther. **106**, 156—165 (1952).

FREEDMAN, A. M., and H. C. HIMWICH: Effect of age on lethality di*iso*propyl fluophosphate. Amer. J. Physiol. **153**, 121—126 (1948).

GARREY, W. E.: Action of acetylcholine on cultures of chick heart. Amer. J. Physiol. **119**, 314 (only) (1937).

GIARMAN, N. U.: Neurohumors in the brain. Yale J. Biol. Med. **32**, 73—92 (1959).

GREEN, J. D.: An hypophysial portal system in certain amphibia, and nerve endings associated with neuro-hypophysial vessels. Anat. Rec. **97**, 416 (only) (1947).

HALL, E. K.: Acetylcholine and epinephrine effects on the embryonic rat heart. J. cell. comp. Physiol. **49**, 187—200 (1957).

HERRICK, C. J.: Internal structure of the thalamus and midbrain of early feeding larvae of Amblystoma. J. comp. Neurol. **70**, 89—135 (1939).

— Optic and postoptic systems in the brain of Amblystoma tigrinum. J. comp. Neurol. **77**, 191—353 (1942).

HOGBEN, L., and D. SLOME: The pigmentary effector system. VI. The dual character of endo-crine coordination in Amphibian color change. Proc. roy. Soc. Lond. B. **108**, 10—53 (1931).

—, and F. R. WINTON: Hypophysis and Amphibian color change. Proc. roy. Soc. Lond. B. **85**, 15—30 (1923).

HOLMSTEDT, B.: Pharmacology of organophosphorus cholinesterase inhibitors. Pharmacol. Rev. **11**, 567—688 (1959).

HOLZ, W.: Wirkung von E 605-f auf Eier verschiedener Insekten. Anz. Schädlingsk. **22**, 134—138 (1949).

JONES, D. S.: The origin of the vagi and the parasympathetic ganglion cells of the viscera of the chick. Anat. Rec. **82**, 185—197 (1942).

— Effects of acetylcholine and adrenalin on experimentally uninnervated heart of the chick embryo. Anat. Rec. **130**, 253—260 (1958).

JONES, J. C.: The heart and associated tissues of Anopheles quadrimaculatus Say (Diptera: Culicidae). J. Morph. **94**, 71—124 (1954).

— The heart and associated tissues of Anopheles quadrimaculatus Say larvae. J. exptl. Zool. **131**, 223—233 (1956a).

— Effects of drugs on Anopheles heart rates. J. exptl. Zool. **133**, 573—588 (1956b).

KARCZMAR, A. G.: Anti-cholinesterase and toxic effects of Parathion (o-o-diethyl p-nitrophenol thiophosphate). Anat. Rec. **101**, 739 (only) (1948).
— Limb regeneration and differentiation of "overt behavior" in urodeles as studied by means of their response to chemical agents. Ann. N. Y. Acad. Sci. **60**, 1108—1135 (1955).
—, and T. KOPPANYI: Action of central nervous system depressants at different growth periods of salamander larvae, II. Anat. Rec. **101**, 713 (only) (1948).
— — Central effects of diisopropylfiurophosphonate (DFP) in Urodele larvae. Naunyn-Schmiedeberg's Arch. exp. Path. Pharmak. **219**, 263—272 (1953).
—, and J. P. LONG: Relationship between peripheral cholinolytic potency and tetraethyl-pyrophosphate antagonism of a series of atropine substitutes. J. Pharmacol. exp. Ther. **123**, 230—237 (1958).
KARNOFSKY, D. A.: The use of the developing chick embryo in pharmacologic research. Stanf. med. Bull. **13**, 247—259 (1955).
— C. Ross and C. G. W. LEAVITT: Effects of quaternary ammonium and cholinergic drugs on skeletal development of chick embryo. Fed. Proc. **13**, 373 (only) (1954).
KLEINHOLZ, L. H.: Studies in reptilian color changes, II. The pituitary and adrenal glands in the regulation of the melanophores of Anolis carolinensis. J. exp. Biol. **15**, 474—491 (1938).
KOELLE, G. B.: Histochemical demonstration of reversible anticholinesterase action at selective cellular sites in vivo. J. Pharmacol. exp. Ther. **120**, 488—503 (1957).
KOPPANYI, T., and A. G. KARCZMAR: Pharmacological methods in the study of overt behavior. Fed. Proc. **6**, 346 (only) (1947).
— — Contribution to the study of the mechanism of action of cholinesterase inhibitors. J. Pharmacol. exp. Ther. **101**, 327—343 (1951).
KRIJGSMAN, B. J.: Contractile and pacemaker mechanism of the heart of arthropods. Biol. Rev. **27**, 320—346 (1952).
—, and N. E. KRIJGSMAN: Heart mechanism of arthropods. Nature (Lond.) **165**, 936—937 (1950).
KHUDOROZHEVA, A. T.: The role of Cerebellum in the development of the functions of skeletal muscles in ontogenesis. Material on Evolut. Physiol. **1**, 333—348 (1956). Available in English Translation in The Central Nervous System and Behavior, U.S. Dept. of Health, Education and Welfare, Bethesda, Md. (1959).
KUSCHINSKY, G., H. LULLMANN and E. MUSCHOLL: Untersuchungen über die Einwirkung von verschiedenen Pharmaka auf die Spontanrhythmik des isolierten Hühneramnion. Naunyn-Schmiedeberg's Arch. exp. Pathol. Pharmakol. **223**, 369—374 (1954).
LANDAUER, W.: Le problème de l'électivité dans les expériences de la tératogenèse biochimique. Arch. Anat. micr. Morph. exp. **38**, 184—189 (1949).
— On teratogenic effects of pilocarpine in chick development. J. exptl. Zool. **122**, 469—483 (1953a).
— Abnormality of down pigmentation associated with experimentally produced skeletal defects of chicks. Proc. nat. Acad. Sci. (Wash.) **39**, 54—58 (1953b).
— On the chemical production of developmental abnormalities and of phenocopies in chicken embryos. J. cell. comp. Physiol. **43**, 261—305 (1954).
LANGLEY, J. N.: On the reaction of the cells and of nerve endings to certain poisons, chiefly as regards the reaction of striated muscle to nicotine and to curari. J. Physiol. (Lond.) **33**, 374—413 (1905).
LEVI-MONTALCINI, R., and F. VISINTIAI: Azione del curare, della stricnina, dell'eserina, dell'acetilcolina sulla transmissione dell'influsso nell' embrione di pollo del 4° all' 8° giorno d'incubazione. Boll. Soc. ital. Biol. sper. **13**, 979—981 (1938).
LEWIS, S. E., and K. S. FOWLER: Effect of diisopropylphosphorofluoridate on the acetylcholine content of flies. Nature (Lond.) **178**, 919—920 (1956).
LORD, K. A., and C. POTTER: Mechanism of action of organo-phosphorus compounds as insecticides. Nature (Lond.) **166**, 893—894 (1950).
— — Studies on the mechanism of insecticidal action of organo-phosphorus compounds with particular reference to their anti-esterase activity. Ann. appl. Biol. **38**, 495—507 (1951).
— — Hydrolysis of esters by extracts of insects. Nature (Lond.) **172**, 679—681 (1953).
MATHEWS, A. P.: The action of pilocarpine and atropine on the embryos of the starfish and the sea-urchin. Amer. J. Physiol. **6**, 207—215 (1902).
MAZUR, A., and O. BODANSKY: Mechanism of *in vitro* and *in vivo* inhibition of cholinesterase activity by di-isopropyl fluorophosphate. J. biol. Chem. **163**, 261—276 (1946).
McCARTY, L. P., W. C. LEE and F. E. SHIDEMAN: Measurement of the inotropic effects of drugs on the innervated and non-innervated embryonic chick heart. J. Pharmacol. exp. Ther. **129**, 315—321 (1960).
MENDEL, B., D. K. MYERS, I. E. MYLDERT, A. C. RUYS and W. M. DEBRUYN: Aliesterase inhibitors and growth. Brit. J. Pharmacol. **8**, 217—224 (1953).
MEHROTRA, K. N., and B. N. SMALLMAN: Ovicidal action of organo-phosphorus insecticides. Nature (Lond.) **180**, 97—98 (1957).

METCALF, R. L., R. B. MARCH and M. G. MAXON: Substrate preferences of insect cholinesterases. Ann. Ent. Soc. Amer. 48, 222—228 (1955).

MICHAELIS, M., J. E. FINESINGER, F. DEBALBIAN VERSTER and R. W. ERICSON: The effect of the intravenous injection of DFP and atropine on the level of free acetylcholine in the cerebral cortex of the rabbit. J. Pharmacol. exp. Ther. 111, 169—175 (1954).

MILBURN, N., E. A. WEIANT and K. D. ROEDER: The release of efferent nerve activity in the roach, *Periplaneta americana*, by extracts of the corpus cardiacum. Biol. Bull. 118, 111 to 119 (1960).

MONRO, J.: Cholinesterase and the secretion of the brain hormone in insects. Aust. J. biol. Sci. 11, 399—406 (1958).

NACHMANSOHN, D., M. A. ROTHENBERG and E. A. FELD: The *in vitro* reversibility of cholinesterase inhibition by di*iso*propyl fluorophosphate (DFP). Arch. Biochem. 14, 197—211 (1947).

O'BRIEN, R. D.: Occurrence of cholinesterase in *Tenebrio* and *Tribolium*. Nature (Lond.) 172, 162—163 (1953).

PARKER, G. H.: On the neurohumors of the color changes in catfish and on fats and oils as protective agents for such substances. Proc. Amer. Philos. Soc. 83, 379—409 (1940).

— Animal color changes and their neurohumors. Quart. Rev. Biol. 18, 205—227 (1943).

PICKERING, J. W.: Observation on the physiology of the embryonic heart. J. Physiol. (Lond.) 14, 383—466 (1893).

— Muscarine on chick embryo hearts. J. Physiol. (Lond.) 18, 470—483 (1895).

POTTER, C.: Report Rothamsted expt. Sta. 131 (only) (1958).

— K. A. LORD, J. KENTEN, E. H. SALKELD and D. V. HOLBROOK: Embryonic development and esterase activity of eggs of *Pieris brassicae* in relation to TEPP poisoning. Ann. appl. Biol. 45, 361—375 (1957).

PROSSER, C. L.: An analysis of the action of acetylcholine on hearts, particularly in arthropods. Biol. Bull. 83, 145—164 (1942).

— Comparative Animal Physiology. Philadelphia: W. B. Saunders Co. 1950.

RINALDI, F., and H. E. HIMWICH: Alerting responses and actions of atropine and cholinergic drugs. Arch. Neurol. Psychiat. (Chicago) 73, 387—395 (1955).

ROEDER, K. D., L. TOZIAN and E. A. WEIANT: Endogenous nerve activity and behavior in the mantis and cockroach. J. Insect Physiol. 4 (1), 45—62 (1960).

RUSSELL, R. W.: Effects of "biochemical lesions" on behavior. Acta Psychol. 14, 281—294 (1958).

SALKELD, H., and C. POTTER: The effect of the age and stage of development of insect eggs on their resistance to insecticides. Bull. ent. Res. 44, 527—580 (1953).

SAWYER, C. H.: Cholinesterase and the behavior problem in Amblystoma. I. The relationship between the development of the enzyme and early motility. II. The effects of inhibiting cholinesterase. J. exptl. Zool. 92, 1—27 (1943a).

— Cholinesterase and the behavior problem in Amblystoma. III. The distribution of cholinesterase in nerve and muscle throughout development. IV. Cholinesterase in nerveless muscle. J. exptl. Zool. 94, 1—31 (1943b).

— Nature of the early somatic movements in Fundulus heteroclitus. J. cell. comp. Physiol. 24, 71—84 (1944).

— Cholinergic stimulation of the release of melanophore hormone by the hypophysis in salamander larvae. J. exptl. Zool. 106, 145—180 (1947).

— Further experiments on cholinesterase and reflex activity in Amblystoma larvae. J. exptl. Zool. 129, 561—578 (1955).

SCHUHMANN, G.: Investigations on the effect of phosphonic acid esters on pests occurring in stone fruit (*Rhagoletis cerasi* L., *Laspeyresia funebrana* Tr., *Hoplocampa minuta* Christ. and *Hoplocampa flava* L.). Höfchen-Briefe VI (5), 233—250 (1953).

SCHWARTZ, E.: Wirkung von E 605-f auf Eier des Kartoffelkäfers. Anz. Schädlingsk. 23, 87 (only) (1950).

SEAMAN, G. R., and H. K. HOULIHAN: Enzyme systems of Tetrahymena gelii (S). II. Acetylcholinesterase activity. Its relation to motility of the organism and to coordinated ciliary action in general. J. cell. comp. Physiol. 37, 309—322 (1951).

SHAPPIRIO, D. G., and C. M. WILLIAMS: The cytochrome system of the Cecropia silkworm. I. Spectroscopic studies of individual tissues. Proc. roy. soc. Lond. B 147, 218—232 (1957).

SHEN, T. C. R.: The mechanism of the melanophore-expanding action of several drugs and its relationship to the internal secretion of the hypophysis in frogs. Arch. int. Pharmacodyn. 62, 295—329 (1939).

SINGER, M., M. H. DAVIS and M. R. SCHEUING: The influence of atropine and other neuropharmacological substances on regeneration of the forelimb in the adult Urodele, *Triturus*. J. exptl. Zool. 143, 33—46 (1960).

SIPPEL, T. O.: The growth of succinoxidase activity in the hearts of rat and chick embryos. J. exptl. Zool. **126**, 205—221 (1954).
— Properties and development of cholinesterase in the hearts of certain vertebrates. J. exptl. Zool. **128**, 165—184 (1955).
SMALLMAN, B. N., and R. W. FISHER: Effect of anticholinesterases on acetylcholine levels in insects. Canad. J. Biochem. **36**, 575—585 (1958).
SMITH, E. H.: Further studies on the ovicidal action of Parathion to eggs of the peach tree borer. J. Econ. Ent. **48**, 727—731 (1955).
—, and A. W. AVENS: The ovicidal action of Parathion in control of the peach tree borer. J. Econ. Ent. **47** (5), 912—917 (1954).
—, and A. C. WAGENKNECHT: The occurrance of cholinesterase in the eggs of the peach tree borer and large milk weed bug and its relation to the ovicidal action of Parathion. J. Econ. Ent. **49**, 777—783 (1956).
SOLLMANN, T. L.: The simultaneous action of pilocarpine and atropine on the developing embryos of the sea-urchin and starfish. A contribution to the study of the antagonistic action of poisons. Amer. J. Physiol. **10**, 352—361 (1904).
SPEYER, W.: Haben die modernen Kontaktgifte eine ovicide Wirkung? Nachrichtenbl. Dtsch. Pflanzenschutzdienst (Berlin) **2**, 2—3 (1950).
STAUDENMAYER, T.: The influence of "E 605" on the respiration of silkworm eggs. Höfchenbr. Wiss. **6**, 158—166 (1953).
— Die Cholinesterase während der Eierentwicklung von *Bombyx mori* und die ovizide Wirkung von Phosphorsäure-ester (E 600 and E 605). Z. vergl. Physiol. **37**, 416—423 (1955).
— Die Wirkung verschiedener Kontaktinsektizide auf die Atmung von Seidenspinnereien. Z. vergl. Physiol. **39**, 262—273 (1957).
STOPPANI, A. O. M.: Pharmacology of color regulation in Amphibia and the importance of endocrine glands. J. Pharm. exp. Ther. **76**, 118—125 (1942).
TEAGUE, R. S., R. O. NOOJIN and E. M. K. GEILING: The hypophysectomized frog (Rana pipiens) as a specific test object for melanophore hormone of the pituitary body. J. Pharm. exp. Ther. **65**, 115—127 (1939).
TSCHERMAK, V. A.: Physiologische Untersuchungen am embryonalen Fischherzen. S.-B. Akad. Wiss. Wien, Abt. III **118**, 17—115 (1909).
VAN ASPEREN, K.: Mode of action of organophosphorus insecticides. Nature (Lond.) **181**, 355—356 (1958).
VAN DER KLOOT, W. G.: The control of neurosecretion and diapause by physiological changes in the brain of the Cecropia silkworm. Biol. Bull. Wood's Hole **109**, 276—294 (1955).
WHITING, H. P.: Functional development in the nervous system. In: H. WAELSH, Ed., Biochemistry of the Developing Nervous System, 85—103. New York: Academic Press Inc. 1955.
WILLIAMS, C. M.: Biochemical mechanisms in insect growth and metamorphosis. Fed. Proc. **10**, 546—552 (1951).
WILSON, I. B.: Acetylcholinesterase. XI. Reversibility of tetraethyl pyrophosphate inhibition. J. biol. Chem. **190**, 111—117 (1951).
WINTERINGHAM, F. P. W., and A. HARRISON: Study of anticholinesterase action in insects by a labelled pool technique. Nature (Lond.) **178**, 81—83 (1956).
WOODBURY, L. A., H. H. HECHT and A. R. CHRISTOPHERSON: Membrane resting and action potentials of single cardiac muscle fibers of the frog ventricle. Amer. J. Physiol. **164**, 307—318 (1951).
YOUNGSTROM, K. A.: On the relationship between cholinesterase and the development of behavior in amphibia. J. Neurophysiol. **1**, 357—363 (1938a).
— Studies on the developing behavior of amura. J. comp. Neurol. **68**, 357—379 (1938b).
— Acetylcholinesterase concentration during the development of the human fetus. J. Neurophysiol. **4**, 473—477 (1941).
ZACKS, S. I.: Esterases in the early chick embryo. Anat. Rec. **118**, 509—537 (1954).
ZINGONI, U.: The effect of acetylcholine and adrenin on inotropism, chronotropism and tonus of the chick embryo heart lacking nervous elements. Arch. Fisiol. **56** (3), 226—236 (1956).
ZWILLING, E.: Carbohydrate metabolism in insulin-treated chick embryos. Arch. Biochem. **33**, 228—242 (1951).

Chapter 18

Toxicological Evaluation
of the Anticholinesterase Agents

By

Kenneth P. DuBois

Contents

Introduction

The toxicology of the anticholinesterase (anti-ChE) agents has received a great deal of attention during the last twenty years. The intense interest exhibited in this aspect of their biological actions has been stimulated by consideration of their potential value as chemical warfare agents and to a greater extent in recent years by their established value and widespread use as agricultural insecticides. The latter practical application of these compounds has prompted investigation of their toxicity to various laboratory animals as a means of evaluating the possible human health hazards to those engaged in the manufacture and use of these compounds and the consumption of food upon which they have been used. The anti-ChE agents have limited medicinal uses. By far the most important use of these agents at the present time, from the standpoint of both the quantities involved and benefits derived, is for the eradication of destructive insects. High toxicity to insects is thus an essential requirement for anti-ChE agents.

Any consideration of available toxicity data on anti-ChE agents must take into account the fact that the conduction of experiments of this type is generally done in connection with some aspect of the practical use of the chemical agents because toxicological studies are costly and time consuming. As a result each group of investigators conducts toxicity tests in which the types of experiments and procedures used are selected with primary consideration's being given to the practical problems at hand. The data originating from various laboratories are thus frequently not strictly comparable. Nevertheless, the available data are sufficiently comprehensive to permit a close estimation of the degree of toxicity exhibited by most of the important anti-ChE agents.

Toxicological studies on anti-ChE agents have benefited from the attention of investigators in several disciplines who have not limited their work to the collection of toxicity data. Thus, the mode of action, the metabolism, and factors governing the toxicity of these compounds are receiving a great deal of attention. This approach to the study of the toxicology of anti-ChE agents has proven fruitful by contributing substantially to an understanding of the details of their biological actions.

At the present time evaluation of the toxicology of anti-ChE agents usually consists in the conduction of a series of experiments which include the measurement of acute toxicity by several routes of administration, subacute toxicity by the repeated injection or by feeding the compounds, and chronic toxicity by feeding various low levels of the compounds in the diet for long periods of time. With this particular group of compounds measurement of the anti-ChE action has become an established part of the toxicity evaluations. This chapter describes the toxicity of a number of anti-ChE agents together with consideration of their mode of action and metabolism as they relate to and govern the toxicology of these chemical agents.

A. Acute toxicity

Acute poisoning by the anti-ChE agents results in characteristic signs and symptoms which are referable primarily to inhibition of cholinesterases (ChE's) with consequent accumulation of acetylcholine (ACh). Thus, the symptoms of acute intoxication are probably due chiefly to ACh, the normal hydrolytic disposal of which is inhibited by the agents. The resultant effects on various organ systems have been described in detail in other chapters of this volume. Only a brief description of the effects that result from acute intoxication in the intact animal will be presented here for the purpose of orientation in connection with subsequent comments concerning the differences in toxicity between individual anti-ChE agents.

In view of the extensive use of anti-ChE agents as insecticides, exposure to vapors or aerosols of these agents is common. This type of exposure causes a local action on the eye and respiratory tract before any systemic effects are noted. The local ocular action consists in miosis, spasm of accommodation, and dimness of vision. The actions on the respiratory tract are characterized by tightness in the chest, a watery nasal discharge, bronchoconstriction, and increased bronchial secretion. Recognition of these symptoms can be extremely important from the standpoint of avoiding systemic intoxication because they occur at dosage levels far below those necessary to produce systemic effects.

The systemic toxic effects of anti-ChE agents may occur after inhalation, contamination and penetration of the skin, or ingestion. The majority of anti-ChE agents to which people are liable to be exposed have a relatively low volatility, but their use generally necessitates dispersion as liquid sprays or dusts thus making inhalation the most frequent route of poisoning for those engaged in the formulation and use of these materials. The majority of important organic phosphates of the anti-ChE series are liquid, fat-soluble compounds which are absorbed appreciably through the intact skin, thus presenting a danger to all those engaged in any aspect of their manufacture and use. With a few exceptions the anti-ChE agents of this chemical class are well absorbed from the gastrointestinal tract, but acute poisoning by this route has occurred largely from intentional, and probably only occasionally from accidental ingestion.

Acute intoxication by the anti-ChE agents always results in the occurrence of at least some symptoms referable to stimulation of the parasympathetically innervated effectors (muscarinic effects), consisting in bronchoconstriction, sweating, salivation and other increased glandular secretions, anorexia, nausea, abdominal cramps, vomiting, diarrhea, involuntary defecation, and increased urination. These effects are of paramount importance because all anti-ChE agents with activity *in vivo* produce some or all of the muscarinic actions of ACh.

The actions of anti-ChE agents on skeletal muscle (nicotinic effects) include muscular twitching, muscular fasciculation, increased fatigability, and weakness of skeletal muscles, including the muscles of respiration.

Among the effects of anti-ChE agents on the central nervous system are anxiety, restlessness, impairment of memory, speech defects, convulsions, and coma.

From a qualitative standpoint the signs and symptoms produced by anti-ChE agents in various mammalian species are essentially the same, which suggests similar tissue distribution patterns. However, the doses required to elicit toxic effects differ considerably in various species; this is probably due largely to differences in the rate and extent of detoxification of the compounds.

I. Fluoride and cyanide-containing organic phosphates

Several hundred phosphorus-containing compounds of widely varying structures were examined as candidate chemical warfare agents during World War II, but only a few, including the dialkyl phosphorofluoridates, the diamidophosphoryl fluorides, the alkyl fluorophosphonates and the alkyl phosphoroamidocyanidates, have merited detailed toxicological evaluation. The phosphorofluoridates have been used extensively in research on the nervous system but their high toxicity, volatility, and instability have prevented their use as insecticides and markedly restricted their medicinal applications. The phosphorofluoridates have been surpassed in toxicological potency and potential value as chemical warfare agents by other agents, including the alkyl phosphoroamidocyanidates and phosphonofluoridates.

In view of the former interest in these anti-ChE agents as potential chemical warfare agents, most of the toxicity studies conducted for the purpose of comparing the potency of various compounds and the measurement of species differences in susceptibility have been done using the inhalation route. Table 1 shows the inhalation toxicity of diisopropyl phosphorofluoridate (DFP) to several species. The data are expressed in terms of the LCt_{50}, which is the product of the airborne vapor concentration (in mg per m³) and the exposure time (in minutes) that causes death of 50% of the exposed animals. Table 2 gives the LCt_{50} values for several of the more important members of this class of compounds under comparable experimental conditions. These data show the extremely high toxicity of ethyl-N-dimethyl phosphoramidocyanidate (Tabun) and the phosphonofluoridates. Species differences

Table 1.
Toxicity of DFP by inhalation

Species	LCt_{50} (mg/m³) × min
Mouse	5,900
Rat	2,800
Guinea pig	8,000
Rabbit	8,000
Dog	5,000
Monkey	800

in susceptibility to the toxicity of these particular compounds are small. It is likely that the high toxicity of these agents to all species is due to their potent anti-ChE activity and to inefficient detoxification mechanisms. The phosphorofluoridates are considerably less toxic and exhibit larger species differences than the cyanidates and phosphonofluoridates.

The parenteral toxicity of some members of this class of compounds has received some attention. HORTON et al. (1946) found that the LD_{50}'s of DFP by the oral route in mg/kg are 37 for mice, 5 to 10 for rats, and 4 to 10 for rabbits. These investigators obtained i.v. LD_{50} values of 1.6 mg/kg for cats, 3.4 for dogs, 0.34 for rabbits, 0.25 for monkeys, and 0.8 for goats. McNAMARA (1946) found the LD_{50} by the i.m. route to be 0.75 mg/kg for rabbits. STREICHER (1951) reported that the LD_{50} for mice given DFP by the s.c. route is 4.7 mg/kg. FRAWLEY et al. (1952) observed a sex difference in the susceptibility of rats to DFP as evidenced by oral

53*

LD_{50} values of 7.7 and 13.5 mg/kg for females and males, respectively. It is clear from these data that there are considerable species differences in the susceptibility of various species to DFP, and that within a given species the LD_{50} is influenced significantly by the route of administration of the compound. The acute toxic actions of DFP are closely associated with its anti-ChE activity. However, if species differences in susceptibility were due only to differences in the reactivity of the compound with ChE's, it would be expected that similar patterns of species susceptibility would be noted with other organophosphorus compounds. However,

Table 2. *Inhalation toxicity of organophosphorus compounds containing fluoride and cyanide*

	Chemical structure	LCt_{50} (mg/m³) × min		
		Mouse	Monkey	Rat
Ethyl-N-dimethyl phos-phoroamidocyanidate (Tabun)	$(CH_3)_2N$ C_2H_5O >P—CN ‖ O	380	250	300
*Iso*propyl-methyl-phosphonofluoridate (Sarin)	i—C_3H_7O CH_3 >P—F ‖ O	250	150	300
*Iso*propyl-ethyl-phos-phonofluoridate	i—C_3H_7O C_2H_5 >P—F ‖ O	330	200	260
Dimethyl phosphoro-fluoridate	CH_3O CH_3O >P—F ‖ O	2,600	...	4,000
Diethyl phosphoro-fluoridate	C_2H_5O C_2H_5O >P—F ‖ O	8,200	...	10,500
Di*iso*propyl phosphoro-fluoridate (DFP)	i—C_3H_7O i—C_3H_7O >P—F ‖ O	5,900	600	2,800

All values were obtained using a 10-minute exposure period.

it will become apparent in this communication that there is no predictable or consistent pattern among the various compounds. Therefore, it seems reasonable to assume that the toxic dose of each compound for various species is influenced to a large extent by the rate and extent of detoxification. Thus, in the case of DFP the "phosphofluorase" activity (MAZUR 1946) of the tissues of various species was shown to influence the toxicity of the compound.

Relatively little information has been published on the parenteral toxicity of the phosphonofluoridates and the phosphoamidocyanidates. HOLMSTEDT (1951, 1959) reported that the i.p. LD_{50} of *iso*propyl methylphosphonofluoridate (Sarin; GB) for mice is 0.42 mg/kg. Unpublished experiments in the reviewer's laboratory have indicated that the i.v. LD_{50} values for this compound in mg/kg are 0.045 for rats and 0.016 for rabbits; the oral LD_{50} for rats is 0.55. The ethyl analogue of Sarin (*iso*propyl-ethylphosphonofluoridate) is slightly less toxic as evidenced by an LD_{50} of 0.69 mg/kg for mice by the i.p. route (HOLMSTEDT 1951, 1959).

The parenteral toxicity of ethyl-N-dimethyl phosphoroamidocyanidate (Tabun) is extremely high. Thus, the i.v. LD_{50} values obtained in the reviewer's laboratory, in mg/kg, are 0.15 for mice, 0.06 for rats, 0.06 for rabbits, and 0.08 for dogs. By the oral route the compound is considerably less toxic as indicated by LD_{50} values of 3.7 for rats, 16.3 for rabbits, and 8 for dogs. The value for mice, i.p., is 0.6 (HOLMSTEDT 1951). The latter author measured also the i.p. toxicity of several similar compounds and found that *iso*propyl-N-dimethyl phosphoroamidocyanidate is more toxic than Tabun, but ethyl substitution of the nitrogen atom or replacement of the ethoxy group with *iso*propyl or methyl groups reduced the toxicity, as evidenced by LD_{50} values in the range of 1 to 5 mg/kg.

In England, three of the fluoride-containing organophosphates have been employed as systemic insecticides. They have properties that are unique among the organophosphates in that they are stable in aqueous solutions, are readily absorbed by plants, and are translocated throughout plants rendering them toxic to several species of insects (SCHRADER and KÜKENTHAL 1941, GREENSLADE 1949,

Table 3. *Chemical structures and toxicities of phosphorodiamidic fluorides to rats*

Compound	Chemical structure	Half-life at pH 7	I.p. LD_{50} for rats (mg/kg)
Tetramethylphosphorodiamidic fluoride (Dimefox; BFPO; Hanane)	$(CH_3)_2N$ $(CH_3)_2N$ $>$P—F ‖ O	>10 years	5
N,N'-Di*iso*propylphosphorodiamidic fluoride (Mipafox; Isopestox)	i—C_3H_7NH i—C_3H_7NH $>$P—F ‖ O	60 days	90
Tetraethylphosphorodiamidic fluoride	$(C_2H_5)_2N$ $(C_2H_5)_2N$ $>$P—F ‖ O	>10 years	3

RIPPER 1952). Table 3 gives the names, chemical structures, and some physical properties of fluoride-containing organophosphorus insecticides. Since the insecticidal use of these compounds requires absorption by plants, their mammalian toxicity is a problem of considerable importance and has resulted in marked restriction of their practical applications.

The acute toxicity of tetramethyl phosphorodiamidic fluoride (BFPO; Dimefox) has been studied by several investigators (DUBOIS and COCHRAN 1951, HOLMSTEDT 1951, ALDRIDGE and BARNES 1952, ALDRIDGE 1953, OKINAKA et al. 1954). Under comparable conditions the LD_{50} values by the i.p. route were found (OKINAKA et al. 1954) to be 5 mg/kg for rats, 1.4 for mice, and 2.5 for guinea pigs. The oral LD_{50} for rats was 7.5 mg/kg and the i.v. LD_{50} for dogs was between 5 and 10. Similar toxicity values have been reported by other investigators as evidenced by i.p. LD_{50} values of 5 mg/kg for rats and 1.2 for mice. Rats exhibit no significant sex difference in susceptibility to this compound. Aqueous solutions of BFPO exhibit the same toxicity when allowed to stand at room temperature for two weeks (OKINAKA et al. 1954). It is pertinent to a discussion of the toxicity of this compound to indicate that the parent compound has extremely low anti-ChE activity *in vitro* (COCHRAN and DUBOIS 1951, ALDRIDGE and BARNES 1952, OKINAKA et al. 1954) but is a highly active inhibitor of ChE's *in vivo* due to oxidation of the parent compound to a metabolite with high anti-ChE activity. It is also noteworthy with respect to the toxicity of this compound that it produces all the cholinergic effects of organophosphorus compounds except signs referable to stimulation of the central nervous system. This selective action is due to the inability of the active metabolite to gain access to brain ChE *in vivo* (OKINAKA et al. 1954). Thus, BFPO produces essentially the same type of actions as DFP and has similar mammalian toxicity, but it differs in its stability in aqueous solutions and in its inability to affect the central nervous system. The toxicity of the ethyl analogue (tetraethylphosphorodiamidic fluoride) of BFPO has received little attention but it appears to be considerably less toxic than BFPO as evidenced by an s.c. LD_{50} of 160 mg/kg for mice (SAUNDERS 1957).

N,N-Di*iso*propylphosphorodiamidic fluoride (Mipafox; Isopestox) has been given a considerable amount of study in connection with its systemic insecticidal action. It has a lower acute toxicity than BFPO as indicated by an i.p. LD_{50} of 90 mg/kg for rats and an oral LD_{50} of 100 for rabbits (GREENSLADE 1949, DAVIES 1954). The acute toxic effects of this compound are typical of anti-ChE agents, with the muscarinic actions predominating. However, it produces also persistent muscular paralysis after a latent interval of approximately two weeks following sublethal doses. Two cases of paralysis in humans have been described in detail by BIDSTRUP et al. (1953) who pointed out the similarity between this compound and the demyelinating action of triorthocresyl phosphate. The biochemical mechanism underlying the ability of Mipafox and some other organophosphate compounds to produce demyelination and a resultant persistent paralysis has not been elucidated. This action is exhibited most often by those agents which have a relatively low toxicity and weak anti-ChE action, or when atropine is given to experimental animals to oppose the acute toxicity and thus increase the dose which can be tolerated (DURHAM et al. 1956). The ability of DFP, when given repeatedly at sublethal doses, to produce a persistent muscular paralysis (KOELLE and GILMAN 1946) might be considered an exception to the concept that the organophosphorus compounds with low toxicity are most apt to produce demyelination; however, the administration of repeated sublethal doses of a highly toxic compound may be equivalent to a single dose of a less toxic compound insofar as the action which causes demyelination is concerned. Thus, the available evidence seems to indicate that demyelination involves a mechanism unrelated to anti-ChE activity. This aspect is discussed in detail in Chapter 19.

II. Derivatives of pyrophosphoric acid

The toxicity and anti-ChE action of alkyl-substituted derivatives of pyrophosphoric acid have attracted the attention of numerous investigators during the past decade. All toxic members of the alkyl-substituted pyrophosphate series gain access to the ChE's of all parts of the body, and thus produce the nicotinic, muscarinic, and central effects of ACh. They are unstable in aqueous solution. Thus, the general characteristics of the individual members of this series are essentially the same, and they differ essentially only in degree of toxicity, which is dependent upon the nature of the alkyl substituent.

The initial toxicity studies on this group of compounds were conducted on tetraethyl pyrophosphate by Prof. EBERHARD GROSS (SCHRADER 1951) and by MANGUN and DUBOIS (1947); the interest of the latter group was a result of indirect evidence that it was the active component of the preparation designated as hexaethyl tetraphosphate (HETP), which is an extremely unstable compound (DUBOIS and MANGUN 1947). The LD_{50} values for tetraethyl pyrophosphate (TEPP) were found to be 0.65 mg/kg for rats and 0.85 for mice by the i.p. route, and 1.4 for rats by the oral route. Other investigators (BRAUER 1948, BURGEN et al. 1949, SALERNO and COON 1949) obtained similar toxicity values for this compound. Numerous studies have been carried out on the details of its cholinergic action.

A comparison of the toxicity and anti-ChE action of several other alkyl pyrophosphates under strictly comparable conditions has been made by DUBOIS and

COON (1952). All the compounds were administered by the i.p. route as solutions in propylene glycol, and the anti-ChE activity was measured manometrically using mouse brain homogenates as the source of ChE. The results of this comparison are summarized in Table 4. From the standpoint of structure-activity relationships, it is interesting to note that TEPP is the most toxic of the group. The methyl substituted compound is about one-half as toxic as TEPP. There are now many other examples among cholinergic organic phosphates of the greater toxicity of ethyl substituted derivatives of phosphoric acid as compared with other alkyl substituents. Another notable feature of these compounds is the close correlation between toxicity and anti-ChE activity *in vitro*.

Table 4. *Toxicity and anti-ChE action of alkyl pyrophosphates*

Compound	Structural formula	I.p. LD$_{50}$ for mice (mg/kg)	I$_{50}$ for ChE *in vitro* (M)
Tetramethyl pyrophosphate	$\begin{array}{c} CH_3O \\ CH_3O \end{array} > P-O-P < \begin{array}{c} OCH_3 \\ OCH_3 \end{array}$, $\parallel$ O O	1.7	1.8×10^{-8}
Tetraethyl pyrophosphate (TEPP)	$\begin{array}{c} C_2H_5O \\ C_2H_5O \end{array} > P-O-P < \begin{array}{c} OC_2H_5 \\ OC_2H_5 \end{array}$, $\parallel$ O O	0.85	4.0×10^{-9}
Dimethyl diethyl pyrophosphate (asym.)	$\begin{array}{c} CH_3O \\ CH_3O \end{array} > P-O-P < \begin{array}{c} OC_2H_5 \\ OC_2H_5 \end{array}$, $\parallel$ O O	1.1	8.0×10^{-9}
Dimethyl di*iso*propyl pyrophosphate (asym.)	$\begin{array}{c} CH_3O \\ CH_3O \end{array} > P-O-P < \begin{array}{c} OCH(CH_3)_2 \\ OCH(CH_3)_2 \end{array}$, $\parallel$ O O	2.5	2.0×10^{-7}
Tetra*iso*propyl pyrophosphate	$\begin{array}{c} (CH_3)_2CHO \\ (CH_3)_2CHO \end{array} > P-O-P < \begin{array}{c} OCH(CH_3)_2 \\ OCH(CH_3)_2 \end{array}$, $\parallel$ O O	16.0	1.4×10^{-6}

Some thiono derivatives of pyrophosphoric acid have been prepared and subjected to a limited amount of toxicological study (TOY 1951).

The effect of replacement of two oxygen atoms by sulfur to form the dithionopyrophosphates is to decrease the toxicity and anti-ChE action as compared with the analogous alkyl-substituted pyrophosphates. Thus the s.c. LD$_{50}$ for tetraethyl dithionopyrophosphate in mice is 8 mg/kg (TOY 1951) and it is, therefore, about one-tenth as toxic as TEPP. The LD$_{50}$ of tetra-*n*-propyl dithionopyrophosphate for rats is 1100 mg/kg, i.p., and 1450 orally (DOULL and DuBOIS 1952, DuBOIS et al. 1953). Tetra*iso*propyl dithionopyrophosphate has a low mammalian toxicity as indicated by an oral LD$_{50}$ exceeding 200 mg/kg for mice (METCALF and MARCH 1950). The monothionopyrophosphates, in which only one oxygen is replaced by sulfur, have not been extensively studied, but SHUGAEV (1955) has recently tested tetraethyl monothiopyrophosphate and found that its toxicity closely resembles that of TEPP (see Chapter 9 for further details). Since the toxicity of pyrophosphates can be varied to suit the intended use of the compound by appropriate alkyl substitution, and since their detoxification results in the formation of non-toxic substances, this group seems worthy of further investigation in connection with current efforts to develop organic phosphorus-containing insecticides with low mammalian toxicity.

The alkyl pyrophosphates have in common the ability to inhibit ChE's *in vitro* and *in vivo*, and to produce both central and peripheral cholinomimetic actions. However, derivatives of pyrophosphoric acid in which amide groups replace the alkoxy linkages differ in several respects from TEPP and other alkyl pyrophosphates, and have thus attracted considerable attention from the standpoint

of their toxicity and pharmacologic actions. Of this group, octamethyl pyrophosphortetramide (OMPA) has been studied most extensively. This compound was
first synthesized by SCHRADER (1950), who stated that it was absorbed from the
soil by plants, rendering them insecticidal. The potential value of systemic insecticides like OMPA that protect plants against insects without exerting a phyto-
toxic action has been discussed by MARTIN (1949). OMPA is one of the organic
phosphates which is now permitted to be used on food crops in most countries,
including the U.S.A. where the residue remaining on treated crops (tolerance level)
may not exceed 0.75 parts per million. The toxicology of OMPA has been studied
extensively by DuBOIS et al. (1950a, 1950b) who found that the LD_{50} by the i.p.
route is 8.5 mg/kg for male rats, 17 for mice, and 10 for guinea pigs. By the oral
route the LD_{50} was 10 mg/kg for rats; an i.v. value of 5 to 10 was obtained for
dogs. No sex or age differences in susceptibility to this compound were noted.
OMPA produces all the muscarinic effects of organophosphates and the nicotinic
action on skeletal muscle, but has no action on the central nervous system.
Although the signs produced by OMPA are typical of those caused by anti-ChE
agents, in vitro studies showed that concentrations above 0.01 M were required
to produce 50% inhibition of the enzyme activity. On the other hand, small doses
(5 mg/kg, i.p.) caused marked inhibition of the ChE activity of the ileum, submaxillary gland, serum and skeletal muscle of rats. No inhibition of brain ChE was noted,
which is consistent with the absence of signs referable to the central nervous
system. A selective peripheral action of this type had not been observed previously
with phosphorus-containing anti-ChE agents. The long duration of action of
OMPA, its stability in aqueous solution, and the absence of central effects prompted
its trial and use in the management of myasthenia gravis (RIDER et al. 1951a,
1951b).

The ineffectiveness of OMPA as an inhibitor of ChE in vitro, in contrast to its
strong anti-ChE action in the intact animal, prompted DuBOIS et al. (1950a, 1950b)
to investigate the possibility that OMPA undergoes a metabolic change and is
transformed into a highly active ChE inhibitor. At that time knowledge of the
enzyme systems which catalyze drug transformations was meager in comparison
with currently available information. The idea that OMPA undergoes metabolic
activation was tested by the relatively simple procedure of incubating the compound
with tissue slices in Krebs-Ringer-phosphate buffer under aerobic and anaerobic
conditions, using glucose as a substrate. The anti-ChE action of the OMPA before
and after incubation with tissue slices was measured, and it was found that OMPA
was transformed under aerobic conditions into a potent anti-ChE agent. This
finding explained the difference between the effects of OMPA on ChE in vitro and
in vivo. It also provided an explanation for the delay in onset of signs, which is
due apparently to the time required for the biotransformation of OMPA to an
active metabolite. The marked difference between the effects in vitro and in vivo
of OMPA clearly demonstrated the limitations of any tests in vitro for screening
compounds for anti-ChE activity. Several subsequent investigations have been
conducted on the metabolic conversion of OMPA to an active metabolite (GAR-
DINER and KILBY 1950, ALDRIDGE and BARNES 1952, CASIDA 1954, CASIDA et al.
1956). DAVISON (1955) demonstrated that a pyridine-linked oxidase in liver microsomes catalyzes the activation of OMPA. Although the active metabolite has not
been identified yet, it seems probable, as a result of the work of several investigators
(CASIDA et al. 1954, TSUYUKI et al. 1955), that an N-oxide of OMPA is the first
product of oxidation, since the anti-ChE activity of the oxidative intermediate
was associated with a group which yielded formaldehyde upon treatment with
acid.

The marked differences between TEPP and OMPA in their anti-ChE actions *in vitro*, and the selective action of the metabolite of OMPA on the ChE's of peripheral tissues *in vivo* stimulated interest in the investigation of pyrophosphates containing both amide and alkoxy linkages. DuBois et al. (1953) measured the toxicity and anti-ChE activity of symmetrical *bis*-dimethyl pyrophosphordiamide and its asymmetrical analogue. The structures of these compounds and a comparison with OMPA and TEPP of their i.p. toxicity to rats and their anti-ChE action *in vitro* are given in Table 5. These results, which were obtained under strictly comparable conditions for all the compounds, demonstrated clearly that both the symmetrical and asymmetrical analogues of *bis*-dimethyl pyrophosphordiamide resemble TEPP in their strong anti-ChE action *in vitro*. The asymmetrical compound resembled TEPP in toxicity and the symmetrical analogue resembled OMPA. Other species exhibited similar susceptibility as evidenced by i.p. LD$_{50}$ values of 5 mg/kg for male mice, and 5 to 7 for male guinea pigs for the

Table 5. *Toxicity and anti-ChE action of some pyrophosphates*

Chemical name	Structural formula	I.p. LD$_{50}$ for male rats (mg/kg)	I$_{50}$ for ChE *in vitro* (M)
Tetraethyl pyrophosphate (TEPP)	$(C_2H_5O)_2{=}P{-}O{-}P{=}(OC_2H_5)_2$ with O, O	0.65	4×10^{-9}
Octamethyl pyro-phosphortetramide (OMPA)	$\left(\begin{smallmatrix}CH_3\\CH_3\end{smallmatrix}{>}N\right)_2{-}P{-}O{-}P{-}\left(N{<}\begin{smallmatrix}CH_3\\CH_3\end{smallmatrix}\right)_2$ with O, O	8.5	1×10^{-2}
Diethyl *bis*-dimethyl pyrophosphordiamide (sym.)	$\begin{smallmatrix}CH_3\\CH_3\end{smallmatrix}{>}N{-}P{-}O{-}P{-}N{<}\begin{smallmatrix}CH_3\\CH_3\end{smallmatrix}$ with C_2H_5O, O, O, OC_2H_5	11.5	4.7×10^{-7}
Diethyl *bis*-dimethyl pyrophosphordiamide (asym.)	$(C_2H_5O)_2{=}P{-}O{-}P{=}\left(N{<}\begin{smallmatrix}CH_3\\CH_3\end{smallmatrix}\right)_2$ with O, O	2.7	2.8×10^{-7}

asymmetrical compound, and values for the symmetrical analogue of 16 for male mice and 13 to 16 for male guinea pigs. Both compounds are well absorbed from the gastrointestinal tract, as evidenced by oral LD$_{50}$ values which closely approximated those obtained by the i.p. route.

An interesting aspect of the toxicology of *bis*-dimethyl pyrophosphordiamide is the resemblance to OMPA in its anti-ChE action *in vivo*. Both the symmetrical and asymmetrical analogues of this compound cause marked inhibition of the ChE activity of all peripheral tissues, but have no effect on brain ChE *in vivo*. The signs are correlated with the anti-ChE action, and consist in muscarinic and nicotinic effects, but there are no signs referable to the central nervous system. Thus, the presence of two amide groups in the alkylpyrophosphate structure limits the action of the resulting compound to peripheral tissues. The extent to which the site of action of other cholinergic organophosphorus compounds could be modified by the addition of amide groups is unknown. Since the phosphoroamidocyanidates produce a generalized cholinergic action and have no selective effect on the ChE of peripheral tissues, it is clear that the presence of one amide group is insufficient to prevent penetration into the central nervous system, at least in that class of compounds. Fluorophosphates containing two amide groups do not inhibit brain ChE *in vivo* as evidenced by the selective action of tetramethylphosphorodiamidic fluoride (BFPO). No systematic studies have been conducted on the extent to which the central actions of cholinergic organic phosphates can be reduced by amide substitution. This would seem to be a worthwhile area for future investigation of new insecticides from the toxicological standpoint, since treatment of casualties could be limited to peripheral signs and symptoms.

III. Phosphorothioates

Numerous derivatives of thiophosphoric acid have been synthesized and tested for insecticidal activity following the report by SCHRADER (1950) of the effectiveness of Parathion (0,0-diethyl 0-[4-nitrophenyl] phosphorothioate). These efforts have resulted in the development of numerous phosphorothioates with cholinergic actions and insecticidal activity. All the prominent compounds of this class bear a remarkable similarity to Parathion in their resultant signs, symptoms, and anti-ChE activities; the toxicity of individual members of the group varies somewhat depending upon the substituent groups.

The acute mammalian toxicity of Parathion was studied by DuBois et al. (1948, 1949) shortly after introduction of the compound into use as an insecticide. The i.p. LD_{50} in mg/kg was found to be 7 for male rats, 4 for female rats, and about 10 for female and male mice. The i.v. LD_{50} for cats was between 3 and 5 mg/kg, and the value for dogs by the same route was 12 to 20. By the oral route the LD_{50} was 6 for female rats and 15 mg/kg for male rats; thus, Parathion is well absorbed from the gastrointestinal tract. A significant sex difference in suscepti-bility to rats was noted when Parathion was given either orally or parenterally. The administration of diethylstilbestrol to male rats and testosterone to female rats nearly abolished the sex difference in response. A similar sex difference in susceptibility of rats to other phosphorothioates has been observed subsequently in every case in which the sexes have been studied individually.

After parenteral administration of Parathion, signs appear in 2 to 5 minutes, and death occurs within 30 minutes after lethal doses (DuBois et al. 1949). The signs are indicative of a generalized cholinergic action with prominent muscarinic, nicotinic, and central nervous system effects. The pattern is similar with all phos-phorothioates, with a few exceptions. All of the technical Parathion samples for insecticidal use have appreciable anti-ChE activity *in vitro* which is now known to be due to impurities, particularly to contamination by the oxygen analogue. This fact was unknown until DIGGLE and GAGE (1951) demonstrated that purified Parathion has no anti-ChE activity *in vitro* but undergoes metabolic oxidative desulfuration to form the oxygen analogue (diethyl-4-nitrophenyl phosphate) *in vivo* which is responsible for the toxicity and anti-ChE action of the parent compound. Several other investigations (MYERS et al. 1952, GAGE 1953, METCALF and MARCH 1953, DAVISON 1955, MURPHY and DuBois 1957) soon firmly estab-lished this important principle for Parathion as well as all other cholinergic phos-phorothioates.

During recent years the mammalian toxicity of several compounds which may be considered as derivatives of Parathion has been studied. Table 6 shows the chemical structures and the i.p. LD_{50} values for several nitrophenyl phosphoro-thioates following administration to rats, using 80% propylene glycol and 20% ethanol as the solvent. Of this group, Methylparathion (0,0-dimethyl 0-[4-nitro-phenyl] phosphorothioate) and EPN (0-ethyl 0-[4-nitrophenyl] phenylphosphono-thioate) are of greatest interest because they are both permitted to be used as insecticides on food crops in the U.S.A. Neither of these compounds exhibits any unique toxicological properties and their acute toxicity does not deviate markedly from that of Parathion. DEICHMANN et al. (1952) compared the toxicity of purified Methylparathion and Parathion to rats by the oral route, and obtained LD_{50} values of 14.8 and 4, respectively, when they were given as 1% corn oil solutions. The use of 2% corn oil solutions of Methylparathion resulted in an LD_{50} of 9.7 mg/kg, which is a noteworthy difference since it suggests that the variety of solvents and concentrations of active ingredient in solutions used for toxicity tests are undoubtedly largely responsible for the different toxicity values obtained by various laboratories. These variations emphasize the necessity of using standard-ized conditions with respect to solvents and drug concentrations when accurate comparison of the toxicity of various organophosphates is desired. The results of these studies as well as those of HECHT and WIRTH (1950) indicate that Methyl-parathion is slightly less toxic than Parathion, but that the presence of small and variable amounts of the oxygen analogues of both these compounds in most commercial samples tends to obscure any differences in their inherent toxicities. The maximum permitted level on food crops has, therefore, been set at 1 part per million for both of these compounds.

Table 6. *Toxicity of nitrophenyl phosphorothioates to female rats*

Chemical name	Synonym	Structural formula	I.p. LD_{50} for female rats (mg/kg)
0,0-Diethyl 0-(4-nitrophenyl) phosphorothioate	Parathion	$(C_2H_5O)_2{=}P{-}O{-}\langle\rangle{-}NO_2$, S	2.0
0,0-Dimethyl 0-(4-nitrophenyl) phosphorothioate	Methylparathion	$(CH_3O)_2{=}P{-}O{-}\langle\rangle{-}NO_2$, S	2.8
0-Ethyl 0-(4-nitrophenyl) phenylphosphonothioate	EPN	$C_2H_5O{-}P{-}O{-}\langle\rangle{-}NO_2$, S	7.2
0,0-Dimethyl 0-(3-chloro-4-nitrophenyl) phosphorothioate	Chlorthion	$(CH_3O)_2{=}P{-}O{-}\langle\rangle{-}NO_2$, S, Cl	750
0,0-Dimethyl 0-(2-chloro-4-nitrophenyl) phosphorothioate	—	$(CH_3O)_2{=}P{-}O{-}\langle\rangle{-}NO_2$, Cl, S	100

The most thorough study of the toxicity of EPN was conducted by HODGE et al. (1954). They found the oral LD_{50} of crystalline EPN to be 14 mg/kg for female and 42 for male rats. Technical EPN was somewhat more toxic as evidenced by oral LD_{50} values of 7 and 33 for male and female rats, respectively. By the i.p. route, the LD_{50} was 24 for females and 64 for males. The lethal range for dogs by the oral route was 20 to 45 mg/kg for the crystalline EPN, and 2 to 75 for the technical material. Similar values were obtained by FRAWLEY et al. (1952), who reported oral LD_{50} values in mg/kg of 14.5 for female rats, 91 for male rats, 45.5 for male and female mice, and 79 for male and female guinea pigs. The sex difference in susceptibility of rats to EPN was larger than that which has been observed with any other phosphorothioate. With respect to the treatment of EPN poisoning, DI STEFANO et al. (1951) made the interesting observation that Coramine (nikethamide) in combination with atropine raised the LD_{50} of EPN for female rats from 7.1 to 86 mg/kg, whereas atropine alone increased the value only to 12.2 mg/kg. A similar but less striking effect by the same combination was obtained in males. Coramine alone was not an effective antidote and did not change the LD_{50} in either sex. The analeptic action of Coramine was probably not responsible for the protective effect because pentylenetetrazol, amphetamine, picrotoxin, and caffeine did not protect and actually increased the mortality rate of EPN-treated animals.

The influence of addition of a chlorine atom to the phenyl group of Parathion on toxicity is illustrated by Chlorthion (0,0-dimethyl 0-[3-chloro-4-nitrophenyl] phosphorothioate) and the analogous 2-chloro derivative.

The LD_{50} of Chlorthion is 750 mg/kg by the i.p. route and 1,500 by the oral route to rats (DuBois et al. 1953). Technical Chlorthion is often contaminated with highly toxic impurities (BAGDON and DuBois 1956). The oral LD_{50} of the 2-chloro analogue has been reported to be 400 mg/kg for mice (HOLMSTEDT 1959). Recent unpublished tests on this compound in the reviewer's laboratory have indicated that the i.p. LD_{50} is 100 mg/kg for rats. Neither of these compounds has been used as an insecticide. Their low mammalian toxicity is apparently paralleled by relatively low toxicity to insects.

Several phosphorothioates have been prepared which resemble Parathion, except for replacement of the p-nitrophenyl group by other aromatic substituents.

The chemical structures of these compounds are presented in a recent review by HOLM-STEDT (1959). The first compound of this type to be subjected to toxicity tests was 0,0-diethyl 0-(4-methylumbelliferyl) phosphorothioate (Potasan, E 838). The i.p. LD_{50} of this compound to female rats was found to be 15 mg/kg (DuBois and COON 1952). FRAWLEY et al. (1952) measured the acute oral toxicity of Potasan and obtained LD_{50} values in mg/kg of 19 for female rats, 42 for male rats, 98.5 for mice, and 25 for guinea pigs. This compound inhibits the ChE activity of all tissues and produces generalized cholinergic actions. It thus exhibits no properties that are appreciably different from those of Parathion except for a somewhat lower mammalian toxicity. Although Potasan has no insecticidal use, the 3-chloro derivative (0,0-diethyl 0-[3-chloro-4-methylumbelliferyl] phosphorothioate), which is known as Resistox in Europe and as Co-Ral in the U.S.A., is used for the control of pests on domestic animals by application of suspensions to the body surface. The LD_{50} of suspensions of Co-Ral to rats by the i.p. route has been reported to be 90 to 110 mg/kg (KLOTZSCHE 1955). Unpublished data from the reviewer's laboratory confirmed this finding when suspensions of Co-Ral were administered, as evidenced by i.p. LD_{50} values in mg/kg of 110 for female rats, 155 for male rats, 200 for male and female mice, and 140 for guinea pigs. However, when the compound was dissolved in an organic solvent (Velsicol AR-60) the i.p. LD_{50} to rats was 9 mg/kg, indicating that Co-Ral is actually a highly toxic compound the insolubility of which prevents detection of its toxicity when suspensions are given, and thus has given the erroneous impression of low inherent mammalian toxicity. Diazinon (0,0-diethyl 0-[3-chloro-4-methylumbelliferyl] phosphorothioate) may be considered as a derivative of Parathion with lower mammalian toxicity. BRUCE et al. (1955) studied the toxicity of this compound and obtained acute oral LD_{50} values of 100 to 150 mg/kg for rats and 82 for mice. Diazinon is permitted for use on certain food crops in the U.S.A. but the residues cannot exceed 0.75 parts per million. Diazinon has a tendency to undergo decomposition on storage with the formation of highly toxic derivatives and different commercial samples, therefore, exhibit marked variations in their toxicity.

A series of phosphorothioates containing an ethyl mercaptoalkyl linkage has been subjected to toxicity tests. The stimulus for the study of compounds of this type came from the development by SCHRADER (1950) of 0,0-diethyl 0-(2-ethio-ethyl) phosphorothioate (Systox, Demeton) which is a widely used topical and systemic insecticide. All toxicological evaluations of Systox have shown that it may be classed among the most toxic organophosphate insecticides. It inhibits the ChE activity of all tissues and thus produces generalized cholinergic actions. WIRTH (1953) obtained an oral LD_{50} for male rats of 7.5 mg/kg for a purified sample of Systox. DEICHMANN and RAKOCZY (1955) measured the toxicity of a purified sample of the compound and reported approximate lethal doses in mg/kg of 117 for female rats and 50 for rabbits by the oral route. By the s.c. route, values of 37 and 120 mg/kg were obtained for dogs and mice, respectively. However, these investigators recognized that commercial Systox preparations usually contain about 60% Systox and 40% of its thiol (P=O) isomer. This mixture is much more toxic than pure Systox as evidenced by approximate lethal doses of 3 to 5 mg/kg for female rats and 5 to 6 for male rats by the i.p. route. The values for mice and guinea pigs by the s.c. route were 10 and 5, respectively. The toxicology of Systox has been complicated by the fact that commercial preparations consist of two compounds. In addition, the mercaptosulfur of the ethylmercaptoethyl portion of both isomers is oxidized to the sulfoxide and sulfone derivatives. Thus in the intact animal the toxicity is the result of the action of several compounds. WIRTH (1958) reported oral LD_{50} values for rats of 100 and 90 mg/kg for Systox sulfoxide and Systox sulfone, respectively, indicating that these metabolites have approximately the same toxicity as the parent compound. Methylsystox (0,0-dimethyl 0-[2-ethioethyl]phosphorothioate) is considerably less toxic than Systox. WIRTH (1958) obtained an LD_{50} of 250 mg/kg for this compound given orally to rats and the values for the sulfoxide and sulfone derivatives of this compound by the same route were 600 and 500, respectively.

IV. Phosphorodithioates

The mammalian toxicology of several phosphorodithioates has been studied. All members of this group have essentially the same pharmacologic actions which are characterized by generalized cholinergic effects and, after metabolic conversion, they all inhibit the cholinesterase activity of both the central and peripheral nervous systems. None of the members of this group is a ChE inhibitor *in vitro*, and their activity *in vivo* requires oxidative desulfuration to form the corresponding phosphates. The individual members of the group differ appreciably in their mammalian toxicity, which is governed by the rate and extent of conversion to the phosphates, the inherent anti-ChE activity of the phosphates, and the rate of detoxification of the active metabolites and the parent compounds.

Table 7. *The acute toxicity of phosphorodithioates to female rats*

Chemical name	Synonym	Chemical structure	Oral LD_{50} (mg/kg)
0,0-Dimethyl S-(1,2-di-carbethoxyethyl) phosphorodithioate	Malathion	$\begin{matrix}CH_3O\\CH_3O\end{matrix}{>}P{-}S{-}CH{-}COOC_2H_5$, $\overset{\|}{S}$ $CH_2{-}COOC_2H_5$	1500
0,0-Dimethyl S-(4-oxo-3-H-1,2,3-benzotriazine-3-methyl) phosphoro-dithioate	Guthion; DBD	$\begin{matrix}CH_3O\\CH_3O\end{matrix}{>}P{-}S{-}CH_2{-}N{-}C$ structure	16.4
0,0-Diethyl S-(2-eththio-ethyl) phosphoro-dithioate	Disyston; Dithio-systox	$\begin{matrix}C_2H_5O\\C_2H_5O\end{matrix}{>}P{-}S{-}CH_2CH_2SC_2H_5$	5.0
0,0-Diethyl S-(2-ethionyl-ethyl) phosphoro-dithioate	Disyston sulfoxide	$\begin{matrix}C_2H_5O\\C_2H_5O\end{matrix}{>}P{-}S{-}CH_2CH_2SC_2H_5$	6.5
0,0-Diethyl S-(2-ethsulfo-nylethyl) phosphoro-dithioate	Disyston sulfone	$\begin{matrix}C_2H_5O\\C_2H_5O\end{matrix}{>}P{-}SCH_2CH_2SC_2H_5$	7.5
0,0-Diethyl S-eththio-methyl phosphoro-dithioate	Thimet	$\begin{matrix}C_2H_5O\\C_2H_5O\end{matrix}{>}P{-}SCH_2SC_2H_5$	2.1
0,0-Diethyl S-eththionyl-methyl phosphoro-dithioate	Thimet sulfoxide	$\begin{matrix}C_2H_5O\\C_2H_5O\end{matrix}{>}P{-}SCH_2SC_2H_5$	2.1
0,0-Diethyl S-ethsulfonyl-methyl phosphoro-dithioate	Thimet sulfone	$\begin{matrix}C_2H_5O\\C_2H_5O\end{matrix}{>}P{-}SCH_2{-}SC_2H_5$	1.7

Table 7 gives a comparison of the structure and toxicity of the most important phosphorodithioates. Of this group, Malathion (0,0-dimethyl S-[1,2-dicarbethoxy-ethyl] phosphorodithioate) is of greatest importance because of its extensive insecticidal use. It is unique among organophosphorus compounds in that it represents the only real success in achieving low toxicity to mammals and high toxicity to insects. The low mammalian toxicity is due to rapid hydrolysis of the ester linkages in the 1,2-dicarbethoxyethyl side-chains (MARCH et al. 1956, COOK et al. 1957,

O'BRIEN 1957). The initial studies on the toxicology of Malathion were conducted by HAZELTON and HOLLAND (1953) who obtained an oral LD$_{50}$ of 1,160 mg/kg for male rats given propylene glycol solutions, and of 5,840 when the compound was given in the undiluted form. Mice exhibited similar susceptibility. Other investigations (DUBOIS et al. 1953) in which Malathion was dissolved in 20% ethanol and 80% propylene glycol showed that the LD$_{50}$ was 750 mg/kg for rats by the i.p. route and 1,500 by the oral route. Rapid detoxification of Malathion by non-specific esterases in the liver and serum of mammals accounts for the low toxicity. The high potential toxicity of this compound was demonstrated recently by MURPHY et al. (1959) who found that the i.p. LD$_{50}$ of Malathion was reduced to 8.2 mg/kg for male rats when detoxification was inhibited by triorthotolyl phosphate. In spite of the low toxicity of Malathion, some cases of poisoning have been reported (PARKER and CHATTIN 1955, GOLDMAN and TEITEL 1958) in young subjects. It is possible that defects in the detoxification system were responsible for these accidents or that the detoxifying esterases are lower in concentration in the young. No studies on the effect of age on the ability of animals to detoxify Malathion have been reported; this would seem to be a worthwhile area of investigation.

The toxicity of 0,0-dimethyl S-(4-oxo-3,H-1,2,3-benzotriazine-3-methyl) phosphorodithioate (Guthion, DBD) has been studied rather extensively by DUBOIS et al. (1957). These investigators obtained i.p. LD$_{50}$ values in mg/kg of 11.6 for male rats, 5.7 for female rats, 5.4 for male mice, 3.4 for female mice, and 40 for guinea pigs. By the oral route the LD$_{50}$ was 16.4 mg/kg for female rats and 80 for male guinea pigs. Because of its stability this compound was used by MURPHY and DUBOIS (1957) as a substrate for the development of a quantitative method for measuring conversion of phosphorothioates and dithioates to their corresponding oxygen analogues and for measuring the influence of various factors on the enzymatic oxidation of these compounds (MURPHY and DUBOIS 1958).

Measurements of the toxicity of Di-syston (0,0-diethyl [2-ethioethyl] phosphorodithioate) (WIRTH 1958, BOMBINSKI and DUBOIS 1958) and Thimet (0,0-diethyl S-eththiomethyl phosphorodithioate) (WIRTH 1958) have shown that these compounds have high mammalian toxicity and the sulfoxide and sulfone derivatives, to which the compounds are changed *in vivo* (MARCH et al. 1955), resemble the parent compounds in acute mammalian toxicity.

V. Phosphates

The development and toxicological evaluation of cholinergic phosphates has not kept pace with research on the chemically related phosphorothioates since the latter group have proven to be more valuable as insecticides. However, since the phosphorothioates must undergo metabolic conversion to the corresponding oxygen analogues, the toxicity and anti-ChE action of all these compounds are due to the metabolically formed phosphates. The cholinergic phosphates exert a direct anti-ChE action *in vitro* and *in vivo* and, therefore, constitute a useful group of compounds for studying the influence of chemical structure on activity. Several phosphates which are the oxygen analogues of important insecticidal thiophosphates have been subjected to toxicological studies. The toxicity of some of these compounds is shown in Table 8. By comparison of these data with values for the corresponding phosphorothioates and dithioates in previous tables it may be seen that the oxygen analogues are considerably more toxic than the parent compounds. Differences in detoxification or incomplete conversion of the parent compounds to their oxygen analogues must account for the variations in toxicity. All of the active members of this group produce the nicotinic, muscarinic, and central nervous system effects of ACh. Their onset of action is extremely rapid, and reversal of inhibition of ChE occurs in a few hours to a few days depending upon the particular compound. No sex difference in susceptibility to these compounds is observed in rats in contrast to the corresponding phosphorothioates, to which females are considerably more susceptible than males.

Table 8. *Acute toxicity of cholinergic phosphates to female rats*

Chemical name	Chemical structure	Oxygen analogue of	I.p. LD$_{50}$ (mg/kg)
Dimethyl 4-nitrophenyl phosphate (Paraoxon-Me)	CH_3O, CH_3O >P—O—⟨ ⟩—NO_2, ‖O	Methyl-parathion	1.0
Diethyl 4-nitrophenyl phosphate (Paraoxon)	C_2H_5O, C_2H_5O >P—O—⟨ ⟩—NO_2, ‖O	Parathion	0.6
O,O-Diethyl O-(3-chloro-4-methylumbelliferyl) phosphate	C_2H_5O, C_2H_5O >P—O—⟨ ⟩ (coumarin ring with C=O, C—Cl, CH_3), ‖O	Co-Ral; Resistox	2.8
O,O-Dimethyl S-(4-oxo-3-H-1,2,3-benzotriazine-3-methyl) phosphate	CH_3O, CH_3O >P—S—CH_2—N (benzotriazine ring with C=O, N=N), ‖O	Guthion	0.45

Only one cholinergic phosphate is currently approved for use on food crops in the U.S.A. It is dimethyl 1-methyl-2-carbomethoxyvinyl phosphate (Phosdrin) which has an oral LD$_{50}$ for mice of 8.9 mg/kg (KODAMA et al. 1955). Several other vinyl phosphates have been subjected to toxicity tests. Of these dimethyl 2,2-dichlorovinyl phosphate (DDVP) has attracted the most attention. DURHAM et al. (1957) obtained oral LD$_{50}$ values of 80 mg/kg for male rats and 56 for females, and cutaneous LD$_{50}$ values of 107 for males and 75 for females. The reported sex differences in response to this compound are unusual; however, examination of the data shows overlapping between the values for the two sexes, and the actual differences might not be as great as the calculated LD$_{50}$ values suggest. The toxicity of diethyl 4-nitrophenyl phosphate (Paraoxon, Mintacol) has been studied thoroughly because of its limited use in the treatment of glaucoma (WIRTH 1949, HECHT and WIRTH 1950, AUGUSTINSSON 1953). These investigators obtained i.v. LD$_{50}$ values in mg/kg of 0.5 for mice, 0.4 for rats, and 0.3 for rabbits. By the s.c. route the values were 0.6 for mice, 0.5 for guinea pigs, 0.4 for rabbits, and 0.7 for cats. These values demonstrate the extremely high toxicity of this compound to mammals.

VI. Phosphonates

Only a limited amount of research has been done on cholinergic phosphonates. As a result only one compound of this type has attracted attention from the toxicological standpoint. It is dimethyl 2,2,2-trichloro-1-hydroxyethylphosphonate, which is commonly known as Dipterex. The toxicology of this compound has been studied by DEICHMANN and LAMPE (1955) and DuBOIS and COTTER (1955). The latter investigators obtained i.p. LD$_{50}$ values in mg/kg of 225 for rats, 500 for mice, and 300 for guinea pigs. The oral LD_{50} for rats was 450. Dipterex exerts a generalized cholinergic action due to inhibition of the ChE of all parts of the nervous system. A notable feature of the mammalian toxicity of this compound is the extremely rapid reversal of the inhibition of ChE activity after single sublethal doses. In view of the high anti-ChE activity of Dipterex and its low mammalian toxicity, further studies on compounds of this type seem warranted from the standpoint of the development of new insecticides.

VII. Organophosphorus compounds containing substituted ammonium ions

It is now generally accepted that the cholinergic phosphorus-containing compounds react at the esteratic site of the ChE molecule. Within the past few years considerable attention has been given to the possibility that compounds which are capable of reacting also with the anionic site of the ChE molecule would exhibit greater potency than those which react with one or the other of the two presumed sites of attachment of ACh to the ChE. Accordingly, a number of compounds containing the ChE inhibiting phosphate moiety plus a substituted ammonium group have been prepared and subjected to toxicological study. The results of these studies have shown clearly that the presence of groups which would permit dual attachment to the enzyme results in increased potency. The LD_{50} values for the most active compounds of this series range from 0.01 to 0.1 mg/kg (HOLMSTEDT 1959). The toxicity of 0,0-diethyl-S-2-trimethylammonium ethyl phosphorothiodate iodide (echothiophate, Phospholine) is of interest in view of its use in the treatment of glaucoma. KOELLE and STEINER (1956) obtained in rabbits an i.v. LD_{50} of 0.087 micromol./kg and demonstrated that this compound does not gain access to brain AChE readily *in vivo*. None of the members of this series has yet become useful as an insecticide.

VIII. Carbamates

The toxicity and anticholinesterase activity of carbamic acid esters is well-known as a result of extensive studies and clinical use of compounds such as physostigmine and neostigmine. It is, therefore, unnecessary to review the toxicology of the older members of this series. It is noteworthy, however, that this group of compounds differs from the organophosphates in their rapidly reversible anti-ChE action and their comparative inability to inhibit brain ChE *in vivo*. Numerous cholinergic carbamic acid derivatives have been prepared and subjected to mammalian toxicity tests with the result that compounds of widely varying toxicity are known. A detailed study of the relation between chemical structure and toxicity of various cholinergic carbamates has been conducted in the reviewer's laboratory. A few of the results of tests which were conducted on more than 300 compounds are presented in Tables 9 and 10.

The influence on toxicity of esterification of substituted phenols with carbamic acid is shown in Table 9, in which it may be seen that the presence of the carbamate group is responsible for a marked enhancement of the toxicity.

Substitution of sulfur for oxygen to form the corresponding thiocarbamates destroys the toxicity. The toxicity of both monomethyl and dimethyl carbamates is enhanced by the addition of a second carbamate group in the ortho position as illustrated by compounds 4 and 5 in Table 9. No increase in toxicity is achieved when the second group is in the *meta* or *para* position. Addition of a third adjacent carbamate group reduces the toxicity. Substitution in the carbamate nitrogen increases the toxicity as shown by compounds 6 and 7 in Table 9. Monomethyl substitution is the most effective regardless of the position of the quarternary nitrogen, its alkyl substituents, or the presence of alkyl additions to the ring. Of 20 pairs of compounds tested, the monomethyl carbamates exceeded the dimethyl carbamates in toxicity in 14 cases by 10 to 40 times and in other cases they were approximately equal.

The addition of a quarternary ammonium group to an unsubstituted phenyl carbamate causes a striking increase in toxicity, as illustrated by compounds 1 and 2 in Table 10.

Table 9. *Comparison of the toxicity of some carbamic acid derivatives to mice*

Compound No.	Chemical name	Chemical structure	S.C LD$_{50}$ (mg/kg)
1	Phenol, 3-(diethylamino) methochloride	⬡—OH, $\overset{+}{N}(C_2H_5)_2$ CH$_3$ Cl$^-$	40
2	Carbamic acid, N-methyl-3-diethylaminophenyl ester, methochloride	⬡—OCONHCH$_3$, $\overset{+}{N}(C_2H_5)_2$ CH$_3$ Cl$^-$	0.09
3	Carbamthiolic acid, N-methyl-3-dimethylamino-4-methyl-phenyl ester, methiodide	⬡—SCONHCH$_3$, $\overset{+}{N}(CH_3)_3$ I$^-$ CH$_3$	>80
4	Carbamic acid, N,N-dimethyl-phenyl ester	⬡—OCON(CH$_3$)$_2$	>80
5	Benzene, 1,2-bis(dimethyl-carbamyloxy)	⬡—OCON(CH$_3$)$_2$ OCON(CH$_3$)$_2$	1.4
6	Carbamic acid, 2-methyl-5-(dimethylamino)-phenyl ester methiodide	CH$_3$—⬡—OCONH$_2$	5.0
7	Carbamic acid, N-methyl-2-methyl-5-dimethylamino-phenyl ester methiodide	CH$_3$—⬡—OCONHCH$_3$, $\overset{+}{N}(CE_3)_3$ I$^-$	0.1

Table 10. *Acute toxicity of some carbamic acid derivatives to mice*

Compound No.	Chemical name	Chemical structure	S.C. LD$_{50}$ (mg/kg)
1	Carbamic acid, N-methylphenyl ester	⬡—OCONHCH$_3$	80
2	Carbamic acid, N-methyl-3-dimethylaminophenyl ester, methiodide	⬡—OCONHCH$_3$, $\overset{+}{N}(CH_3)_3$ I$^-$	0.27
3	Carbamic acid, N-methyl-3-methylthiophenyl ester methosulfate	⬡—OCONHCH$_3$, $\overset{+}{S}(CH_3)_2SO_4CH_3^-$	0.37
4	Carbamic acid, N,N-dimethyl-3-dimethylarsinophenyl ester, methiodide	⬡—OCON(CH$_3$)$_2$, $\overset{+}{As}(CH_3)_3$ I$^-$	1.0

The quarternary ammonium group is much more effective than the primary or tertiary amino group. In the absence of alkyl substituents on the ring, the quarternary nitrogen is at least 100 times as effective in the *meta* position as in the *ortho* or *para* position. In the presence of a methyl or *iso*-propyl group on the ring, the *meta* position is still the most effective position for the quarternary nitrogen. Both sulfonium and arsonium groups endow carbamates with relatively high toxicity but do not equal quarternary ammonium groups as shown by compounds 2, 3 and 4 in Table 10. Numerous other variations in structure of carbamates have been studied but all of them support the conclusion that the most active compounds are those containing carbamic acid and quarternary ammonium groups with the latter group *meta* to the carbamic acid group. A considerable number of additions can be made to this basic structure without greatly decreasing the toxicity.

B. Subacute toxicity

Acutely toxic single doses of the anticholinesterase agents cause a precipitous decrease in the ChE activity of the tissues of animals. The maximum inhibition of enzyme activity usually occurs within a few hours but occasionally requires up to three days with those compounds that are slowly absorbed. With sublethal doses, reversal of the inhibition of enzyme activity occurs at a rate which depends upon the type of alkylphosphorylation, but with most compounds reversal is complete or nearly so within two weeks. Information on the rate at which animals recover from sublethal doses of organophosphorus compounds has been obtained by studying their subacute toxicity. This has been done for some of those agents that are used as pesticides by repeated daily injection of sublethal doses and by feeding various levels in the diet for several months. The present discussion will be limited to those experiments in which the agents were injected daily at various dosage levels for a period of 60 days, since the effects of various dietary levels have been discussed in another chapter (10) of this volume.

The stimulus for investigating the subacute toxicity of anticholinesterase agents was provided by the realization that those engaged in the manufacture and use of these compounds could receive repeated exposure to small doses. One of the early published studies on the subacute i.p. toxicity of insecticidal organophosphorus compounds was conducted on Parathion (DuBois et al. 1949) using a sample which had an acute LD_{50} of 4 mg/kg. When rats were given daily i.p. doses of 3 mg/kg, 100% mortality occurred within 5 days. A daily dose of 2 mg/kg caused 87% mortality, and 1 mg/kg caused 46% mortality. Animals were able to tolerate repeated daily injection of 0.5 mg/kg (1/8 of the acute LD_{50}) of this compound without the occurrence of mortality. The signs which accompanied subacute poisoning were the same as those observed after acutely toxic doses, suggesting that appropriate repeated doses gradually depressed the ChE activity to a level which caused the manifestations of ACh poisoning.

A similar study was performed with OMPA except that it was expanded to include some ChE assays on tissues of animals given repeated daily doses (DuBois et al. 1950). The daily i.p. injection of 1 mg/kg (1/8 of the acute LD_{50}) and higher doses caused 100% mortality within 10 days but rats were able to tolerate 0.5 mg/kg daily for 60 days with the occurrence of no mortality. Cholinesterase assays demonstrated 26% inhibition of activity at 24 hours after the first dose of 1 mg/kg of OMPA, and after each successive dose a progressively greater amount of the enzyme was inhibited until at 24 hours after the fifth dose 70% inhibition of enzyme activity was observed. Assays were performed also on rats given a dose which they could tolerate for 60 days (0.5 mg/kg). Groups of animals were sacrificed at weekly intervals 24 hours after the last dose of OMPA. In one week after beginning the treatment the ChE activity of the submaxillary gland was 52% inhibited and the amount of inhibition was only a few per cent greater at 4 weeks. Maintenance of the inhibition at a constant level appeared to provide an explanation for the ability of animals to withstand repeated exposure to sublethal doses of anti-ChE agents. A similar subacute toxicity study (DuBois et al. 1953) demonstrated that the maximum daily doses of Chlorthion, tetrapropyl dithionopyrophosphate, and Malathion that could be tolerated by rats were 50, 100, and 100 mg/kg, respectively which amounted to between 5% and 15% of the acute single LD_{50}'s for the compounds. Assays performed at daily intervals during the first 5 days of treatment showed a progressive decrease in ChE activity of the tissues during this period.

Measurements of the subacute toxicity of Dipterex (DuBois and Cotter 1955) demonstrated that the maximum daily i.p. dose that rats can tolerate for 60 days is 50 mg/kg, which is approximately 25% of the acute LD_{50}. The higher fraction of the acute LD_{50} of this compound that could be tolerated repeatedly as compared with other compounds is consistent with the extremely rapid reversibility of the inhibitory effects of Dipterex on ChE. Assays performed at intervals during the period of treatment with 50 mg/kg daily of Dipterex again demonstrated a progressive decrease in the enzyme activity during the first 5 days in all tissues, as was noted with other compounds. At subsequent intervals, however, the enzyme activity was maintained at essentially the same level in the range of 30 to 60% of normal for the various tissues that were assayed. From this and previous experiments it appeared that some as yet unexplained physiological change occurred during the first week of treatment which permitted maintenance of the enzyme activity at a constant level. This effect was observed in a more striking manner by BOMBINSKI and DuBOIS (1958) in a recent study on Di-syston. The typical results obtained with other organophosphorus compounds were observed after repeated daily doses, and the animals were able to tolerate 0.5 mg/kg (1/4 of the acute LD_{50}) for 60 days without mortality. However, close observation of the animals at all dosage levels resulted in extremely interesting findings that were most evident at the dosage level of 1 mg/kg daily, which 80% of the initial group were able to tolerate for 60 days. During the first seven days of treatment, typical cholinergic effects occurred after each dose of the compound, with a parallel decrease in body weight. However, at 7 to 10 days after the initial dose the animals began to recover in spite of continued daily treatment with the compound. It was apparent from the absence of signs after the first 10 days of injection of the compound that the critical period with respect to survival or mortality occurs during the first 10 days. Cholinesterase assays on animals receiving daily doses of 1 mg/kg of Di-syston showed that the enzyme activity of brain and serum fell progressively during the first week to about 20% of normal, and that that level was maintained throughout the remainder of the 60-day observation period. With lower daily doses the enzyme activity fell to a lesser extent during the first week and was maintained at that level thereafter. The apparent ability of animals to adjust to organophosphate-induced depression of ChE has been observed with Systox by BARNES and DENZ (1954) in feeding studies. However, the rapidity with which adjustment can occur was less apparent in the feeding experiments than when repeated doses were given i.p. The mechanism responsible for this response to anti-ChE agents is an interesting problem which remains for future investigation.

C. Potentiation of Toxicity

Until recently there was no evidence that more than additive toxic effects result from combinations of anticholinesterase agents. However, FRAWLEY et al. (1957) undertook experiments to ascertain whether potentiation of toxicity results from the simultaneous administration of combinations of organophosphorus insecticides to animals. The conduction of this experiment was suggested by the realization that people may ingest several food products, each containing a different organophosphate, at the same meal, and workers may be exposed to two or more compounds on the same or successive days during their manufacture or use. The results of this study demonstrated that the combination of EPN and Malathion, both of which are permitted to be used on food crops, caused marked potentiation of acute toxicity. Thus, when the two compounds were given orally in an approximately equitoxic ratio of 25 parts of Malathion to 1 part of EPN, the LD_{50} was 167 mg/kg for Malathion and 6.6 for EPN, which represented a 10-fold increase in the toxicity of each agent. If the two compounds had exerted strictly additive toxicity the LD_{50} of this particular mixture should have been 700 mg/kg of Malathion plus 32.5 of EPN (one-half of the LD_{50} of each compound). Following these observations subacute toxicity tests were undertaken in which rats and dogs were fed this combination of compounds in the diet for a period of 8 weeks, and blood ChE measurements were used to estimate whether greater than additive toxicity occurred. The results of these measurements on rats indicated that dietary levels of 25 parts per million (p.p.m.) of EPN and 50 p.p.m. of Malathion caused a degree of inhibition of ChE which was much greater than would be expected on the basis of strictly additive effects. Similar studies on dogs indicated that even the tolerance levels of each compound for fruits and vegetables (3 p.p.m. of EPN and 8 p.p.m. of Malathion) caused potentiated toxicity which was detectable by erythrocyte AChE measurements. These experiments formed the basis for the existing requirement of the U.S. Food and Drug Administration that the toxicological evaluation of all new organophosphorus insecticides include potentiation tests in which the new compound is given in combination with each of the other organophosphates for which tolerance levels have been established, and with all other new compounds which are at a similar stage of development.

The detection of potentiation by acute toxicity tests may be accomplished by comparing the observed LD_{50} with the expected values on the basis of strict additivity for various pairs of compounds. The simplest method of detecting potentiation acutely involves the simultaneous administration of equivalent fractions of the LD_{50} of each compound. If the administration of one-half of the LD_{50} of each of two compounds results in additive (50%) or less than additive mortality, it is apparent that no potentiation has occurred. In cases where potentiation does occur an indication of the magnitude of the effect can be obtained by further toxicity tests. There are several methods which can be used for measuring the degree of potentiation of toxicity. The most satisfactory procedure is to measure the LD_{50} of equitoxic mixtures. This is done by mixing the two compounds using concentrations of each which are related to their comparative toxicities. Thus, if the LD_{50} of one component of the mixture is 10 mg/kg and the LD_{50} of the other component is 90, a mixture containing 10% of one and 90% of the other compound respectively would be employed for the toxicity tests. Comparison of the observed LD_{50} with the value that would be expected on the basis of strictly additive effects provides an indication of the degree of potentiation.

Experiments have been conducted on a number of pairs of organophosphorus compounds to ascertain whether potentiation of toxicity occurs. These tests have revealed that strict additivity, less than additive toxicity, and potentiation of toxicity can occur. The experience in the reviewer's and in other laboratories has been that most pairs of organophosphates produce either additive or less than additive acute toxic effects. With respect to acute toxicity tests it is important to recognize that the dose of each compound is necessarily limited by its toxicity. For this reason the use of intact animals is superior to *in vitro* systems for potentiation tests from the standpoint of assessing the practical hazard, since with the latter method evidence of potentiation can sometimes be obtained at dosage levels which could never be achieved in mammalian organisms.

When one-half of the LD_{50} of each of two compounds having the same mode of action, parallel dosage-mortality curves, and a similar time of onset of toxic effects is administered simultaneously, mortality in the neighborhood of 50% is the expected response. It is noteworthy, however, that the requirements for strict additivity are rather rigid, in contrast to the apparent assumption by many investigators that strict additivity is an expected response from two compounds having the same mode of action. The data presented in Table 11 show results of tests conducted in the reviewer's laboratory in which 21 pairs of organophosphorus compounds were found to exhibit strictly additive toxicity. Less than additive acute toxicity was obtained with 18 pairs of organophosphorus compounds as shown by the data in Table 12. It is noteworthy that these pairs of compounds have the same mechanism of action and that their LD_{50} regression lines are parallel, but additional factors prevent the occurrence of strictly additive toxicity. In this connection the time of occurrence of maximal depression of ChE activity by each compound is important. Some organophosphorus compounds must undergo metabolic conversion to active metabolites, and the onset of effects depends upon the rate of this reaction. The rate at which this conversion takes place differs for various compounds. Consequently, the time after administration at which each one exerts its maximal toxic effect varies from one compound to another. In addition, the rates of absorption and detoxification are different for various cholinergic organophosphates. Some compounds exhibit rather pronounced differences in one or both of these factors, and consequently their simultaneous administration does not result in the occurrence of the maximal toxic effects of each compound at the same time. Thus strict additivity of the toxic actions does not occur.

In the studies which have been conducted in the reviewer's laboratory, only four of a total of 43 pairs of organophosphorus insecticides caused potentiation of acute toxicity. The degree of acute potentiation produced by these combinations, as indicated by measurements of the LD_{50} of equitoxic mixtures, is shown in Table 13. In each case the ratio of the expected LD_{50} to the observed value exceeded unity. Recent studies by ROSENBERG and COON (1958) have shown that EPN, Malathion, Chlorthion and Phostex in all possible paired combinations produce potentiated toxicity in mice. In addition MURPHY et al. (1959) found that triorthotolyl phosphate (TOTP) markedly potentiates

Table 11. *Additive acute toxicity by various combinations of organophosphates*

Organophosphate	Second organophosphate	% Mortality
Parathion	EPN	45
Parathion	Dipterex	55
Parathion	Systox	50
Systox	EPN	45
Systox	Malathion	60
Guthion	EPN	60
Co-Ral	Systox	45
Co-Ral	Disyston	60
Co-Ral	Parathion	50
Co-Ral	Guthion	60
Co-Ral	Trithion	50
Co-Ral	Diazinon	65
Co-Ral	EPN	65
Dipterex	Phosdrin	40
Disyston	Parathion	55
Disyston	Systox	45
Disyston	Malathion	55
Disyston	EPN	40
Disyston	Trithion	45
Disyston	Diazinon	50

One-half of the LD_{50} of each compound was given simultaneously to groups of 20 female rats.

Table 12. *Less than additive acute toxicity by combinations of organophosphorus anticholinesterase agents*

Organophosphate	Second organophosphate	% Mortality
Parathion	Malathion	10
Parathion	Guthion	10
Dipterex	EPN	30
Dipterex	Systox	10
Malathion	Guthion	10
Systox	Guthion	5
Co-Ral	Dipterex	30
Co-Ral	Methylparathion	30
Co-Ral	Phosdrin	30
Dipterex	Systox	15
Dipterex	Methylparathion	20
Dipterex	Trithion	10
Dipterex	Diazinon	10
Dipterex	Disyston	25
Disyston	Methylparathion	20
Disyston	Guthion	15

One-half of the LD_{50} of each compound was given simultaneously to groups of 20 female rats.

gewichten entspricht, quantitativ verschieden, wie es ja auch bei den verschiedenen Endresultaten beider Reaktionen der Fall sein muß.

Beispielsweise fand SCHREINER für die Reaktion (d), daß sich die EMK (in Volt) bei Zimmertemperatur (t in Celsiusgraden) durch die Formel:

$$E = - 0{,}62892 + 0{,}0006882 \cdot t \qquad (\text{I})$$

wiedergeben läßt. (Das negative Vorzeichen soll bedeuten, daß beim Ablaufen der Reaktion im Sinne der Gleichung (d) elektrische Arbeit nach außen abgegeben wird.) Für $t = 17^0$, $T = 290^0$, folgt also $E = -0{,}61722$ V, $\mathfrak{K} = -0{,}61722 \cdot 2 \cdot 23062 = -28470$ cal (da 2 Mol H+-Ionen bei der Reaktion entladen werden.)   Ferner [nach (13), § 16] $-\dfrac{\mathfrak{L}}{T} = 2\mathscr{F}\dfrac{\partial E}{\partial T} = +6{,}882 \cdot 10^{-4} \cdot 2 \cdot 23062$, $\mathfrak{L} = -9206$ cal, endlich $\mathfrak{W} = \mathfrak{K} + \mathfrak{L} = -37676$ cal.

Sind nun die Absolutentropien der beiden festen Stoffe bei der Reaktionstemperatur aus Messungen der spezifischen Wärmen und unter Annahme des NERNSTschen Theorems bekannt, so kann auch die des Wasserstoffgases bei dieser Temperatur berechnet werden, da

$$\mathfrak{L} = T\mathfrak{S} = T \sum \nu_i s^{(i)} \qquad (2)$$

ist. Nach den von SCHREINER gegebenen, auf Messungen von F. LANGE[1] beruhenden Tabellen[2] finden wir $s_{(290)} = s_{(0)} + \displaystyle\int_0^{290} \dfrac{c_p}{T}\, dT$, mit $s_{(0)} = 0$, für

$$\begin{aligned}
\text{Chinhydron:} &\quad s_{(290)} = 68{,}38; \\
\text{Hydrochinon:} &\quad s_{(290)} = 33{,}05; \\
\text{Chinon:} &\quad s_{(290)} = 39{,}12.
\end{aligned}$$

Wir erhalten also für die Reaktion (d):

$$s^{(\mathrm{H_2})} = -\frac{\mathfrak{L}}{T} - s^{(\mathrm{Chinh.})} + 2\, s^{(\mathrm{Hydroch.})} = +\frac{9206}{290} - 68{,}38 + 2 \cdot 33{,}05 = 29{,}47. \quad (3)$$

Andererseits gilt für die Entropie eines idealen Gases (und das ist der Wasserstoff bei 290^0 und 1 Atm.) nach (26), § 13:

$$s^{(t)} = \frac{5+r}{2} R \ln T + \int_0^T \frac{c_2}{T}\, dT - R \ln p + R\left(i + i_r + \frac{5+r}{2} + \ln g_{(0)}\right) \quad (4)$$

oder, wenn man den Druck in Atmosphären mißt:

$$s^{(t)} = c_p^0 \ln T + \int_0^T \frac{c_2}{T}\, dT - R \ln p_{\mathrm{Atm.}} + c_p^0 + 4{,}573 \cdot \overline{C}. \qquad (4a)$$

---

[1] Z. f. physik. Chem. Bd. 110, S. 343, 1924.

[2] Tabelliert sind von SCHREINER: $\displaystyle\int_0^T c_p\, dT$ und $\displaystyle\int_0^T \frac{dT}{T^2}\int_0^T c_p\, dT$; daraus findet man nach (7), § 11, und (6), S. 101, s zu:

$$s = \int_0^T \frac{c_p}{T}\, dT = \frac{1}{T}\int_0^T c_p\, dT + \int_0^T \frac{dT}{T^2}\int_0^T c_p\, dT.$$

wobei wir noch, wie schon beim 3. Beispiel, c_p^0 statt $\frac{5+r}{2}R$ und [Gleichung (2),
S. 547] $\overline{C} = 0{,}4343\,(i + i_r + \ln g_{(0)}) - 6{,}0057$ eingeführt und für $\frac{R}{0{,}4343}$ den Zahlen-
faktor 4,573 geschrieben haben. Da für Wasserstoff die Rotationswärme für
tiefe Temperaturen verschwindet, setzt SCHREINER $r = 0$, also $c_p^0 = \frac{5}{2}R$ und
zählt die Molwärme der Rotation dem temperaturveränderlichen Teil der Molwärme c_z zu (s. S. 565 unten). Er tabelliert ferner, nach Auswertung der über
die spezifische Wärme des Wasserstoffs vorliegenden Messungen, die Funktionen

$$w - w_{(0)} = \int\limits_0^T c_p\,dT = T c_p^0 + \int\limits_0^T c_z\,dT \quad \text{(mit } U - U_0 \text{ bezeichnet) sowie}$$

$$c_p^0 \ln T + \int\limits_0^T \frac{dT}{T^2}\int\limits_0^T c_z\,dT$$

(die in Analogie zu der bei kondensierten Stoffen üblichen Bezeichnungsweise

mit $-\dfrac{A - A_0}{T}$ oder $\int\limits_0^T \dfrac{dT}{T^2}\int\limits_0^T c_p\,dT$ bezeichnet wird). Nun ist (da $c_p = c_p^0 + c_z$):

$$\frac{1}{T}\int\limits_0^T c_p\,dT + c_p^0 \ln T + \int\limits_0^T \frac{dT}{T^2}\int\limits_0^T c_z\,dT = c_p^0 + c_p^0 \ln T + \int\limits_0^T \frac{c_z}{T}\,dT \tag{5}$$

[nach Gleichung (7), § 11], also sind die von SCHREINER tabellierten Funktionen
Bestandteile von $s^{(g)}$ nach (4a), so daß wir ihre Zahlenwerte direkt zum Aufbau
von $s^{(g)}$ benutzen können. Es wird angegeben für $T = 290^0$: „$U - U_0$" $= 1704$,

also ist $\dfrac{1}{290}\int\limits_0^{290} c_p\,dT = 5{,}88$; ferner „$-\dfrac{A - A_0}{T}$" $= 28{,}63$. Wir finden, wenn

wir diese Zahlen in (4a) einsetzen und noch $p = 1$ Atm. berücksichtigen:

$$s^{(H_2)} = 5{,}88 + 28{,}63 + 4{,}573\,\overline{C}. \tag{6}$$

Da nun nach dem experimentellen $\mathfrak{S}$-Wert gemäß (3) $s^{(H_2)} = 29{,}47$ sein soll,
folgt für $\overline{C}$ aus (g):

$$\overline{C} = \frac{29{,}47 - 5{,}88 - 28{,}63}{4{,}573} = -1{,}10.$$

Ganz analog läßt sich die Rechnung für Reaktion (c) durchführen. Für $\overline{C}$
ergab sich hier das gleiche Resultat $-1{,}09$ bis $1{,}11$, das mit dem aus dem Ver-
dampfungsgleichgewicht (analog der von uns als Beispiel 3 gebrachten Rechnung
am Wasserdampf) gefundenen Wert $-1{,}09$ vollständig übereinstimmt. Es ist
das anscheinend eine der besten bisher beigebrachten Bestätigungen des NERNST-
schen Theorems. Dazu ist allerdings zu bemerken, daß man gerade im Fall des
Wasserstoffs, wie in § 13 und besonders § 17, S. 317, erörtert, Grund zu der
Annahme hat, daß das (effektive) Quantengewicht $g_{(0)}$ im festen Zustand bei
$T = 0$ von 1 verschieden ist. Der hier erhaltene Befund würde also nicht,
die in § 12 erwähnte nächstliegende Deutung des NERNSTschen Theorems zu-
lassen, wonach sich bei $T = 0$ die beteiligten festen Körper im Zustand völliger
Ordnung befinden (Quantengewicht 1), sondern es müßte durch Kondensation
des Wasserstoffs sowohl am Chinhydron unter Bildung von Hydrochinon, wie
auch am Chinon unter Bildung von Chinhydron jedesmal das (bei der Extrapolation der spezifischen Wärme im Effekt auftretende) Quantengewicht dieser

for the various compounds differ considerably. The time at which maximal inhibition of ChE's occurred varied from 15 minutes to 3 hours. In some cases the AChE activity of the brain and parasympathetic nervous system, as indicated by the submaxillary gland, and the non-specific ChE of serum were inhibited to the same extent by a particular compound. However, a notable exception was seen in the case of the phosphoramides which do not gain access to brain AChE, and Guthion which does not inhibit non-specific ChE. Marked differences in the rate of reversal of the inhibitory effects on ChE's *in vivo* were noted. Various anti-ChE agents differ more in this respect than in any other aspect of their actions *in vivo*. In view of the variable durations of action of various anti-ChE agents, the performance of assays on the tissues of animals at intervals after acutely toxic doses provides a great deal of useful information relative to the toxicity of these compounds.

Summary

The development and toxicological evaluation of anti-ChE agents have been stimulated within recent years by their widespread use as agricultural insecticides. Some medicinal uses and the applicability of the compounds for studying the nervous system have also stimulated interest in their toxicology. The acute toxicity of various compounds of the anti-ChE class covers a wide range. Among the more toxic anti-ChE agents which have been studied are the fluoride and cyanide-containing organophosphates and phosphorus compounds containing substituted ammonium ions. The LD_{50} values of some members of this series are as low as 0.01 mg/kg. Most of the anti-ChE agents which are employed as insecticides have acute LD_{50} values ranging from 1 to 10 mg/kg. Many attempts have been made to develop compounds of this class having low mammalian toxicity and high toxicity to insects. Most efforts along this line have been unsuccessful, with the notable exception of Malathion, the low mammalian toxicity of which apparently depends upon its efficient detoxification through an enzymatic mechanism that is absent from insect species.

The majority of anti-ChE agents produce the muscarinic and nicotinic actions of ACh, as well as its effects on the central nervous system. The carbamates and some phosphoramides lack the central actions due to an inability of the compounds to gain access to the central nervous system. The effects of acute toxic doses of anti-ChE agents are reversible. After single doses all of the members of this series produce death or apparently complete recovery within a period of 10 days after the administration of single doses. The rate of recovery of the inhibition of ChE's varies from a few hours to several days for different compounds.

It is now apparent that the organophosphorus anti-ChE agents may serve either as substrates for enzymes which catalyze their degradation and loss of toxicity, or as inhibitors of these detoxifying enzymes. The latter action can result in potentiation of acute toxicity when a second compound, the detoxification of which depends upon an enzyme, is administered simultaneously with an inhibitor of the corresponding enzyme. Several combinations of organophosphorus compounds have been found to exhibit potentiated toxicity when administered simultaneously. The most marked potentiation observed thus far was noted with EPN and Malathion, in which the detoxification of the latter compound is markedly inhibited by EPN. Further studies on this aspect of the toxicological evaluation of anti-ChE agents will undoubtedly contribute substantially to knowledge of the detoxification pathways for these compounds. Since the toxicity *in vivo* of these agents is due not only to the inherent anti-ChE activity of the parent compound or active metabolites but also to the rate of detoxification, a more complete understanding of the latter process for various compounds would greatly advance our knowledge of their mammalian toxicity.

Literature

AUGUSTINSSON, K. B.: Mintacol (diethyl p-nitrophenyl phosphate). Svensk farm. T. **57**, 261 to 267 (1953).

ALDRIDGE, W. N.: The differentiation of true and pseudocholinesterase by organophosphorus compounds. Biochem. J. **53**, 62—67 (1953).

—, and J. M. BARNES: Some problems in assessing the toxicity of the "organophosphorus" insecticides towards mammals. Nature (Lond.) **169**, 345—352 (1952).

BAGDON, R. E., and K. P. DUBOIS: Pharmacologic effects of Chlorthion, Malathion and tetra-propyl dithionopyrophosphate in mammals. Arch. int. Pharmacodyn. **103**, 192—199 (1955).

BARNES, J. M., and F. A. DENZ: The reaction of rats to diets containing octamethyl pyro-phosphoramide (Schradan) and 0,0-diethyl-S-ethylmercaptoethanol thiophosphate ("Systox"). Brit. J. industr. Med. **11**, 11—19 (1954).

BIDSTRUP, P. L., J. A. BONNELL and A. G. BECKETT: Paralysis following poisoning by a new organic phosphorus insecticide (Mipafox). Brit. med. J. **1**, 1068—1072 (1953).

BOMEINSKI, T. J., and K. P. DUBOIS: Toxicity and mechanism of action of Di-Syston. A. M. A. Arch. industr. Hlth **17**, 192—199 (1958).

BRAUER, R. W.: Inhibition of the cholinesterase activity of human blood plasma and ery-throcyte stromata by alkylated phosphorus compounds. J. Pharmacol. exp. Ther. **92**, 162—172 (1948).

BRUCE, R. B., J. W. HOWARD and J. R. ELSEA: Toxicity of 0,0-diethyl 0-(2-isopropyl-6-methyl-4-pyrimidyl phosphorothioate (Diazinon). J. Agric. food Chem. **3**, 1017—1021 (1955).

BURGEN, A. S. V., C. A. KEELE and D. SLOME: Pharmacological actions of tetraethylpyro-phosphate and hexaethyltetraphosphate. J. Pharmacol. exp. Ther. **96**, 396—409 (1949).

CASIDA, J. E.: Metabolism of organophosphorus insecticides in relation their antiesterase activity, stability, and residual properties. J. Agric. food Chem. **4**, 772—785 (1956).

— T. C. ALLEN and M. A. STAHMANN: Mammalian conversion of octamethyl pyrophosphor-amide to a toxic phosphoramide-N-oxide. J. biol. Chem. **210**, 607—616 (1954).

COOK, J. W., J. R. BLAKE and M. W. WILLIAMS: The enzymic hydrolysis of Malathion and its inhibition by EPN and other organic phosphorus compounds. J. Ass. Off. Agric. Chem. **40**, 664—665 (1957).

DAVIES, D. R.: Cholinesterases and the mode of action of some anticholinesterases. J. Pharmacol. **6**, 1—26 (1954).

DAVISON, A. N.: The conversion of Schradan (OMPA) and Parathion into inhibitors of cholinesterase by mammalian liver. Biochem. J. **61**, 203—209 (1955).

DEICHMANN, W. B., and K. LAMPE: Dipterex: Its pharmacologic action and an appraisal of the hazard associated with its use. Univ. Miami School med. Bull. **9**, 7—12 (1955).

— W. PUGLIESE and J. CASSIDY: Effects of dimethyl and diethyl paranitrophenyl thio-phosphate on experimental animals. A. M. A. Arch. industr. Hyg. **5**, 44—51 (1952).

—, and R. RAKOCZY: Toxicity and mechanism of action of Systox. A. M. A. Arch. industr. Hlth **11**, 324—331 (1955).

DIGGLE, W. M., and J. C. GAGE: Cholinesterase inhibition in vivo by 0,0-diethyl 0-p-nitro-phenyl thiophosphate (Parathion, E 605). Biochem. J. **49**, 491—494 (1951).

DISTEFANO, V., L. HURWITZ, W. F. NEUMAN and H. C. HODGE: Coramine (Nikethamide) as adjuvant to atropine in treatment of poisoning by EPN (ethyl p-nitrophenyl thionobenzene-phosphonate). Proc. Soc. exp. Biol. (N. Y.) **78**, 712—713 (1951).

DOULL, J., and K. P. DUBOIS: Toxicity and anticholinesterase action of tetra-n-propyl dithionopyrophosphate. J. Pharmacol. exp. Ther. **106**, 382 (1952).

DUBOIS, K. P.: Potentiation of the toxicity of organophosphorus compounds. Advances in Pest Control Research, Vol. 4. In press. New York: Interscience Publishers 1961.

—, and K. W. COCHRAN: Inhibition of cholinesterase by dimethylamino fluorophosphate. Fed. Proc. **10**, 292 (1951).

—, and J. M. COON: Toxicology of organic phosphorus-containing insecticides to mammals. Arch. industr. Hyg. **6**, 9—13 (1952).

—, and G. J. COTTER: Studies on the toxicity and mechanism of action of Dipterex. A. M. A. Arch. industr. Hlth **11**, 53—60 (1955).

— J. DOULL and J. M. COON: Toxicity and mechanism of action of p-nitro-phenyl-diethyl-thionophosphate (E 605). Fed. Proc. **7**, 216 (1948).

Chapter 19

Neurotoxicity of Organophosphorus Compounds

By

D. R. Davies

With 16 Figures

Contents

Introduction

Although many attempts have been made to find pharmacological actions of organo-phosphorus compounds other than those resulting from the inactivation of acetylcholinesterase (AChE), [e.g., the inactivation of trypsin, chymotrypsin, and ali-esterase (MOUNTER et al. 1957), or the interference with ion transfer across a membrane (GREIG and HOLLAND 1949)], with but one exception, none of these has been shown to be of any great physiological significance. Certain compounds

verwiesen. Im ganzen ergibt sich also $\left(\text{mit } \dfrac{0,4343}{R} = \dfrac{1}{4,573}\right)$ aus (6), (7) und (8), analog zu (27c), § 13, und ähnlich (6), § 16:

$$
\begin{aligned}
\frac{\mathfrak{K}}{4,573 \cdot T} = \frac{\mathfrak{W}(0)}{4,573 \cdot T} &- \nu^{(\mathrm{g})} \frac{c_p^0}{R} \cdot \log T \\
&- \sum \nu_i \int_0^T \frac{dT}{4,573 \cdot T^2} \int_0^T c^{(i)} \cdot dT + \nu^{(\mathrm{g})} \cdot \log p - \nu^{(\mathrm{g})} \cdot \bar{C},
\end{aligned} \right\} \quad (9)
$$

wobei $c^{(i)} = c_z$ für das Gas, $c^{(i)} = c_p^{(i)}$ für die kondensierten Phasen ist. Für das Zersetzungsgleichgewicht $(\mathfrak{K} = 0, \ p = \pi)$ folgt endlich:

$$
\nu^{(\mathrm{g})} \log \pi = - \frac{\mathfrak{W}(0)}{4,573 \cdot T} + \nu^{(\mathrm{g})} \frac{c_p^0}{R} \log T + \sum \nu_i \int_0^T \frac{dT}{4,573 \cdot T^2} \int_0^T c^{(i)} \cdot dT + \nu^{(\mathrm{g})} \cdot \bar{C}. \quad (10)
$$

Um $\mathfrak{W}_{(0)}$ aus $\mathfrak{W}_{(298)}$ zu bestimmen [analog (3)], brauchen wir außer dem in (5) schon berechneten Integral über $c_p^{(\mathrm{CO}_2)}$ $(= 2070 + 180 \text{ cal})$ noch die Werte $w_{(298)} - w_{(0)}$ für $\mathrm{CaCO_3}$ und CaO, die nach den Tabellen von MIETHING 3710[1] bzw. 1610 cal betragen. Dann ist also:

$$
\begin{aligned}
\mathfrak{W}_{(0)} &= \mathfrak{W}_{(298)} - \sum \nu_i \left(w_{(298)}^{(i)} - w_{(0)}^{(i)} \right) \\
&= 42\,600 + 3710 - 1610 - 2250 = 42\,450 \text{ cal.}
\end{aligned} \right\} \quad (11)
$$

$\bar{C}$ ist von EUCKEN, KARWAT und FRIED aus Messungen des Verdampfungsgleichgewichts der Kohlensäure bestimmt worden, auf demselben Wege, den wir oben im 3. Beispiel an der Wasserverdampfung dargestellt haben. Man erhält $\bar{C} = 0,91$. Bei Gültigkeit des NERNSTschen Theorems müßte man mit diesem Werte auch die Dissoziationsdrucke des $\mathrm{CaCO_3}$ befriedigend darstellen können.

Für die Auswertung des Doppelintegrals in (10) reichen bei hohen Temperaturen die MIETHINGschen Tabellen nicht aus, wir müssen daher von irgendeiner Temperatur T_0 ab Interpolationsformeln für die Molwärmen der Kondensate benutzen. Da jedoch von BÄCKSTRÖM (s. o.) eine Interpolationsformel für die ganze Summe $\sum \nu_i c_p^{(i)}$ unserer Reaktion im Bereich von 0—1000° C aufgestellt worden ist, und zwar:

$$
\sum \nu_i c_p^{(i)} = 3,34 - 1,378 \cdot 10^{-2} \cdot T + 4,13 \cdot 10^{-6} T^2, \quad (12)
$$

so ist es am bequemsten, eine Zerlegung des Aufbaus (9) in zwei Temperaturgebiete nicht nur für die beiden kondensierten Phasen [für $\mathrm{CO_2}$ würde ja die bis zu sehr hohen Temperaturen ausreichende Formel (4) zur Verfügung stehen], sondern für die ganze Reaktion durchzuführen und als Zwischentemperatur $T_0 = 298°$ zu wählen, da für diese Temperatur der $\mathfrak{W}$-Wert der Reaktion bekannt ist.

Wir benutzen demgemäß Gleichung (9) direkt nur zur Bestimmung von $\left(\dfrac{\mathfrak{K}}{T}\right)_{(p,\,T_0)}$ und gehen dann zur Temperatur T bei konstantem Druck nach (6b), § 11 weiter, indem wir setzen ($\mathfrak{W}_0$ abgekürzt für $\mathfrak{W}_{(p,\,T_0)}$):

$$
\left(\frac{\mathfrak{K}}{T}\right)_{(p,\,T)} = \left(\frac{\mathfrak{K}}{T}\right)_{(p,\,T_0)} - \frac{\mathfrak{W}_0}{T_0} + \frac{\mathfrak{W}_0}{T} - \int_{T_0}^T \frac{dT}{T^2} \int_{T_0}^T \sum \nu_i c_p^{(i)} \, dT. \quad (13)
$$

---

[1] Mit einer Abänderung nach EUCKEN: Z. f. physik. Chem. Bd. 100, S. 159, 1922.

Die direkten Messungen ergeben ziemlich auseinandergehende Werte. Aus den wohl genauesten (von JOHNSTON, J. Am. Ch. Soc. Bd. 32, S. 938, 1910, sowie SMYTH und ADAMS, J. Am. Ch. Soc. Bd. 45, S. 1167, 1923) folgt der Wert 0,0208. Die Ursache der Diskrepanzen ist nach HÜTTIG und LEWINTER[1] darin zu suchen, daß die Zusammensetzung der festen Phasen etwas variabel ist. Hierdurch werden gewisse Voraussetzungen unserer Berechnung hinfällig; zwar nicht die Existenz eines nur von der Temperatur abhängigen Zersetzungsdruckes und die nach § 31 ganz allgemeine Gültigkeit von Gleichung (1), wohl aber die Extrapolation von $\mathfrak{W}$ nach (3) mittels der spezifischen Wärmen der reinen Substanzen. Ferner ist auch zu berücksichtigen, daß bei Beginn der Zersetzung des Calcits möglicherweise eine CaO-Anreicherung der $CaCO_3$-Phase ohne sofortiges Auftreten einer dritten (CaO-) Phase vorliegen kann; dann wird natürlich der Zersetzungsdruck nicht mehr eine bloße Temperaturfunktion sein. Auch wird, wenn variable Zusammensetzungen der festen Phasen möglich sind, die Herstellung des Gleichgewichts in ganz anderer Weise durch langsame Diffussionsvorgänge in den Festphasen verzögert als bei invariabeln Festphasen. Allgemein zeigt sich immer häufiger, daß Systeme, die früher als aus „reinen Stoffen" bestehend angenommen wurden, dies doch nicht in Strenge sind.

b) Bestimmung des absoluten Zersetzungsdruckes nach dem NERNST schen Theorem. Wir wollen am Beispiel der $CaCO_3$-Dissoziation noch eine etwas andere Aufgabe studieren, indem wir zunächst wieder von der Komplikation durch die Veränderlichkeit der Festphasen absehen. Es handelt sich darum, bei einer vorgegebenen Temperatur den Zersetzungsdruck seiner Absolutgröße nach zu berechnen, oder zu einem vorgegebenen Zersetzungsdruck — z. B. 1 Atm. — die Gleichgewichtstemperatur zu finden. Würde man die Gleichung (2) integrieren, indem man $\mathfrak{W}$ mit Hilfe der spezifischen Wärmen als Funktion von T ausdrückt, so würde jedoch noch ein Faktor (eine Chemische Konstante) unbekannt bleiben.

Zu einer vollständigen Bestimmung des Zersetzungsdruckes gelangen wir auf Grund von Wärmemessungen und der Konstante $\bar{C}$ des CO_2-Gases mit Hilfe des NERNST schen Theorems, indem wir von der Gleichung

$$\mathfrak{K} = \sum \nu_i \mu^{(i)} \tag{6}$$

ausgehen und für die beiden festen Reaktionsteilnehmer

$$\frac{\mu}{RT} = \frac{w_{(0)}}{RT} - \int_0^T \frac{dT}{RT^2} \int_0^T c_p \, dT \tag{7}$$

setzen [mit Vernachlässigung der Druckabhängigkeit, s. § 12, (8b)]. Für die gasförmige Komponente, bei der wir Gültigkeit der idealen Gasgesetze annehmen, ist nach (27a), § 13:

$$0{,}4343 \cdot \frac{\mu^{(g)}}{RT} = 0{,}4343 \cdot \frac{u_{(0)}^{(g)}}{RT} - \frac{c_p^0}{R} \log T - 0{,}4343 \int_0^T \frac{dT}{RT^2} \int_0^T c_z \cdot dT + \log p_{\text{Atm.}} - \bar{C}, \tag{8}$$

wobei wir sogleich die Umformungen vorgenommen haben, die mit der Zählung von p in Atmosphären und der Einführung dekadischer Logarithmen verbunden sind. Wegen der Bedeutung von c_p^0 und $\bar{C}$ sei auf S. 547 Gleichung (2) und S. 555 oben

---

[1] Z. f. angew. Chem. Bd. 41, S. 1034, 1928.

of this type however can give rise to neurotoxic effects in man of a particularly unpleasant and long-lasting nature. These consist in a polyneuritis with a flaccid paralysis of the distal muscles of the upper and lower extremities, accompanied by degeneration of the myelin sheaths and axons of the spinal cord, sciatic nerve, and medulla.

Historical

From 1896 to the present time about 40,000 cases of neurotoxicity have occurred in humans due to poisoning with triarylphosphates.

The earliest recorded cases were six which occurred in 1896. They arose out of treatment of 41 tuberculosis patients with phosphocreosote (LOROT 1899). This remedy appears to have been fashionable during the ensuing 35 years, for during this period more than 50 additional cases due to this same cause were reported (ROGER and RECORDIER 1934).

The classical outbreak occurred early in 1930 when symptoms of paralysis were observed in thousands of people in the Southern States of the U.S.A. These were shown to have arisen through the ingestion of certain varieties of "Jamaica Ginger" during prohibition (GOLDFAIN 1930, MILLIS 1931). Owing to the enormous demand for this extract as a beverage, a variety of oily like substances were added to impart added potency. As a result no fewer than 20,000 cases of intoxication were recorded (KIELY and RICH 1932, WEBER 1937). SMITH and his colleagues, in a now classical series of researches, showed that in all the preparations which caused paralysis, triorthocresylphosphate (TOCP) was the adulterant (SMITH, M. I. et al. 1930), a discovery which shed light upon those cases poisoned with phosphocreosote, since this substance was known to contain TOCP as an impurity.

During 1931, TER BRAAK reported 40 cases which occurred in Holland due to the use of an adulterated extract of parsley, called apiol, which was used as an abortifacient. A further 50 cases were reported during 1932 from Germany, France, Switzerland and Yugoslavia (GERMON 1932). The adulterant was TOCP which was present to the extent of 28 to 50%. The reason for the use of such an adulterant is unknown, since TOCP does not resemble in taste, colour or odour the original extract; neither is its intended function in the extract clear (HUNTER et al. 1944). Between 1936 and 1940 a new hazard arose due to the accidental or deliberate addition of tricresylphosphates to edible and cooking oils (MEDNIKYAN and MIRZOYAN 1936). A typical example of the accidental contamination of edible oils occurred in Natal where 68 people were affected through partaking of soya bean oil containing 0.4% TOCP. The victims developed a lower motor neuron paralysis of both hands and feet (SAMPSON 1938, 1942).

The deliberate use of mineral oils containing tricresylphosphate (TCP) as cooking oils became common in Germany during the 1939—1945 war (HENSCHLER 1958). Torpedo oil (Igelheit) and machine gun oil were used extensively and each contained significant amounts of crude TCP. Although the actual number of cases which occurred is not known, the resulting outbreak of ataxia and paralysis must have reached serious proportions, for the authorities made quite strenuous attempts to prevent the use of such substitutes. Even so the outbreak subsided only when normal vegetable oils and cooking fats became available. Such outbreaks were not, however, confined to Germany, for in 1940, 80 men of the Swiss Army were poisoned when TOCP was accidentally used as a cooking oil (WALTHARD 1946), and several cases, due to a very similar cause, occurred sporadically in Liverpool (HOTSON 1946).

The insidious character of the intoxication is well illustrated by eleven cases which occurred in Durban in 1955 (SUSSER and STEIN 1957). The victims were poisoned by drinking water stored in drums which they had removed from the paint factory in which some of the victims worked and which formerly contained TOCP.

More recently an outbreak of epidemic proportions occurred in Meknes, N. Africa (SMITH, H. V. and SPALDING 1959). About 10,000 people have been estimated to have been affected. The cause of the epidemic seems to have been the widespread use of a mixture of olive oil and lubricating oil. The latter, which was normally used in jet engines, contained considerable amounts of TCP.

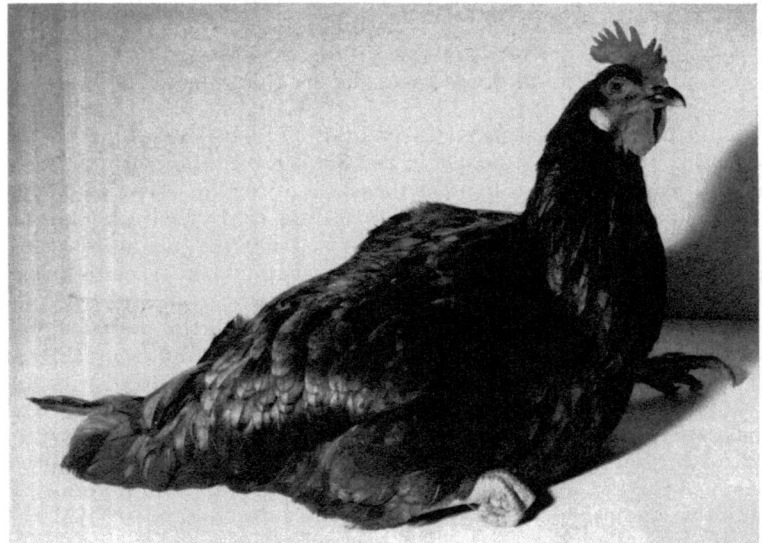

Fig. 1

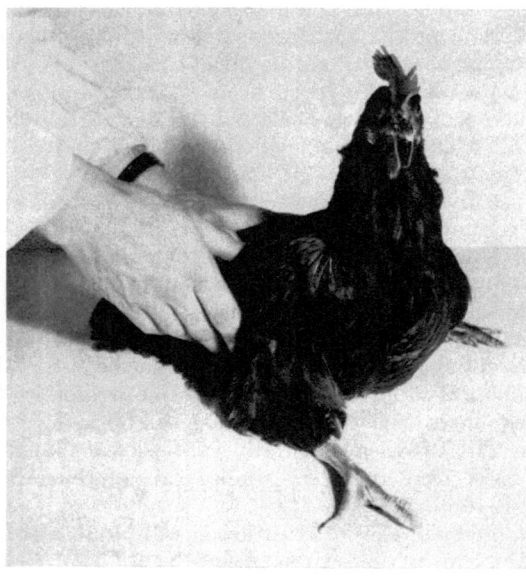

Fig. 2

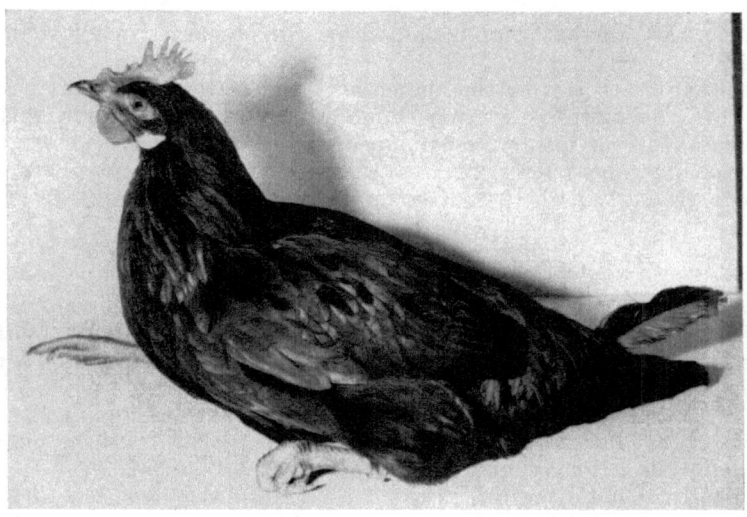

Fig. 3

Plate 1 (Figs. 1 to 3). Typical posture of hens exhibiting neurotoxic signs following DFP poisoning

Tricresylphosphate is important in the plastics industry, particularly in the preparation of polyvinyl chloride. Since it is fairly readily soluble in fat solvents, it may be absorbed by careless handling of the finished product. Three such cases of toxic polyneuritis occurred in 1942 (HUNTER et al. 1944) and in more recent years a considerable number of cases of industrial intoxication has been reported in East Germany (HENSCHLER 1958).

A new neurotoxic hazard was discovered in 1951 when a man and a woman were accidentally poisoned with an entirely different type of organophosphorus compound, NN'-di*iso*propylphosphoro-diamidic fluoride (Mipafox), an insecticide which was being developed because it exhibited a low toxicity to mammals but a high one to insects. The course of the poisoning differed from that following TOCP, in that the victims experienced immediate acute signs of anticholinesterase (anti-ChE) poisoning before the delayed onset of ataxia and paralysis (BIDSTRUP et al. 1953).

A The experimental production of neurotoxicity in animals

I. Species differences

The experimental production of neurotoxic effects in animals is complicated by the existence of marked species differences, and it is only in the chicken and the cat that the clinical syndrome bears any close resemblance to that seen in man (SMITH, M. I. and LILLIE 1931, HENSCHLER 1958; FRIES et al. 1959). These species differences are particularly evident with TOCP (SMITH, M. I. et al. 1932). For example, the response of the rodent is quite atypical. Even with quite large doses no demonstrable effect can be produced in the albino rat; in the rabbit and the guinea pig general stimulation of the CNS occurs, followed by a paralysis of the respiratory centre 6 to 48 hr later. These effects are not, however, followed by the delayed effects seen in man.

A partial motor paralysis of the upper, but predominently of the lower extremities occurs in the monkey, but it is of short duration only. The calf and the dog both exhibit signs which resemble those seen in man, but so little work has been done on the calf that a rigid comparison with the human clinical picture is not justified.

Absorption of TOCP from the alimentary tract of the dog occurs only with difficulty, consequently it is not easy to produce neurotoxic effects by this route. After subcutaneous or intramuscular injections, however, a flaccid paralysis of the posterior extremities develops after an unusually long latent period of 4 to 6 weeks (SMITH, M. I. et al. 1932, KOELLE and GILMAN 1946, FRIESS et al. 1959).

II. Neurotoxicity in the cat and the chicken

The cat behaves similarly to man but the development of the various phases of the malady are dose-dependant (KIDD and LANGWORTHY 1933). With large doses the latent period is short, 7 to 14 days. At the end of this period a rapidly ascending paralysis, beginning at the tail and hind legs, develops and quickly involves the muscles of the forelegs and the trunk. Death follows in 36 to 72 hr and is due to respiratory (bulbar) paralysis. With smaller doses the interval to onset of paralysis is longer, the clinical picture is more "spread out," and the different phases do not overlap. Thus, the first sign is drooping of the tail followed rather later by a moderate hind leg ataxia. The forelegs are affected only about a fortnight later. Death occurs only after a significantly longer period than with larger doses, and may be due either to bulbar paralysis or to cachexia secondary to the prolonged lower motor neuron paralysis.

The chicken is the species which behaves most consistently, and because they are so convenient have been used most for experimental purposes.

After the administration of TOCP to chickens, there follows a latent and completely symptom-free period in which the birds appear to be normal. This interval, which is virtually diagnostic in the chicken, is about 8 to 14 days. At the end of this period the birds tire easily on standing and spend most of their time squatting on their haunches in a quite characteristic pose (FENTON 1955). After exercise a decided broadening and clumsiness of gait can be seen, and on the day following these first signs of incipient paralysis, overt weakness and clumsiness are obvious even without exercise. The feet slap heavily on the floor, are clumsy and irregular in action, and widely spread to maintain balance. Ankle jerks are uniformly depressed and the legs are hypotonic; power is severely reduced in the ankle and knee movements but the upper parts of the limbs are still able to perform quite strong actions though these are poorly co-ordinated. Although the wings are sometimes noticeably weakened, they are never affected to the same degree as the legs (CAVANAGH 1954).

At the end of fifteen or sixteen days, the birds are severely paralysed in the legs, and once the condition has reached this stage there is no evidence of further functional damage. If the dose is suitably chosen the birds survive, and after an initial setback during the onset of nervous damage gain weight and maintain good general health (Plate 1, Figs. 1—3).

III. The effect of age upon the susceptibility to paralysis

Age is a significant factor in the development of neurotoxic effects (BARNES and DENZ 1953). Ataxia and paralysis cannot be produced in young chicks. At 40 mg/kg, orally, Mipafox produced ataxia and paralysis in 2-year old hens, but when this dose was given to 1-year old birds no such effects developed; if, however, the same dose was given subcutaneously, ataxia and paralysis followed.

One mg/kg of di*iso*propyl phosphorofluoridate (DFP) given i.m. is a certain paralysing dose in adult hens, but 10 successive doses of this size, given weekly, failed to produce any such changes in hens of less than 8 weeks of age.

This phenomenon has been examined in greater detail by BARNES (personal communication), and he has shown that there is a critical age at which the chick becomes susceptible. With both DFP and TOCP this is between 55 and 70 days.

B. The histology of neurotoxicity in hens

I. The general character of the lesion

Demyelination is always found in the sciatic nerves, spinal cord, and medulla in paralysed hens, but these changes are seldom found until the clinical signs are well developed (CAVANAGH 1954, FENTON 1955). M. I. SMITH and LILLIE (1931) described the condition as a "specific demyelinating" disease, but it is not too clear what they meant, since they made no special investigation into the integrity of the axon. It is probable that the term was used in a descriptive rather than a causal sense, for the criterion of demyelination is that loss of myelin should be in excess of axon damage. That axon damage does occur was noted by KIDD and LANGWORTHY (1933) and later by AHRING (1942), but neither of these authors commented upon this fact.

The selection of the tracts and the general distribution of the changes closely resemble those seen in thiamine-deficient birds (SWANK and PRADOS 1942). Although SWANK (1940) considered that the axons were the first to degenerate in thiamine deficiency, ZIMMERMAN (1943) held a contrary view.

This same problem exists in the present case, and it is of importance to decide whether the organophosphorus compounds are cytotoxic, i.e., they produce their effects by virtue of toxic action upon specific cells, or whether they are poisonous because they interfere directly with myelin metabolism. This issue has been investigated very carefully in recent years by a number of workers (CAVANAGH 1954, FENTON 1955, SILVER 1960). CAVANAGH and FENTON are in agreement that there is no evidence for believing that disintegration of myelin precedes axis cylinder fragmentation by any significant interval of time. They are also in agreement that the timing and the sequence of events closely follow those seen in Wallerian degeneration. More recently these interpretations have been questioned (SILVER 1960).

In view of these differing opinions it is therefore of importance to describe the experimental findings in some detail.

II. Experimental methods

1. The preparation of tissues prior to staining

The various methods for demonstrating demyelination are very liable to artifact, consequently technique, particularly in the preparation of tissues prior to staining, is of paramount importance. The major problem is the risk of damaging the tissue during manipulation, and different authors have employed varying procedures to prevent this. M. I. SMITH and LILLIE (1931) killed their birds with chloroform and immediately removed the entire central nervous system and sciatic nerves, which they fixed by immersion in 10% formalin. BARNES and DENZ (1953) sacrificed their birds with nembutal and immediately perfused them through the aorta with about 2 l of physiological saline solution, followed by about 6 to 8 l of formalin-saline solution. The brain, spinal cord, and sciatic nerves were then dissected out and fixed further in formalin-saline solution overnight. FENTON (1955) used almost precisely the same technique; it differed only in more prolonged periods of perfusion and immersion in formalin-saline solution.

CAVANAGH (1954) killed his birds by decapitation, and after the skin had been stripped off, each sciatic nerve was exposed from the trochanter of the femur to the ankle joint and portions from both distal and proximal regions were allowed to adhere to perforated cardboard to prevent shrinkage. The tissues were then dropped into 1% osmic acid for 48 hr. This combined fixing and staining. The brain and spinal cord, together with dorsal root ganglia at various levels, were exposed and fixed for 48 hr in formalin-saline solution before being dissected out. The peripheral nerves which had been fixed in osmic acid were dissociated in glycerine, washed, and mounted in glycerine jelly. By this method it was judged that minimal distortion of the myelin sheaths had been incurred and at the same time quite considerable lengths of individual fibres, sometimes including four or five consecutive modes of Ranvier, could be readily examined.

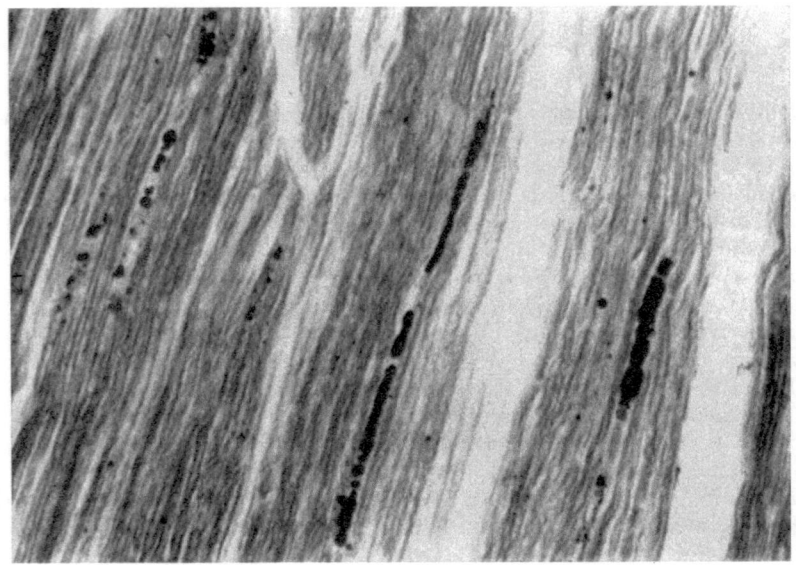

Fig. 4. Sciatic nerve of chicken. Demyelination following Mipafox. Marchi. × 64

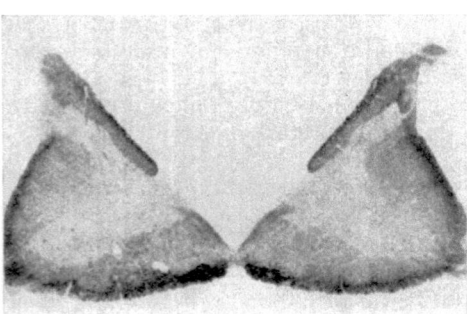

Fig. 5. Sacral segment of spinal cord of chicken. Demyelination of anterior columns. Marchi. × 24

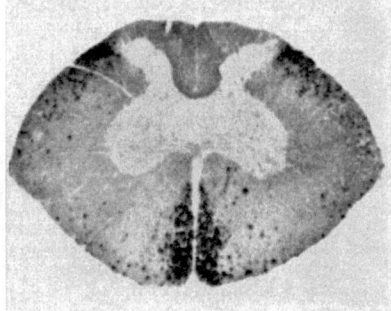

Fig. 7. Lower lumbar cord of chicken. Demyelination of anterior and lateral columns. Marchi. × 24

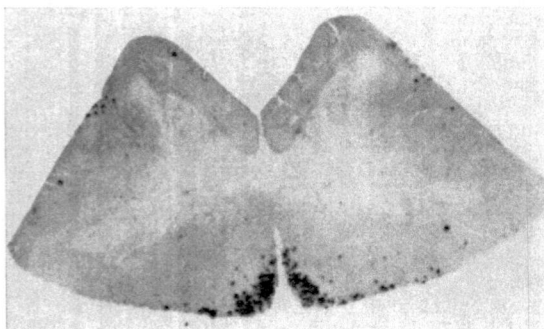

Fig. 6. Lumbo-sacral cord of chicken. Demyelination in anterior columns and a few damaged fibres in lateral columns. Marchi. × 24

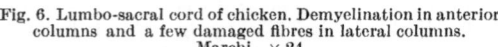

Fig. 8. Lumbo-dorsal cord of chicken. Demyelination of anterior and lateral columns. Marchi. × 24

Plate 2 (Figs. 4 to 8). Demyelination of peripheral nerve and spinal cord of chicken following Mipafox.
(From BARNES and DENZ 1953)

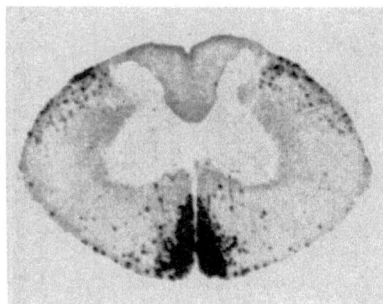

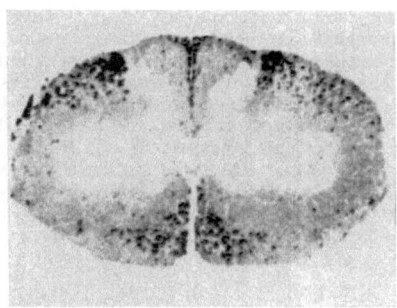

Fig. 9. Mid-dorsal cord of chicken. Demyelination of anterior columns most extensive in this region. Marchi. × 24

Fig. 10. Upper dorsal cord of chicken. Demyelination of fasciculus gracilis in posterior columns as well as in anterior and lateral columns. Marchi. × 24

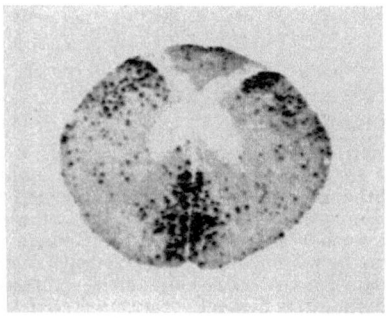

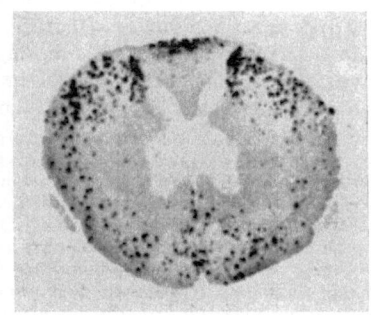

Fig. 11. Lower cervical cord of chicken. Demyelination in anterior, lateral and posterior columns. Marchi. × 24

Fig. 12. Mid-cervical cord of chicken. Damaged fibres in anterior columns reduced in number and less well localised. Marchi. × 24

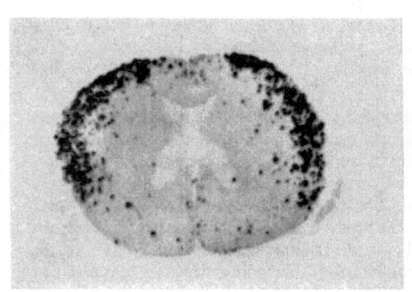

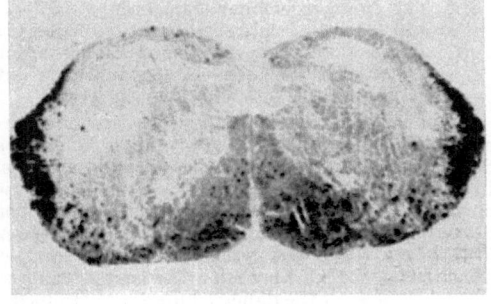

Fig. 13. Upper cervical cord of chicken. Damaged fibres grouped in lateral columns. Very few damaged fibres in anterior columns. Marchi. × 24

Fig. 14. Medulla of chicken. Demyelinated fibres grouped in lateral angles. Marchi. × 24

Plate 3 (Figs. 9 to 14). Demyelination of spinal cord and medulla of chicken following Mipafox. (From BARNES and DENZ 1953)

2. Staining methods used

The staining techniques of individual workers varied quite markedly, but none gave reasons for the choice of any given method.

For the detection of myelin degeneration, the Marchi stain or some more recent modification has been used by every investigator. Thus, M. I. SMITH and LILLIE (1931) used the original technique; BARNES and DENZ (1953) used Glee's modification (GATENBY and BEAMS 1950); whilst both CAVANAGH (1954) and FENTON (1955) employed the SWANK and DAVENPORT (1935) form of the Marchi method.

Axon degeneration was studied by CAVANAGH (1954) and FENTON (1955). The former employed the silver impregnation method of GLEES and MARSLAND (1952) and the latter, *Holmes*' method.

Nissl granules and nerve cells were examined by the well established techniques of SWANK and DAVENPORT (1935), EINARSON's gallocyanin, and also buffered thionine.

III. The demyelinated pathways in TOCP poisoned hens

There is general agreement that demyelination is confined to the sciatic nerve, spinal cord, and medulla oblongata. The cord is the most sensitive to damage and the first tissue to show signs of damage (BARNES and DENZ 1953, LANCASTER 1960). Demyelination appears later in the sciatic nerve and medulla but these tissues appear to be equally sensitive.

The distribution of myelin damage in the nervous system has been mapped by several authors (BARNES and DENZ 1953, CAVANAGH 1954, FENTON 1955) and their results agree closely. The following account is due to BARNES and DENZ (1953).

Peripheral Nerves (see Plate 2). There is great variation in the number of demyelinated fibres seen in the sciatic nerves of different birds but in all cases the damage is more extensive in the distal part of the nerve, an observation confirmed by other authors (CAVANAGH 1954, FENTON 1955). There are very few damaged fibres seen in the lumbosacral plexus, but in the anterior or posterior tibial nerves up to half the fibres show some degeneration. In an attempt to determine whether motor or sensory fibres were injured, the dorsal and ventral spinal roots in the lumbosacral region were examined in continuity with the cord. The almost complete absence of damage at this level, even when there was extensive demyelination in the sciatic or tibial nerves, makes it difficult to answer the question.

In the upper limb there is always some damage in the radial and ulnar nerves and less in the branchial plexus, but the lesions are never so extensive as in the leg.

Spinal cord. Three tracts are involved in the spinal cord (see Plates 2 and 3).

1. The posterior columns in the cervical region.

2. The spinocerebellular tract occupying a superficial position in the dorsal portions of the lateral column. (Increasing damage to this tract is found as the cord is ascended, and is especially heavy at its termination in the posterior lobe of the cerebellum.)

3. An anterior tract on either side of the anterior median fissure. The damage to this tract increases as it is followed down the cord.

The changes consist in demyelination of some of the tracts in the cord, the position and extent of which can be traced forward from the sacral lesion. At this level the majority of damaged fibres are found in the anterior columns close to the midline, while a few are seen in the posterolateral columns. In the lumbar region more damaged fibres are seen distributed chiefly in the sulco-marginal fasciculus on either side of the anterior median fissure and extending deeply towards the grey matter. Some can be seen crossing the cord to become lost among the anterior horn cells. The damaged fibres in the lateral columns are more numerous in the lumbar than in the sacral region and they continue to increase as the cord is ascended. Most of the damaged fibres are grouped on the lateral borders of the posterior horns but a few are scattered in the superficial layers of the lateral columns.

In the mid-dorsal region the damaged fibres in the ventral column are sharply localised in the form of a triangular tract, but in the upper dorsal region this becomes frayed as the damaged fibres spread laterally. The number of damaged fibres in the lateral columns is increased and in the upper dorsal region a new set of demyelinated fibres is found. These fibres lie in the posterior columns on either side of the posterior median fissure and correspond in distribution to the septo-marginal fasciculus; they are probably the homologue of the fasciculus gracilis in man.

In the cervical region there is a further change in the distribution of the damaged fibres in the anterior columns which start in the lower part as a diamond-shaped tract. From these the fibres spread laterally through the posterior columns of the cord and the damaged fibres gradually disappear as the cord is ascended. By the time the upper cervical cord is reached, only a few damaged fibres can be seen in the anterior columns.

The number of damaged fibres in the lateral columns increases in the upper part of the cervical cord. In the posterior columns the demyelinated fibres become more superficial in position and damaged fibres gradually disappear from the ventral columns. By the time the medulla is reached all the damaged tracts are concentrated in the lateral angles. The demyelinated fibres in the dorsal columns fade away, presumably to end in the inconspicuous nucleus gracilis in the lower medulla. From the medulla, the damaged fibres sweep forward and upward and pass through the restiform body into the cerebellum, where they are widely distributed to all parts of the cerebellar cortex. Above the level of the cerebellar peduncles no damaged fibres have ever been found. All damaged fibres either end in the cord or medulla, or pass into the cerebellum.

IV. Axonal degeneration in poisoned hens

Axonal damage is an invariable finding 8 to 10 days after poisoning. The axons undergo segmentation and swelling, and finally break into fine granular debris (CAVANAGH 1954, FENTON 1955) (see Plate 4). These changes appear at the same time as those seen in the myelin, and at this stage individual axons show ballooning, nodularity, and fragmentation. As with the demyelinated fibres the damage is more extensive distally than proximally to the neuron (CAVANAGH 1954). In the spinal cord and brain stem, silver-impregnated preparations show that in all regions where there is myelin fragmentation there can also be seen evidence of axis cylinder disintegration. The greatest amount of degeneration in the ventral tract occurs caudally, and in the dorsal-lateral tract rostrally, indicating that the same peripheral progression of changes takes place in these tracts as has been observed in peripheral nerves.

V. Cellular changes in poisoned hens

No visible alteration in the appearance of the Schwann cells can be seen during the first week after poisoning, but following the disintegration of the axon and myelin sheath the cells of the affected fibres begin to proliferate and become conspicuous. Macrophages appear in these fibres after about 12 to 14 days, but foam cells do not make their appearance until about the 20th day onwards. The normal process of cell proliferation occurs but on a reduced scale.

No changes either of a primary or secondary nature occur in the nerve cells of the damaged fibres, and examination of the spinal cord even 35 days after poisoning shows no changes in the nerve cells which could account for the damage.

The Golgi apparatus, too, is undamaged up to 3 weeks after poisoning.

Both the appearance and the numbers of the glial and oligodendroglial cells of the spinal cord and brain stem are normal during the first 10 days, although later there is a slight increase in the neuro- and astroglia (CAVANAGH 1954).

A search for damaged neurones has been quite unsuccessful, the only cells found to be regularly damaged being the anterior horn cells in the lumbar region of the cord. These exhibit chromatolysis, beginning at the periphery and extending inwards.

VI. The relationship between degeneration of the myelin sheath and axon cylinder

Both CAVANAGH (1954) and FENTON (1955) state that there is no evidence to support the belief that demyelination of the sheath occurs significantly before damage to the axon can be detected. FENTON made a specific attempt to investigate this point using a technique described by SWANK (1940).

The sciatic nerve from its origin down to its main branches — approximately 4 inches in length — was removed and cut into five equal segments. The whole of segments 1, 3, and 5 were embedded, cut and stained in block by the Marchi method, and then frozen sections were cut from the whole of each segment, all sections being cut along the longitudinal axis of the nerve. Because the degeneration begins at the periphery and runs centrally, if myelin degeneration were the primary event this process might be expected to appear at a higher level in the nerve sheath than in the axon. Neither myelin degeneration nor axonal damage was found to be in excess of the other.

If the disintegration of the myelin were consequent upon some local metabolic change, then it might be expected that the breakdown of the sheath might occur segmentally, at least

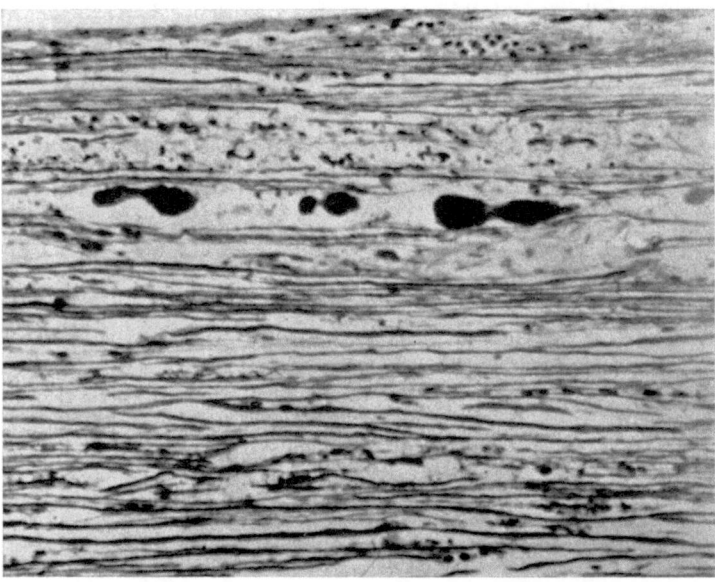

Fig. 15. Longitudinal section of chicken cervical cord, showing swelling and fragmentation of axons. Holmes's silver stain. × 220

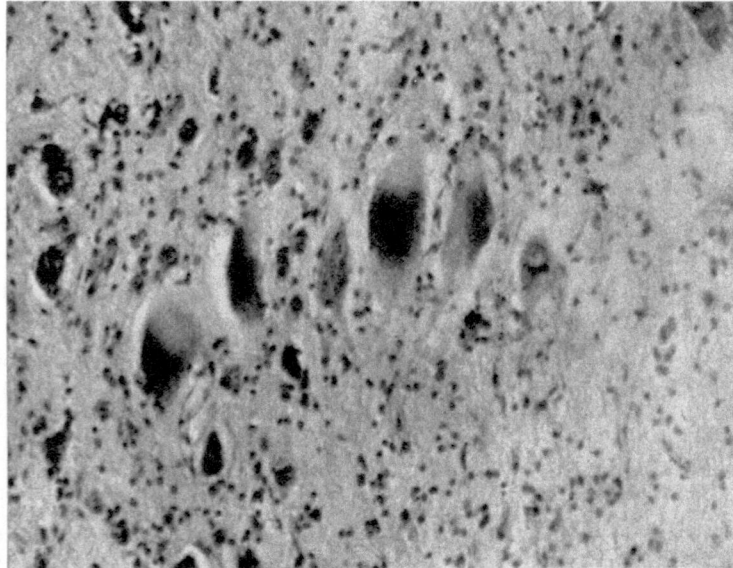

Fig. 16. Motor neurons from chicken lumbar cord, showing chromatolysis. Thionin. × 220

Plate 4 (Figs. 15 and 16). Neuronal damage in spinal cord of chicken following organophosphorus poisoning. (From FENTON 1955)

during the early stages of the process, since it is probable that the internodal stretches of the sheath are isolated units controlled by adjacent Schwann cells. Such focal lesions have never been observed, even in the early stages of degeneration (CAVANAGH 1954).

Again, it is doubtful that myelin degeneration *per se* can produce such a rapid and uniform effect upon its enclosed axon as has been observed. Three different lines of evidence tend to support this view.

1. The axons frequently persist in plaques of disseminated sclerosis even when they have been stripped of their myelin covering,

2. Segments of nerve may break down during the development of amphibian nerve without any apparent adverse effect upon the nerve fibre (SPEIDEL 1933),

and finally,

3. In starving rats the myelin may undergo fragmentation whilst the axon remains intact (SWANK 1940).

There is a close similarity between the histopathological picture in the poisoned nerves and in nerves undergoing Wallerian degeneration. In the former condition it is claimed by both CAVANAGH and FENTON that the axon and myelin sheath deteriorate together.

Indeed it is difficult, when all the evidence is weighed, to arrive at any other conclusion but that the axon is the primary seat of damage. No other process can explain the striking predilection for such damage to occur maximally at those regions which are furthest removed from their parent nerve cell body. Thus, the spinocerebellar pathways with their neurons in the thoraco-lumbar region are principally affected in the medulla and cervical sections; the ventral tract, which is a pure descending path (CAVANAGH 1954), is virtually involved only in the lumbar and thoracic regions though its nerve cells are probably located in the tectal region of the brain stem (PAPEZ 1929). As mentioned, a similar distal distribution can be found in peripheral nerves. While the structure which ultimately suffers is thus located, the manner in which it is damaged is not known, nor is the reason for the selective vulnerability of these pathways apparent. It should be recalled, however, that these same pathways are damaged in chronic thiamine -deficiency (beri-beri), and both CAVANAGH and FENTON are agreed on this similarity.

C. The relationship between chemical structure and neurotoxicity

I. General

Neurotoxicity is a more general property of organophosphorus compounds than has hitherto been appreciated. Two types of compounds are neurotoxic:

1. Certain triarylphosphates, which are active at about 50 to 2000 mg/kg, and

2. Certain alkyl organophosphorus compounds which are extremely neurotoxic, being active at approximately 0.5 to 2.5 mg/kg.

The triarylphosphates produce few if any acute effects at doses which cause ataxia and paralysis. The first signs of toxicity are not apparent for several days. Cholinesterase (ChE) inhibition in blood, brain, etc. occurs *in vivo*, but if as a class the compounds behave similarly to TOCP, this arises only after metabolic transformation in the body (ALDRIDGE 1954).

The alkyl phosphorus compounds on the other hand are potent inhibitors of ChE's both *in vitro* and *in vivo*. The administration of these substances gives rise to acute symptoms of acetylcholine (ACh) poisoning which can be brought under control by oximes and atropine (DAVIES and GREEN 1959). This phase is then followed by a completely symptom-free period of some days, followed by the development of ataxia and paralysis.

The demonstration of neurotoxic effects is more difficult with alkyl than with triaryl compounds, since the paralysing dose and the lethal dose of the former are similar. Indeed, in many instances the lethal dose is less than the paralysing, and with such compounds the neurotoxic dose must either be given in sublethal aliquots over a period, or to animals protected by previous administration of prophylactic agents such as oxime and atropine (DAVIES, HOLLAND and RUMENS 1960).

II. The neurotoxicity of the triarylphosphates

Not all triarylphosphates are neurotoxic, but despite the fact that no really comprehensive investigation into the relationship between chemical structure and neurotoxic activity has been made some generalisations are still possible. Table 1 lists the triarylphosphates which have been tested.

Table 1. *The neurotoxicity of triarylphosphates*

Substituents			Neurotoxic activity	Dose[1] mg/.kg	Reference
1	2	3			
o-methyl	o-methyl	o-methyl	Positive	25	b and c
m-methyl	m-methyl	m-methyl	Negative	5000	b
p-methyl	p-methyl	p-methyl	Negative	5000	b
o-ethyl	o-ethyl	o-ethyl	Negative	5 × 500	a and b
m-ethyl	m-ethyl	m-ethyl	Negative	2500	a
p-ethyl	p-ethyl	p-ethyl	Positive	200	a
o-n-propyl	o-n-propyl	o-n-propyl	Negative	5 × 500	a
2:3-dimethyl	2:3-dimethyl	2:3-dimethyl	Negative	1000	a
2:5-dimethyl	2:5-dimethyl	2:5-dimethyl	Negative	2500	b
2:6-dimethyl	2:6-dimethyl	2:6-dimethyl	Negative	2500	b
3:4-dimethyl	3:4-dimethyl	3:4-dimethyl	Negative	2500	a
3:5-dimethyl	3:5-dimethyl	3:5-dimethyl	Negative	1000	b
o-methyl	o-methyl	m-methyl	Positive	50	b
o-methyl	o-methyl	p-methyl	Positive	25—50	b and c
o-ethyl	o-ethyl	p-methyl	Positive	100	a
o-n-propyl	o-n-propyl	p-methyl	Positive	100	a
p-ethyl	p-ethyl	p-methyl	Negative	4 × 1000	a
p-methyl	p-methyl	p-ethyl	Negative	7 × 1000	a
o-methyl	phenyl	phenyl	Positive	500	b
o-methyl	p-methyl	p-methyl	Positive	25	b and c
o-methyl	m-methyl	m-methyl	Positive	25	c
o-methyl	m-methyl	p-methyl	Positive	25	c
o-ethyl	p-methyl	p-methyl	Positive	50	c
o-n-propyl	p-ethyl	p-ethyl	Positive	100	a

[1] The doses quoted are (1) in the case of positive compounds, the minimum dose at which it has been claimed to produce ataxia and (2) with inactive compounds the maximum dose at which it has been tested.

References: a BONDY et al. (1960); b HINE et al. (1956); c HENSCHLER (1958).

Of the seven symmetrical derivatives which have been examined, only two are toxic, TOCP and tri-*p*-ethylphenyl phosphate (T*p*EPP). The functional picture in T*p*EPP poisoning differs from that seen after TOCP and appears to be atypical

(SILVER 1960). It will be referred to later. The remaining active compounds contain at least one substituent in the *ortho* position. Replication of *ortho*-substitution does not seem to enhance neurotoxicity; rather, the reverse is true.

HENSCHLER (1958) claimed that the mono *o*-ester is more toxic than the di-*ortho* and the di-*ortho* more toxic than the tri-*ortho* analogue. This is not very well substantiated for *o*-tolyl derivatives but appears to have some truth in the case of *o*-ethyl and *o*-*n*-propyl derivatives (BONDY et al. 1960). It is however not a very good working rule. On the other hand replication of *ortho*-substitution in the same ring, e.g., as in xylenyl derivatives, results in almost complete disappearance of neurotoxicity, for none of the trixylenylphosphates is active at less than 1 g/kg.

There are three exceptions to the foregoing, but two of the compounds, T*p*EPP (SILVER 1960) and triphenylphosphate (TPP) (SMITH et al. 1932), behave atypically, either clinically or histologically. The remaining compound, di-*o*-*n*-propylphenyl-*p*-methylphenylphosphate, is active only at very high doses, and since the purity of the specimen examined was not firmly established, some doubt must exist as to its activity.

III. Atypical neurotoxic effects of some triarylphosphates

Because T*p*EPP and TPP are exceptions, in any attempted correlation of the chemical structure of triarylphosphates and neurotoxic activity it is desirable to discuss the effects they produce in some detail.

In TOCP poisoned hens ataxia is associated with very marked flexion of the joints of the leg and with curling of the toes. In contrast, in T*p*EPP poisoning, extensor tone is greatly, increased, the hens stand on tiptoe, and walk with an exaggerated extension of the legs (SILVER 1960). The time course of the two conditions is also different. In TOCP poisoning changes in gait are never seen before the seventh day after dosing, but once signs appear, the condition progresses rapidly and many birds become moribund during the 3rd or 4th week. Only those birds with relatively mild signs survive and even then recovery is slow. In T*p*EPP poisoning, the signs appear as early as the 4th day but they develop more slowly and less steadily than in TOCP poisoning. Recovery is quicker and although some birds die, others have shown obvious improvement after the 4th or 5th week (SILVER 1960, CAVANAGH et al. 1960), and in some less affected birds recovery has almost been complete in 7 weeks after dosing. T*p*EPP differs from all the other active triarylphosphates in not inhibiting ChE either *in vitro* or *in vivo* (ALDRIDGE and BARNES 1961).

Triphenylphosphate is atypical in its behaviour in producing ataxia and paralysis in the cat but not in the hen (SMITH, M. I. et al 1930). In the cat, 0.1 ml to 0.2 ml produces a typical flaccid paralysis in 4 to 26 days, the interval depending upon the dose. The paralysis changes in character, within a few days of onset, to a spastic form affecting the muscles of the neck, with foot and toe drop and rigidity in the posterior limbs. This lasts a relatively short time—about three weeks.

Thus, it would seem that not all organophosphorus compounds manifest their toxic effects in the same way, and it is possible that those seen after T*p*EPP and TPP may arise from different actions at different sites from those following TOCP poisoning.

IV. Structure and neurotoxic activity amongst alkyl organophosphorus compounds

Alkyl organophosphorus compounds have been studied more systematically than the triarylphosphates (DAVIES, HOLLAND and RUMENS 1960). These compounds are lethal at very small doses, consequently protective treatment with 100 mg/kg of 2-hydroxyiminomethyl-N-methylpyridinium methanesulphonate (P2S) plus 1 mg/kg of atropine sulphate was a standard procedure in testing them.

Table 2. *The neurotoxicity of alkyl organophosphorus compounds*[1]
Active compounds

Type of compound	R_1	R_2	Minimum dose producing ataxia mg/kg
Phosphorofluoridates R_1O, R_2O, P, $=O$, F	CH_3	CH_3	30
	C_2H_5	C_2H_5	0.75
	C_3H_7	C_3H_7	0.25
	$i\text{-}C_3H_7$	$i\text{-}C_3H_7$	0.3
	C_4H_9	C_4H_9	0.5
	$i\text{-}C_4H_9$	$i\text{-}C_4H_9$	1.5
	$\text{sec } C_4H_9$	$\text{sec } C_4H_9$	1.5
	C_5H_{11}	C_5H_{11}	2.5
	$\text{sec } C_5H_{11}$	$\text{sec } C_5H_{11}$	2.5
	$\text{cyclo-}C_6H_{11}$	$\text{cyclo-}C_6H_{11}$	2.5
	C_2H_5	$n\text{-}C_3H_7$	1.0
Phosphonofluoridates R_1O, R_2, P, $=O$, F	$i\text{-}C_3H_7$	CH_3	1.0
	$i\text{-}C_3H_7$	C_2H_5	1.0
	CH_3	$i\text{-}C_3H_7$	5.0
	C_2H_5	CH_3	3.0
	$i\text{-}C_4H_9$	CH_3	3.0
Phosphorfluorido-thionates R_1O, R_2O, P, $=S$, F	C_2H_5	C_2H_5	5.0

Type of compound	R_1	R_2	X	Minimum dose producing ataxia mg/kg
Miscellaneous R_1, R_2, P, $=O$, X	$i\text{-}C_3H_7O$	$i\text{-}C_3H_7O$	N_3	5.0
	C_2H_5O	$(CH_3)_2N$	F	5.0

Inactive compounds

Type of compound	R_1	R_2	X	Max. dose investigated mg/kg
Miscellaneous compounds of the type of the phosphorofluoridates, where F is replaced by other groups R_1O, R_2O, P, $=O$, X	C_2H_5	C_2H_5	Cl	100
	C_2H_5	C_2H_5	CN	50
	C_2H_5	C_2H_5	OC_2H_5	10
	$n\text{-}C_3H_7$	$n\text{-}C_3H_7$	O—phenyl—CH_3	10
	$i\text{-}C_3H_7$	$i\text{-}C_3H_7$	HNC_6H_5	50
	$n\text{-}C_4H_9$	$n\text{-}C_4H_9$	Cl	20
	$i\text{-}C_4H_9$	$i\text{-}C_4H_9$	Cl	20
	C_2H_5	C_2H_5	$SC_2H_4N(C_2H_5)_2$	20
	phenyl—O (—CH_3)	phenyl—O (—CH_3)	CH_3	50

[1] DAVIES, HOLLAND and RUMENS 1960.

Inactive compounds (continued)

Type of compound	R_1	R_2	Max. dose investigated mg/kg
Phosphinofluoridates R_1 — P(=O)(F) — R_2	C_2H_5 $n\text{-}C_3H_7$ $i\text{-}C_3H_7$ $n\text{-}C_4H_9$	C_2H_5 $n\text{-}C_3H_7$ $i\text{-}C_3H_7$ $n\text{-}C_4H_9$	5.0 5.0 5.0 2.5

Type of compound	R_1	R_2	R_3	R_4	Max. dose investigated mg/kg
Pyrophosphonates R_1 — P(=O) — O — P(=O) — R_3	C_2H_5O C_2H_5O $n\text{-}C_4H_9O$ C_2H_5O $i\text{-}C_3H_7O$ C_2H_5O	C_2H_5O CH_3 CH_3 CH_3 CH_3 CH_3	C_2H_5O $n\text{-}C_3H_7O$ $n\text{-}C_4H_9O$ C_2H_5O $i\text{-}C_3H_7$ C_2H_5O	C_2H_5O CH_3 CH_3 C_2H_5 CH_3 CH_3	100 10 10 10 10 10

This did not influence the (1) incidence, (2) onset, or (3) severity of neurotoxic signs, but did permit the administration of many times an otherwise lethal dose. This was very important in defining a negative response (DAVIES and HOLLAND, unpublished results).

A wide variety of phospho-fluoridates and closely related structures were examined (see Table 2). The following generalisations may be made as a result (see Table 3).

1. All the neurotoxic alkyl organophosphorus compounds contain fluorine, but not all compounds containing this atom are active.

2. The nature of the alkyl groups attached to the ester oxygen or directly to the phosphorus atom in phosphoro- and phosphonofluoridates is not critical.

Table 3. *General relationship between structure of alkyl organophosphorus compounds and neurotoxicity* [1]

Type of compound	Number tested	Number positive	Type of compound	Number tested	Number positive
R_1O — P(=O)(F) — R_2O	11	11	R_1 — P(=O)(F) — R_2	4	0
R_1O — P(=O)(F) — R_2	5	5	R_1O — P(=O) — O — P(=O) — OR_3 / R_2 ... R_4	6	0
R_1O — P(=S)(F) — R_2O	1	1	R_1O — P(=O)(X) — R_2O	9	0
R_1A — P(=O)(F or N$_3$) — R_2B	3	3	R_1R_2 etc. = alkyl groups X = miscellaneous groups A = oxygen or secondary amino groups B = oxygen or secondary or tertiary amino groups (see Table 2).		

[1] DAVIES, HOLLAND and RUMENS (1960).

3. At least one ester oxygen appears to be necessary, since phosphinic fluorides are inactive (III).

$$\begin{array}{c} R_1 \\ \diagdown \\ P \diagup ^O \\ \diagup \quad \diagdown \\ R_2 \qquad F \end{array} \quad \text{(III)}$$

4. The ester oxygen may under certain circumstances be replaced by a secondary amino group, for compounds of the type IV and V are active.

$$\begin{array}{c} i\text{-}C_3H_7NH \\ \diagdown \\ P \diagup ^O \\ \diagup \quad \diagdown \\ i\text{-}C_3H_7NH \qquad F \end{array} \qquad \text{and} \qquad \begin{array}{c} EtO \\ \diagdown \\ P \diagup ^O \\ \diagup \quad \diagdown \\ (CH_3)_2N \qquad F \end{array}$$

$$\text{IV. (Mipafox)} \qquad\qquad\qquad \text{V. (Fluortabun).}$$

It is not clear how completely interchangeable are the amino groups and ester oxygen.

V. The effects of repeated sub-neurotoxic doses

The continued absorption of relatively small sub-neurotoxic doses may well be the main industrial hazard, yet few attempts have been made to determine with any degree of reliability the relationship between total dose, size of sub-paralysing dose, and interval between doses in the production of neurotoxic effects. TOCP fed in small quantities to chickens gave rise to ataxia and paralysis, but there was a threshold dose below which no effects were produced, despite the fact that the total dose administered was far in excess of that required to produce ataxia when given as a single dose (SMITH et al. 1932).

This problem has been investigated more carefully using DFP (DAVIES and HOLLAND, unpublished observations). Dose-response curves were constructed following dosing with (1) single doses and (2) 20% aliquots of these given daily. The 50% paralysing dose when given as in (2) was twice that when given as in (1), but the interval between completion of dosing and onset of ataxia was not altered, nor were the signs any less severe in the affected birds.

D. Organophosphorus neurotoxicity in man

I. Early manifestations of neurotoxicity

Although thousands of human beings have suffered from neurotoxic effects from tricresylphosphate poisoning, none of them appeared to have been poisoned by a single substance, for the detailed clinical signs have varied from outbreak to outbreak (HENSCHLER 1958). This might have been due to the fact that various preparations contained greater proportions of mixed as compared with homogeneous triarylphosphate esters, or it might have been due to the toxic properties of the substances with which the TCP was associated, e.g., alcoholic extract of ginger, torpedo oil, apiol, or aircraft cleaning oils. Whatever the reason, the detailed clinical picture undoubtedly must have been influenced.

The only well established cases in which poisoning was due to a comparatively pure substance were those due to the insecticide, Mipafox, which occurred in Cambridge (England) in 1951.

Fortunately, the more serious case was fully reported and the following account, which is due to BIDSTRUP and BONNELL (1954), concerns a research chemist (female) aged 28 who had been employed in the manufacture of this substance on a small scale. She had been engaged on the development of various organophosphorus compounds for 21 months prior to her admission to hospital on 21st August 1951. During that time she had handled a number of compounds, and although her exposure to them had been mainly in the laboratory she was occasionally concerned in the manufacture of small amounts of new compounds in pilot plants. She first developed acute signs of anti-ChE poisoning on 20th August. These were controlled by atropine and she was given 58 mg over a period of four days. The ChE levels of both red blood cells (acetylcholinesterase, AChE) and plasma (butyrocholinesterase, BuChE) were reduced almost to zero. However, she was apparently well by the 14th day after poisoning, and was discharged from the hospital. During the third week after the acute episode, she noticed weakness of the legs and this became worse after exertion. The patient was readmitted to the hospital 25 days after the onset of the acute symptoms, and she was found to be suffering from a flaccid paralysis of both legs together with tenderness and weakness of the thigh muscles. The knee jerks were diminished and the ankle jerks absent. There was no change in cutaneous sensation to pinprick or light touch. Five days later the paralysis of the lower limbs was complete, both knee and ankle jerks were absent, and no plantar response could be elicited. Tone and power in the forearms and hands were greatly reduced. The biceps jerk was just present, but neither the supination nor the triceps jerk could be elicited. There was weakness of the trunk muscles, but cranial nerves were normal and no signs of central nervous system involvement or disturbance of cutaneous sensation could be demonstrated. All leg muscles, particularly those of the calf, were tender to palpation, and muscle twitchings were observed in the deltoid and facial muscles and in the muscles of the legs.

Power returned gradually, over a period of weeks, to the muscles of the thighs, arms, and forearms. Sixty-five days after the acute episode, power and tone were normal in the upper arm muscles, and the biceps and triceps jerks were present and brisk. There was weakness of the long extensors of the fingers and the small muscles of the hands were wasted and completely paralysed. Power had returned to the thigh muscles, the knee jerks were exaggerated, and patellar clonus was elicited without difficulty but there was no spasticity. The leg muscles and the small muscles of the feet were completely paralysed and wasted. The ankle jerks were absent. Fasciculation was still present in the deltoids, facial muscles, and muscles of the legs. The patient complained of cramp-like pains affecting particularly the muscles of the lower limbs.

Four to seven months after poisoning, a slow improvement occurred in those groups of muscles which had begun to regain their normal function, but the muscles of the legs and feet remained completely paralysed. The wasting of the small muscles of the hand continued, but nine months after the initial incident they began to recover. Power returned slowly to the lumbricals, interossei, and opponens pollicis, and a month later the wasting was much less marked. Two years later the upper limbs were normal. After nine months the ankle jerks were first elicited, followed quite quickly, i.e., in a few days, by a return of movement of the toes. From this time on progress was steady although slow.

The development of paralysis in man following Mipafox and TOCP is very similar. The disease is manifested clinically as a severe polyneuritis with disability evident in the motor functions. Histological studies complement the clinical findings, the lesions are limited to the nerves and the anterior horn cells of the spinal cord and in some instances to the motor cells in the medulla. The pyramidal tracts in the cord appear to be involved early in TOCP poisoning.

II. The late stages of neurotoxic effects in man

AHRING (1942) examined over 100 patients in the late stage of the disease.

The usual pattern after the advent of the paralysis was of a gradual return of strength over several months until a stationary stage was reached, usually about 1 year or more after the onset of the disease. The upper extremities improved more rapidly and to a greater degree than the lower. Age did not influence the signs. Gait during this stage of the disease was of the spastic rather than of the flaccid type of paralysis, which is typical of the early phase of the condition. Atrophy of muscles was generalized in the extremities, but much more obvious in the distal than in the proximal. The hands were clawed, the fingers resting in a position of moderate or extreme flexion. The foot had assumed the shape usually associated with Friedrich's familial ataxia. The arch was high and the proximal joints were fixed in moderate dorsiflexion and there was contracture of the Achilles tendon. Despite the atrophy and deformity of the hand the grip usually was strong. Extension of the fingers and hands was slightly weakened, and there was still bilateral foot drop and inability to move the ankles and toes through more than a 15 to 25-degree arc.

The late pathology may be divided into neural and extraneural signs.

The main neural lesions consisted in spotty loss of muscle fibres and replacement by connective tissue and fat. The small arteries and particularly the capillaries showed marked thickening of the walls with corresponding narrowing of the lumina. The larger arteries were relatively normal.

Degeneration was always found in the nerves; the axons were of irregular width and were decreased in number. There was a marked patchy loss of myelin in the nerves and a heavy overgrowth of connective tissue in the nerve trunks.

In the spinal cord the leptomeninges were always thickened though there was little nuclear increase. Degeneration in the white matter varied in severity from case to case, but was invariably present. There was no exception to involvement of the lateral pyramidal tracts. This degeneration was most severe in the lower segments of the cord and was not found above the upper segments. The myelin of the direct pyramidal tracts usually appeared to be affected, but this may have been part of the rim of degeneration that circled the cord. This rim resembled the vacuolated type most often seen in subacute combined degeneration. The lateral pyramidal degeneration on the other hand differed in that it was not vacuolated and there was intense gliosis in the degenerated area. The degeneration of the white matter always stopped short of the medulla; in no case was there white matter degeneration in the cerebrum.

In the grey matter of the anterior horns many of the nerve cells were affected. They were markedly reduced in numbers, and those remaining were pyknotic and many had lost their outline. The segments in which the grey matter was most severely involved were the lower dorsal and upper lumber.

A minor degree of neuronal change occurred in the brain stem and cerebrum, but in no case was the loss and deterioration of nerve cells as obvious as in the spinal cord.

E. The mechanism of neurotoxic action of organophosphorus compounds

I. General considerations

Any complete theory of the neurotoxic action of organophosphorus compounds must be capable of explaining four typical features of the intoxication:

1. The characteristic delay in the onset of clinical signs.
2. The marked species differences in response to such compounds.
3. The highly specific sites in which the histological lesions are found.
4. Why, although all the active neurotoxic agents with but one exception are anti-ChE agents, there are many anti-ChE agents which are inactive.

No hypothesis has yet been produced which will account for all of these. However, it is tempting to suggest that the biochemical lesion occurs very quickly after poisoning, and the delay in the appearance of neurotoxic signs is associated with the turnover of a metabolite which is gradually being depleted as a result of the metabolic block which constitutes the biochemical lesion. Species differences could well arise on this basis.

The biochemical lesion may occur outside the nervous system, but this is unlikely. If, as is more probable, it occurs within the nervous system, it might be found at the same site at which the histological lesion is seen, or alternatively it might occur in the cell—possibly the neuron—which controls the metabolism of the nerve fiber.

II. The role of cholinesterases in the production of neurotoxic effects

Investigations of the biochemical actions of the poisons themselves, together with studies into the relationship between chemical structure and neurotoxicity, have been more profitable, and the fact that known neurotoxic agents are nearly all anti-ChE agents has been the basis of a provocative hypothesis.

In 1941 BLOCH, considering only TOCP, suggested that the inactivation of the ChE at the motor end plate might be the cause of the paralysis. In this form the hypothesis was untenable for a number of reasons. Not only was this idea incapable of explaining the delayed onset of signs, or why the lesions occurred so specifically in the nervous system but later work showed that TOCP is nearly totally inactive towards AChE, the enzyme which destroys ACh at the motor endplate. Triorthocresylphosphate is in fact an inhibitor of BuChE only.

Thompson and his colleagues modified this idea. They showed that BuChE is associated with the white matter in those areas in the brain and spinal cord where demyelination occurs (Ord and Thompson 1952). Furthermore, the only known neurotoxic agents at that time, TOCP, Mipafox, and DFP, were all specific inhibitors of BuChE, and thus it was suggested that it was the inactivation of this enzyme which possibly contributed to demyelination (Earl and Thompson 1952a). Additional support for this hypothesis came from a series of later investigations. Thus, the BuChE of the plasma, brain, and spinal cord of hens is markedly inhibited after TOCP poisoning and it remains at a low level for at least 10 days afterwards. The AChE of the various tissues is relatively unaffected (Earl and Thompson 1952b). Triorthocresylphosphate exhibits marked differences in its action upon the BuChE of the tissues of different species. It is highly selective towards the enzyme of human cerebrum, spinal cord, and sciatic nerve; it is less selective towards that of the corresponding tissues of the chicken and rabbit, but towards the corresponding enzyme of the nervous tissues of the rat it is virtually inactive, even in high concentrations (Earl and Thompson 1952a).

The effect of TOCP upon a wide variety of other enzyme systems has been examined (Earl, Thompson and Webster 1953). The oxidation of glucose and pyruvate by brain homogenates, and trypsin, brain amine oxidase, pancreatic lecithinase, and brain cephalinase were not affected.

In the poisoned hen only two enzyme systems were effectively inactivated, the BuChE and the ali-esterase of the spinal cord. The ChE, however, was always more markedly inhibited than the ali-esterase.

If the conclusion of Earl and Thompson (1952b), that inactivation of BuChE is the prelude to demyelination, be true, then any potent inhibitor of this enzyme should be neurotoxic. This however is not so, for a number of selective inhibitors of BuChE have been examined and shown to be inactive. Davison (1953) examined DFP, TOCP, Mipafox, o,o-diisopropyl-o-p-nitrophenylphosphate, N,N′,N′′,N′′′-tetraisopropylpyrophosphoramide, and tetraisopropylpyrophosphate. The first three of these produced paralysis whilst the last three did not. With the exception of TOCP, the pattern of inhibition was the same for both neuro- and non-neurotoxic agents. It consisted in a rapid depression of the BuChE of the central nervous system (CNS), within 2 hrs, followed by a steady and almost complete restoration of enzyme activity during the next 6 to 8 days. With TOCP, the inhibition was more prolonged and the level of enzymic activity remained low for 10 days. In other experiments the BuChE of the CNS was kept at a very low level with repeated injections of inhibitor for 10 to 14 days, but no neurotoxic effects resulted (Austin and Davies 1954). Thus, neither prolonged nor short-period inactivation of the BuChE of the CNS appears to be a prerequisite for the production of paralysis.

The possible role of ChE has, however, been given a different significance by the recent work of Davies, Holland and Rumens (1960). This work emphasizes the significance of fluorine in alkyl organophosphorus neurotoxic compounds. It is postulated that the biochemical lesion arises from the liberation of fluorine in situ and that it then blocks some, as yet unidentified, metabolic pathway. The role of ChE is therefore a primary but not necessarily the main one, in that by rupture of

the $>\overset{\parallel}{P}$—X bond it liberates the toxic moiety and so effects a toxic biosynthesis.

It should be clearly understood that any process whereby the $>\overset{\parallel}{P}$—X bond is broken in situ to liberate a fluoride ion will achieve the same end-result.

The main deficiency of this theory is that it does not embrace the triaryl-phosphates, and although it is possible that a substituted alkylphenyl group or its metabolic product may function as the toxophore, in our present state of knowledge this must remain only a provocative speculation.

III. Vitamin E and neurotoxicity

Because TCP (tricresylphosphate) produced testicular atrophy, haemorrhagic pneumonia, and muscular effects in dogs, in addition to neurotoxic effects, it has been suggested that TOCP as well as TCP interfere with vitamin E utilisation (CARPENTER et al. 1959). This possibility had been investigated earlier.

MEUNIER et al. (1947) showed that TOCP caused a pronounced fall in the rabbit plasma level of tocopherol, and they then inferred that TOCP has an anti-vitamin E action. However, vitamin E does not prevent the inhibition of BuChE nor the paralysis caused by TOCP in chickens (MYERS and MULDER 1953). When tocopherol and TOCP are given to chickens, the latter is absorbed from the intestine but the former is not. When they are given simultaneously, the BuChE is only partially inhibited and the chickens do not become paralysed even after a second dose of TOCP. This interesting finding has not been followed up, and the mechanism by which TOCP prevents the absorption of tocopherol is not yet clear. In addition the utilisation of other fat-soluble alcohols may be interfered with.

These observations would be most significant if they could be repeated using DFP as the neurotoxic agent.

IV. The problem of therapy in organophosphorus neurotoxicity

Although oximes and atropine are effective antidotes to the lethal effects, no chemotherapy for the treatment of organophosphorus neurotoxicity is known. Treatment consists largely in physiotherapy, in attempts to aid the progress of natural recovery or readjustment.

The approach to therapy, however, presents a number of interesting issues. The characteristic delay period before neurotoxic signs are evident raises the important question as to "what to treat". Ideally an attack on the biochemical lesion would constitute the most fundamental approach and indeed the most satisfying. Attempts to repair the lesion several days after it has been produced would seem to be optimistic, and therefore the practical approach may well lie in attempts to accelerate the recovery of the sheath and axon after damage.

The direction of future research should be (1) the elucidation of the toxic processes which result in delayed damage to the nerve, and (2) the characterization of this damage, with the specific object of accelerating the recovery of the damaged nerve.

Literature

AHRING, C. D.: The systemic nervous affinity of triorthocresyl phosphate (Jamaica Ginger Palsy). Brain 65, 34—47 (1942).
ALDRIDGE, W. N.: Tricresyl phosphates and cholinesterase. Biochem. J. 56, 185 (1954).
—, and J. M. BARNES: Neurotoxic and biochemical properties of some tri-aryl phosphates. In the press.
AUSTIN, L., and D. R. DAVIES: The part played by inhibition of cholinesterase of the CNS in producing paralysis in chickens. Brit. J. Pharmacol. 9, 145—152 (1954).
BARNES, J. M.: Personal communication.
—, and F. A. DENZ: Experimental demyelination with organophosphorus compounds. J. Path. Bact. 65, 597—605 (1953).
BIDSTRUP, P. L., and J. A. BONNELL: Anticholinesterases. Paralysis in man following poisoning by cholinesterase inhibitors. Chem. and Indust. 1954, 674.
— — and A. G. BECKETT: Paralysis following poisoning by a new organic phosphorus insecticide. (Mipafox). Brit. med. J. 1953, I, 1068—1072.

BLOCH, H.: Specificity of inhibitors in esters inhibited by tri-*ortho*-cresyl phosphate. Helv. chim. Acta. **26**, 733 (1943).

BONDY, H. F., E. J. FIELD, A. N. WORDEN and J. P. W. HUGHES: A study on the acute toxicity of the tri-aryl phosphates used as plasticisers. Brit. J. industr. Med. **17**, 190 (1960).

CARPENTER, H. W., D. J. JENDEN, N. R. SHULMAN and J. R. TURENAN: Toxicology of a tri-aryl phosphate oil. (1) Experimental toxicology. A.M.A. Arch. industr. Hlth. **20**, 234—252 (1959).

CAVANAGH, J. B.: The toxic effects of tri-*ortho*-cresyl phosphate on the nervous system; experimental study in hens. J. Neurol. Neurosurg. Phychiat. **17**, 163—172 (1954).

—, D. R. DAVIES, P. HOLLAND and M. LANCASTER: Comparison of the functional effects of Dyflos, Tri-o-cresyl phosphate and tri-p-ethylphenyl phosphate in chickens. Brit. J. Pharmacol. **17**, 21—27 (1961).

DAVIES, D. R., and A. L. GREEN: The chemotherapy of poisoning by organophosphate anti-cholinesterases. Brit. J. industr. Med. **16**, 128 (1959).

—, and P. HOLLAND: Unpublished results.

— — and M. J. RUMENS: The relationship between the chemical structure and neurotoxicity of alkyl organophosphorus compounds. Brit. J. Pharmacol. **15**, 271—278 (1960).

DAVISON, A. N.: Some observations on the cholinesterases of the central nervous system after the administration of organophosphorus compounds. Brit. J. Pharmacol. **8**, 212—216 (1953).

EARL, C. J., and R. H. S. THOMPSON: The inhibitory action of tri-*ortho*-cresyl phosphate on cholinesterases. Brit. J. Pharmacol. **7**, 261—269 (1952a).

— — Cholinesterase levels in the nervous system in tri-*ortho*-cresyl phosphate poisoning. Brit. J. Pharmacol. **7**, 685—692 (1952b).

— — and G. R. WEBSTER: Observations on the specificity of the inhibition of cholinesterases by tri-*ortho*-cresyl phosphate. Brit. J. Pharmacol. **8**, 110—114 (1953).

FENTON, J. C. B.: The nature of the paralysis in chickens following organophosphorus poisoning. J. Path. Bact. **69**, 181—189 (1955).

FRIESS, S. L., D. J. JENDEN and J. R. TURENAN: Toxicology of a tri-aryl phosphate oil. (II) A quantitative study of toxicity in different production batches. A.M.A. Arch. industr. Hlth. **20**, 253—257 (1959).

GATENBY, J. B., and H. W. BEAMS: Bolles Lees. The Microtomists Vademecum. 573. 11th Edit. London 1950.

GERMON, C.: Intoxication Mortelle par Apiol. Thèse de Paris 1932.

GLEES, P., and T. A. MARSLAND: Degeneration of pyramidal fibres studied by a paraffin silver method. J. Physiol. (Lond.) **118**, 51 P (1952).

GOLDFAIN, E.: Jamaica ginger multiple neuritis. J. Okla. St. med. Ass. **23**, 191 (1930).

GREIG, M. E., and W. C. HOLLAND: Studies on the permeability of erythrocytes. Proc. Soc. exp. Biol. (N. Y.) **71**, 189—192 (1949).

HENSCHLER, D.: Die Trikresylphosphatvergiftung. Experimentelle Klärung von Problemen der Atiologie und Pathogenese. Klin. Wschr. **36**, 663 (1958).

HINE, C. H., M. K. DUNLAP, E. G. RICE, M. M. COURSEY, R. M. GROSS and H. H. ANDERSON: Neurotoxicity and anticholinesterase properties of some substituted phenyl phosphates (and related compounds). J. Pharmacol. exp. Ther. **116**, 227—236 (1956).

HOTSON, R. D.: Outbreak of Polyneuritis due to *ortho*-tricresyl phosphate poisoning. Lancet **1946 I**, 207.

HUNTER, D., K. M. A. PERRY and R. B. EVANS: Toxic polyneuritis arising during the manufacture of tricresyl phosphate. Brit. J. industr. Med. **1**, 227 (1944).

KIDD, J. G., and C. G. LANGWORTHY: Jake paralysis. Bull. John Hopk. Hosp. **52**, 39—66 (1933).

KIELY, C. E., and M. L. RICH: An epidemic of motor neuritis in Cincinnati, Ohio, due to drinking adulterated Jamaica Ginger. Publ. Hlth. (Wash.), **47**, 2039 (1932).

KOELLE, G. B., and A. GILMAN: The chronic toxicity of D.F.P. in dogs, monkeys and rats. J. Pharmacol. exp. Ther. **87**, 435—448 (1946).

LANCASTER, M.: A note on the demyelination produced in hens by dialkylfluoridates. Brit. J. Pharmacol. **15**, 279—281 (1960).

LOROT, C.: Les combinaisons de la créosote dans le traitement de la tuberculose pulmonaire. Thèse de Paris (1899).

MEDNIKYAN, G. A., and S. A. MIRZOYAN: Toxicology of tritolyl phosphate. II. Arch. intern. Pharmacodyn. **53**, 248 (1936).

MEUNIER, P., A. VINET and J. JOUANNETEAU: Antagonistic actions of vitamin E and fish liver oil on the growth of rabbits. Bull. Soc. clin. Biol. **29**, 507 (1947).

MILLIS, E. R.: Cause of "Jake Paralysis". J. Kans. med. Ass. **31**, 359 (1932).

MOUNTER, L. A., H. C. ALEXANDER, K. D. TUCK and LIEN TIEN H. DIEN: The reactivity of esterases and proteases in the presence of organophosphorus compounds. J. biol. Chem. **226**, 873—879 (1957).

MYERS, D. K., and H. E. W. MULDER: Effect of tri-*ortho*-cresyl phosphate on the absorption of Tocopherol. Nature (Lond.) **172**, 773 (1953).

ORD, M. G., and R. H. S. THOMPSON: Pseudo-cholinesterase activity in the central nervous system. Biochem. J. **51**, 245 (1952).

PAPEZ, J. W.: Comparative Neurology. New York: Thomas and Crowell 1929.

ROGER, H., and M. RECORDIER: Les polynévrites phosphocréosotiques (phosphate) de créosote, ginger paralysis, apiol). Ann. Méd. **35**, 44 (1934).

SAMPSON, B. F.: The strange Durban epidemic of 1937. S. Afr. med. J. **16**, 1 (1942).

SILVER, A.: Ataxia in hens poisoned with tri-*para*-ethylphenyl phosphate. Nature (Lond.) **185**, 247—248 (1960).

SMITH, HONOR V., and J. M. K. SPALDING: Outbreak of paralysis in Morocco due to *ortho*-cresyl phosphate poisoning. Lancet **1959**, **II**, 1019—1021.

SMITH, M. I., R. ELVOVE and W. H. FRAZIER: The pharmacological actions of certain phenol esters, with special reference to the etiology of so-called ginger paralysis. Publ. Hlth. Repr. (Wash.) **45**, 2509 (1930).

— E. W. ENGEL and H. F. STOHLMAN: Further studies on the pharmacology of certain phenol esters with special reference to the relation of chemical constitution and physiologic action. Nat. Inst. Hlth Bull. **160**, 1 (1932).

—, and R. D. LILLIE: The histopathology of tri-*ortho*-cresyl phosphate poisoning; Etiology of so-called ginger paralysis (Third Report). Arch. Neurol. Psychiat. (Chicago) **26**, 976—992 (1931).

SPEIDEL, C. C.: Studies of living nerves; activities of ameboid growth cones, sheath cells, and myelin segments, as revealed by prolonged observation of individual nerve fibers in frog tadpoles. Amer. J. Anat. **52**, 1—80 (1933).

SUSSER, M., and Z. STEIN: An outbreak of tri-*ortho*-cresyl phosphate (T.O.C.P.) poisoning in Durban. Brit. J. industr. Med. **14**, 111 (1957).

SWANK, R. L.: Avian thiamine deficiency. J. exp. Med. **71**, 683—702 (1940).

—, and H. A. DAVENPORT: Chlorate-osmic-formalin method for staining degenerating myelin. Stain Technol. **10**, 87 (1935).

—, and M. PRADOS: Avian thiamine deficiency. II. Pathologic changes in the brain and cranial nerves (especially the vestibular) and their relation to the clinical behaviour. Arch. Neurol. Psychiat. (Chicago) **47**, 97—131 (1942).

TER BRAAK, J. W. C.: Een epidemie van polyneuritis van bijzondere oorsprong: A polyneuritis epidemic of peculiar origin. Ned. T. Geneesk. **75**, 2329 (1931).

WALTHARD, K. M.: Aperçu des résultats obtenus lors des derniers examens des malades intoxiqués en 1940 par le phosphate triorthocrésilique. Schweiz Arch. Neurol. Psychiat. **58**, 189 (1946).

WEBER, M. L.: A follow-up study of thirty-five cases of paralysis caused by adulterated Jamaica-ginger extract. Med. Bull. Veterans' Adm. (Wash.) **13**, 228 (1937).

ZIMMERMAN, H. M.: Pathology of vitamin B group deficiencies. Res. Publ. Ass. nerv. ment. Dis. **22**, 51 (1943).

Chapter 20

Pharmacological Antagonists of the Anticholinesterase Agents

By

J. H. WILLS

Contents

A. Dangerous functional changes induced by anticholinesterase (anti-ChE) agents

Chapters 11 through 14 have set forth in some detail the functional changes induced by anticholinesterase (anti-ChE) agents. Those most dangerous to life are probably the following:

56*

I. Sialorrhea and bronchorrhea

These two effects are typical muscarinic ones, the importance of which arises from the fact that accumulation of fluids in the upper airway can interfere seriously with pulmonary ventilation. The sialogogic have been studied more thoroughly than the bronchorrheic actions, but there is little doubt that poisoning with anti-ChE compounds of either the reversible type (e.g., physostigmine, neostigmine), or the organophosphorus type (e.g., DFP, Sarin), can result in relatively large increases in the rates of secretion by both the bronchial glands (GREEN et al. 1947) and the salivary glands (SECKER 1934, GROB, LILIENTHAL et al. 1947). The effects on salivary and other oral and nasal glands seem to be considerably greater than that on bronchial glands (CULLUMBINE and DIRNHUBER 1955).

II. Bradycardia and hypotension

Initially the anti-ChE agents frequently produce an increase in heart rate and a rise in blood pressure, followed by a reversal of these two effects. The initial increases in heart rate and blood pressure, when they occur, seem to arise from a combination of nicotinic activity, leading to the peripheral release of catecholamines from the adrenal glands and sympathetic fibers (KROP and KUNKEL 1954, PAULET 1954, DEBURGH DALY and WRIGHT 1956), and of a central stimulating action (VARAGIC 1955, DIRNHUBER and CULLUMBINE 1955, HORNYKIEWICZ and KOBINGER 1956, POLET and DESCHAEPDRYVER 1959). In addition, physostigmine may have a direct peripheral effect (VON EICKSTEDT et al. 1955). The eventual slowing of the heart and the associated fall in blood pressure appear to be typical muscarinic effects, but they depend, at least in part, on anoxia (WILLS 1957, unpubl.[1]).

Anoxia contributes also to increased activity by the sympathetic nervous system (TURPAEV and PUTINCEVA 1955). The bradycardia involves both A-V and bundle-branch block (HOLMSTEDT 1951, KROP and KUNKEL 1954) and precedes any noticeable alteration in blood pressure (DEBURGH DALY 1957).

III. Stimulation and depression of brain stem and cerebral cortex

Desynchronization of the EEG is the first sign of action by anti-ChE compounds (BRADLEY et al. 1953, RINALDI and HIMWICH 1955a) on the ascending reticular activating system of MORUZZI and MAGOUN (1949). Convulsions resulting from the stimulatory action of anti-ChE agents on diencephalic structures are manifested in the curarized animal by the appearance of seizure patterns in the EEG (GROB, HARVEY et al. 1947, FREEDMAN et al. 1949); doses of anti-ChE compounds greater than those required to produce electrical convulsions result in the disappearance of the seizure pattern and the appearance of small voltage waves of extremely high frequency (WESCOE et al. 1948). In uncurarized animals, increasing doses of the anti-ChE compounds produce a sequence of tremor, convulsion, and flaccid paralysis.

Anticholinesterase compounds affect also spinal reflex activity and some medullary functions. The effects on spinal reflexes usually involve initial augmentation of reflex activity followed by decrease to abolition of such activity (CALMA 1949, HOLMSTEDT and SKOGLUND 1953). The latter authors found this generalization to apply to Tabun as well as to other anti-ChE agents, but HAASE et al. (1957) reported that Tabun always decreases only the response to sensory excitation of the monosynaptic flexor reflex arc. ERDMANN and SCHAEFER (1954) reported that Parathion induces only decreased response to sensory stimulation within the multisynaptic flexor reflex pathway.

A medullary site of action for anti-ChE compounds in altering ventilation is suggested by the findings that anti-ChE compounds: 1) can alter medullary reflexes (SCHWEITZER and WRIGHT 1937a, SCHWEITZER and WRIGHT 1937b, GESELL and FREY 1950, METZ 1958); 2) can alter impulse traffic over the phrenic nerves (KRIVOY et al. 1951, DOUGLAS and MATTHEWS 1952, DECANDOLE et al. 1953, WRIGHT 1954, SAKAI et al. 1958); 3) administered intracisternally can produce the same effect on ventilatory activity as peripheral applications of these compounds (MILLER 1949, HALEY 1957, METZ 1958); and 4) can produce the same changes in the respiratory rate following denervation of the aortic and carotid chemoreceptors as before this operation (PAULET 1956). WILLS and BORISON (1959) have found that Sarin elevates the voltage threshold of a medullary inspiratory site without altering clearly those of a nearby expiratory area or of a rostral cough-inducing area. The last findings show a direct effect on the properties of one part of the central regulator of ventilatory activity and contradict, therefore, the conclusion that anti-ChE compounds do not alter the properties of the respiratory center (HEYMANS et al. 1946, HEYMANS and JACOB 1947).

---

[1] References in the text without corresponding entries in the bibliography, such as here, refer to reports given limited distribution only.

Physostigmine and neostigmine, but not DFP, have been found to enhance the convulsogenic actions of several compounds, including pentamethylenetetrazol, picrotoxin, and strychnine (HYDE et al. 1949). However, atropine in moderate doses does not antagonize the actions of strychnine on the brain and spinal cord of the cat (WESCOE and GREEN 1948). Diisopropyl phosphorofluoridate enhances the central depressant action of sodium pentobarbital (BAYLISS et al. 1957); OMPA, EPN, Malathion, Chlorothion, or Phostex (a mixture of bis-(dialkoxy phosphinothioyl) disulfides) increases that of hexobarbital (ROSENBERG and COON 1958). Diisopropyl phosphorofluoridate had no effect on the response to pentamethylenetetrazol (BAYLISS et al. 1957); TEPP or BFP (bis-dimethylamido phosphorofluoridate) had no effect on hexobarbital sleeping time (ROSENBERG and COON 1958), and TEPP did not alter the tremor induced by a standard dose of 1,4-dipyrrolidino-2-butyne (Tremorine) (BAKER and McPHILLIPS 1956, unpubl.). It appears, therefore, that the enhancement of central activity by the anti-ChE agents noted above does not necessarily depend directly on their anti-ChE activities, and in some cases may be dependent upon peripheral effects.

The enhancement of the central activity of an appropriate chemical by an anti-ChE compound may be another example of an incidental action, similar to the production of demyelinization by certain anti-ChE agents (SMITH and LILLIE 1931, PETRY 1951, BARNES and DENZ 1953, BIDSTRUP et al. 1953, AUSTIN and DAVIES 1954, CAVANAUGH and THOMPSON 1954, DURHAM et al. 1956, PETTY 1958; see Chapter 19. As such, these actions may have no connection with the major mechanism of toxicity of the anti-ChE agents for the central nervous system, but may be significant factors in the prophylactic or therapeutic employment of other chemicals in poisoning by anti-ChE's.

IV. Hypopnea and apnea

The previously mentioned effects on the central control of ventilatory activity and on the secretory activity of glands within the mouth and the respiratory tract are only two of the possible mechanisms whereby anti-ChE compounds may lead to diminished or completely abolished ventilation. Other possible sources of embarrassment of pulmonary gas exchange arise from airway obstruction by a retroverted tongue, by possible laryngospasm or by bronchoconstriction (DIXON and BRODIE 1903, MODELL et al. 1946), or from failure of neuromuscular transmission (ECCLES et al. 1942). EVANS (1951) has shown that the neuromuscular blockade established by physostigmine or neostigmine is easily reversible, but that that established by DFP, TEPP, Tabun, Sarin, Soman, or other organophosphorus anti-ChE agents is overcome only with difficulty.

Alterations of ventilatory activity have been reported following parenteral administration of DFP (LUNDHOLM 1949, VERBEKE 1949, KRIVOY et al. 1951, DECANDOLE et al. 1953, McNAMARA et al. 1954, PAULET 1956, POCHET 1957), OMPA (PAULET 1956), TEPP (BURGEN et al. 1949, DECANDOLE et al. 1953, McNAMARA et al. 1954, WRIGHT 1954, PAULET 1956), neostigmine (ERDMANN, KEMPE and LÜHNING 1955, PAULET 1956), Paraoxon (BARNES 1953, DECANDOLE et al. 1953, SAKAI et al. 1958), Parathion (SALLÉ 1950, ERDMANN, KEMPE and LÜHNING 1955, SAKAI et al. 1958), physostigmine (GESELL and HANSEN 1943, MILLER 1949, DECANDOLE et al. 1953, McNAMARA et al. 1954, PAULET 1956), Sarin (DECANDOLE et al. 1953, KROP and KUNKEL 1954, WRIGHT 1954, HEYMANS et al. 1956, OBERST et al. 1956, POCHET 1957), Soman (DECANDOLE et al. 1953), and Tabun (HOLMSTEDT 1951, DECANDOLE et al. 1953, HEYMANS et al. 1956, POCHET 1957). GESELL and FREY (1950) found that i.v. injection of either physostigmine or DFP increased the depth of the ventilatory response to electrical stimulation of the carotid nerve.

HOLMSTEDT (1951) found that Tabun in the cat began to raise bronchial resistance at an intravenous dose of 0.08 mg/kg, and that bronchoconstriction was complete at a dose of 0.12. In atropinized cats, paralysis of the diaphragm began at a dose of 0.09 mg/kg and was complete after 0.17. The muscles of the chest and abdominal walls were able to maintain some air exchange until respiratory paralysis occurred at a mean dose of Tabun of 0.25 mg/kg. DECANDOLE et al. (1953) have shown that bronchoconstriction following anti-ChE agents in the monkey and the rabbit is slight but is marked in the cat. In both the rabbit and the cat neuromuscular block in the phrenic-diaphragm system is marked, and is greater than that in the intercostal-thoracic wall systems; in the monkey, neuromuscular block does not appear to contribute to respiratory failure. In the last species central failure appears to be the principal cause of cessation of ventilation; in the rabbit and the cat, central failure is an important component of the paralysis of respiration. The dog resembles the cat in general, with marked bronchoconstriction (BERMAN 1953, unpubl.). Man is thought, on the basis of studies of mild intoxication with organophosphorus anti-ChE agents, to undergo less marked bronchoconstriction than the dog (JOHNSON et al. 1958), although one of the complaints in intoxication by vaporized anti-ChE agents is a sensation of tightness of the chest. Central respiratory failure and neuromuscular paralysis both contribute to apnea in man (GROB 1956). Thus, the problem of treating the apneic man with severe poisoning from anti-ChE agents is probably very similar to that of treating apneic dogs or cats.

B. Means for antagonizing functional changes induced by anticholinesterase agents

Non-specific effects (i.e., effects not resulting from inhibition of ChE's) of certain anti-ChE compounds, in enhancing the central action of a number of other chemicals and in producing demyelination of neurons within the central or peripheral nervous systems, have been mentioned. Other nonspecific effects of certain individual agents include stimulation of denervated muscle upon close-intra-arterial injection (RIKER and WESCOE 1946, GROBLEWSKI et al. 1956) and changes in the concentrations in the blood of factors concerned with clotting (HOLMES and GAON 1956). Despite the occurrence of miscellaneous effects apparently unrelated to the ability to inhibit ChE's, the most important acute toxic actions of the anti-ChE agents seem to result from the inhibition of acetylcholinesterase (AChE) and the consequent accumulation of acetylcholine (ACh).

Acetylcholine is released at cholinergic nerve endings following the arrival of impulses conducted along the axons, and smaller amounts are probably liberated during the resting stage (Chapter 6); the ACh is replaced in the terminals through synthesis by choline acetylase (ChAc) (NACHMANSOHN 1946, ZAWADZKI 1955). According to EMMELIN and MacINTOSH (1956) the superior cervical ganglion of the cat releases 25 $\mu\mu g$ ACh per preganglionic volley. Such minute bursts of ACh are believed to diffuse across the narrow space separating the nerve ending and the structure innervated and to unite with a receptor substance at the surface of the latter. This union initiates the activity characteristic of the particular structure innervated. The AChE or ChE's present in about the same places as the cholinergic nerve endings catalyse the hydrolysis of ACh, so that the duration of action of the transmitter substance is quite brief in normal tissues.

Inhibition of the ChE's in the vicinities of nerve terminations allows the ACh released by nerves to accumulate (STEWART 1952), so that local concentrations of ACh rise progressively to levels limited only by the ability of ACh to diffuse from the site of its release to the blood and lymph channels draining the local area. At the same time, inhibition of the ChE's in blood allows the development of increased blood levels of ACh, which may exert significant effects on organs and tissues far from the site of ACh release (DOUGLAS and PATON 1954).

Considering, from the above discussion, 1) that the ACh acting locally originates largely by release from vicinal nerve endings (HOLMES 1953, EMMELIN and MAC-INTOSH 1956), 2) that there may be some contribution from an elevated circulating level of ACh (DOUGLAS and PATON 1954), 3) that ChAc, AChE, and receptor protein all may be involved in originating the discreet effects composing the syndrome of anti-ChE poisoning, particularly in establishing the four types of dangerous functional effects mentioned above, it is apparent that there are the following general possibilities for using chemicals to antagonize the toxic effects of anti-ChE agents:

I. Prophylaxis

When the protective drug can be administered before the poison enters the body:

1. Destruction of the anti-ChE agent before it reaches functional sites.
2. Protection of AChE from inhibition.
3. Prevention of access of ACh to the receptor site.

II. Therapy

When the protective drug must be used after ChE's have been inhibited and ACh has accumulated near receptor sites:

1. Reduction of local accumulation of ACh by decreasing its release at nerve endings.
2. Prevention of access of ACh to receptor sites.
3. Reactivation of inhibited AChE.

C. Chemicals that destroy anticholinesterase agents

I. Externally

The skin is the principal locus of impaction on the body at which anti-ChE agents might be destroyed by chemical reaction. The reversible types of anti-ChE agents (e.g., physostigmine, neostigmine, benzpyrinium, and edrophonium) seem not to be absorbed in any significant amount from the skin surface, but the organophosphorus anti-ChE agents have been known to penetrate intact human skin since the work of HODGE and STERNER (1943) with triorthocresyl phosphate. This applies to both the alkyl esters of halogenated, cyanidated, or otherwise substituted organophosphates, and to the phosphorylcholines and thiocholines of TAMMELIN (1957a, b, 1958) and of GHOSH and NEWMAN (1955).

The mechanism of percutaneous absorption of Sarin and two homologs has been studied by BLANK et al. (1957, 1958), GRIESEMER et al. (1958), and FREDRIKSSON (1958). BLANK and his group found, with both rabbit skin *in situ* and excised human skin, that penetration of Sarin is primarily transepidermal (BLANK et al. 1958, GRIESEMER et al. 1958); FREDRIKSSON found in the hair follicles of cat skin an accumulation of P^{32} from labeled Sarin, or its 1-methyl-butoxy and 1-methyl-hexoxy homologs, 30 min after the labeled material had been spread on the skin. The latter author pointed out, however, that accumulation of radioactive material in the hair follicles does not mean necessarily that these structures are its main route of absorption; thus, FREDRIKSSON concluded that transepidermal absorption is as likely as transfollicular absorption. In intact rabbit skin the rate of penetration of Sarin was found to lie in the range of 50 to 500 $\mu g/cm^2/hr$ (GRIESEMER et al. 1958); in intact cat skin this rate of penetration was 60 to 120 $\mu g/cm^2/hr$ (FREDRIKSSON 1958).

Intact skin appears, therefore, to have a definite penetrability for Sarin and other organophosphorus anti-ChE agents, the magnitude of which may depend largely on the integrity of a thin layer of cells near the base of the stratum corneum (BLANK et al. 1957). The accumulation of P^{32} in the superficial portions of the hair follicles (FREDRIKSSON 1958) suggests that decontamination of skin would be aided by surface-active substances that would facilitate penetration of the decontaminant chemical into these potential reservoirs of lethal material. Furthermore, the findings that unchanged organophosphorus anti-ChE agents can penetrate skin (BLANK et al. 1957, FREDRIKSSON 1958, GRIESEMER et al. 1958), despite the fact that the agent is hydrolyzed partially within the skin (FREDRIKSSON 1958, GRIESEMER et al. 1958), and that there is a diffuse distribution of P^{32} throughout the dermis (BLANK et al. 1958, FREDRIKSSON 1958) suggest that a decontaminant capable of penetrating into the dermis would be more effective than one restricted to the surface of the skin.

The earliest methods for decontaminating skin splashed with anti-ChE compounds involved the use of water or alkaline solutions for washing the skin (COLLOMP 1949, WOOD et al. 1951). Washing with soap and water was recommended as an alternative procedure. In experiments with guinea pigs, FREDRIKSSON (1958) found that washing with alkaline soap, of pH 10.5, 10 min after the skin was contaminated with Sarin saved none of the animals but did prolong the mean time to death. Washing with the same soap 5 min after application of Sarin to the skin saved 30% of the guinea pigs; washing 2 min after contamination saved 80%. It is apparent, therefore, that the time lag between contamination of the skin and the performance of decontamination procedures is quite critical. Using rabbits and guinea pigs and applying Sarin to the clipped abdomens of the animals, KON-DRITZER et al. (1959), found that flushing the contaminated area with cool water 2 min after application of the Sarin increased the rabbit percutaneous LD_{50} from 43 to 415 cu mm/kg; the percutaneous LD_{50} for the guinea pig was raised from 104 to 674 cu mm/kg. The same group of workers found that flushing a rabbit's eyes with water one min after application of Sarin to the eyes had hardly any effect on the lethality of Sarin by this route. When irrigation of the eye was started within 30 sec after contamination, the perconjunctival LD_{50} of Sarin was raised from 35 to 47 $\mu g/kg$; irrigation of the eye within 10 sec after its contamination raised this value to 94.

The derivatives of anionically substituted phosphorus acids are known to be hydrolyzed by water as follows (KILPATRICK and KILPATRCK 1949), using Sarin as the model:

$$CH_3-\overset{\overset{O}{\|}}{\underset{\underset{F}{|}}{P}}-O-CH\overset{CH_3}{\underset{CH_3}{<}} + H_2O \longrightarrow CH_3-\overset{\overset{O}{\|}}{\underset{\underset{OH}{|}}{P}}-O-CH\overset{CH_3}{\underset{CH_3}{<}} + HF$$

The phosphorylcholines (phosphoro- or phosphono-cholinates) undergo a similar hydrolysis (TAMMELIN 1957a, LARSSON 1957):

$$CH_3-\overset{\overset{O}{\|}}{\underset{\underset{F}{|}}{P}}-O-CH_2-\overset{+}{N}\overset{CH_3}{\underset{CH_3}{<}} + H_2O \longrightarrow CH_3-\overset{\overset{O}{\|}}{\underset{\underset{OH}{|}}{P}}-O-CH_2-CH_2-\overset{+}{N}\overset{CH_3}{\underset{CH_3}{<}} + HF$$

In the phosphorylthiocholines (phosphoro- or phosphono-thiocholinates), the thiocholine moiety acts as the cation during hydrolysis (TAMMELIN 1958a);

$$\begin{array}{c} CH_3-\overset{\overset{O}{\|}}{\underset{\underset{S-CH_2-CH_2\overset{+}{N}\overset{CH_3}{\underset{CH_3}{<}}}{|}}{P}}-OC_2H_5 \end{array} + H_2O \longrightarrow CH_3-\overset{\overset{O}{\|}}{\underset{\underset{OH}{|}}{P}}-OC_2H_5 + HS-CH_2-CH_2-\overset{+}{N}\overset{CH_3}{\underset{CH_3}{<}}$$

These hydrolyses are catalyzed by both hydronium and hydroxyl ions (KILPATRICK and KILPATRICK 1949), by undissociated metallic salts (KILPATRICK and KILPATRICK 1949, EPSTEIN and ROSENBLATT 1958, LARSSON 1958c), and by metal chelates (WAGNER-JAUREGG et al. 1955, COURTNEY et al. 1957). The hypochlorite ion is one of the most effective agents in promoting hydrolysis of Sarin (EPSTEIN, ROSENBLATT and DEMEK 1956); hypochlorite ion, although less effective than for Sarin, is active at pH values of 5 and above in promoting hydrolysis of triethyl-phosphorothiolate, a model of the phosphorylthiocholines (LORDI and EPSTEIN 1958), but is consumed in this hydrolysis by reacting with the ethyl mercaptan freed during the hydrolysis. Similarly, hypochlorite is consumed during the hydrolysis of Tabun by reacting with the cyanide thus freed (EPSTEIN 1956). Compounds containing combined chlorine, e.g., chloramides, have little catalytic effect on the hydrolysis of Sarin or Tabun (EPSTEIN 1956); chloramides may react directly with phosphorylthiocholines.

Table 1 summarizes data from several sources on the relative catalytic efficiencies of representative compounds of various types known to catalyze the hydrolysis of organophosphorus anti-ChE agents. The anionic resins in the table (Amberlites IRA-400 and IRA-401) are more effective than the single cationic resin listed (Dowex 50), which was the most effective of 4 cationic resins studied by CHASANOV and EPSTEIN (1958). However, the anionic resins not only function as catalysts but also exchange hydroxyl groups for the anions of the acids released by the hydrolysis. In this latter way the anionic resins lose gradually their catalytic potency.

Either anionic or cationic resins in contact with solutions containing solutes in addition to the organophosphorus anti-ChE agents exchange their catalytic moieties for corresponding ions of the solutes and thereby lose their effectiveness as catalysts. This means that such resins are not applicable to decontamination of large supplies of ground water. A possible use for the ion-exchange resins would be for decontamination in the stomach of residues of ingested organophosphorus anti-ChE agents not removed by prior gavage or vomiting.

Table 1. *Relative efficacies, derived from velocity constants, of substances as catalysts of hydrolysis of derivatives of phosphorofluoridate*

Substance	Relative efficacy	Reference
Crosslinked Dowex 50 . . .	1	CHASANOV and EPSTEIN 1958
CrO_4^-	10	LARSSON 1958c
MoO_4^-	13	LARSSON 1958c
WO_4^-	15	LARSSON 1958c
Amberlite IRA-400	15	CHASANOV and EPSTEIN 1958
Amberlite IRA-401	19	CHASANOV and EPSTEIN 1958
Histidine	24	WAGNER-JAUREGG and HACKLEY 1953
Imidazole	26	WAGNER-JAUREGG and HACKLEY 1953
OH^-	100	EPSTEIN, DEMEK and ROSENBLATT 1956
H^+	100	EPSTEIN 1956
Cu^{++} imidazole	280	WAGNER-JAUREGG et al. 1955
Cu^{++} l-histidine	500	WAGNER-JAUREGG et al. 1955
$Cu(H_2O)^{++}$	580	EPSTEIN and ROSENBLATT 1958
$Ce(H_2O)^{+++}$	810	EPSTEIN and ROSENBLATT 1958
Cu^{++} α,α'-dipyridyl	810	WAGNER-JAUREGG et al. 1955
ClO^-	1000	EPSTEIN, DEMEK and ROSENBLATT 1956

Table 1 shows that hypochlorite is a highly effective catalyst of hydrolysis. As such, it may be used either for decontamination of skin or of water supplies. Particularly in the latter application, control of pH is important: at pH 9, one-fourth the concentration of free chlorine used at pH 6 yielded a nine-fold more rapid decontamination of Sarin. At constant pH, the rate of hydrolysis in the presence of hypochlorite approximately doubles with a $10°C$ rise in temperature (EPSTEIN 1956). Hypochlorite used for decontamination of skin or water supplies must be kept from contact with ammonia or either tertiary or quaternary amines, all of which form chloramides. The latter are almost inactive in catalyzing the hydrolysis of derivatives of anionically-substituted phosphorus acids, even though they do react with phosphorylthiocholine derivatives.

Alkali alone may be used for decontaminating water supplies or skin of derivatives of anionically-substituted phosphorus acids. As shown in Table 2, alkaline hydrolysis is not uniformly effective, however; it is particularly ineffective against phosphonocholinates and phosphorocholinates (TAMMELIN 1958b) and less so against the corresponding thiocholine salts. Mild alkali (sodium bicarbonate) may be used to decontaminate the skin of derivatives of phosphoro- or phosphono-halidates, of phosphonocyanidates, and of other organophosphorus anti-ChE agents susceptible to alkaline hydrolysis (LARSSON 1958d); strong alkali or organic solvents are to be avoided, as well as mechanical irritation of the skin by rough friction (KONDRITZER 1956). Alkaline decontamination of water may be carried out by raising the pH to 10 with soda ash, slaked lime, or magnesium hydroxide, followed after an appropriate interval by coagulation with ammonium alum or ferric chloride, filtration, and normal chlorination (EPSTEIN 1956).

For decontamination of skin spattered with organophosphorus anti-ChE agents, preparations liberating free chlorine may be particularly advantageous because chlorine has been shown to penetrate and pervade the entire epidermis (FERGUSON and SILVER 1947). Thus, the hypochlorite ion may catalyze hydrolysis of the phosphoro- or phosphono-compounds not only on the skin surface but actually

Table 2. *Second order velocity constants for the alkaline hydrolysis at 25° C of representative P-containing anticholinesterase agents*

Compound	k_2 (1 mole^{-1} sec^{-1})	Reference
Diisopropyl phosphorofluoridate (DFP)	0.8	KILPATRICK and KILPATRICK 1949
Methyl isopropyl phosphonofluoridate (Sarin)	26	LARSSON 1957
Methyl ethyl phosphonofluoridate	61	LARSSON 1957
Methyl cholinyl phosphonofluoridate	935	LARSSON 1957
Dimethylamino ethyl phosphonocyanidate (Tabun) .	7.5	LARSSON 1958b
Methyl ethyl phosphonocholinate	0.03	TAMMELIN 1958b
Methyl ethyl phosphonothiocholinate	0.2	TAMMELIN 1958b

throughout the epidermis to the basement membrane. This property of chlorine of penetration into the epidermis would be of particular value in the use of chlorine -liberating preparations for decontamination of skin from substances absorbed slowly from the skin surface.

In addition to hydrolysis, simple or catalysed, certain organophosphorus anti-ChE agents have been found to react with such reagents as amines, amino acids, phenols, catechols, vicinal trihydroxybenzene derivatives, hydrogen peroxide, hydroxylamine, hydroxamic acids, and oximes.

Because the organophosphorus compounds were known to react rapidly with such proteins as the ChE's and chymotrypsin, the reactivity of DFP with several amines and amino acids has been studied (WAGNER-JAUREGG et al. 1951). Although DFP itself was found not to react readily with amino acids, its chloro-analog, diisopropyl phosphorochloridate, was found to phosphorylate benzylamine and cyclohexylamine as well as ethyl glycinate, glycineamide, and methyl threoninate. Benzylamine reacted only slightly with DFP, cyclohexylamine to a considerable extent, and dodecylamine almost quantitatively. Phenol was phosphorylated at room temperature by both DFP and its chloro-analog. Tetraethylpyrophosphate phosphorylated cyclohexylamine and ethyl glycinate. All these phosphorylations, except those of phenol, took place on the amino nitrogen. Ethyl tyrosinate was phosphorylated by diisopropyl phosphorochloridate on both the α-amino group and the hydroxyl group. It is apparent, therefore, that either the amino nitrogen or the phenolic hydroxyl group in protein may be a point of primary reaction with the organophosphorus anti-ChE agents. Dihydroxy phenylalanine (DOPA) was found to react rapidly with DFP, Sarin, and Tabun (JANDORF et al. 1952, AUGUSTINSSON 1952, BERRY et al. 1955).

Table 3 shows the relative rates of reaction with DFP of a small series of poly-hydroxybenzene derivatives. It is apparent that introduction of an alcoholic hydroxyl group into the molecule has a fairly striking effect on the reactivity with DFP, but that introduction of a third vicinal phenolic hydroxyl has an even more marked effect. Catechol was found to react also with Sarin; the rate of reaction was proportional to both the Sarin and the monocatecholate ion concentrations (EPSTEIN, ROSENBLATT and DEMEK 1956). This finding of the importance of an undissociated phenolic hydroxyl group in the reaction between Sarin and catechols is mirrored in the findings (JANDORF et al. 1952) that pyrogallol in the presence of excess DFP reacts with approximately 2 moles of DFP per mole of pyrogallol, that the reaction product of equimolar amounts of pyrogallol and DFP yields ARNOW's

(1937) test for o-dihydroxyphenols, and that the reaction product of 2 moles of DFP with one of pyrogallol still yields a test for the phenolic hydroxyl but not Arnow's test. It seems likely, therefore, that pyrogallol reacts with the organophosphorus anti-ChE agents after dissociation of a single hydroxyl group, probably in the 2-position. There is evidence that the polyhydroxybenzene derivatives do not react appreciably with the phosphoro- and phosphono-cholinates (Epstein 1959, unpubl.).

Hydrogen peroxide reacts with organophosphorus anti-ChE agents, such as Sarin and Paraoxon, to produce perhydroxylated intermediates that react further to yield the hydrolyzed substrates and molecular oxygen (Epstein, Demek and Rosenblatt 1956, Larsson 1958d). The initial reaction is due to the perhydroxyl ion and the succeeding ones to either unionized hydrogen peroxide or, to a small extent, to the hydroxyl ion.

Jandorf (1951) found that hydroxylamine reacts rapidly with DFP and Sarin to detoxify the organophosphorus compounds. This finding was confirmed by Augustinsson (1952). Study of the mechanism of the reaction (Jandorf 1956) has

Table 3. *Relative reaction velocities of polyhydroxy benzene derivatives (1,2-dihydroxy-4-R-benzene) with DFP*

R	Relative velocity
H	100
—C(O)CH(CH₃)NHCH(CH₃)₂ . .	100
—CH(NH₂)CH₂NHCH₃	150
—CH(OH)CH(CH₃)NHCH(CH₃)₂	210
—CH(OH)CH₂NHCH₃	210
1,2,3-trihydroxy benzene	420

Data of Jandorf B. J. (unpublished).

shown that it consists probably of two steps: 1) one molecule of organophosphate reacts with one of hydroxylamine to yield both an acid, derived from the anion of the organophosphate, and the oxamine of the original substrate, 2) the latter molecule reacts with two additional hydroxylamine molecules to yield an hydroxylated organophosphorus product plus nitrogen and ammonia gases.

The search for a modification of the hydroxylamine molecule that would react more rapidly with organophosphorus anti-ChE agents led to recognition of the effectiveness of the hydroxamic acids (Hackley et al. 1955). Studies of the reaction rates of various hydroxamic acids with Sarin have been reported (Swidler and Steinberg 1956, Steinberg and Bolger 1956, Stolberg and Mosher 1957, Green et al. 1958, Swidler et al. 1959). The most rapidly reactive of all the hydroxamic acids seems to be cishexahydrophthalohydroxamic acid (Stolberg and Mosher 1957).

The reactivity of the hydroxamic acids with Sarin can be predicted reasonably accurately from the ionization constant alone (Stolberg and Mosher 1957, Green et al. 1958, Swidler et al. 1959) by the equation $\log k = 0.8\ pK_a - 5.65$ (Swidler et al. 1959), where k is the specific rate constant in $1\ \text{mole}^{-1}\ \text{sec}^{-1}$. Steinberg et al. (1957, unpubl.) showed that for maximal reactivity at physiological pH there is an optimal ionization constant corresponding to a pK_a of about 8. Reactions between the hydroxamic acids and Sarin occur in two distinct steps: an initial phosphorylation of the hydroxamate ion, followed by a Lossen rearrangement of the product (Hurd and Bauer 1954, unpubl., Swidler and Steinberg 1956). The first step was found to be the rate limiting one.

Green and Saville (1956) showed that oximes, like the hydroxamic acids, react with Sarin by a rate-controlling phosphorylation of the oxamate ion, followed by rapid splitting of the oxime phosphonate into acidic products. In comparing the rates of reaction of several hydroxamic acids and oximes with various organophosphorus anti-ChE agents, Green et al. (1958) found that the rate of reaction varies with the anti-ChE agent as well as with the hydroxamic acid or oxime. In general, the order of increasing reactivity of the organophosphorus compounds with oximes or hydroxamic acids was Paraoxon, DFP, TEPP, Tabun, and Sarin. This is also the order of increasing toxicity of these anti-ChE compounds. Furthermore, GREEN et al. found that certain hydroxamic acids react directly with the organophosphorus compounds at a greater rate than any oximes tested. Despite the fact that a number of oximes and hydroxamic acids react with organophosphorus compounds at greater rates than the hypochlorite ion (Table 4), they have not replaced the latter for use in decontaminating water supplies or skin contaminated with organophosphorus anti-ChE agents. The relative ease with which an excess of hypochlorite ion can be removed from a water supply is the probable explanation for this situation in the first instance; the instability of the lowermost compounds in Table 4 has militated against their inclusion in pharmaceutical preparations (solutions or ointments) for use in decontaminating skin some months or years after manufacture.

Table 4. *Relative reaction rates of some nucleophilic reagents with Sarin at 25° C*

Substance	Relative rate	Reference
Hydroxylamine	1	JANDORF 1956
Salicylhydroxamic acid	100	GREEN et al. 1958
2-Formyl N-methylpyridinium iodide oxime (P-2-AM).	110	GREEN and SAVILLE 1956
Pyruvaldoxime (MINA)	220	GREEN and SAVILLE 1956
2,3-Butanedione 2-oxime (DAM)	360	GREEN and SAVILLE 1956
ClO⁻	530	EPSTEIN, DEMEK and ROSENBLATT 1956
Benzhydroxamic acid	900	STOLBERG and MOSHER 1957
o-Dimethylamino-benzhydroxamic acid . . .	1300	STOLBERG and MOSHER 1957
Salicylaldoxime	1300	GREEN and SAVILLE 1956
2-Formyl pyridine oxime (P-2-A)	1500	GREEN and SAVILLE 1956
cis-Hexahydrophthalohydroxamic acid	5700	STOLBERG and MOSHER 1957

II. Internally

The first compound found to react with organophosphorus anti-ChE agents at a sufficiently high rate *in vitro* to justify its experimental trial in intoxication by these chemicals was hydroxylamine (JANDORF 1951, AUGUSTINSSON 1952). Because of the possible value of hydroxylamine in detoxifying absorbed organophosphorus anti-ChE agents before they have had an opportunity to react with ChE's at important sites within the body, the histotoxic properties of hydroxylamine were studied (WILLS and STABILE 1951, unpubl.).

Sixty rabbits were divided into 5 groups; each group received uniquely an intravenous injection of one of the following five dosages of hydroxylamine: 5, 10, 20, 30, and 40 mg/kg. Only three histotoxic effects appeared to be related to increasing dosage of hydroxylamine: pulmonary congestion, renal congestion, and appearance of tubular casts and petechial hemorrhages within the kidneys. There were no effects on liver histology attributable to hydroxylamine. Congestion of the lungs appeared in 87% of the rabbits given 5 mg/kg of hydroxylamine and in 100% of those given 10 mg/kg; renal congestion appeared in only 1/3 of the rabbits given the lowest dose, but in 93% of those given 10 mg/kg; tubular casts and petechial hemorrhages were not seen in the kidneys until 10 mg/kg had been given, and appeared in only 25% of the animals given 40 mg/kg. Furthermore, intravenous injection of hydroxylamine produced precipitous falls in blood pressure and heart rate. Acute death after a lethal dose of the compound resulted from a profound and prolonged lowering of blood pressure.

Despite the finding that intravenous injection of 10 mg of hydroxylamine/kg into an anesthetized dog will prevent the usual toxic effects of a subsequent intravenous injection of 1 mg of DFP/kg (WILLS and STABILE 1951, unpubl.), the toxicity of the compound, the fact that its protective effect lasted for less than 30 min, and the finding that it had comparatively little therapeutic value in DFP -poisoning were held to rule out practical use of hydroxylamine. These results with hydroxylamine proved that chemicals can antagonize, in a presumably specific manner, the toxic effects of organophosphorus anti-ChE agents, even though hydroxylamine appeared not to be suitable for actual use.

Hydroxamic acids and oximes also have prophylactic value as antagonists of anti-ChE agents (CHILDS et al. 1955, STEWART 1955, unpubl., EPSTEIN and FREEMAN 1956). The first two reports stated that mono*iso*nitrosoacetone (MINA) is more effective as a prophylactic of lethal effects by TEPP or Sarin in the rat than several other oximes and three hydroxamic acids. The oximes tested by CHILDS et al. (1955) included 2-formyl-pyridine-oxime (P-2-A), which was the least toxic and also one of the weakest prophylactic compounds. Another active oxime in protecting the rat against Sarin was 2,3-butanedione-2-oxime (DAM), according to CHILDS et al. (1955). EPSTEIN and FREEMAN (1956) found that a number of hydroxamic acids protected mice against 2 to 3 LD_{50}'s of Sarin; the best of 13 compounds studied by them seemed to be lact-hydroxamic acid and nicotine-hydroxamic acid. The methodide of the latter compound was less effective in preserving life than its tertiary parent, but was less toxic. In a subsequent study (DULTZ et al. 1957), the same group found that a number of oximes protected mice from 2 to 3 LD_{50}'s of Sarin and rats from up to 15 LD_{50}'s; DAM was their most effective prophylactic compound.

ASKEW (1956) found that DAM is much more effective as a prophylactic against the lethal actions of Sarin in the rat than it is in the guinea pig, monkey, mouse, or rabbit. In the last 4 species an i.p. injection of 150 mg of DAM/kg 15 min before the s.c. injection of Sarin protected against 1.7 to 3.0 LD_{50}'s of the anti-ChE agent; in the rat, the same dosage of DAM protected against 26.5 LD_{50}'s of Sarin. Administration of atropine with the oxime to the rat increased the prophylactic value of the pre-treatment by 1.7 times (ASKEW 1957). Equimolar doses of MINA or, especially, of 1-methyl-2-formylpyridinium iodide oxime (P-2-AM) were less actively prophylactic than DAM; administration of atropine with MINA or P-2-AM did not improve the protective value of the prophylaxis, in contradistinction to the finding with DAM.

KING and POULSEN (1958) examined the protective value in mice of P-2-AM (75 mg/kg, i.p.) given 20 min before s.c. injection of Parathion, DFP, Paraoxon, or Sarin. They found that P-2-AM is effective in raising the LD_{50} of Paraoxon to about 2.7 times that in mice not protected by P-2-AM; it had only a slight protective effect against DFP and barely detectable protective effects against Sarin and Parathion. WILSON and SONDHEIMER (1957) found that P-2-AM, given 5 min before the poison, was a more potent protective agent against Sarin than against Tabun. BAY et al. (1958) found that 1,3-*bis*(4-formylpyridinium bromide)-propane dioxime (TMB-4) is more actively prophylactic than P-2-AM against Sarin in rabbits, cats, and dogs. In man, P-2-AM and DAM have been found to protect against blockade of neuromuscular transmission by not only organophosphorus anti-ChE agents but also neostigmine (GROB and JOHNS 1958). In the mouse, TMB-4 protects against DFP, TEPP, diethyl-phosphostigmine, and neostigmine, but not against *bis*-neostigmine or *bis*-pyridostigmine (HOBBIGER and SADLER 1588, HOBBIGER and SADLER 1959).

Prophylaxis with atropine (1 mg/kg, i.p.), in addition to TMB-4 (27.2 mg/kg, i.p.), increased the degree of protection afforded to mice (HOBBIGER and SADLER 1959). Use of atropine with 1-methyl-2-formyl-pyridinium methanesulfonate oxime (P 2 S) also increased the effectiveness of protection afforded to mice or rats against TEPP or Sarin (DAVIES et al. 1959). Compounds of these groups are discussed in detail in Chapter 21.

D. Chemicals that protect cholinesterase by competitive occupation

I. Choline esters

Protection from the lethal effects of dimethylphosphorofluoridate with large doses of methacholine (MeCh), but not of ACh, was reported in 1943 (HUTCHENS et al., unpubl.). In a further study of this effect, MCNAMARA et al. (1946) added MeCh (20 mg/kg) to a mixture of atropine sulfate (20 mg/kg) and magnesium sulfate (800 mg/kg) injected i.m. into rabbits 15 to 30 min before intravenous injection of 0.5 mg of DFP/kg. Addition of the MeCh to the prophylactic mixture increased its protective effect by 1.6 times. Two possible explanations for this protective action of MeCh are that it combines with the receptor site of the cell surface, thereby blocking access of ACh to this point, or that it competitively occupies the reactive center of the ChE, thereby preventing its inactivation by DFP or other anti-ChE agents.

ROEPKE (1937), STRAUS and GOLDSTEIN (1943), and GOLDSTEIN (1944) had shown that addition of ACh to a physostigmine-ChE complex results in gradual displacement of the inhibitor from the enzyme. KOELLE (1946) found, however, that neither ACh nor MeCh, incubated with a homogenate of rat brain before addition of DFP, was significantly capable of preventing inactivation of the AChE by the DFP; carbamylcholine did prevent phosphorylation of the enzyme by DFP. On the other hand, ACh added to AChE from the electric eel simultaneously with physostigmine, neostigmine, DFP, or TEPP protected the enzyme against inactivation by the anti-ChE agent (AUGUSTINSSON and NACHMANSOHN 1949). Butyrylcholine (BuCh), propionylcholine, carbamylcholine, succinylcholine, and N-acetyl-p-aminobenzoyl-choline also protected ChE in vitro against inactivation by TEPP; benzoylcholine and salicyl-choline were almost inactive (AUGUSTINSSON 1953b).

STOVNER (1956) found that choline (0.002 to 0.021 M) partially protected the isolated rat diaphragm preparation from neuromuscular block induced by either physostigmine or DFP. Acetylcholine has been found (FLEISHER et al. 1958) to promote reactivation of ChE on the surfaces of the fibers in isolated frog's muscle. Thus, there is evidence in vitro that carbamylcholine and, less surely, ACh, MeCh, or other choline esters are able to compete successfully with organophosphorus anti-ChE agents for the active site on ChE's. It seems possible that this competitive behavior explains the protective effect that choline esters have been reported to exert against lethal actions by anti-ChE agents. It should be noted, however, that COHEN et al. (1951) found that BuCh did not protect rats against the lethal effect of DFP although it protected AChE in vitro from inhibition by DFP.

On the other hand, COHEN and POSTHUMUS (1955) have presented evidence that BuCh is capable of sensitizing frog muscle to ACh even in the presence of an excess of DFP. These authors presented the idea that DFP, and Sarin, combine with an esterase-like grouping in the receptor surface with which ACh also combines normally. Acetylcholine and BuCh, but not DFP or Sarin, combine also with a specific anionic site, this latter combination triggering muscular contraction. If this idea is correct, the antagonism by choline esters of the failure of neuromuscular transmission induced by DFP or Sarin, and presumably that initiated by other organophosphorus anti-ChE agents, would be the result of protection or reactivation of esteratic groupings in the end-plate region, with displacement of the phosphorylating moiety, and of increased sensitivity of the end-plate to ACh through sequestration of some of the specific anionic sites by the choline ester applied as an antagonist.

THESLEFF's (1955) finding that ACh (5 to 20×10^{-6}M) in the presence of neostigmine produces a persistent neuromuscular block in isolated nerve-muscle preparations from the frog, but a non-persistent depolarization in the end-plate region, and that of MEETER (1958) that DFP (0.33 μg/ml) produces a slowly waxing and waning depolarization of the endplate region of isolated diaphragm from the rat, correlated in intensity with the duration of the refractory period of the end-plate, suggest that neuromuscular block induced by DFP is not due entirely to the impingement of a high concentration of ACh on the end-plate region. The important point from our present standpoint, however, is that some choline esters do appear to have a mild antagonistic effect against the lethal actions of DFP, Sarin, and probably other similar chemicals, whatever the mechanism of that effect may be.

II. Reversible inhibitors and local anesthetics

The reversible ChE inhibitors are compounds belonging to the physostigmine-neostigmine group; the majority are substituted carbamic acid esters containing a basic substituent (AESCHLIMANN and REINERT 1931) (see Chapter 8). These compounds and local anesthetics will be considered together because local anesthetics of the benzoic acid ester type have been found to be inhibitors of ChE's, as well as being cholinolytic and locally anesthetic compounds (AKOPYAN and SAMVELYAN 1958). In the series studied by AKOPYAN and SAMVELYAN, cholinolytic and locally anesthetic effects ran parallel in double-peaked curves generated by plotting effectiveness against substituting groups; anti-ChE activity had a single-peaked curve nearly congruent with one of the peaks of the other curves. KALOW and MAYKUT (1956) had found a parallelism between locally anesthetic effectiveness and anti-ChE potency in two other series of compounds related chemically to procaine.

The competitive nature of the reactions of physostigmine and ACh with ChE was proved first by LOEWI and NAVRATIL (1926); this competitive relationship was shown to extend to neostigmine by ROEPKE (1937). KOSTER (1946) seems to have been the first person to use a reversible anti-ChE agent to prevent "irreversible" inactivation of ChE by an organophosphorus anti-ChE agent *in vivo*, and to protect animals against the lethal effects of DFP. KOELLE (1946) showed that both physostigmine and neostigmine protect AChE *in vitro* from inactivation by DFP; he found procaine also to be slightly active in this respect. Previously HAZARD et al. (1945) had found that procaine antagonizes the bradycardiac and parvisystolic effects of ACh and of physostigmine.

SALERNO and COON (1949) used the isolated rabbit's ileum to show that procaine (5×10^{-6}M) maintains pendular activity when applied to the intestinal segment before addition to the bath fluid of effective doses of physostigmine, neostigmine, DFP, HETP, or TEPP. Physostigmine has been found to prevent almost entirely the development of spontaneous activity by isolated skeletal muscles of the frog following their immersion in TEPP (10^{-6} M) (HOBBIGER 1950, KIRSCHNER and STONE 1951). Cocaine and procaine were found to have the same sort of action against TEPP (KRAATZ 1957, unpubl.). AUGUSTINSSON and GRAHN (1952) found that procaine protects BuChE *in vitro* against Tabun; AUGUSTINSSON (1953a) reported that physostigmine also protects the ChE of cobra venom *in vitro* against inhibition by Paraoxon. In an extension of these studies, AUGUSTINSSON (1953b) found that procaine, tetracaine, tutocaine, or physostigmine is able to protect the ChE's of human plasma, human red cells, or cobra venom from inactivation *in vitro* by TEPP or Tabun. Ethylaminobenzoate and dibucaine had very little, if any, protective activity; amylocaine and lidocaine had only moderate activity. Examination of these compounds leads to the conclusion that the maximal protective effect *in vitro* is related to the existence in the molecule of the local anesthetic of both an ester and a dimethyl- or diethyl-amino group.

Following earlier work by ATANACKOVIC and DALGAARD-MIKKELSEN (1951), in which procaine was found to block ganglionic transmission as well as muscarinic and nicotinic phenomena elicited by ACh, physostigmine, DFP, or 1-dimethyl-carbaminoyl, 4-phenyl, 6-trimethyl-ammonomethyl-benzene bromide (Nu-683), BHATTACHARYA and ATANACKOVIC (1956), studied the effects of procaine on the responses of the isolated lung of the guinea pig. They found that procaine can block almost completely the bronchoconstriction induced by ACh and, less completely, that induced by pilocarpine, physostigmine, or neostigmine.

Although the mechanisms involved in the foregoing findings are uncertain, these findings do indicate that local anesthetics might be effective antagonists of poisoning by anti-ChE compounds *in vivo*. WILLS (1955) reported that procaine amide hydrochloride is a moderately effective adjunct to atropine in the prophylaxis of poisoning by Sarin in the rabbit. Table 5 shows that a large dose of this compound is as effective an adjunct to atropine as a forty-fold smaller dose of physostigmine; both of these doses are much more effective than the smaller dose of MeCh. All drugs used as adjuncts to atropine in Table 5 were used in the maximal dose that could be given without obvious deleterious effect on the rabbits.

A number of other local anesthetics have been studied as adjuncts to atropine in preventing experimental poisoning with Sarin in the rabbit. The most effective of these compounds was dimethylaminopropyl-*p*-(dimethylamino)-benzoate; the corresponding amide was almost as active as the ester. Both of these compounds were about as effective adjuncts to atropine in a dose of 2 mg/kg as procaine amide was in a dose of 20 mg/kg.

Trimethylammonopropyl-*p*-(dimethylamino)-benzoate iodide is more toxic than its parent, but, in a dose of 0.5 mg/kg, it was still an effective adjunct to atropine in preventing poisoning by Sarin. Trimethylammonoproyl-*p*-(trimethylammono)-benzoate diiodide is much more toxic than any of the previously mentioned compounds (the intravenous LD_{50} for the mouse is 1/193 that of procaine amide hydrochloride) and, in

Table 5. *Effects of intravenous drug injections two minutes prior to intravenous injection of 30 μg/kg of Sarin on mortality in the rabbit*

Atropine sulfate mg/kg	Methacholine chloride mg/kg	Physostigmine hydrochloride mg/kg	Procaine amide hydrochloride mg/kg	Mortality
—	—	—	—	9/9
2	—	—	—	4/5
2	0.2	—	—	4/6
2	—	0.5	—	0/5
2	—	—	20	0/6

WILLS, unpublished

the maximum tolerated dose (0.08 mg/kg, i.v.), it is inactive as an adjunct to atropine in the rabbit. The triethylammono homolog of procaine amide is about 3 times as toxic as its parent and is almost inactive as an adjunct to atropine in preventing poisoning by i.v. injection of Sarin.

BAY (1959, unpubl.) found that dibucaine is an effective adjunct to a mixture of atropine and an oxime, not only in preventing but also in treating poisoning by organophosphorus anti-ChE agents in the rabbit, despite Augustinsson's report that the compound is almost inactive in protecting ChE against inactivation *in vitro* by TEPP or Tabun. The therapeutic activity of local anesthetics may be related either to their ability to reduce the release of ACh by nerve endings (JACO and WOOD 1944) or to their antagonism of the change in the permeability of the cell membrane to K^+ and Na^+ that usually accompanies the arrival of an action or transmitter potential at some particular point on the membrane (FLECKENSTEIN 1955). The membrane becomes less sensitive, therefore, to depolarizing substances, such as ACh. The precise mechanism of action of the local anesthetics as adjuncts to atropine in the prophylaxis or therapy of poisoning by anti-ChE compounds is unknown at present.

In view of the high protective activity shown by physostigmine in Table 5, a number of synthetic, reversible inhibitors of ChE have been studied as adjuncts to atropine in the treatment of poisoning by Sarin in the rabbit. The most active compounds, other than physostigmine, all contain the dimethyl carbaminoyl group in the *meta* or *para* position of a benzene or pyridine ring, with respect to a quaternary nitrogen atom, either attached to, or included within, the ring. Closely related compounds having a configuration in the carbaminoyl group other than dimethyl, containing no quaternary nitrogen atom, or having the two side chains on the ring in the *ortho* relationship were relatively inactive.

The most active adjunct to atropine among the reversible inhibitors of ChE studied was 1-dimethylcarbaminoyl-3-methyl-4-trimethylammono-6-*iso*propyl-benzene. A mixture of 0.025 mg/kg of this compound and 2 mg/kg of atropine sulfate injected i.v. into rabbits two min before i.v. injection of 0.09 mg/kg of Sarin protected one-half the animals from death; the atropine alone protected one-half the animals from a dose of only about 0.040 mg/kg of Sarin.

Not only do the reversible inhibitors of ChE prevent some of the toxic effects of organophosphorus compounds but also certain of them antagonize some toxic effects of others of the same group. BAKER and CAPLAN (1957, unpubl.) have reported that the isolated frog's heart is stimulated by neostigmine but is depressed by physostigmine. Depression induced by the latter compound is antagonized by neostigmine. In the intact animal, however, these two anti-ChE compounds do not have contrasting effects except on the central nervous system, where neostigmine is predominantly a depressant and physostigmine predominantly a stimulant (SCHWEITZER and WRIGHT 1937b).

E. Chemicals that block receptor sites outside the central nervous system

The toxic effects of the anti-ChE compounds all come under the three categories of muscarinic, nicotinic and central neuronal effects. Chemicals that antagonize the actions of anti-ChE compounds will be discussed under these same three headings.

I. Antimuscarinic drugs[1]

1. Optimal conditions for employment of antimuscarinic drugs

The antagonism between atropine and physostigmine was found (KLEINWÄCHTER 1864, FRASER 1870) long before physostigmine had been shown to be an anti-ChE compound (LOEWI and NAVRATIL 1926). BARRETT et al. (1942, unpubl.) reported that atropine given after DFP decreased the severity of the toxic effects and prolonged, but did not preserve, life. HUTCHENS et al. (1943, unpubl.) reported that the protection against the lethal actions of dimethyl phosphorofluoridate afforded by atropine was questionable. McNAMARA et al. (1946) found that 800 mg/kg of Mg SO$_4$, i.m., was almost ineffective in protecting rabbits against 0.5 mg/kg of DFP; when the same dose of Mg SO$_4$ was injected along with 20 mg/kg of atropine sulfate, the mixture preserved life in about 2/3 of the group of rabbits. DuBOIS et al. (1949) found that atropine protects cats and dogs against 2 to 3 lethal doses of Parathion. SALERNO and COON (1949) reported that physostigmine, neostigmine, DFP, and TEPP have similar effects on blood pressure, heart rate, the electrocardiographic record, the isolated heart, and the isolated ileum. Atropine was found to reverse all these effects except those on the isolated heart.

The isolated heart was found to be relatively insensitive to all four anti-ChE agents studied by SALERNO and COON. MURTHA and WILLS (1955. unpubl.) found that papillary muscle from the cat's heart undergoes only a slight reduction in the amplitude of contraction after being exposed for 2 hrs to an initial concentration of 133 μg/ml of DFP, and is unaffected by exposure for 2 hrs in an initial concentration of 13 μg/ml of TEPP or for 3 hrs to initial concentrations of 10 μg/ml of Tabun or 3 μg/ml of Sarin. Furthermore, Sarin was found not to potentiate the action of ACh on isolated papillary muscle. Anti-ChE compounds appear, therefore, to have no direct action on ventricular muscle related to their ability to inhibit ChE, so that it is not remarkable that atropine is unable to overcome toxic effects of anti-ChE agents on the isolated heart.

Atropine has been found, on the other hand, to overcome in the intact animal or man the bradycardia and hypotension induced by a variety of anti-ChE agents, the hyperactivity of glands and smooth muscles of the respiratory and gastrointestinal tracts, the constriction of the pupil, and the mortality resulting from 2 to 3 LD$_{50}$ doses (UHDE and MOORE 1945, unpubl., BURGEN et al. 1947, GROB and

[1] This section (pages 897—901) was prepared in collaboration with Dr. JOHN F. O'LEARY, whose help is gratefully acknowledged.

HARVEY 1949, MUIR and BURGESS 1949, unpubl., GROB 1950, GROB et al. 1950, SILVER et al. 1950, unpubl., HOLMSTEDT 1951, CULLUMBINE et al. 1952, DOUGLAS and MATTHEWS 1952, DECANDOLE et al. 1953, MEYER 1953, MUIR and CLEMENTS 1953, unpubl., KROP and KUNKEL 1954, PUNTE et al. 1954, unpubl., LOOMIS and KROP 1955, unpubl., GROB 1956, HEYMANS et al. 1956, HOLMES and GAON 1956, OBERST et al. 1956, DECANDOLE and MCPHAIL 1957, HOLMES et al. 1957).

The conditions for optimal employment of atropine in cases of poisoning by organophosphorus compounds have been summarized by GROB and HARVEY (1953) and by FREEMAN and EPSTEIN (1955), and are discussed in detail in Chapter 22. Laboratory data support qualitatively the conclusion of FREEMAN and EPSTEIN (1955) that early and vigorous use of atropine is a *sine qua non* in the successful treatment of anti-ChE poisoning. They demonstrate also that for every dose of an anti-ChE compound there is a maximally effective dosage of atropine; dosages of atropine above this level accomplish nothing additional therapeutically, although they may exercise effectiveness for longer periods of time than do maximally effective dosages. In addition, dosages of atropine greater than that maximally effective present the possibility of intoxication by atropine itself.

Atropine intoxication is characterized by dilated pupils, dry and flushed skin, tachycardia (heart rate increased to 140 to 165 beats per min), restlessness, disorientation, hallucination, and maniacal behavior. The physical activity associated with the last effect may be interpreted incorrectly as being convulsive in nature; if the other signs of atropine intoxication are not recognized, struggling by the overatropinized patient poisoned originally by an anti-ChE compound may be considered to be a manifestation of central cholinergic effects and may lead to administration of additional atropine to the already over-atropinized subject. Fortunately, overatropinization is incapacitating but of little danger to life, except in elevated environmental temperatures (GORDON and FRYE 1955).

The findings that atropine is absorbed within guinea pig muscle more rapidly from a concentrated solution than from a more dilute one and more rapidly from a solution containing hyaluronidase than from a simple solution of the same concentration of atropine sulfate (SCHRIFTMAN and KONDRITZER 1957) indicate ways in which the absorption of atropine from the intramuscular site of injection can be accelerated. The finding of SEIFTER and BAEDER (1954) that partially depolymerized hyaluronic acid also enhances the absorption of atropine from an intramuscular site of injection proves that enhancers of the absorption of intramuscularly injected atropine more stable than hyaluronidase can be found. In addition, the finding that man excretes in his urine more unchanged atropine than the cat, guinea pig, rat, or mouse (KALSER et al. 1957, GOSSELIN et al. 1960) suggests that compounds may be found that prolong the biological half-life of atropine by blocking its excretion through the kidneys. Thus, there are several possibilities for increasing the speed of absorption of atropine from an intramuscular site of injection or for prolonging the activity of a dose of atropine once it has been absorbed. Successful research on these possibilities could result in provision for individual use in anti-ChE intoxication of a more rapidly and lastingly effective anticholinergic preparation than the presently available buffered solution of atropine sulfate.

2. Structure-activity relationships

In a series of studies in the mouse using TEPP as the lethal agent, KARCZMAR and LONG (1958) found that 14 of 29 esters were more active than the most potent of 6 aminoalcohols studied. They found also that the administration of 1.26 mg/kg of methylatropinium nitrate, along with a tertiary anticholinergic drug and 0.3 mg/kg of benzoquinonium, did not alter appreciably the prophylactic efficacy of the mixture of tertiary anticholinergic drug and benzoquinonium; the dose of the anticholinergic drug required to protect one-half the mice was used as the measure of activity. KARCZMAR and LONG considered that the ineffectiveness of methylatropinium nitrate in this situation is an indication that the protection afforded by tertiary anticholinergic compounds is exerted chiefly centrally; however, in the same paper they showed that peripheral cholinolytic effectiveness, graded on the basis of comparative mydriatic activities, and protective efficacy against TEPP are nearly exactly proportional to one another. On the other hand, DAHLBOM et al. (1953) found that the protective effects against Tabun in the rabbit and guinea pig of a group of acyl derivatives of phenothiazine are not strictly parallel to their antimuscarinic effects.

KAGAN (1956), in discussing the protective effects against Parathion of the diphenylacetic acid ester of tropinol and of the phenylcyclopentylcarboxylic acid ester of 2-diethylaminoethanol, concluded that both muscarinic and nicotinic actions are involved in the lethal effect of Parathion, so that compounds antagonizing both of these types of action are better antidotes than such predominantly antimuscarinic drugs as atropine. Similarly, SPENCER (1953, unpubl.) found that the protective activity against Sarin in the rat and the guinea pig of a series of basic amides had only a rough relationship to their ability to block the effect of ACh on isolated guinea pig's ileum. BHATTACHARYA (1956) found that 2,2-diphenyl-4-di*iso*propyl-butyramide methiodide was more effective in antagonizing bronchoconstriction induced in the isolated lung of the guinea pig by ACh than it was in antagonizing that induced by neostigmine.

Study in the author's laboratory of a large number of anticholinergic compounds as prophylactic or therapeutic agents in unanesthetized rats and rabbits and in anesthetized dogs and monkeys poisoned by Sarin led to the following general conclusions:

a) There is a general, but not precise, agreement between the prophylactic and therapeutic efficacies of anticholinergic compounds.

b) The most effective and safest antagonists of the lethal actions of Sarin within the anticholinergic group are esters of aminoalcohols containing the diethylamino, or equivalent, grouping.

c) Diethylamino compounds were more active than dimethylamino ones; piperidine-3 derivatives were more active than corresponding piperidine-1 compounds, but both sorts of piperidine derivatives were more toxic and less effective than corresponding dimethylamino or diethylamino compounds.

d) Replacement of piperidine-1 by morpholine-1 in two cases increased the lethal activity and reduced markedly the protective activity against Sarin; two pyrrolidine-1 compounds were less lethal and considerably more effective than the corresponding piperidine-1 derivatives.

e) In esters or ketones, replacement of one hydrogen on the α-carbon atom to the carbonyl group by a hydroxyl group increased potency and lethality by about the same fraction.

f) Quaternization increased lethal activity and decreased effectiveness against Sarin.

g) A small group of synthetic anticholinergic drugs rank in man in roughly the same order of activity as in experimental animals (GROB 1955); in man, no synthetic drug tested was more active than atropine, although 3 of them seemed to be superior in some respects to atropine in the animal experiments.

O'BRIEN and DAVISON (1958) studied antagonists to seven organophosphorus compounds, including OMPA, Parathion, and Guthion. The last three compounds must all be converted in the body to other compounds to have significant anti-

ChE activity. Adiphenine and chlorpromazine, along with a number of other compounds, were ineffective in protecting mice against intraperitoneal injections of 25 mg/kg of OMPA, 10 mg/kg of Parathion, or 12 mg/kg of Guthion, when the possible antagonists were injected i.p. before injection of the organophosphorus compound. Iproniazid, p-diethylaminoethyl diphenylpropyl acetate (SKF 525 A), and 3-acetylpyridine were found to prevent death from OMPA, but were not particularly effective against Parathion or Guthion. This latter finding is particularly striking because SKF 525 A has been found to inhibit oxidation *in vitro* of Parathion to Paraoxon (DAVISON 1955) and of Guthion to its corresponding phosphorothioate (MURPHY and DuBois 1957). The greater sensitivity of OMPA to antagonism by iproniazid, SKF 525 A, or 3-acetylpyridine indicates presumably that it has less affinity for some active metabolic system than the other two.

3. Inter-effectual relationships

The correlation between antagonistic action against poisoning by anti-ChE compounds and anticholinergic effectiveness has been discussed above. The work of O'BRIEN and DAVISON (1958) has shown that the capacities of SKF 525 A, iproniazid, and 3-acetylpyridine to prevent poisoning by OMPA parallel closely their capacities to interfere with detoxication of pentobarbital. It is likely, therefore, that these three compounds are effective antagonists to poisoning by OMPA because they inhibit the metabolic system that converts OMPA into an active inhibitor of ChE's.

TODRICK (1954) studied the abilities of 46 substances to inhibit the ChE's in a homogenate of rat's brain (chiefly AChE) and in a homogenate of mucosa from rat's small intestine (chiefly butyrocholinesterase BuChE), relating the results to the functional effects induced by the chemicals. His general conclusion was that the ratio of the concentration of chemical inhibiting brain ChE by 50% to that inhibiting similarly intestinal mucosal ChE has a value of less than 0.2 for most compounds that block neuromuscular transmission, lies between 5 and 60 for antimuscarinic compounds, and between 40 and 3000 for drugs effective in Parkinsonism. GYERMEK (1955a), in a somewhat similar study of 13 quaternary tropinol esters, found that increasing antimuscarinic activity tends to be associated with increasing specificity for BuChE, whereas interference with both neuromuscular and ganglionic transmissions seems to be correlated positively with increasing specificity for AChE.

In an attempt to elucidate further the relationship between antagonism to the lethal effect of Sarin and other functional effects of anticholinergic substances, the reviewer has studied 41 compounds, mostly esters and amides, on which information was available concerning their abilities to produce local anesthesia by intradermal injection into the guinea pig, to block the pressor effect of nicotine in the dog, to block the carotid occlusion reflex in the dog, to block the stimulatory effect of ACh on the isolated ileum, to block the stimulatory effect of barium chloride on the isolated ileum, and to block the stimulatory effect of histamine on the isolated ileum (WILLS, unpubl.). In brief, the only consistent covariance between protective activity against Sarin and one of the other functional activities was that with ability to block the stimulatory effect of ACh on the isolated ileum. Even this correlation was a general one, with wide variations from the trend in individual cases.

4. Limitations of antimuscarinic compounds

We use the term "antimuscarinic" to refer to activity antagonizing the effects of ACh on peripheral effectors innervated by the autonomic nervous system. Intoxication by anti-ChE compounds includes also paralysis of skeletal muscle and abolition of respiratory discharges over the phrenic nerves (DOUGLAS and MATTHEWS 1952). DOUGLAS and MATTHEWS, DECANDOLE et al., (1953) and WRIGHT (1954), among others, have shown that atropine, hyoscine, and other tertiary anticholinergic compounds do not antagonize significantly the block of neuromuscular transmission induced by anti-ChE compounds. Quaternary anticholinergic compounds, because of poor penetration of the blood-brain barrier, have little central activity and that little becomes evident only slowly (FARQUHARSON and JOHNSTON 1959); tertiary anticholinergic compounds can overcome the silencing of the phrenic outflow caused by ChE inhibitors (KRIVOY et al. 1951, DOUGLAS and MATTHEWS 1952). Thus, the principal limitation on the effectiveness of atropine and other tertiary antimuscarinic compounds is their inability to restore neuromuscular transmission.

Some quaternary analogs have the latter action, so that they have value as adjuncts to atropine in prevention or treatment of poisoning by anti-ChE agents. Thus, N-benzyl-atropinium chloride, which prevents stimulation of skeletal muscle by ACh injected into the arterial supply of the muscle, has been found to increase the survival ratio when administered along with atropine to rabbits prior to injection of Sarin (KUNKEL et al. 1957).

The foregoing limitation is illustrated by an experiment of MUIR and CLEMENTS (1953, unpubl.) in the monkey exposed to vapor of Sarin and then treated either by i.m. injection of atropine sulfate, by artificial ventilation, or by a combination of both procedures. Intramuscular injection of atropine (0.0285 mg/kg) was found to save monkeys from not more than 3 LD_{50}'s of inhaled Sarin; the combination of the same dose of atropine sulfate and artificial ventilation saved the animals following exposure to 80 LD_{50}'s of vaporized Sarin. Similarly, OBERST et al. (1956) found that treatment with both i.m. injection of atropine sulfate and artificial ventilation raised the LD_{50} of inhaled Sarin vapor for the dog by at least 35 times when treatment was instituted within 2 minutes after the end of the 60-sec period of exposure.

II. Ganglionic blocking agents

The limited effectiveness of atropine and other antimuscarinic compounds in preventing death from multiple lethal doses of anti-ChE agents has led to a search for adjunctive compounds to be given along with atropine to supplement the latter's life-saving value. Because ganglia are among the structures in which abnormal activity is induced by the nicotine-like phenomena of poisoning by anti-ChE compounds, one obvious possibility was compounds having the ability to modify ganglionic transmission. Certain barbiturates, local anesthetics, and quaternary amines are known to have this type of action.

Table 6. *Effectiveness of ganglion-blocking compounds as adjuncts to atropine sulfate (2 mg/kg, i.v.) in preventing lethal effects of Sarin (30 µg/kg, i.v.) when both drugs are administered 2 min before Sarin*

Adjunct and dose (i. v.)	Rabbits dead/total
None	3/6
Amobarbital, 20 mg/kg	0/6
Procaine amide, 20 mg/kg	2/6
Propantheline, 2 mg/kg	2/6

WILLS, unpublished.

Examples of these groups which possess adjunctive activity when administered along with atropine in anti-ChE poisoning in experimental animals are given in Table 6.

Of particular potency in blocking ganglionic transmission are the *bis*quaternary amines of moderate chain length (PATON and ZAIMIS 1952). Study of a series of such compounds as adjuncts to atropine in the antagonism of poisoning by Sarin in the rabbit has shown that the optimal chain length between the two quaternary nitrogen atoms is 5 carbon atoms. Alteration of the composition of the chain without significant change in chain length, as by replacing one of the methylene groups with an oxygen, a sulfur, or a nitrogen atom, reduces the adjunctive efficacy. Changes in the constitution of the quaternary head also alter adjunctive potency; the pentamethylene derivative with triethyl ammonium heads is more effective than those with trimethyl or dimethyl-ethyl ammonium heads.

Examples of the effectiveness of *bis*quaternary amines used with atropine in the prevention of death among rabbits given approximately 4 LD_{50}'s of Sarin are given in Table 7. PARKES and SACRA (1954) have reported that hexamethonium can increase the protective limit of atropine against anti-ChE agents from about 2 LD_{50} for atropine alone to about 10 LD_{50} for atropine plus hexamethonium. A study of 22 *bis*quaternary amines for potency in reducing transmission of vagal impulses to the heart, in reducing transmission of impulses through the superior cervical ganglion, and in enhancing the protective efficacy of atropine against Sarin has shown that the last

Table 7. *Effectiveness of bisquaternary compounds as adjuncts to atropine sulfate (2 mg/kg, i.v.), both given 2 min before poisoning, in saving rabbits poisoned with Sarin (60 µg/kg, i.v.)*

Adjunct and dose (i. v.)	Mortality
None	6/6
Azamethonium, 5 mg/kg	1/6
Pentamethonium, 5 mg/kg	0/6

WILLS, unpublished.

activity parallels the first one more exactly than it does the second. All three sorts of activity reach their maximal values in compounds with a 5-carbon chain between two quaternary heads (KUNKEL et al. 1952).

Other types of ganglion-blocking compounds studied as adjuncts to atropine in prevention of lethality from Sarin administration belong to either the 2-chlorethylamine group studied by LOEW and MICETICH (1948a, 1948b, 1949), STONE and LOEW (1948), and by NICKERSON and NOMAGUCHI (1951), or the tertiary amine group related to mecamylamine. In general, these compounds are less effective adjuncts than the *bis*quaternary amines; Table 8 gives examples of the adjunctive effectiveness of three of the most potent chemicals in these two classes. The last compound in the table, which is more effective than mecamylamine in this test, is less active than the two *bis*quaternary compounds illustrated in Table 7.

Table 8. *Effectiveness of adrenolytic and tertiary ganglion-blocking compounds as adjuncts to atropine (2 mg/kg, i.v.), both drugs being administered 2 min before poisoning, in preventing death in rabbits poisoned with Sarin (30 or 60 µg/kg, i.v.)*

Adjunct and dose (i. v.)	Mortality	
	30 µg/kg	60 µg/kg
None	3/6	6/6
N-butyl, N-(2-phenylphenoxy)-ethyl, 2-chlorethylamine, 2 mg/kg .	2/6	—
N-benzyl, N-phenyl*iso*propyl, 2-chlorethylamine, 5 mg/kg	2/6	6/6
5-Amino, 6-phenyl, 1,4-endomethylene-2-cyclohexene, 2 mg/kg. . .	—	3/6
5-Amino, 6-phenyl, 1,4-endomethylene-2-cyclohexene, 5 mg/kg. . .	1/6	3/6

WILLS, unpublished.

III. Curarizing and other musculotropic drugs

The most important of the nicotinic actions of anti-ChE compounds is paralysis of skeletal muscle. The ganglion-blocking and cholinolytic compounds just discussed have comparatively little effect on neuromuscular transmission. Six di- to hexa-methylene and two azapentylene *bis*quaternary compounds studied by GYERMEK (1955b) had approximately 1/20 as much effect on transmission across the neuromuscular junction in frog muscle as on transmission across the synapse in the superior cervical ganglion of the cat. The most active of these compounds with respect to the neuromuscular junction had only about one-quarter the activity of d-tubucurarine.

Studies of chemical means for overcoming neuromuscular block induced by Sarin showed that N-methyl and N-*iso*propyl atropinium salts have temporary effects of the kind sought. Atropine quaternized with more weighty radicals, e.g., benzyl or phenacyl, was found to be capable of increasing the response of skeletal muscle to single stimuli applied to the motor nerve in cats poisoned with Sarin (KUNKEL et al. 1956). Many other compounds containing quaternary nitrogen atoms, of which a few examples are given in Table 9, have been found to be capable of increasing sharply the response of skeletal muscle to indirect stimulation at low frequency (Fig. 2 of KUNKEL et al. 1956). Apparently the N atom in the

Table 9. *Effectiveness of adjuncts to atropine sulfate (0.5 mg/kg, i.v.) in promoting recovery of twitch response of the gastrocnemius-soleus muscle of the cat to sciatic nerve stimulation following injection of 220 μg/kg of Sarin. Atropine given before, adjuncts after, Sarin*

Treatment compound	Dose mg/kg	Minutes for	
		50% recovery	85% recovery
None	—	19.6	27.1
Atropine sulfate	2.0	16.1	22.3
Benzylatropinium chloride	5.0	6.4	8.3
N-2-Chlorobenzylatropinium chloride	5.0	6.4	11.8
N-2-Chlorobenzylnoratropine chloride	5.0	14.2	18.6
N-Methylpromethazinium iodide	2.0	6.3	7.0
Dibutoline	5.0	6.6	10.7
Gallamine triethiodide	0.25	7.1	16.9
d-Tubocurarine chloride	0.3	6.7	8.1
Decamethonium iodide	0.01	25.4	30.0
Benzoquinonium chloride	0.05	9.5	16.8
4632	0.17	10.2	15.0
Ambenonium chloride	0.05	25.2	38.4
6043	0.5	6.5	9.0
7502	1.0	6.4	8.0
6277	0.5	7.0	8.9
5372	0.5	6.3	8.3
5669	0.5	6.4	8.0

N4632 = *bis*(N-ethyl bromide) analog of benzoquinonium chloride;
N6043 = *bis*(N-2-methoxybenzyl) analog of ambenonium chloride;
N7502 = *bis*(N-dipropyl) homolog of ambenonium chloride;
N6277 = *bis*(ammonopropyl) homolog of ambenonium chloride;
N5372 = *bis*(N-benzyl) analog of 6277;
N5669 = *bis*(N-3-chlorobenzyl-pyrrolidinium) analog of 6277.

WILLS and KUNKEL, unpublished.

tropinol ring requires a comparatively large quaternizing group (larger than *iso*-propyl) to prevent the charged atom from being hindered sterically within the tropinol structure; when the N atom is in the periphery, as it is in the molecule of promethazine, a small quaternizing group suffices. Some support for this idea may be seen in the efficacy of Dibutoline, which has both an exposed N atom and a fairly small quaternizing group (ethyl).

The findings that competitive inhibitors (e.g., d-tubocurarine and gallamine triethiodide) of the response of muscle to ACh enhance the rate of recovery of responsiveness of muscle to slowly repetitive stimulation of the motor nerve after a large dose of Sarin, and that the depolarizing inhibitors (e.g., decamethonium iodide) actually prolong the recovery from Sarin-induced neuromuscular blockade are not unexpected. While it is true that Sarin and DFP, like neostigmine (RIKER and WESCOE 1946), have a direct stimulatory effect on skeletal muscle (GROBLEW-SKI et al. 1956), this effect is not related to the anti-ChE actions of the compounds and is of little practical importance. The major actions of the organophosphorus compounds on the neuromuscular junction are due almost certainly to ACh accumulation; ACh is known to be both depolarizing and desensitizing (THESLEFF 1955, KRIVOY and WILLS 1956). Thus it is not surprising that the neuromuscular block established by an anti-ChE agent is intensified by other depolarizing compounds and mitigated by competitive antagonists to ACh.

It is evident from Table 9 that benzoquinonium chloride is considerably more active in restoring neuromuscular transmission after a large dose of Sarin than is its *bis* (N-ethyl bromide) analog (4632). This finding, coupled with the greater effectiveness of benzylatropinium chloride than of methyl- or *iso*propylatropinium salts, suggests that the benzyl radical has some comparatively specific effect in directing the entire molecule to the neuromuscular junction.

The 2-chlorobenzyl radical seems not to be remarkably different from the benzyl radical. This conclusion seems to be supported by the findings with the analogs and homologs of ambenonium. Thus, 6043 (the 2-methoxybenzyl analog of ambenonium) in a dose 10 times that of ambenonium produced about 4 times as rapid recovery as the latter. Compound 7502, which has the 2-chlorobenzyl radical but not the bilateral diethylamino configuration of ambenonium, is effective in restoring the response of the muscle to indirect stimulation, but in a dose twice that of 6043 and 20 times that of ambenonium. The other 3 compounds in Table 9 all contain propyl, instead of ethyl, chains be-

Table 10. *Musculotropic compounds as adjuncts to atropine sulfate (2 mg/kg, i.v.), both compounds being given 2 min before poisoning, in preventing death in rabbits given Sarin intravenously*

Adjunct	I. V. dose (mg/kg)	I. V. LD50 of Sarin (μg/kg)
None.	—	30
Benzylatropinium chloride . .	2.0	45
Gallamine triethiodide	0.25	60
d-Tubocurarine chloride . . .	0.13	38
Benzoquinonium chloride . . .	0.005	60
Ambenonium chloride	0.025	90
6043[1]	0.125	60
7502[1]	1.0	79
6277[1]	0.5	90

[1] See Table 9 for identification of this compound.

WILLS, unpublished.

tween the quaternary heads and the oxamide nucleus. Here, the compound with the benzyl radical (5372) seems to be slightly more rapidly effective than the one with the 2-chlorobenzyl radical (6277). The compound with 3-chlorobenzyl-pyrrolidinium quaternary heads in place of ammonium ones was as rapidly active as any compound tested.

The most interesting point in Table 9 is that 6043 is slightly more rapidly acting than 6277, but is known to be less potent as a ChE inhibitor, as an antagonist to d-tubocurarine, and as a relaxant of skeletal muscle. Three measures of affinity for functional systems in muscle indicate, therefore, that 6277 is more musculotropic than 6043; yet 6043 has a more rapid effect in restoring transmission of nerve stimulation to muscle than 6277. KARCZMAR (1957) found that 6043 sensitizes to ACh without appreciable anti-ChE effect. It may be that the rapid recovery of the twitch response induced by some of the oxamide derivatives in Table 9 (ambenonium and subsequent compounds in the table) depends on this ability to sensitize the muscle previously desensitized by the ACh accumulated subsequent to inhibition of AChE.

To study the effectiveness of musculotropic drugs as adjuncts to atropine in prophylaxis of poisoning by Sarin, the dose of drug that could be injected intravenously into rabbits without obvious incapacitation was injected intravenously along with 2 mg/kg of atropine SO_4 into groups of rabbits 2 minutes before intravenous injections of graded doses of Sarin. An estimate of the LD_{50} for Sarin with each prophylactic regimen was obtained; some results are given in Table 10. These show that the most effective of the adjuncts studied are capable of increasing the protective efficacy of atropine sulfate alone by only three-fold. This is similar to the benefit found with the *bis*quaternary amines (Table 7).

F. Centrally acting drugs

Effects of the anti-ChE compounds on the central apparatus of respiration and on several other functions of the central nervous system have been mentioned previously. An interesting effect seen in laboratory animals is the compulsive turning ("adversive syndrome") induced by injection of an anti-ChE agent into one carotid artery (FREEDMAN and HIMWICH 1949).

I. Anticholinergic drugs

Atropine and other predominantly anticholinergic compounds have been found by most investigators to antagonize the effects of anti-ChE agents on the central respiratory apparatus (GESELL and HANSEN 1943, SALLÉ 1950, KRIVOY et al. 1951, DOUGLAS and MATTHEWS 1952, WRIGHT 1954, ERDMANN, KEMPE and LÜHNING 1955, PAULET 1956), on preconvulsive and convulsive phenomena (GROB et al. 1947, WESCOE et al. 1948, FREEDMAN et al. 1949, ESSIG et al. 1950, SALLÉ 1950, HIM-WICH et al. 1950, DOUGLAS and MATTHEWS 1952, BRADLEY et al. 1953, ERDMANN, DUENSING and SCHAEFFER 1955, RINALDI and HIMWICH 1955a, b, c), on reflex activities (BÜLBRING and BURN 1941, ERDMANN, DUENSING and SCHAEFFER 1955, SCHAEFFER 1955), and on the adversive syndrome (FREEDMAN and HIMWICH 1949, DIAMANT 1954, NATHAN et al. 1955).

The reviewer's laboratory has studied about 40 compounds, most of which were anti-cholinergic drugs, for ability to speed return of the knee-jerk reflex following its abolition after intramuscular injection of 800 μg/kg of Sarin into the cat anesthetized with sodium pento-barbital (WILLS, unpubl.). Atropine, although it had some effectiveness in shortening the recovery time of the knee-jerk (from a mean of 41 to one of 30 min), was not especially active in this regard, in agreement with previous findings (ERDMANN, DUENSING and SCHAEFFER 1955, SCHAEFFER 1955). More effective was d-hyoscyamine camphor sulfonate; still more effective were Amethone, benactyzine, D-2 (2,2-diphenyl-4-dimethylaminomethyl-1,3-di-oxolane), 6371 [2-N-(2-chloro-2-butenyl)-N-(2-dimethylaminoethyl)-aminopiperidine], 8350 [1-(5-methyl-3-phenylhexyl) piperidine] and 6724 (1,1-dimethyl-2-dimethyl-aminoethyl diphenylacetate). The most active of these drugs reduced the recovery time for the knee-jerk to about 6 min. The compounds mentioned above were given i.v. in a dose of 2 mg/kg, except that doses of up to 4 mg/kg of atropine SO$_4$ were administered. With atropine, the dose made very little difference within the range from 1 to 4 mg/kg; for benactyzine, however, increasing the dose from 1 to 2 mg/kg shortened the recovery time of the knee-jerk to 1/5 of its value with the lower dose. Morphine (1 mg/kg, i.v.) was found to prolong the recovery time of the knee-jerk.

When a medullary reflex was studied by recording the contraction of the diaphragm in response to interruption of artificial ventilation in an anesthetized (sodium pentobarbital) cat with open chest, i.v. injection of 50 μg/kg of Sarin was found to change the response from a smooth inspiratory apneusis to a series of brief, repetitive contractions of the diaphragm. Intravenous injection of 2 mg/kg of atropine sulfate at 2 min after the injection of Sarin aborted the repetitive response seen after Sarin alone.

Intravenous injection of 2 mg/kg doses of three compounds found to be more active than atropine in antagonizing the action of Sarin on the knee-jerk disclosed no activity against the action of Sarin on this medullary reflex greater than that of atropine itself. Drugs tested in this way include N-benzhydryl-tropylamine binoxalate, benzhexol, and diethazine, the first approaching the closest to atropine in activity. Thus, atropine is effective in antagonizing the effects of anti-ChE compounds on the medullary respiratory mechanisms, but is not particularly effective in antagonizing the actions of these compounds on spinal reflexes, such as the knee-jerk.

HIMWICH and his associates (1952, unpubl.) studied a group of synthetic anticholinergic compounds for their ability to stop the adversive syndrome in rabbits after unilateral intracarotid injection of DFP. The most effective compounds were 8315 (1-methyl-4-α-propylbenzylidene piperidine), 6456 (1-methyl-α,α-diphenyl-2-piperidine-butyronitrile), 4607 (3-quinuclidinyl benzilate), 4608 (3-quinuclidinyl diphenylacetate), and benzhexol. By means of the inverse matrix (FISHER 1950), the correlation coefficient and the multiple correlation coefficients between the prophylactic values of 35 compounds against death following intravenous injection of Sarin and their therapeutic values against the adversive syndrome were calculated. All coefficients were found to lie between 0.32 and 0.47; this indicates that there is no significant relation between the ability of a compound to abort compulsive turning and its ability to combat the lethal effects of an anti-ChE agent.

Table 11. *The adjunctive effectiveness in preventing death in rabbits from intravenous injections of the indicated doses of Sarin of centrally-active compounds injected intravenously with 2 mg/kg of atropine sulfate 2 min before poisoning*

Adjunct and Dose (i. v.)	Mortality	
	30 μg/kg	60 μg/kg
None.	3/6	6/6
Atropine sulfate (2 mg/kg) . .	3/6	5/6
Benactyzine (2 mg/kg)	0/6	1/6
Benzhexol (2 mg/kg)	4/6	—
Diethazine (2 mg/kg)	0/6	5/6
6371[1] (5 mg/kg)	4/6	—

[1] 2-N-(2-chloro-2-butenyl)-N-(2-dimethylaminoethyl) amino piperidine.

WILLS, unpublished.

Table 11 shows the effectiveness of some of the compounds mentioned in this section as adjuncts to atropine in preserving life in rabbits given Sarin i.v. Of the 4 compounds in this table, only diethazine and benactyzine appear to be adjunctive. The greater effectiveness of the latter might be related to its powerful depressant action on the reticular formation (HIMWICH and RINALDI 1957), although benzhexol also is a potent depressant of the arousal reaction (STUMPF 1957).

II. Antihistaminic and antiepileptic drugs

SCHIFF et al. (1950) reported that the adversive syndrome in rabbits can be terminated by injection of 5 mg/kg, i.v., of dimenhydrinate. In similar experiments, JOHNS and HIMWICH (1950) found that diphenhydramide, dimenhydrinate, and promethazine were more active than tripelennamine, antazoline, mepyramine, phenindamine, or chlorprophenpyridamine. HIMWICH and associates (1952, unpubl.) found that prophenpyridamine had about the same activity as phenindamine. DIAMANT (1954) compared a group of phenothiazine derivatives, including ethopropazine, with diphenhydramine and dimenhydrinate for efficacy against the adversive syndrome induced by Tabun. He found the phenothiazine derivatives studied to be more effective than diphenhydramine and dimenhydrinate, and to be approximately as active as atropine. The centrally acting muscular relaxant, mephenesin, was found to be completely inactive in a dose of 100 mg/kg, i.v. HIMWICH et al. (1952, unpubl.) found that neither barbiturates (phenobarbital and methylphenobarbital) or anticonvulsants (phenytoin, phenacemide, mephenytoin, trimethadione and paramethadione) are capable of either preventing or aborting compulsive turning. Although the barbiturates may produce prostration, the animal turns until prostrated; upon recovery of mobility, it turns again in the same direction as before.

Table 12 shows the adjunctive values of representatives of the types of compound discussed in this section when given along with atropine in the prophylaxis of mortality induced by i.v. injection of Sarin. The most potent of these adjuncts are chlorpromazine and sodium pentobarbital. The antiepileptic drugs have little, if any, value in increasing the effectiveness of drug prophylaxis of anti-ChE poisoning. The mixture of atropine sulfate and chlorpromazine shown in the table raises the intravenous LD_{50} of Sarin for the rabbit to about 150 μg/kg, which is

Table 12. *Adjunctive effectiveness, when given by the indicated routes in the indicated doses, of various compounds administered with atropine sulfate (2 mg/kg, i.v.) before intravenous injection into rabbits of the indicated doses of Sarin*

	Route	Dose	Mortality		
			30 μg/kg	60 μ/kg	90 μg/kg
None	—	—	3/6	6/6	—
Mepazine.	I.V.	2 mg/kg	1/6	5/6	—
Chlorpromazine	I.V.	2 mg/kg	1/6	6/6	—
Chlorpromazine	I.V.	4 mg/kg	0/6	1/6	1/6
8297[1]	I.V.	4 mg/kg	0/6	5/6	6/6
Na pentobarbital	I.V.	15 mg/kg	0/6	0/6	6/6
Na phenytoin.	P.O.[2]	50 mg/kg	6/6	—	—
Trimethadione	P.O.[2]	300 mg/kg	6/6	—	—
Paramethadione	P.O.[2]	150 mg/kg	3/6	—	—

[1] Diethylaminoethyl-10-phenothiazine carboxylate.
[2] Given 30 min prior to intravenous injection of Sarin. Atropine and other intravenously administered drugs given 2 min before injection of Sarin in all experiments.

WILLS, unpublished.

nearly 10 times the normal value. This is a considerably greater increase than can be effected with even a large dose of atropine alone. Thus, the adjunctive effect of chlorpromazine to atropine in these experiments can not depend simply upon the addition of more atropine-like activity. It is possible that the lowered metabolism established by chlorpromazine plays an important role in its adjunctive capacity; the addition of sodium pentobarbital to the mixture of atropine and chlorpromazine raises still higher the intravenous LD_{50} of Sarin, to about 210 μg/kg.

III. Analeptic drugs

One important effect of anti-ChE compounds has been known to be a central stimulation of respiration followed by paralysis of the respiratory center (HEUBNER 1905), associated with transitory hypertension followed by hypotension (KOBERT 1886, STEWART and ROGOFF 1921). Sympathomimetic amines other than epinephrine and norepinephrine were known to stimulate the respiratory center (ALTSCHULE and IGLAUER 1940); sympathomimetic amines in general induce marked increases in blood pressure (OLIVER and SCHÄFER 1895, GUNN 1939). On this basis a sympathomimetic amine, 1-(4-hydroxyphenyl)-2-methylaminoethanol (Sympatol), was a component of the "BS Solution" supplied to the German Army during World War II for treatment of anti-ChE poisoning.

Other respiratory stimulants have been studied also. For instance, nikethamide (Coramine) has been reported (DI STEFANO et al. 1951) to increase by six-fold the LD_{50} of ethyl-p-nitrophenyl-thionobenzenephosphonate (EPN) in female rats treated with atropine also. In male rats, nikethamide increased the LD_{50} of EPN by less than twice. ROSENBERG and COON (1960) found that nikethamide was an effective adjunct to atropine in treating poisoning by EPN in the female guinea pig also, and had a detectable adjunctive effect in the female mouse. Nikethamide was inactive as an adjunct to atropine in preventing death or prolonging survival among female mice poisoned with DFP, OMPA, Parathion, or TEPP, and among female rats poisoned with any of these 4 compounds or physostigmine. Nikethamide injected alone into female rats 90 min prior to oral administration of EPN in corn oil was equally as protective against EPN as a mixture of atropine and nikethamide injected immediately after the oral administration of EPN. Metabolites of nikethamide, nicotinamide and N'-methylnicotinamide, also were effective adjuncts to atropine in treating poisoning by EPN. Nicotinamide exerted some protection against DFP, OMPA, Parathion, and TEPP also.

The results of these experiments of ROSENBERG and COON show apparently that the adjunctive effect of nikethamide against EPN is not dependent upon the analeptic molecule but resides in simpler molecules, such as nicotinic acid and nicotinamide. ROSENBERG and COON found further that 6-aminonicotinamide, a potent competitor with nicotinamide for union with pentose in the formation of DPN and TPN, enhanced, instead of decreasing, the protective activity of nicotinamide when the two compounds were administered simultaneously; alone, the 6-amino compound prolonged survival time. This experiment seems to show clearly that the protective action of nicotinamide against anti-ChE poisoning is a direct action of some sort, not related to the usual metabolic role of the compound. The effectiveness of nicotinamide against DFP, OMPA, Parathion, and TEPP, compounds not antagonized by nikethamide, may indicate that the rate and extent of metabolic conversion of the last molecule into the first are important factors in the effectiveness of nikethamide against various organophosphorus anti-ChE agents. The protective effect of nicotinamide may be related to WILSON's (1952) finding that this molecule is capable of reactivating ChE inhibited by TEPP *in vitro*; ROSENBERG and COON have found that nicotinamide protects ChE in brain, spinal cord, heart, lung, diaphragm, intercostal muscle, RBC, and blood plasma from inhibition by EPN *in vivo*.

The author's laboratory has studied the values of several hypertensive (e.g., ephedrine, naphazoline, and paredrine) and respiratory stimulant compounds (e.g., pentylenetetrazol) as adjuncts to atropine in treating organophosphorus anti-ChE poisoning in the anesthetized (sodium pentobarbital) dog. When atropine was supplemented by respiratory stimulants or hypertensive agents, the most effective adjuncts were pentylenetetrazol and ephedrine. The most effective of a group of hypertensive agents as an adjunct to a mixture of atropine and pentylenetetrazol was ephedrine. Supplementation of a mixture of atropine SO_4 (0.5 mg/kg, i.v.), pentylenetetrazol (50 mg/kg, i.v.), and ephedrine HCl (2.5 mg/kg, i.v.) by other hypertensive compounds or respiratory stimulants decreased rather than improved therapeutic effectiveness.

If administration of atropine alone to anesthetized dogs poisoned severely with organophosphorus anti-ChE agents nearly sufficed to restore effective spontaneous respiration, administration of a mixture of ephedrine and pentylenetetrazol would institute effective cyclic respiration lasting for at least several hours. If, on the other hand, i.v. injection of atropine produced only a few feeble respiratory efforts, administration of the ephedrine-pentylenetetrazol mixture did not induce spontaneous respiration of any useful duration. Analeptic compounds appear, therefore, to play a fairly small role in the chemical treatment of poisoning by anti-ChE compounds; certainly, the initiation of effective artificial ventilation is a much more life-saving procedure that the administration of an analeptic drug or mixture. Atropine administration facilitates artificial ventilation by stopping secretion by the glands of the mouth and upper respiratory tract.

G. Chemicals that prevent ACh synthesis and release

If the toxic effects of the anti-ChE agents are caused primarily by accumulation of ACh, any material that would lessen this accumulation should improve the condition of the poisoned subject. There are two general approaches to the desired end: reduction of synthesis of ACh by neural tissue and reduction of its release.

I. Chemicals that reduce the synthesis of ACh by neural tissue

Many compounds are known to inhibit the ChAc system that is concerned in the synthesis of ACh in neural tissue (REISBERG 1957). One of the most active compounds *in vitro* is copper sulfate; other inhibitors of the sulfhydryl group are active also. Other compounds reported to be effective *in vitro* are flavonoids (BEILER et al. 1950), dibenamine and vitamin K_2 (KUMOGAI et al. 1953), physostigmine and neostigmine (SHELLEY 1956), hemicholinium-3 (α,α-dimethylethanolamino-4,4'-biacetophenone) (MacINTOSH et al. 1956) and mecamylamine (MICHEL et al. 1959, unpubl.). DESMEDT (1958) reported that hemicholinium-3, injected into a cat in a dose of 1.5 mg/kg, i.v., had no effect on the response of skeletal muscle to stimulation of its motor nerve until the nerve had been stimulated repetitively for sufficiently long to deplete the stock of preformed ACh. After faradization, there was a brief facilitation of the muscle's contraction followed by a "post-tetanic exhaustion" lasting for about 15 minutes.

These effects of hemicholinium-3 *in vivo* encouraged the reviewer's laboratory to study six compounds of the same group as antagonists of the neuromuscular block induced by large doses of Sarin. Hemicholinium-3, in a dose of 0.05 to 0.1 mg/kg, i.v., prolonged slightly the times for recovery of the twitch response to 50 and 85% of its original value after inhibition by Sarin. The only hemicholinium with any beneficial effect was N^{21}-diethyl, N^{21}-benzyl-N^1-(α-diethylamino-*p*-phenylene-dimethylene) eicosakis [diethyl (*p*-phenylene-dimethylene)]-heneicosakis (ammonium bromide). This compound, in a dose of 0.5 to 2.0 mg/kg, i.v., reduced to an average of 8.1 min the recovery time of the twitch response to 50% of its original value, from the mean of 19.6 min for spontaneous recovery (Table 9). After treatment with this compound, however, the twitch response never exceeded about 80% of its original magnitude and then regressed. Repetition of the dose of hemicholinium did not improve the response of the muscle to stimulation of its motor nerve.

One of the most active inhibitors of ChAc among the flavonoids studied by BEILER et al. (1950) was morin (2',3,4',5,7-pentahydroxyflavone). This compound has been studied by BALOTIN and COON (1960) as an antagonist to the lethal effects of TEPP, both alone and with atropine sulfate. Injected into mice in a dose of 50 mg/kg, i.p., in an oil-in-water emulsion, morin alone raised the LD_{50} dose of TEPP by an insignificant amount; atropine alone in the dose employed did not alter the LD_{50} dose of TEPP. A mixture of atropine and morin elevated the LD_{50} dose of TEPP by about 30%. In atropinized, anesthetized (sodium pentobarbital) rats, morin sustained respiration, suppressed muscular fasciculation and increased by nearly two-fold the mean survival time. Morin antagonized also the actions of TEPP on the isolated frog heart and the isolated rabbit ileum, but did not combat the effects of ACh on these organs.

Thus, results with one hemicholinium compound and morin indicate that compounds which interfere with synthesis of ACh may have some effectiveness as antagonists to the lethal actions of anti-ChE agents. The benefits seen thus far from such compounds are modest, but more effective chemicals of this functional type may be found.

II. Chemicals that reduce the release of ACh by neural tissue

Any chemical that blocks transmission of the excitation wave in the small preterminal nerve fibers near a neuro-effector junction presumably would prevent release of ACh or other transmitter substance by the neural components of the junction; local anesthetics and botulinum toxin are known particularly to possess this activity. The local anesthetics act upon any type of nerve, but this effect of botulinum toxin is restricted to cholinergic nerves (AMBACHE 1949). The prophylactic and therapeutic values of local anesthetics have been discussed previously in this chapter (D-II). Addition of 1 mg/kg of dibucaine to an atropine-oxime mixture, that alone saved one of six rabbits from death following administration of 10 LD_{50} doses of an anti-ChE agent, saved three of a similar group when given before the anti-ChE agent, and all six when the drug mixture was given after the anti-ChE compound (BAY 1959, unpubl.).

It has been reported that botulinum toxin prevents release of ACh by motor nerves (GUYTON and MacDONALD 1947, BURGEN et al. 1949), and that it does this neither by affecting the synthesis of ACh (BURGEN et al. 1949, STEVENSON and GIRVIN 1953) nor by inactivating the ACh-release mechanism *per se* (BROOKS 1954). However, its effect on the neuromuscular junction is not antagonized by eserine, neostigmine, or TEPP (EDMUNDS and KEIPER 1924, GUYTON and MacDONALD 1947, BURGEN et al. 1949). Conversely, botulinum toxin had no useful antagonistic effect in experimental poisoning by Parathion (WOODARD 1952, unpubl.) or Sarin.

GIOIA and MORPURGO (1958) have reported a series of substituted biphenylacetic acids that reduce markedly the release of ACh and block stimulation of guinea pig ileum *in vitro* by eserine, neostigmine, or pyridostigmine; they do not block stimulation by ACh. Apparently, this group of compounds has not been studied *in vivo* as antagonists to lethal effects of anti-ChE agents.

H. Chemicals that reactivate phosphorylated ChE's

So long as the organophosphorus anti-ChE agents were considered to be irreversible inhibitors or inactivators of ChE's, there seemed to be no possibility of specific therapy for intoxication by these compounds. With the reversible inhibitors, time alone was needed to terminate their effects. WILSON (1951) and HOBBIGER (1951) first showed that ChE's inhibited by certain organophosphorus anti-ChE agents can be reactivated slowly by water. More rapid reactivation is obtained with hydroxylamine and choline (WILSON 1951). The development of more effective reactivators and their properties are described in Chapter 21; only a few points pertinent to the present subject will be discussed here.

Oximes of the monoquaternary (e.g., P-2-AM) or the *bis*quaternary (e.g., TMB-4) types are the most potent reactivators now known. These two types of oximes are also the most effective chemical adjuncts to atropine in the treatment of organophosphorus anti-ChE poisoning. For example, 5 dogs poisoned by subcutaneous injection of Sarin and then treated, when the signs of poisoning became severe, by i.v. injection of a mixture containing 1 mg/kg of atropine sulfate, 7.5 mg/kg of P-2-AM and 7.5 mg/kg of TMB-4 Cl survived 70 LD_{50} doses of Sarin. The same treatment in dogs poisoned with 70 LD_{50} of Tabun saved 4 of the group of 5 animals (O'LEARY 1960, unpubl.). No other type of adjunct to atropine has a therapeutic effect which approaches this magnitude.

Evidence has been presented recently (WILLS 1959) that the monoquaternary type of oxime has its major effect at the neuromuscular junction. One of this group of oximes (P-2-AM) has been found to produce functional effects that are interpretable as arising from an immediate depolarization at the neuromuscular junction (WILLS et al. 1959), and also to produce a slowly developing decrement in the response of skeletal muscle to electrical stimulation of its motor nerve. This latter effect may be an indication of a slowly developing competitive desensitization of the neuromuscular junction to ACh, similar to the immediate effect of the *bis*quaternary oxime TMB-4 (BAY 1959). The tertiary oxime DAM also has been reported to resemble d-tubocurarine in its effects on the response of skeletal muscle to stimulation (EDERY 1959).

The actions of the oximes to desensitize muscle to ACh could be an important facet of their activity at the neuromuscular junction; the more rapid action of TMB-4 than of P-2-AM in overcoming lethal effects of Sarin (BAY et al. 1958) fits qualitatively the findings mentioned above, that TMB-4 has an immediate desensitizing effect whereas P-2-AM has a more delayed one. The ability of the oximes to reactivate inhibited ChE's may relate also to their effectiveness as antagonists to paralysis of neuromuscular transmission. By comparison of the illustrations in two of KOELLE's papers, it seems that P-2-AM is a more potent reactivator *in vivo* of AChE inhibited by DFP (KOELLE 1957) than is either MINA or DAM (RAJAPURKAR and KOELLE 1958). Although the quaternary oximes reactivate AChE *in vivo* in ganglia as well as in muscle (KOELLE 1957, RAJAPURKAR and KOELLE 1958) and in blood (HOBBIGER and SADLER 1959, WILLS 1959), they produce no significant reactivation of AChE in brain (HOBBIGER and SADLER 1959, WILLS 1959), nor do they antagonize significantly the toxic effects of anti-ChE agents on brain functions (SAKAI et al. 1958, WILLS and BORISON 1959, BROWN 1960). This is true especially of the quaternized oximes; DAM in an i.v. dose greater than about 60 mg/kg does exert a definite, but small, antagonism to the effects of Sarin on medullary function in the cat (WILLS and BORISON 1959, unpubl.) Furthermore, DAM in an intravenous dose of 60 mg/kg in the rat induced within 90 min reactivation of 9% of the AChE of brain inhibited by Sarin; TMB-4 in a parallel experiment caused reactivation of only about 2% of the inhibited AChE (FLEISHER et al. 1960).

It should be noted that none of the usable reactivators of phosphorylated ChE's known today has a striking effect *in vivo* on phosphorylated ChE of brain, so that any anti-ChE compound having important cerebral effects will probably require the adjunctive use of atropine for its central effects. The greater the action of the anti-ChE agent on neuromuscular junctions, the more important is the use of a quaternary oxime in conjunction with atropine in the therapy of the intoxication.

If the anti-ChE agent has important non-specific effects, i.e., effects not related to inhibition of ChE's, neither atropine nor oximes nor any of the other substitutes or adjuncts for atropine mentioned in this chapter will necessarily constitute effective therapy. Nothing is known about methods for treating the non-specific effects of the anti-ChE compounds; this is an important field for investigation, because chemicals are now known that have such effects as their principal mechanisms of intoxication. Some of the non-specific actions are discussed in detail in Chapter 18. If what has been said in this paragraph and in Chapter 18 arouses an interest in developing antagonists for the non-specific actions of anti-ChE compounds, this may lead to an important forward step in the prevention of fatality and possible crippling or other persistent incapacitation by certain of these compounds.

Literature

AESCHLIMANN, J. A., and M. REINERT: The pharmacological action of some analogues of physostigmine. J. Pharmacol. exp. Ther. **43**, 413—444 (1931).

AKOPYAN, N. E., and V. M. SAMVELYAN: Relationship between local anesthetic, cholinolytic and anticholinesterase activity of benzoic acid esters (in Russian). Farmakol. i Toksikol. **21**, No. 5, 38—42 (1958).

ALTSCHULE, M. D., and A. IGLAUER: The effect of benzedrine and paredrine on the circulation, metabolism and respiration in normal man. J. clin. Invest. **19**, 497—502 (1940).

AMBACHE, N.: The peripheral action of Clostridium botulinum toxin. J. Physiol. (Lond.) **108**, 127—141 (1949).

ARNOW, L. E.: Colorimetric determination of the components of 3,4-dihydroxyphenylalanine-tyrosine mixtures. J. biol. Chem. **118**, 531—537 (1937).

ASKEW, B. M.: Oximes and hydroxamic acids as antidotes in anticholinesterase poisoning. Brit. J. Pharmacol. **11**, 417—423 (1956).

— Oximes and atropine in sarin poisoning. Brit. J. Pharmacol. **12**, 340—343 (1957).

ATANACKOVIC, D., and S. DALGAARD-MIKKELSEN: Contributions à la pharmacologie de la procaine. Arch. int. Pharmacodyn. **85**, 1—16 (1951).

AUGUSTINSSON, K.-B.: Reaction of organophosphorus compounds with dihydroxyphenyl derivatives. Acta chem. scand. **6**, 959—961 (1952).

— Enzyme studies with diethyl-p-nitrophenylphosphate (Mintacol). Acta pharmacol. (Kbh.) **9**, 245—252 (1953a).

— Biochemical studies with tabun and allied compounds. Ark. Kemi. **6**, 331—350 (1953b).

—, and M. GRAHN: Protection of cholinesterases by procaine against inactivation by tabun in vitro. Acta physiol. scand. **27**, 10—17 (1952).

—, and D. NACHMANSOHN: Studies on cholinesterase. VI. Kinetics of the inhibition of acetylcholine esterase. J. biol. Chem. **179**, 543—559 (1949).

AUSTIN, L., and D. R. DAVIES: The part played by inhibition of cholinesterases of the CNS in producing paralysis in chickens. Brit. J. Pharmacol. **9**, 145—152 (1954).

BALOTIN, N. M., and J. M. COON: The antagonism of some actions of TEPP by morin. Arch. int. Pharmacodyn. **123**, 395—405 (1960).

BARNES, J. M.: The reactions of rabbits to poisoning by p-nitrophenyldiethylphosphate (E600). Brit. J. Pharmacol. **8**, 208—211 (1953).

—, and F. A. DENZ: Experimental demyelination with organophosphorus compounds. J. Path. Bact. **65**, 597—605 (1953).

BAY, E.: Pharmacodynamics of 1,1'trimethylene bis (4-formylpyridinium bromide) dioxime (TMB-4). Fed. Proc. **18**, 366 (1959).

— S. KROP and L. F. YATES: Chemotherapeutic effectiveness of 1,1'-trimethylene bis (4-formyl-pyridinium bromide) dioxime (TMB-4) in experimental anticholinesterase poisoning. Proc. Soc. exp. Biol. (N. Y.) **98**, 107—110 (1958).

BAYLISS, B. J., J. ELKES, S. G. SPANNER and A. TODRICK: The effect of DFP on the sensitivity of rats to centrally-acting drugs. Brit. J. Pharmacol. **12**, 536—539 (1957).

BEILER, J. M., R. BRENDEL, M. GRAFF and G. J. MARTIN: Effect of vitamin P compounds on choline acetylase. Arch. Biochem. **26**, 72—76 (1950).

BERRY, W. K., K. P. FELLOWES, P. J. FRASER, J. P. RUTLAND and A. TODRICK: The in vitro protection of cholinesterases against some organophosphorus inhibitors. Biochem. J. **59**, 1—5 (1955).

BHATTACHARYA, B. K.: Antispasmodic properties of certain quaternary derivatives of 2,2-diphenyl-4-diisopropylamino-butyramide and other compounds in the isolated perfused guinea pig lung. Arch. int. Pharmacodyn. **104**, 285—292 (1956).

—, and D. ATANACKOVIC: On the pharmacology of procaine and its antagonists on the bronchial musculature. Arch. int. Pharmacodyn. **104**, 275—284 (1956).

BIDSTRUP, P. L., J. A. BONNELL and A. G. BECKETT: Paralysis following poisoning by a new organic phosphorus insecticide (mipafox): report on two cases. Brit. med. J. **1953I**, 1068—1072.

BLANK, I. H., R. D. GRIESEMER and E. GOULD: The penetration of an anticholinesterase agent (sarin) into skin. I. Rate of penetration into excised human skin. J. invest. Derm. **29**, 299—309 (1957).

— — — The penetration of an anticholinesterase agent (sarin) into skin. II. Autoradiographic studies. J. invest. Derm. **30**, 187—191 (1958).

BRADLEY, P. B., S. CERQUIGLINI and J. ELKES: Some effects of diisopropylfluorophosphate on the electrical activity of the brain of the cat. J. Physiol. (Lond.) **121**, 51P—52P (1953).

BROOKS, V. B.: The action of botulinum toxin on motor-nerve filaments. J. Physiol. (Lond.) **123**, 501—515 (1954).

Brown, R. V.: The effects of intracisternal sarin and pyridine-2-aldoxime methyl methanesulfonate in anesthetized dogs. Brit. J. Pharmacol. 15, 170—174 (1960).

Bülbring, E., and J. H. Burn: Observations bearing on synaptic transmission by acetylcholine in the spinal cord. J. Physiol. (Lond.) 100, 337—368 (1941).

Burgen, A. S. V., F. Dickens and L. J. Zatman: The action of botulinum toxin on the neuromuscular junction. J. Physiol. (Lond.) 109, 10—24 (1949).

— C. A. Keele, M. Chennells, J. delCastillo, W. F. Floyd, D. Slome and S. Wright: Physiological effects of alkyl polyphosphates. Nature (Lond.) 160, 760—761 (1947).

— — and D. Slome: Pharmacological actions of tetraethylpyrophosphate and hexaethyltetraphosphate. J. Pharmacol. exp. Ther. 96, 396—409 (1949).

Calma, I.: Observations on the action of prostigmine on the spinal cord of the cat. J. Physiol. (Lond.) 108, 282—291 (1949).

Candole, C. A. de, W. W. Douglas, C. L. Evans, R. Holmes, K. E. v. Spencer, R. W. Torrance and K. M. Wilson: The failure of respiration in death by anticholinesterase poisoning. Brit. J. Pharmacol. 8, 466—475 (1953).

—, and M. K. McPhail: Sarin and paraoxon antagonism in different species. Canad. J. Biochem. 35, 1071—1083 (1957).

Cavanagh, J. B., and R. H. S. Thompson: Demyelination. Brit. med. Bull. 10, 47—51 (1954).

Chasanov, M. G., and J. Epstein: Ion exchange resins as catalysts in the decomposition of sarin. J. Polym. Sci. 31, 399—414 (1958).

Childs, A. F., D. R. Davies, A. L. Green and J. P. Rutland: The reactivation by oximes and hydroxamic acids of cholinesterase inhibited by organophosphorus compounds. Brit. J. Pharmacol. 10, 462—465 (1955).

Cohen, J. A., and C. H. Posthumus: The mechanism of action of anticholinesterases. Acta physiol. pharmacol. neerl. 4, 17—36 (1955).

— M. G. P. J. Warringa and B. R. Bovens: Protection of true cholinesterase against DFP by butyrylcholine. Biochim. biophys. Acta 6, 469—476 (1951).

Collomp, J.: Les trilons. Bull. d'Inf. Tech. Sci. No. 23/G, 1 (1949).

Couetney, R. C., R. L. Gustafson, S. J. Westerback, H. Hyytiäinen, S. C. Chaberek, jr. and A. E. Martell: Metal chelate compounds as catalysts in the hydrolysis of isopropyl methylphosphonofluoridate and diisopropylphosphorofluoridate. J. Amer. chem. Soc. 79, 3030—3036 (1957).

Cullumbine, H., and P. Dirnhuber: Oral and bronchial fluids in poisoning with anticholinesterases. J. Pharm. (Lond.) 7, 580—585 (1955).

Dahlbom, R., H. Diamant, T. Edlund, T. Ekstrand and B. Holmstedt: Protective effect of phenothiazine derivatives against poisoning by the irreversible cholinesterase inhibitor dimethylamidoethoxy-phosphoryl cyanide (tabun). Acta pharmacol. (Kbh.) 9, 163—167 (1953).

Dale, H. H.: The action of certain esters and ethers of choline and their relation to muscarine. J. Pharmacol. 6, 147—190 (1914).

Davies, D. R., A. L. Green and G. L. Willey: 2-hydroxyiminomethyl-N-methylpyridinium methanesulfonate and atropine in the treatment of severe organophosphate poisoning. Brit. J. Pharmacol. 14, 5—8 (1959).

Davison, A. N.: The conversion of schradan (OMPA) and parathion into inhibitors of cholinesterase by mammalian liver. Biochem. J. 61, 203—209 (1955).

DeBurgh Daly, M.: The cardiovascular effects of anticholinesterases in the dog with special reference to hemodynamic changes in the pulmonary circulation. J. Physiol. (Lond.) 139, 250—272 (1957).

—, and P. G. Wright: The effects of anticholinesterases upon peripheral vascular resistance in the dog. J. Physiol. (Lond.) 133, 475—497 (1956).

Desmedt, J. E.: Myasthenic-like features of neuromuscular transmission after administration of an inhibitor of acetylcholine synthesis. Nature (Lond.) 182, 1673—1674 (1958).

Diamant, H.: Cholinesterase inhibitors and vestibular function. Acta otolaryng. (Stockh.) Suppl. 111, 1—84 (1954).

Dirnhuber, P., and H. Cullumbine: The effect of anticholinesterase agents on the rat's blood pressure. Brit. J. Pharmacol. 10, 12—15 (1955).

DiStefano, V., L. Hurwitz, W. F. Neuman and H. C. Hodge: Coramine (Nikethamide) as adjuvant to atropine in treatment of poisoning by EPN. Proc. Soc. exp. Biol. (N. Y.) 78, 712—713 (1951).

Dixon, W. E., and T. G. Brodie: Contributions to the physiology of the lungs. I. The bronchial muscles, their innervation and the action of drugs upon them. J. Physiol. (Lond.) 29, 97—173 (1903).

Douglas, W. W., and P. B. C. Matthews: Acute tetraethylpyrophosphate poisoning in cats and its modification by atropine or hyoscine. J. Physiol. (Lond.) 116, 202—218 (1952).

914   Literature

DOUGLAS, W. W., and W. D. M. PATON: The mechanisms of motor end-plate depolarization
    due to a cholinesterase-inhibiting drug. J. Physiol. (Lond.) **124**, 325—344 (1954).
DUBOIS, K. P., J. DOULL, P. R. SALERNO and J. M. COON: Studies on the toxicity and mecha-
    nism of action of p-nitrophenyl diethyl thionophosphate (parathion). J. Pharmacol. exp.
    Ther. **95**, 79—91 (1949).
DULTZ, L., M. A. EPSTEIN, G. FREEMAN, E. H. GRAY and W. B. WEIL: Studies on a group of
    oximes as therapeutic compounds in sarin poisoning. J. Pharmacol. exp. Ther. **119**,
    522—531 (1957).
DURHAM, W. F., T. B. GAINES and W. J. HAYES, jr.: Paralytic and related effects of certain
    organic phosphorus compounds. Arch. industr. Hlth. **13**, 326—330 (1956).
ECCLES, J. C., B. KATZ and S. W. KUFFLER: Effect of eserine on neuromuscular transmission.
    J. Neurophysiol. **5**, 211—230 (1942).
EDERY, H.: Effects of diacetyl monoxime on neuromuscular transmission. Brit. J. Pharmacol.
    14, 317—322 (1959).
EDMUNDS, C. W., and G. F. KEIPER: Further studies on the action of botulinus toxin. J. Amer.
    med. Ass. **83**, 495—501 (1924).
EICKSTEDT, K.-W. VON, W.-D. ERDMANN u. K.-P. SCHAEFER: Über die blutdrucksteigernde
    Wirkung von Esteraseblockern (E 605, eserin und prostigmin). Naunyn-Schmiedeberg's
    Arch. exp. Path. Pharmak. **226**, 435—441 (1955).
EMMELIN, N., and F. C. MACINTOSH: The release of acetylcholine from perfused sympathetic
    ganglia and skeletal muscles. J. Physiol. (Lond.) **131**, 477—496 (1956).
EPSTEIN, J.: Nerve gas in public water. Publ. Hlth. Rep. **71**, 955—962 (1956).
— M. M. DEMEK and D. H. ROSENBLATT: Reaction of paraoxon with hydrogen peroxide in
    dilute aqueous solution. J. org. Chem. **21**, 796—797 (1956).
—, and D. H. ROSENBLATT: Kinetics of some metal ion-catalyzed hydrolyses of isopropyl
    methylphosphonofluoridate (GB) at 25°. J. Amer. chem. Soc. **80**, 3596—3598 (1958).
— — and M. M. DEMEK: Kinetics of the reaction of isopropyl methylphosphonofluoridate
    with catechols at 25°. J. Amer. chem. Soc. **78**, 341—343 (1956).
EPSTEIN, M. A., and G. FREEMAN: Toxicity of hydroxamic acid analogues: prophylactic and
    therapeutic efficacy against nerve gas poisoning in mice. Proc. Soc. exp. Biol. (N. Y.) **92**,
    660—662 (1956).
ERDMANN, W.-D., F. DUENSING u. K.-P. SCHAEFFER: Zentralnervöse Wirkungen von E 605
    am Warmblüter. Naunyn-Schmiedeberg's Arch. exp. Path. Pharmak. **225**, 114—115 (1955).
— H. D. KEMPE u. W. LÜHNING: Über die Wirkung von Esteraseblockern (E605, Eserin und
    Prostigmin) auf das Atemzentrum von Katze und Hund. Naunyn-Schmiedeberg's Arch.
    exp. Path. Pharmak. **225**, 359—368 (1955).
—, and K. P. SCHAEFER: Über die Wirkung von Diäthylnitrophenylthiophosphat (E605) auf
    Rückenmarksreflexe an der Katze. Naunyn-Schmiedeberg's Arch. exp. Path. Pharmak.
    223, 519—532 (1954).
ESSIG, C. F., J. L. HAMPSON, P. D. BALES, A. WILLIS and H. E. HIMWICH: Effect of panparnit
    on brain wave changes induced by diisopropyl fluorophosphate (DFP). Science **111**, 38—39
    (1950).
EVANS, C. L.: Neuromuscular block by anticholinesterases. J. Physiol. (Lond.) **114**, 6P (1951).
FARQUHARSON, M. E., and R. G. JOHNSTON: Antagonism of the effects of tremorine by tropine
    derivatives. Brit. J. Pharmacol. **14**, 559—566 (1959).
FERGUSON, R. L., and S. D. SILVER: Demonstration in skin of active chlorine from chlorine-
    liberating ointments. Amer. J. clin. Path. **17**, 35—36 (1947).
FISHER, R. A.: Statistical methods for research workers, 11th ed. Edinburgh: Oliver and Boyd
    (1950). Section 29.
FLECKENSTEIN, A.: Der Kalium-Natrium-Austausch als Energieprinzip in Muskel und Nerv.
    Berlin-Göttingen-Heidelberg: Springer 1955.
FLEISHER, J. H., J. P. CORRIGAN and J. W. HOWARD: Potentiation of the response of frog
    rectus muscle to acetylcholine by isopropyl methyl phosphonofluoridate and its modifi-
    cation by pyridine-2-aldoxime methiodide. Brit. J. Pharmacol. **13**, 291—295 (1958).
— J. HANSA, P. J. KILLOS and C. S. HARRISON: Effects of 1,1'trimethylene bis (4-formyl-
    pyridinium bromide) dioxime (EA 1814) on cholinesterase activity and neuromuscular
    block in rats following poisoning with sarin and DFP. J. Pharmacol. exp. Ther. **130**,
    461—468 (1960).
FRASER, T. R.: An experimental research on the antagonism between the actions of physostigma
    and atropia. Trans. roy. Soc. Edinb. **26**, 529—713 (1870).
FREDRIKSSON, T.: Studies on the percutaneous absorption of sarin and two allied organo-
    phosphorus cholinesterase inhibitors. Acta derm.-venereol. (Stockh.) Suppl. **41**, 1—83
    (1958).
FREEDMAN, A. M., P. D. BALES, A. WILLIS and H. E. HIMWICH: Experimental production of
    electrical major convulsive patterns. Amer. J. Physiol. **156**, 117—124 (1949).

FREEDMANN, A. M., and H. E. HIMWICH: DFP: site of injection and variation in response. Amer. J. Physiol. **156**, 125—128 (1949).

FREEMAN, G., and M. A. EPSTEIN: Therapeutic factors in survival after lethal cholinesterase inhibition by phosphorus insecticides. New Engl. J. Med. **253**, 266—271 (1955).

GESELL, R., and J. S. FREY: Temporal summation of stimuli studied with the aid of anticholinesterases. Amer. J. Physiol. **160**, 375—384 (1950).

—, and E. T. HANSEN: Eserine, acetylcholine, atropine and nervous integration. Amer. J. Physiol. **139**, 371—385 (1943).

GHOSH, R., and J. F. NEWMAN: A new group of organophosphorus pesticides. Chem. Ind. 29 January 1955, 118.

GIOIA, A., and C. MORPURGO: Effect of inhibitors of choline acetylation on acetylcholine output and motility in response to anticholinesterases and to distension of the lumen of isolated guinea-pig ileum. Brit. J. Pharmacol. **13**, 467—470 (1958).

GOLDSTEIN, A.: The mechanism of enzyme-inhibitor-substrate reactions. Illustrated by the cholinesterase-physostigmine-acetylcholine system. J. gen. Physiol. **27**, 529—580 (1944).

GORDON, A. S., and C. W. FRYE: Large doses of atropine; low toxicity and effectiveness in anticholinesterase intoxication. J. Amer. med. Ass. **159**, 1181—1184 (1955).

GOSSELIN, R. E., J. D. GABOUREL and J. H. WILLS: The fate of atropine in man. Clin. Pharmacol. Therap. **1**, 597—603 (1960).

GREEN, A. L., G. L. SAINSBURY, B. SAVILLE and M. STANSFIELD: The reactivity of some active nucleophilic reagents with organophosphorus anticholinesterases. J. chem. Soc. **1958**, 1583—1587.

—, and B. SAVILLE: The reaction of oximes with isopropyl methylphosphonofluoridate (sarin). J. chem. Soc. **1956**, 3887—3892.

GREEN, R. E., E. A. McKAY and S. KROP: The action of DFP on the caliber of the bronchial tree in isolated lungs. Fed. Proc. **6**, 334 (1947).

GRIESEMER, R. D., I. H. BLANK and E. GOULD: The penetration of an anticholinesterase agent (sarin) into skin. III. A method for studying the rate of penetration into the skin of the living rabbit. J. invest. Derm. **31**, 255—258 (1958).

GROB, D.: Uses and hazards of the organic phosphate anticholinesterase compounds. Ann. intern. Med. **32**, 1229—1234 (1950).

— The manifestations and treatment of poisoning due to nerve gas and other organic phosphate anticholinesterase compounds. Arch. intern. Med. **98**, 221—239 (1956).

— W. L. GARLICK and A. McG. HARVEY: The toxic effects in man of the anticholinesterase insecticide parathion (p-nitropenyl diethyl thionophosphate). Bull. Johns Hopk. Hosp. **87**, 106—129 (1950).

—, and A. McG. HARVEY: Observations on the effects of tetraethyl pyrophosphate (TEPP) in man, and on its use in the treatment of myasthenia gravis. Bull. Johns Hopk. Hosp. **84**, 532—567 (1949).

— — The effects and treatment of nerve gas poisoning. Amer. J. Med. **14**, 52—63 (1953).

— — O. R. LANGWORTHY and J. L. LILIENTHAL, jr.: The administration of diisopropyl fluorophosphate (DFP) to man. III. Effect on the central nervous system with special reference to the electrical activity of the brain. Bull. Johns Hopk. Hosp. **81**, 257—266 (1947).

—, and R. J. JOHNS: Use of oximes in the treatment of intoxication by anticholinesterase compounds in normal subjects. Amer. J. Med. **24**, 497—511 (1958).

— J. L. LILIENTHAL, jr., A. M. HARVEY and B. F. JONES: The administration of diisopropyl fluorophosphate (DFP) to man. I. Effect on plasma and erythrocyte cholinesterase; general systemic effects; use in study of hepatic function and erythropoiesis; and some properties of plasma cholinesterase. Bull. Johns Hopk. Hosp. **81**, 217—244 (1947).

GROBLEWSKI, G. E., B. P. McNAMARA and J. H. WILLS: Stimulation of denervated muscle by DFP and related compounds. J. Pharmacol. **118**, 116—122 (1956).

GUYTON, A. C., and M. A. MacDONALD: Physiology of botulinus toxin. Arch. Neurol. Psychiat. (Chicago) **57**, 578—592 (1947).

GYERMEK, L.: Studies on cholinergic blocking substances. VII. Correlations between anticholinergic and cholinesterase-blocking effects. Acta Physiol. **8**, 43—48 (1955a).

— Studies on cholinergic blocking substances. VIII. Pharmacological actions of certain polymethylene bis- and azapentylene bis-pyrrolidine and piperidine derivatives. Acta Physiol. **8**, 49—60 (1955b).

HAASE, J., D. LÜCKE, F. SCHELER, R. SCHÜTZ, B. MÜHLBERG u. W. KOLL: Die Wirkung von Cholinesterasegiften auf Reflexsysteme der tiefspinalen Katze. Naunyn-Schmiedeberg's Arch. exp. Path. Pharmak. **232**, 274—276 (1957).

HACKLEY, B. E., jr., R. PLAPINGER, M. STOLBERG and T. WAGNER-JAUREGG: Acceleration of the hydrolysis of organic fluorophosphates and fluorophosphonates with hydroxamic acids. J. Amer. chem. Soc. **77**, 3651—3653 (1955).

HALEY, T. J.: Intracerebral injection of neostigmine and eserine in conscious mice. J. Amer. pharm. Ass. sci. Ed. **46**, 252—254 (1957).

HAZARD, R., E. CORTEGGIANI and J. CHEYMOL: Différenciation par la novocaine des effets dépresseurs de l'ésérine sur le coeur et de son action sensibilisante à l'acétylcholine. C. R. Acad. Sci. (Paris) **220**, 627—628 (1945).

HEUBNER, W.: Pharmakologisches und Chemisches über das Physostigmin. Naunyn-Schmiedeberg's Arch. exp. Path. Pharmak. **53**, 313—330 (1905).

HEYMANS, C., and J. JACOB: Sur la pharmacologie du di-isopropyl-fluorophosphonate (D.F.P.) et le rôle des cholinestérases. Arch. int. Pharmacodyn. **74**, 233—252 (1947).

— R. PANNIER and R. VERBEKE: Influence des anticholinestérases prostigmine, ésérine et di*iso*propylfluorophosphate, et de l'atropine, sur la transmission centrale et périphérique des excitations nerveuses. Arch. int. Pharmacodyn. **72**, 405—429 (1946).

— A. POCHET and H. VAN HOUTTE: Contributions à la pharmacologie du sarin et du tabun. Arch. int. Pharmacodyn. **104**, 293—332 (1956).

HIMWICH, H. E., C. F. ESSIG, J. L. HAMPSON, P. D. BALES and A. M. FREEDMAN: Effect of trimethadione (tridione) and other drugs on convulsions caused by di*iso*propyl fluorophosphate (DFP). Amer. J. Psychiat. **106**, 816—820 (1950).

—, and F. RINALDI: The antiparkinson activity of benactyzine. Arch. int. Pharmacodyn. **110**, 119—127 (1957).

HOBBIGER, F.: The action of carbamic esters and tetraethylpyrophosphate on normal and curarized frog rectus muscle. Brit. J. Pharmacol. **5**, 37—48 (1950).

— Inhibition of cholinesterases by irreversible inhibitors *in vitro* and *in vivo*. Brit. J. Pharmacol. **6**, 21—30 (1951).

—, and P. W. SADLER: Protection by oximes of bis-pyridinium ions against lethal DFP poisoning. Nature (Lond.) **182**, 1672—1673 (1958).

— — Protection against lethal organophosphate poisoning by quaternary pyridine aldoximes. Brit. J. Pharmacol. **14**, 192—201 (1959).

HODGE, H. C., and J. H. STERNER: The skin absorption of triorthocresyl phosphate as shown by radioactive phosphorus. J. Pharmacol. **79**, 225—234 (1943).

HOLMES, J. H., and M. D. GAON: Observations on acute and multiple exposures to anticholinesterase agents. Trans. Amer. clin. climat. Ass. **68**, 86—101 (1956).

— E. J. KINZER and R. W. HIBBERT: Parathion poisoning case report. Rocky Mtn. med. J. **54**, 1022—1031 (1957).

HOLMES, R.: The physiological mechanisms involved in poisoning with anticholinesterases. Proc. roy. Soc. Med. **46**, 799—800 (1953).

HOLMSTEDT, B.: Synthesis and pharmacology of dimethylamidoethoxy-phosphoryl cyanide (Tabun) together with a description of some allied anticholinesterase compounds containing the N—P bond. Acta physiol. scand. suppl. **90**, 1—120 (1951).

—, and C. R. SKOGLUND: The action on spinal reflexes of dimethylamidoethoxy-phosphoryl cyanide, "Tabun," a cholinesterase inhibitor. Acta physiol. scand. **29**, 410—427 (1953).

HORNYKIEWICZ, O., and W. KOBINGER: Über den Einfluß von Eserin, Tetraäthylpyrophosphat (TEPP) und Neostigmin auf den Blutdruck und die pressorischen Carotissinusreflexe der Ratte. Naunyn-Schmiedeberg's Arch. exp. Path. Pharmak. **228**, 493—500 (1956).

HYDE, J., S. BECKETT and E. GELLHORN: Acetylcholine and convulsive activity. J. Neurophysiol. **12**, 17—27 (1949).

JACO, N. T., and D. R. WOOD: The interaction between procaine, cocaine, adrenaline and prostigmine on skeletal muscle. J. Pharmacol. **82**, 63—73 (1944).

JANDORF, B. J., 1951, quoted by W. H. SUMMERSON: Progress in the biochemical treatment of nerve gas poisoning. U.S. armed Forces chem. J. **9**, No. 1, 24—26 (1955).

— Chemical reactions of nerve gases in neutral solution. I. Reactions with hydroxylamine. J. Amer. chem. Soc. **78**, 3686—3691 (1956).

— T. WAGNER-JAUREGG, J. J. O'NEILL and M. A. STOLBERG: The reaction of phosphorus-containing enzyme inactivators with phenols and polyphenols. J. Amer. chem. Soc. **74**, 1521—1523 (1952).

JOHNS, R. J., and H. E. HIMWICH: A central action of some antihistamines. Amer. J. Psychiat. **107**, 367—373 (1950).

JOHNSON, R. P., A. J. GOLD and G. FREEMAN: Comparative lung-airway resistance and cardiovascular effects in dogs and monkeys following parathion and sarin intoxication. Amer. J. Physiol. **192**, 581—584 (1958).

KAGAN, Y. S.: Experimental data on the therapy of intoxication with the organophosphorus insecticide thiophos (in Russian). Farmakol. i Toksikol. **19**, No. 2, 49—52 (1956).

KALOW, W., and M. O. MAYKUT: The interaction between cholinesterases and a series of local anesthetics. J. Pharmacol. exp. Ther. **116**, 418—432 (1956).

KALSER, S. C., J. H. WILLS, J. D. GABOUREL, R. E. GOSSELIN and C. F. EPES: Further studies of the excretion of atropine-alpha-C¹⁴. J. Pharmacol. exp. Ther. **121**, 449—456 (1957).

KARZCMAR, A. G.: Antagonism between a bis-quaternary oxamide, WIN 8078, and depolarizing and competitive blocking agents. J. Pharmacol. exp. Ther. **119**, 39—47 (1957).

—, and J. P. LONG: Relationship between peripheral cholinolytic potency and tetraethylpyrophosphate antagonism of a series of atropine substitutes. J. Pharmacol. exp. Ther. **123**, 230—237 (1958).

KILPATRICK, M., and M. L. KILPATRICK: The hydrolysis of di*iso*propyl fluorophosphate. J. phys. coll. Chem. **53**, 1371—1385 (1949).

KING, T. O., and E. POULSEN: The action of an aldoxime (2-pyridine aldoxime methiodide) on acute alkylphosphate poisoning in mice. Arch. int. Pharmacodyn. **114**, 118—121 (1958).

KIRSCHNER, L. B., and W. E. STONE: Action of inhibitors at the myoneural junction. J. gen. Physiol. **34**, 821—834 (1951).

KLEINWÄCHTER, L.: Beobachtung über die Wirkung des Calabar-Extracts gegen Atropin-Vergiftung. Berl. klin. Wschr. **1**, 369—371 (1864).

KOBERT, R.: Über die Deutung der Muscarinwirkung am Herzen. Naunyn-Schmiedeberg's Arch. exp. Path. Pharmak. **20**, 92—115 (1886).

KOELLE, G. B.: Protection of cholinesterase against irreversible inactivation by DFP *in vitro*. J. Pharmacol. exp. Ther. **88**, 232—237 (1946).

— Histochemical demonstration of reactivation of acetylcholinesterase *in vivo*. Science **125**, 1195—1196 (1957).

KONDRITZER, A. A.: Chemistry, detection and decontamination of nerve gases. U.S. armed Forces med. J. **7**, 791—796 (1956).

— W. H. MAYER and P. ZVIRBLIS: Removal of sarin from skin and eyes. Arch. industr. Hlth. **20**, 50—52 (1959).

KOSTER, R.: Synergisms and antagonisms between physostigmine and di-*iso*propyl fluorophosphate in cats. J. Pharmacol. exp. Ther. **88**, 39—46 (1946).

KRIVOY, W. A., E. R. HART and A. S. MARRAZZI: Further analysis of the actions of DFP and curare on the respiratory center. J. Pharmacol. exp. Ther. **103**, 351 (1951).

—, and J. H. WILLS: Adaptation to constant concentrations of acetylcholine. J. Pharmacol. exp. Ther. **116**, 220—226 (1956).

KROP, S., and A. M. KUNKEL: Observations on the pharmacology of the anticholinesterases sarin and tabun. Proc. Soc. exp. Biol. (N. Y.) **86**, 530-533 (1954).

KUMAGAI, H., S. EBASHI and F. TAKEDA: Studies on choline acetylase (in Japanese). Folia pharmacol. jap. **49**, 477—484 (1953).

KUNKEL, A. M., A. H. OIKEMUS and J. H. WILLS: Studies on bisquaternary aliphatic compounds. Fed. Proc. **11**, 365 (1952).

— J. H. WILLS and J. S. MONIER: Antagonists to neuromuscular block produced by sarin. Proc. Soc. exp. Biol. (N. Y.) **92**, 529—532 (1956).

— — and A. H. OIKEMUS: Effect of a quaternary derivative of atropine, N-benzyl atropinium chloride. Proc. Soc. exp. Biol. (N. Y.) **96**, 791—794 (1957).

LARSSON, L.: The alkaline hydrolysis of isopropoxy-methyl-phosphoryl fluoride (sarin) and some analogues. Acta chem. scand. **11**, 1131—1142 (1957).

— A kinetic study of the reaction of isopropoxy-methyl-phosphoryl fluoride (sarin) with hydrogen peroxide. Acta chem. scand. **12**, 723—730 (1958a).

— The alkaline hydrolysis of two sarin analogues and of tabun. Acta chem. scand. **12**, 783—785 (1958b),

— The catalytic effect of CrO_4^{2-}, MoO_4^{2-} and WO_4^{2-} on the hydrolysis of isopropoxy-methylphosphoryl fluoride (sarin). Acta chem. scand. **12**, 1226—1230 (1958c).

— Studies on the chemical reactivity of organic phosphorus compounds. Svensk. kem. Tidskr. **70**, 405—427 (1958d).

LOEW, E. R., and A. MICETICH: Adrenergic blocking drugs. I. Comparisons of effectiveness in decreasing epinephrine toxicity in mice. J. Pharmacol. exp. Ther. **93**, 434—443 (1948a).

— — Adrenergic blocking drugs. II. Antagonism of histamine and epinephrine with N-(2-haloalkyl)-1-naphthalene-methylamine derivatives. J. Pharmacol. exp. Ther. **94**, 339—349 (1948b).

— — Adrenergic blocking drugs. IV. Antagonism of epinephrine and histamine with 2-(2-biphenyloxy) 2'-chlorodiethylamine derivatives. J. Pharmacol. exp. Ther. **95**, 448—454 (1949).

LOEWI, O., u. E. NAVRATIL: Über humorale Übertragbarkeit der Herznervenwirkung. XI. Über den Mechanismus von Physostigmin und Ergotamine. Pflügers Arch. ges. Physiol. **214**, 689—696 (1926).

LORDI, N. G., and J. EPSTEIN: Kinetics and mechanism of chlorination of triethyl-phosphorothiolate in dilute aqueous media at 25°. J. Amer. chem. Soc. **80**, 509—515 (1958).

LUNDHOLM, L.: The effect of DFP on respiration, blood pressure and muscular function in the rabbit. Acta physiol. scand. **16**, 345—366 (1949).

MacIntosh, F. C., R. I. Birks and P. B. Sastry: Pharmacological inhibition of acetylcholine synthesis. Nature (Lond.) **178**, 1181 (1956).

McNamara, B. P., G. B. Koelle and A. Gilman: The treatment of DFP poisoning in rabbits. J. Pharmacol. exp. Ther. **88**, 27—33 (1946).

— E. F. Murtha, A. D. Bergner, E. M. Robinson, C. W. Bender and J. H. Wills: Studies on the mechanism of action of DFP and TEPP. J. Pharmacol. exp. Ther. **110**, 232—240 (1954).

Meeter, E.: The relation between end-plate depolarization and the repetitive response elicited in the isolated rat phrenic nerve-diaphragm preparation by DFP. J. Physiol. (Lond.) **144**, 38—51 (1958).

Metz, B.: Brain acetylcholinesterase and a respiratory reflex. Amer. J. Physiol. **192**, 101—105 (1958).

Meyer, F.: Untersuchungen über 17 neue Dialkyl-dihalogenvinyl- und Tetrahalogenäthylphosphate. Thesis, Hamburg University (1953).

Miller, F. R.: Effects of eserine and acetylcholine on the respiratory centers and hypoglossal nuclei. Canad. J. Res. E. **27**, 374—386 (1949).

Modell, W., S. Krop, P. Hitchcock and W. F. Riker, jr.: General systemic actions of di-isopropyl fluorophosphate (DFP) in cats. J. Pharmacol. exp. Ther. **87**, 400—413 (1946).

Moruzzi, G., and H. W. Magoun: Brain stem reticular formation and activation of the EEG. Electroenceph. clin. Neurophysiol. **1**, 455—473 (1949).

Murphy, S. D., and K. P. DuBois: Enzymatic conversion of the dimethoxy ester of benzotriazine dithiophosphoric acid to an anticholinesterase agent. J. Pharmacol. exp. Ther. **119**, 572—583 (1957).

Nachmansohn, D.: Chemical mechanism of nerve activity. Ann. N. Y. Acad. Sci. **47**, 395—428 (1946).

Nathan, P., M. H. Aprison and H. E. Himwich: A comparison of the effects of atropine with those of several central nervous system stimulants on rabbits exhibiting forced circling following the intracarotid injection of diisopropyl fluorophosphate. Confin. neurol. (Basel) **15**, 1—10 (1955).

Nickerson, M., and G. M. Nomaguchi: Adrenergic blocking action of phenoxyethyl analogues of dibenamine. J. Pharmacol. exp. Ther. **101**, 379—396 (1951).

Oberst, F. W., R. S. Ross, M. K. Christensen, J. W. Crook, P. Cresthull and C. W. Umland, II: Resuscitation of dogs poisoned by inhalation of the nerve gas GB. Mil. Med. **119**, 377—386 (1956).

O'Brien, R. D., and A. N. Davison: Antagonists to schradan poisoning in mice. Canad. J. Biochem. **36**, 1203—1210 (1958).

Oliver, G., and E. A. Schäfer: The physiological effects of extracts of the suprarenal capsules. J. Physiol. (Lond.) **18**, 230—276 (1895).

Parkes, M. W., and P. Sacra: Protection against the toxicity of cholinesterase inhibitors by acetylcholine antagonists. Brit. J. Pharmacol. **9**, 299—305 (1954).

Paton, W. D. M., and E. J. Zaimis: The methonium compounds. Pharmacol. Rev. **4**, 219—253 (1952).

Paulet, G.: Nouvelle contribution à l'étude de l'action pharmacologique du tétraéthylpyrophosphate (TEPP). Arch. int. Pharmacodyn. **97**, 157—185 (1954).

— Activité cholinestérasique et fonctionnement des centres respiratoires. J. Physiol. Path. gén. **48**, 915—936 (1956).

Petry, H.: Polyneuritis durch E 605. Zbl. Arbeitsmed. **1**, 86—89 (1951).

Petty, C. S.: Organic phosphate insecticide poisoning. Amer. J. Med. **24**, 467—470 (1958).

Pochet, A.: Action des neurotoxiques phosphorés sur la respiration. Acta belg. mil. **110**, 153—165 (1957).

Polet, H., and A. F. de Schaepdryver: Effect of sarin on the cardio-inhibitory vasomotor and respiratory centers of the isolated head in dogs. Arch. int. Pharmacodyn. **118**, 231—247 (1959).

Rajapurkar, M. V., and G. B. Koelle: Reactivation of DFP-inactivated acetylcholinesterase by monoisonitroso-acetone (MINA) and diacetylmonoxime (DAM) in vivo. J. Pharmacol. exp. Ther. **123**, 247—253 (1958).

Reisberg, R. B.: Properties and biological significance of choline acetylase. Yale J. Biol. Med. **29**, 403—435 (1957).

Riker, W. F., jr.: and W. C. Wescoe: The direct action of prostigmine on skeletal muscle; its relationship to the choline esters. J. Pharmacol. exp. Ther. **88**, 58—66 (1946).

Rinaldi, F., and H. E. Himwich: Alerting responses and actions of atropine and cholinergic drugs. Arch. Neurol. Psychiat. (Chicago) **73**, 387—395 (1955a).

— — Cholinergic mechanism involved in function of mesodiencephalic activating system. Arch. Neurol. Psychiat. (Chicago) **73**, 396—402 (1955b).

— — Drugs affecting psychotic behavior and function of mesodiencephalic activating system. Dis. nerv. Syst. **16**, 133—141 (1955c).

ROEPKE, M. H.: A study of choline esterase. J. Pharmacol. exp. Ther. **59**, 264—276 (1937).

ROSENBERG, P., and J. M. COON: Increase of hexobarbital sleeping time by certain anti-cholinesterases. Proc. Soc. exp. Biol. (N. Y.) **98**, 650—652 (1958).

— — Nikethamide, nicotinamide and some related compounds in anticholinesterase poisoning. J. Pharmacol. exp. Ther. **128**, 289—298 (1960).

SAKAI, F., H. DAL RI, W. D. ERDMANN u. G. SCHMIDT: Über die Atemlähmung durch Parathion oder Paraoxon und ihre antagonistische Beeinflußbarkeit. Naunyn-Schmiedeberg's Arch. exp. Path. Pharmak. **234**, 210—219 (1958).

SALERNO, P. R., and J. M. COON: A pharmacologic comparison of hexaethyl tetraphosphate (HETP) and tetraethyl pyrophosphate (TEPP) with physostigmine, neostigmine and DFP. J. Pharmacol. exp. Ther. **95**, 240—255 (1949).

SALLÉ, J.: Etude pharmacologique sur le thiophosphate de diéthyle et de paranitrophényle (Thiophos). Arch. int. Pharmacodyn. **82**, 181—191 (1950).

SCHAEFFER, K.-P.: Wirkung von E 605 und anderen Esteraseblockern auf Körperstell- und -haltereflexe. Naunyn-Schmiedeberg's Arch. exp. Path. Pharmak. **226**, 505—517 (1955).

SCHIFF, M., W. G. ESMOND and H. E. HIMWICH: Forced circling movements (adversive syndrome). Correction with dimenhydrinate ("Dramamine"). Arch. Otolaryng. (Chicago) **51**, 672—677 (1950).

SCHRIFTMAN, H., and A. A. KONDRITZER: Absorption of atropine from muscle. Amer. J. Physiol. **191**, 591—594 (1957).

SCHWEITZER, A., and S. WRIGHT: The action of eserine and related compounds and of acetylcholine on the central nervous system. J. Physiol. (Lond.) **89**, 165—197 (1937a).

— — Further observations on the action of acetylcholine, prostigmine and related substances on the knee jerk. J. Physiol. (Lond.) **89**, 384—402 (1937b).

SECKER, J.: The humoral control of the secretion by the submaxillary gland of the cat following chorda stimulation. J. Physiol. (Lond.) **81**, 81—92 (1934).

SEIFTER, J., and D. H. BAEDER: Partially depolymerized hyaluronic acid (PDHA) as a spreading agent. Proc. Soc. exp. Biol. (N. Y.) **85**, 160—162 (1954).

SHELLEY, H.: The inhibition of acetylcholine synthesis in guinea-pig brain slices by eserine and neostigmine. J. Physiol. (Lond.) **131**, 329—340 (1956).

SMITH, M. I., and R. D. LILLIE: Histopathology of triorthocresyl phosphate poisoning: etiology of so-called ginger-paralysis. Arch. Neurol. Psychiat. (Chicago) **26**, 976—992 (1931).

STEINBERG, G. M., and J. BOLGER: N-hydroxy aryl carbamates. A class of hydroxamic acids which form stable phosphorylated and sulfated derivatives. J. org. Chem. **21**, 660—662 (1956).

STEVENSON, J. W., and G. T. GIRVIN: The effect of botulinum toxin on the bacterial acetylation of choline. Atti VI. Congr. int. Microbiol. **4**, 133—134 (1953).

STEWART, G. N., and J. M. ROGOFF: The action of drugs upon the output of epinephrin from the adrenals. VII. Physostigmine. J. Pharmacol. exp. Ther. **17**, 227—248 (1921).

STEWART, W. C.: Accumulation of acetylcholine in brain and blood of animals poisoned with cholinesterase inhibitors. Brit. J. Pharmacol. **7**, 270—276 (1952).

STOLBERG, M. A., and W. A. MOSHER: Rates of reaction of vicinally substituted hydroxamic acids with isopropyl methylphosphonofluoridate (sarin). J. Amer. chem. Soc. **79**, 2618—2620 (1957).

STONE, C. A., and E. R. LOEW: Adrenergic blocking drugs. III. Effects of 2-halogenated ethylamines on pressor responses to epinephrine, nicotine and adrenergic nervous reflexes. J. Pharmacol. exp. Ther. **94**, 350—358 (1948).

STOVNER, J.: Effect of choline on the action of anticholinesterases. Acta pharm. tox. (Kbh.) **12**, 175—186 (1956).

STRAUS, O. H., and A. J. GOLDSTEIN: Zone behavior of enzymes. Illustrated by the effect of dissociation constant and dilution on the system cholinesterase-physostigmine. J. gen. Physiol. **26**, 559—585 (1943).

STUMPF, C.: Pharmakologie des aszendierenden retikulären Systems. Wien. klin. Wschr. **69**, 298—303 (1957).

SWIDLER, R., R. E. PLAPINGER and G. M. STEINBERG: The kinetics of the reaction of isopropyl methylphosphonofluoridate (sarin) with substituted benzohydroxamic acids. II. J. Amer. chem. Soc. **81**, 3271—3274 (1959).

—, and G. M. STEINBERG: The kinetics of the reaction of isopropyl methylphosphonofluoridate (sarin) with benzohydroxamic acid. J. Amer. chem. Soc. **78**, 3594—3598 (1956).

TAMMELIN, L.-E.: Methyl-fluoro-phosphorylcholines. Two synthetic cholinergic drugs and their tertiary homologues. Acta chem. scand. **11**, 859—865 (1957a).

— Dialkoxy-phosphorylthiocholines, alkoxy-methyl-phosphorylthiocholines and analogous choline esters. Syntheses, pKa, of tertiary homologues and cholinesterase inhibition. Acta chem. scand. **11**, 1340—1349 (1957b).

— Organophosphorylcholines and cholinesterases. Ark. Kemi **12**, 287—298 (1958a).

TAMMELIN, L.-E.: Choline esters. Substrates and inhibitors of cholinesterases. Svensk. kem. T. **70**, 157—181 (1958b).

THESLEFF, S.: Neuromuscular block caused by acetylcholine. Nature (Lond.) **175**, 594—595 (1955).

TODRICK, A.: The inhibition of cholinesterases by antagonists of acetylcholine and histamine. Brit. J. Pharmacol. **9**, 76—83 (1954).

TURPAEV, T. M., and T. G. PUTINCEVA: Compensatory reactions of the sympathetic nervous system in asphyxia due to bronchial spasm (in Russian). Fiziol. Z. (Mosk.) **41**, 71—77 (1955).

VARAGIC, V.: The action of eserine on the blood pressure of the rat. Brit. J. Pharmacol. **10**, 349—353 (1955).

VERBEKE, R.: Nouvelles contributions à la pharmacologie du di-isopropylfluorophosphonate (DFP). Arch. int. Pharmacodyn. **79**, 1—31 (1949).

WAGNER-JAUREGG, T., and B. E. HACKLEY jr.: Model reactions of phosphorus-containing enzyme inactivators. III. Interaction of imidazole, pyridine and some of their derivatives with dialkyl halogeno-phosphates. J. Amer. chem. Soc. **75**, 2125—2130 (1953).

— — T. A. LIES, O. O. OWENS and R. PROPER: Model reactions of phosphorus-containing enzyme inactivators. VI. The catalytic activity of certain metal salts and chelates in the hydrolysis of di*iso*propyl fluorophosphate. J. Amer. chem. Soc. **77**, 922—929 (1955).

— J. J. O'NEILL and W. H. SUMMERSON: The reaction of phosphorus-containing enzyme inhibitors with amines and amino acid derivatives. J. Amer. chem. Soc. **73**, 5202—5206 (1951).

WESCOE, W. C., R. E. GREEN, B. P. McNAMARA and S. KROP: The influence of atropine and scopolamine on the central effects of DFP. J. Pharmacol. exp. Ther. **92**, 63—72 (1948).

— — On the mechanism of the convulsant action of strychnine; the lack of atropine antagonism. J. Pharmacol. exp. Ther. **94**, 78—84 (1948).

WILLS, J. H.: Substitutes for and adjuncts to atropine in nerve gas poisoning. U.S. armed Forces med. J. **6**, 1329—1332 (1955).

— Recent studies of organic phosphate poisoning. Fed. Proc. **18**, 1020—1025 (1959).

—, and H. L. BORISON: Modification by sarin and antagonists of medullary respiratory activities. Fed. Proc. **18**, 459 (1959).

— A. M. KUNKEL, J. F. O'LEARY and A. H. OIKEMUS: Effect of 2-PAM on neuromuscular blockade induced by certain chemicals. Proc. Soc. exp. Biol. (N. Y.) **101**, 196—197 (1959).

WILSON, I. B.: Acetylcholinesterase. XI. Reversibility of tetraethyl pyrophosphate inhibition. J. biol. Chem. **190**, 111—117 (1951).

— Acetylcholinesterase. XIII. Reactivation of alkyl phosphate-inhibited enzyme. J. biol. Chem. **199**, 113—120 (1952).

—, and F. SONDHEIMER: A specific antidote against lethal alkyl phosphate intoxication. V. Antidotal properties. Arch. Biochem. **69**, 468—474 (1957).

WOOD, J. R., P. F. DICKENS, jr., J. RIZZOLO and M. W. BAYLISS: Treatment of nerve-gas casualties. U.S. armed Forces med. J. **2**, 1609—1617 (1951).

WRIGHT, P. G.: An analysis of the central and peripheral components of respiratory failure produced by anticholinesterase poisoning in the rabbit. J. Physiol. (Lond.) **126**, 52—70 (1954).

ZAWADZKI, B.: The site of origin of acetylcholine (ACh) liberated from the motor nerve endings during stimulation (in Polish). Acta physiol. pol. **6**, 15—32 (1955).

Chapter 21

Reactivation of Phosphorylated Acetylcholinesterase

By

F. Hobbiger

With 4 Figures

Contents

Introduction

The active centre of acetylcholinesterase (AChE) contains two subsites which are generally called the anionic and esteratic sites. Hydrolysis of acetylcholine (ACh) by AChE involves the following sequence of reactions:

Binding of the ester to the two subsites of the enzyme → hydrolysis of the ester with release of choline into solution and binding of the acetyl group to a basic group of the esteratic site → hydrolysis of the acetylated enzyme.

Formation of the acetylated enzyme is considered to be the rate-determining step in this sequence of reactions. The acetylated enzyme is extremely unstable and has a half-life of a fraction of a millisecond.

Acetylcholinesterase also reacts with organophosphorus compounds, referred to from now on as organophosphates, having the general structure (I).

$$X—P{\overset{R_1}{\underset{R_2}{<}}}$$
$$\underset{O}{\|}$$

(I)

In many organophosphates of this type, R_1 is an alkoxy group, R_2 an alkoxy, alkyl, or dialkylamido group, and X a halogen, cyanide, phenoxy, or di-substituted phosphoryloxy group. The reaction between organophosphates and AChE is analogous to the reaction between ACh and AChE and can be represented as follows:

$$\underset{..}{G}—H + X—\underset{\underset{O}{\|}}{P}{\overset{R_1}{\underset{R_2}{<}}} \rightarrow G—\underset{\underset{O}{\|}}{P}{\overset{R_1}{\underset{R_2}{<}}} + XH \qquad (1)$$

$$G—\underset{\underset{O}{\|}}{P}{\overset{R_1}{\underset{R_2}{<}}} + HOH \xrightarrow[\text{extremely slow}]{} \underset{..}{G}—H + HO—\underset{\underset{O}{\|}}{P}{\overset{R_1}{\underset{R_2}{<}}} \qquad (2)$$

where G—H represents a part of the esteratic site of AChE and the electron pair (..) and H are symbols for a basic and a protonated acidic group, respectively. Phosphorylated AChE, unlike acetylated AChE, is extremely stable, i.e., reaction (2) proceeds at a very low rate, and for this reason organophosphates are inhibitors and not substrates of AChE.

Nearly all the work which we shall discuss in Section A has been carried out with three types of phosphorylated AChE:

　　a) diethylphosphoryl-AChE, where R_1 and R_2 are ethoxy groups,
　　b) di*iso*propylphosphoryl-AChE, where R_1 and R_2 are *iso*propoxy groups, and
　　c) *iso*propyl methylphosphonyl-AChE, where R_1 is an *iso*propoxy and R_2 a methyl group.

Amongst the better known organophosphates which form a) are tetraethyl pyrophosphate (TEPP) and diethyl-4-nitrophenyl phosphate (Paraoxon). Di*iso*-

propyl phosphorofluoridate (DFP) and *iso*propyl methylphosphonofluoridate (Sarin) form b) and c), respectively. These and many other organophosphates are *per se* phosphorylating agents of AChE.

A second group of organophosphates consists of compounds which are *per se* only weak anticholinesterase (anti-ChE) agents but are converted into highly potent phosphorylating agents *in vivo* (see CASIDA 1956). To this group belong the majority of organophosphate insecticides used at present, e.g., 0,0-diethyl 0-(4-nitrophenyl) phosphorothioate (Parathion) which is converted into Paraoxon.

In 1951, WILSON reported that choline and hydroxylamine reactivate diethylphosphoryl-AChE considerably faster than water alone. Information gained in these studies has led to the discovery of the high reactivating potency of hydroxamic acids and oximes. The most potent reactivators of the phosphorylated AChE of types a), b), and c) are oximes, some of which are useful antidotes in organophosphate poisoning. This is of considerable practical importance because the widespread use of organophosphate insecticides frequently leads to accidental, homicidal, or suicidal poisoning of man in some countries (e.g., NAMBA 1958a, TOIVONNEN et al. 1959), and an effective treatment of organophosphate poisoning is urgently needed.

A. Biochemical studies of the reactivation of phosphorylated acetylcholinesterase

The rates of spontaneous reactivation, i.e., dephosphorylation, of different types of phosphorylated AChE by water (reaction 2) vary considerably. Spontaneous reactivation of dimethylphosphoryl-AChE, where R_1 and R_2 are methoxy groups, proceeds faster than that of any other type of dialkoxyphosphoryl-AChE (BURGEN and HOBBIGER 1951), and at 37° and pH 7.6 amounts to approximately 50% in 90 min when rabbit erythrocytes are used as enzyme source (ALDRIDGE 1953, ALDRIDGE and DAVISON 1953). With diethylphosphoryl-AChE (prepared from human erythrocytes) 25 to 40% spontaneous reactivation takes place at pH 7.45 and 37° in 24 hours (BURGEN and HOBBIGER 1951, HOBBIGER 1951). In the case of di*iso*propylphosphoryl-AChE and *iso*propyl methylphosphonyl-AChE no spontaneous reactivation can be recorded.

In the following text an account is given of the reactivation of various types of phosphorylated AChE by nucleophilic reagents. For simplicity the term "phosphorylation" will be used when the reference applies to phosphorylation as well as phosphonylation and reactions involving phosphoramides. For references which apply solely to phosphonylation the term "phosphonylation" will be retained. The rates of reactivation of phosphorylated AChE obtained in different laboratories with the more potent reactivators, i.e., oximes, sometimes vary considerably. This seems to be attributable largely to the enzyme source used for preparation of phosphorylated AChE. WILSON and his co-workers used highly purified AChE of electric eel tissue whereas work carried out in other laboratories, unless otherwise stated, was done with washed human erythrocytes. For simplicity, reference to the enzyme source is omitted from the text except in places where it is essential.

Reactivators of phosphorylated AChE restore also the activity of those types of phosphorylated butyrocholinesterase (BuChE) and phosphorylated chymotrypsin which are formed by organophosphates which yield a reactivatable phosphorylated AChE. This in discussed briefly.

Only certain types of phosphorylated AChE and BuChE are reactivatable, and those which possess this property become non-reactivatable on ageing; the experiments to be discussed were all carried out with freshly prepared phosphorylated AChE and BuChE unless stated otherwise.

A key to abbreviations used for hydroxamic acids and oximes is given in the Appendix, while abbreviations used for organophosphates are listed in Table 9. The Appendix also contains references to papers which describe the synthesis of hydroxamic acids and oximes and a list of short review articles on reactivation of phosphorylated AChE. Figures and tables are reproduced by kind permission of the authors and journals concerned.

I. Reactivation of dialkoxyphosphoryl- and *iso*propyl methylphosphonyl-acetylcholinesterase

1. Reactivation by choline, hydroxylamine, and other weak reactivators

Acylated AChE reacts with hydroxylamine or choline to give hydroxamic acids or choline esters, respectively (WILSON et al. 1950). Hydroxylamine and choline also act as acceptors of phosphoryl groups and thus reactivate phosphorylated AChE.

WILSON (1951, 1952) studied reactivation of diethylphosphoryl-AChE by hydroxylamine and choline and reported that at pH 7 and 31°, 0.25 M choline produces 60% reactivation in 4 hours, whereas at the same pH and 30°, 0.1 M hydroxylamine produces 50% reactivation in 30 min.

The rate of reactivation obtained with choline approaches a maximum with 0.1 M concentration of the reactivator, increases markedly when the pH is raised from 6 to 8, and approaches a constant value in the pH range between 8 and 9. The rate of reactivation obtained with hydroxylamine increases with increasing concentration of the reactivator and shows a maximum at pH 7. Reactivation by choline and hydroxylamine is temperature-dependent and has an energy of activation of 14.5 and 7 kcal./mole, respectively.

Di*iso*propylphosphoryl-AChE is far more difficult to reactivate than diethylphosphoryl-AChE and the ratios of the rate constants for reactivation of diethylphosphoryl-AChE to those of di*iso*propylphosphoryl-AChE are over 100 and 40 for choline and hydroxylamine, respectively (WILSON 1952, 1955a).

WILSON (1955a) has interpreted these results as follows. Reactivation by choline involves a combined acid-base attack by the two atoms of the hydroxyl group. This can be represented as:

$$G—P{<}^{R_1}_{R_2} + (CH_3)_3\overset{+}{N}C_2H_4OH \rightarrow G{\cdot\cdot}H + (CH_3)_3\overset{+}{N}C_2H_4O—P{<}^{R_1}_{R_2} \qquad (3)$$
$$\overset{\|}{O} \qquad\qquad\qquad\qquad\qquad\qquad\qquad\qquad \overset{\|}{O}$$

The nucleophilic activity of the alcoholic group of choline can hardly be high enough to account fully for the observed rates of reactivation. It is necessary to assume that bonding of the quaternary ammonium group of choline to the anionic site of phosphorylated AChE greatly contributes to reactivation. This interpretation is supported by the finding that quaternary ammonium ions competitively inhibit reactivation by choline (WILSON 1952). The affinity of choline for the anionic site of diethylphosphoryl-AChE is approximately 1/60 of that for the anionic site of AChE because the former is shielded by the ethyl groups of the phosphoryl moiety. Shielding of the anionic site by *iso*propyl groups is greater than that by ethyl groups, and thus choline reactivates diethylphosphoryl-AChE at a much higher rate than di*iso*propylphosphoryl-AChE.

Amongst the interpretations put forward for the reactivation of phosphorylated AChE by hydroxylamine (WILSON 1955a, 1959, WILSON et al. 1955), the following appears to be the most likely. Unionized hydroxylamine or its zwitterion, if it exists, is the active species which reacts with a protonated form of phosphorylated AChE, hence the pH dependence of reactivation (WILSON et al. 1955). This can be represented as:

$$\text{G—P}{<}^{R_1}_{R_2} + \text{HOH} \rightleftarrows \text{H—G—P}{<}^{R_1}_{R_2} + \text{OH}^- \qquad (4)$$

with O double-bonded to each P.

$$\text{H—G—P}{<}^{R_1}_{R_2} + \text{H}_2\text{NOH} \rightarrow \underset{\cdot\cdot}{\text{G}}\text{—H} + \text{H}_2\text{NO—P}{<}^{R_1}_{R_2} + \text{H}^+ \qquad (5\,a)$$

$$\text{or H—G—P}{<}^{R_1}_{R_2} + \text{H}_3\text{N}^+\text{O}^- \rightarrow \underset{\cdot\cdot}{\text{G}}\text{—H} + \text{H}_2\text{NO—P}{<}^{R_1}_{R_2} \qquad (5\,b)$$

Such an interpretation is supported by results obtained in studies of the *reaction between organophosphates and hydroxylamine*. JANDORF (1956) found that the rate-determining step in the hydrolysis of organophosphates by hydroxylamine is the formation of phosphorylated hydroxylamine, and that the active species of hydroxylamine is its (electrically) neutral form. According to JANDORF the overall reaction between DFP or Sarin and hydroxylamine, when the latter is present in excess, can be represented as:

$$\text{X—P}{<}^{R_1}_{R_2} + 3\,\text{H}_2\text{NOH} \rightarrow \text{HO—P}{<}^{R_1}_{R_2} + \text{HX} + \text{N}_2 + \text{NH}_3 + 2\,\text{H}_2\text{O} \qquad (6)$$

Other weak reactivators: Nucleophilic or basic reagents such as pyridine and compounds with an amino, amidino, guanidino or hydroxyl group also reactivate diethylphosphoryl-AChE but are less effective than hydroxylamine or choline (WILSON 1952).

2. Reactivation by hydroxamic acids

Hydroxamic acids are more potent than hydroxylamine as reactivators of phosphorylated AChE, whereas O-substituted hydroxylamines are devoid of reactivating properties and simple N-substituted hydroxylamines are less potent than hydroxylamine (WILSON 1955a, 1959). The same applies to the rates at which they hydrolyse organophosphates (WAGNER-JAUREGG 1956).

The best reactivators amongst hydroxamic acids at pH 7 to 8 are nicotine-hydroxamic acid methiodide (NHAM, II), picolinehydroxamic acid (III), and pyrimidine-2-hydroxamic acid (IV).

$$\begin{array}{ccc}
\text{(II)} & \text{(III)} & \text{(IV)}
\end{array}$$

(II) pyridinium ring with CONHOH substituent, $\overset{+}{\text{N}}$—CH$_3$ I$^-$; (III) pyridine ring with CONHOH; (IV) pyrimidine ring with CONHOH.

The superiority of these three hydroxamic acids over hydroxylamine as reactivators of various types of phosphorylated AChE is illustrated by the following results.

WILSON and MEISLICH (1953) compared reactivation of phosphorylated AChE by $0.1\,M$ hydroxylamine and NHAM at 24° (pH not stated but probably 7) and obtained results which are summarized in Table 1.

Picolinehydroxamic acid, in $0.05\,M$ concentration, reactivates within 2 min 60 and 21% of diethyl- and di*iso*propyl-phosphoryl-AChE, respectively, at 25° and pH 8 (WILSON and GINSBURG 1955a). Pyrimidine-2-hydroxamic acid is approximately 1.5 times more potent than picolinehydroxamic acid as a reactivator of diethylphosphoryl-AChE at pH 7.4 (CHILDS et al. 1955).

Reactivation of diethylphosphoryl-AChE by hydroxamic acids shows a first order dependence on the concentration of phosphorylated AChE. The time-course of reactivation of freshly prepared diisopropyl-phosphoryl-AChE and isopropyl methylphos-phonyl-AChE also follows or approaches first oder kinetics during the first 30 to 60 min, but then usually slows down considerably (WILSON et al. 1955, WILSON and GINSBURG 1955a, CHILDS et al. 1955,

Table 1. *Reactivation of phosphorylated AChE by 0.1 M hy-droxylamine and nicotinehydroxamic acid methiodide (NHAM) at 24° (WILSON and MEISLICH 1953)*

Type of phosphorylated AChE	Reactivator	Period of reactivation in min	% reactivation
diethylphosphoryl-	Hydroxylamine	30	40
	NHAM	15	63
diisopropylphosphoryl-	Hydroxylamine	240	17
	NHAM	240	38

Phosphorylated AChE was prepared from highly purified AChE of electric eel tissue.

HOBBIGER 1956). Formation of a second type of phosphorylated AChE (by ageing) which cannot be reactivated by hydroxamic acids and which will be discussed later (see page 941) probably accounts for the slowing down.

Factors determining the rate of reactivation. The rate of reactivation of different types of phosphorylated AChE by individual hydroxamic acids is mainly deter-mined by four factors:

a) The concentration of the hydroxamate ion which is the active species of the reactivator.

b) The nucleophilic activity of the hydroxamate ion, which increases with increasing pK_a of the hydroxamic acid.

c) The extent to which an acidic group at the esteratic site of phosphorylated AChE is in a protonated form.

d) The degree of complimentariness and strength of bonding between hydrox-amate ion and phosphorylated AChE. Formation of a complex between phos-phorylated AChE and hydroxamate ion accounts for rates of reactivation which are greater than those expected from the nuc-leophilic activity of the hydroxamate ion.

This conclusion is based on the following findings.

Hydrolysis of organo-phosphates. Valuable in-formation concerning the mechanism of reactiva-tion of phosphorylated AChE by hydroxamic acids is obtained from studies of the hydrolysis of organophosphates.

The half-times of hy-drolysis of 1.7 mM DFP and 2.3 mM Sarin by var-

Table 2. *Hydrolysis of organophosphates by hydroxamic acids at pH 7.6 and 30° (DFP: HACKLEY et al. 1955; Sarin: WAGNER-JAUREGG 1956)*

Hydroxamic acid	pK_a	Time for 50% hydrolysis in min	
		DFP	Sarin
Benzhydroxamic acid	8.8	22 (1.3)	2 (0.12)
Nicotinehydroxamic acid	8.3	20 (3.3)	3.4 (0.57)
Nicotinehydroxamic acid methiodide (NHAM)	6.5	68 (64)	5 (4.7)
Picolinehydroxamic acid	8.7	20 (1.4)	1.5 (0.11)
Picolinehydroxamic acid methiodide	7.5	65 (35)	2.3 (1.2)
Isonicotinehydroxamic acid	7.8	28 (11)	2.8 (1.1)
Isonicotinehydroxamic acid methiodide	6.3	73 (69)	7.3 (6.9)

The figures in brackets represent the time (in min) required for 50% hydrolysis when the acid is fully dissociated; these figures were calculated from the data provided by the authors.

ious hydroxamic acids, used in a five-fold excess, have been reported by HACKLEY et al. (1955) and WAGNER-JAUREGG (1956), and are summarized in Table 2.

Under comparable conditions the half-times of hydrolysis of DFP and Sarin by hydroxylamine are 108 and 11 to 12 min, respectively (WAGNER-JAUREGG 1956, JANDORF 1956). The superiority of hydroxamic acids over hydroxylamine (pK_a 6.3) as reactivators of phosphorylated AChE is thus partly accounted for by a difference in the nucleophilic activity of the active species of these compounds.

The hydrolysis of diethyl phosphorofluoridate by hydroxamic acids has not been investigated. Results summarized in Table 2, and the observation that under identical conditions nucleophilic reagents hydrolyze diethyl phosphorochloridates approximately 5 to 10 times faster than their corresponding di*iso*propyl derivatives (DOSTROVSKY and HALMANN 1953) indicate that the ease of hydrolysis of organophosphates which share a common substituent group X (see I), and which can thus be considered to be simple models of the various types of phosphorylated AChE, shows the order *iso*propyl methylphosphonate $\geq$ diethyl phosphate $>$ di*iso*propyl phosphate.

The active species of the hydroxamic acids are their anions, as shown by the effect of pH on the hydrolysis of organophosphates by hydroxamic acids (HACKLEY et al. 1955, SWIDLER and STEINBERG 1956). Differences between the rates at which an individual organophosphate is hydrolyzed by various hydroxamic acids at a given pH (as shown in Table 2) arise mainly from two sources, firstly the different degrees of dissociation of the various hydroxamic acids at a given pH, and secondly the differences between nucleophilic activities of the hydroxamate ions. The latter is illustrated in Table 2 by the figures in brackets, and also by results of GREEN et al. (1958) who calculated the rate constant (expressed as $l. mole^{-1} min^{-1}$) for the reaction of anions of the following two hydroxamic acids with organophosphates at 25° as:

Hydroxamic acid	Sarin	TEPP	DFP	Paraoxon
Salicylhydroxamic acid (pK_a 7.43)	114	19	4.9	0.071
Benzhydroxamic acid (pK_a 8.75)	1020	160	36	1.0

Hydrolysis of organophosphates by hydroxamic acids yields as an intermediate a phosphorylated hydroxamate ion which undergoes a Lossen rearrangement to give a hydrolyzed organophosphate $\left(HO\!-\!\underset{\underset{O}{\|}}{P}\!\!<^{R_1}_{R_2} \right)$ and an isocyanate. When hydroxamate ions are present in excess a carbamyl-hydroxamate is formed, and thus 2 moles of hydroxamate ions are consumed during the hydrolysis of one mole of organophosphate. The rate-determining step in this reaction is the formation of the phosphorylated hydroxamate ion (HACKLEY et al. 1955, SWIDLER and STEINBERG 1956).

Reactivation of phosphorylated AChE. Rates of reactivation of phosphorylated AChE by hydroxamic acids vary with pH and have a narrow pH optimum as is illustrated in Fig. 1. The position of the pH optimum is directly related to the pK_a of the hydroxamic acid, and the pH dependence of reactivation at a pH below the pH optimum is accounted for largely by variations in the concentration of the hydroxamate ion with pH. The pH dependence of reactivation at a pH above the pH optimum indicates that hydroxamate ions react with a protonated form of phosphorylated AChE. The ionizing group involved is assumed to be the acidic group in the esteratic site, which loses a proton during phosphorylation (see reaction 1). Reactivation of phosphorylated AChE by hydroxamic acids, therefore, can be represented as follows (WILSON et al. 1955):

$$\text{G--P}{<}^{R_1}_{R_2} + \text{HOH} \rightleftharpoons \text{H--G--P}{<}^{R_1}_{R_2} + \text{OH}^- \tag{4}$$
$$\underset{\text{O}}{\parallel} \qquad\qquad\qquad \underset{\text{O}}{\parallel}$$

$$\text{H--G--P}{<}^{R_1}_{R_2} + \text{RCONHO}^- \rightarrow \text{H--\overset{..}{G}} + \text{RCONHO--P}{<}^{R_1}_{R_2} \tag{7}$$
$$\underset{\text{O}}{\parallel} \qquad\qquad\qquad\qquad\qquad \underset{\text{O}}{\parallel}$$

The pK_a of the acidic group at the esteratic site of diethylphosphoryl-AChE has been calculated as 7.6 on the assumption that the optimum pH for reactivation equals $^1/_2$ ($pK_{a1} + pK_{a2}$), where K_{a1} is the dissociation constant of the hydroxamic acid and K_{a2} that of the acidic group of the esteratic site of the phosphorylated enzyme (DAVIES and GREEN 1956).

There are two ways in which reactivation can occur. It can either be a simple chemical displacement reaction or involve complex formation between phosphorylated AChE and hydroxamate ion before dephosphorylation occurs.

In the former case, and provided that steric hindrance plays only a very small part, the rate of reactivation of phosphorylated AChE will be proportional to the concentration and nucleophilic activity of the hydroxamate ion and the percentage of phosphorylated AChE which is in a protonated form. Under these conditions a similar relationship must exist between the rates of hydrolysis of an organophosphate by different hydroxamic acids and the rates of reactivation of phosphorylated AChE (formed by the same organophosphate) by these hydroxamic acids if both types of experiment are carried out at the same pH. The same must apply to the relationship between the rates at which a given hydroxamic acid hydrolyses different organophosphates with a common substituent group, X, and the rates at which it reactivates the various types of phosphorylated AChE formed by them, provided that the pH is the same in each type of experiment.

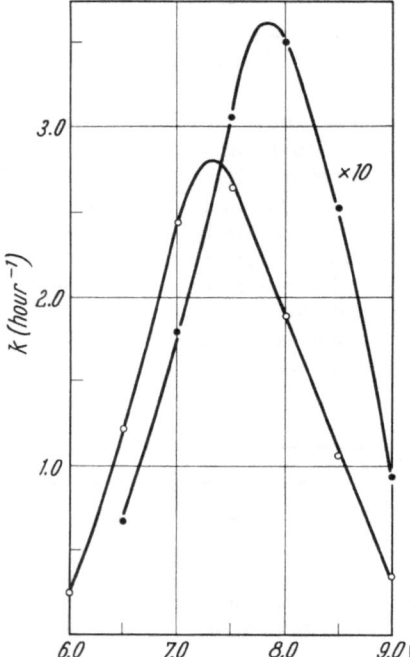

Fig. 1. pH-*dependence of reactivation of diethyl-phosphoryl-AChE by hydroxamic acids at 25°* (WILSON *et al. 1955*). *k* is the first order constant of reactivation. ●, nicotinehydroxamic acid, 0.05 *M*; ○ nicotinehydroxamic acid methiodide (NHAM), 0.05 *M*. Enzyme used for preparation of phosphorylated AChE: highly purified electric eel AChE

With many hydroxamic acids which have been investigated in greater detail it was found that the relationships outlined above do not hold. This has led to the interpretation that reactivation by hydroxamic acids which are potent reactivators is not a simple chemical displacement reaction, but that hydroxamic acids form a complex with phosphorylated AChE which promotes reactivation. In any individual case the degree of promotion is determined by the dissociation constant of the complex formed between protonated phosphorylated AChE and hydroxamate ion, and the orientation of the nucleophilic oxygen atom of the hydroxamate ion relative to the phosphorus atom of the phosphoryl group at the esteratic site of the enzyme.

This interpretation is supported by the finding that at a given pH the ratio $k/[R]$[1], where k is the first order constant of reactivation and $[R]$ the molar concentration of hydroxamic acid used, for reactivation of diethylphosphoryl-AChE by NHAM and its tertiary base decreases with increasing $[R]$, whereas a linear relationship exists between k^{-1} and $[R]^{-1}$ (WILSON et al. 1955). Similar studies have not been carried out with other hydroxamic acids or other types of phosphorylated AChE, but it must be pointed out that in cases where the bonding of the reactivator is not sterically affected by the phosphoryl moiety a constant ratio, $k/[R]$, does not disprove complex formation. There is not sufficient information available which would enable us to assess the promoting effect on reactivation arising from complex formation between phosphorylated AChE and many of the hydroxamate ions, but it is certainly justifiable to conclude that at pH 7 to 8 a low reactivating potency of hydroxamic acids with pK_a's of 6 to 9 is attributable to the absence or a low order of the promoting effect.

Results obtained with pairs of quaternary hydroxamic acids and their tertiary bases have been used to locate bonding sites. Quaternary hydroxamic acids, like choline, reactivate diethylphosphoryl-AChE 20 to 100 times faster than di*iso*propylphosphoryl-AChE, whereas with their tertiary bases the ratio varies only between 2 and 9 (WILSON 1955a). The latter is in reasonable agreement with the ratio observed when model compounds, i.e., organophosphates of the type $(RO)_2 - P - X$, where R is an ethyl or *iso*propyl group and X a halogen (see page 927),
$$\overset{\|}{O}$$
are hydrolyzed by hydroxamic acids but the former is greatly in excess of it. WILSON (1955a), therefore, concluded that quaternary hydroxamic acids form a complex with phosphorylated AChE by bonding of the quaternary ammonium group of the hydroxamic acid to the anionic site of phosphorylated AChE (before dephosphorylation takes place), since the anionic site of diethylphosphoryl-AChE is shielded to a smaller extent than the anionic site of di*iso*propylphosphoryl-AChE. This interpretation is supported by two findings. Trimethylamine inhibits reactivation of diethylphosphoryl-AChE by NHAM, and NHAM in concentrations required for reactivation inhibits ACh hydrolysis (HOBBIGER 1956). According to WILSON et al. (1955), complex formation plays a considerable part in the reactivation of diethylphosphoryl-AChE by quaternary hydroxamic acids but it is not certain to what extent, if at all, it contributes to reactivation of di*iso*propylphosphoryl-AChE. Neutralization of the charge on the anionic site in acid media is, according to WILSON et al. (1955), an additional factor which contributes to the pH dependence of reactivation by those hydroxamic acids which form a complex with phosphorylated AChE by bonding to the anionic site.

The high reactivating potency of picolinehydroxamic acid must be attributed to formation of a complex with phosphorylated AChE which promotes reactivation of both diethyl- *and* di*iso*propyl-phosphoryl-AChE. The bonding site involved in this case, however, cannot be the anionic site, and cations which reduce bonding to the anionic site (MYERS 1950, BERGMAN and SHIMONI 1952) accelerate reactivation by picolinehydroxamic acid (GREEN and SMITH 1958a). GREEN and SMITH (1958c) proposed that a hydrogen bond is formed between phosphorylated AChE and the ring-nitrogen atom of picolinehydroxamic acid. The high reactivating potency of pyrimidine-2-hydroxamic acid was explained similarly by these authors.

Reactivating potency at pH 7 to 8. In view of the practical importance of reactivation of phosphorylated AChE *in vivo*, it is important to have some

---

[1] $k/[R]$ is frequently referred to in the literature as "rate constant".

measure of reactivating potencies which apply to dilute solutions of hydroxamic acids at pH 7 to 8. Such purpose is served by the ratio $k/[R]$, calculated from the percentage reactivation obtained by using an $[R]$ which gives a submaximal rate of reactivation, and Table 3 shows such ratios for some hydroxamic acids. When comparing the ratios $k/[R]$ presented in Table 3 it must be remembered that they are not necessarily constant when $[R]$ is varied, and that they vary with pH.

Table 3. *Reactivation of phosphorylated AChE at 25° by those hydroxamic acids which are most effective at pH 7 to 8*

Hydroxamic acid	pH	$k/[R]$ in l. mol^{-1} min^{-1}			
		Type of phosphorylated AChE			
		diethyl-phosphoryl-	di*iso*propyl-phosphoryl-	*iso*propyl methyl-phosphonyl-	
Nicotinehydroxamic acid methiodide (NHAM)	8	0.74	0.025	—	} see a)
Picolinehydroxamic acid	8	9.2	1.8	—	
Nicotinehydroxamic acid methiodide (NHAM)	7.4	0.3	<0.05	0.3	} Reported by DAVIES and GREEN (1956)
Picolinehydroxamic acid	7.4	2.9	0.6	0.2	
Pyrimidine-2-hydroxamic acid	7.4	4.5	—	—	Calculated from results obtained by CHILDS et al. (1955)

a) Ratios calculated from results reported by WILSON (1955), WILSON et al. (1955), and WILSON and GINSBURG (1955a); they used highly purified AChE of electric eel tissue as enzyme source.

DAVIES and GREEN (1956), and CHILDS et al. (1955) used human erythrocytes as enzyme source.

Nicotinehydroxamic acid has approximately 20% of the activity of its methiodide (NHAM) as a reactivator of diethylphosphoryl-AChE at pH 7.4, but both are approximately equiactive at pH 7.4 in reactivating di*iso*propylphosphoryl-AChE (WILSON et al. 1955). Picolinehydroxamic acid methiodide, unlike NHAM, is less active as a reactivator than its tertiary base (WILSON 1955a).

Salicylhydroxamic acid, furohydroxamic acid, benzhydroxamic acid, 4-aminobenzhydroxamic acid, 4-methylbenzhydroxamic acid, hippurohydroxamic acid, *iso*nicotinehydroxamic acid, and tropohydroxamic acid have been screened for potential reactivating properties at pH 7.4 by CHILDS et al. (1955). At this pH the reactivating potency of the first two hydroxamic acids approaches that of NHAM, whereas all the other hydroxamic acids are less effective.

3. Reactivation by oximes

Many oximes are more potent reactivators than hydroxamic acids at pH 7 to 8. Reactivation of phosphorylated AChE by oximes and hydroxamic acids is controlled by the same factors, i.e., the concentration of the anion of the reactivator and its nucleophilic activity, protonation of an acidic group at the esteratic site of phosphorylated AChE, and the degree of complementariness and strength of bonding between the anion of the reactivator and phosphorylated AChE. If we substitute the anion of an oxime for the hydroxamate ion, reactivation can be represented as shown in reactions (4) and (7). The nucleophilic activities of anions of oximes and hydroxamic acids with a common pK_a are similar (GREEN and SAVILLE 1956, GREEN et al. 1958), but at any given pH oximes often produce much higher rates of reactivation than hydroxamic acids with similar pK_a's. In the case of the oximes which have a very high reactivating potency at pH 7 to 8, complementariness with phosphorylated AChE and complex formation play an even greater part in the reactivation than they do in the case of the hydroxamic acids listed in Table 3.

Only few detailed investigations of the relationship between pH and rates of reactivation have been carried out, and amongst them that of DAVIES and GREEN (1956) is the most detailed one. Figure 2 is an illustration taken from their paper, and as can be seen the shape of the pH-activity curve of an oxime closely resembles that shown in Fig. 1 for NHAM and its tertiary base.

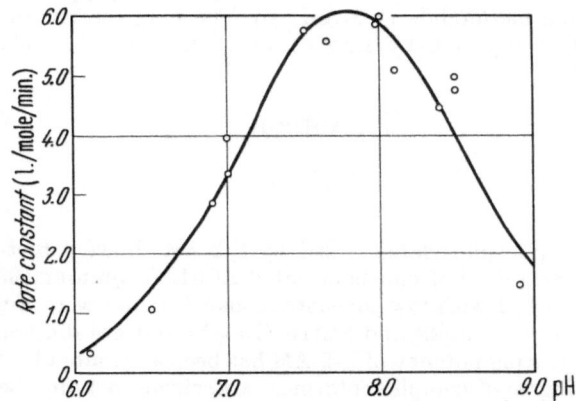

Fig. 2. *pH-dependence of reactivation of diethylphosphoryl-AChE by monoisonitrosoacetone (MINA) at 25°* (DAVIES and GREEN 1956). The ordinate shows the ratio $k/[R]$ where k is the first order constant of reactivation and $[R]$ a fixed concentration of MINA. The open circles represent the observed ratios and the curve is derived on the assumption that reactivation is a reaction between the anion of MINA (pK_a 8.3) and a protonated form of the phosphorylated enzyme with a pK_a of 7.3 of the acidic group in the esteratic site. Enzyme used for preparation of phosphorylated AChE: human erythrocytes

Hydrolysis of organophosphates by 2-oxo-oximes was investigated by GREEN and SAVILLE (1956) who found that for Sarin the reaction is kinetically first order in the presence of excess of oxime and that phosphonylation of the oxime is the rate-determining step in the hydrolysis. These authors also identified the anion of oximes as the active species. Hydrolysis of Sarin by the oximes can be presented as follows (GREEN and SAVILLE 1956):

$$\text{F---P}{<}^{R_1}_{R_2} + \text{RCOCR'NOH} + \text{H}_2\text{O} \rightarrow \text{HO---P}{<}^{R_1}_{R_2} + \text{HF} + \text{RCOOH} + \text{R'CN} \qquad (9)$$
$$\underset{\text{O}}{\|} \qquad\qquad\qquad\qquad\qquad\qquad \underset{\text{O}}{\|}$$

The hydrolysis of Sarin by mono- and *bis*-quaternary pyridine aldoximes was investigated by HACKLEY (1956) who found that the reaction initially conforms with first order kinetics. The hydrolysis involves the formation of a phosphonylated anion of the oxime and the release of HF. The stability of the phosphonylated anions of isomeric pyridine aldoxime methiodides varies, and at pH 7.6 and 30° the 4-isomer has a half-life of 200 min; the corresponding 2-isomer is more stable and has a half-life of 5 to 20 min under the same conditions (HACKLEY et al. 1959).

The hydrolysis of organophosphates (see I) with different substituent groups for R_1, R_2, and X by three 2-oxo-oximes and two hydroxamic acids was investigated by GREEN et al. (1958) with the aim of gaining information on the relationship between structure and reactivity.

Reactivation at pH 7 to 8. In the following three subsections some of the features of reactivation of phosphorylated AChE by oximes will be discussed in greater detail, particularly the complex which is formed between phosphorylated AChE and the anion of the reactivator. All experiments were carried out at pH 7 to 8, and the ratio $k/[R]$, for $k \ll k_{max}$, will be used for comparison of reactivating potencies. As in the case of hydroxamic acids, these ratios in cases where k is not linearly related to $[R]$ are valid only for a narrow range of $[R]$ and for the pH at which they were determined.

a) Mono-quaternary pyridine aldoximes and closely related oximes

The most potent reactivator amongst mono-quaternary pyridine aldoximes is pyridine-2-aldoxime methiodide (P-2-AM; V). The high reactivating potency of this oxime was first reported by DAVIES and GREEN (1955) and WILSON and GINSBURG (1955b).

$$\underset{(V)}{\underset{\underset{CH_3 \quad I^-}{|}}{\overset{\displaystyle\bigcirc}{N}}\text{CHNOH}}$$

Reactivation of phosphorylated AChE by P-2-AM shows a first-order dependence on the concentration of phosphorylated AChE (HOBBIGER 1956). The rates of reactivation obtained with low concentrations of oxime were investigated by HOBBIGER (1957b) and GREEN and SMITH (1958b) and are illustrated in Fig. 3.

The high reactivating potency of P-2-AM has been attributed by WILSON et al. (1958) to a high degree of complimentariness and strong bonding between oxime and phosphorylated AChE. The findings of these authors and the conclusions which they have drawn form their work are as follows:

Mono-quaternary pyridinoyl formaldoximes (VI) and pyridine-aldoximes (VII), like nicotinehydroxamic acid methiodide (NHAM), are with the exception of pyridine-3-aldoxime methiodide (P-3-AM) considerably more potent than their tertiary bases as reactivators of diethylphosphoryl-AChE (Table 4).

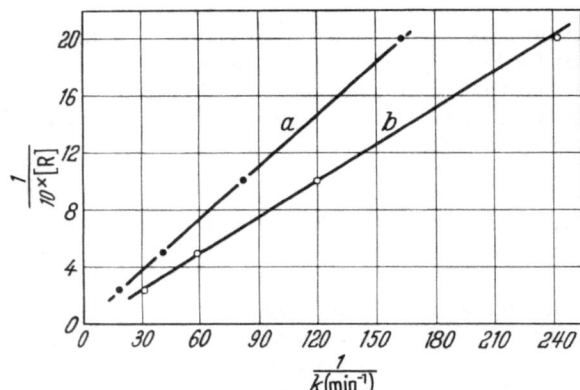

Fig. 3. *Reactivation of phosphorylated AChE by low concentrations of P-2-AM* (HOBBIGER *1957b*). a = diethylphosphoryl-AChE ($x = 4$), b = diisopropylphosphoryl-AChE ($x = 3$); both were prepared from human erythrocytes. Reactivation at 37° and pH 7.45. k is the first order constant of reactivation and $[R]$ the concentration of P-2-AM

$$\underset{(VI)}{\underset{\underset{CH_3 \quad I^-}{|}}{\overset{\displaystyle\bigcirc}{N}}\text{COCHNOH}}$$

$$\underset{(VII)}{\underset{\underset{CH_3 \quad I^-}{|}}{\overset{\displaystyle\bigcirc}{N}}\text{CHNOH}}$$

The marked differences between the reactivating potencies of the three isomeric mono-quaternary pyridine aldoximes at pH 7 (see Table 4) are not attributable to differences between the concentrations of the anions of the three oximes and their nucleophilic activities, since the rates of hydrolysis of 4-nitrophenyl acetate and of Sarin by the three isomeric mono-quaternary pyridine aldoximes differ only by a factor of 2, and since the rates of reactivation of diethylphosphoryl-chymotrypsin obtained with them are also very similar. The high reactivating potency of P-2-AM and P-4-AM, therefore, must be attributed to formation of a complex with phosphorylated AChE which promotes reactivation. As in the case of quaternary hydroxamic acids, the complex seems to involve bonding of the quaternary ammonium group of the oxime to the anionic site of phosphorylated AChE, since the relative potency of P-2-AM as a reactivator of diethyl- and diisopropyl-phosphoryl-AChE, and of isopropyl methylphosphonyl-AChE is 100,

Table 4. *Reactivation of diethylphosphoryl-AChE by mono-quaternary oximes and their tertiary bases at 25° (ratios are calculated from results reported by* WILSON et al. *1958)*

Oxime	pK_a	pH	$k/[R]$ in l.mole^{-1} min^{-1}
Nicotinoyl formaldoxime	7.8	7.9	83
Nicotinoyl formaldoxime methiodide	7.2	7.9	2,500
*Iso*nicotinoyl formaldoxime	7.8	7.9	22
*Iso*nicotinoyl formaldoxime methiodide	7.1	7.9	2,300
Pyridine-2-aldoxime	10.4	7	0.28
Pyridine-2-aldoxime methiodide (P-2-AM)	8.0	7	14,000
Pyridine-3-aldoxime	10.2	7	0.16
Pyridine-3-aldoxime methiodide (P-3-AM)	9.2		0.01
Pyridine-4-aldoxime	10.2	7	0.48
Pyridine-4-aldoxime methiodide (P-4-AM)	8.6	7	300

Highly purified AChE of electric eel tissue was used for preparation of the phosphorylated AChE. For information concerning differences (between ratios) which are attributable to variations between concentrations of the anions of the oximes and their nucleophilic activities see text.

1, and 2, respectively. Amongst the oximes listed in Table 4, P-2-AM has the most rigid structure. Resonance between the oxygen and the ring, and steric hindrance by the methyl group tend to fix the oxygen in the plane of the ring in the position shown in (VIII). The 4- and 3-isomers of P-2-AM (P-4-AM and P-3-AM) are also planar molecules because of resonance but their oxygen can be in two positions, one of which is shown in (IX) and (X). The distance between

(VIII)   (IX)   (X)

the anionic site and the basic group of the esteratic site which is phosphorylated can be calculated from results obtained in studies of the relationship between structure and anti-AChE activity of neostigmine and related compounds (WILSON and QUAN 1958). The spatial relationship between the oxygen atom of the oximes and the phosphorus atom of phosphorylated AChE during reactivation must be as shown in (VIII), (IX), and (X), where the position of the phosphorus atom is labelled ℗. As can be seen, the nucleophilic oxygen atom of P-2-AM and of P-4-AM is in close proximity to the phosphorus atom. This accounts for the exceptionally high potency of these two oximes as reactivators of diethyl-phosphoryl-AChE. Slight modification of the structure of P-2-AM reduces the complimentariness between oxime and phosphorylated AChE, as shown by the finding that introduction of an alkyl group in the 3, 5, or 6 position in the pyridine ring, which affects the pK_a of the oxime only slightly, is associated with a loss of reactivating potency. The orientation of P-3-AM on the enzyme surface is unsatisfactory and, therefore, the oxime is a poor reactivator.

Phosphorylated AChE prepared from human erythrocytes. As pointed out previously, WILSON and his co-workers used highly purified AChE of electric eel tissue as the enzyme source for the preparation of phosphorylated AChE, whereas in most other laboratories washed human erythrocytes were used for this purpose.

Although the results obtained with the two preparations are qualitatively in agreement, there are considerable quantitative differences which either arise from differences between the purity of the enzyme preparations or which reflect genuine differences between the AChE of electric eel tissue and that of mammalian tissues.

Table 5. *Reactivation by P-2-AM of phosphorylated AChE prepared from different sources*

$k/[R]$ in l. mole^{-1}min^{-1}				
Type of phosphorylated AChE		pH	Temp.	Source of AChE
diethyl-phos-phoryl-	diisopropyl-phosphoryl-			
14,000	140	7.0	25°	electric eel tissue (WILSON et al. 1958)
1,450	115	7.4	37°	human erythrocytes (HOBBIGER et al. 1960)
500	17	7.4	25°	human erythrocytes (DAVIES and GREEN 1955, GREEN and SMITH 1958b)

The differences between the rates of reactivation by P-2-AM of phosphorylated AChE prepared from the highly purified AChE of electric eel tissue and that prepared from human erythrocytes are shown in Table 5.

Kinetic studies by GREEN and SMITH (1958b) show that after formation of a complex between phosphorylated AChE and reactivator has taken place, the anionic form of P-2-AM dephosphorylates diethylphosphoryl-AChE 5 times faster than diisopropylphosphoryl-AChE; this finding is in agreement with the results of DOSTROVSKY and HALMANN (1953), who found that nucleophilic reagents hydrolyze diethyl phosphorochloridate 5 to 10 times faster than diisopropyl phosphorochloridate. P-2-AM reactivates diethylphosphoryl-AChE 30 times faster than diisopropylphosphoryl-AChE under the experimental conditions used by GREEN and SMITH, and thus they concluded that the contribution towards reactivation attributable to bonding of the anionic form of the oxime to phosphorylated AChE is 6 times greater for diethyl- than for diisopropyl-phosphoryl-AChE. Promotion of reactivation by complex formation plays also a considerable part in the reactivation of diisopropylphosphoryl-AChE and isopropyl methylphosphonyl-AChE, since at pH 7.4, P-2-AM (pK_a 8.0) is much more potent than a hydroxamic acid with a similar pK_a, e.g., nicotinehydroxamic acid (pK_a 8.3), as a reactivator of these two types of phosphorylated AChE.

At pH 7.45 and 37° the observed reactivating potencies of P-4-AM and P-3-AM, relative to that of P-2-AM, are 6% and 0.03%, respectively, for diethylphosphoryl-AChE prepared from human erythrocytes; if there were no differences between concentrations of oxime anions and their nucleophilic activities, the percentages would be 17 and 0.3, respectively (HOBBIGER et al., 1960). These findings and results obtained by GREEN and SMITH (1958b) suggest that the superiority of

P-2-AM over P-4-AM as a reactivator of diethylphosphoryl-AChE is mainly attributable to differences in their bonding to phosphorylated AChE.

Supporting the interpretation that the quaternary ammonium group of P-2-AM is bound to the anionic site of phosphorylated-AChE is the observation that Na^+, K^+, and NH_4^+ ions, choline, and high concentrations of ACh inhibit reactivation of diethylphosphoryl-AChE and *iso*propyl methylphosphonyl-AChE by this oxime (HOBBIGER 1957b, GREEN and SMITH 1958a, SCAIFE 1959).

The importance of complimentariness between reactivator and phosphorylated AChE for reactivation is stressed by the observation that quaternary quinoline aldoximes and 3,3-dimethyl indolenine-2-aldoxime methiodide are less potent reactivators than P-2-AM, and that enlarging or lengthening the N-alkyl group of P-2-AM leads to a loss of reactivating potency which is not attributable to differences between concentrations of the anions of the oximes or their nucleophilic activities (HOBBIGER et al. 1960).

b) Bis-quaternary pyridine aldoximes

The most potent reactivators of phosphorylated AChE belong to a group of oximes with the general structure (XI):

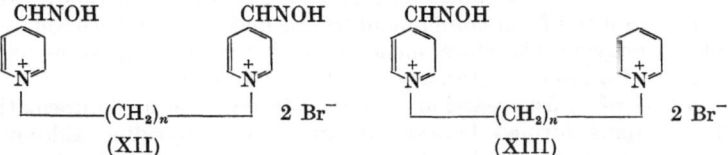

where $\overset{+}{R}$ is a pyridinium aldoxime, pyridinium, isoquinolinium, trialkylammonium, or thiouronium group (HOBBIGER and SADLER 1958, 1959, HOBBIGER et al. 1958, 1960, POZIOMEK et al. 1958, WILSON and GINSBURG 1958, BERRY et al. 1959, SCAIFE 1959).

The reactivating potencies of many of these *bis*-quaternary pyridine aldoximes, e.g., the oximes with structures (XII) and (XIII), are considerably greater than that of P-2-AM when comparisons are based on the rates of reactivation obtained during short periods of incubation of the oximes with phosphorylated AChE.

Oximes with structure (XII) will be referred to generally as 4,4'-dioximes of N,N'-polymethylene*bis*(pyridinium bromide), and oximes with structure (XIII) as 4-monoximes of N,N'-polymethylene*bis*(pyridinium bromide).

The time-courses of reactivation (by *bis*-quaternary pyridine aldoximes) of diethyl- and di*iso*propyl-phosphoryl-AChE and of *iso*propyl methylphosphonyl-AChE, generally deviate from first order kinetics. In many cases reactivation is rapid initially but then slows down considerably and proceeds only at a very low rate. The relationship between percentage reactivation obtained after a given period of reactivation, and concentration of *bis*-quaternary pyridine aldoxime is similar to that obtained in experiments with mono-quaternary pyridine aldoximes.

HOBBIGER et al. (1960) showed that deviations of the time-course of reactivation from first order kinetics were much greater with diethylphosphoryl-AChE prepared from human erythrocytes than with di*iso*propylphosphoryl-AChE prepared from the same source or diethylphosphoryl-AChE prepared from partly purified bovine erythrocyte AChE. They also showed that ACh prevented the deviation in all cases. Various possible sources of interference with reactivation were ruled out, and the conclusion was reached that phosphorylation of AChE by the phosphorylated anion of the oxime which is formed during reactivation accounts for the anomalous time-course of reactivation. Phosphonylating properties of the phosphonates formed between Sarin and P-2-AM or P-4-AM have been demonstrated by SOMERS and BAY (1959) and HACKLEY et al. (1959). The latter found also that phosphonylated P-4-AM is $\geq$ 10 times more stable than phosphonylated P-2-AM. An extension of these studies to phosphorylated and phosphonylated *bis*-quaternary pyridine aldoximes is urgently needed.

SCAIFE (1959) studied the reactivation of *iso*propyl methylphosphonyl-AChE (prepared from highly purified AChE of electric eel tissue) by *bis*-quaternary pyridine aldoximes, and the effect of AChE on it. His results show that reactivation of *iso*propyl methylphosphonyl-AChE by *bis*-quaternary pyridine aldoximes can be represented as

$$\text{E—P} + \text{oxime} \underset{k_2}{\overset{k_1}{\rightleftharpoons}} \text{E} + \text{oxime-phosphonate} \tag{8}$$

where E is AChE, and E—P phosphonylated AChE.

Reaction (8) is obviously generally applicable to reactivation of phosphorylated AChE by all the *bis*-quaternary pyridine aldoximes. In any individual case the constant k_2 will be proportional to the concentration, phosphorylating potency, and stability in aqueous solution of the phosphorylated oxime which is formed during reactivation, and the higher the ratio k_1/k_2 the closer the time-course of reactivation of phosphorylated AChE by *bis*-quaternary pyridine aldoximes approaches first order characteristics. In the case of mono-quaternary pyridine aldoximes and 2-oxo-oximes, k_1 is $\gg k_2$.

The initial rates of reactivation of phosphorylated AChE obtained with many *bis*-quaternary pyridine aldoximes are greater than those obtained with their mono-quaternary parent oximes, P-2-AM, P-3-AM, and P-4-AM. This is, on the whole, not attributable to differences between concentrations of the anionic forms of the oximes and their nucleophilic activities (HOBBIGER et al. 1960). Promotion of reactivation resulting from complimentariness and bonding between oxime and phosphorylated enzyme, therefore, must be greater with *bis*-quaternary pyridine aldoximes than with mono-quaternary pyridine aldoximes.

Measurements of k_1 (see reaction 8) obviously give the best information concerning the complex formed between *bis*-quaternary pyridine aldoximes and phosphorylated AChE, but such data are unfortunately not available at present. HOBBIGER et al. (1960) measured the reactivating potencies of *bis*-quaternary pyridine aldoximes and P-2-AM by incubating phosphorylated AChE for 30 min with an oxime, and then allowing reactivation to continue for 35 min in the presence of ACh; AChE-activity between 5 and 35 min after addition of the substrate was used for assessing reactivation. The authors showed that results obtained by this method closely approach those obtained by incubating phosphorylated AChE with oximes in the presence of ACh (which prevents rephosphorylation of AChE by the phosphorylated oxime). Table 6 summarizes the results obtained by HOBBIGER et al. (1960) and also shows relative reactivating potencies calculated from results published by POZIOMEK et al. (1958), WILSON and GINSBURG (1958), and BERRY et al. (1959). POZIOMEK et al. reported rate constants, and in the latter two cases, the relative potencies were calculated from the percentages of reactivation reported by the authors by assuming that the ratio $k/[R]$ for reactivation by P-2-AM is constant over the range of concentrations which are required to give the same percentage reactivation as was obtained with the *bis*-quaternary pyridine aldoximes. Relative potencies calculated by this method are, therefore, only approximations. To what extent the ratios $k/[R]$ calculated from results reported by WILSON and GINSBURG (1958) and POZIOMEK

Table 6. *Reactivation of phosphorylated AChE by bis-quaternary pyridine aldoximes with the general structure (XI)*

Position of oxime group	R+	n	pK$_a$	diethylphosphoryl- a	diethylphosphoryl- b	diethylphosphoryl- c	diisopropylphosphoryl- d	diisopropylphosphoryl- e	isopropyl methylphosphonyl- f
2	[ring] N–CHNOH	3	7.8		0.5	0.074			
		4	7.8			0.65			
		5	7.9			2.4		5.2	
		6	7.8		15	0.57			
	*iso*quinolinium	3	7.8		2				
	trimethyl-ammonium	5	7.8			0.15		0.6	
3	[ring] CHNOH	3				0.27			
		6				0.33			
	*iso*quinolinium	3				<0.2			
4	CHNOH [ring]	1	7.6	2.8 (1.1)		0.2			
		2	7.8	17 (11)	12	0.7	22 (7)		
		3	8.2	22 (20)	12	3.9	52 (26)		3
		4	8.2	18 (18)	8.6	3.9	38 (20)		5
		5	8.3	16 (18)		3.9	36 (20)	37	
		6	8.3		2.4	2.8			
		10	8.4		<0.2	3.3			
	trimethyl-ammonium	3	8.0*	8 (14)		4.6	11 (11)		
		4	8.0*	6.7 (13)			10 (11)		
		5	8.2	7.5 (16)		1.2	11 (12)	78	
		5	8.3			1.6		8.2	
	triethyl-ammonium	3				0.46			
	thiouronium	3				<0.2			
	*iso*quinolinium	3			4				

a) and d) Results reported by HOBBIGER et al. (1960). Enzyme source: human erythrocytes; 37°, pH 7.45. The figures in brackets are the relative reactivating potencies which would be observed if all oxime groups were functional and if there were no differences between the concentrations of oxime anions and their nucleophilic activities.

b) Relative potencies are calculated from results reported by BERRY et al. (1959) who measured the time required for 25% reactivation by 0.02 mM concentrations of the oximes. Enzyme source: human erythrocytes; 25°, pH 7.4.

c) and e) Relative potencies calculated from results reported by WILSON and GINSBURG (1958) who used 6 min for reactivation and variable oxime concentrations. Enzyme source: highly purified AChE of electric eel tissue; 25°, pH 7.8.

f) Relative potencies calculated from rate constants reported by POZIOMEK et al. (1958). Enzyme source: highly purified AChE of electric eel tissue; 25°, pH 7.4.

The pK$_a$'s are those reported by WILSON and GINSBURG (1958) except in two cases (*). The latter were reported by HOBBIGER et al. (1960).

For further explanations see text.

et al. (1958) and some of the results reported by BERRY et al. (1959) are affected by rephosphorylation is not known.

According to WILSON et al. (1958) and WILSON (1959), reactivation of phosphorylated AChE by P-2-AM and P-4-AM involves bonding of their quaternary ammonium group to the anionic site of phosphorylated AChE, as discussed previously. It seems logical to assume that mono- and *bis*-quaternary pyridine aldoximes share a common bonding site, and if we accept the interpretation of WILSON for the bonding site of mono-quaternary pyridine aldoximes, the common bonding site is the anionic site of phosphorylated AChE. Additional bonding of the second quaternary ammonium group of *bis*-quaternary pyridine aldoximes to another site would raise the affinity of these oximes (relative to that of mono-quaternary pyridine aldoximes) for phosphorylated AChE, and consequently raise the reactivating potency of *bis*-quaternary pyridine aldoximes over that of mono-quaternary pyridine aldoximes. The interpretation that *bis*-quaternary pyridine aldoximes are bonded to two sites of phosphorylated AChE is strongly supported by the finding that a minimum distance between the two quaternary nitrogens of the reactivator is required for maximum reactivating potency. According to the results obtained by HOBBIGER et al. (1960) with 4-monoximes and 4,4'-dioximes of N,N'-polymethylene*bis*(pyridinium bromide), the distance between the two bonding sites is approximately 5 Å. The results of other authors, obtained with the corresponding 3,3'- and 2,2'-dioximes (see Table 6), indicate a larger distance, but since the part played by steric hindrance or rephosphorylation of AChE or both in the reactivation by these oximes is not known, we cannot put too much emphasis on these findings at present. The anti-AChE potency of many of the *bis*-quaternary pyridine aldoximes which have the highest reactivating potency is of the same order as that of P-2-AM (HOBBIGER et al. 1960). To explain this we have to postulate that if *bis*-quaternary pyridine aldoximes are bonded to two sites of phosphorylated AChE, one of which is the anionic site, the strength of bonding to the anionic site must vary, and the spatial relationship between the nucleophilic oxygen atom of *bis*-quaternary pyridine aldoximes and the phosphorus atom must be better than that in the complex formed by P-2-AM. There is at present no direct evidence to support this interpretation. The high reactivating potency of 3,3'-dioximes of N,N'-polymethylene*bis*(pyridinium bromide) relative to P-3-AM is also surprising, since bonding of the quaternary ammonium group of P-3-AM to the anionic site gives such an unfavourable orientation for the nucleophilic oxygen atom of P-3-AM (see X). Although there can be no doubt that *bis*-quaternary pyridine aldoximes are bonded to two sites of phosphorylated AChE, more information is required before we can give a generally acceptable interpretation of the bonding and complimentariness between phosphorylated AChE and mono- and *bis*-quaternary pyridine aldoximes. Until then, the conclusions of WILSON et al. (1958) and WILSON (1959) concerning reactivation of phosphorylated AChE by mono-quaternary pyridine aldoximes should be considered only as a working hypothesis.

The importance of two positively charged groups for high reactivating potency is also illustrated by results obtained with oximes with the general structure (XIV).

CHNOH

$n = 2, 3,$ or 4

$(CH_2)_n \overset{\delta+}{C}H_2Br$ Br^-

(XIV)

The contribution towards reactivation attributable to bonding and complimentariness of the anionic form of these oximes is 4 to 25 times higher than that obtained with the anionic form of their parent oxime, P-4-AM (HOBBIGER et al. 1960).

It has been pointed out previously that the rates of reactivation of phosphorylated AChE by mono-quaternary pyridine aldoximes vary according to the source of enzyme which is used for the preparation of phosphorylated AChE (see Table 5). Similar discrepancies are found when *bis*-quaternary pyridine aldoximes are used as reactivators (see Table 6). HOBBIGER et al. (1960), who used phosphorylated AChE prepared from human erythrocytes, found that the reactivating potencies of oximes of N,N'-polymethylene*bis*(pyridinium bromide) relative to P-2-AM are very similar for diethyl- and di*iso*propyl-phosphoryl-AChE's when allowance is made for differences between concentrations of the anionic forms of these oximes and their nucleophilic activities (Table 6; figures in brackets); this also applies to reactivation of phosphorylated AChE prepared from partly purified AChE of bovine erythrocytes, as recorded by these authors. WILSON and GINSBURG (1958), on the other hand, prepared phosphorylated AChE from the highly purified enzyme of electric eel tissue, and found that the rates of reactivation of di*iso*propylphosphoryl-AChE relative to that of diethylphosphoryl-AChE are considerably greater with *bis*-quaternary pyridine aldoximes than with P-2-AM. These observations indicate that phosphorylated AChE's prepared from the two sources differ in behaviour.

c) 2-Oxo-oximes

A large number of 2-oxo-oximes with the general formula (XV)

RCOCR'NOH

(XV)

reactivate phosphorylated AChE (CHILDS et al. 1955). The most potent reactivators amongst them are:

Oxime	R	R'
di*iso*nitrosoacetone (DINA)	CHNOH	H
mono*iso*nitrosoacetone (MINA). . .	CH$_3$	H
*iso*nitrosoacetophenone	phenyl	H
*iso*nitrosoacetylacetone	CH$_3$	acetyl

Table 7 shows the reactivating potency of these oximes at pH 7.4 and also that of diacetylmonoxime (R and R' = CH$_3$; referred to later as DAM). The latter is included because of its marked antidotal action in Sarin poisoning of rats (ASKEW 1956, 1957).

In screening a large number of related oximes, CHILDS et al. (1955) found that at pH 7.4 phenylglyoxime and 4-methoxy*iso*nitrosoacetophenone have reactivating potencies similar to those of the most potent 2-oxo-oximes listed in Table 7, whereas glyoxime, methylglyoxime, acetoxime, salicylaldoxime, α- and β-furfuralaldoximes, 4-hydroxybenzaldoxime, di*iso*nitrosocyclohexanone, *iso*nitrosoacetylfuran, isatin-β-oxime, tri*iso*nitrosopropane, 2-chlorobenzaldoxime, pyrogallol aldoxime, cyclohexane-1:2 dione dioxime, gallacetophenone oxime, 3- and 4-hydroxybenzaldoximes, *iso*nitrosodimedone, pentane-2:3:4-trione-2:3-dioxime, and pyrrole-2-aldoxime are either less effective than the first four oximes listed in Table 7 or devoid of reactivating properties at the concentrations used.

Kinetic studies of the reactivation of phosphorylated AChE by 2-oxo-oximes indicate that formation of a complex between the anions of these oximes and phosphorylated AChE, which promotes reactivation, is essential for the high reactivating potency of the oximes listed in Table 7 (GREEN and SMITH 1958c). K⁺, Na⁺, and NH₄⁺ ions accelerate reactivation (GREEN and SMITH 1958a), and thus the bonding site involved cannot be the anionic site of phosphorylated AChE. Variation of the alkyl group (R) has only little effect on the reactivating potency of 2-oxo-oximes. This indicates that the carbonyl oxygen atom of the oximes is linked by a hydrogen bond to phosphorylated AChE in the complex; since the ring-nitrogen atom of picolinehydroxamic acid (III) is in a position analogous to

Table 7. *Reactivation of phosphorylated AChE by oximes with the general structure (XV) at 25° and pH 7.4*

Oxime	pK$_a$	$k/[R]$ in l. mole^{-1} min^{-1}		
		Type of phosphorylated AChE		
		diethyl-phosphoryl-	di*iso*propyl-phosphoryl-	*iso*propyl methyl-phosphonyl-
di*iso*nitrosoacetone (DINA)		8.4	0.8	24.3
mono*iso*nitrosoacetone (MINA).	8.3	6.8	0.7	22.1
*iso*nitrosoacetophenone	8.3	10.7	5.1	4.4
*iso*nitrosoacetylacetone	7.4	0.7	—	1.1
diacetylmonoxime (DAM)	9.3	approx.0.2	—	5.2
pyridine-2-aldoxime methiodide (P-2-AM) .	8.0	500	17	200

Results obtained by DAVIES and his co-workers and mainly based on work published by DAVIES and GREEN (1956). Human erythrocytes were used for the preparation of phosphorylated AChE. All oximes with structure (XV) are less potent than P-2-AM as reactivators, and results obtained with P-2-AM are included for comparison.

that of the carbonyl oxygen atom in 2-oxo-aldoximes, it seems likely that the complex formed between phosphorylated AChE and picolinehydroxamic acid involves hydrogen bonding of the ring-nitrogen atom of the latter (GREEN and SMITH 1958c). Kinetic studies of GREEN and SMITH (1958b) suggest that the complimentariness (arising from orientation) between reactivator and diethylphosphoryl-AChE in the complex formed between the phosphorylated AChE and P-2-AM or MINA is of a similar order, and that the higher reactivating potency of P-2-AM (relative to that of MINA) arises mainly from stronger bonding of the former. The findings of these authors indicate also that the orientation of MINA in the complex which it forms with *iso*propyl methylphosphonyl-AChE is better than that of P-4-AM in the corresponding complex, whereas the reverse is true for the strength of bonding of the two oximes to the phosphonylated AChE.

The apparent energy of reactivation of diethylphosphoryl-AChE and *iso*propyl methylphosphonyl-AChE by di*iso*nitrosoacetone is approximately 11.5 kcal/mole, according to results obtained by DAVIES and GREEN (1956).

4. Reactivation by ammonium molybdate

Ammonium molybdate hydrolyses organophosphates (HOBBIGER 1956, AUGUSTINSSON 1958, LARSSON 1958) and reactivates phosphorylated AChE (HOBBIGER 1956). Ammonium molybdate has approximately 1/100 of the potency of P-2-AM as a reactivator of diethyl- and di*iso*propyl-phosphoryl-AChE at pH 7.45 and 37°. Reactivation by ammonium molybdate does not involve the formation of a complex between reactivator and anionic site of phosphorylated AChE, since it is not inhibited by trimethylamine.

5. Formation of a phosphorylated acetylcholinesterase which cannot by reactivated by hydroxamic acids or oximes

Phosphorylated AChE formed by reaction (1) is converted into a non-reactivatable form on ageing.

The conversion is acid-catalysed and follows a first order law (DAVIES and GREEN 1956, HOBBIGER 1956, MICHEL 1958). To obtain complete or near complete reactivation of di*iso*propylphosphoryl-AChE or *iso*propyl methylphosphonyl-AChE, as described in the preceeding text, it is essential to use enzyme samples (freshly prepared in the case of erythrocytes) which have been exposed to organophosphates for only short periods. With diethylphosphoryl-AChE, on the other hand, near complete reactivation is still obtained when the phosphorylated enzyme is several hours old (JANDORF et al. 1955a, b, WILSON et al. 1955, DAVIES and GREEN 1956, HOBBIGER 1956).

The conversion of reactivatable into non-reactivatable phosphorylated AChE occurs both *in vitro* and *in vivo* (HOBBIGER 1956), and at pH 7.2 to 7.5 and 37° the approximate half-lives of reactivatable phosphorylated AChE's are diethylphosphoryl-AChE: 40 hr (HOBBIGER 1956), di*iso*propylphosphoryl-AChE and *iso*propyl methylphosphonyl-AChE: 2 to 3 hr (HOBBIGER 1956, DAVIES and GREEN 1956). The experiments of HOBBIGER (1956) were carried out in a medium containing only 0.025 M NaHCO$_3$, whereas DAVIES and GREEN (1956) used a buffer consisting of 0.01 M sodium diethylbarbiturate (veronal), 0.002 M KH$_2$PO$_4$, and 0.3 M KCl. It was shown by HOBBIGER (1956) that the rate of conversion (relative to that obtained in 0.025 M NaHCO$_3$) is slightly less if a medium of 0.075 M NaCl and KCl and 0.025 M NaHCO$_3$ is used, and that the addition of 0.04 M MgCl$_2$ to 0.025 M NaHCO$_3$ approximately halves it.

Organophosphates react with butyrocholinesterase (BuChE) in the same way as with AChE (reactions 1 and 2), and phosphorylated BuChE is also subject to "ageing" (HOBBIGER 1955). The conversion of reactivatable di*iso*propylphosphoryl-BuChE into a non-reactivatable phosphorylated BuChE has been studied by BERENDS et al. (1959), who showed that there is a parallelism between the rate of conversion and the rate at which one *iso*propyl group is lost from the di*iso*propylphosphoryl group of the phosphorylated enzyme. This suggests that conversion of dialkoxyphosphoryl-AChE and *iso*propyl methylphosphonyl-AChE into a monoalkoxyphosphoryl-AChE and methylphosphonyl-AChE, respectively, is responsible for the loss of reactivatability. Since *iso*propyl methylphosphonyl-chymotrypsin, formed by the reaction between Sarin and chymotrypsin, is not converted into a non-reactivatable form (GREEN and NICHOLLS 1959), the elimination of one alkyl group from reactivatable phosphorylated AChE might be catalyzed by the phosphorylated AChE itself. It is possible that the conversion leads to additional bonding, e.g., of the type enzyme-P-O-enzyme.

II. Reactivatability of the phosphorylated acetylcholinesterases formed by Tabun, OMPA, and methylfluorophosphorylcholines

Only a few investigations have been carried out on the reactivation of phosphorylated AChE with is formed by organophosphates which possess other than a dialkoxyphosphoryl or *iso*propyl methylphosphonyl group.

Phosphorylated AChE (with purified electric eel AChE as the enzyme source) formed by ethyl-N-dimethyl phosphoramidocyanidate (Tabun) at low temperatures can be reactivated by *bis*-quaternary pyridine aldoximes (SCAIFE 1959). At pH 7.4 these oximes reactivate the phosphorylated AChE formed by Tabun at approximately 1/10 of the rate at which they reactivate *iso*propyl methylphosphonyl-AChE. Reactivation by P-2-AM and N,N'-trimethylene*bis*(pyridine-4-aldoxime bromide) [4 D (3), TMB-4] of the phosphorylated AChE formed by the reaction between purified electric eel AChE and Tabun was reported recently also by FLEISHER et al. (1960). WILSON and SONDHEIMER (1957), on the other hand, were unable to reactivate with P-2-AM the phosphorylated AChE formed by incubation of purified electric eel AChE with Tabun; these authors did not state what interval elapsed between preparation of the phosphorylated AChE and attempted reactivation, and in view of the results obtained by SCAIFE (1959) and FLEISHER et al. (1960) we must assume that the phosphorylated AChE formed by Tabun is speedily converted into a non-reactivatable form.

Octamethyl pyrophosphortetramide (OMPA) is an organophosphate which is not *per se* a phosphorylating agent. The phosphorylated AChE formed by its active metabolite, which contains presumably a phosphoramido-N-oxide group (CASIDA et al. 1954), could not be reactivated by concentrations of P-2-AM which readily reactivate diethyl- and di*iso*propyl-phosphoryl-AChE, and *iso*propyl methylphosphonyl-AChE (KEWITZ 1957a). These experiments do not rule out the possibility that initially a reactivatable phosphorylated AChE is formed which is rapidly converted into a non-reactivatable form.

The phosphonylated AChE formed by a 10 min incubation of washed human erythrocytes with methylfluorophosphorylcholines cannot be reactivated by 0.004 M P-2-AM, di*iso*nitrosoacetone (DINA), diacetylmonoxime (DAM), or nicotinehydroxamic acid methiodide (NHAM) (ENANDER 1958).

III. Reactivation of phosphorylated butyrocholinesterase

Information concerning reactivation of phosphorylated BuChE is limited to diethyl- and di*iso*propyl-phosphoryl-BuChE.

The rate of spontaneous reactivation of these two types of phosphorylated BuChE was investigated by HOBBIGER (1951), DAVISON (1953), and ALDRIDGE and DAVISON (1953) and found to be species-dependent. This indicates that the BuChE's of different species are not identical but represent a group of enzymes with closely related substrate-characteristics. Spontaneous reactivation of diethyl-phosphoryl-BuChE of a given species is faster than that of diethylphosphoryl-AChE. In some cases the difference is small but in others it is considerable, e.g., the diethylphosphoryl-BuChE prepared from rat BuChE regains at 37° and pH 7.6 50% activity in 5 hours (DAVISON 1953). Spontaneous reactivation of di*iso*propylphosphoryl-BuChE's is negligible (HOBBIGER 1951, 1955, DAVISON 1953).

The reactivation of diethyl- and di*iso*propyl-phosphoryl-BuChE by hydroxamic acids and oximes has not been studied in great detail, but as far as is known the kinetics of reactivation are the same as those oberserved in experiments with the corresponding types of phosphorylated AChE.

On ageing, dialkoxyphosphoryl-BuChE is converted into a form which cannot be reactivated; in a $MgCl_2$-containing medium the rate of conversion of human di*iso*propylphosphoryl-BuChE into a non-reactivatable form is 20 to 40 times faster than that of di*iso*propylphosphoryl-AChE, and a similar difference applies to diethyl derivatives (HOBBIGER 1955).

Reactivating potencies at pH 7 to 8. Nicotinehydroxamic acid methiodide reactivates human diethyl- and di*iso*propyl-phosphoryl-BuChE (prepared from plasma) approximately 5 times faster than the corresponding types of phosphorylated AChE (HOBBIGER 1955), but this difference is not observed when fraction IV-6-3 of human plasma is used as enzyme source (WILSON 1955); it is possible that a difference between the media in which reactivation was carried out (HOBBIGER used a solution containing $NaHCO_3$, NaCl, KCl, and $MgCl_2$ whereas WILSON used only $NaHCO_3$) accounts for this. WILSON (1955b) also observed that quaternary hydroxamic acids are generally more potent reactivators than their tertiary bases. Pyridine-2-aldoxime methiodide reactivates human diethylphosphoryl-BuChE at 0.05 to 0.1 % of the rate at which it reactivates diethylphosphoryl-AChE (WILSON et al. 1958), and N,N'-trimethylene*bis*(pyridine-4-aldoxime bromide) [4 D (3), TMB-4] is slightly more potent than P-2-AM as a reactivator of diethylphosphoryl-AChE (prepared from highly purified horse serum BuChE) (SCAIFE 1959). The reactivating potency of P-2-AM at pH 7 is approximately 15 times greater than that of P-3-AM, and the reactivating potency of P-4-AM is intermediate between that of P-2-AM and of P-3-AM (WILSON et al. 1958).

These results show that promotion of reactivation by complex formation plays a part in the reactivation of phosphorylated BuChE, although in the case of oximes promotion is much less than that obtained during reactivation of phosphorylated AChE. This is not unexpected since both the anionic and the esteratic sites of AChE are different from those of BuChE (see DAVIES and GREEN 1958).

IV. Reactivation of phosphorylated chymotrypsin

Organophosphates also phosphorylate proteolytic enzymes with esterase activity, e.g., chymotrypsin, and the reaction can be presented as in (1) and (2).

Neither diethyl- nor di*iso*propyl-phosphoryl-chymotrypsin appears to be subject to any significant spontaneous reactivation, but *iso*propyl methylphosphonyl-chymotrypsin shows 48% reactivation at 25° and pH 7.4 when incubated for 96 hr in a sodium acetate-acetic acid buffer. The rate of spontaneous reactivation of *iso*propyl methylphosphonyl-chymotrypsin in different buffers varies considerably (GREEN and NICHOLLS 1959). *Iso*propyl methylphosphonyl-chymotrypsin is not converted into a non-reactivatable form on ageing (GREEN and NICHOLLS 1959).

Diethyl- and di*iso*propyl-phosphoryl-chymotrypsin, and *iso*propyl methylphosphonyl-chymotrypsin can be reactivated by hydroxylamine, hydroxamic acids, and oximes (CUNNINGHAM and NEURATH 1953, CUNNINGHAM 1954, JANDORF et al. 1955a, b, WILSON et al. 1958, GREEN and NICHOLLS 1959). The most detailed studies are those by GREEN and NICHOLLS (1959) who found that hydroxamic acids and oximes reactivate *iso*propyl methylphosphonyl-chymotrypsin faster

Table 8. *Reactivation of* iso*propyl methylphosphonyl-chymotrypsin at 25°* (GREEN and NICHOLLIS 1959)

Oxime or hydroxamic acid	pH	pK_a	$k/[R]$ in l.mole^{-1} min^{-1}
Mono*iso*nitrosoacetone (MINA) .	7.5	8.3	0.02
P-2-AM	7.5	8.0	0.008
Picolinehydroxamic acid	8.0	8.7	0.02
Salicylhydroxamic acid	7.4	7.4	0.05

than diethyl- or di*iso*propyl-phosphoryl-chymotrypsin. The reactivating potencies of some oximes and hydroxamic acids at pH 7.4 to 8 are shown in Table 8. Reactivation of *iso*propyl methylphosphonyl-chymotrypsin, which shows a first order dependence on the concentration of phosphonylated enzyme, is markedly pH dependent (similar to that illustrated in Figs. 1 and 2). This indicates that reactivation, as in the case of phosphorylated AChE, is due to a reaction between the anion of the reactivator and a protonated form of phosphonylated chymotrypsin. The observed differences between the reactivating potencies of different hydroxamic acids and oximes are of a similar order as those expected to arise under the experimental conditions from the difference between the concentrations of the anions of the reactivators and their nucleophilic activities. Promotion of reactivation by formation of a complex between reactivator and phosphonylated chymotrypsin does not seem to play any significant part in the reactivation.

Similar conclusions were reached by WILSON et al. (1958) who determined the rate of reactivation of diethylphosphoryl-chymotrypsin by the three isomeric mono-quaternary pyridine aldoximes.

B. *In vivo* actions of reactivators of phosphorylated acetylcholinesterase

Acetylcholinesterase plays a vital part at those sites where ACh acts as a transmitter of nerve impulses. To meet the requirements for a chemical transmitter it is essential that the action of ACh be short-lasting. The latter is accomplished by AChE which speedily hydrolyzes the ester. Organophosphates interfere with the hydrolysis of ACh by inhibiting AChE by phosphorylation. The symptoms of organophosphate poisoning in animals and man are, therefore, the same as those which result from inhibition of AChE by other anti-ChE agents, e.g., physostigmine (eserine) or neostigmine, and similar to those produced by appropriate injection of ACh. The severity of the symptoms, which are generally long-lasting, is dependent upon the extent to which AChE is phosphorylated (RIKER and WESCOE 1949, KAMIJO and KOELLE 1952), and death occurs when sufficient ACh has accumulated at strategic sites.

Symptoms of sub-lethal organophosphate poisoning can be prevented or reversed by substances which compete with ACh for those sites at which the ester acts as a chemical transmitter. For example, atropine antagonizes the actions of ACh on smooth muscles, glands, heart and blood vessels, i.e., the so-called "muscarinic" actions of ACh, and probably also those at some sites within the central nervous system. *d*-Tubocurarine and ganglion-blocking agents antagonize the "nicotinic" actions of ACh at motor endplates in striped muscle and on ganglion cells, respectively. Protection of animals against several lethal doses of organophosphates can be obtained only by a combination of atropine, *d*-tubocurarine and a ganglion-blocking agent (PARKES and SACRA 1954). The intrinsic hazard of such treatment is considerable. Details of this approach are discussed in chapters 20 and 22.

An alternative method of treating or preventing organophosphate poisoning is the reactivation of phosphorylated AChE. During the past few years the antidotal action of hydroxamic acids and oximes which reactivate diethyl- and di*iso*propylphosphoryl-AChE, and *iso*propyl methylphosphonyl-AChE has been studied extensively in animals. One of the oximes, pyridine-2-aldoxime methiodide (P-2-AM), has also been used successfully in the treatment of Parathion poisoning of man. The following account deals with the antidotal action of hydroxamic acids and oximes in organophosphate poisoning, its relation to reactivation of phosphorylated AChE, and information obtained in related studies. To make a direct comparison between biological and biochemical data possible, all doses and concentrations of hydroxamic acids and oximes are expressed on a molar basis. Information concerning the action of P-2-AM in organophosphate poisoning of man is dealt with extensively in chapter 22 because of its great clinical importance.

I. Protection against lethal organophosphate poisoning

Many hydroxamic acids and oximes raise the LD_{50} of those organophosphates which form initially a reactivatable phosphorylated AChE, and most of the oximes can completely reverse various symptoms of poisoning caused by sub-lethal doses of

Table 9. *Organophosphates used for studies of the antidotal action of hydroxamic acids and oximes*

Chemical name and code used in text	Chemical formula $\left(X - P \overset{R_1}{\underset{O\,(S)}{\overset{\|}{<}} R_2}\right)$	Type of phosphorylated AChE formed
Group I		
tetraethyl pyrophosphate (TEPP)		diethylphosphoryl-
diethyl 4-nitrophenyl phosphate (Paraoxon)		diethylphosphoryl-
3-(diethylphosphato)-N-trimethylanilinium methyl-sulphate (Ro 3-0340)		diethylphosphoryl-
3-(diethylphosphato)-N-methylquinolinium methyl-sulphate (Ro 3-0422)		diethylphosphoryl-
di*iso*propyl phosphorofluoridate (DFP)		di*iso*propyl-phosphoryl-
3-(di*iso*propylphosphato)-pyridine (Ro 3-0351)		di*iso*propyl-phosphoryl-
*iso*propyl methylphosphono-fluoridate (Sarin)		*iso*propyl methyl-phosphonyl-
ethyl-N-dimethyl phosphoramidocyanidate (Tabun)		? dimethylamido ethylphosphoryl-
Group II		
0,0-dimethyl 0-(4-nitrophenyl) phosphorothioate (Methyl-Parathion)		dimethylphosphoryl

Table 9. (Continued)

Chemical name and code used in text	Chemical formula $\left(X-P<^{R_1}_{R_2} \,\,\|\,\, O\,(S) \right)$	Type of phosphorylated AChE formed
0,0-dimethyl 0-(2-ethylthio-ethyl) phosphorothioate (Metasystox)	$H_5C_2SH_2CH_2C-O-P<^{OCH_3}_{OCH_3}$ ‖ S	dimethylphos-phoryl-
0,0-dimethyl S-(N-methyl-carbamyl-methyl) phosphorodithioate (Dimethoate)	$H_3CHNOCH_2C-S-P<^{OCH_3}_{OCH_3}$ ‖ S	dimethylphos-phoryl-
0,0-dimethyl S-(4-oxo-3-H-1,2,3-benzotriazine-3-methyl) phosphoro-dithioate (Guthion)	benzotriazine ring—N—CH$_2$—S—P$<^{OCH_3}_{OCH_3}$ ‖ S	dimethylphos-phoryl-
0,0-diethyl 0-(4-nitrophenyl) phosphorothioate (Parathion)	O_2N-⟨phenyl⟩$-O-P<^{OC_2H_5}_{OC_2H_5}$ ‖ S	diethylphosphoryl-
0,0-diethyl 0-(2-*iso*propyl-6-methyl-4-pyrimidyl) phosphorothioate (Diazinon)	H_3C, H_3C, HC-, pyrimidyl ring (CH$_3$, N) $-O-P<^{OC_2H_5}_{OC_2H_5}$ ‖ S	diethylphosphoryl-
0,0-diethyl 0-(2-ethylthio-ethyl) phosphorothioate (Systox)	$H_5C_2SH_2CH_2C-O-P<^{OC_2H_5}_{OC_2H_5}$ ‖ S	diethylphosphoryl-
0,0-diethyl S-(2,5-dichloro-phenylthiomethyl) phosphorodithioate (Phenkaptone)	Cl, dichlorophenyl—S—CH$_2$—S—P$<^{OC_2H_5}_{OC_2H_5}$ ‖ S, Cl	diethylphosphoryl-
octamethyl pyrophosphor-tetramide (OMPA)	$(CH_3)_2N$, $(CH_3)_2N$ ⟩P$-O-P<^{N(CH_3)_2}_{N(CH_3)_2}$ ‖ ‖ O O	?
tetramethylphosphoro-diamidic fluoride (Dimefox)	$F-P<^{N(CH_3)_2}_{N(CH_3)_2}$ ‖ O	?

Group I: These organophosphates are *per se* phosphorylating agents and have a short half-life *in vivo* since they are speedily hydrolysed by phosphoryl-phosphatases. Ro 3-0340 and Ro 3-0351 are known exceptions and are not hydrolysed by these enzymes.

Group II: These organophosphates only become phosphorylating agents after metabolic conversion. Metabolism of phosphorothioates yields the corresponding oxo-derivatives $\left(X-P<^{R_1}_{R_2} \,\,\|\,\, S \to X-P<^{R_1}_{R_2} \,\,\|\,\, O \right)$. Metabolism of octamethyl pyrophosphortetramide probably in-volves formation of one phosphoramido-N-oxide group. The latent period of intoxication following administration of an organophosphate of Group II is generally greater than that following administration of organophosphates of Group I.

these organophosphates. Organophosphates used for studies of the antidotal action of hydroxamic acids and oximes are listed in Table 9, which also gives information concerning the type of phosphorylated AChE formed by individual organophosphates.

As can be seen from this Table several of the organophosphates form dimethylphosphoryl-AChE. So far no studies of the reactivation *in vitro* of this type of phosphorylated AChE have been published. Unpublished work by HOBBIGER showed the following. The rate of reactivation of dimethylphosphoryl-AChE by quaternary pyridine aldoximes is $^1/_{10}$ to $^1/_5$ of that of diethyl-phosphoryl-AChE, and 50 per cent of dimethylphosphoryl-AChE is converted into a non-reactivatable form at 37° and pH 7.45 (0.025 M NaHCO$_3$ was used as medium) in approximately 7 hr when spontaneous reactivation is reduced by the continued presence of free organophosphate. VANDEKAR and HEATH (1957) observed that recovery *in vitro* of AChE activity following the injection of organophosphates which *per se* form dimethylphosphoryl-AChE was marked during the first 24 hr but afterwards continued at only a slow rate; the initial phase of speedy spontaneous reactivation was missing if the organophosphate used was one of those which require metabolic conversion for activity.

Hydroxamic acids are only weak antidotes, and insufficient information is available for comparisons between their antidotal activity[1] and reactivating potency[2].

Oximes are much more effective antidotes than hydroxamic acids, and most of the published work deals with the antidotal action of quaternary pyridine aldoximes. The relationship between antidotal activity and reactivating potency of oximes is complex and its main characteristics can be summarized as follows:

a) The reactivating potency (see Section A) is a rough guide to antidotal activity against a given organophosphate only when closely related oximes, e.g., quaternary pyridine aldoximes, are used.

b) Oximes with a high lipid solubility, e.g., MINA, are more effective antidotes of the lipid-soluble organophosphate Sarin than are oximes with a low lipid solubility, e.g., quaternary pyridine aldoximes.

c) The antidotal activity of an individual oxime against organophosphates which are *per se* phosphorylating agents of AChE and which form the same type of phosphorylated AChE varies greatly.

d) The antidotal activity of oximes (given in the form of a single injection) against organophosphates which become phosphorylating agents after metabolic conversion is generally lower than that against organophosphates which are *per se* phosphorylating agents but form the same type of phosphorylated AChE as the former.

A maximum antidotal activity is obtained when hydroxamic acids or oximes are injected shortly before the organophosphate. The majority of results, summarized below, were obtained when the hydroxamic acids and oximes were injected up to 15 min before the organophosphate. In nearly all cases alternate routes, usually i.p. or s.c., were used for the injections of hydroxamic acids or oximes and organophosphates, to minimize direct interaction between the two compounds, i.e., hydrolysis of the organophosphate.

1. Hydroxamic acids

EPSTEIN and FREEMAN (1956) reported that large amounts of glycinehydroxamic acid, lacthydroxamic acid, nicotinehydroxamic acid, its methiodide, and serinehydroxamic acid, i.e., near-lethal doses (approx. 4 to 12 mmole/kg), given i.p., raise the LD$_{50}$ of Sarin, s.c., in mice 2.5- to 2.9-fold. Nicotinehydroxamic

---

[1] Antidotal activity is assessed by the ratio: Rise of the LD$_{50}$ of organophosphate observed (called antidotal action)/mole of hydroxamic acid or oxime injected per kg.

[2] As determined *in vitro* by the ratio $k/[R]$ (see Section A).

acid methiodide, glycinehydroxamic acid, and other hydroxamic acids, however, when given i.p., in amounts which just fail to produce toxic actions on their own, do not prevent death in rats injected s.c. with 2 LD_{50}'s of Sarin (ASKEW 1956).

BETHE et al. (1957) raised the lethal dose of Parathion, given by i.v. infusion, in anaesthetized guinea pigs approximately two-fold with a single i.v. injection of 0.11 mmole nicotinehydroxamic acid methiodide/kg given during the infusion. In mice a similar degree of protection against Parathion poisoning was obtained with 1.3 mmole 3-pyridine acethydroxamic acid methiodide/kg when the two compounds were given i.p. (CONLEY 1958).

Protection against lethal poisoning by DFP, given s.c., was investigated by FUNKE et al. (1955), who found that s.c. injections of the 2- and 4-trimethyl-ammonium benzhydroxamic acid iodides protect mice to a greater extent than equimolar amounts of nicotinehydroxamic acid methiodide, given s.c. The 2-isomer is the most effective antidote, and in doses of 0.78 mmole/kg raises the LD_{50} of DFP in mice approximately two-fold.

2. Oximes

a) Pyridine-2-aldoxime methiodide (P-2-AM)

The antidotal action of P-2-AM has been investigated much more extensively than that of hydroxamic acids. KEWITZ and WILSON (1956), KEWITZ et al. (1956), HOBBIGER (1957a), EDERY and SCHATZBERG-PORATH (1958), and KING and POUL-SEN (1958) reported that 0.1 to 0.4 mmole P-2-AM/kg, s.c., raises the LD_{50} of Paraoxon, s.c., in mice two[1]- to five[1]-fold, and comparable results were obtained in anaesthetized guinea pigs by BETHE et al. (1957). Protection of mice against lethal poisoning by Guthion, i.p., appears to be of a similar order (EDERY and SCHATZBERG-PORATH 1959). Pyridine-2-aldoxime methiodide, i.p., is more effective in protecting mice against lethal poisoning by Ro 3-0340, s.c., than in protecting them against lethal poisoning by Paraoxon, s.c., (HOBBIGER 1957a) but in doses up to 0.4 mmole P-2-AM/kg raises the LD_{50} at best only two-fold, and in some cases fails to give any protection to mice or rats against lethal poisoning by TEPP, Ro 3-0422, Parathion, Metasystox, Sarin, DFP, Ro 3-0351, Tabun, OMPA or Dimefox if the oxime and organophosphate are given by alternate routes (ASKEW 1956, KEWITZ and WILSON 1956, LOOMIS 1956, FOURNEL 1957, HOBBIGER 1957a, WILSON and SONDHEIMER 1957, EDERY and SCHATZBERG-PORATH 1958, KING and POULSEN 1958). Protection of mice by P-2-AM, i.p., against lethal poisoning by Systox and Metasystox, given s.c., is greater than protection against lethal poisoning by TEPP or DFP, given s.c., (JAQUES et al. 1957), but the published results do not allow a quantitative assessment of the antidotal action. KARLOG (1960) found that in rats 0.29 mmole P-2-AM/kg, i.p., raises the LD_{50} of Systox, Metasystox and Paraoxon, given s.c., three- to four-fold but is less effective against Parathion.

b) Bis-quaternary pyridine aldoximes

The most effective antidotes of TEPP and DFP are the 4-monoximes and 4,4'-dioximes of N,N'-polymethylene*bis*(pyridinium bromide) (XII and XIII; HOBBIGER et al. 1958, HOBBIGER and SADLER 1958, 1959). Several of these oximes are better antidotes than P-2-AM, particularly N,N'-trimethylene*bis*-(pyridine-4-aldoxime bromide), which in a dose of 0.095 mmole/kg, i.p., raises the LD_{50} of TEPP and DFP, s.c., in mice approximately twenty- and five-fold,

---

[1] i.e., $\dfrac{LD_{50} \text{ of organophosphate in animals pretreated with oxime}}{LD_{50} \text{ of organophosphate in control animals}} = 2 \text{ to } 5.$

respectively (Table 10). The same oxime is much less effective in Sarin poisoning but nevertheless gives greater protection than P-2-AM (BAY et al. 1958).

N,N'-Trimethylene*bis*(pyridine-4-aldoxime bromide) [4 D(3), TMB-4], like P-2-AM, raises the LD_{50} of Ro 3-0340, s.c., to a greater extent than the LD_{50} of TEPP, s.c. (HOBBIGER and SADLER 1958).

Table 10. *Protection by quaternary pyridine aldoximes against lethal poisoning of mice by TEPP and DFP* (HOBBIGER and SADLER 1959)

Oxime	TEPP (mg/kg)							DFP (mg/kg)					
	0.4	0.8	1.6	3.2	6.4	12.8	25.6	5	7.5	10	20	40	80
None	11/12	0/12	0/6	0/6	0/6	0/6		6/6	2/6	0/6	0/6	0/6	
P-2-AM		0/6	0/18	0/12					6/6	2/6	0/6	0/6	
4 M (3)			6/6	3/6	3/6	1/7				6/6	6/6	2/6	0/6
4 M (4)			6/6	5/6	3/6	1/7				6/6	4/6	0/6	
4 M (5)			6/6	5/6	6/6	5/9	2/9			6/6	5/6	0/6	
4 D (2)			6/6	2/6	1/6	0/7				6/6	3/6	0/6	
4 D (3)[1]			6/6	6/6	6/6	9/11	7/15	0/6		6/6	6/6	3/6	0/6
4 D (4)			6/6	6/6	5/6	8/9	1/9			6/6	5/6	1/6	0/6

Mice received 0.095 mmole oxime/kg, i.p., 5 to 10 min before TEPP or DFP (given s.c.). Ratios represent number of mice surviving for 24 hr/number of mice injected. The oximes used are P-2-AM and oximes of N,N'-polymethylene*bis*(pyridinium bromide). The latter are referred to by a code. Oximes labelled 4 M and 4 D are 4-monoximes and 4,4'-dioximes, respectively [see (XII) and (XIII)]; the figures in brackets give the number of carbon atoms of the polymethylene chain.

[1] TMB-4.

Protection of rats by P-2-AM and N,N'-trimethylene*bis*(pyridine-4-aldoxime bromide) against lethal poisoning by six commonly used organophosphate insecticides, administered orally, was studied by SANDERSON and EDSON (1959), who found that when 0.38 mmole/kg and 0.055 mmole/kg, respectively, of the oximes are injected three times (15 min before the organophosphate and 4 hr later, i.p., and after another 4 hr, s.c.) approximately equal degrees of protection are obtained with the two oximes. The results of these authors show that protection against Parathion and Methyl-Parathion is greater than protection against Diazinon and Phenkaptone, and least against Dimethoate and Dimefox. The published data are not suitable for quantitative assessment of the antidotal action of the oximes used.

c) Mono*isonitrosoacetone (MINA) and diacetylmonoxime (DAM)*

The antidotal actions of these two oximes were investigated by ASKEW (1956), DULTZ et al. (1957), and COHEN and WIERSINGA (1959). ASKEW found that 0.4 mmole MINA or DAM/kg raises the LD_{50} of Sarin, given s.c., in rats approximately 4.6- and 5.6-fold, respectively, when the oxime is injected i.p. 15 min before the organophosphate. MINA is, however, considerably more effective than DAM if the oximes are injected after the organophosphate. The antidotal activity of DAM, injected i.p., before Sarin, is much greater in rats than in other species, and 1.5 mmole/kg raises the LD_{50} of Sarin 26.5-fold in rats but only 1.6- to threefold in mice, guinea pigs, rabbits, and monkeys (ASKEW 1956); the monkeys were given Sarin i.v. whereas all other species received Sarin s.c. MINA and DAM, i.p., are both much less effective antidotes in poisoning by TEPP and DFP, given s.c., than in poisoning by Sarin, given s.c. (ASKEW 1956). In TEPP poisoning P-2-AM, i.p., is a better antidote than DAM, i.p. (EDERY and SCHATZBERG-PORATH 1958).

d) Other oximes

A large number of oximes in addition to those mentioned under a) to c) has been screened for an antidotal action in Sarin poisoning of rats and mice (ASKEW 1956, DULTZ et al. 1957). The most effective amongst these oximes are glyoxime, *iso*nitrosodiethylketone, 2-methyl-3-oximino-4-oxopentane, 2-oxo-3-oximinopentane, salicylaldoxime, tri*iso*nitrosopentane, α-oximinoacetamide, tri*iso*nitrosopropane, and 2-oximino-3-pentanone, which when used in large doses, given i.p., raise the LD_{50} of Sarin, given s.c., between two- and five-fold.

Effects of prophylactic[1] and therapeutic[2] injections of antidote. The interval separating the injection of hydroxamic acid or oxime and organophosphate greatly affects antidotal activity. For example, mice which are first injected i. p. with 0.16 mmole P-2-AM/kg and 30,60, 90 or 120 min later s.c. with 1 mg Paraoxon/kg showed a percentage survival of 100, 40, 30, and 25, respectively (KEWITZ et al. 1956). The protection which is obtained when oximes are injected i.p. or s.c. after the administration of an organophosphate, usually given s.c., is always less than that observed with the reverse sequence of injections.

Oral administration of oximes. Pyridine-2-aldoxime methiodide, administered orally in large doses to rats or mice, raises the LD_{50} of TEPP and Guthion, given i.p., for several hours (EDERY and SCHATZBERG-PORATH 1959). No information on the duration and extent of the antidotal action following oral administration of other oximes is at present available. Since oral administration of the antidote appears to be the ideal approach for prevention of organophosphate poisoning, more work on these lines should be undertaken.

II. Enhancement of the antidotal action by atropine

Atropine is a useful adjuvant to hydroxamic acids and oximes, and in most cases the antidotal action of combinations of atropine and an oxime is considerably greater than that attributable to a summation of individual antidotal actions (obtained when the two compounds are used singly). The degree of enhancement of the antidotal action of oximes which is obtained with atropine varies between species and with the oxime (see Table 11).

CONLEY (1958) reported that a combination of atropine and 1.3 mmole 3-pyridine acethydroxamic acid methiodide/kg, given i.p., raises the LD_{50} of i.p. Parathion in mice and rats three- to four-fold. In poisoning by DFP, given s.c., the antidotal action of combinations of atropine and trimethylammonium benzhydroxamic acid iodides, given s.c., is greater than that of the hydroxamic acids alone (FUNKE et al. 1955).

---

[1] The antidote is given before the organophosphate.
[2] The antidote is given after the organophosphate.

Legend for Table 11:

The phosphorylated AChE's formed by the various organophosphates are all reactivatable under the experimental conditions.

[1] In these experiments the antidotal treatment was given within 1 min after the organophosphate. In all other cases oximes and/or atropine were given before the organophosphate.

[2] P2S: pyridine-2-aldoxime methyl methanesulphonate. This oxime is approximately 10 times more soluble in water than P-2-AM. The solubility of P-2-AM in water at 25° is approximately 4%. P-2-AM and P2S have identical biochemical and biological actions.

Bis-quaternary pyridine aldoximes (see XI and XII) are referred to by the following Code: D stands for dioximes, the first figure gives the position of the oxime group in the ring, and the second figure, which is in brackets, gives the number of carbon atoms of the polymethylene chain. The oxime 4 D (3) [N,N'-trimethylene*bis*(pyridine-4-aldoxime bromide), TMB-4] is readily soluble in water.

Table 11. *Protection against lethal organophosphate poisoning by prophylactic injections of oximes and its enhancement by atropine*

Oxime and route	Dose of oxime in mmole/kg	Atropine sulphate in mg/kg and route	LD₅₀ of organophosphate in treated group relative to that in control group (taken as 1) — Oxime + atropine	Oxime	Atropine	Organophosphate and route	Species	Results obtained by
P-2-AM, i.p.	0.19	10, i.p.	>15			Paraoxon, s.c.	Mouse	KEWITZ et al. (1956)
P-2-AM, i.p.	0.19	10, i.p.	approx. 19			DFP, s.c.	Mouse	
P-2-AM, i.v.	0.23	10, i.v.	21	3.5	1.8	DFP, i.v.	Guinea-pig	BETHE et al. (1957)
P-2-AM, i.p.	0.095	50, i.p.	32	2	1—2	TEPP	Mouse	HOBBIGER (1957a)
			8—16	2	1—2	Ro 3-0422		
			>120	2—4	2	Paraoxon ⎬ s.c.		
			32—64	8	1—2	Ro 3-0340		
			16—32	1—2	2	DFP		
			8	1—2	1—2	Ro 3-0351		
P-2-AM, i.v.	0.019	2, i.v.	21	1.5	3.2	Sarin, i.v.	Rabbit	WILLS et al. (1957)[1]
P-2-AM, i.p.	0.34	10, i.p.	9.3			TEPP, s.c.	Mouse	WILSON and SONDHEIMER (1957)
P-2-AM, i.p.	0.34	10, i.p.	approx. 2			Sarin, s.c.	Mouse	
P-2-AM, i.p.	⎱0.38	⎱17.4, i.p.	11.3	1.4	1.2		Mouse	ASKEW (1957)
P-2-AM, i.p.	⎰	⎰	13.8	1.3	1.3		Rat	
MINA, i.p.	0.4		11.6	4.6	1.3		Rat	
MINA, i.m.	0.12	⎱0.029, i.m.	6.8		3.0	Sarin, s.c.	Monkey[1]	
MINA, i.m.	0.23	⎰	14.0		3.0		Mouse	
DAM, i.p.	⎱1.5	⎱17.4, i.p.	9.0	5.3	1.2		Mouse	
DAM, i.p.	⎰	⎰	48.3	25.8	1.3		Rat	
DAM, i.p.			2.6	2.5	1.0		Guinea-pig	
P2S[2], i.m.	0.12	17.4, i.m.	35			TEPP, s.c.	Mouse	DAVIES et al. (1959)
			45				Rat	
			50				Guinea-pig	
			28				Rabbit	
			3.7				Mouse	
			3.2			Sarin, s.c.	Rat	
			73				Guinea-pig	
			120				Rabbit	
P2S, i.m.	0.019		approx. 8			TEPP, s.c.	Rat	BERRY et. al. (1959)
4 D (3), i.m.	0.011		>100					
2 D (6), i.m.	0.01	17.4, i.m.	>100					
4 D (3), i.m.	0.011		approx. 3			Sarin, s.c.		
2 D (6), i.m.	0.01		4					
4 D (3), i.p.	0.0095	1, i.p.	4—8	approx. 2	1	TEPP	Mouse	HOBBIGER and SADLER (1959)
			32—64	8—16	1	Ro 3-0340 ⎬ s.c.		
			approx. 3	1—2	1	DFP		
P-2-AM, i.p.	0.34	10, i.p.	approx. 1.6	<1.6	<1.6	Tabun, s.c.	Mouse	WILSON and SONDHEIMER (1957)
P-2-AM, i.v.	0.06	4, i.v.	1.5			Tabun, i.v.	Rat	FLEISHER et al. (1960)[1]
4 D (3), i.v.	0.06	4, i.v.	10					
P-2-AM, i.v.	0.06	4, i.v.	2.3			Sarin, i.v.		
4 D (3), i.v.	0.06	4, i.v.	12					

The highest degree of protection against lethal organophosphate poisoning is obtained with a combination of atropine and an oxime. When the oximes are injected up to 15 min before the organophosphate and atropine is given either at the same time as the oxime or earlier, the LD_{50} of several organophosphates can be raised at least ten-fold and in some cases more than hundred-fold (Table 11). As can be seen from the results summarized in Table 11, combinations of oximes of N,N'-polymethylene*bis*(pyridinium bromide) and atropine are particularly effective. Not included in Table 11 are results obtained by BAY et al. (1958) and O'LEARY et al. (1958), since it is not possible to express their results quantitatively. These authors showed that combinations of N,N'-trimethylene*bis*(pyridine-4-aldoxime bromide) and atropine, given i.v., give a greater degree of protection against lethal poisoning of rabbits and cats by Sarin, i.v. or s.c., than combinations of P-2-AM and atropine, given i.v. Enhancement of the antidotal action of P-2-AM, s.c., by atropine, i.v. and s.c., in poisoning of cattle by Parathion, given orally, has been reported by WOODARD (1957).

The antidotal action of combinations of atropine and P-2-AM can be enhanced by artificial respiration (BETHE et al. 1957) but not by analeptic drugs (HOBBIGER 1957a).

III. Effect on individual actions of organophosphates

Death in animals injected with an organophosphate and a hydroxamic acid or oxime is always preceded by signs and symptoms typical of accumulation of ACh.

In all cases where a significant rise of the LD_{50} of an organophosphate is obtained, the oximes shorten the duration of signs produced by a sub-lethal dose of the organophosphate. The greater the effect of the oxime on the LD_{50} of the organophosphate, the speedier is the disappearance of signs in animals injected with the oxime and a sub-lethal dose of the organophosphate. The persistance of signs in rats injected with Sarin, s.c., and DAM, i.p., (RUTLAND 1958) is the only known exception.

More detailed studies of the effect of hydroxamic acids and oximes on individual actions of organophosphates clearly illustrate the therapeutic action of the former in sub-lethal organophosphate poisoning.

Organophosphates, by virtue of their phosphorylating action on AChE, enhance the effectiveness of injected ACh, produce bradycardia, reduce the ability of indirectly stimulated striped muscle to sustain a tetanus, and depress respiration. All these changes are relatively long-lasting.

In dogs which are first injected i.v. with Sarin, 0.38 mmole P-2-AM/kg, given i.v., restores a normal heart rate and a normal sensitivity to injected ACh (LOOMIS 1956). In guinea pigs which are first injected i.v. with 0.11 mmole Parathion/kg, P-2-AM, given i.v., rapidly restores the heart rate and electrocardiogram to normal but has less effect on respiration, which it improves only gradually (BETHE et al. 1957).

In anaesthetized cats the tension of limb muscles developed in response to indirect stimulation is reduced by i.v. Sarin and recovers only slowly. The rate of recovery is slightly enhanced by an i.v. injection of 0.13 to 0.25 mmole nicotinehydroxamic acid methiodide/kg (KUNKEL et al. 1956).

Pyridine-2-aldoxime methiodide and MINA, given i.v., restore the ability of striped muscle to sustain a tetanus in response to indirect stimulation in animals previously injected i.v. with organophosphates. This was observed by HOLMES and ROBINS (1955) in anaesthetized cats which were first injected with TEPP and then with 0.28 to 1.1 mmole MINA/kg, by FOURNEL (1957) who injected anaesthetized dogs first with Parathion and then with 0.048 mmole P-2-AM/kg, and by

BROWN et al. (1957) and WILLS et al. (1957) who injected anaesthetized cats and dogs first with Sarin or Tabun and then with 0.019 mmole P-2-AM/kg. The latter group found also that P-2-AM has identical effects on the recovery of limb muscles and the diaphragm. On the other hand, a slow i.v. infusion of 0.18 mmole DAM/kg, which is much less potent than P-2-AM or MINA as a reactivator of phosphorylated AChE (see Table 7), fails to reverse neuromuscular block produced in anaesthetized cats by i.v. TEPP (EDERY 1959).

Pyridine-2-aldoxime methiodide, 0.019 mmole/kg, i.v., speeds the return of spontaneous respiration in atropinized and anaesthetized cats and dogs injected i.v. first with Tabun or Sarin (BROWN et al. 1957), and 0.038 mmole P-2-AM/kg restores effective spontaneous respiration in anaesthetized dogs previously injected i.v. with Sarin and kept alive by artificial respiration (LOOMIS 1956). The improvement of respiration obtained with P-2-AM, i.v., appears to arise from a peripheral action of the oxime since an intracisternal injection of up to 0.004 mmole pyridine-2-aldoxime methyl methanesulphonate (P2S) fails to initiate respiration in dogs previously injected by the same route with Sarin (BROWN 1960).

IV. Reactivation of phosphorylated acetylcholinesterase

The rise of the LD_{50} of organophosphates and the improvement or complete reversal of signs of organophosphate poisoning which are obtained with hydroxamic acids and oximes can be attributed, either in part or fully, to reactivation of phosphorylated AChE only if we can show that the latter does indeed occur under the experimental conditions.

Very little information is available on reactivation obtained with hydroxamic acids. Oximes, when injected in amounts which raise the LD_{50} of an organophosphate, reactivate phosphorylated AChE (i.e., those forms which are reactivatable) in blood and peripheral tissues, but a good reactivation of phosphorylated AChE in brain is on the whole obtained only with lipid-soluble oximes. The most conclusive results are obtained when oximes are injected some time after a sublethal dose of an organophosphate, given either alone or in combination with atropine. Under these conditions reactivation is often considerable and can be detected by manometric assay or by titration. Small degrees of reactivation can be demonstrated with certainty only by KOELLE's histochemical method (KOELLE 1950, 1951).

1. Reactivation in blood, striped muscle, and ganglia

Since tissues contain a mixture of AChE and BuChE, the activity of the former must be assessed by the rate of hydrolysis of a specific substrate, e.g., acetyl-β-methylcholine (ALLES and HAWES 1940, MENDEL and RUDNEY 1943). In some cases, ACh and acetylthiocholine, both of which are hydrolysed by both types of cholinesterase (ChE), have been used as substrates, and we shall call enzyme activity determined by the rate of hydrolysis of these two substrates ChE activity. Increases of ChE activity obtained after treatment with oximes are valid qualitative evidence for reactivation of phosphorylated AChE. RUTLAND (1958) showed that in experiments with MINA the percentage reactivation calculated from the rates of hydrolysis of ACh and acetyl-β-methylcholine are very similar. Pyridine-2-aldoxime methiodide and bis-quaternary pyridine aldoximes, on the other hand, reactivate phosphorylated BuChE at a much lower rate than a corresponding phosphorylated AChE (WILSON et al. 1958, SCAIFE 1959), and in many tissues reactivation of phosphorylated AChE obtained with these oximes is greater than is indicated by the change in ChE activity.

a) Hydroxamic acids

PAULET and ANDRÉ (1956) reported that in guinea pigs, 1 mmole glycolhydrox-amic acid or picolinehydroxamic acid/kg, injected i.p. 24 hr after TEPP, given s.c., reactivated the phosphorylated AChE in erythrocytes to a considerable extent, whereas equimolar doses of nicotinehydroxamic acid or nicotinehydroxamic acid methiodide, i.p., produced no reactivation.

b) Oximes

KEWITZ (1957a) injected mice with Paraoxon, s.c., and 1 hr later with 0.095 mmole P-2-AM/kg, i.p. Twenty-four hours after the injection of Paraoxon, ChE activity in the diaphragm of such mice was 97% of normal whereas ChE activity in the diaphragm of mice injected with Paraoxon only was approximately 70% of normal. Seven hours after s.c. injection of DFP, ChE activity in the dia-phragm of mice which were injected i.p. with 0.34 mmole P-2-AM/kg 90 min after DFP had been injected was 28% of normal as compared with 6 to 9% of normal in mice injected with DFP only. The antidotal action of a combination of atropine and P-2-AM against OMPA is negligible compared with that against Paraoxon and DFP, and similarly no reactivation is obtained when mice are first injected s.c. with OMPA and then i.p. with 0.57 mmole P-2-AM/kg.

HOBBIGER (1957a) injected mice s.c. with TEPP, Paraoxon, Ro 3-0340 or Ro 3-0422 (all of which form diethylphosphoryl-AChE) and 30 min later i.p. with 0.095 mmole P-2-AM/kg. Thirty, 60 and 120 min after the injection of P-2-AM, AChE activity in the blood of these animals was considerably higher than AChE activity in the blood of mice injected with organophosphate only. The differences in enzyme activity between the two groups represented a reactivation of phosphoryl-ated AChE amounting to 31 to 39, 45 to 52, and 49 to 56%, respectively. Under the same conditions 0.095 mmole P-2-AM/kg failed to raise the AChE activity in the blood of mice previously injected with DFP or other organophosphates with form di*iso*propylphosphoryl-AChE.

RUTLAND (1958) found that in rats the AChE activity of erythrocytes rose within 1 hr from 6 to 26% of normal if 0.4 mmole MINA/kg was injected i.p. 3 to 5 min after Sarin, s.c. Ninety min after the i.p. injection of 1.5 mmole DAM/kg, given 30 min after Sarin, s.c., ChE activity in blood had risen from 15 to 50% of normal. Pyridine-2-aldoxime methiodide, 0.38 mmole/kg, injected i.p. 3 to 5 min after Sarin, s.c., raised ChE activity in blood and striped muscle in 1 hr from 3 to 35% of normal, and from 15 to 66% of normal, respectively.

Acetylcholinesterase activity in the blood of mice injected s.c. with TEPP, and 30 min later i.p. with 0.0095 or 0.095 mmole of the 4-monoximes or 4,4'-dioximes of N,N'-trimethylene- and N,N'-tetramethylene-*bis*(pyridinium bromide)/kg, or 0.095 mmole P-2-AM/kg, rose within 1 hr to 47 to 56% of normal as compared with 12% of normal in mice which were injected with TEPP only. Pyridine-2-aldoxime methiodide, 0.0095 mmole/kg, i.p., produced a smaller effect and raised AChE activity within 1 hr from 12 to 29% of normal (HOBBIGER and SADLER 1959).

A speedy increase of AChE activity in erythrocytes from approximately 25% of normal to 80% of normal or more was obtained by NAMBA and HIRAKI (1958) in rabbits which were injected i.v. with 0.11 to 0.68 mmole P-2-AM/kg several hours after Parathion had been given s.c. In some cases reactivation was only transient, probably because Paraoxon was still being formed from Parathion, and phosphorylation of AChE continued when the concentration of P-2-AM had fallen below effective levels. Speedy recovery of AChE activity in erythrocytes was also obtained by KARLOG (1960) who injected rabbits first i.p. with Paraoxon or Parathion and then with 0.29 mmole P-2-AM/kg, i.p.

O'LEARY et al. (1959) reported that P-2-AM reactivated phosphorylated AChE in striped muscle but not in salivary glands (organophosphate used not stated).

Histochemical studies. KOELLE (1957a) investigated reactivation by using his histochemical method. He injected atropine-protected cats first with DFP, 0.02 mmole/kg, i.v., and 5 to 64 min later with 0.02 to 0.04 mmole P-2-AM/kg, i.v. The cats were killed 15 to 30 min after the injection of P-2-AM and sections of the ciliary and stellate ganglia and of the motor endplate region in striped muscle were examined histochemically for ChE activity. The sections obtained from cats injected with DFP and P-2-AM showed considerably more staining, i.e., higher ChE activity, than sections obtained from cats which had been injected with DFP only. In the case of the former, staining was particularly pronounced at cell membranes and terminations of nerve fibres.

RAJAPURKAR and KOELLE (1958) extended this work on cats injected first with DFP and then with an oxime, both i.v. They showed that staining of sections of the superior cervical and stellate ganglia and of motor endplate regions in striped muscle was considerably increased following the injection of 0.04 mmole MINA/kg. Injections of 0.4 mmole DAM/kg produced an effect similar to that obtained with 0.04 mmole MINA/kg, but 0.04 mmole DAM/kg had hardly any detectable effect. Acetylcholinesterase activity in cervical and stellate ganglia was also measured manometrically in parallel experiments. An enzyme activity of 6 to 9% of normal was found in cats injected with DFP and then with 0.4 mmole MINA/kg as compared with 1.5% in cats injected with DFP only. No reactivation could be detected manometrically following the injection of 0.04 mmole MINA/kg or 0.4 mmole DAM/kg.

Acetylthiocholine is hydrolysed by P-2-AM, P-4-AM, and DAM (BERGNER and O'NEILL 1958), and thus precautions have to be taken to exclude false positive results when reactivation *in vitro* of phosphorylated AChE by oximes is assessed histochemically.

2. Reactivation in brain and spinal cord

Reactivation of phosphorylated AChE in brain does not always go parallel with reactivation in blood and peripheral tissues. The entrance of quaternary ammonium compounds from blood into the brain is restricted, and P-2-AM and oximes of N,N'-polymethylene*bis*(pyridinium bromide), given i.p. or i.m., have either very little or no effect on phosphorylated AChE in the brain of animals previously injected s.c. or i.p. with TEPP, DFP, Sarin, or other lipid-soluble organophosphates (HOBBIGER 1957a, KEWITZ and NACHMANSOHN 1957, RUTLAND 1958, EDERY and SCHATZBERG-PORATH 1959, HOBBIGER and SADLER 1959). Only by using large doses of P-2-AM, i.e., 0.95 mmole/kg, i.p., were KEWITZ and NACHMANSOHN (1957) able to raise the ChE activity, in the brain of mice which had previously been injected s.c. with Paraoxon, by 25% of normal above the level of ChE activity in the brain of mice which had been injected with Paraoxon only. This effect is much smaller than that observed in the diaphragm or in the blood of mice which are first injected s.c. with Paraoxon and then i.p. with 0.095 mmole P-2-AM/kg.

In all these experiments the enzymic activity of homogenates of the total brain or spinal cord was used to assess reactivation of phosphorylated AChE. The possibility that considerable reactivation occurred in some small areas with a higher permeability for quaternary ammonium compounds (MAYER and BAIN 1956) and escaped detection must be considered.

Approximately 15 to 50% reactivation of phosphorylated ChE in the cerebellum was reported in cats which were given an intracisternal injection of 0.038 mmole P-2-AM after the i.v. administration of Parathion (SAKAI et al. 1958). It is possible that the reactivation observed in these experiments is an artifact arising from reactivation *in vitro* (HOBBIGER 1957a).

MINA and DAM are lipid-soluble, and 0.4 mmole MINA/kg, i.p., raises AChE activity in the brain of rats to the same extent as in erythrocytes when the oxime is injected after Sarin, s.c. DAM is less effective than MINA, and 1.5 mmole DAM/kg, injected i.p. after Sarin, s.c., raises AChE activity in brain only by approximately 10% of normal (RUTLAND 1958).

Time-course of reactivation. With doses used in the experiments described, reactivation of phosphorylated AChE at central and peripheral sites either reaches or approaches a maximum within 1 hr after the injection of an oxime (HOBBIGER 1957a, RUTLAND 1958).

3. The effect of prophylactic or simultaneous[1] administration of oximes on acetylcholinesterase activity

Oximes not only reactivate phosphorylated AChE but also hydrolyze organophosphates, and in concentrations required for reactivation inhibit AChE reversibly. Both these actions can mimic reactivation when oximes are injected prophylactically or together with an organophosphate. Differences between the activity of AChE in animals which receive oximes either prophylactically or together with organophosphates, and that in animals injected with organophosphates only, are not necessarily entirely due to reactivation of phosphorylated AChE.

The AChE activity in the blood of mice injected first i.p. with 0.095 mmole P-2-AM/kg and 5 min later s.c. with TEPP, Paraoxon, Ro 3-0340, or Ro 3-0422 remains at a considerably higher level than the activity of AChE in the blood of mice which are injected with organophosphates only (HOBBIGER 1957a). The same is the case with the AChE activity in the blood and brain of rats injected first i.p. with 0.4 mmole MINA/kg and 10 min later s.c. with Sarin (RUTLAND 1958).

The AChE activity in erythrocytes of rats which received 0.38 mmole P-2-AM/kg or 0.055 mmole N,N'-trimethylene*bis*(pyridine-4-aldoxime bromide)/kg, i.p., 15 min before the oral administration of an organophosphate insecticide, and 4 hr and 8 hr later were injected with an identical dose of the same oxime (i.p. at 4 hr and s.c. at 8 hr), was investigated by SANDERSON and EDSON (1959). Their results show that AChE activity in rats treated with Parathion, Diazinon, and Phenkaptone (the active metabolite of which forms diethylphosphoryl-AChE) and oxime was, after 24 hr, considerably higher than AChE activity in rats treated with organophosphate only. The oximes had no effect on AChE activity in rats injected with Dimethoate, Methyl-Parathion, or Dimefox; this was attributed by the authors to extensive conversion of reactivatable dimethylphosphoryl-AChE into a non-reactivatable form (owing to prolonged presence of the phosphorylating metabolite) in the case of Dimethoate and Methyl-Parathion, and lack of reactivatability of the phosphorylated AChE formed by Dimefox.

Rats injected first i.p. with 0.4 mmole DAM/kg and 10 min later s.c. with Sarin retain their normal AChE activity in brain (RUTLAND 1958). This finding is characteristic for rats and is not obtained with mice (EDERY and SCHATZBERG-PORATH 1958).

The level of AChE activity in erythrocytes of rabbits which received prophylactic oral administration of a large dose of P-2-AM before Parathion, s.c., remained

---

[1] With organophosphate.

at a much higher level than that of rabbits injected with Parathion only (NAMBA and HIRAKI 1958).

V. Actions on isolated organs and tissue sections which have previously been exposed to organophosphates

Hydroxamic acids and oximes reverse the effects of certain organophosphates on isolated organs and the following results can be attributed either to a large extent or entirely (in some cases) to reactivation of phosphorylated AChE.

Nicotinehydroxamic acid methiodide, in a concentration of 11 mM, has no atropine-like action but reverses the effect of TEPP on isolated auricles and intestine of rabbits (ROY and KUPERMAN 1955). The bradycardia of isolated rabbit and guinea pig auricles produced by Paraoxon is reversed by 0.38 mM P-2-AM (BETHE et al. 1957).

Neuromuscular block produced in the isolated rat nerve-diaphragm preparation by TEPP and Sarin is reversed by 1 mM MINA or di*iso*nitrosoacetone, and 1 mM MINA, di*iso*nitrosoacetone, or P-2-AM, respectively. Reversal of neuromuscular block produced by DFP is obtained when the concentrations of the oximes are above 10 mM (HOLMES and ROBINS 1955). Neuromuscular block produced in the same preparation by TEPP cannot be reversed by 10 mM DAM (EDERY 1959) which at pH 7 to 8 has only approximately 1/30 of the potency of MINA as a reactivator of diethylphosphoryl-AChE. Depolarization of motor endplates in the isolated rat diaphragm following exposure to DFP is reversed by P-2-AM and at the same time normal behaviour of the motor endplates is restored (MEETER 1958).

The potentiation of the ACh response of the isolated frog rectus abdominis muscle produced by Sarin is greatly reduced by bathing the muscle for 8 min in 0.2 mM P-2-AM, and a loss of 88% of the potentiation is concurrent with an increase in the activity of total and functional AChE by 35 and 71%, respectively, of normal (FLEISHER et al. 1958).

Reactivation of phosphorylated ChE's by 1 mM P-2-AM was demonstrated histochemically by BERGNER and WAGLEY (1958) in sections of frog iliofibularis muscle previously exposed to TEPP.

VI. Relationship between antidotal action of hydroxamic acids and oximes and reactivation of phosphorylated acetylcholinesterase

The question which arises now is to what extent does reactivation of phosphorylated AChE account for the antidotal action of hydroxamic acids and oximes in organophosphate poisoning when they are injected singly or in combination with atropine.

The actions of the quaternary pyridine aldoximes and of MINA and DAM have been investigated in much greater detail than those of other oximes or hydroxamic acids, and our discussion is by necessity limited to results obtained with the former. Good protection against lethal organophosphate poisoning is obtained with quaternary pyridine aldoximes, MINA, and DAM, used singly or in combination with atropine, if the organophosphates used form a reactivatable phosphorylated AChE, whereas protection against lethal poisoning by organophosphates which form a non-reactivatable phosphorylated AChE is negligible by comparison with the former situation. In some cases the percentage reactivation is small and can be detected only histochemically. The concentration of AChE which is required to keep an animal alive, especially when atropine also has been injected, represents only a small fraction of the total AChE present in tissues, and it seems reasonable to assume that reactivation of a few percent of phosphorylated AChE will raise the LD_{50} of organophosphates and reduce the severity of symptoms of organophosphate poisoning.

KOELLE and his co-workers (KOELLE and STEINER 1956, KOELLE 1957b, RAJAPURKAR and KOELLE 1958, FUKUDA and KOELLE 1959, KOELLE and KOELLE 1959, McISAAC and KOELLE 1959) and FLEISHER et al. (1958a) have shown that AChE in tissues is located at cell membranes and at intracellular sites, and that only the former, for which the name functional AChE was suggested, hydrolyzes ACh at sites of cholinergic transmission. At present we have no quantitative information concerning percentage reactivation of phosphorylated functional AChE in tissues, and in the case of quaternary pyridine aldoximes it must be greater than the percentage reactivation of total phosphorylated AChE decribed previously.

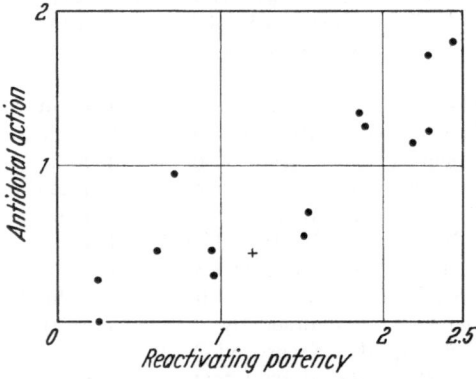

Fig. 4. *Relationship between antidotal action and reactivating potency of* bis-*quaternary pyridine aldoximes* (BERRY et al. 1959). Full circles: various bis-quaternary pyridine aldoximes [structure (XI)]; +: pyridine-2-aldoxime methyl methanesulphonate (P2S). Abscissa: $\log_{10}$ of reactivating potency of the oximes for diethylphosphoryl-AChE expressed in arbitrary units and calculated from the time required to obtain 25% reactivation with equimolar concentrations of the oximes. Ordinate: $\log_{10}$ of the LD_{50} of TEPP (mg/kg) in rats injected first i.m. with 17.4 mg/kg atropine sulphate and 5 mg oxime/kg and 10 min later with TEPP (s.c.). — Differences between molecular weights of the bis-quaternary oximes are small and the relationship between antidotal activity and reactivating potency of bis-quaternary oximes is, therefore, similar to that shown in the Figure. P2S has only approx. half the molecular weight of the other oximes and if we use the ordinate as a measure of antidotal activity, the value for P2S on the ordinate is approx. half that shown

BERRY et al. (1959) showed that the *in vitro* reactivating potency of P2S and *bis*-quaternary pyridine aldoximes for diethylphosphoryl-AChE, prepared from human erythrocytes, and their antidotal activity against TEPP in atropinized rats are undoubtedly related, although some discrepancies exist which appear to be outside the limits of experimental error (Fig. 4). The same applies to the relationship between the reactivating potency *in vitro* of intraperitoneally injected P-2-AM and 4-monoximes and 4,4'-dioximes of N,N'-polymethylene*bis*(pyridinium bromide) and their antidotal activity in mice injected s.c. with TEPP or DFP (HOBBIGER and SADLER 1959).

MINA and DAM are considerably less potent than P-2-AM as reactivators of *iso*propyl methylphosphonyl-AChE (Table 7), but more effective than the latter as antidotes in Sarin poisoning. MINA and DAM are highly lipid-soluble and reactivate phosphorylated AChE in brain as well as in peripheral tissues (RUTLAND 1958), whereas quaternary pyridine aldoximes have a low lipid solubility (HOBBIGER et al. 1960) and in doses of 0.1 mmole/kg or less act more or less solely on the latter. RUTLAND proposed that reactivation of phosphonylated AChE in brain plays an essential part in the antidotal action of MINA and DAM against Sarin. This interpretation is supported by the following findings. Atropine is far more effective in enhancing the antidotal action of P-2-AM than in enhancing the antidotal action of MINA or DAM (Table 11; ASKEW 1957), and the lipid-soluble reactivator pyridine-2-aldoxime dodecyl iodide (PAD) greatly enhances the antidotal action of P-2-AM in Sarin poisoning (WILSON 1958).

HACKLEY et al. (1959) reported that the phosphonylated anion of P-2-AM, formed by interaction of P-2-AM with Sarin, is a potent phosphonylating agent of AChE. It is tempting, therefore, to speculate that rephosphonylation of AChE is at least in part responsible for the low antidotal activity of P-2-AM in

Sarin poisoning. Further light would be thrown on this problem by an investigation of the properties of the phosphonylated anion of MINA.

The antidotal activity of DAM in rats injected first with the oxime and then with Sarin is greater than that of MINA, although the opposite is true for their re-activating potencies. This discrepancy is explained by results obtained by MYERS (1959). DAM speedily reactivates phosphonylated aliesterase[1] in the plasma of rats injected with Sarin. Large quantities of Sarin react with aliesterase in the plasma, and DAM, by reactivating the phosphonylated aliesterase, enables the enzyme to remove still more Sarin and to lower the concentration of Sarin which is available for phosphonylation of AChE. After inhibition of aliesterase by tri-o-cresyl-phosphate, DAM has only a small effect on the LD_{50} of Sarin in rats. Reactivation of phosphonylated aliesterase largely accounts, therefore, for the marked antidotal activity of prophylactic injections of DAM in Sarin poisoning of rats. In mice the phosphonylated aliesterase formed by Sarin is relatively resistant to reactivation by DAM. This explains why the antidotal activity of prophylactic injections of DAM is greater in rats than in mice.

It is known that anti-ChE agents which do not phosphorylate, e.g., physo-stigmine, protect AChE from phosphorylation and raise the LD_{50} of organo-phosphates (KOSTER 1946, KOELLE 1946). Quaternary pyridine aldoximes are weak reversible inhibitors of AChE, and the possibility that such an action con-tributes to their antidotal action must be considered. The same applies to hy-drolysis of the organophosphates by oximes. To what extent these two actions contribute to the antidotal action of individual oximes is impossible to decide. In the case of quaternary pyridine aldoximes there is no correlation between anti-AChE activity or rate of hydrolysis of organophosphates by the oximes at pH 7 to 8 and antidotal activity (HOBBIGER, unpublished). On the whole it seems justifiable to conclude that in the absence of reactivation, an anti-AChE action of oximes and hydrolysis of organophosphates by oximes would at best produce only a very small antidotal action.

Additional information concerning the specificity of the antidotal action of oximes comes from studies of their antidotal action against anti-ChE agents which are not phosphorylating agents of AChE. Pyridine-2-aldoxime methiodide, injected i.p. in doses up to 0.19 mmole/kg, does not raise the LD_{50} of physostigmine or neostigmine, given s.c., in mice (KEWITZ et al. 1956, HOBBIGER and SADLER 1959). The same result was obtained with i.v. injection in guinea pigs (BETHE et al. 1957). N,N'-Trimethylene*bis*(pyridine-4-aldoxime bromide) [4 D (3), TMB-4], at 0.0095 mmole/kg i.p., does not raise the LD_{50} of neostigmine, given s.c., in mice (HOBBIGER and SADLER 1959) but at 0.095 mmole/kg, i.p., raises the LD_{50} of neostigmine, given s.c., in mice approximately three-fold, protects to a smaller extent against lethal poi-soning by s.c. *bis*pyridostigmine (N,N'-hexamethylene*bis*{3-(N-methylcarbamoyl-oxy)-N-methylpyridinium bromide}; BC 51), but does not affect the LD_{50} of s.c. *bis*neostigmine (N,N'-decamethylene*bis*{3-(N-methylcarbamoyloxy)-N,N,N-tri-methylanilinium bromide}; BC 48) (HOBBIGER and SADLER 1959). These effects are considerably smaller than those observed in mice injected with the organo-phosphates TEPP or Ro 3-0340. Since protection against lethal poisoning by the three non-phosphorylating anti-ChE agents is variable, and the action of organo-phosphates is generally much longer-lasting than that of the non-phosphorylating anti-ChE agents, it is impossible to say to what extent the mechanism which is responsible for protection against lethal poisoning by some non-phosphorylating anti-ChE agents does contribute to protection against lethal organophosphate

---

[1] Aliesterase is an esterase which hydrolyzes predominantly aliphatic esters but not choline esters.

poisoning. It might well be that this mechanism will not raise the LD_{50} of organophosphates in the absence of reactivation, but allows reactivation to continue for a longer period by delaying death.

No information is available on the antidotal action of MINA and DAM against non-phosphorylating anti-ChE agents.

The evidence which we have discussed indicates that with the exceptions to be stated later, reactivation of phosphorylated AChE plays a vital part in the antidotal action of quaternary pyridine aldoximes (P-2-AM, P2S, and bis-quaternary pyridine aldoximes) and MINA, and that these oximes would have a considerably smaller or no antidotal activity if they were devoid of reactivating properties. The antidotal action solely attributable to reactivation of phosphorylated AChE cannot be determined experimentally since other actions of the oximes which themselves (i.e., in the absence of reactivation) can raise the LD_{50} of organophosphates or non-phosphorylating anti-ChE's only slightly or fail to affect it, might enable them to produce a higher degree of protection against lethal organophosphate poisoning than would be obtained without them. The contribution of "other" actions towards the antidotal action is obviously variable and will depend on the oxime, organophosphate, and perhaps also the species of animals used; the experimental evidence suggests that it is greater with bis-quaternary oximes than with P-2-AM when both are used in equimolar doses. The marked enhancement of the antidotal action of oximes by atropine is probably mainly due to the anti-ACh action of atropine (SCHAUMANN 1959).

Protection against lethal organophosphate poisoning which is largely attributable to actions other than reactivation is obtained in Sarin poisoning of rats injected prophylactically with DAM. The antidotal actions of DAM against other organophosphates (in rats) and in other species probably involve reactivation together with a marked contribution from other actions. Protection by oximes against lethal poisoning by organophosphates which, according to the results available, form a non-reactivatable type of phosphorylated AChE, e.g., OMPA or Dimefox, is small, even when the oximes are given with atropine, and obviously not the consequence of reactivation.

In the case of the oximes mentioned on page 950 (Section d) and of hydroxamic acids, no conclusion can be reached since the available data are too scanty, but it seems reasonable to assume that reactivation contributes to the antidotal action of the more effective compounds.

Two findings have so far not been discussed. Firstly, the antidotal activity in mice of an individual quaternary pyridine aldoxime, injected either singly or in combination with atropine, varies considerably when different organophosphates are used which form the same type of phosphorylated enzyme (HOBBIGER 1957a, HOBBIGER and SADLER 1959). Secondly, protection of mice by a combination of atropine and P-2-AM against lethal poisoning by DFP is greater than protection against lethal poisoning by TEPP, although the rate of reactivation of diethylphosphoryl-AChE by P-2-AM in vivo must be at least ten times higher than that of diisopropylphosphoryl-AChE (KEWITZ et al. 1956, HOBBIGER 1957a, WILSON and SONDHEIMER 1957). We are unable at present to explain these findings satisfactorily but two observations are worth mentioning in connection with them.

Death in organophosphate poisoning is caused primarily by respiratory failure, but circulatory failure may also contribute (HOLMSTEDT et al. 1957). Bronchoconstriction and bronchial secretion, neuromuscular block in respiratory muscles, and central respiratory failure all contribute to the respiratory failure. Which of these factors predominates depends on the species of animal and the organophosphate (CANDOLE et al. 1953, HOLMES 1953). There is no reason why the nature of the respiratory failure should not be one of the factors which control species variations of the antidotal activity of oximes and the degree of enhancement of the antidotal action of oximes obtained with atropine. The same applies to variations of the antidotal activity shown by an individual oxime against different organophosphates which form the same type of phosphorylated AChE.

The antidotal activity of oximes in mice injected with organophosphates which form diethylphosphoryl-AChE, and which are *per se* phosphorylating agents, appears to be related directly to the stability of the organophosphates *in vivo*. The significance of this observation is at present unknown, and its analysis might contribute to a better understanding of the various factors which determine the antidotal activity of oximes.

Sub-lethal poisoning. The complete and sustained reversal of signs obtained with oximes in animals which have previously been injected with a sub-lethal dose of an organophosphate can be attributed mainly or entirely to reactivation of phosphorylated AChE. The rate of reversal, however, might be enhanced by actions described in the following Section.

VII. Actions which are not due to reactivation of phosphorylated acetylcholinesterase

The specificity of the actions of hydroxamic acids and oximes is determined by the dose or concentration in which they are used. In addition to reactivation of phosphorylated AChE and actions attributable to it, a variety of other actions can be demonstrated with these compounds in the absence of organophosphates.

Pyridine-2-aldoxime methiodide, in concentrations of 0.05 to 1 mM, sensitizes the isolated frog rectus abdominis muscle to ACh by inhibiting ChE's, and in higher concentrations it antagonizes ACh (BETHE et al. 1957. FLEISHER et al. 1958b). Similar effects are obtained with P-2-AM on the isolated intestine and atrium of the rabbit. Nicotinehydroxamic acid methiodide in higher concentrations has the same properties as P-2-AM (BETHE et al. 1957).

The actions of P-2-AM on neuromuscular transmission are a mixture of AChE inhibition and depolarization. In a concentration of 1 mM, P-2-AM blocks neuromuscular transmission in the rat nerve-diaphragm preparation (HOLMES and ROBINS 1955) and enhances the endplate potential in frog muscle (WAGLEY 1957). The i.v. injection of 0.02 mmole P-2-AM/kg produces a slight anticurare action and enhances neuromuscular block produced by depolarizing drugs in cats (WILLS et al. 1959). In a concentration of 1 mM, P-2-AM reverses neuromuscular block in the rat nerve-diaphragm preparation produced by methylfluorophosphorylcholines (which form a non-reactivatable phosphonylated AChE (ENANDER 1958)) as well as neuromuscular block produced by Sarin (which forms a reactivatable phosphonylated AChE); the former proceeds at 1/4 to 1/2 of the rate of the latter (FREDRIKSSON and TIBBLING 1959).

Pyridine-2-aldoxime methiodide has a slight and very transient atropine-like action when cats are injected i.v. with 0.38 mmole oxime/kg (KEWITZ et al. 1956, LOOMIS 1956), and 0.11 mM P-2-AM is required to reduce the sensitivity of the isolated guinea pig ileum to low concentrations of ACh by 50% (HOBBIGER and SADLER 1959).

One mM MINA, like P-2-AM, enhances the endplate potential in frog muscle, but DAM, at 10 mM, reduces and lengthens it (WAGLEY 1957). Ten mM MINA has no effect on neuromuscular transmission in the rat nerve-diaphragm preparation (HOLMES and ROBINS 1955), whereas 10 mM DAM acts like *d*-tubocurarine on the same preparation. One mM MINA and di*iso*nitrosoacetone, like P-2-AM, reverse neuromuscular block in the rat nerve-diaphragm preparation produced by methyl-fluorophosphorylcholines as well as that produced by Sarin (FREDRIKSSON and TIBBLING 1959). One mmole/kg DAM produces flaccid paralysis in hens and frogs (EDERY 1959). A ganglionic blocking action of 1 to 2 mmole MINA/kg, i.v., in rats and dogs was described by FOULHOUX (1958).

The atropine-like and neuromuscular blocking activities of oximes of N,N'-poly-methylene*bis*(pyridinium bromide) were investigated by HOBBIGER and SADLER (1959). No correlation was found between either of these two activities and antidotal activity in organophosphate poisoning. The atropine-like action was most pronounced with N,N'-trimethylene*bis*(pyridine-4-aldoxime bromide), and a 50% reduction in sensitivity of the isolated guinea pig ileum to low concentrations of ACh was obtained with 0.013 mM solutions of the oxime.

Since P-2-AM in doses up to 0.19 mmole/kg does not raise the LD_{50} of physostigmine and neostigmine, it seems unlikely that any of the actions described above can themselves protect animals against lethal organophosphate poisoning when P-2-AM is used in doses not exceeding 0.2 mmole/kg. The same applies to the actions of MINA when the oxime is used in doses below 1 mmole/kg. In the case of DAM and N,N'-trimethylene*bis*(pyridine-4-aldoxime bromide), a neuromuscular blocking action and an atropine-like action, respectively, must be considered as factors which can contribute to the antidotal action particularly when higher doses of the oximes are used. As far as other actions of these two oximes and the actions of other oximes are concerned, it seems likely that they will not affect the LD_{50} of organophosphates directly but they could delay the onset of death and thus promote the antidotal action by enabling reactivation to continue for longer periods.

VIII. Distribution, excretion, and metabolism

Oximes are quickly and widely distributed throughout the body. Even after i.v. injection, the amount found in plasma rapidly falls below 10% of the administered dose. The half-life of oximes in plasma depends on both the species and the oxime. Extensive conversion of oximes into inactive products occurs, mainly in the liver.

Distribution. The highest concentrations reached in the blood of rats after i.p. injections of 0.4 mmole MINA/kg or 1.5 mmole DAM/kg are approximately $0.6\,mM$ and $2\,mM$, respectively; in dogs injected i.p. with 0.68 mmole MINA/kg or 5 mmole DAM/kg the highest concentrations in blood are approximately $1.5\,mM$ and $7\,mM$, respectively (ASKEW et al. 1956, RUTLAND 1958). The concentrations in human plasma shortly after i.v. injection of 0.057 mmole P-2-AM/kg or 0.15 mmole DAM/kg are $0.076\,mM$ and $0.25\,mM$, respectively (JAGER et al. 1958).

DAM freely enters the central nervous system whereas P-2-AM does not. Neither of the oximes enters into erythrocytes or is bound to plasma proteins (JAGER et al. 1958).

In vivo half-life in blood. When P-2-AM is determined by the Blum reaction, which is not specific for P-2-AM but measures also some of its metabolite(s), the half-life of "P-2-AM" in man and rats can be calculated as 54 and 25 min, respectively; kidney disease and nephrectomy were found to prolong it considerably (JAGER et al. 1958).

The half-life of DAM in rats and dogs is given as 137 and 270 min, respectively, by DULTZ et al. (1957), and in man as 430 min by JAGER et al. (1958). A considerably shorter half-life in rats and dogs is indicated by the results of ASKEW et al. (1956) and RUTLAND (1958). The reason for this discrepancy is unknown.

Metabolism is mainly responsible for the disappearance of DAM and nephrectomy has little effect on its half-life (DULTZ et al. 1957).

The half-life of MINA in rats and dogs is similar to that of DAM (ASKEW et al. 1956, RUTLAND 1958).

Metabolism. Minces or slices of liver metabolize P-2-AM, P2S, and DAM (DULTZ et al. 1957, JAGER et al. 1958, CREASEY and GREEN 1959). The urinary excretion product of P-2-AM appears to be an aldehyde, probably pyridine-2-aldehyde (JAGER et al. 1958), and the metabolism of MINA and di*iso*nitroso-acetone yields cyanide (ASKEW et al. 1956).

IX. Toxicity

In view of the potential usefulness of oximes in the treatment of organophosphate poisoning of man, studies of their toxicity are of great importance. Most of these studies were carried out in mice and other small laboratory animals.

Toxic signs produced by hydroxamic acids and oximes are on the whole very similar. Animals injected with near-lethal doses of these compounds show reduced activity and slight respiratory impairment. Lethal doses produce prostration, muscular tremor, clonic convulsions, loss of reflexes, cyanosis, dyspnoea, and finally respiratory arrest while the heart still continues to beat. After the i.v. injection of 2 LD_{50}'s or larger doses, death can occur in less than 5 min.

The metabolism of MINA and di*iso*nitroso-acetone yields cyanide. Death in animals injected with one of these oximes is due to cyanide poisoning and can be prevented by suitable prophylactic treatment (ASKEW et al. 1956). In the case of 4-monoximes

Table 12. *Toxicity of oximes (i.p.injection)*

Oxime	Species	LD_{50} in mmole/kg	
MINA	Mouse	1.7	DULTZ et al. (1957)
	Rat (male)	0.57	DAVIES and WILLEY (1958)
	Rat (female)	0.85	
DAM	Mouse	9	DULTZ et al. (1957)
	Mouse	0.5	KEWITZ and WILSON (1956)
	Mouse	0.84	LOOMIS (1956)
P-2-AM	Mouse	0.88	DAVIES and WILLEY (1958)
	Rat	1.12	
	Mouse	0.6	NAMBA (1958b)
	Mouse	1.0	HOBBIGER and SADLER (1959)
P2S	Mouse	0.76	DAVIES and WILLEY (1958)
	Rat	1.05	
4 M (3)		0.5	
4 M (4)		0.36	
4 M (5)	Mouse	0.16	HOBBIGER and SADLER (1959)
4 D (2)		0.62	
4 D (3)[1]		0.29	
4 D (4)		0.19	

Oximes of N,N'-polymethylene*bis*(pyridinium bromide) with the structure (XII) and (XIII) are referred to by a code. Oximes labelled 4 M and 4 D are 4-monoximes and 4,4'-dioximes, respectively; the figures in brackets give the number of carbon atoms of the polymethylene chain.

[1] TMB-4.

and 4,4'-dioximes of N,N'-polymethylene*bis*(pyridinium bromide), a good correlation exists between the LD_{50} in mice and the ability to block neuromuscular transmission in the rat nerve-diaphragm preparation (HOBBIGER and SADLER 1959).

Plots of percentage mortality against dose show a steep regression, and when 50% of an LD_{50} dose is injected few or no signs are noted. The LD_{50} of individual oximes is somewhat variable between species but in the case of P2S, given i.m., differs only by a factor of 1.6 between mice, rats, rabbits, guinea pigs, and monkeys

(DAVIES and WILLEY 1958). The toxicity depends on the route of administration and in the case of P-2-AM and P2S is of the order i.v. > i.m., i.p. > s.c. ≫ oral (DAVIES and WILLEY 1958, NAMBA 1958b).

The LD$_{50}$'s of oximes which have been shown to possess a marked antidotal activity in organophosphate poisoning when used alone or in combination with atropine (see Table 11) are summarized in Table 12. Information on the toxicity of other oximes is given by ASKEW (1956), DULTZ et al. (1957) and HOBBIGER and SADLER (1959), and data on the toxicity of hydroxamic acids have been reported by ASKEW (1956) and EPSTEIN and FREEMAN (1956).

Post mortem analyses of mice injected with lethal doses of P-2-AM showed edema in brain, lungs, kidneys, and spleen, and generalized vasodilatation (NAMBA 1958b). In rats injected with a lethal dose of P2S, venous congestion of the lungs and kidneys and collapse of the lungs together with slight haemorrhages were observed (DAVIES and WILLEY 1958).

X. Therapeutic action of P-2-AM in organophosphate poisoning of man

The only oxime which has so far been used therapeutically in man suffering from organophosphate poisoning is P-2-AM. In each case poisoning was caused by Parathion and the oxime was always given, usually after atropine, when poisoning was well established.

NAMBA and HIRAKI (1958) and NAMBA (1958c) used P-2-AM in 39 cases of Parathion poisoning. In 13 of these patients poisoning was severe and caused dizziness, profuse sweating, salivation, dyspnoea, nausea, vomiting, slurred speech, blurred vision, miosis, loss of reflexes, muscular fasciculation, urinary and faecal incontinence, and in the later stages unconsciousness. Pyridine-2-aldoxime methiodide injected i.v. in a dose of 3.8 to 7.6 mmole, i.e., 1 to 2 g, speedily reactivated the diethylphosphoryl-AChE in erythrocytes; e.g., in a particular case enzyme activity rose from 13% of normal to normal values within 10 min; at the same time consciousness was restored and all other signs and symptoms of poisoning disappeared speedily. Only one of the 13 patients with severe poisoning could not be saved by treatment with P-2-AM, but of course it is not known how many patients would have survived if they had been treated with atropine alone. The finding that P-2-AM restored consciousness is remarkable since studies in animals show that P-2-AM does not cross freely the blood-brain barrier. Perhaps penetration into the brain is higher in some areas than in others and the animal experiments are misleading in this respect, as pointed out previously. It is interesting in this connection that LONGO et al. (1960) found that 0.19 mmole PAM/kg, injected i.v. before 20 μg Sarin/kg, given by the same route, prevents the appearance of a "grand mal" pattern of the EEG in rabbits.

Reactivation of diethylphosphoryl-ChE in blood and improvement of respiration by P-2-AM in a single case of Parathion poisoning has been reported by ERDMANN et al. (1958), and the successful use of P-2-AM in the treatment of Parathion poisoning has also been described by FUKUHARA (1957), YAMADA (1957), and KARLOG et al. (1958).

Reactivation of phosphorylated AChE by P-2-AM in patients with Parathion poisoning is sometimes only transient (NAMBA and HIRAKI 1958, ERDMANN et al. 1958), due to further conversion of Parathion into Paraoxon after the concentration of P-2-AM has fallen below effective levels. In such cases repeated injections of P-2-AM are more effective than single injections.

Eight mmole (2 g) of P-2-AM, the dose recommended by NAMBA and HIRAKI (1958), produces negligible effects in healthy man when injected slowly (GROB and

JOHNS 1958a, JAGER and STAGG 1958, NAMBA 1958b). Five to 20 mmole of DAM, on the other hand, produces drowsiness, giddiness, and if injected more rapidly, transient unconsciousness and sometimes convulsions (GROB and JOHNS 1958a, JAGER and STAGG 1958). Nineteen to 38 mmole, i.e., 5 to 10 g, of P-2-AM has been given orally and was well tolerated (LADELL 1958, NAMBA 1958b).

The work of GROB and JOHNS (1958a, b, c) shows that P-2-AM and DAM have additional actions in man which are not accomplished by reactivation of phosphorylated AChE. Pyridine-2-aldoxime methiodide, 0.0002 mmole, or 0.001 mmole DAM, injected i.a., reduces the amplitude of evoked action potentials of striped muscle and reverses the effect on neuromuscular transmission produced by i.a. injections of neostigmine, *bis*neostigmine, pyridostigmine (3-(N,N-dimethyl-carbamoyloxy)N-methylpyridinium bromide), *bis*pyridostigmine, and ambenonium (N,N'-*bis*(diethyl-2-chlorobenzyl-ammoniumethyl) oxamide dichloride), which are potent anti-ChE agents but not phosphorylating agents, just as it modifies the similar actions of Sarin. Two to 7.6 mmole P-2-AM or 5 to 20 mmole DAM, injected i.v., reduces fasciculation and generalized muscular weakness produced by a preceding i.v. injection of any of the foregoing anti-ChE agents and at the same time AChE activity transiently increases. The effect of P-2-AM is greater than that of DAM, and the increase of AChE activity is most marked and lasts longest in subjects previously injected with Sarin.

These findings support the interpretation that the lasting therapeutic effects of P-2-AM in Parathion poisoning are principally due to reactivation of phosphorylated AChE, but they indicate also that other actions of P-2-AM which themselves might not raise the LD_{50} of organophosphates could contribute to the antidotal action of P-2-AM.

Atropine is a useful adjuvant to oximes and greatly raises the antidotal action of the latter in laboratory animals (Table 11). Atropine is more toxic to man (GORDON and FRYE 1955) than to small animals and thus can be given to man only in doses considerably below those generally used in animals. Enhancement of the antidotal action of N,N'-trimethylene*bis*(pyridine-4-aldoxime bromide) (4 D (3), TMB-4) by 1 mg atropine sulphate/kg, i.p., in mice and of MINA by 0.029 mg atropine sulphate/kg, i.m., in monkeys (see Table 11) strongly indicates that atropine should be used in combination with oximes for the treatment of organophosphate poisoning of man.

This topic is discussed fully in Chapter 22.

Concluding remarks

Biochemical studies. Diethyl- and di*iso*propyl-phosphoryl-AChE and *iso*propyl methylphosphonyl-AChE can be reactivated, i.e., dephosphorylated[1], by nucleophilic reagents amongst which hydroxamic acids and oximes are the most potent. Reactivation by hydroxamic acids and oximes is a reaction between a protonated form of phosphorylated AChE and the anion of the reactivator, and thus a function of the pK_a of the reactivator and of the pH of the medium used for reactivation. The rate of reactivation is greatly enhanced (promoted) by formation of a complex between the anion of the reactivator and phosphorylated AChE. The strength of bonding and degree of complimentariness between phosphorylated AChE and reactivator determine the degree of promotion and accounts to a large extent for differences between rates of reactivation observed with individual hydroxamic acids and oximes with similar pK_a's. At pH 7 to 8, mono-quaternary

---

[1] The term phosphorylation is used for simplicity and includes both phosphorylation and phosphonylation.

pyridine aldoximes, e.g., P-2-AM, are more potent reactivators than hydroxamic acids, and *bis*-quaternary pyridine aldoximes are the most potent reactivators known at present. Mono-quaternary pyridine aldoximes[1] and quaternary hydroxamic acids are thought to form a complex by bonding of their quaternary ammonium group to the anionic site of phosphorylated AChE; it seems reasonable to assume that *bis*-quaternary pyridine aldoximes share a bonding site with mono-quaternary pyridine aldoximes but are subject also to additional bonding. The time-course of reactivation obtained with *bis*-quaternary pyridine aldoximes is determined by the rates of reactivation and rephosphorylation. The latter is attributed to the phosphorylated anion of the oxime which is formed during reactivation. Rephosphorylation does not appear to play any part in the interaction between hydroxamic acids or other oximes and phosphorylated AChE.

Dialkoxyphosphoryl- and *iso*propyl methylphosphonyl-AChE undergo "ageing," probably by being converted into monoalkoxyphosphoryl- and methylphosphonyl-AChE, respectively. The latter type is not reactivatable and is formed much more speedily from di*iso*propylphosphoryl-AChE and *iso*propyl methylphosphonyl-AChE than from diethylphosphoryl-AChE.

Hydroxamic acids and oximes, in their anionic forms, reactivate also dialkoxy-phosphoryl-BuChE, and dialkoxyphosphoryl- and *iso*propyl methylphosphonyl-chymotrypsin. Oximes reactivate phosphorylated BuChE's at much lower rates than corresponding phosphorylated AChE's, but formation of a complex still seems to play some part in the reactivation. The rates of reactivation of phosphorylated chymotrypsin are considerably lower than those of phosphorylated AChE or BuChE, and are determined solely by the concentration of the anion of the reactivator and its nucleophilic activity.

Information concerning reactivation of those types of phosphorylated AChE which are formed by organophosphates (or their metabolites) which do not possess a dialkoxyphosphoryl or an *iso*propyl methylphosphonyl group is very scanty. The available results indicate that the various types of phosphorylated AChE formed by them are either less easily reactivatable, e.g., the phosphorylated AChE formed by TABUN, than the various dialkoxyphosphoryl-AChE's, and subject to rapid "ageing," or are resistant to reactivation from the start, e.g., the phosphorylated AChE's formed by OMPA or Dimefox.

Antidotal actions. The toxic actions of organophosphates which are *per se* phosphorylating agents of AChE or become such after metabolic conversion are mainly due to accumulation of ACh following phosphorylation of AChE. Many oximes and some hydroxamic acids raise the LD_{50} of organophosphates which form a reactivatable phosphorylated AChE, and the former reverse or ameliorate signs and symptoms of sub-lethal poisoning produced by them. Hydroxamic acids are much weaker antidotes than oximes and have to be used in large doses to produce an antidotal action. They are, therefore, of no practical importance.

The antidotal action of mono- and *bis*-quaternary pyridine aldoximes, MINA, and DAM against organophosphates which form a dialkoxyphosphoryl-AChE or *iso*propyl methylphosphonyl-AChE has been investigated in considerable detail. The relationship between antidotal activity and reactivating potency of these oximes is a complex one; the former can rarely be predicted from the latter and varies even when organophosphates are used which form the same type of phosphorylated AChE. Protection by the oximes against lethal poisoning by organophosphates in most cases is enhanced greatly by atropine, and the LD_{50} of some

---

[1] This view is no longer acceptable for reasons discussed on pages 975 and 976.

organophosphates can be raised more than one hundred-fold by the combination of bis-quaternary pyridine aldoximes with atropine. Protection is associated with reactivation of phosphorylated AChE in peripheral tissues. Only the lipid-soluble oximes, e.g., MINA and DAM, reactivate phosphorylated AChE in brain to any great extent, and the superiority of MINA over quaternary pyridine aldoximes as an antidote in Sarin poisoning has been attributed to this property; quaternary pyridine aldoximes form potent phosphonylating agents on interaction with Sarin and this might be another factor responsible for the relatively low antidotal activity of the quaternary pyridine aldoximes in Sarin poisoning.

The results obtained with the various oximes indicate that protection obtained with mono- and bis-quaternary pyridine aldoximes and MINA against lethal poisoning by organophosphates which form a reactivatable phosphorylated AChE is essentially due to reactivation of phosphorylated AChE. Other actions of these oximes which in themselves (i.e., in the absence of reactivation) would raise the LD_{50} of organophosphates only to a small extent or fail to affect it, might enable these oximes to give a considerably higher degree of protection against lethal organophosphate poisoning than would be obtained without them. To what extent this applies in any individual case will depend on the oxime, organophosphate, and possibly the species of animals used. The experimental evidence suggests that actions other than reactivation contribute more to the antidotal action of bis-quaternary pyridine aldoximes than to that of P-2-AM when both are given in equimolar doses. In spite of this limitation, the main factor responsible for the superiority of bis-quaternary over mono-quaternary pyridine aldoximes seems to be the difference between their reactivating potencies. Protection against lethal organophosphate poisoning which is largely attributable to an action other than reactivation is obtained in Sarin poisoning of rats injected prophylactically with DAM; the experimental evidence also suggests that in addition to reactivation other actions play a considerable part in the antidotal action of DAM against organophosphates in general.

Pyridine-2-aldoxime methiodide has been used in the treatment of Parathion poisoning of man and has been found to be an effective antidote. Since bis-quaternary pyridine aldoximes are considerably more potent as antidotes than P-2-AM, and have a greater therapeutic ratio than P-2-AM in animals, trials of these oximes in man should be carried out as soon as possible. Routine protection of man by prophylactic injections of oximes against lethal organophosphate poisoning is at present impracticable since the protection obtained with single injections is only of a transient nature. For the same reason repeated injections of oximes must be given when poisoning is caused by organophosphates which are not per se phosphorylating agents but become such after metabolic conversion.

Very little or no protection is obtained with oximes or combinations of oximes with atropine against lethal poisoning by organophosphates which form a non-reactivatable type of phosphorylated AChE from the start. Unfortunately, some of the organophosphate insecticides which are used at present belong to this group of organophosphates.

Symptoms of acute sub-lethal poisoning by organophosphates which form a reactivatable phosphorylated AChE can now be speedily terminated by repair of the biochemical lesion. This represents a major progress in the therapy of organophosphate poisoning of man. Certain types of phosphorylated AChE are reactivatable initially but quickly converted into a non-reactivatable form; in all such cases treatment with oximes must be started without delay to secure an effect.

Appendix

Key to abbreviations

a) *Hydroxamic acids and oximes:*

NHAM   nicotinehydroxamic acid methiodide (used in Section A only)
P-2-AM   pyridine-2-aldoxime methiodide
P-3-AM   pyridine-3-aldoxime methiodide
P-4-AM   pyridine-4-aldoxime methiodide
P2S   pyridine-2-aldoxime methyl methanesulphonate
MINA   mono*iso*nitrosoacetone
DAM   diacetylmonoxime
4 D (3) ⎱   N,N'-trimethylene*bis*(pyridine-4-aldoxime bromide), or 1,1'-trimethyl-
TMB-4 ⎰   ene*bis*(4-formylpyridinium bromide) dioxime

b) *Organophosphates:*

See Table 9.

c) *Symbols:*

k first order constant of reactivation of phosphorylated acetylcholin-
           esterase,
$[R]$ concentration of reactivator, i.e., hydroxamic acid or oxime,
LD_{50} amount of compound required to produce 50% mortality in a group
           of animals.

Detailed descriptions of the synthesis and chemical properties of hydroxamic acids and oximes are found in the following publications:

nicotinehydroxamic acid and its methiodide	WILSON et al. (1955)
other hydroxamic acids	HACKLEY et al. (1955)
mono-quaternary pyridine aldoximes, their tert. bases and related oximes	GINSBURG and WILSON (1957) POZIOMEK et al. (1958) WILSON and GINSBURG (1958) WILSON et al. (1958) HOBBIGER et al. (1960)
pyridine-2-aldoxime methyl methanesulphonate	CREASEY and GREEN (1959)
bis-quaternary pyridine aldoximes	POZIOMEK et al. (1958) WILSON and GINSBURG (1958) BERRY et al. (1959) HOBBIGER and SADLER (1959)

Reviews: Short review articles dealing with limited aspects of the reactivation of phosphorylated AChE and based mainly on work conducted by individual groups have been published by KEWITZ (1957b), DAVIES and GREEN (1959), and WILSON (1959). Review articles covering a wider field and including small sections on reactivation of phosphorylated AChE have been written by ALDRIDGE (1956), NACHMANSOHN (1957), ERDMANN and LENDLE (1958), DAVIES and GREEN (1958), and HOLMSTEDT (1959). These publications are listed in the Section *Literature*.

Literature

ALDRIDGE, W. N.: The inhibition of erythrocyte cholinesterase by tri-esters of phosphoric acid: 3. The nature of the inhibitory process. Biochem. J. **54**, 442—448 (1953).
— Organophosphorus compounds and esterases. A. R. Chem. Soc. **53**, 294—305 (1956).
—, and A. N. DAVISON: The mechanism of inhibition of cholinesterases by organophosphorus compounds. Biochem. J. **55**, 763—765 (1953).
ALLES, G. A., and R. C. HAWES: Cholinesterase in blood of man. J. biol. Chem. **133**, 375—390 (1940).
ASKEW, B. M.: Oximes and hydroxamic acids as antidotes in anticholinesterase poisoning. Brit. J. Pharmacol. **11**, 417—423 (1956).
— Oximes and atropine in sarin poisoning. Brit. J. Pharmacol. **12**, 340—343 (1957).
— D. R. DAVIES, A. L. GREEN and R. HOLMES: The nature of the toxicity of 2-oxo-oximes. Brit. J. Pharmacol. **11**, 424—427 (1956).
AUGUSTINSSON, K. B.: Enzymic hydrolysis of organophosphorus compounds. VIII. Effect of anions. Acta chem. scand. **12**, 1286—1291 (1958).
BAY, E., S. KROP and L. F. YATES: Chemotherapeutic effectiveness of 1,1'-trimethylenebis-(4-formylpyridinium bromide) dioxime (TMB-4) in experimental anticholinesterase poisoning. Proc. Soc. exp. Biol. (N. Y.) **98**, 107—110 (1958).
BERENDS, F., C. H. POSTHUMUS, I. v. d. SLUYS and F. A. DEIERKAUF: The chemical basis of the "ageing process" of DFP-inhibited pseudocholinesterase. Biochim. biophys. Acta **34**, 576—579 (1959).
BERGMAN, F., and A. SHIMONI: Quaternary ammonium salts as inhibitors of acetylcholinesterase. II. pH dependence of the inhibitory effects and the dissociation constant of the anionic site. Biochim. biophys. Acta **9**, 473—477 (1952).
BERGNER, A. E., and J. J. O'NEILL: A modification of the Koelle technique for use with oximes. J. Histochem. Cytochem. **6**, 72—74 (1958).
BERGNER, A. D., and P. F. WAGLEY: An effect of pyridine-2-aldoxime methiodide (2-PAM) on cholinesterase at motor end-plates. Proc. Soc. exp. Biol. (N. Y.) **97**, 90—92 (1958).
BERRY, W. K., D. R. DAVIES and A. L. GREEN: Oximes of αω-diquaternary alkane salts as antidotes to organophosphate anticholinesterases. Brit. J. Pharmacol. **14**, 186—191 (1959).
BETHE, K., W. D. ERDMANN, L. LENDLE u. G. SCHMIDT: Spezifische Antidot-Behandlung bei protrahierter Vergiftung mit Alkylphosphaten (Paraoxon, Parathion, DFP) und Eserin an Meerschweinchen. Naunyn-Schmiedeberg's Arch. exp. Path. Pharmak. **231**, 3—22 (1957).
BROWN, R. V.: The effects of intracysternal sarin and pyridine-2-aldoxime methyl methanesulphonate in anaesthetized dogs. Brit. J. Pharmacol. **15**, 170—174 (1960).
— A. M. KUNKEL, L. M. SOMERS and J. H. WILLS: Pyridine-2-aldoxime methiodide in the treatment of Sarin and Tabun poisoning, with notes on its pharmacology. J. Pharmacol. exp. Ther. **120**, 276—284 (1957).
BURGEN, A. S. V., and F. HOBBIGER: The inhibition of cholinesterase by alkylphosphates and alkylphenylphosphates. Brit. J. Pharmacol. **6**, 593—605 (1951).
CANDOLE, C. A. DE, W. W. DOUGLAS, C. LOVATT EVANS, R. HOLMES, K. E. V. SPENCER, R. W. TORRANCE and K. M. WILSON: The failure of respiration in death by anticholinesterase poisoning. Brit. J. Pharmacol. **8**, 466—475 (1953).
CASIDA, J. E.: Metabolism of organophosphorus insecticides in relation to their antiesterase activity, stability and residual properties. J. agric. Food Chem. **4**, 772—785 (1956).
— T. C. ALLEN and M. A. STAHMANN: Mammalian conversion of octamethyl-pyrophosphoramide to a toxic phosphoramide-N-oxide. J. biol. Chem. **210**, 607—616 (1954).
CHILDS, A. F., D. R. DAVIES, A. L. GREEN and I. P. RUTLAND: The reactivation by oximes and hydroxamic acids of cholinesterase inhibited by organophosphorus compounds. Brit. J. Pharmacol. **10**, 462—465 (1955).
COHEN, E. M., and H. WIERSINGA: Oximes in treatment of nerve gas poisoning. Acta physiol. pharmacol. neerl. **8**, 40—51 (1959).
CONLEY, B. E.: Studies on chemical protection against the lethal action of Parathion. Arch. int. Pharmacodyn. **116**, 375—388 (1958).
CREASEY, H. N., and A. L. GREEN: 2-hydroxyiminomethyl-N-methylpyridinium methanesulphonate (P2S), an antidote to organophosphorus poisoning. Its preparation, estimation and stability. J. Pharm. (Lond.) **8**, 485—490 (1959).
CUNNINGHAM, L. W. jun.: Reactivation of diethyl-p-nitrophenyl phosphate-inhibited α-chymotrypsin by hydroxylamine. J. biol. Chem. **207**, 443—458 (1954).
—, and H. NEURATH: Reactivation of α-chymotrypsin inhibited by organic phosphates. Biochim. biophys. Acta **11**, 310 (1953).
DAVIES, D. R., and A. L. GREEN: Results quoted under Contributions to the general discussion. In: The Physical Chemistry of Enzymes. Disc. Faraday Soc. No. 20, 269. Aberdeen University Press Ltd. 1955.

DAVIES, D. R., and A. L. GREEN: The kinetics of reactivation, by oximes, of cholinesterase inhibited by organophosphorus compounds. Biochem. J. **63**, 529—535 (1956).
— — The mechanism of hydrolysis by cholinesterase and related enzymes. In: F. F. NORD, Ed.: Advanc. Enzymol. **20**, 283—318 (1958).
— — The chemotherapy of poisoning by organophosphate anticholinesterases. Brit. J. industr. Med. **16**, 128—134 (1959).
— — and G. L. WILLEY: 2-hydroxyiminomethyl-N-methylpyridinium methanesulphonate and atropine in the treatment of severe organophosphate poisoning. Brit. J. Pharmacol. **14**, 5—8 (1959).
—, and G. L. WILLEY: The toxicity of 2-hydroxyiminomethyl-N-methylpyridinium methane-sulphonate (P2S). Brit. J. Pharmacol. **13**, 202—207 (1958).
DAVISON, A. N.: Return of cholinesterase activity in the rat after inhibition by organophosphorus compounds. Biochem. J. **54**, 583—590 (1953).
DOSTROVSKY, I., and M. HALMANN: Kinetic studies in the phosphinyl chloride and phosphoro chloridate series. Part IV. General discussion. J. chem. Soc. **1953**, 516—519.
DULTZ, L., M. A. EPSTEIN, G. FREEMAN, E. H. GRAY and W. B. WEIL: Studies on a group of oximes as therapeutic compounds in sarin poisoning. J. Pharmacol. exp. Ther. **119**, 522—531 (1957).
EDERY, H.: Effects of diacetyl monoxime on neuromuscular transmission. Brit. J. Pharmacol. **14**, 317—322 (1959).
—, and G. SCHATZBERG-PORATH: Pyridine-2-aldoxime methiodide and diacetyl monoxime against organophosphorus poisoning. Science **128**, 1137—1138 (1958).
— — Prophylactic and therapeutic effects of pyridine-2-aldoxime methiodide and diacetyl monoxime against poisoning by organophosphorus compounds. Arch. int. Pharmacodyn. **121**, 104—109 (1959).
ENANDER, I.: Experiments with methyl-fluorophosphorylcholine-inhibited cholinesterase. Acta chem. scand. **12**, 780—781 (1958).
EPSTEIN, M. A., and G. FREEMAN: Toxicity of hydroxamic acid analogues; prophylactic and therapeutic efficacy against nerve gas poisoning in mice. Proc. Soc. exp. Biol. (N. Y.) **92**, 660—662 (1956).
ERDMANN, W. D., u. L. LENDLE: Vergiftungen mit esteraseblockierenden Insecticiden aus der Gruppe der organischen Phosphorsäureester (E 605 und Verwandte). In: L. HEILMEYER, R. SCHOEN, E. GLANZMANN and B. DE RUDDER, Eds.: Ergebn. inn. Med. Kinderheilk. **10**, 103—184 (1958).
— F. SAKAI u. F. SCHELER: Erfahrungen bei der spezifischen Behandlung einer E 605-Vergiftung mit Atropin und dem Esteraseaktivator PAM. Dtsch. med. Wschr. **83**, 1359 bis 1362 (1958).
FLEISHER, J. H., J. P. CORRIGAN and J. W. HOWARD: Potentiation of the response of frog rectus muscle to acetylcholine by *iso*propyl methyl phosphonofluoridate and its modification by pyridine-2-aldoxime methiodide. Brit. J. Pharmacol. **13**, 291—295 (1958).
— H. O. MICHEL, L. YATES and C. S. HARRISON: 1,1'-trimethylene bis(4-formylpyridinium bromide) dioxime (TMB-4) and 2-pyridine aldoxime methiodide (2-PAM) as adjuvants to atropine in the treatment of anticholinesterase poisoning. J. Pharmacol. exp. Ther. **129**, 31—35 (1960).
— J. W. HOWARD and J. P. CORRIGAN: Effect of pyridine aldoximes on response of frog rectus muscle to acetylcholine. Brit. J. Pharmacol. **13**, 288—290 (1958).
FOULHOUX, N.: L'action antinicotinique d'une oxime. C. R. Soc. Biol. (Paris) **152**, 1116—1118 (1958).
FOURNEL, J.: Action antidote de l'iodométhylate de l'α-pyridylaldoxime vis-à-vis des intoxications expérimentales provoquées par les insecticides organophosphorés. C. R. Soc. Biol. (Paris) **151**, 1373—1377 (1957).
FREDRIKSSON, T., and G. TIBBLING: Reversal of effects on the rat nerve-diaphragm preparation produced by methylfluorophosphorylcholines. Biochem. Pharmacol. **2**, 63—67 (1959).
FUKUDA, T., and G. B. KOELLE: The cytological localization of intracellular neuronal acetylcholinesterase. J. biophys. biochem. Cytol. **5**, 433—440 (1959).
FUKUHARA, A.: Parathion poisoning. III. Effect of sulfhydryl compounds and 2-pyridine aldoxime methiodide on Parathion-poisoning. Okayama Igakkai Zasshi **69**, 945—958 (1957) (in Japanese, quoted by HOLMSTEDT 1959).
FUNKE, A., G. BENOIT et J. JACOB: Ammoniums quaternaires dans la série des acides hydroxamiques. I. Synthèse d'iodométhylates d'acides diméthylaminobenzoylhydroxamiques, antagonistes du diisopropylfluorophosphate (DFP). C. R. Acad. Sci. (Paris) **240**, 2575 à 2577 (1955).
GINSBURG, S., and I. B. WILSON: Oximes of the pyridine series. J. Amer. chem. Soc. **79**, 481—485 (1957).

GORDON, A. S., and C. W. FRYE: Large doses of atropine. Low toxicity and effectiveness in anticholinesterase intoxication. J. Amer. med. Ass. 159, 1181—1184 (1955).

GREEN, A. L., and J. D. NICHOLLS: The reactivation of phosphorylated chymotrypsin. Biochem. J. 72, 70—75 (1959).

—, and B. SAVILLE: The reaction of oximes with isopropyl methylphosphonofluoridate (Sarin). J. chem. Soc. 1956, 3887—3892.

—, and H. J. SMITH: The effect of electrolytes on the reactivation of phosphorylated cholinesterase. Biochim. biophys. Acta 27, 212—213 (1958a).

— — The reactivation of cholinesterase inhibited with organophosphorus compounds. II. Reactivation by pyridine aldoxime methiodides. Biochem. J. 68, 32—35 (1958b).

— — The reactivation of cholinesterase inhibited with organophosphorus compounds. I. Reactivation by 2-oxoaldoximes. Biochem. J. 68, 28—31 (1958c).

— G. L. SAINSBURY, B. SAVILLE and M. STANSFIELD: The reactivity of some active nucleophilic reagents with organophosphorus anticholinesterases. J. chem. Soc. 1958, 1583—1587.

GROB, D., and R. J. JOHNS: Use of oximes in the treatment of intoxication by anticholinesterase compounds in normal subjects. Amer. J. Med. 24, 497—511 (1958a).

— — Use of oximes in the treatment of intoxication by anticholinesterase compounds in patients with myasthenia gravis. Amer. J. Med. 24, 512—518 (1958b).

— — Treatment of anticholinesterase intoxication with oximes. J. Amer. med. Ass. 166, 1855—1858 (1958c).

HACKLEY, B. E. jun.: Ph. D. Dissertation, University of Delaware (1956). (Quoted by HACKLEY, B. E. jun., STEINBERG, G. M. and J. C. LAMB 1959.)

— R. PLAPINGER, M. STOLBERG and T. WAGNER-JAUREGG: Acceleration of the hydrolysis of organic fluorophosphates and fluorophosphonates with hydroxamic acids. J. Amer. chem. Soc. 77, 3651—3653 (1955).

— G. M. STEINBERG and J. C. LAMB: Formation of potent inhibitors of AChE by reaction of pyridinaldoximes with isopropyl methylphosphonofluoridate (GB). Arch. Biochem. 80, 211—214 (1959).

HOBBIGER, F.: Inhibition of cholinesterase by irreversible inhibitors in vitro and in vivo. Brit. J. Pharmacol. 6, 21—30 (1951).

— Effect of nicotinhydroxamic acid methiodide on human plasma cholinesterase inhibited by organophosphates containing a dialkylphosphato group. Brit. J. Pharmacol. 10, 356—362 (1955).

— Chemical reactivation of phosphorylated human and bovine true cholinesterases. Brit. J. Pharmacol. 11, 295—303 (1956).

— Protection against the lethal effects of organophosphates by pyridine-2-aldoxime methiodide. Brit. J. Pharmacol. 12, 438—446 (1957a).

— Reactivation of phosphorylated acetocholinesterase by pyridine-2-aldoxime methiodide. Biochim. biophys. Acta 25, 652—654 (1957b).

— D. G. O'SULLIVAN and P. W. SADLER: New potent reactivators of acetocholinesterase inhibited by tetraethyl pyrophosphate. Nature (Lond.) 182, 1498—1499 (1958).

—, and P. W. SADLER: Protection by oximes of bis-pyridinium ions against lethal diisopropyl phosphonofluoridate poisoning. Nature (Lond.) 182, 1672—1673 (1958).

— — Protection against lethal organophosphate poisoning by quaternary pyridine aldoximes. Brit. J. Pharmacol. 14, 192—201 (1959).

— M. PITMANN and P. W. SADLER: Reactivation of phosphorylated acetocholinesterases by pyridinium aldoximes and related compounds. Biochem. J. 75, 363—372 (1960).

HOLMES, R.: The physiological mechanisms involved in poisoning with anticholinesterases. Proc. roy. Soc. Med. 46, 799—800 (1953).

—, and E. L. ROBINS: The reversal by oximes of neuromuscular block produced by anticholinesterases. Brit. J. Pharmacol. 10, 490—495 (1955).

HOLMSTEDT, B.: Pharmacology of organophosphorus cholinesterase inhibitors. Pharmacol. Rev. 11, 567—688 (1959).

— L. KROOK and J. R. ROONEY: The pathology of experimental cholinesterase-inhibitor poisoning. Acta pharmacol. (Kbh.) 13, 337—344 (1957).

JAGER, B. V., and G. N. STAGG: Toxicity of diacetyl monoxime and of pyridine-2-aldoxime methiodide in man. Johns Hopk. Hosp. Bull. 102, 203—211 (1958).

— — N. GREEN and LOUISE JAGER: Studies on distribution and disappearance of pyridine-2-aldoxime methiodide (PAM) and of diacetyl monoxime (DAM) in man and in experimental animals. Johns Hopk. Hosp. Bull. 102, 225—234 (1958).

JANDORF, B. J.: Chemical reactions of nerve gases (organophosphorus anticholinesterases) in neutral solution. I. Reactions with hydroxylamine. J. Amer. chem. Soc. 78, 3686—3691 (1956).

— E. A. CROWELL and A. P. LEVIN: Role of hydroxamic acids in prevention and reversal of cholinesterase inactivation by DFP and Sarin. Fed. Proc. 14, 231 (1955a).

JANDORF, B. J., H. O. MICHEL, N. K. SCHAFFER, R. EGAN and W. H. SUMMERSON: The mechanism of reaction between esterases and phosphorus-containing anti-esterases. In: The Physical Chemistry of Enzymes, Disc. Faraday Soc. No. 20, 134—142. Aberdeen University Press Ltd. 1955 b.

JAQUES, R., H. I. BEIN and R. MEIER: Therapeutische Möglichkeiten bei Vergiftung durch phosphororganische Anti-Esterasen. Schweiz. med. Wschr. 87, 1096—1098 (1957).

KAMIJO, K., and G. B. KOELLE: The relationship between cholinesterase inhibition and ganglionic transmission. J. Pharmacol. exp. Ther., 105, 349—357 (1952).

KARLOG, O.: Experimental studies on the effect of P-2-AM in acute poisoning with alkyl phosphates. Nord. Vet.-Med. 12, 37—46 (1960).

— M. NIMB and E. POULSEN: Treatment of Parathion (Bladan) poisoning with 2-PAM (pyridyl-(2)-aldoxime-N-methyliodide). Ugeskr. Laeg. 120, 177—183 (1958) (in Swedish, quoted by HOLMSTEDT 1959).

KEWITZ, H.: A specific antidote against lethal alkyl phosphate intoxication. III. Repair of chemical lesion. Arch. Biochem. 66, 263—270 (1957a).

— Die Wiederherstellung der Cholinesteraseaktivität bei der Alkylphosphat-Vergiftung durch ein spezifisches Antidot. Klin. Wschr. 35, 521—526 (1957b).

—, and D. NACHMANSOHN: A specific antidote against lethal alkyl phosphate intoxication. IV. Effects in brain. Arch. Biochem. 66, 271—283 (1957).

—, and I. B. WILSON: A specific antidote against lethal alkylphosphate intoxication. Arch. Biochem. 60, 261—263 (1956).

— — and D. NACHMANSOHN: A specific antidote against lethal alkylphosphate intoxication. II. Antidotal properties. Arch. Biochem. 64, 456—465 (1956).

KING, T. O., and E. POULSEN: The action of an aldoxime (2-pyridine aldoxime methiodide) on acute alkylphosphate poisoning in mice. Arch. int. Pharmacodyn. 114, 118—121 (1958).

KOELLE, G. B.: Protection of cholinesterase against irreversible inactivation by DFP in vitro. J. Pharmacol. exp. Ther. 88, 232—237 (1946).

— The histochemical differentiation of types of cholinesterases and their localizations in tissues of the cat. J. Pharmacol. exp. Ther. 100, 158—179 (1950).

— The elimination of enzyme diffusion artifacts in the histochemical localization of cholinesterases and a survey of their cellular distributions. J. Pharmacol. exp. Ther. 103, 153—171 (1951).

— Histochemical demonstration of reactivation of acetylcholinesterase in vivo. Science 125, 1195—1196 (1957a).

— Histochemical demonstration of reversible anticholinesterase action at selective cellular sites in vivo. J. Pharmacol. exp. Ther. 120, 488—503 (1957b).

—, and E. C. STEINER: The cerebral distributions of a tertiary and a quaternary anticholinesterase agent following intravenous and intraventricular injection. J. Pharmacol. exp. Ther. 118, 420—434 (1956).

KOELLE, WINIFRED A., and GEORGE B. KOELLE: The localization of external or functional acetylcholinesterase at the synapses of autonomic ganglia. J. Pharmacol. exp. Ther. 126, 1—8 (1959).

KOSTER, R.: Synergisms and antagonisms between physostigmine and di-isopropyl fluorophosphate in cats. J. Pharmacol. exp. Ther. 88, 39—46 (1946).

KUNKEL, A. M., J. H. WILLS and J. S. MONIER: Antagonists to neuromuscular block produced by Sarin. Proc. Soc. exp. Biol. (N. Y.) 92, 529—532 (1956).

LADELL, W. S. S.: Treatment of anticholinesterase poisoning. Brit. med. J. 1958 II, 141 to 142.

LARSSON, L.: The catalytic effect of CrO_4^{2-}, MoO_4^{2-} and Wo_4^{2-} on the hydrolysis of iso-Propoxy-methyl-phosphoryl fluoride (Sarin). Acta chem. scand. 12, 1226—1230 (1958).

LONGO, V. G., D. NACHMANSOHN and D. BOVET: Aspects électroencéphalographiques de l'antagonisme entre le iodométhylate de 2-pyridine aldoxime (PAM) et le méthylfluorophosphate d'isopropyle (Sarin). Arch. int. Pharmacodyn. 123, 282—290 (1960).

LOOMIS, T. A.: The effect of an aldoxime on acute Sarin poisoning. J. Pharmacol. exp. Ther. 118, 123—128 (1956).

MAYER, S. E., and J. A. BAIN: Localization of the haematoencephalic barrier with fluorescent quaternary acridones. J. Pharmacol. exp. Ther. 118, 17—25 (1956).

MCISAAC, R. J., and G. B. KOELLE: Comparison of the effect of inhibition of external, internal and total acetylcholinesterase upon ganglionic transmission. J. Pharmacol. exp. Ther. 126, 9—20 (1959).

MEETER, E.: The relation between end-plate depolarization and the repetitive response elicited in the isolated rat phrenic nerve-diaphragm preparation by DFP. J. Physiol. (Lond.) 144, 38—51 (1958).

MENDEL, B., and H. RUDNEY: The cholinesterases in the light of recent findings. Science 100, 499—500 (1944).

MICHEL, O. H.: Development of resistance of alkylphosphorylated cholinesterase to reactivation by oximes. Fed. Proc. 17, 275 (1958).

MYERS, D. K.: Effects of electrolytes on cholinesterase inhibition. Arch. Biochem. 27, 341 to 347 (1950).

— Mechanism of the prophylactic action of diacetylmonoxime against Sarin poisoning. Biochim. biophys. Acta 34, 555—557 (1959).

NACHMANSOHN, D.: Etudes sur la conduction de l'influx nerveux au niveau moléculaire. Bull. Soc. Chim. biol. (Paris) 39, 1021—1035 (1957).

NAMBA, T.: PAM (pyridine-2-aldoxime methiodide) as a prophylactic for Parathion poisoning. Naika no Ryôiki 6, 442—445 (1958a) (in Japanese).

— Toxicity of PAM (pyridine-2-aldoxime methiodide). Naika no Ryôiki 6, 437—441 (1958b) (in Japanese).

— The effectiveness of pyridine-2-aldoxime methiodide (PAM) against Parathion poisoning in thirty-nine human cases. Naika no Ryôiki. 6, 84—95 (1958c) (in Japanese).

—, and K. HIRAKI: PAM (pyridine-2-aldoxime methiodide) therapy for alkylphosphate poisoning. J. Amer. med. Ass. 166, 1834—1839 (1958).

O'LEARY, J. F., J. H. WILLS and L. A. CARLSTROM: Relative efficacy of various prophylactic adjuncts to atropine in Sarin poisoning. Fed. Proc. 17, 401 (1958).

— B HARRISON, G. GROBLEWSKI and J. H. WILLS: The effect of 2-formyl-1-methylpyridinium iodide oxime (2-PAM) on reactivation of tissue cholinesterase following poisoning by a certain phosphate anticholinesterase. Fed. Proc. 18, 430 (1959).

PARKES, M. W., and P. SACRA: Protection against the toxicity of cholinesterase inhibitors by acetylcholine antagonists. Brit. J. Pharmacol. 9, 299—305 (1954).

PAULET, G., et P. ANDRÉ: De l'action de certains dérivés de l'acide hydroxamique sur la réactivation des cholinéstérases du sang inhibées in vivo par les composés organophosphorés. C. R. Soc. Biol. (Paris) 150, 1716—1720 (1956).

POZIOMEK, E. J., B. E. HACKLEY jun. and G. M. STEINBERG: Pyridinium aldoximes. J. org. Chem. 23, 714—717 (1958).

RAJAPURKAR, M. V., and G. B. KOELLE: Reactivation of DFP-inactivated acetylcholinesterase by monoisonitrosoacetone (MINA) and diacetylmonoxime (DAM) in vivo. J. Pharmacol. exp. Ther. 123, 247—253 (1958).

RIKER, W. F., and W. C. WESCOE: The relationship between cholinesterase inhibition and function in a neuroeffector system. J. Pharmacol. exp. Ther. 95, 515—527 (1949).

ROY, B. B., and A. S. KUPERMAN: Reversal of the actions of tetraethylpyrophosphate in surviving mammalian tissue. Proc. Soc. exp. Biol. (N. Y.) 89, 255—258 (1955).

RUTLAND, J. P.: The effect of some oximes in Sarin poisoning. Brit. J. Pharmacol. 13, 399 to 403 (1958).

SAKAI, F., H. RI dal., W. D. ERDMANN u. G. SCHMIDT: Über die Atemlähmung durch Parathion oder Paraoxon und ihre antagonistische Beeinflußbarkeit. Naunyn-Schmiedeberg's Arch. exp. Path. Pharmakol. 234, 210—219 (1958).

SANDERSON, D. M., and E. F. EDSON: Oxime therapy in poisoning by six organophosphorus insecticides in the rat. J. Pharm. (Lond.) 11, 721—728 (1959).

SCAIFE, J. F.: Oxime reactivation studies of inhibited true and pseudo cholinesterase. Canad. J. Biochem. 37, 1301—1311 (1959).

SCHAUMANN, W.: Über den Einfluß von Atropin auf die zentrale Hemmung der Atmung durch Anticholinesterasen. Naunyn-Schmiedeberg's Arch. exp. Path. Pharmak. 236, 415—420 (1959).

SOMERS, L., and E. BAY: Pharmacological studies of 4-formyl-1-methylpyridinium iodide, σ-(isopropoxymethylphosphinyl) oxime (4-PPAM). Fed. Proc. 18, 446 (1959).

SWIDLER, R., and G. M. STEINBERG: The kinetics of the reaction of isopropyl methylphosphonofluoridate (Sarin) with benzohydroxamic acid. J. Amer. chem. Soc. 78, 3594—3598 (1956).

TOIVONEN, T., K. OKELA and W. J. KAIPAINEN: Parathion poisoning increasing frequency in Finland. Lancet 1959 II, 175—176.

VANDEKAR, M., and D. F. HEATH: The reactivation of cholinesterase after inhibition in vivo by some dimethyl phosphate esters. Biochem. J. 67, 202—208 (1957).

WAGLEY, P. F.: A study of end-plate potentials. II. Observations on the actions of certain oximes. Johns Hopk. Hosp. Bull. 100, 287—293 (1957).

WAGNER-JAUREGG, T.: Experimentelle Chemotherapie von durch phosphorhaltige Anti-Esterasen hervorgerufene Vergiftungen. Arzneimittel-Forsch. 6, 194—196 (1956).

WILLS, J. H., A. M. KUNKEL, R. V. BROWN and G. E. GROBLEWSKI: Pyridine-2-aldoxime methiodide and poisoning by anticholinesterases. Science 125, 743—744 (1957).

— — J. F. O'LEARY, and A. H. OIKEMUS: Effect of 2-PAM on neuromuscular blockade induced by certain chemicals. Proc. Soc. exp. Biol. (N. Y.) 101, 196—197 (1959).

WILSON, I. B.: Acetylcholinesterase. XI. Reversibility of tetraethyl pyrophosphate inhibition. J. biol. Chem. **190**, 111—117 (1951).
— Acetylcholinesterase. XIII. Reactivation of alkyl phosphate-inhibited enzyme. J. biol. Chem. **199**, 113—120 (1952).
— Promotion of acetylcholinesterase activity by the anionic site. In: The Physical Chemistry of Enzymes. Disc. Faraday Soc. No. 20, 119—125. Aberdeen University Press Ltd. 1955a.
— Reactivation of human serum esterase inhibited by alkyl phosphates. J. Amer. chem. Soc. **77**, 2383—2386 (1955b).
— Designing of a new drug with antidotal properties against the nerve gas Sarin. Biochim. biophys. Acta **27**, 196—199 (1958).
— Molecular complementarity and antidotes for alkyl phosphate poisoning. Fed. Proc. **18**, 752—758 (1959).
— F. BERGMANN and D. NACHMANSOHN: Acetylcholinesterase. X. Mechanism of the catalysis of acylation reactions. J. biol. Chem. **186**, 781—790 (1950).
—, and S. GINSBURG: Reactivation of acetylcholinesterase inhibited by alkyl phosphates. Arch. Biochem. **54**, 569—571 (1955a).
— — A powerful reactivator of alkyl phosphate-inhibited acetylcholinesterase. Biochim. biophys. Acta **18**, 168—170 (1955b).
— — Reactivation of alkyl phosphate-inhibited acetylcholinesterase by bis-quaternary derivatives of 2-PAM and 4-PAM. Biochem. Pharmacol. **1**, 200—206 (1958).
— —, and E. K. MEISLICH: The reactivation of acetylcholinesterase inhibited by tetraethyl pyrophosphate and diisopropyl fluorophosphate. J. Amer. chem. Soc. **77**, 4286—4291 (1955).
— — and C. QUAN: Molecular complementariness as basis for reactivation of alkyl phosphate-inhibited enzyme. Arch. Biochem. **77**, 286—296 (1958).
—, and E. K. MEISLICH: Reactivation of acetylcholinesterase inhibited by alkyl phosphates. J. Amer. chem. Soc. **75**, 4628 (1953).
—, and C. QUAN: Acetylcholinesterase studies on molecular complementariness. Arch. Biochem. **73**, 131—143 (1958).
—, and F. SONDHEIMER: A specific antidote against lethal alkyl phosphate intoxication. V. Antidotal properties. Arch. Biochem. **69**, 468—474 (1957).
WOODARD, G. T.: The treatment of organic phosphate insecticide poisoning with atropine sulphate and 2-PAM (2-pyridine aldoxime methiodide). Vet. Med. **52**, 571—578 (1957).
YAMADA, M.: Alkylphosphate poisoning. III. Effect of 2-pyridine-aldoxime methiodide in the therapy of parathion poisoning. Okayama-Igakkai-Zasshi, **69**, 525—539 (1957) (in Japanese, quoted by HOLMSTEDT 1959).

Addendum

During the period which has elapsed since Chapter 21 was written a considerable number of papers dealing with reactivation of phosphorylated AChE and related studies have been published. The more important aspects of these papers are summarized below and only those findings which are of particular interest are dealt with more extensively. Whenever the term "previously" is used it refers to Chapter 21, and new references are listed at the end of the Addendum.

Contents

A. Biochemical studies of the reactivation of phosphorylated AChE

I. Hydrolysis of organophosphates by reactivators

SWIDLER et al. (1959) have extended their work on the hydrolysis of Sarin by benz-hydroxamic acids and have confirmed the correctness of the sequence of reactions reported previously (page 927; SWIDLER and STEINBERG 1956).

Reactivators of phosphorylated AChE can be considered as simplified models of AChE in all those cases where the phosphorylation process is not preceded by bonding between AChE and organophosphate. This is illustrated by the results of ASKNES (1960) who found that the relative rates of hydrolysis of three organophosphates (with a common substituent group X) by MINA are comparable to the relative rates at which the former react with AChE. The findings of SWIDLER et al. (1959) and ASKNES (1960) together with those discussed previously show that the rate of hydrolysis of different organophosphates by an individual nucleophilic reagent increases with increasing charge of the phosphorus atom (of the organophosphate) and that the increase in the rate of hydrolysis of an organophosphate which is obtained by increasing the basicity of the nucleophilic reagent is greatest for those organophosphates which have the highest positive charge on the phosphorus atom.

II. Reactivation of phosphorylated AChE by hydroxamic acid and oximes

GILBERT et al. (1961) studied the reactivation of *iso*propyl methylphosphonyl-AChE and the inhibition of AChE by fifteen hydroxamic acids. Their findings support the interpretation (pages 928 and 929) that potent reactivators are bonded to phosphorylated AChE before reactivation takes place and that in the case of hydroxamic acids with structures II and III (see page 925) or related hydroxamic acids, two different bonding sites are involved. The number of available bonding sites is probably greater than two because the esteratic site of AChE must be surrounded by a three-dimensional array of groups which vary in size, charge, polarity, and chemical affinity, since the majority of proteins retain a helical arrangement in solution (DOTY et al. 1954).

Additional evidence that the order of potency for reactivation of *iso*propyl methyl-phosphonyl-AChE is P-2-AM > MINA ≫ DAM has been obtained by COHEN and WIERSINGA (1960) who used as enzyme source homogenized brain, diaphragm, and ileum of rats and erythrocytes and homogenized brain of guinea pigs.

GINSBURG and WILSON (1957) reported two methods for the synthesis of mono-quaternary pyridine aldoximes. They compared the melting points, acidities, and solubilities of the oximes obtained by the two methods with those of oximes derived from pyrrole and benzene and arrived at the conclusion that mono-quaternary pyridine aldoximes can be obtained in a *syn*[1]

---

[1] *syn* and *anti* refer to the steric relationship between hydrogen and oxygen atom; in the case of P-4-AM the two geometrical isomers are:

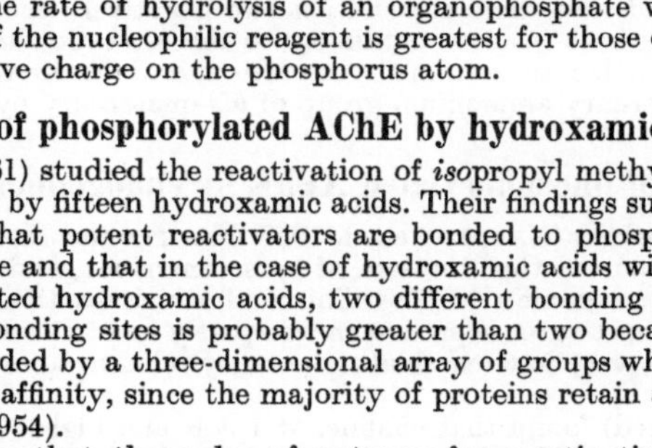

   syn   *anti*

and *anti*[1] configuration and that in solution most oximes with a *syn* configuration are converted rapidly into oximes with an *anti* configuration. Poziomek et al. (1961a) repeated the preparation and characterization of mono-quaternary pyridine aldoximes to which Ginsburg and Wilson assigned a *syn* configuration and came to the conclusion that these compounds are not oximes but carbinolamines. Poziomek et al. (1961b) also reported the synthesis of genuine geometrical isomers of P-4-AM of which the *syn* isomer is approximately three times more potent than the *anti* isomer in reactivating *iso*propyl methylphosphonyl-AChE. According to Wilson et al. (1958), Wilson and Ginsburg (1958), and Wilson (1959), bonding of the quaternary ammonium group of isomeric quaternary pyridine aldoximes to the anionic site (of phosphorylated AChE) is essential for high rates of reactivation, and differences between the reactivating potencies of P-2-AM, P-3-AM, P-4-AM, and their *bis*-quaternary derivatives arise mainly from differences in the alignment of the nucleophilic oxygen of the oxime and the phosphorus atom of the phosphoryl group after bonding of the *anti* isomer of the oxime to the anionic site has taken place (see VIII, IX and X; page 933). If this interpretation were correct the *syn* isomer of P-4-AM should have a considerably lower reactivating potency than the *anti* isomer of P-4-AM. Exactly the opposite is the case, as shown by the results of Poziomek et al. (1961b), and we must conclude, therefore, that the *syn* isomer of P-4-AM does not share a bonding site with the *anti* isomer of P-2-AM but is bonded to another negatively charged site. In view of this it is impossible to say which site serves for bonding of the *anti* isomer of P-4-AM. Spectroscopic analysis of oximes (Sadler 1961) indicates that the configuration (assessed by the steric relationship between the ring nitrogen and the nucleophilic oxygen) of mono- and *bis*-quaternary pyridine 3- and 4-aldoximes which have been used for studying reactivation of phosphorylated AChE *in vitro* and antidotal activity and other actions *in vivo* corresponds to that which is illustrated as *syn* on the previous page. Since it is very likely that *bis*-quaternary pyridine aldoximes share a common bonding site with their corresponding mono-quaternary pyridine aldoximes, and since the *anti* isomer of P-2-AM and the *syn* isomer of P-4-AM are not bonded to the same site, it is now easy to understand why the optimum lengths of the polymethylene chains of *bis*-quaternary derivatives of P-2-AM and P-4-AM are different. In conclusion we can say that the unitarian theory of Wilson and his coworkers for bonding of quaternary pyridine aldoximes to the anionic site of phosphorylated AChE is unacceptable and that there are at least two negatively charged bonding sites for quaternary pyridine aldoximes in close proximity to the esteratic site of AChE, and other negatively charged sites further away from the esteratic site which serve as additional bonding sites for the second quaternary ammonium group of *bis*-quaternary pyridine aldoximes.

III. Reactivation of phosphorylated AChE by endogenous reactivators

Kewitz and his coworkers (Neubert et al. 1958, Kewitz and Neuhoff 1960, Neuhoff and Kewitz 1961a, b) reported that the sera of horse, man, rat, and mouse, and the brain and liver of rats contain an organic acid (?levulinic acid) which reactivates diethylphosphoryl-AChE. This endogenous reactivator is present *in vivo* partly in a free and partly in an inactive form but seems to have a very low reactivating potency relative to most of the oximes described previously.

Hobbiger (unpublished) found that choline, at 1 mM and higher concentrations, reactivates dimethylphosphoryl-AChE, whereas choline, 0.01 M, does not reactivate diethyl- or di*iso*propyl-phosphoryl-AChE.

To what extent choline and the reactivator found by Kewitz and his coworkers reactivate dialkoxyphosphoryl-AChE's and -BuChE's at various sites *in vivo* is not known.

IV. Ageing of phosphorylated AChE and BuChE

The rate of ageing of diethyl- and di*iso*propyl-phosphoryl-AChE and -BuChE, i.e., their conversion from a reactivatable into a non-reactivatable form, is temperature-dependent and considerably reduced by lowering the temperature from 37° to 4° (Latki and Erdmann 1961).

V. Reactivation of carbamylated AChE by hydroxylamine

Hobbiger (1954) suggested that the inhibition of ChE's by anti-ChE agents which contain a carbamyl group, e.g., neostigmine and physostigmine, involves carbamylation but that the extent to which carbamylation occurs is uncertain.

Wilson et al. (1960, 1961) showed that on dilution of a mixture of AChE and a carbamate, the rate of return of enzymic activity was the same when different carbamates were used which had a common carbamyl group. According to these authors, the rate of spontaneous reactiva-

---

[1] See [1] p. 975.

tion of different types of carbamyl-AChE is dimethylcarbamyl-AChE $>$ monomethylcarb-amyl-AChE $\gg$ carbamyl-AChE's formed by *bis*-quaternary carbamates. Hydroxylamine, 0.1 M, reactivates all three types of carbamyl-AChE and the order of reactivatability is monomethyl-carbamyl-AChE $>$ dimethylcarbamyl-AChE $\gg$ carbamyl-AChE's formed by *bis*-quaternary carbamates.

Quaternary pyridine aldoximes raise the LD_{50} of carbamates but not of other non-phosphorylating anti-ChE agents *(vide infra)*, and it is thus tempting to attribute the former to an interference by the oximes with the process of carbamylation or decarbamylation of AChE or both. However, at present this is not possible for several reasons. Firstly, the effect of quaternary pyridine aldoximes on the system AChE-carbamate is unknown. Secondly, WILSON et al. stated neither what level of carbamylation was obtained with different carbamates nor the interval used for incubation of AChE with carbamates; in view of this, the extent to which carbamylation occurs under various conditions *in vitro* and *in vivo* remains unknown. Thirdly, it has been claimed also that in a system containing AChE (or other esterases)-ACh-carbamate, the inhibition arises in the majority of cases mainly from competition and not from carbamylation (MYERS et al. 1957, CASIDA et al. 1960); the results obtained by these authors too are not as conclusive as one might think, since protection by substrate against inhibition of the enzyme by a carbamate must vary with the carbamate and its concentration. Thus, much more work is needed before we can explain why quaternary pyridine aldoximes are antidotes of many carbamates but not of other non-phosphorylating anti-ChE agents.

B. Actions of reactivators of phosphorylated AChE in vivo and related studies

I. Protection by oximes against lethal organophosphate poisoning

A considerable amount of new information is available on the antidotal action of oximes, particularly of P-2-AM and N,N'-trimethylene*bis*(pyridine-4-aldoxime bromide)[1]. Some of this work has been carried out with organophosphates which are not included in Table 9 and which are listed below. In all cases where it is known that the organophosphate is not *per se* a phosphorylating agent but becomes such during its metabolism *in vivo*, the first name is preceded by an asterisk.

Organophosphates which form dimethylphosphoryl-AChE: Dipterex [0,0-dimethyl 0-(2,2,2-tri-chloro-1-hydroxyethyl) phosphate], *Malathion [0,0-dimethyl S-(1,2-dicarbethoxyethyl) phosphorodithioate], *Methyl-Diazinon [0,0-dimethyl 0-(2-*iso*propyl-6-methyl-4-pyrimidyl) phosphorothioate], *Methyl-Phenkapton [0,0-dimethyl S-(2,5-dichlorophenylthiomethyl) phosphorodithioate], Phosphamidon [0,0-dimethyl 0-(2-diethylcarbamyl-2-chloro-1-methylvinyl) phosphate], Phosdrin [0,0-dimethyl 0-(2-carbmethoxy-1-methylvinyl) phosphate], *Morphothion [0,0-dimethyl S-(morpholinocarbonylmethyl) phosphorodithioate].

Organophosphates which form diethylphosphoryl-AChE: 217 AO [0,0-diethyl S-(2-dimethyl-aminoethyl) phosphorothioate acid oxalate], Phospholine (echothiophate) [0,0-diethyl S-(2-tri-methylammonium-ethyl) phosphorothioate iodide], *Thimet [0,0-diethyl S-(eththiomethyl) phosphorodithioate], *Ethyl-Guthion [0,0-diethyl S-(4-oxo-3-H-1,2,3-benzotriazine-3-methyl) phosphorodithioate], *DSDP [0,0-diethyl S-(2-diethylaminoethyl) phosphorodithioate], Iso-Systox [0,0-diethyl S-(2-eththioethyl) phosphorothioate], Vinylphosphate (OS 1836) [0,0-di-ethyl 2-chlorovinyl phosphate].

Organophosphate which forms another type of phosphorylated-AChE: *EPN [0-ethyl 0-(4-nitrophenyl) 0-phenyl phosphonothioate].

Pyridine-2-aldoxime methiodide and TMB-4 raise the LD_{50} of most of the organophosphates listed above when given either shortly before, together with, or shortly after the organophosphate. Information concerning the antidotal action of oximes, given by injection, against the organophosphates listed above and extension of work with organophosphates listed in Table 9 can be summarized as follows:

1. Poisoning by organophosphates which form dimethylphosphoryl-AChE

Pyridine-2-aldoxime methiodide, 0.3 to 0.4 mmole/kg, i.v., raised the LD_{50} in mice of Methyl-Parathion, Malathion, and Dipterex, given by injection (NAMBA et al. 1959 b, d) and of

---

[1] This oxime is frequently referred to as TMB-4 and because of its simplicity this Code is used throughout the *Addendum;* it must be remembered, however, that throughout *Chapter 21* itself N,N'-trimethylene*bis*(pyridine-4-aldoxime bromide) and the Code 4 D (3) were used in text and tables, respectively, instead of the Code TMB-4. A frequently used chemical name for TMB-4 is 1,1'-trimethylene*bis*(4-formylpyridinium bromide) dioxime.

Methyl-Parathion and Metasystox, given orally (STENGER 1960). N,N-Trimethylene*bis*-(pyridine-4-aldoxime bromide), 0.056 to 0.11 mmole/kg, i.p., raised the LD_{50} in mice of Phosphamidon, Metasystox, and Dipterex, s.c. (MILOŠEVIĆ et al. 1959). The LD_{50} of Phosphamidon, s.c., in mice was raised also by 0.1 to 0.4 mmole P-2-AM/kg, i.p. (JAQUES and BEIN 1960), and in rats P-2-AM, 0.4 mmole/kg, i.p., raised the LD_{50} of Phosdrin, Guthion, and Phosphamidon, given orally (SANDERSON 1961).

Little or no antidotal action was obtained with P-2-AM, 0.4 mmole/kg, i.v., in mice against Methyl-Diazinon or Methyl-Phenkaptone, given orally (STENGER 1960) or with P-2-AM, 0.4 mmole/kg, i.p., in rats against Morphothion, given orally (SANDERSON 1961).

2. Poisoning by organophosphates which form diethylphosphoryl-AChE

Oximes are particularly effective in reducing the toxicity of Phospholine: 0.3 mmole P-2-AM/kg and 0.08 mmole TMB-4/kg, i.p., raised in mice the LD_{50} of Phospholine, i.p., 24- and 220-fold, respectively (LEHMAN et al. 1960). Phospholine does not cross easily the blood-brain barrier and shares this property with Ro 3-0340 and Ro 3-0422 (see Table 9) which also form diethylphosphoryl-AChE. Quaternary pyridine aldoximes have a high antidotal activity against Phospholine and Ro 3-0340 but not against Ro 3-0422 (Table 11), and thus the high antidotal activity of quaternary pyridine aldoximes against Phospholine and Ro 3-0340 cannot be attributed solely to the fact that these two organophosphates do not cross easily the blood-brain barrier.

In mice TMB-4, 0.056 to 0.11 mmole/kg, i.p., raised the LD_{50} of Paraoxon and Parathion, s.c. (MILOŠEVIĆ et al. 1959); P-2-AM, 0.32 mmole/kg, i.v., raised the LD_{50} of Parathion, TEPP, and Diazinon, given by injection (NAMBA et al. 1959 b, d); P2S, 0.2 mmole/kg, i.p., raised the LD_{50} of DSDP, s.c. (SCAIFE 1960), and P-2-AM, 0.4 mmole/kg, i.v., raised the LD_{50} of Diazinon, Phenkaptone, Parathion, and Systox (STENGER 1960).

In rats the LD_{50} of Ethyl-Guthion and Systox, but not of Thimet, was raised when P-2-AM, 0.4 mmole/kg, i.p., was given shortly after the oral administration of the organophosphate (SANDERSON 1961), and a rise of the LD_{50} of Systox, Isosystox, Paraoxon, and Parathion, s.c., was obtained with 0.3 mmole P-2-AM/kg, i.p. (KARLOG 1958).

SVETLICIC and VANDEKAR (1960) found that P-2-AM, 0.2 to 0.6 mmole/kg, i.p. or i.v., raised the LD_{50} of Parathion in mice, rats, and rabbits, and confirmed that the antidotal activity of P-2-AM is species-dependent. NAMBA et al. (1959 b, d) compared in mice the antidotal activity of P-2-AM, MINA, and DAM, i.v., against various organophosphates which form dimethyl- and diethyl-phosphoryl-AChE; the authors observed that on the whole the order of antidotal activity is P-2-AM > MINA > DAM, which is in agreement with previous observations.

3. Poisoning by Sarin and Tabun

O'LEARY et al. (1961) carried out a detailed analysis of the antidotal action of i.v. and orally administered P-2-AM (and its methanesulphonate [P2S], lactate, and chloride equivalents), MINA, DAM, and TMB-4 (bromide or chloride), and mixtures of these oximes in dogs and rabbits injected i.v. with Sarin or Tabun. The results obtained by these authors are in line with those discussed previously, but one aspect of the work requires special attention. O'LEARY et al. found that in the presence of atropine, mixtures of P-2-AM, 0.02 mmole/kg, i.v., and TMB-4, 0.011 mmole/kg, i.v., or their chloride equivalents gave a degree of protection against lethal poisoning by Sarin and Tabun which was greater than that obtained when atropine was given with only one of the two oximes in the dose stated. The toxicity of TMB-4 (bromide or chloride) was not increased by P-2-AM (or its chloride equivalent), and since the mixture of the chlorides of the two oximes has a high solubility and stability the authors recommended the use of this mixture in preference to the use of a single oxime. O'LEARY et al. did not show, however, that under their conditions the antidotal activity of the mixture was indeed greater than that of a single oxime, since the oxime concentration in the mixture was greater than that of the single oxime. The recommendation made by O'LEARY et al. must be followed with caution in view of results obtained by MILOŠEVIĆ et al. (1961). These authors found that in mice P-2-AM, 0.1 to 0.2 mmole/kg, i.p., did not increase the antidotal action of TMB-4, 0.028 mmole/kg, i.p., against Phosphamidon, s.c., and with higher doses of the oximes, 0.056 mmole TMB-4/kg and 0.4 mmole P-2-AM/kg, the antidotal action of the combination was less than that which was obtained when either of the two oximes was given singly in the dose stated.

The time-course of the antidotal action in rats of a single dose of DAM, i.p., against Sarin is illustrated by the results of WILLS (1959). An antidotal action in mice was obtained with TMB-4, 0.05 mmole/kg, i.p. (STERN and BOŠKOVIĆ 1960 b).

The work summarized under 1, 2, and 3 is in line with that discussed previously. It illustrates further that single injections of quaternary pyridine aldoximes in suitable doses raise the LD_{50} of most organophosphates which form dimethyl- or diethyl-phosphoryl-AChE and of Sarin and Tabun, and that in many cases the antidotal action of P-2-AM corresponds to a two-fold or smaller rise of the LD_{50} of an organophosphate. The antidotal activity of the oximes is not predictable from the type of phosphorylated AChE one deals with even when the organophosphate is *per se* a phosphorylating agent, and since much of the work quoted above deals with organophosphates which are not *per se* phosphorylating agents, the existence of variations in the antidotal activity of an individual oxime against different organophosphates which form the same type of phosphorylated AChE is not surprising. Failures to obtain any antidotal action against some organophosphates which form a reactivatable phosphorylated AChE can arise from an unfavourable combination of the time-course of the antidotal activity of a single dose of the oxime, given by injection, and the time-course of entry of the organophosphate or its active metabolite(s) into the circulation. These two parameters probably played a decisive part in the experiments of SANDERSON (1961), who observed that in rats the antidotal activity of P-2-AM, i.p., against orally administered organophosphate insecticides which form the same type of phosphorylated AChE was related directly to the speed of onset of poisoning. Of particular interest are the results of STENGER (1960) who found that in mice the antidotal activity of P-2-AM, i.v., against orally administered Diazinon, Phenkaptone, Parathion, and Systox was considerably greater than that against the methyl-derivatives of these organophosphate insecticides. Pyridine-2-aldoxime methiodide reactivates dimethyl-phosphoryl-AChE faster than diethylphosphoryl-AChE (page 947), and this together with differences between the rates at which the organophosphates are converted into active metabolites could account for the results obtained by STENGER.

In agreement with previous observations are the findings that TMB-4 has a higher antidotal activity (LEHMAN et al. 1960, O'LEARY et al. 1961) and therapeutic ratio than P-2-AM, and that the antidotal activity of oximes is species-dependent (SVETLICIC and VANDEKAR 1960, COLEMAN et al. 1961). The same applies to the frequent observation that in the case of organophosphates which form a reactivatable type of phosphorylated AChE, the antidotal action of a combination of atropine (or atropine-like drug) with an oxime is greater than that given by either the oxime or atropine alone, and in some cases exceeds greatly that expected from an additive behaviour of the two antidotes (WILLS 1959, JAQUES and BEIN 1960, SCAIFE 1960, STERN and BOŠKOVIĆ 1960a, b, COLEMAN et al. 1961, MILOŠEVIC et al. 1961, O'LEARY et al. 1961). STERN and BOŠKOVIĆ (1960a, b) reported that in mice the antidotal action of a combination of P-2-AM or TMB-4 and atropine, i.p., against Tabun and DFP, i.m. or s.c., is increased by substances which are known to inhibit the microsomal metabolism of drugs.

4. Poisoning by organophosphates which form a phosphorylated AChE for which reactivatability has not yet been demonstrated *in vitro*

No antidotal action was obtained in mice with TMB-4, 0.11 mmole/kg, i.p., against OMPA and Dimefox, s.c. (MILOŠEVIĆ et al. 1959), but in the same species P-2-AM, 0.32 mmole/kg, i.v., approximately doubled the LD_{50} of Pestox 3, which is a preparation containing OMPA, the pentadimethylamide of triphosphoric acid, and wetting agents (NAMBA et al. 1959a, d). EPN forms a phosphonylated AChE which can be reactivated *in vivo*, and P-2-AM, 0.32 mmole/kg, i.v., approximately doubles its LD_{50} in mice (NAMBA et al. 1959b).

5. Poisoning by anti-ChE agents which are not phosphorylating agents

Quaternary pyridine aldoximes raise the LD_{50} of some non-phosphorylating anti-ChE agents (page 959) but not of others, and the antidotal activity of TMB-4 is greater than that of P-2-AM. This has been confirmed by several authors; the non-phosphorylating anti-ChE agents used by them but not referred to previously include:
Ro 2-1250 [N-methyl-N-(4-chlorophenyl)-carbamoyloxy-3(trimethylammoniumphenyl) bromide], BW 284c51 [1,5-*bis*(N-allyl-N,N-dimethyl-4-ammoniumphenyl) pentane-3-one dibromide], edrophonium (Tensilon) [3-hydroxy N,N,-dimethyl-N-ethylammoniumphenyl chloride], Isolan [5-(N',N'-dimethylcarbamoyloxy)-3-methyl-1-*iso*propyl pyrazole], Dimetilan [5-(N',N'-dimethylcarbamoyloxy)-3-methyl-2-(N'',N''-dimethylcarbamoyl) pyrazole], and Sevin [1-(N-methylcarbamoyloxy) naphthalene].
MILOŠEVIĆ et al. (1959) raised in mice the LD_{50} of Ro 2-1250, neostigmine, and physostigmine but not of BW 284c51, s.c., with TMB-4, 0.11 mmole/kg, i.p.; LEHMAN et al. (1960) raised in mice with P-2-AM, 0.3 mmole/kg, i.p., and TMB-4, 0.08 mmole/kg, i.p., the LD_{50} of pyridostigmine and BC 48 but not of edrophonium and ambenonium, i.p.; SANDERSON (1961) raised in rats with P-2-AM, 0.4 mmole/kg, i.p., the LD_{50} of orally administered Isolan and Dimetilan but not of Sevin, and STENGER (1960) also raised the LD_{50} of orally administered Dimetilan in mice with P-2-AM, 0.4 mmole/kg, i.v.

The non-phosphorylating anti-ChE agents which have been used in work summarized above and discussed previously can be grouped as follows: dimethylcarbamates: neostigmine, pyridostigmine, Isolan and Dimetilan; monomethylcarbamates: physostigmine and Sevin; *bis*quaternary carbamates: BC 48 (*bis*neostigmine) and 51 (*bis*pyridostigmine); other carbamates: Ro 2-1250; and anti-ChE agents which are not carbamates: edrophonium, ambenonium, and BW 284c51.

The greatest antidotal action observed in any experiment is that of TMB-4, 0.08 to 0.1 mmole/kg, i.p., against neostigmine, which represents a three- to four-fold increase of the LD_{50} of the carbamate (HOBBIGER and SADLER 1959, LEHMAN et al. 1961). Many of the available data are not suitable for quantitative assessment of the change in LD_{50} produced by quaternary pyridine aldoximes, but it appears that the antidotal activity of the oximes against carbamates which produce, according to WILSON et al. (1961), the same type of carbamyl-AChE is not uniform although there is a tendency for it to be greatest against dimethyl-carbamates.

Inspection of all available results shows that quaternary pyridine aldoximes fail to raise the LD_{50} of non-phosphorylating anti-ChE agents which are not carbamates. If we accept the interpretation that these agents produce death by inhibiting AChE, then we must conclude that anti-ACh actions of the oximes and other actions which are demonstrable in the absence of anti-ChE agents can not play a major part in the mechanism(s) by which the quaternary pyridine aldoximes raise the LD_{50} of carbamates. At present, however, there is no experimental evidence in support of the interpretation that a decarbamylating property of the oximes is involved and that the mechanism of antidotal action of quaternary pyridine aldoximes against carbamates is analogous to that against organophosphates.

6. Antidotal action of orally administered quaternary pyridine aldoximes

The half-life *in vivo* of oximes given in the form of a single injection is relatively short, and investigations of the antidotal action obtained by oral administration of oximes and its time-course are of considerable importance for evaluation of the suitability of oximes for the prophylaxis against organophosphate poisoning in man. Work on this line has been carried out by LEHMAN and NICHOLLS (1960) who gave mice first an oral dose of either the chloride equivalent of P-2-AM (which is much more soluble than P-2-AM), in amounts up to 12 mmole/kg, or TMB-4, in amounts up to 4.5 mmole/kg, and at different intervals afterwards injected Phospholine, i.p. A maximum antidotal action of the oximes was observed 30 to 60 min after their administration. When the highest doses of the chloride equivalent of P-2-AM or of TMB-4 were given, the maximum antidotal action represented a 50- and 280-fold rise, respectively, of the LD_{50} of Phospholine and a considerable antidotal action was still present ten hours after the administration of the oximes. Using the oximes in amounts which raise the LD_{50} of Phospholine ten-fold, the therapeutic index for oral administration relative to that for injection is of the same order for TMB-4 and higher for the chloride equivalent of P-2-AM.

The findings of COLEMAN et al. (1961) merit also a more detailed presentation. These authors made the following observations. The LD_{50} of DSDP in rats could be raised 44-fold by giving P2S, 0.13 mmole/kg, and atropine sulphate, 12.5 mg/kg, i.m., 15 min before DSDP, s.c. By giving P2S, 0.84 mmole/kg, orally 15 min before DSDP, s.c., and atropine sulphate, 12.5 mg/kg, i.m., $^1/_2$ min after DSDP, s.c., the LD_{50} of DSDP in rats was raised 14-fold and it took 4 hours for a 50% decrease of the antidotal action; the same antidotal treatment (when the organophosphates were given s.c.) raised the LD_{50} of DSDP in mice and guinea pigs 10- and 17-fold, respectively, raised in rats the LD_{50} of TEPP 9-fold, of Vinylphosphate 25-fold, of Isosystox 16-fold, of Paraoxon 55-fold, of Tabun 1.6-fold, and of Sarin 1.8-fold, and raised in mice the LD_{50} of DFP 6-fold, and of OMPA 4-fold.

The time-course of the antidotal action in mice of TMB-4, 0.056 mmole/kg, given orally, against Phosphamidon, i.p., has been studied by MILOŠEVIĆ et al. (1961). SCAIFE (1960) reported first that the chloride equivalent of P-2-AM, 0.12 mmole/kg, given orally, is an effective antidote against DSDP, s.c., in the same species.

II. Reversal by oximes of the symptoms of organophosphate poisoning

Reversal of the symptoms of organophosphate poisoning by oximes (page 952) is further illustrated by the following findings. LEHMAN et al. (1960) reversed in cats the effect of Phospholine on heart rate, blood pressure, respiration, and neuromuscular transmission by giving 0.025 mmole P-2-AM/kg, i.v.; muscarinic and nicotinic symptoms of Parathion poisoning in dogs and horses were reversed with P-2-AM, 0.2 mmole/kg, i.p., and 0.08 mmole/kg, i.v., respectively (SVETLICIC and VANDEKAR 1960); SCHAUMAN (1960a) reversed neuromuscular block produced in the rat with the organophosphate 217 AO by giving 0.08 mmole P-2-AM/kg, i.v., and O'LEARY et al. (1961) demonstrated in cats a reversal of Sarin-induced neuromuscular block by giving i.v. 0.06 mmole P2S/kg, 0.01 mmole TMB-4/kg, or a mixture of the two oximes, containing 0.03 mmole/kg of the former and 0.01 mmole/kg of the latter.

The potency of different oximes, given i.v., for reversing Sarin-induced neuromuscular block in cats was of the order P-2-AM>P-4-AM>MINA≫pyridine-2-aldoxime, P-3-AM, DAM (WILLS 1959); no reversal could be demonstrated with the last three oximes when they were given in doses of 0.1, 0.02, and 0.3 mmole/kg, respectively.

III. Reactivation of phosphorylated AChE *in vivo*

1. Peripheral tissues and blood

In peripheral tissues and erythrocytes, reactivation of phosphorylated AChE can be detected frequently manometrically or by titration when oximes are given in doses which raise the LD_{50} of organophosphates and produce a reversal of symptoms of organophosphate poisoning (pages 953 to 956). This is illustrated further by the following observations. KARLOG (1958), NAMBA (1959a, b, d), and ROSSI and ROSSI (1960) found that reactivation of phosphorylated AChE took place in erythrocytes of rabbits when P-2-AM, 0.3 to 0.4 mmole/kg, was given i.v. after Parathion; the same was observed in dogs and horses with P-2-AM, 0.2 mmole/kg, i.p., and 0.08 mmole/kg, i.v., respectively (SVETLICIC and VANDEKAR 1960). NAMBA et al. (1959b, d) demonstrated reactivation of phosphorylated AChE in erythrocytes of rabbits when P-2-AM, 0.4 mmole/kg, i.v., was given after Methyl-Parathion, EPN, TEPP, Diazinon, Dipterex, or DFP, but not after Malathion; comparisons of the reactivating potencies of different oximes *in vivo* (NAMBA et al. 1959d) showed the general order P-2-AM>MINA>DAM. Reactivation by P-2-AM, 0.3 mmole/kg, s.c., of phosphorylated ChE in the blood of mice treated with Phospholine was demonstrated by LEHMAN et al. (1960), and MILOŠEVIĆ et al. (1961) observed that the AChE activity in the blood of mice injected simultaneously with Phosphamidon, s.c., and TMB-4, 0.056 mmole/kg, i.p., was higher than that of mice injected with Phosphamidon only. FLEISHER et al. (1960) found that 0.056 mmole TMB-4/kg, given i.v. after Sarin, reactivated the phosphonylated AChE in erythrocytes of rats.

The work of NAMBA et al. (1959c) showed that P-2-AM, 0.32 mmole/kg, i.v., and TMB-4, 0.09 mmole/kg, i.v., reactivated the phosphorylated AChE in striped muscle of mice injected previously with Methyl-Parathion or TEPP but failed to do so when given after EPN, Malathion, or Dipterex; at the dose level stated, only TMB-4 reactivated the phosphorylated AChE in striped muscle of mice injected previously with Diazinon. The same authors also measured changes in the ChE activity of liver and kidney which occurred concurrently with those in striped muscle and reported that the reactivating potencies *in vivo* of MINA, DAM, and pyridine-2-aldoxime dodecyl iodide (PAD) were less than those of P-2-AM and TMB-4.

All organophosphates referred to so far (under B, III, 1) form an initially reactivatable phosphorylated AChE and, as discussed previously, a failure to observe reactivation by the methods used does not exclude the existence of reactivation of phosphorylated functional AChE at strategic sites at a time when the oximes exert an antidotal action.

No reactivation, as shown previously, is obtained when oximes are given after OMPA which forms a non-reactivatable phosphorylated AChE, and this has been confirmed by NAMBA et al. (1959b, d).

2. Brain

In brain, reactivation is a function of the lipid solubility of the oxime, and with quaternary pyridine aldoximes it is at best small by comparison with that observed in peripheral tissues or blood (page 955). This is further illustrated by the following observations. FLEISHER et al. (1960) found no reactivation of phosphorylated AChE in the brain of rats when TMB-4, 0.056 mmole/kg, was given i.v. after Sarin, i.v.; the same applies to mice injected with Phosphamidon, s.c. (MILOŠEVIĆ et al. 1961). Reactivation of phosphorylated AChE in the brain of rats which were given an intracardiac injection of Sarin and 90 sec later an i.p. injection of an oxime was found to be a function of the lipid solubility and reactivating potency of the oxime; a high degree of reactivation was obtained with MINA, 0.4 mmole/kg, much less with DAM, 1.5 mmole/kg, and none with 0.2 to 0.4 mmole P-2-AM/kg (COHEN and WIERSINGA 1960). NAMBA et al. (1959c), on the other hand, reported that when P-2-AM, 0.32 mmole/kg, or TMB-4, 0.09 mmole/kg, was given i.v. after an organophosphate, reactivation of phosphorylated AChE in brain occurred when the organophosphate was TEPP or Parathion, but not when the organophosphate was Methyl-Parathion, EPN, Malathion, Dipterex, or Diazinon; in cases where reactivation occurred in brain it was less than that which took place in peripheral tissues.

SCHAUMAN (1960a) found that mice which were first injected with 0.4 mmole P-2-AM/kg, s.c., and later with Paraoxon or the organophosphate 217 AO, s.c., had a higher AChE activity of the brain than mice injected with the organophosphates only. As pointed out on page 956, such results might not be attributable entirely to reactivation of phosphorylated AChE. The same applies to the findings of METZ (1961) who observed that AChE activity in the pons and medulla of dogs injected intracysternally with a mixture of P-2-AM or P2S, 0.02 mmole, and TEPP was higher than that of dogs injected with TEPP only.

A more detailed analysis of the reactivation of phosphorylated-AChE was carried out by ROSENBERG (1960) who gave rabbits Paraoxon and $^1/_2$ to 2 hours later 0.4 to 1 mmole P-2-AM/kg, i.v. He found that P-2-AM reactivated the phosphorylated AChE in all parts of the brain but that reactivation in different areas was not uniform and could be presented in the order: area postrema > medulla > pons > cerebellar cortex > cerebellum. Provided that there are no species differences, one might conclude from the results obtained by ROSENBERG that some reactivation of phosphorylated AChE takes place always at areas which control respiration and circulation when P-2-AM is given in doses which produce an antidotal action, and that this reactivation, which might not be detectable in homogenates, would contribute significantly to the mechanism by which P-2-AM raises the LD_{50} of an organophosphate. Contrary to such an interpretation are two findings, firstly, atropine greatly enhances the antidotal action of quaternary pyridine aldoximes but not of MINA; secondly, WILLS and BORISON (1959) observed that quaternary pyridine aldoximes, given in doses up to 0.2 mmole/kg, did not reverse a Sarin-induced elevation of the threshold for electrical stimulation of centres for inspiration and expiration in cats. In view of this we must conclude that at present there is insufficient support for the interpretation that reactivation of phosphorylated AChE in the brain plays an important part in the antidotal action obtained with doses of quaternary pyridine aldoximes which can be given to man and which have been used most frequently in animal studies.

The AChE activity in the brain of atropinized mice could be reduced to less than 0.5% of normal without killing the animal if 0.2 mmole P-2-AM/kg and 10 mg atropine/kg were given i.p. before the administration of certain organophosphates (SCHAUMAN 1960b). This might explain, at least in part, why it is possible to obtain such remarkable degrees of protection against organophosphates as illustrated in Table 11.

C. Reactivation of phosphorylated AChE in isolated organs and tissue sections

FLEISHER et al. (1960) showed that the rate of reversal of DFP-induced neuromuscular block in the isolated diaphragm of the rat by TMB-4, 0.006 mM, was closely related to the rate of reactivation of functional phosphorylated AChE.

Benzoyl 2- and 4-aldoxime, but not P-2-AM, 0.01 M, restored electrical excitability abolished by Paraoxon in isolated frog sartorius muscle (HINTERBUCHNER and NACHMANSOHN 1960). The authors believed that reactivation of phosphorylated AChE by benzoyl 2- and 4-aldoxime and failure of P-2-AM to do so accounted for the results, but no experimental evidence in support of this conclusion was given.

Reactivation of diethyl- and di*iso*propyl-phosphoryl ChE and *iso*propyl methylphosphonyl-ChE and of the phosphorylated ChE formed by Tabun was demonstrated histochemically in striped muscle of rats by BERGNER (1959). In these experiments the muscle was excised up to 2 hours after the administration of an organophosphate and then incubated with 1 mM P-2-AM or TMB-4; the degree of reactivation obtained with the latter was greatly in excess of that obtained with P-2-AM.

D. Reactivation of phosphorylated BuChE and other esterases *in vivo*

Reactivation of phosphorylated BuChE in plasma of rabbits was obtained by injecting P-2-AM, 0.3 to 0.5 mmole/kg, i.v., or TMB-4, 0.09 mmole/kg, i.v., after Parathion (KARLOG 1958, ROSSI and ROSSI 1960, NAMBA et al. 1959a, b, d) and Methyl-Parathion, EPN, TEPP, and Malathion, but not after OMPA, Diazinon, Dipterex, or DFP (NAMBA et al. 1959b, d). In Parathion poisoning of horses, on the other hand, P-2-AM, 0.08 mmole/kg, i.v., failed to reactivate phosphorylated BuChE in plasma (SVETLICIC and VANDEKAR 1960).

Anaphylactic shock in rabbits can be prevented by injecting sensitized animals with DFP before the antigen is given. Normal anaphylactic shock was obtained when P-2-AM, 0.3 mmole/kg, i.v., was given between the injections of DFP and antigen (LECOMTE and SCHOFFENIELS 1961). This indicates that an esterase plays an essential part in the sequence of reactions which follow the injection of antigen in sensitized animals.

Reactivation of phosphorylated BuChE in brain, spinal cord, and sciatic nerve of chickens was obtained when pyridine-2-aldoxime dodecyl iodide (PAD) was given i.m. in doses of 0.25 mmole/kg 6 and 10 hr, and then once daily for 6 days after the oral administration of a demyelinating dose of tri-*o*-cresylphosphate (HENSCHLER 1959). At the same time, the severity of symptoms was reduced and their onset retarded. There is overwhelming evidence for a lack of a causal relation between phosphorylation of BuChE in the central nervous system and demyelination (DAVISON 1953), and the antidotal activity of the oxime, which has a broad spectrum of actions *(vide infra)*, is hardly attributable to the observed reactivation of phosphorylated BuChE.

E. Specificity of the antidotal action of oximes against organophosphates

The evidence discussed previously (pages 957 to 961) showed that reactivation of phosphorylated AChE plays a vital part in the antidotal action of P-2-AM (and other salts of N-methyl pyridine-2-aldoxime), *bis*-quaternary pyridine aldoximes, and MINA, and that other actions of the oximes which themselves, i.e., in the absence of reactivation, would raise the LD_{50} of organophosphates only to a small extent or fail to affect it, might enable the oximes to give a considerably higher degree of protection against lethal organophosphate poisoning than would be obtained without them. In the case of DAM, however, reactivation of phosphorylated AChE usually plays only a subordinate part in the antidotal action. The following new information on the specificity of the actions of oximes supports these conclusions.

COHEN and WIERSINGA (1960) compared the levels of ChE activity in the brain of rats which were given P-2-AM, MINA, or DAM, i.v., after an intracardiac injection of Sarin. Their results showed that DAM very effectively protected the ChE in brain from phosphonylation and produced only a small degree of reactivation, whereas the reverse was the case with MINA, and P-2-AM lacked both actions.

N,N'-Trimethylene*bis*(pyridine-4-aldoxime bromide), P-2-AM, and DAM, 0.01 M, had no effect *in vitro* on the activity of the fluorophosphatase which hydrolyses DFP, or on the activating effect of Mn^{++} or Co^{++} ions on this enzyme (EDERY and SCHATZBERG-PORATH 1961).

In concentrations used to obtain an antidotal action, DAM protected rats from lethal convulsions induced by pentylenetetrazol (4 mmole DAM/kg, i.p.; GABOUREL 1961), reduced the motility of cilia of the isolated frog oesophagus (1 mM DAM; RAJAPURKAR and PANJWANI 1961), and in cats depressed respiration and the response of striped muscle to direct and indirect stimulation (0.5 mmole DAM/kg, i.v.; WISLICKI 1960). WISLICKI also made the following observations. The effect of DAM on the excitability of striped muscle was reversed by neostigmine, and the respiratory depression caused by DAM was associated with a reduction of spontaneous centrifugal impulses in the phrenic nerve. Pyridine-2-aldoxime methiodide, 0.04 mmole/kg, i.v., on the other hand, had no effect on the response of striped muscle to direct or indirect stimulation and increased the respiratory volume without affecting the respiratory rate; in larger doses P-2-AM also depressed respiration. Neuromuscular block produced in cats by d-tubocurarine was reversed by P-2-AM, 0.05 mmole/kg and higher, i.v., whereas the reverse applied to neuromuscular block produced by depolarizing dugs.

ERDMANN and HEYE (1958) showed, that on the isolated rabbit intestine, P-2-AM, 0.23 mM, rapidly reversed the increase in tone of longitudinal muscle produced by Parathion, Paraoxon, or Systox; this effect was not maintained when the bath fluid was changed shortly after addition of the oxime, and was attributed to an anti-ACh action of the oxime. In the absence of organophosphates, P-2-AM, 0.15 mM, enhanced the spontaneous activity of the isolated rabbit intestine, and in large concentrations, 3.8 mM, it reduced it. Nicotinehydroxamic acid methiodide in concentrations comparable to those of P-2-AM had the same actions. Since nicotinehydroxamic acid methiodide and P-2-AM have a comparable anti-ACh activity, and the antidotal activity of P-2-AM is much higher than that of the hydroxamic acid, it is very unlikely that in the absence of reactivation the anti-ACh action of P-2-AM would raise the LD_{50} of organophosphates. An atropine-like property of quaternary pyridine aldoximes was confirmed by LINDGREN and SUNDWALL (1960) who showed that in the cat TMB-4, 0.056 mmole/kg, i.v., blocked vagal impulses to the heart and small intestine. Pyridine-2-aldoxime methiodide had the same action, but its potency was only approximately 1/8 of that of TMB-4, whereas DAM in doses up to 0.5 mmole/kg lacked such an action. The quaternary pyridine aldoximes had no or only very little effect on ganglionic transmission.

COLEMAN et al. (1960) showed that in Sarin poisoned rats the antidotal action of MINA or DAM in combination with P2S and atropine was much greater than that attributable to an additive action of the oximes when the oximes were given orally and atropine i.p. Under the same conditions, P2S had little antidotal action on its own, enhanced the antidotal action of MINA and DAM in mice only slightly, and failed to increase the antidotal action of *bis*-quaternary pyridine aldoximes in Sarin poisoning of rats and mice. The authors concluded from these results that the action of P2S under the experimental conditions was not attributable to reactivation of phosphorylated AChE.

Mono- and *bis*-quaternary pyridine aldoximes, when used in concentrations of 0.001 or 0.01 mM, are bound to solubilized "receptor" proteins which have a high affinity for ACh or d-tubocurarine or both (EHRENPREIS 1960, EHRENPREIS and FISHMAN 1960, EHRENPREIS and KELLOCK 1960). Such high concentrations of the oximes are never reached *in vivo*, and the findings of EHRENPREIS and his coworkers, therefore, throw no light on the mode(s) of action of oximes in organophosphate poisoning.

The *specificity of the antidotal action of pyridine-2-aldoxime dodecyl iodide* (PAD) has become very doubtful since it has a variety of actions in concentrations which are required for reactivation and in lower concentrations. The oxime, 0.1 μM and 1 μM, increased and decreased, respectively, the amplitude and duration of the spike potential at the Ranvier nodes in frog sciatic nerves (DETTBARN 1960), and at 0.01 to 0.1 mM it depolarized these sites (DETTBARN 1959). The last mentioned effect is attributable probably to an action on cell metabolism, since 0.1 mM PAD inhibited microsomal ATP-ase and its activation by Na$^+$ ions (JÄRNEFELT 1961).

F. Distribution, excretion, and metabolism of oximes

The concentration of P-2-AM in brain, kidney, striped muscle, liver, lung, heart, spleen, stomach, intestine, bile, serum, urine, and gastric and intestinal contents of rabbits was measured at $^1/_2$, 2, and 5 hr after the oral or i.v. administration of 0.28 mmole P-2-AM/kg by NAMBA et al. (1959a). Similar peak concentrations were obtained in most tissues with both routes of administration. Some of the results of NAMBA et al. are rather puzzling, e.g., after i.v. injection the concentration of P-2-AM increased over a period of 2 hr in all organs other than the kidneys; furthermore, at 2 hr the concentration of P-2-AM in brain was similar to that in peripheral organs, and continued to increase throughout a period of 5 hr; finally, 2 hr after oral administration the brain level was much higher than 2 hr after i.v. administration. In view of these results, the specificity of the method used for measuring P-2-AM and the significance of the findings are doubtful.

SUNDWALL (1960) recorded the concentration of P2S in plasma and urine after oral, i.v., or i.m. administration of the oxime to man. He used a UV-absorption method for measuring P2S and showed that the method gives reproducible results and does not measure metabolites of P2S. According to SUNDWALL, the half-life of P2S in plasma is less than 30 min when P2S, 0.08 mmole/kg, is given i.v. After i.m. administration of 0.12 mmole/kg, a maximum plasma level of 0.06 mM (mean of several experiments) was obtained at 15 min, after which time the concentration in plasma declined gradually; one hour after administration of the oxime the plasma levels were the same for both the i.v. and i.m. route of administration. After oral administration of P2S, 0.02 mmole/kg in gelatin capsules, a maximum plasma concentration of approximately 0.02 mM was reached within 30 to 90 min and maintained over 4 hr. SUNDWALL concluded that concentrations required for an antidotal action against organophosphates are reached with the doses given i.v. or i.m., but not orally. Under the experimental conditions 23% of the administered dose appeared in urine within 4 hours. Results in dogs were similar to those in man, and in the former it could be demonstrated that P2S is absorbed from the proximal jejunum and duodenum but not from the stomach (SUNDWALL and ELVIN 1960).

The major pathway for the degradation of P-2-AM in aqueous solutions at pH 7 to 13 is, according to ELLIN (1958), P-2-AM → 2-cyanopyridine methiodide → 2-hydroxypyridine methiodide → N-methylpyridone. Pyridine-2-aldoxime methiodide and its degradation products can be separated paper-chromatographically by using as solvent butanol: acetic acid: water (5:1:3), water-saturated butanol, or a water-saturated mixture of acetic acid (4 ml) and butanol (100 ml) (ELLIN and EASTERDAY 1961).

In vivo studies of the metabolism of P2S by ENANDER et al. (1961a, b) showed that rats which were given P2S, 0.12 mmole/kg, i.m., or 0.4 mmole, orally, and man treated with P2S, 13 mmole, orally, excreted thiocyanate in the urine, because the oxime was converted into cyanopyridine methyl methanesulphonate which in turn yielded cyanide and a metabolite which has not yet been identified. Cyanide is rapidly converted into inorganic thiocyanate which is excreted in urine. Only 3 to 4% and 0.4% of the administered dose of the oxime was converted into cyanide in rat and man, respectively, and thus the toxicity of P2S is not attributable to the formation of cyanide. Cyanopyridine methyl methanesulphonate, however, is slightly more toxic than P2S.

G. Toxicity of oximes

The toxicity of the chloride equivalents of P-2-AM and TMB-4, given singly or as a mixture, was investigated in mice and rabbits (O'LEARY et al. 1961), and it was concluded that the chlorides should be used in preference to the other halides for several reasons. Firstly, the chlorides have a slightly lower toxicity than the iodides and bromides when comparisons are made on a molar basis. Secondly, oximes have to be given in relatively large doses in order to produce an antidotal action against organophosphates, and the iodide and bromide anions of the oximes have undesirable actions on their own. Finally, the solubility of the chloride equivalent of P-2-AM is considerably greater than that of the iodide.

H. Therapeutic action of P-2-AM in organophosphate poisoning of man

Several reports of the beneficial effect of P-2-AM in organophosphate poisoning of man have been published recently. They concern the antidotal action of P-2-AM in Parathion poisoning (NAMBA et al. 1959a, ERDMANN 1960, SCHUCHTER et al. 1960, JACOBZINER and RAYBIN 1961) and in poisoning with EPN (NAMBA et al. 1959a). The use of the P-2-AM in combination with atropine is now generally recommended for the treatment of organophosphate poisoning in man. Pralidoxime iodide has become the official name (B.P.) of P-2-AM.

WILLS (1959) reported the side effects of P-2-AM, TMB-4, and DAM in man. The experiments with TMB-4, 0.043 mmole/kg, i.v., were carried out on hemiplegic subjects, and profound hypotension and temporary anuria were observed. It is possible that for this reason the oxime has not yet been tried in the treatment of organophosphate poisoning of man. In healthy man, however, TMB-4 does not seem to produce anuria (WILLS, personal communication); as far as its hypotensive action is concerned, it shares this property with P-2-AM but is a more potent hypotensive agent than the latter.

I. Oximes which possess reactivating properties together with marked atropine-like properties

In view of the high antidotal activity (against organophosphates) obtained with combinations of atropine and some oximes it should be of interest to study the antidotal activity of oximes which possess reactivating properties together with marked atropine-like properties. Two oximes which have a relationship to atropine have so far been synthesized. These oximes are:

Oxime 1   Oxime 2   Atropine

Oxime 1 was synthesized by TAMMELIN and FLORMARK (1961) but nothing is known about its reactivating and antidotal potency. Oxime 2 was synthesized by HOBBIGER and SADLER (unpublished) and found to have, at pH 7.45, 1% of the reactivating potency of P-2-AM; in a dose of 0.1 mmole/kg, i.p., the oxime failed to protect mice against death from 2 LD_{50}'s of TEPP, s.c.

Future work will be necessary to show whether it is possible to obtain an oxime which when given alone has an antidotal activity comparable to that obtained with a combination of atropine and an oxime.

Literature

Applicable to the Addendum only and not listed previously

ASKNES, G.: Nucleophilic displacements on phosphorus. Reaction of hydroxyl ion and *iso*-nitroso acetone with organofluorophosphorus compounds. Acta chem. scand. 14, 1515—1525 (1960).

BERGNER, A. D.: Histochemical detection of fatal anticholinesterase poisoning. II. Reactivation of cholinesterase in cadavers of rats. Amer. J. Path. 35, 807—817 (1959).

CASIDA, J. E., K. B. AUGUSTINSSON and G. JONSSON: Stability, toxicity and reaction mechanism with esterases of certain carbamate insecticides. J. econ. Ent. **53**, 205—212 (1960).

COHEN, E. M., and H. WIERSINGA: Oximes in the treatment of nerve gas poisoning. II. Acta physiol. pharmacol. neerl. **9**, 276—302 (1960).

COLEMAN, I. W., P. E. LITTLE and G. A. GRANT: Oxime mixtures and atropine in the protection of mice and rats from Sarin poisoning. Canad. J. Biochem. **38**, 1035—1043 (1960).

— — — Oral prophylaxis for anticholinesterase poisoning. Canad. J. Biochem. **39**, 351—363 (1961).

DAVISON, A. N.: Some observations on the cholinesterases of the central nervous system after the administration of organophosphorus compounds. Brit. J. Pharmacol. **8**, 212—216 (1953).

DETTBARN, W. D.: Action of lipid-soluble quaternary ammonium ions on the resting potential of myelinated nerve fibres of the frog. Biochim. biophys. Acta **32**, 381—386 (1959).

— New evidence for the role of acetylcholine in conduction. Biochim. biophys. Acta **41**, 377—386 (1960).

DOTY, P., A. M. HOLTZER, J. H. BRADBURY and E. R. BLOUT: Polypeptides. II. The configuration of polymers of γ-benzyl-L-glutamate in solution. J. Amer. chem. Soc. **76**, 4493—4494 (1954).

EDERY, H., and G. SCHATZBERG-PORATH: Phosphorylphosphatase and oximes. Brit. J. Pharmacol. **17**, 276—277 (1961).

EHRENPREIS, S.: Isolation and identification of the acetylcholine receptor protein of electric tissue. Biochim. biophys. Acta **44**, 561—577 (1960).

—, and M. M. FISHMAN: The interaction of quaternary ammonium compounds with chondroitin sulfate. Biochim. biophys. Acta **44**, 577—585 (1960).

—, and M. G. KELLOCK: The interaction of quaternary ammonium compounds with hyaluronic acid. Biochim. biophys. Acta **45**, 525—528 (1960).

ELLIN, R. I.: Stability of pyridine-2-aldoxime methiodide. I. Mechanism of breakdown in aqueous alkaline solution. J. Amer. chem. Soc. **80**, 6588—6590 (1958).

—, and D. E. EASTERDAY: Chromatographie separation of the degradation products of pralidoxime iodide (pyridine-2-aldoxime methiodide). J. Pharm. (Lond.) **13**, 370—373 (1961).

ENANDER, I., A. SUNDWALL and B. SÖRBO: Metabolic studies on N-methylpyridinium-2-aldoxime. I. The conversion to thiocyanate. Biochem. Pharmacol. **7**, 226—231 (1961a).

— — — Metabolic studies on N-methylpyridinium-2-aldoxime. II. The conversion to N-methylpyridinium-2-nitrile. Biochem. Pharmacol. **7**, 232—236 (1961b).

ERDMANN, W. D.: Klinische Erfahrungen mit dem Antidot Pyridine-2-aldoxime-methyljodid (PAM) bei E 605-Vergiftungen. Ausgewählte Kasuistik. Dtsch. med. Wschr. **85**, 1014 bis 1016 (1960).

—, u. D. HEYE: Analyse der erregenden und lähmenden Wirkung von Alkylphosphaten (Parathion, Paraoxon, Systox) am isolierten Kaninchendarm. Naunyn-Schmiedeberg's Arch. exp. Path. Pharmak. **232**, 507—521 (1958).

FLEISHER, J. H., J. HANSA, P. J. KILLOS and C. S. HARRISON: Effects of 1,1'-trimethylene bis(4-formylpyridinium bromide) dioxime (TMB-4) on cholinesterase activity and neuromuscular block following poisoning with Sarin and DFP. J. Pharmacol. exp. Ther. **130**, 461—468 (1960).

GABOUREL, J. D.: Anticonvulsant properties of diacetylmonoxime (DAM). Biochem. Pharmacol. **5**, 283—286 (1961).

GILBERT, G., T. WAGNER-JAUREGG and G. M. STEINBERG: Hydroxamic acids: relationship between structure and ability to reactivate phosphonate-inhibited acetylcholinesterase. Arch. Biochem. **93**, 469—475 (1961).

HENSCHLER, D.: Antidotische Wirkung von Pyridin-2-aldoximdodecyljodid bei der Trikresylphosphatlähmung. Naunyn-Schmiedeberg's Arch. exp. Path. Pharmak. **236**, 503—509 (1959).

HINTERBUCHNER, L. P., and D. NACHMANSOHN: Electrical activity evoked by a specific chemical reaction. Biochim. biophys. Acta **44**, 554—560 (1960).

HOBBIGER, F.: Anticholinesterases. The *in vitro* inhibition of cholinesterases by physostigmine, neostigmine and other related (non-phosphorus) compounds. Chem. and Ind. **1954**, 415 to 418.

JACOBZINER, H., and H. W. RAYBIN: Parathion poisoning successfully treated with 2-PAM (pralidoxime chloride). New Engl. J. Med. **265**, 436—437 (1961).

JÄRNEFELT, J.: Mechanism of sodium transport in cellular membranes. Nature (Lond.) **190**, 694—697 (1961).

JAQUES, R., and H. J. BEIN: Toxikologie und Pharmakologie eines neuen systemisch wirksamen Insektizids der Phosphorsäureester-Reihe, Phosphamidon (2-Chlor-diäthylcarbamoyl-1-methylvinyldimethylphosphat). Arch. Toxikol. **18**, 316—330 (1960).

KARLOG, O.: Reactivators of cholinesterase. Arch. Pharm. Chemi. **65**, 467—475 (1958) (in Swedish with English summary).

KEWITZ, H., u. V. NEUHOFF: Herstellung eines Trockenpräparates alkylphosphatvergifteter Acetylcholinesterase für Reaktivierungsversuche. Naunyn-Schmiedeberg's Arch. exp. Path. Pharmak. **240**, 126—133 (1960).

LATKI, O., u. W. D. ERDMANN: Hemmung und Reaktivierung von Cholinesterasen nach der Vergiftung mit Paraoxon und DFP in vitro. Naunyn-Schmiedeberg's Arch. exp. Path. Pharmak. **240**, 514—522 (1961).

LECOMTE, J., and E. SCHOFFENIELS: Action du 2-PAM et des inhibiteurs de l'acetylcholinesterase sur le choc anaphalactique du lapin. Biochem. Pharmacol. **5**, 305—310 (1961).

LEHMAN, R. A., and M. E. NICHOLLS: Antagonism of phospholine (echothiophate) iodide by certain quaternary oximes. Proc. Soc. exp. Biol. (N. Y.) **104**, 550—554 (1960).

— H. M. FITCH, L. P. BLOCH, H. A. JEWELL and M. E. NICHOLLS: Antidotes and potentiating agents for phospholine iodide. J. Pharmacol. exp. Ther. **128**, 307—317 (1960).

LINDGREN, P., and A. SUNDWALL: Parasympatholytic effects of TMB-4 (1,1-trimethylene-bis(4-formylpyridinium bromide)-dioxime) and some related oximes in the cat. Acta Pharmacol. (Kbh.) **17**, 69—83 (1960).

METZ, B.: The brain ACh-AChE-ChA system in respiratory control. Neurology **11**, 37—45 (1961).

MILOŠEVIĆ, M., V. VOJVODIĆ and V. MILOŠEVIĆ: The action of N,N'-trimethylenebs(4-hydroxy-iminomethyl-pyridinium bromide) (TMB-4) on acute lethal anticholinesterase poisoning in mice. Arh. hig. rada **10**, 213—216 (1959).

— M. TERZIĆ and V. VOJVODIĆ: Protection against lethal phosphamidone poisoning by N,N'-trimethylenebis(4-hydroxyiminomethyl-pyridinium bromide) (TMB-4). Arch. int. Pharmacodyn. **132**, 180—188 (1961).

MYERS, D. K., A. KEMP jun., J. W. TOL and M. H. T. DE JONGE: Studies on aliesterases. 6. Selective inhibitors of the aliesterases of brain and saprophytic mycobacteria. Biochem. J. **65**, 232—241 (1957).

NAMBA, T., Y. TANIGUCHI, S. OKAZAKI, Y. UEMATSU, H. NAGAMATSU, T. WAKIMOTO, S. HAMA and H. NISHISHITA: Use of large doses of PAM in severe alkylphosphate poisoning. Naika no Ryôiki **7**, 709—713 (1959a) (in Japanese).

— Y. UEMATSU, Y. TANIGUCHI, S. OKAZAKI, H. NAGAMATSU and T. WAKIMOTO: Use of PAM in poisoning due to various alkylphosphates, with special reference to EPN poisoning. Naika no Ryôiki **7**, 714—720 (1959b) (in Japanese).

— S. OKAZAKI, Y. TANIGUCHI, Y. UEMATSU, N. NAGAMATSU and T. WAKIMOTO: Inhibition of tissue cholinesterase by alkylphosphates and its reactivation by oximes. Naika no Ryôiki **7**, 680—683 (1959c) (in Japanese).

— Y. UEMATSU, S. OKAZAKI, Y. TANIGUCHI, H. NAGAMATSU and T. WAKIMOTO: Effectiveness of oximes against poisoning by alkylphosphates. Naika no Ryôiki **7**, 684—690 (1959d) (in Japanese).

NEUBERT, D., J. SCHAEFER u. H. KEWITZ: Reaktivierung der Acetylcholinesterase durch körpereigene Stoffe. Naturwissenschaften **12**, 290 (1958).

NEUHOFF, V., u. H. KEWITZ: Reinigung eines endogenen Reaktivators der alkylphosphorylierten Cholinesterase. Naunyn-Schmiedeberg's Arch. exp. Path. Pharmak. **241**, 548—549 (1961a).

NEUHOFF, L. V., and H. KEWITZ: Reactivation of alkylphosphorylated cholinesterase by a constituent of liver. Biochem. Pharmacol. **8**, 118 (1961b).

O'LEARY, J. F., A. M. KUNKEL and A. H. JONES: Efficacy and limitations of oxime-atropine treatment of organophosphorus anticholinesterase poisoning. J. Pharmacol. exp. Ther. **132**, 50—57 (1961).

POZIOMEK, E. J., D. N. KRAMER, B. W. FROMM and W. A. MOSHER: Observations on the geometrical isomerism of formyl-1-methylpyridinium iodide oximes; carbinolamine intermediates. J. org. Chem. **26**, 423—427 (1961a).

— — W. A. MOSHER and H. O. MICHEL: Configurational analysis of 4-formyl-1-methyl-pyridinium iodide oximes and its relationship to a molecular complimentarity theory on the reactivation of inhibited acetylcholinesterase. J. Amer. chem. Soc. **83**, 3916—3917 (1961b).

RAJAPURKAR, M. V., and M. H. PANJWANI: Action of diacetylmonoxime (DAM) on ciliary activity. Arch. int. Pharmacodyn. **131**, 107—115 (1961).

ROSENBERG, P.: In vivo reactivation by PAM of brain cholinesterase inhibited by paraoxon. Biochem. Pharmacol. **3**, 212—219 (1960).

ROSSI, L., and A. ROSSI: Therapeutic effect of pyridine-2-aldoxime methiodide (PAM) in experimental Parathion poisoning. Boll. Soc. ital. Biol. sper. **36**, 1230—1233 (1960) (in Italian).

SADLER, P. W.: Spectroscopic studies of quaternary aldoximes and ketoximes. J. chem. Soc. 1961, 2162—2165.

SANDERSON, D. M.: Treatment of poisoning by anticholinesterase insecticides in the rat. J. Pharm. (Lond.) 13, 435—442 (1961).

SCAIFE, J. F.: Protection of human red cell cholinesterase against inhibition by Tabun and 0,0-diethyl-S-2-diethylaminoethyl phosphorothiolate. Canad. J. Biochem. 38, 301—303 (1960).

SCHAUMANN, W.: Beziehungen zwischen den peripheren und zentralen Wirkungen von Cholinesterase-Hemmern und der Inaktivierung der Cholinesterase. Naunyn-Schmiedeberg's Arch. exp. Path. Pharmak. 239, 96—113 (1960a).

— Maximal inhibition of cholinesterase in the central nervous system. Brit. J. Pharmacol. 15, 432—435 (1960b).

SCHUCHTER, A., H. G. KAWEL u. J. SCHNEIDER: Kombinierte Behandlung einer Vergiftung durch Diäthyl-p-nitrophenylthiophosphat mit Pyridin-aldoxim-(2)-methojodid und Atropin. Arzneimittel-Forsch. 10, 399—400 (1960).

STENGER, E. G.: Beitrag zur Antidotwirkung des Pyridin-2-aldoxim-N-methyljodid (PAM). Med. exp. 3, 143—149 (1960).

STERN, P., and B. BOŠKOVIĆ: Contribution to the treatment of poisoning by diisopropyl fluorophosphate. Voj. San. Pregled 17, 792—794 (1960a) (in Serbo-Croat).

— — Contribution to the treatment of Tabun poisoning. Voj. San. Pregled 17, 1008—1011 (1960b) (in Serbo-Croat).

SUNDWALL, A.: Plasma concentration curves of N-methylpyridinium-2-aldoxime methane sulphonate (P2S) after intravenous, intramuscular and oral administration in man. Biochem. Pharmacol. 5, 225—230 (1960).

—, and C. E. ELWIN: Absorption studies on N-methylpyridinium-2-aldoxime methanesulphonate (P2S) in dog and man. Acta physiol. scand. 50, 146—147 (1960).

SVETLICIC, B., and M. VANDEKAR: Therapeutic effect of pyridine-2-aldoxime methiodide in Parathion poisoned mammals. J. comp. Path. 70, 257—271 (1960).

SWIDLER, R., R. E. PLAPINGER and G. M. STEINBERG: The kinetics of the reaction of isopropyl methylphosphonofluoridate (Sarin) with substituted benzohydroxamic acids. II. J. Amer. chem. Soc. 81, 3271—3274 (1959).

TAMMELIN, L. E., and A. FLORMARK: Synthesis of an oxime analogue to atropin. Acta chem. scand. 15, 1207—1208 (1961).

WILLS, J. H.: Recent studies of organic phosphate poisoning. Fed. Proc. 18, 1020—1025 (1959).

—, and H. L. BORISON: Modification by Sarin and antagonists of medullary respiratory activities. Fed. Proc. 18, 102 (1959).

WILSON, I. B., M. A. HATCH and S. GINSBURG: Carbamylation of acetylcholinesterase. J. biol. Chem. 235, 2312—2315 (1960).

— M. A. HARRISON and S. GINSBURG: Carbamyl derivatives of acetylcholinesterase. J. biol. Chem. 236, 1498—1500 (1961).

WISLICKI, L.: Differences in the effect of oximes on striated muscle and respiratory centre. Arch. int. Pharmacodyn. 129, 1—17 (1960).

Chapter 22

Anticholinesterase Intoxication in Man and its Treatment

By

DAVID GROB

With 6 Figures

Contents

A. Anticholinesterase (anti-ChE) compounds that have produced intoxication in man

I. Organophosphorus anti-ChE compounds

Intoxication has resulted from absorption of toxic amounts of organophosphorus anticholinesterase (anti-ChE) compounds during preparation or use as insecticides or chemical warfare agents, or as pharmaceutical agents.

1. Insecticides

Parathion, Malathion, EPN, Phosdrin, Mipafox, TEPP, and OMPA (Table 1) have been used widely as agricultural insecticides and their indiscriminate dispersal has resulted in a number of instances of poisoning, some of them fatal (GROB et al. 1949, 1950a, b; FAUST 1949; MILLES and SALT 1950; GROB 1950a, b; BARNES 1953; HAMBLIN and GOLZ 1955; KLIMMER 1957; ERDMANN and LENDLE 1958; FREDERIKSSON 1958). Until recently Parathion was the most widely used of the organophosphorus insecticides, and most intoxications, including

6,000 in Japan alone, have been caused by this compound. In recent years there has been increasing use of Malathion, which is less toxic to mammals, but has produced poisoning after ingestion (SNYDER 1956, WALTERS 1957, GOLDMAN and TEITEL 1958).

The organophosphorus insecticides may be marketed as concentrated liquids, which are diluted prior to use, or they may be adsorbed on attapulgus or Bentonite clay to form wettable powders containing 15 to 25% of the active ester (THOMPSON 1955; METCALF 1955, 1957; KOSOLAPOFF 1959). These may be blended with inert material to a concentration of 1 to 2%, or diluted with water for use as aqueous sprays. Methods of applying dusts and sprays include mechanical spraying from tractors, hand spraying, and dusting from airplanes. Aerosols or smoke cannisters containing insecticide have also been used in greenhouses. Poisoning has occurred during the production, packaging, or handling of any of these compounds by chemists,

Table 1. *Organophosphorus anti-ChE agents that have produced intoxication in man*
(see Chapter 9 for structural formulae)

General formula:
$$\begin{array}{c} R_1 \quad\; O \\ \diagdown P \diagup \\ \diagup \quad \diagdown \\ R_2 \qquad X \end{array}$$

Symbol or common name	Chemical name
A. *Compounds where X = halogen or CN*	
Sarin (GB)	*Iso*propyl methyphosphonofluoridate
DFP	Di*iso*propyl phosphorofluoridate
Tabun (GA).	Ethyl-N-dimethyl phosphoramidocyanidate
Mipafox (Isopestox)	N,N'-Di*iso*propylphosphorodiamidic fluoride
B. *Compounds where X = alkyl, alkoxy or aryloxy*	
Phosdrin	Dimethyl 1-methyl-2-carbomethoxyvinyl phosphate
Paraoxon	Diethyl 4-nitrophenyl phosphate
C. *Thiol- and thionophosphorus compounds*	
EPN	0-Ethyl 0-(4-nitrophenyl)phenylphosphono-thioate
Parathion.	0,0-Diethyl 0-(4-nitrophenyl)phosphorothioate
Malathion	0,0-Dimethyl S-(1,2-dicarbethoxyethyl) phosphorodithioate
D. *Derivatives of pyrophosphorus acid*	
TEPP	Tetraethyl pyrophosphate
OMPA	Octamethyl pyrophosphortetramide
E. *Compound containing a quaternary nitrogen*	
Phospholine (echothiophate).	0,0-Diethyl-S-2-trimethylammonium-ethyl phosphonothiolate iodide

formulators, packers, or men employed on maintenance in manufacturing plants. Poisoning has also occurred in agricultural workers, such as field sprayers, entomologists, dusting pilots, fruit pickers, and nurserymen. Some of the most serious intoxications have occurred following accidental exposure or ingestion, particularly by children, or ingestion with suicidal or homicidal intent (CONLEY 1953, CHAMBERLIN et al. 1953). Parathion is very slowly hydrolyzed in water at pH less than 10, 120 days being required for 50% hydrolysis at 25°. The volatility at 25° and 76 mm of mercury is also low, being 0.0025 mg/l of air. For these reasons, Parathion is very persistent and after it is sprayed in fields and orchards there is left a residue that declines in potency rapidly on most crops for the first few days and then more gradually over a period of weeks. Significant percutaneous absorption has occurred in workers engaged in irrigating, cultivating, thinning, or picking in fields or orchards sprayed one month before. Absorption is most likely to occur if protective clothing is not worn, or if contaminated clothing is worn persistently, particularly if there is considerable sweating. Elevated atmospheric temperature and humidity, which promote sweating, and light rain before exposure increase the likelihood of absorption (QUINBY et al. 1958).

2. Chemical warfare agents

The organophosphorus chemical warfare agents have been termed nerve gases because of their effects on the central nervous system. Sarin and Tabun are among the more important of these, and several instances of intoxication have occurred following exposure to these compounds (GROB 1956a, b, WILLS and BROWN 1957). Sarin and Tabun are colorless liquids which are volatile at ordinary temperatures. They may be dispersed as liquids, aerosols, or vapors. While they have a faint, sweetish odor, this is not sufficiently intense or distinctive to enable detection under field conditions.

3. Pharmaceutical agents

Dilute solutions of DFP, TEPP, and echothiophate (Phospholine) have been used locally in the management of glaucoma (MARR and GROB 1950, LEHMAN et al. 1960). DFP has been administered intramuscularly in doses of 1 to 2 mg in the management of paralytic ileus (GROB et al. 1947a, b). Dilute solutions of DFP, TEPP, HETP (hexaethyl tetraphosphate), OMPA, Sarin, and Phospholine have been administered orally or intramuscularly in clinical trials in the management of myasthenia gravis (HARVEY et al. 1947, RIDER et al. 1951, ARANOW et al. 1958, GROB 1958). Intoxication has occurred following inadvertent overdose with these compounds, or following absorption of concentrated material during manufacture or handling (MOORE 1956).

II. Quaternary ammonium anti-ChE compounds

These compounds are used mainly in the management of myasthenia gravis, and, to a lesser extent, of glaucoma and paralytic ileus. Drugs used in myasthenia gravis include neostigmine (Prostigmine), pyridostigmine (Mestinon) (OSSERMAN et al. 1954), and ambenomium (Mytelase) (SCHWAB et al. 1955). Clinical trials have also been carried out with *bis*-neostigmine (BC-40) (PATEISKY et al. 1955, 1957) and *bis*-pyridostigmine (Hexamarium, BC-51). Neostigmine and edrophonium (Tensilon) are also used in the diagnosis of myasthenia gravis. Fatal toxic reaction to neostigmine, while rare, has been reported in a non-myasthenic patient who received this drug without prior administration of atropine (MERRILL 1948). The effects of edrophonium are due not only to its transient anti-ChE action, but also to a direct cholinomimetic effect (GROB et al. 1956c). There is evidence that neostigmine may also have a direct cholinomimetic action on skeletal muscle in addition to its anti-ChE action (RIKER and WESCOE 1946). Neostigmine is also used in the management of paralytic ileus, and it has been employed, with equivocal results, in an attempt to relieve muscle spasticity in a variety of disorders, including poliomyelitis, upper motor neuron lesions, and rheumatoid arthritis.

III. Tertiary amine anti-ChE compounds

Physostigmine (eserine) is employed in the management of glaucoma by instillation into the conjunctival sac. It was at one time employed in the management of myasthenia gravis (WALKER 1934), but was replaced by neostigmine. Intoxication by physostigmine is now rarely encountered.

B. Properties and toxic doses of anti-ChE compounds

I. Anti-ChE activity

Human plasma cholinesterase (chiefly butyrocholinesterase, BuChE) is slightly less sensitive *in vitro and in vivo* to inhibition by Sarin than the cholinesterases (ChE's) (chiefly acetylcholinesterase, AChE) present in red blood cells, muscle, and brain, which are approximately equally sensitive (GROB 1950c, GROB and HARVEY 1958). Tetraethyl pyrophosphate, DFP, neostigmine, and Parathion, on the other hand, inhibit plasma BuChE more readily than the AChE's of red cells, brain, or muscle. Tabun inhibits these enzymes equally effectively. The inhibitory activity of Sarin against the AChE of the red cells, muscle, and brain is greater than that of the other well known anti-ChE compounds, being approximately 5 times that of Tabun, 10 times that of TEPP, 100 times that of DFP or neostigmine, and 4,000 times that of Parathion. Sarin, Tabun, and DFP combine with ChE's *in vitro* almost irreversibly during the first hour of their reaction. In contrast, the combination of TEPP or Parathion with ChE is slowly reversible, while the combination of neostigmine with the enzyme is readily reversible.

II. Lipoid solubility

Sarin, DFP, and Parathion are highly soluble in lipoid medium, while TEPP, OMPA, Phospholine, and neostigmine are only slightly soluble (GROB and HARVEY 1958); Tabun is intermediate. There is good correlation between lipoid solubility of these compounds and the degree of their effect on the central nervous system, the less soluble compounds having less central neural effect. This is presumably owing to their inability to cross the blood-brain barrier, as they are effective inhibitors of homogenized brain AChE *in vitro* (KOELLE and STEINER 1956, FREDRIKSSON 1957, 1958).

III. Routes of absorption and toxic and lethal doses

Most of the organophosphorus anti-ChE compounds are liquids, and many are volatile at ordinary temperatures. Most react slowly with water and rapidly with strong alkali, yielding products of hydrolysis which are either non-toxic or less toxic than the compounds themselves. When dispersed as a vapor, spray, or aerosol, or adsorbed on dust, most are readily absorbed through the respiratory tract or conjunctivae, while the liquid compounds or solutions may be absorbed through the conjunctivae, skin, or gastrointestinal tract. If the agent comes in contact with the eyes or respiratory tract, local effects on these tissues ensue. Local effects occur also in the skin and gastrointestinal tract. If absorption is sufficiently great, generalized systemic effects follow.

The commonest routes of absorption are the skin, respiratory tract, gastrointestinal tract, and, following exposure to liquid, the eyes. The respiratory tract is the most rapid and most complete of these routes of absorption. Penetration through the skin occurs more rapidly at elevated temperature and in the presence of superficial trauma to the skin (BLANK et al. 1957, GRIESEMER et al. 1958, FREDRIKSSON 1958). Some solvents, particularly amines, increase the rate of absorption through the skin. Elevated temperature not only increases percutaneous absorption, but may also increase inhalation of vapor and perhaps toxicity (BAETJER et al. 1956).

Table 2. *Comparison between the anti-ChE activity (against human red blood cell AChE) in vitro of Sarin and other organophosphorus anti-ChE compounds, and the effects in rats and man of the intramuscular (I.M.), intra-arterial (I.A.), and oral administration of these compounds* (from GROB and HARVEY 1958)

Relative anti-ChE activity *in vitro*	In rats LD$_{50}$ (mg/kg)		In man Dose (mg/kg) that produced 50% depression of RBC AChE		In man Dose (mg/kg) that produced moderate symptoms		Estimated lethal dose (mg/kg)	
	I. M.	oral	I. M. or I. A.	oral	I. M. or I. A.	oral	I. M.	oral
Sarin 1	0.17	0.6	0.003 (I.A.)	0.01	0.006 (I.A.)	0.028	0.03	0.14
Tabun 1/5	0.80	3.7						
TEPP 1/10	0.65	1.4	0.025 (I.M.)	0.10	0.083 (I.M.)	0.35	0.38	1.7
DFP 1/100	1.8	6	0.07 (I.M.)	0.28	0.083 (I.A.)	?0.32	0.48	2.1
Parathion 1/4,000	6	10						
Malathion		1375 (males) 1000 (females)				?150		?600

The estimated toxic and lethal doses of some organophosphorus anti-ChE compounds in man, and comparison with their anti-ChE activities *in vitro* and LD$_{50}$ values in rats, are recorded in Table 2. There is a relatively narrow margin between doses that produce mild and those which cause moderately severe symptoms. Thus, for Sarin, the most toxic of the compounds listed here, these doses are 0.02 and 0.03 mg/kg, orally, respectively. The least toxic is Malathion, which is less injurious to mammals than to insects, owing to rapid breakdown in the mammalian body (MARCH et al. 1956).

The quaternary ammonium anti-ChE compounds are, for the most part, nonvolatile solids of low lipoid solubility and therefore poorly absorbed through the skin. Exposure to these compounds is usually the result of oral, intramuscular, or intravenous administration for medicinal purposes, or the result of accidental ingestion. The toxic doses by these routes are of the same order of magnitude as those of many of the organophosphorus anti-ChE compounds, including DFP and Parathion, and some quaternary ammonium anti-ChE compounds have been synthesized which are toxic in much smaller doses (FUNKE et al. 1952). However, since the quaternary ammonium compounds are not absorbed through the skin and respiratory tract, and are seldom accidentally ingested, they rarely produce intoxication except when administered in overdose.

C. Manifestatations of anti-ChE intoxication in man (Table 3)

I. Mechanism of action

The acute actions of anti-ChE compounds are due mainly to their ability to inhibit or inactivate ChE's (KOELLE and GILMAN 1949, HOLMSTEDT 1959). Those organophosphorus compounds which are absorbed through the respiratory tract, conjunctivae, or skin produce local effects on these tissues. Anticholinesterase compounds absorbed through the gastrointestinal tract probably produce some local gastrointestinal symptoms. If absorption is sufficiently great by any route, generalized systemic effects result (GROB and HARVEY 1953, 1958).

The effects of inhibition of ChE's, whether local or systemic, are attributable to the accumulation in nervous tissue or effector organs of excessive concentrations of endogenous acetylcholine (ACh). This compound accumulates at the endings of the parasympathetic cholinergic nerves to the smooth muscle of the iris, ciliary body, bronchial tree, gastrointestinal tract, bladder, and blood vessels, to the secretory glands of the respiratory tract and to cardiac muscle, and of the cholinergic sympathetic nerves to the sweat glands and possibly blood vessels. The accumulation of ACh at these sites results in characteristic "muscarinic" signs and symptoms. The accumulation of ACh at the endings of motor nerves to voluntary muscle and in the autonomic ganglia results in "nicotinic" signs and symptoms, and accumulation in the central nervous system is believed to be responsible for the central effects. All anti-ChE compounds produce muscarinic and nicotinic effects. Organophosphorus compounds of high lipoid solubility, such as Sarin, Parathion, DFP, Malathion, EPN, Phosdrin, and Tabun also produce marked central neural effects, while those of low lipoid solubility, such as TEPP, OMPA, and Phospholine (JEWELL and LEHMAN 1958, SCHAUMANN et al. 1958), and the quaternary ammonium inhibitors, have less effect on the central nervous system.

The duration of symptoms depends in part on the rate of reversibility of the combination of anti-ChE compounds with the ChE's. Sarin and DFP produce practically irreversible inhibition of ChE's, so that restoration is dependent upon synthesis of new enzyme. Although there is no strict correlation between duration of symptoms and measurable restoration of ChE activity, the effects of Sarin and DFP are most prolonged, lasting from several hours to several days, depending upon the severity of the exposure. In contrast, neostigmine produces reversible inhibition of ChE's, and its duration of action is relatively short; i.e., two to four hours. Parathion, TEPP, and OMPA produce partially reversible inhibition of ChE, and the duration of action of these compounds is intermediate between that of the other two groups (GROB and HARVEY 1949, GROB et al. 1950, DUBOIS et al. 1950, GROB and HARVEY 1958).

II. Local effects

Within a few minutes after local exposure to an organophosphorus anti-ChE compound in the form of a vapor, dust, or aerosol there appear local effects on

Table 3. *Signs and symptoms of anti-ChE intoxication*

Site of action	Signs and symptoms
	Following Local Exposure
Muscarinic	
Pupils	Miosis, marked, usually maximal (pin-point), sometimes unequal
Ciliary body	Frontal headache; eye pain on focusing; slight dimness of vision; occasional nausea and vomiting
Conjunctivae.	Hyperemia
Nasal mucous membranes	Rhinorrhea; hyperemia
Bronchial tree	Tightness in chest, sometimes with prolonged, wheezing expiration suggestive of bronchoconstriction or increased secretion; cough
Sweat glands.	Sweating at site of exposure to liquid
Nicotinic	
Striated muscle.	Fasciculation at site of exposure to liquid
	Following Systemic Absorption
Muscarinic	
Bronchial tree	Tightness in chest, with prolonged, wheezing expiration suggestive of bronchoconstriction or increased secretion; dyspnea; slight pain in chest; increased bronchial secretion; cough; pulmonary edema; cyanosis
Gastrointestinal	Anorexia; nausea; vomiting; abdominal cramps; epigastric and substernal tightness (? cardiospasm) with "heartburn" and eructation; diarrhea; tenesmus; involuntary defecation
Sweat glands.	Increased sweating
Salivary glands.	Increased salivation
Lacrimal glands	Increased lacrimation
Heart	Slight bradycardia
Pupils.	Slight miosis, occasionally unequal; later, more marked miosis
Ciliary body	Blurring of vision
Bladder	Frequency; involuntary micturition
Nicotinic	
Striated muscle.	Easy fatigue; mild weakness; muscular twitching; fasciculation; cramps; generalized weakness, including muscles of respiration, with dyspnea and cyanosis
Sympathetic ganglia . .	Pallor; occasional elevation of blood pressure
Central nervous system . . .	Giddiness; tension; anxiety; jitteriness; restlessness; emotional lability; excessive dreaming; insomnia; nightmares; headache; tremor; apathy; withdrawal and depression; bursts of slow waves of elevated voltage in EEG, especially on overventilation; drowsiness; difficulty in concentrating; slowness of recall; confusion; slurred speech; ataxia; generalized weakness; coma, with absence of reflexes; Cheyne-Stokes respiration; convulsions; depression of respiratory and circulatory centers, with dyspnea, cyanosis, and fall in blood pressure

the smooth muscle of the eye and respiratory tract and on the secretory glands of the latter. Liquid splash may also affect the eyes. The earliest of the *ocular effects* is pupillary constriction.

This is an invariable sign of ocular exposure to a concentration of vapor sufficient to produce symptoms, and it is also the last ocular manifestation to disappear. The two eyes may or may not be equally affected. The conjunctival instillation of 0.3 μg of Sarin produces within ten minutes local miosis which is marked but not quite maximal, and which diminishes gradually over a period of 60 hours (GROB and HARVEY 1958). Three times this amount produces maximal miosis which disappears over a period of 90 hours, and which is accompanied by symptoms of "pressure" in the eye, conjunctival hyperemia, increase or even spasm of accomodation, and dimness of vision, especially in the peripheral fields and in dim or artificial light. The miosis may result in a decrease in light perception, but there is no inability to judge distance unless there is unilateral miosis (UPHOLT 1956). The latter may be of particular difficulty to pilots applying insecticides from aircraft.

The earliest effects on the *respiratory tract* following minimal exposure to organophosphorus anti-ChE compounds are watery nasal discharge, nasal hyperemia, a sensation of tightness in the chest, and occasionally prolonged, wheezing expiration, suggestive of bronchoconstriction, or increased bronchial secretion (GROB 1956a, b).

Approximately four times the minimal symptomatic exposure results in extreme miosis, aching in and behind the eyes, slight blurring of distant vision attributed to spasm of accommodation, and more severe rhinorrhea and frontal headache. The aching, which is attributable to ciliary spasm, becomes worse on attempting to focus or to look at a bright light. Some twitching of the eyelids may occur. There is also intermittently more marked tightness in the chest, and there may be some cough. Occasionally there is nausea and vomiting, which, in the absence of systemic absorption, may be due to a reflex initiated by the ocular effects. These local effects may result in moderate discomfort and some loss of efficiency, but they do not produce serious incapacitation. Following minimal symptomatic exposure the miosis lasts for about 24 hours and the rhinorrhea lasts for a few hours. After four times the minimal symptomatic exposure miosis is well established within half an hour, remains maximal for at least 24 hours, and then diminishes gradually over a period of 3 to 14 days. The conjunctival suffusion, eye pain, and headache may last up to two to five days. The rhinorrhea lasts usually for several hours after minimal exposure, and for about one day after more marked exposure. The respiratory symptoms are usually intermittent and of several hours' duration after mild exposure; they may last for one to two days after greater exposure.

III. Systemic effects

1. Time course

The systemic effects are, in general, similar following absorption of anti-ChE compounds by any route, but there are some differences in their sequence and time course. Respiratory and ocular symptoms are the first to appear after inhalation, gastrointestinal symptoms after ingestion, and localized sweating after percutaneous absorption. In severe intoxication by any route most of the muscarinic effects eventually develop, concomitantly with the nicotinic and central neural effects. Marked miosis is consistently present only if there has been local ocular exposure to vapor or liquid; it is usually less severe, or may be absent, if there has been no local exposure, even in patients who have received lethal exposures.

The interval between exposure and onset of systemic effects is shortest after inhalation or ocular exposure to liquid (several minutes), longer after ingestion (one-fourth to two hours), and longest after cutaneous exposure (one-fourth to four hours). The time interval between exposure and occurence of maximal severity of moderate symptoms is of the same order (approximately one-half, two, and six hours) (GROB et al. 1950, GROB and HARVEY 1958). However, after lethal or near-lethal exposure, the time intervals to onset and maximal severity of symptoms are shorter, and may be but a few minutes after overwhelming exposure by any route.

The duration of symptoms produced by quaternary ammonium anti-ChE compounds is generally a few hours, while that of most organophosphorus anti-ChE compounds is generally one to five days, although mild effects may last only several hours. During the period of recovery symptoms may recur intermittently, especially after exertion. After exposure to lethal concentrations the time interval to death depends upon the degree and route of exposure. Most deaths due to organophosphorus compounds have occurred within 1 to 21 hours (average 9 hours) after exposure (GROB et al. 1950), but overwhelming exposure may be fatal within 5 minutes (KELENSKY 1952). The time interval to death, like that to development of symptoms, tends to be shortest after inhalation, longer after ingestion, and longest after cutaneous absorption.

2. Muscarinic effects

a) Respiratory manifestations

Respiratory manifestation are usually the first to appear after inhalation. The "tightness" in the chest, which may be an early local symptom, increases as the anti-ChE compound is absorbed into the systemic circulation. After moderate or marked exposure, excessive bronchial secretion occurs, and this may become very profuse, causing coughing, airway obstruction, and respiratory distress. Audible wheezing may occur, with prolonged expiration and difficulty in moving air into and out of the lungs, owing to increased bronchial secretion, or bronchoconstriction, or both. There may be some pain referred to the lower thorax. Salivation increases to an even greater extent than bronchial secretion (CULLUMBINE and DIRNHUBER 1955), and watery secretions run out of the sides of the mouth. If postural drainage or suction is not employed, airway obstruction and pulmonary edema may ensue. Laryngeal spasm may add to the respiratory difficulties. If the upper airway becomes obstructed by secretions or by laryngeal spasm, or if the bronchial tree becomes obstructed by secretion or bronchoconstriction, little ventilation may occur in spite of respiratory movements. The casualty may gasp for breath, froth at the mouth, and become cyanotic. He may be seized with panic in his struggle for air, thrash about, and then fall unconscious.

The degree of bronchoconstriction produced by anti-ChE compounds varies in different species (DE CANDOLE et al. 1953). It is marked in the dog (KROP and KUNKEL 1954) and may be accompanied by laryngospasm (HEYMANS et al. 1956). It is less than one-fourth as great in the monkey, which like man has far less peribronchial smooth muscle than the dog (JOHNSON et al. 1958). In man, small increases in airway resistance have been observed in mild anti-ChE intoxication. Deeper intoxication may increase airway resistance as a result of bronchorrhea, but signs suggestive of bronchoconstriction and laryngospasm have only occasionally been severe. The decrease in ventilatory exchange that is the most important manifestation of anti-ChE intoxication appears in man to be due mainly to central depression of respiration, secondly to neuromuscular block, thirdly to increased bronchial and salivary secretions, and fourthly to bronchoconstriction and, occasionally, laryngospasm. Respiratory manifestations are likely to be severest in older persons and in those with a history of respiratory disease, particularly bronchial asthma (GROB 1956a, GROB and HARVEY 1958).

b) Gastrointestinal manifestations

Gastrointestinal manifestations are usually the first to appear after ingestion, and consist of anorexia, nausea, vomiting, abdominal cramps, epigastric and substernal tightness suggestive of cardiospasm, "heartburn," eructation, diarrhea, tenesmus, and, in severe intoxication, involuntary defecation. Bloody diarrhea and peptic ulceration have been observed in the dog (JACQUES 1954, SLEISENGER et al. 1958). The symptoms suggestive of cardiospasm that occur in man contrast with esophageal aperistalsis and achalasia in the dog. This difference may be due to the predominance in the human esophagus of smooth muscle, which undergoes increased activity following ChE inhibition, and in the canine esophagus of skeletal muscle, which becomes paralyzed. There is evidence that even smooth muscle (of rabbit intestine) may become paralyzed in severe anti-ChE intoxication following the initial increase in tonus and peristalsis (SHELLY 1955). Unlike the latter, the paralytic effect is unaltered by administration of atropine or oxime and appears, therefore, to be due to some action of the anti-ChE agent on smooth muscle other than inhibition of ChE's.

c) Other muscarinic manifestations

Other muscarinic manifestations include sweating, lacrimation, bradycardia, urinary frequency, and in severe intoxication involuntary micturition and sometimes a variable degree of miosis and slight blurring of distant vision, attributed to spasm of accomodation. The heart rate is slowed in severe intoxication, in some instances following an initial period of sinus tachycardia. Electrocardiographic changes, which have been studied mainly in severely intoxicated experimental animals, consist of progressive prolongation of the P-R interval, widening of the QRS interval, complete heart block with diminution and then disappearance of the P wave, and inconstant changes in the T wave, including increased duration

and voltage (HOLMSTEDT 1951, KROP and KUNKEL 1954). The muscarinic manifestations are reversible by administration of atropine (GROB et al. 1947b). They
are affected to a lesser and variable extent by oximes (GROB and JOHNS 1958a,
NAMBA and HIRAKI 1958, ERDMANN and LENDLE 1958).

3. Nicotinic effects

a) Skeletal muscle

Simultaneously with the appearance of moderate muscarinic systemic effects,
the casualty begins to have increased fatiguability and mild generalized weakness
which is increased by exertion. This is followed by involuntary muscular twitching,
scattered muscular fasciculation, and sometimes muscle cramps. If the exposure
has been sufficiently marked, the fascicular twitchings, which usually appear first
in the eyelids and in the facial and calf muscles, become generalized. Innumerable
rippling movements are seen under the skin, and twitching movements appear in
all parts of the body. This is followed by severe weakness, which is generalized
and includes the muscles of respiration. The respiratory movements become more
labored, shallow, and rapid; then slow, and finally intermittent. The exchange of
air, which has already been interfered with as a result of central depression of
respiration, increased bronchial secretion, bronchoconstriction, and occasionally
laryngeal spasm, is further reduced, and cyanosis increases. Weakness of the
muscles of the tongue and pharynx may aggravate upper airway obstruction. The
weakness of the respiratory muscles may become so profound that all respiratory
efforts cease, and death occurs within a few minutes unless artificial respiration
is promptly instituted.

Anticholinesterase compounds cause an increase in amplitude and frequency of spontaneously occurring miniature end-plate potentials, resulting in the spontaneous appearance of
propagated action potentials which cause twitches in individual muscle fibers (fibrillation)
and in groups of fibers (fasciculation) (FATT 1954). When a nerve impulse reaches the myoneural
junction, there is increased amplitude and striking prolongation of the end-plate potential,
and repetitive firing may occur (DEL CASTILLO and KATZ 1956). The muscle action potential
response to a single nerve stimulus is only slightly affected, but the responses to subsequent
stimuli of a train are progressively reduced (Fig. 5) and muscle contraction is not sustained
(GROB et al. 1956a, b, c).

The neuromuscular block produced by anti-ChE compounds is attributable mainly to the
local accumulation of ACh resulting from inhibition of muscle AChE (GROB 1957). Originally
it was believed that ACh, like other "depolarizing" agents such as decamethonium and
succinylcholine, produced neuromuscular block as a result of persistent depolarization of the
endplate membrane (BURNS and PATON 1951). However, it is now known that the depolarization produced by these compounds is briefer than the neuromuscular block, which continues
despite complete repolarization of the membrane (KATZ and THESLEFF 1957). The neuromuscular block has been attributed to refractoriness to ACh, due perhaps to alteration of the
receptor substance in the endplate.

There is recovery from neuromuscular block produced by TEPP or DFP before there has
been measurable restoration of AChE activity, suggesting that junctional transmission either
is not related solely to AChE activity, or is influenced by recovery that is within the limits
of experimental error (BERRY and LOVETT 1951, BURGEN and HOBBIGER 1951).

Some anti-ChE compounds appear to affect neuromuscular transmission by mechanisms
in addition to ChE inhibition (see Chapter 13). Neostigmine has a direct excitatory action
on cat muscle even after complete inactivation of ChE's by DFP (RIKER and WESCOE 1946).
Ambenomium has more excitatory action than most other anti-ChE compounds, presumably
as a result of direct action. On the other hand, very large doses of DFP produce further
reduction in the muscle response to a single nerve stimulus even after complete inactivation
of ChE's. Furthermore, this block is accentuated by d-tubocurarine, which antagonizes more
moderate degrees of anti-ChE neuromuscular block (BARSTAD 1956).

b) Sympathetic ganglia

Moderate or severe intoxication by Parathion, Sarin, DFP, or TEPP may
cause tachycardia, pallor, mild to moderate elevation of blood pressure (GROB et al.

1950, GROB 1956 a), and occasionally hyperglycemia and glycosuria (CHAMBERLIN et al. 1953). There is evidence that anti-ChE compounds can produce stimulation of cholinergic preganglionic fibers to sympathetic ganglia and to the adrenal medulla (PAULET 1954), as well as a central increase in sympathetic vasoconstrictor tone (VARAGIC 1955, DIRNHUBER and CULLUMBINE 1955).

An increase in blood-borne sympathomimetic substances has been observed in experimental animals (DE BURGH DALY and WRIGHT 1956). The dog and man are most prone to elevation of blood pressure during organophosphorus anti-ChE intoxication. In all species the blood pressure falls when intoxication becomes profound (HOLMSTEDT 1951, DELGA 1957, ERDMANN and LENDLE 1958). In dogs and monkeys chronically exposed to DFP, no change in blood sugar concentration could be detected (KOELLE and GILMAN 1946).

4. Central nervous system effects

The earliest systemic manifestations of organophosphorus anti-ChE poisoning usually include tension, anxiety, jitteriness, restlessness, emotional lability, and giddiness. There may be insomnia and excessive dreaming, occasionally with nightmares. If the exposure is more marked, there follow headache, tremor, drowsiness, difficulty in concentrating, impairment of memory with slow recall of recent events, and slowing of reactions. In some persons there is apathy, withdrawal, and depression.

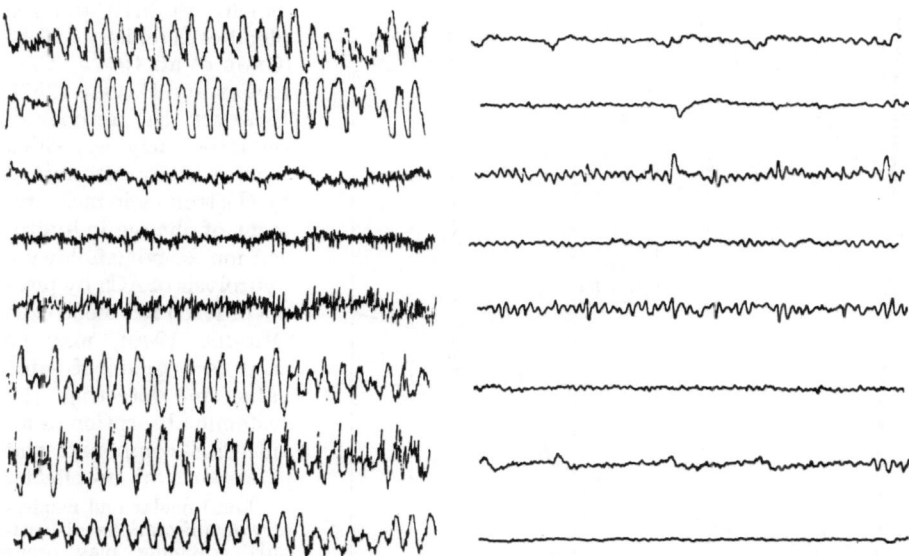

Fig. 1. Effect of marked exposure to Sarin on the electroencephalogram. Left, following exposure to Sarin, showing high-voltage slow waves in temporofrontal and temporocentral leads. Right, two weeks later, showing return to normal. Bipolar leads: left prefrontal to left anterior temporal (top), left anterior temporal to left low central, left low central to left low occiput, left occiput to right low occiput, right occiput to right low central, right low central to right anterior temporal, right anterior temporal to right prefrontal, right prefrontal to left prefrontal (bottom). (From: GROB 1956a)

Elevation of dark adaptation and of the absolute scotopic threshold has been reported to occur after systemic, but not local exposure (RUBIN et al. 1957), and has been attributed to a central effect (RUBIN and GOLDBERG 1957, 1958). With the appearance of moderate symptoms there occur abnormalities of the electroencephalogram, characterized by irregularities in rhythm, variation and increase in potential, and intermittent bursts of abnormally slow waves of elevated voltage similar to those seen in patients with epilepsy (Fig. 1) (GROB et al. 1947c, GROB 1956a). These abnormal waves become more marked after one or more minutes of hyperventilation, which, if prolonged, may occasionally precipitate a generalized convulsion.

If absorption of the anti-ChE compound has been sufficiently great, the casualty then becomes confused and ataxic, and he may have changes in speech, consisting of slurring, difficulty in forming words, and multiple repetition of the last syllable. He may then become comatose. Reflexes may disappear, and respiration may become Cheyne-Stokes in character. Finally, generalized convulsions may ensue. With the appearance of severe central neural symptoms, depression of respiration, central in origin, may occur, adding to the respiratory embarrassment caused by weakness and airway obstruction (KRIVOY et al. 1951). Depression of the circulatory center may also occur, particularly in the presence of anoxia, resulting in a fall of blood pressure some time before death.

5. Depression of plasma and red blood cell cholinesterase activity

The signs and symptoms produced by anti-ChE compounds are due to inhibition of the ChE's of the nervous system, striated and smooth muscle, and secretory glands (RIKER and WESCOE 1949), and not to the coincident inhibition of the cholinesterase enzymes of the plasma (chiefly BuChE) and red blood cells (chiefly AChE) (GROB et al. 1947a, CALLAWAY and DAVIES 1957). However, the activity of the latter enzymes, which is most easily determined by electrometric measurement of change in hydrogen ion activity following hydrolysis of ACh by plasma or lysed red blood cells (MICHEL 1949), may be used as a guide of some value in detecting the systemic absorption of an anti-ChE compound and persistence of its effects.

Local ocular and respiratory manifestations of anti-ChE poisoning may occur without any inhibition of plasma BuChE or red blood cell AChE activity, but systemic manifestations are invariably accompanied by depression of the activity of these enzymes. The depression accompanying the onset of systemic symptoms is less marked following rapid than following gradual absorption of anti-ChE compounds,

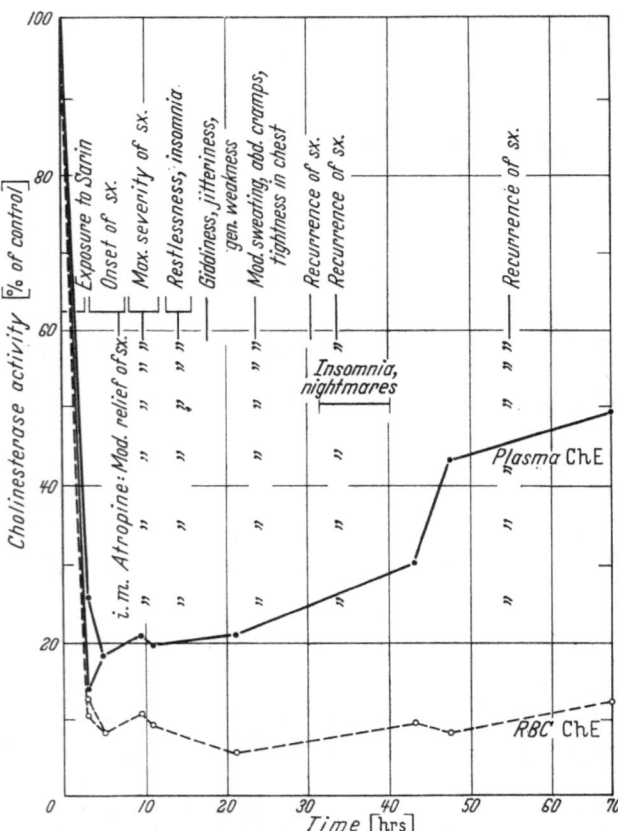

Fig. 2. Time course of symptoms, atropine administration, and depression and restoration of plasma BuChE and red blood cell AChE activities following percutaneous exposure to Sarin liquid. Cholinesterase activities prior to exposure were 0.83 Δ pH/hour (plasma) and 0.56 Δ pH/hour (red blood cells). (From: GROB 1956a)

presumably because rapid absorption results in briefer contact with plasma and red blood cell ChE's and hence more access to the ChE's of other tissues. The plasma BuChE and red blood cell AChE at the time of onset of systemic symptoms due to a single exposure to Sarin are depressed to approximately 60% and 50%, respectively, of initial activity after inhalation of vapor, to 35% and 25% after ingestion of liquid, and to 15% and 10% after percutaneous exposure to liquid (Fig. 2) (GROB 1956a, GROB and HARVEY 1958, CRAIG and WOODSON 1958).

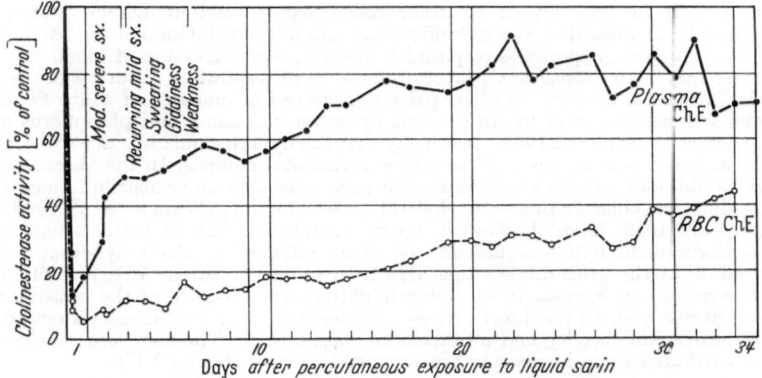

Fig. 3. Further restoration of plasma BuChE and red blood cell AChE activities following depression by percutaneous exposure to Sarin. Same patient as Fig. 2. (From: GROB 1956a)

Restoration of plasma BuChE activity begins 3 to 10 hours after cessation of exposure to most organophosphorus anti-ChE compounds, and restoration of red blood cell AChE activity begins 24 to 48 hours after exposure (Fig. 2). After marked depression, plasma BuChE returns to the original level of activity over a period of 30 to 40 days and red blood cell AChE over a period of 80 to 100 days (Figs. 3 and 4). Repeated exposure to any of these compounds

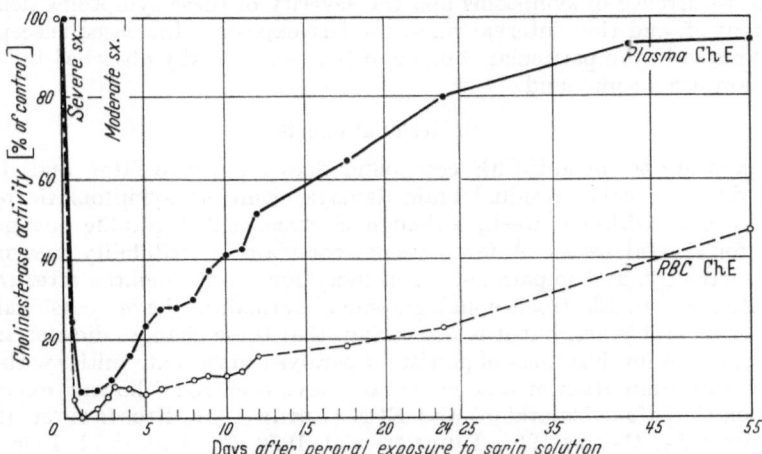

Fig. 4. Time course of symptoms and of depression and restoration of plasma BuChE and red blood cell AChE activities following peroral exposure to an aqueous solution of Sarin. Cholinesterase activities prior to exposure were 1.02 Δ pH/hour (plasma) and 0.80 Δ pH/hour (red blood cells). (From: GROB 1956a)

at intervals of hours or days may result in progressive depression of plasma and red blood cell ChE activity, since there may be insufficient time between exposures for restoration of activity to occur. Following repeated exposure there is no predictable correlation between the onset of symptoms and the precise level of ChE activity of the plasma or red cells, except that this is depressed considerably below normal. The AChE activity of the red blood cells may be gradually depressed to near zero by repeated exposures over a period of several days without systemic symptoms necessarily ensuing, or without any relation to the severity of the symptoms that occur. The red blood cell AChE and, to a lesser extent, the plasma BuChE remain at a low level of activity long after the disappearance of symptoms.

6. Other chemical effects

In severe anti-ChE intoxication, some species such as the horse develop metabolic acidosis, probably secondarily to tissue anoxia resulting from anoxemia and circulatory failure, with increase in blood lactic acid, decrease in buffer base, and fall in pH (GOLD et al. 1957). Other species, such as the goat, experience respiratory acidosis, with elevation of blood pCO_2 occurring concurrently with decreased O_2 saturation owing to respiratory failure, and resulting in fall in pH. In man, a decrease in blood pH was observed in one case of acute Parathion poisoning and was accompanied by an increase in serum potassium and phosphorus and a decrease in calcium (ANNIS et al. 1953). It is likely that the hyperkalemia was due to anoxemia and acidosis, as this has been observed also in experimental animals. In the absence of anoxemia, ChE inhibition was found to have no effect on concentration or distribution of water, potassium, sodium, or chloride in serum, skeletal muscle, or liver (WELLER et al. 1955).

HOLMES et al. (1956) have observed in approximately one-half of patients exposed to Parathion or Sarin slight hypercoagulability of blood, followed by slight hypocoagulability with prolongation of the prothrombin time due to reduction in factor VII, and prolonged thrombin time due to an increase in thrombin inhibitors. In one-third of the patients there was increased fibrinolysis. In one-fourth there was increased coagulation associated with an increase in prothrombin activity and prothrombin consumption. The increased prothrombin activity was attributed to an increase in pro-convertin activity (Factor VII).

7. Cumulative effects of repeated exposure

Daily exposure to concentrations of an organophosphorus anti-ChE compound which are insufficient to produce symptoms following a single exposure may result in the onset of symptoms after several days. Continued daily exposure may be followed by increasingly severe effects. After symptoms subside, increased susceptibility persists for one to several days. The degree of exposure required to produce recurrence of symptoms and the severity of these symptoms depend on the extent of, and time interval since, the last exposure. Increased susceptibility is not limited to the particular compound that was initially absorbed but applies to any anti-ChE compound.

8. Residual effects

If exposure to an anti-ChE compound does not prove fatal, and if severe anoxia does not cause residual brain damage, complete symptomatic recovery usually occurs within a week, although electroencephalographic changes may persist for several weeks. A few patients complain of irritability, nervousness, fatigue, lethargy, and impairment of memory for several months after recovery from intoxication. Electroencephalographic abnormalities have occasionally persisted for several years, but it is not certain that these changes did not antedate the exposure. A few instances of persistent paralysis of the extremities with muscle atrophy and diminution of tendon reflexes have occurred following exposure to Parathion, Mipafox, Malathion, and EPN (PETRY 1951, BIDSTRUP et al. 1953, BIDSTRUP 1954, DAVIES 1954, DURHAM et al. 1956, GLASSON et al. 1956, PETTY 1958).

Electromyographic studies have shown no evidence of neuromuscular block, but have revealed changes similar to those seen in peripheral neuritis. This residual weakness and atrophy, attributed to peripheral neuritis, resembles the peripheral neuritis and demyelinization that occurs more frequently after acute or chronic exposure to triorthocresylphosphate (Ginger Jake paralysis) (SUSSER and STEIN 1957, SMITH and SPALDING 1959). Demyelinization has been observed in the peripheral nerve and spinal cord of experimental animals following the administration of Mipafox, DFP, or other dialkylfluoridates, or triorthocresylphosphate (BARNES et al. 1953, LANCASTER 1960). It has so far not been possible to correlate this effect of organophosphorus compounds with inhibition of any type of ChE, or with any other specific chemical effect (HOTTINGER and BLOCH 1943, BARNES and DENZ 1953, DAVIES 1954). In the case of alkyl organophosphorus compounds containing fluorine, which are the most neurotoxic, it has been suggested that this action may result from liberation of ionic fluorine following rupture of the P—F bond by AChE in the nervous system (DAVIES et al. 1960) (see Chapter 19).

9. Time of death

The time interval between exposure and death varies with the degree of exposure, and to a lesser extent with the route of administration. Death has been reported within five minutes after drinking concentrated TEPP insecticide (KELENSKY et al. 1952). Following the ingestion of bread contaminated by Parathion, symptoms began in 15 to 60 minutes (average 28 minutes), and death occurred 4 to 9 hours (average 6 hours) after the onset of symptoms (WISHAHI et al. 1958). After percutaneous absorption of Parathion, symptoms began $^1/_2$ to 8 hours (average 3 hours) after exposure, and death occurred 1 to $21^1/_2$ hours (average $10^1/_2$ hours) after exposure, and 1 to $13^1/_2$ hours (average 9 hours) after onset of symptoms (GROB et al. 1950).

10. Cause of death

Death from poisoning by organophosphorus anti-ChE compounds is caused by respiratory failure resulting from weakness of the muscles of respiration, central depression of respiration, and airway obstruction by bronchial and salivary secretions and perhaps bronchoconstriction. In overwhelming exposure, when respiration fails rapidly, the circulation is usually relatively unimpaired until terminally (OBERST et al. 1956). When exposure is less acute and death delayed, forward circulatory failure, due at least in part to anoxia, may complicate the respiratory failure (POLET et al. 1959). Most instances of fatal intoxication in man have appeared to be primarily asphyxial; in some, failure of both respiration and circulation have occurred together. It seems likely that a sub-lethal degree of respiratory depression may be made lethal by associated reduction in blood pressure and cardiac output (DE CANDOLE et al. 1953). In fatal poisoning by quaternary ammonium anti-ChE compounds there may be earlier onset of forward circulatory failure (MERRILL 1948).

The relative importance of central depression of respiration, peripheral neuromuscular block, and bronchoconstriction varies in different species and with different anti-ChE compounds and routes of administration (BARNES and DUFF 1953, DE CANDOLE et al. 1953, DOUGLAS and MATTHEWS 1952, WRIGHT 1954, WIRTH 1958). There generally occurs a decrease in tidal volume and respiratory rate and an increase in airway resistance. In man, it is likely that failure of the central drive of respiration is the most important factor, with peripheral neuromuscular block next in importance. Bronchoconstriction appears to be less important in man than in most experimental animals, although airway obstruction due to inspissated secretions may occur and may seriously impair ventilatory exchange.

Many fatalities have occurred in infants and children, but since the amount of agent absorbed is seldom known, it is not possible to compare susceptibility to intoxication with that of adults. However, greater susceptibility to DFP intoxication has been found in the infant rat compared to the adult, and this has been attributed to a lower concentration of brain AChE in the infant (FRIEDMAN and HIMWICH 1948).

11. Postmortem findings

The ChE activities of the plasma and red blood cells of patients who have died of organophosphorus anti-ChE poisoning have been found to be reduced to below 20% of normal, and have usually been close to zero activity (GROB et al. 1950). The AChE activity of brain and muscle has been found to be depressed, usually to below 30% of normal. The latter may be demonstrated not only by manometric analysis of tissue homogenates, but also by staining tissue slices for ChE activity

by the Koelle-Friedenwald technique (BERGNER and DURLACHER 1951). In experimental animals central neural signs of intoxication with anti-ChE agents of
moderate or greater lipoid solubility do not begin until brain AChE has been
reduced to 20 to 50% of normal, and death does not occur until brain AChE has
been depressed to below 10% of normal (KOELLE and GILMAN 1946, OBERST and
CHRISTENSEN 1956). In patients who have died of Parathion poisoning, this compound has been found in blood, brain, liver, and kidneys in concentration of 0.01
to 0.17 mg/100 g of tissue (GROB et al. 1950).

The postmortem changes observed by ordinary gross or histologic examination
have not been of a specific nature. In most patients there has been pulmonary
vascular dilatation, plugging of bronchioles, localized emphysema, and pulmonary
edema, and often vascular dilatation and edema of the brain, gastrointestinal
tract, liver, spleen, kidneys, and subcutaneous tissue (GROB et al. 1950, MARESCH
1957, HOLMSTEDT et al. 1957). Some observers have not noted pulmonary edema
or have ascribed this to postmortem changes (DURLACHER et al. 1949/50). Localized
alveoler emphysema, attributable to bronchosecretion and possibly bronchoconstriction, has been regarded by some to be a more significant change.

D. Diagnosis of anti-ChE intoxication

I. Signs and symptoms

Identification of anti-ChE intoxication can be made from the characteristic
signs and symptoms. If exposure to vapor has occurred, the pupils will be very
small, usually pinpoint, even in the absence of systemic signs of intoxication.
After cutaneous exposure, ingestion, or injection, the pupils may be normal
(DIXON 1957), or, in the presence of severe systemic symptoms, slightly to moderately reduced in size (SANDERSON 1957). In this event, the circumstances of the
exposure and the other manifestations of poisoning must be relied on to establish
the diagnosis. No other group of toxic agents produces pinpoint pupils (in the
absence of severe conjunctival inflammation), muscular twitching and fasciculation, and the characteristic train of muscarinic, nicotinic, and central nervous
system manifestations.

II. Effects of atropine and oxime administration

The administration of atropine alleviates the muscarinic and central neural
manifestations of anti-ChE poisoning, even though, in severe poisoning, such relief
may be transient and repeated administration of atropine may be required. The
amount of atropine required to alleviate these manifestations varies directly, and
the duration of the relief afforded by the atropine varies inversely with the severity
of the poisoning. The administration of a single dose of 2 mg of atropine by any
route to a subject who has absorbed little or no anti-ChE compound produces
mild symptoms of atropinization in most subjects, and repetition of this dose
within one or two hours produces moderate symptoms of atropinization, including
tachycardia, pupillary dilatation, and dryness of the mouth and skin. In contrast,
a subject who is having moderate manifestations of anti-ChE poisoning will not
develop symptoms of atropinization after 2 mg of atropine, and one who is having
severe manifestations may not develop symptoms of atropinization even after the
second dose of atropine.

The pupils alone cannot be used as a guide to the efficacy of atropine in the
management of anti-ChE intoxication. If the pupils are constricted owing to local
exposure, the systemic administration of atropine is usually insufficient to dilate
the pupils; local instillation is required to achieve this effect. The effect of atropine

on sweating, bronchial and salivary secretion, and gastrointestinal and central neural symptoms of anti-ChE intoxication is a better index of therapeutic efficacy. If miosis is not present, the administration of atropine may occasionally induce mydriasis even before the systemic effects of anti-ChE poisoning have been relieved.

Improvement in strength following the intravenous administration of oxime occurs only in the presence of weakness due to anti-ChE intoxication, and hence may aid in confirming the diagnosis.

III. Determination of plasma and red blood cell cholinesterase activity

This determination is seldom essential for establishment of the diagnosis when the clinical manifestations of anti-ChE intoxication are full blown, but it can be of great help in detecting subclinical exposure or mild poisoning, in confirming the diagnosis, or in establishing the cause of death. In attempting to evaluate the significance of determination of plasma and red blood cell ChE activities, it must be kept in mind that the range of normal activity is fairly wide, $1.0 \pm 0.5 \Delta$ pH/hour for plasma by the electrometric method (MICHEL 1949) and $0.8 \pm 0.4 \Delta$ pH/hour for red blood cells (AUGUSTINSSON 1955). In addition, plasma BuChE activity may be moderately reduced in many acute or chronic illnesses, particularly those affecting liver function, as well as following absorption of anti-ChE compounds. On the other hand, red blood cell AChE activity is reduced only by anti-ChE compounds or in relatively uncommon blood diseases such as pernicious anemia or leukemia (GROB et al. 1947a).

IV. Chemical determination of anti-ChE compounds

Some of the anti-ChE compounds, or their degradation products, can be detected in the urine, e.g., p-nitrophenol, a product of Parathion (LEIBMAN et al. 1952, WALDMAN and KRAUSE 1952).

E. Prevention of anti-ChE intoxication and handling of casualties

The use of protective clothing is mandatory during the bulk handling of organophosphorus anti-ChE compounds.

The type and extent of protection required varies with the nature of the exposure, but usually includes rubber gloves and boots, rubber apron, coveralls, antisplash visors, and, when volatile compounds or dusts are handled, a protective mask or respirator. Butyl rubber offers more protection than natural rubber, although the latter is superior to certain synthetic rubbers. Charcoal filter respirators afford good protection if properly fitted, but the filter may have to be changed after prolonged use. Liquid organophosphorus anti-ChE compounds penetrate rapidly through ordinary clothing or impregnated permeable clothing, which offer very little protection to the skin against liquid splash. However, absorption through the skin occurs over a period of minutes, so that, unless the exposure is overwhelming, there should be sufficient time to remove contaminated clothing and to blot and wash the liquid from the skin. Impermeable protective clothing, individual protective covers, and rubber gloves and aprons protect the skin against liquid. Since the liquid, or solution, is more readily absorbed through abraded than intact skin, breaks in the skin should be covered with adhesive tape prior to anticipated exposure. Absorption of the liquid through the conjunctivae is very rapid, and a drop of undiluted liquid may be lethal; consequently, protection of the eyes against splash and immediate washing away of ocular contamination are of the greatest importance. Care must be exercised during the removal of contaminated clothing, and separate showers should be available for use before and after such removal. Some emulsifiers reduce the cutaneous absorption of organophosphorus compounds (DEICHMANN et al. 1952) and may prove useful in the preparation of insecticides.

Casualties who have been contaminated with liquid agent may endanger unprotected personal, particularly since most of the agents are volatile. Attendants in a heavily contaminated area should wear a gas mask and, if possible, protective heavy rubber gloves and aprons. When rubber gloves and aprons have been in contact with liquid, they should be washed off with water as often as is practicable and replaced by fresh ones after several hours of continual use, since the liquid agent slowly penetrates rubber. Ambulances and other vehicles used for the transportation of casualties contaminated with liquid must have their interiors washed with soap and water and be aired before reuse. Contaminated objects should be washed with copious amounts of soap and water, preferably with added alkali, which accelerates hydrolysis of most organophosphorus anti-ChE compounds. Objects which cannot be adequately washed should be buried or burned.

Containers of organophosphorus anti-ChE compounds should be clearly labelled, carefully stored, and used only by trained personnel. Used or broken containers should be carefully disposed of. Many tragic accidents, particularly those involving children, have been the result of careless handling or disposition of these compounds.

It is now regularly accepted practice for industrial and agricultural workers exposed to organic phosphorus insecticides to receive periodic determinations of plasma BuChE and red blood cell AChE activities (WILLIAMS and GRIFFITHS 1951, MARCHAND 1952, KAY et al. 1952, SUMMERFORD et al. 1953). Absorption of sufficient agent to cause significant reduction of ChE activity necessitates transfer to safer duties for at least two to four weeks to enable the ChE activity of the tissues to be restored. Plants that have been sprayed are also periodically tested for insecticide by methods that permit the detection of concentrations as low as 0.1 part per million (ppm) of plant material (NOLAN et al. 1950).

F. Treatment of anti-ChE intoxication

This consists in removal of the toxic agent, administration of atropine and oxime, removal of oral secretions, maintenance of a patent airway, and artificial respiration if needed (GROB 1956, ELAM et al. 1956, ERDMANN and HEYE 1958).

I. Removal of toxic agent

Liquid organophosphorus compound that has come in contact with skin or clothing must be promptly removed.

Liquid on the skin should be blotted with a handkerchief, cloth, or piece of outer clothing. The blotting should be done without spreading the contamination and without rubbing the skin, which may increase absorption (KONDRITZER 1956). A fresh cloth or piece of outer clothing should then be soaked with water and rubbed over the contaminated area firmly enough to remove any remaining liquid contamination, as well as dirt, but not so hard as to abrade the skin or produce reddening. The cloth should be turned over to expose clean wet cloth to the skin with each rubbing. The skin should be washed with copious amounts of water and with soap, if possible. Addition to the water of standard decontaminating agents, such as 50 ppm of chlorine or chloramine, or diluted Chlorox (3% sodium hypochlorite) may have some value. Contaminated clothing should then be quickly removed or cut away, and discarded. When heavy contamination of a limb by concentrated liquid has occurred, a tourniquet may be applied about the limb just proximal to the contaminated area in order to reduce systemic absorption. It should be tied tightly enough to occlude the pulse, loosened for about half a minute at 10-minute intervals over a period of 30 minutes, and then removed. If the tourniquet is allowed to remain in place continuously for more than 15 minutes there will be danger of nerve damage and of gangrene of the ends of fingers or toes, especially in older subjects. When the temperature is near or below freezing, use of the tourniquet to delay absorption should be omitted.

If liquid should get into the eye, instant action is necessary to prevent absorption of a lethal dose.

The head should be tilted back so that the eyes look directly upward, and water poured slowly into the contaminated eye, which is held open with the fingers. The water should be poured slowly, so that the irrigation will last at least 30 seconds. This irrigation must be done even if there is organophosphorus vapor in the atmosphere, in which case the breath should be held as much as possible during the procedure, and a protective respirator put on as soon as the irrigation is completed. The pupil of the contaminated eye should be watched during the next minute. If it rapidly constricts, 2 mg of atropine should be injected intramuscularly at once, and administered again, with intravenously injected oxime, when systemic manifestations of anti-ChE poisoning begin. If the pupil does not constrict, the ocular contamination was not by an anti-ChE agent, and atropine or oxime is not needed.

If the atmosphere is contaminated with organophosphorus vapor, the casualty should be promptly removed to an uncontaminated area. If this is not possible the casualty should be protected with a mask, if available, or by covering his face loosely with a cloth saturated with water.

If ingestion of anti-ChE compound is known to have occurred, gastric lavage with water should be carried out.

II. Administration of atropine

The appearance of any local or systemic signs or symptoms of anti-ChE poisoning calls for the immediate injection of atropine. This drug inhibits the action of ACh at its many sites of action, with the exception of the voluntary muscles. As a result, it has a moderate inhibitory effect on the muscarinic and central neural effects (Fig. 1) of anti-ChE compounds, but no appreciable influence on muscular weakness and fasciculation. The pharmacology of atropine and related drugs as antagonists to the effects of anti-ChE agents is discussed in Chapter 20.

In patients with severely impaired breathing due to anti-ChE poisoning, atropine administration facilitates respiratory exchange by suppressing bronchial and salivary secretion and bronchoconstriction, and perhaps by diminishing central depression of respiration, but it does not appreciably restore strength to paralyzed respiratory muscles. In such patients artificial respiration is of more immediate importance than atropine administration.

1. Rate of action

The action of 2 mg of atropine sulfate or tartrate begins 1, 8, or 20 minutes after intravenous, intramuscular, or oral administration, and becomes maximal in 6, 35, or 50 minutes, respectively. The effects of the drug administered in the same dose by any of these routes are approximately the same once absorption has occurred. In patients with severe anti-ChE intoxication, absorption of orally or intramuscularly administered atropine may be delayed owing to decreased peripheral blood flow. Absorption following inhalation of a solution of atropine (aerosolized) or injection into the lung parenchyma has been found in animals to be nearly as rapid as that following intravenous injection, and administration by the former route has been recommended by some for man.

2. Dose

Atropine should be injected immediately after the appearance of any local or systemic signs or symptoms of anti-ChE poisoning in much larger doses than are employed for other purposes. If appreciable absorption of anti-ChE compound is known to have occurred, 2 mg of atropine may be injected intramuscularly before the effects of poisoning appear, but it is best to avoid administration of atropine when absorption is merely suspected. Atropine should not be administered for preventive purposes prior to contemplated exposure to anti-ChE vapor or aerosol, as this may increase absorption by the respiratory tract as a result of inhibition of bronchial secretion and bronchoconstriction.

When signs or symptoms produced by an anti-ChE compound are mild, 2 mg of atropine should be injected intramuscularly and repeated, if necessary, at 30-minute intervals until muscarinic symptoms are relieved and signs of mild atropinization (dry mouth and skin) appear. A mild degree of atropinization should then be maintained for at least 24 hours by the intramuscular or oral administration of 1 or 2 mg of atropine, as needed, at intervals of several hours.

When symptoms of anti-ChE poisoning are moderately severe, 2 to 4 mg of atropine should be injected intravenously, or, if this is not feasible, intramuscularly, and repeated in doses of 2 mg at 10-minute intervals until muscarinic symptoms are relieved and signs of mild atropinization appear. The site of intramuscular injection may be massaged for several minutes to hasten absorption. A mild degree of atropinization should be maintained for at least 48 hours.

When severe symptoms are present, particularly respiratory distress or convulsions, 4 to 6 mg of atropine should be injected intravenously, or, if this is not feasible, intramuscularly, and repeated in doses of 2 mg at 3 to 8 minute intervals until bronchial secretions and salivation decrease and convulsions cease. In severe anti-ChE poisoning the effect of each injection of atropine may be transient, lasting only 10 to 30 minutes. Therefore, the patient must be observed as closely as possible for recurrence of signs of poisoning, and atropine must be repeated at appropriate intervals to relieve the muscarinic and central neural effects of the anti-ChE compound and to maintain a mild degree of atropinization for at least 48 hours (GROB 1956a). Severely intoxicated patients who have received more than 3 mg of atropine during the first five hours have had a lower mortality than those who have received smaller doses (FREEMAN et al. 1955). In severe poisoning as much as 24 to 48 mg of atropine may be required during the first day.

3. Symptoms produced by atropine

In the presence of systemic evidence of anti-ChE poisoning there is increased tolerance for atropine (GROB and HARVEY 1958), so that fairly large doses may be administered before signs of atropinization appear. In severe anti-ChE poisoning as much as 24 to 48 mg of atropine may be administered in a day without producing more than transient mild symptoms attributable to atropine (GROB 1956a). The absence of increased tolerance for atropine would indicate that anti-ChE poisoning is probably either not present or is mild.

In subjects who have absorbed little or no anti-ChE compound, the administration of a single dose of 2 mg of atropine by any route produces mild symptoms of atropinization, including dryness of the mouth and pharynx, which may cause slight difficulty in swallowing, subjective warmth due to 40% reduction in sweating, slight flushing, slight tachycardia, some hesitancy of urination, and occasional desire to eructate. The pupils may be slightly dilated, but they react to light. In some subjects there may be mild drowsiness, slowness of memory and recall, subjective slowing of motor activity, and blurring of near vision, particularly after the intravenous administration of atropine. Some subjects may have mild postural hypotension. These symptoms should not interfere with ordinary activity except in the occasional person who proves to be unusually reactive to the central neural effects of atropine, and except in hot environments, where interference with sweating and elevation of body temperature may occur. If the environment is cool or the subject at rest, there is no increase in skin or rectal temperature, but if the atmospheric temperature rises to 40°C there is difficulty in regulation of body temperature, particularly during exercise, resulting in a rise in skin and rectal temperature. Some subjects may be unable to work in hot weather for more than one or two hours unless their skin and clothing are periodically wetted.

If a second dose of 2 mg of atropine is given within an hour, or if the initial dose is 3 to 4 mg, the symptoms become moderate in degree and most subjects will be drowsy and have some blurring of near vision, but almost all will be able to continue ordinary activity at reduced efficiency. The skin temperature rises owing to a 70% reduction in sweating, but the rectal temperature does not rise so long as the environment is cool (about 26°C). A third dose of atropine administered within an hour will result in more marked symptoms, which will interfere with ordinary activity in many subjects but will usually not be totally incapacitating except in a warm environment. Further administration of atropine at frequent intervals will result in severe and incapacitating symptoms of over-atropinization, including very dry mouth, thirst, hoarseness, dry flushed skin, dilated pupils, blurring of near vision, tachycardia, urinary retention requiring catheterization of the bladder, constipation, slowing of mental and physical activity, restlessness, headache, giddiness, disorientation, hallucinations, increasing drowsiness, and sometimes, maniacal behavior. Acceleration of the heart rate cannot be used as an index of degree of atropinization, as after a rate of 160 per minute has been produced by about 4 mg, further administration of atropine has little additional effect. Abnormal behavior may require restraint. Body temperature may increase, particularly in a warm environment or after exercise.

The effects of atropine are fairly prolonged, lasting 3 to 5 hours after one or two injections of 2 mg each, 6 to 12 hours after four injections at close intervals, and 12 to 24 hours after marked over-atropinization. Over-atropinization may be incapacitating, but fortunately only extremely high doses endanger life. A single dose of 10 mg of atropine has been inadvertently administered intravenously to normal adults without endangering life, even in the absence of any prior absorption of anti-ChE compound, although it has, of course, produced very marked signs of overdose (GROB 1956a). As much as one-half to one gram of atropine has been ingested with complete recovery (GORDON and FRYE 1955). Doses of 10 to 25 mg have been administered intramuscularly in attempted management of some serious psychiatric disorders (FORRER 1956 and 1958). Death has occasionally occurred, particularly in hot weather and often with manifestations of hyperthermia, following the intramuscular or hypodermic administration of 25 to 32 mg of atropine, or following the oral administration of 200 to 500 mg. However, of 11 patients whose death was attributed to atropine administration, there were some extenuating circumstances in all but three (BAKER and FARLEY 1958). Children, and particularly infants, may be more prone to serious effects of over-atropinization, as death has occasionally occurred following the administration of doses as low as 2 mg.

4. Conjunctival instillation of atropine

Ocular symptoms produced by the local absorption of an anti-ChE compound do not respond to the systemic administration of atropine, but are relieved by the local instillation of 2% homatropine, or 0.5% atropine, repeated as needed at intervals of several hours for one to three days. If local ocular effects of an anti-ChE agent are present, the size of the pupil cannot be used as an indicator of the systemic effects of the agent or of atropine. In one patient the pupils remained constricted following the administration of 354 mg of atropine over 25 hours, despite systemic evidence of atropine poisoning (KARLOG et al. 1958).

The use of concentrations of atropine greater than 0.5% in eye drops is inadvisable, as it may lead to absorption of sufficient drug to cause signs of over-atropinization in patients who do not have anti-ChE poisoning. Acute confusional psychosis has been reported following the repeated instillation of a 1% solution, each drop of which contains 0.6 mg atropine sulphate. This is believed to be due to swallowing of atropine-laden tears, rather than to transconjunctival absorption. It is therefore recommended that compression of the internal angle of the eye be employed to obstruct the lachrymal duct during instillation if a purely local effect is desired (BAKER and FARLEY 1958).

III. Administration of oxime

The administration of large doses of atropine ameliorates the muscarinic effects of anti-ChE compounds, and to a lesser extent the central neural effects, but has no influence on weakness due to neuromuscular block (GROB 1956a). In severe anti-ChE intoxication death occurs as a result of paralysis of the muscles of respiration and of the pharynx and tongue, unless artificial respiration and an open airway are maintained until spontaneous recovery occurs. Until recently, there has been no clinically useful means of accelerating recovery from the neuromuscular block. However, during the past several years, WILSON and others have demonstrated that ChE's inhibited by organophosphorus anti-ChE compounds may

$$O$$

be reactivated *in vitro* by derivatives of hydroxamic acid (R—$\overset{\|}{C}$—$NHOH$), and to a greater extent by a number of oximes (R—$\overset{\|}{C}$—R) (WILSON and MEISLICH 1953,

$$NOH$$

KEWITZ and NACHMANSOHN 1957). Both groups of compounds also react with these inhibitors to inactivate them directly. The action of organophosphorus anti-ChE agents on smooth, cardiac, and skeletal muscle of experimental animals can be reversed by hydroxamic acid derivatives (KEWITZ and NACHMANSOHN 1957) and oximes (HOLMES and ROBINS 1955, BROWN et al. 1957) and their lethal effects reduced (WILLS et al. 1957, ASKEW 1956, KEWITZ et al. 1956), although species differences are wide. A full account of this class of compounds is presented in Chapter 21. Some of the major factors related to their present clinical use are summarized below.

1. Protection and reactivation by oximes of cholinesterase enzymes inhibited by various anti-ChE compounds in vitro

The oximes, pyridine-2-aldoxime methiodide (P-2-AM), pyridine-2-aldoxime methane sulfonate (P2S), 1,1'-trimethylene-bis-(4-formylpyridinium bromide)-dioxime (TMB-4, EA 1814), diacetyl monoxime (DAM), and monoisonitroso acetone (MINA) (Table 4) cause moderate protection and reactivation of ChE's inhibited by organophosphorus compounds such as Sarin, as described in Chapter 21 (WILSON et al. 1955, CHILDS et al. 1955, WILSON 1958, RUTLAND 1958, RAJAPURKAR and KOELLE 1958, HOBBIGER 1958, POZIOMEK et al. 1958, GROB and JOHNS 1958a to e, GREEN and SMITH 1958a, b, DAVIES and GREEN 1959). Reactivation by oxime is less after prolonged contact of organophosphorus inhibitor with enzyme (HOBBIGER 1955, 1956). Pyridine-2-aldoxime methiodide, TMB-4, and to a lesser extent DAM cause slight protection and very slight reactivation of human ChE's inhibited by quaternary ammonium compounds such as neostigmine and pyridostigmine, but not ambenomium (GROB and JOHNS 1958a, e) or physostigmine (KEWITZ et al. 1956).

Table 4. *Reactivators of phosphorylated cholinesterase which have been studied clinically*

Compound	Structural formula
Pyridine-2-aldoxime methiodide (P-2-AM)	
Pyridine-2-aldoxime methane-sulfonate (P2S)	
1,1'-Trimethylene-bis-(4-formyl-pyridinium bromide)-dioxime (TMB-4, EA 1814)	
Diacetyl monoxime (DAM)	$CH_3-C-C-CH_3$ with O and NOH
Monoisonitroso acetone (MINA)	$CH_3-C-CN = NOH$ with O

The inhibition of ChE's by organophosphorus compounds has been considered to occur by direct phosphorylation of some group at the active center of the enzyme, and reversal of this inhibition by oximes to be due to displacement of the alkyl phosphate group from the enzyme (WILSON 1958). Since the quaternary ammonium anti-ChE compounds do not contain a phosphorus atom, it is evident that the oximes may reverse ChE inhibition by a more general mechanism than displacement of phosphorus-containing groups.

2. Inhibition of cholinesterase enzymes by oximes

These enzymes are inhibited *in vitro* by P-2-AM and TMB-4 in concentrations above 10^{-4} M, but not by DAM in concentrations to 10^{-2} M (HOLMES and ROBINS 1955, LOOMIS 1956, BETHE et al. 1957, GROB and JOHNS 1958a, e). However, following the intravenous administration to man of 2,000 mg of P-2-AM or 250 mg of TMB-4, there is no alteration of plasma or red blood cell ChE activity.

3. Reversal by oximes of neuromuscular block produced by various anti-ChE compounds

The neuromuscular block produced in man by the intra-arterial injection of organo-phosphorus anti-ChE compounds such as Sarin, or quaternary ammonium compounds such as neostigmine, *bis*-neostigmine, pyridostigmine, *bis*-pyridostigmine, or ambenomium, is promptly and strikingly reversed in the injected extremity immediately after the intra-arterial injection of 0.05 mg of P-2-AM or DAM, or 0.005 mg of TMB-4 (GROB and JOHNS 1958a, e) (Fig. 5). The oximes also protect against the neuromuscular blocking action of these anti-ChE compounds. The effects of each of these oximes on neuromuscular block produced by organophosphorus and quaternary ammonium anti-ChE compounds are striking and equal, in contrast to the marked differences in their abilities to protect and reactivate ChE's, including that of muscle, *in vitro*. This suggests that either the enzyme in intact muscle may be

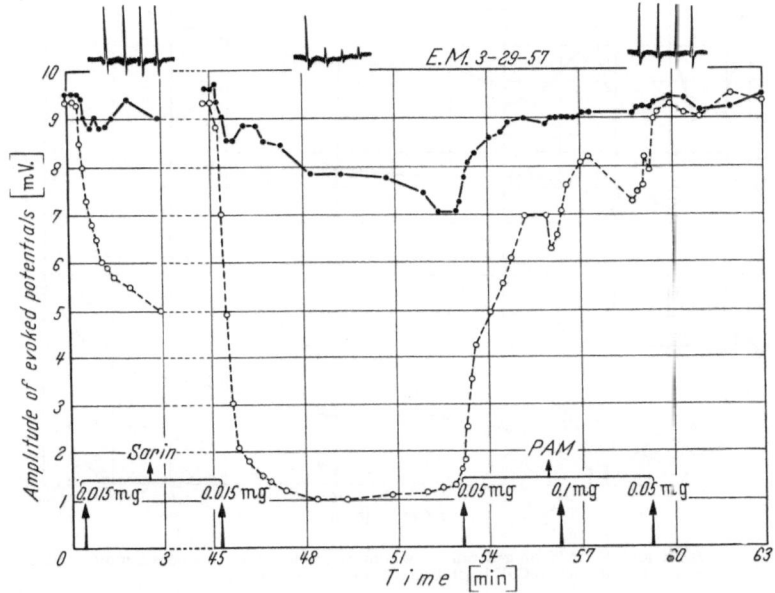

Fig. 5. Reversal by P-2-AM of the depressant effect of Sarin on evoked muscle action potentials. The amplitudes of the first (●———●) and fourth (○----○) muscle action potentials in response to a train of four nerve stimuli (40 msec apart) evoked every five seconds have been plotted, and illustrative potentials recorded above. Injections were intra-arterial. (From GROB and JOHNS 1958)

particularly accessible to the action of the oximes, or the oximes may restore or protect neuro-muscular transmission by another mechanism than restoration or protection of muscle AChE activity. Pyridine-2-aldoxime methiodide, in a concentration of 5×10^{-3} M, has been found to produce reversible inhibition of the action of ACh on isolated frog muscle (FLEISCHER et al. 1958a, b). Lower concentrations of P-2-AM potentiate the action of ACh, perhaps as a result of ChE inhibition. It is possible that the reversal by oximes of anti-ChE neuromuscular block may be due not only to reversal of ChE inhibition, but also to inhibition of the action of ACh.

4. Neuromuscular block produced by oximes

The intra-arterial administration to man of more than 40 mg of P-2-AM or 5 mg of TMB-4 produces a transient neuromuscular block, while DAM has no apparent effect (GROB and JOHNS 1958a, e). The block does not alter the effect of ACh on neuromuscular transmission, and is not reversed by ACh or neostigmine, but is increased by the prior administration of neostigmine. While the latter finding suggests that the blocking action may be due to ChE inhibition, studies in experimental animals indicate that these oximes may also have a direct action on the muscle fiber (HOLMES and ROBINS 1955).

5. Reversal by oximes of generalized weakness due to anti-ChE compounds

The intravenous administration to man of 500 to 2,000 mg of P-2-AM or DAM, or 150 to 250 mg of TMB-4, ameliorates to a moderate degree generalized weakness due to organophosphorus anti-ChE compounds such as Sarin or quaternary ammonium compounds such as neostigmine, *bis*-neostigmine, pyridostigmine, *bis*-pyridostigmine, or ambenomium (GROB and JOHNS 1958a to e) (Fig. 6). Muscular fasciculation is usually reduced to a lesser degree, but may be unchanged. Improvement begins within 30 seconds after injection of oxime, and is maximal in 5 to 10 minutes. Approximately 20 minutes later there is usually some return

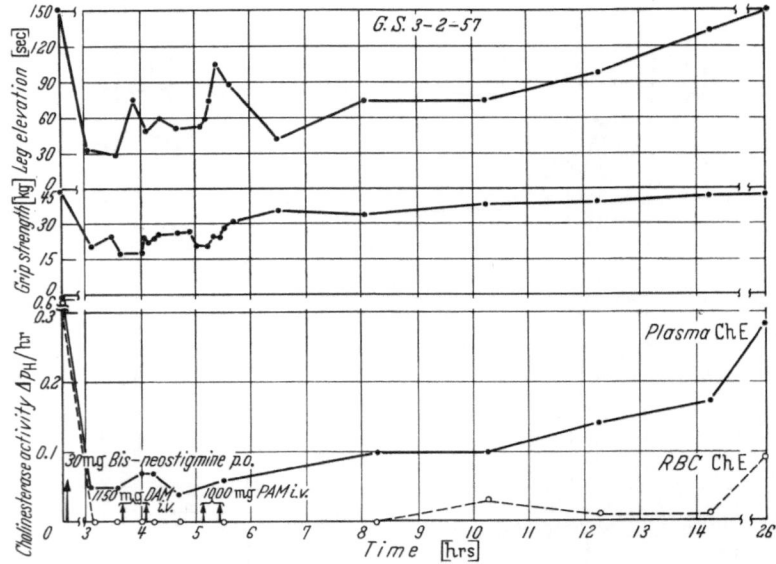

Fig. 6. Reversal by DAM and P-2-AM of generalized weakness produced by *bis*-neostigmine, and transient reversal of plasma BuChE inhibition. (From: GROB and JOHNS 1958a)

of weakness and fasciculation, but not to the original level (Fig. 6). A second injection of oxime then results in further improvement. The more severe the weakness and fasciculation, the less striking is the improvement following oxime administration. The increase in strength is not as dramatic as the reversal in neuromuscular block that occurs following the intra-arterial injection of much smaller doses of oxime.

6. Effect of oximes on other manifestations of anti-ChE intoxication

GROB and JOHNS (1958a to e) found that the intravenous administration of 2,000 mg of P-2-AM or DAM did not appreciably affect the muscarinic symptoms produced by Sarin or quaternary ammonium anti-ChE compounds (sweating, nausea, vomiting, abdominal cramps, diarrhea, and bradycardia). In contrast, the administration of atropine sulfate (1 mg i.v.) promptly ameliorated these symptoms, but had no effect on muscular weakness or fasciculation. The effect of oximes on central neural symptoms due to anti-ChE compounds was more difficult to evaluate, but these did not seem to be affected as much as the muscular weakness.

NAMBA and HIRAKI (1958), on the other hand, reported that P-2-AM relieved not only weakness, fasciculation, and muscle cramps due to Parathion poisoning, but also disturbances of consciousness and some muscarinic signs such as salivation and excessive bronchial secretion. Signs and symptoms of Parathion intoxication which persisted after P-2-AM administration included headache, miosis, pallor, tachypnea, slurred speech, vertigo, nausea, and paresthesias in the extremities. In some patients who had previously received atropine, the administration of P-2-AM and relief of anti-ChE intoxication were sometimes followed by the appearance of signs of atropinization. KARLOG et al. (1958) and YAMADA (1957) also observed clearing of consciousness following the administration of P-2-AM to patients who had swallowed Parathion with suicidal intent.

The ability of oximes to reverse the muscarinic and central neural effects of anti-ChE intoxication appears to be limited, and is clearly less than their ability to reverse neuromuscular block. Reactivation by P-2-AM of ganglionic ChE's inhibited by DFP has been demonstrated (KOELLE 1957a, RAJAPURKAR and KOELLE 1958), but little reactivation of brain ChE inhibited by OMPA or Para-oxon could be shown (KEWITZ and NACHMANSOHN 1957). The latter finding may be due to failure of quaternary ammonium compounds such as P-2-AM to penetrate into the central nervous system.

7. Reversal by P-2-AM and DAM of plasma and red blood cell cholinesterase inhibition produced by anti-ChE compounds

The intravascular administration of 200 to 2,000 mg of P-2-AM or DAM, or of 150 to 250 mg of TMB-4, produces slight to moderate reversal of plasma and red blood cell ChE inhibition by organophosphorus compounds such as Sarin or OMPA, or quaternary ammonium compounds such as neostigmine, bis-neostigmine, pyridostigmine, bis-pyridostigmine, or ambenomium (GROB and JOHNS 1958a, e) (Fig. 6). The increase is usually transient, and is shorter and less marked than the increase in strength. In some instances the ChE activity remains elevated, although this may be due at least in part to spontaneous restoration. The degree and dura-tion of restoration of ChE activity varies inversely with the degree of ChE in-hibition and is slight when the latter is nearly complete. Red blood cell AChE inhibition produced by Parathion poisoning has been reported to be completely reversed within 10 minutes after the injection of P-2-AM (NAMBA and HIRAKI 1958). Plasma BuChE inhibition is only transiently reversed, but returns to normal twice as rapidly as in untreated patients. Pyridine-2-aldoxime methiodide is said to reactivate AChE's, such as those of red cells, brain, and muscle, to a greater extent than the BuChE of plasma (KEWITZ et al. 1956).

8. Use of oximes in the management of anti-ChE intoxication

In contrast to atropine, intravenous administration of 1,000 to 2,000 mg of P-2-AM (500 mg/min) or DAM (200 mg/min), or of 250 mg TMB-4 (25 mg/min), improves muscular strength, and prompt administration of adequate doses di-minishes the necessity for, or duration of mechanical measures to sustain respira-tion. In severe anti-ChE intoxication the initial injection of oxime may not adequately relieve weakness, or the relief may be transient, necessitating a second injection in about 20 minutes.

Since weakness may develop rapidly in the course of severe anti-ChE intoxica-tion, mechanical measures to sustain respiration are still needed in some patients. The intravenous administration of adequate doses of atropine also remains an important adjunct in treatment, since the oximes do not appear to reverse the muscarinic manifestations of anti-ChE intoxication, and their ability to reverse central neural effects remains to be demonstrated (GROB and JOHNS 1958a, LADELL

1958). In experimental animals the prophylactic and therapeutic effects of oxime in anti-ChE poisoning are greatly enhanced by the addition of atropine; in fact, combined action of the two drugs is more than additive (KEWITZ et al. 1956, WILLS et al. 1957, BROWN et al. 1957). Oxime or atropine alone protects most species against approximately 2 LD_{50}'s of Sarin, while the combination protects guinea pigs and rabbits against 40 LD_{50}'s, and mice and rats against 4 to 8 LD_{50}'s, depending on the oxime exployed (DAVIES et al. 1959).

On the other hand, NAMBA and HIRAKI (1958) have questioned the necessity of administering atropine in addition to oxime. They treated 39 patients with Parathion poisoning with P-2-AM, in most instances without atropine. In all but five of the more severe cases, signs of Parathion poisoning almost completely disappeared after the intravenous injection of about 1 gram of P-2-AM. In the more severe cases, further improvement occurred following the injection of additional P-2-AM, except for one patient who died 8 hours after onset of symptoms despite the prompt intravenous administration of 2 grams of P-2-AM and 2 mg of atropine. NAMBA and HIRAKI (1958) observed in almost all instances the disappearance not only of weakness, fasciculation, and skeletal muscle cramps, but also of salivation, bronchial secretions, vomiting, pulmonary rales, and disturbance of consciousness. In spite of these encouraging reports, however, it seems advisable to administer atropine in conjunction with oxime in the management of anti-ChE poisoning, particularly in severe cases.

It is desirable that oxime be administered as soon after onset of symptoms as possible, to enhance the efficacy of treatment and to prevent progression of intoxication. However, the time-limit for maximal efficacy of injected drug is not known. Reversal of neuromuscular block has occurred when oxime was administered as long as four hours after absorption of the anti-ChE compound (GROB and JOHNS 1958a).

Rapidity of intravascular injection of oxime also appears to be advantageous in reversing anti-ChE neuromuscular block. Although slow infusion has been employed by some (NAMBA and HIRAKI 1958), it may not be the optimal mode of administration. The reversal of neuromuscular block that occurs locally following the intra-arterial injection of as little as 0.05 mg of P-2-AM or DAM, or 0.001 mg of TMB-4, is more striking than the general improvement that follows the intravenous injection at a much slower rate of 2,000 mg of P-2-AM or DAM or 250 mg of TMB-4. Since the peak concentration of oxime reaching the affected muscles is believed to be many times higher after intravenous injection of these doses, it appears that the rapidity of intra-arterial administration may be a factor in its greater efficacy, and that rapid intravenous injection may therefore be desirable. However, injection of P-2-AM more rapidly than 500 mg/min may result in transient weakness, and injection of DAM more rapidly than 200 mg/min may produce central neural symptoms and reduction in blood pressure.

Pyridine-2-aldoxime methiodide has proved to be more effective than DAM because it can be injected more rapidly, and most experience in clinical management has been gained with this compound. The former compound has the disadvantage that very high local concentrations produce neuromuscular block, which is enhanced by prior exposure to an anti-ChE compound. The systemic dose of P-2-AM that will produce generalized weakness is not known, but is probably several times the therapeutic dose. Pyridine-2-aldoxime methiodide and DAM are not highly soluble in water and hence are available in aqueous concentration of only 50 mg/ml. While this helps insure against too rapid administration, it necessitates the injection of 20 to 40 ml of solution. Pyridine aldoxime lactate, chloride, and methane sulfonate (P2S) are more soluble than P-2-AM and can be prepared in higher concentration. However, there is no reason to believe that these derivatives are more effective than P-2-AM. There is no evidence that the intramuscular or oral administration of any oxime is effective in the clinical management of anti-ChE intoxication, although the former route has had limited efficacy in experimental animals. Furthermore, in severe intoxication reduction of peripheral blood flow may further slow absorption by these routes. It is possible that intra-muscular or oral administration of oxime may prove to be of some value in preventing anti-ChE intoxication in individuals who are exposed without adequate protective measures. NAMBA and HIRAKI (1958) have observed that farmers who received 1 gram of P-2-AM orally daily excreted more *p*-nitrophenol in the urine after spraying Parathion than did those not receiving P-2-AM. Since P-2-AM is poorly absorbed from the gastrointestinal tract, possibly owing to its limited solubility, pyridine aldoxime lactate, chloride, or methanesulfonate (P2S), or TMB-4, would appear to be more suitable for trial as prophylactic agents.

9. Symptoms produced by oximes

The intravenous administration of 2,000 mg of P-2-AM to man at the rate of 100 to 300 mg/min, or of 260 mg of TMB-4 at the rate of 20 mg/min, produces no signs or symptoms, and no change in blood pressure or cardiac rate (GROB and JOHNS 1958a to e). More rapid injection of P-2-AM may result in transient mild weakness, diplopia, blurred vision, dizziness, impairment of accommodation, and occasionally headache, nausea, and tachycardia (JAGER and STAGG 1958). The oral administration of 1 to 10 g of P-2-AM produces a bitter taste beginning 30 minutes after ingestion and lasting one to two hours (NAMBA and HIRAKI 1958). This appears even after administration by gastric tube. Occasionally there is also rhinitis and a sensation of fatigue of the jaws.

The intravenous administration of 500 to 2,000 mg of DAM at the rate of 60 to 300 mg/min produces a burning sensation at the site of injection radiating up the injected vein, followed by moderate giddiness, drowsiness, a sensation of warmth and tingling in the abdomen and chest, tachycardia, slight increase or decrease in blood pressure, and mild postural hypotension (GROB and JOHNS 1958). Bitter taste, paresthesias and decreased position sense in the extremities, decreased sweating, transient loss of consciousness, clonic movements of the head, and decreased amplitude of the electroencephalogram and of the T wave of the electro-cardiogram may also occasionally occur (JAGER and STAGG 1958). These effects last from one to five minutes after cessation of injection.

The doses of oximes that are lethal for man are not known.

The intraperitoneal LD_{50} of P-2-AM in mice is 190 mg/kg and in rats 75 mg/kg, while that of DAM is 900 mg/kg in mice and 25 mg/kg in rats (DULTZ et al. 1957). The LD_{50} of TMB-4 is approximately half that of P-2-AM. Toxic effects occur following repeated daily administration of half the median lethal doses. The nature of the acute toxicity of these com-pounds is still obscure even in experimental animals (ASKEW et al. 1956, DAVIES and WILLEY 1958). Death from DAM appears to result from central nervous system depression, and TMB-4 causes depression of respiration and blood pressure, and, to a lesser extent, of neuro-muscular transmission. No consistent pathologic changes have yet been noted. It seems likely that in man, as in most experimental animals, there may be about a five-fold difference between the doses effective in anti-ChE intoxication (15 to 30 mg/kg of P-2-AM or DAM, or 3 to 4 mg/kg of TMB-4, i.v.) and the lethal doses. It is not known whether the maximally tolerated doses of oxime are higher in the presence of anti-ChE intoxication, as is the case with atropine.

10. Blood levels and renal excretion of oximes

The intravenous administration of 1,000 mg (15 mg/kg) of P-2-AM or DAM produces a plasma concentration of approximately 2 mg/100 ml (JAGER et al. 1958). Pyridine-2-aldoxime methiodide is removed primarily by renal excretion, and at this dose has a half-life in the blood of 0.9 hour. The renal clearance of P-2-AM is almost three times that of creatinine, with 80% of the injected material appearing in the urine as an altered derivative within six hours. In contrast, DAM is removed more slowly, primarily by means other than renal excretion, and has a half-life of 7.2 hours. The renal clearance of DAM is only 6% that of creatinine, and less than 10% of the injected material appears in the urine in six hours. Observations in experimental animals indicate that the liver is the main site of destruction of DAM (Dultz et al. 1957). Both P-2-AM and DAM appear to be widely dispersed in total body water except that P-2-AM, like most quaternary ammonium compounds, does not enter the spinal fluid; DAM, a tertiary amine, does.

Following intramuscular injection of P-2-AM or DAM, the maximal plasma concentration is reached in 10 minutes, after which the plasma level declines at approximately the same rate as after intravenous injection.

The intravenous administration of 260 mg (4.3 mg/kg) of TMB-4 results in a plasma level of 1.9 mg/100 ml, which declines to half this level in approximately an hour (Sprague et al. 1958).

IV. Other drugs that have been studied

A large number of anticholinergic drugs, including hyoscine, scopolamine (Wescoe et al. 1948), Panparnit (Wilhelmi and Domenjoz 1951), and Buscopan (Deichmann and Rakoczy 1953), has been studied, but none has proved superior to atropine in the management of anti-ChE intoxication (Parkes and Sacra 1954, Karczmar and Long 1958, O'Leary et al. 1958). Ganglionic blocking agents such as hexamethonium and pentamethonium, and magnesium salts (Murtha et al. 1955), thiosulfate, and chlorocobalamin have limited efficacy as adjuncts to atropine in experimental animals, but have not been shown to be of practical value in man. d-Tubocurarine and N-benzyl atropinium can be shown to antagonize anti-ChE neuromuscular block, but the danger of paralytic overdose precludes their use for this purpose (Grob et al. 1956c). Centrally depressant drugs such as barbiturates, and anticonvulsants such as diphenylhydantoin (Dilantin) and trimethadione (Tridione), may rarely be needed to control convulsions due to anti-ChE intoxication that are unrelieved by atropine (Himwich et al. 1950), but their value as adjuncts to atropine and oxime has not been demonstrated (see Chapter 20).

When the ChE's are combined with reversible quaternary ammonium inhibitors, they are protected from inhibition by organophosphorus compounds (Koster 1946, Koelle 1946, Depierre and Martin 1958). However, following exposure to the latter, there is enhanced reactivity to any subsequently administered anti-ChE agent, so that quaternary inhibitors would be harmful as therapeutic agents, and have no practical value in the prophylaxis of anti-ChE poisoning.

The injection of preparations of ChE's has no effect on anti-ChE intoxication, presumably because the enzymes do not reach the sites of local accumulation of ACh in muscle, glands, or nervous tissue (Beck 1951). Chlorinated hydrocarbons (Ball et al. 1954), vitamin B_{12}, and numerous other substances have also been ineffective (see Chapter 20).

V. Removal of secretions and maintenance of patent airway

In severe anti-ChE intoxication there is increased bronchial secretion and salivation, which may become very profuse and interfere with respiratory exchange, particularly in patients who develop some airway obstruction as a result of weakness of the pharyngeal, tongue, and respiratory muscles and, to a lesser extent, of bronchoconstriction. If the casualty is having excessive bronchial secretion and salivation, he should be placed in the prone position with the head to one side, and the foot of the litter or bed elevated to promote drainage. If airway obstruction occurs, the collar should be loosened, the mandible elevated and pulled forward, the tongue pulled forward, and saliva and mucus cleared periodically from the mouth and pharynx with cloth-covered fingers and, if possible, by means of suction through a catheter introduced through the mouth or nose. An oropharyngeal or nasopharyngeal airway may then be inserted and suction carried out intermittently as needed through and around the airway, which will generally be tolerated only by unconscious or flaccid patients (Grob 1956a, Elam et al. 1960).

If the upper airway remains obstructed and adequate exchange of air does not occur in spite of good efforts to carry out artificial respiration, an endotracheal catheter may be inserted.

This should be attempted only in a casualty who is cyanotic because of airway obstruction and who is also either unconscious or flaccid and therefore unable to struggle and resist efforts at intubation. The subject is placed on his back, with the head lifted straight up until the shoulders are slightly elevated, and under direct vision a laryngoscope is passed down the dorsum of the tongue until the epiglottis is visualized. It is then passed under the epiglottis, which is lifted to visualize the vocal cords. The endotracheal tube, lubricated with water-soluble jelly, is inserted into the glottis with a rolling motion and gently passed into the larynx and trachea for a distance of about 3 inches. A cuffed tube is preferable, as this prevents aspiration of secretions more completely than does an ordinary tube or a tracheotomy. When the tube is in place, a roll of gauze is inserted between the teeth to prevent the tube from being bitten as the patient recovers, and adhesive is tied about the endotracheal tube and gauze roll (separately) and taped to the face. Suction may then be carried out by means of a No. 16 catheter passed through the endotracheal tube. If air exchange through the endotracheal tube is not evident, the tube should be removed and, if the airway is still obstructed, another attempt to pass it should be made. If the subject is able to struggle and resist passage of the endotracheal tube, attempts to pass it should be discontinued, as this procedure will be difficult and attempts to carry it out may result in injury and edema of the larynx. The endotracheal tube may be removed when the casualty regains consciousness and is breathing spontaneously.

It should not be left in place more than 48 hours, as this produces edema of the larynx and results in airway obstruction when the tube is removed. In the rare patient who requires an artifical airway for more than 48 hours, a tracheotomy should be performed prior to withdrawal of the endotracheal tube.

VI. Artificial respiration

If respiration is severely impaired, death may occur in a matter of minutes unless an effective method of artificial respiration is begun immediately and maintained continuously until spontaneous respiration is resumed. In severe casualties this may take several hours. In spite of the concomitant administration of atropine to reduce secretions and bronchoconstriction and careful attention to patency of the airway, increased airway resistance usually renders artificial respiration more difficult, requiring greater inspiratory pressure than in respiratory failure due to most other causes. Fortunately, airway resistance may diminish following initial inflation of the lungs, making subsequent exchange less difficult (ELAM et al. 1956). Care must be taken to avoid delivery of excessive inspiratory pressure against high airway resistance, as this favors movement of air into the esophagus and gastric dilatation. If the gastric contents are not removed by stomach tube, aspiration and pneumonia may occur.

Obstruction of the airway above the larynx is the commonest cause of failure of artificial respiration. It is essential that this be prevented by extending the head at the atlanto-occipital joint (sniffing position) and displacing the lower jaw forward. The hands are placed at the angle of the mandibles, which are pulled up and forward, and the head tilted back as far as possible, in order to prevent the base of the tongue from blocking the airway. In the absence of a mechanical aid to artificial respiration, the only way in which the airway can be held open in this manner, and respiration maintained simultaneously by a single attendant, is by means of mouth-to-nose, or mouth-to-mouth respiration.

1. Mouth-to-nose and mouth-to-mouth respiration

As indicated above, these are the most effective means of manual artificial respiration and the only methods that permit the attendant's hands to be free to pull the mandibles forward and up and to tilt the head back while respiratory exchange is being maintained (ELAM et al. 1960). They also permit the attendant more easily to evaluate airway obstruction and adequacy of exchange. In the paralyzed patient these methods achieve better exchange than other manual procedures (ELAM et al. 1954; GORDON et al. 1958; SAFAR 1957, 1958; SAFAR et al. 1958). Mouth-to-nose respiration, in which the rescuer breathes into the patient's nose, is preferable to the mouth-to-mouth procedure, as it is less likely to cause gastric dilatation. In mouth-to-nose respiration the rescuer exhales into the patient's nose while the mouth is sealed with the thumbs, and the remaining fingers pull the mandibles forward and up. The uvula acts as a flap valve to prevent entry of air into the stomach. In the small proportion of persons who have bilateral nasal obstruction, mouth-to-mouth respiration can be employed. The attendant peels the lips back and exhales into the mouth, sealing the nostrils with the thumbs. Difficulty in this procedure may be encountered in early asphyxia, before consciousness is lost, as the increase in blood pCO_2 that occurs may increase the tone of skeletal muscle, including that of the jaws, and result in trismus. If this occurs, mouth-to-nose respiration must be employed. In late asphyxia, the muscles become relaxed, particularly if the patient is unconscious, so that breathing into the mouth becomes feasible. In an atmosphere that is contaminated, mask-to-mask artificial respiration may be carried out, with the attendant respiring the casualty by means of a tube connecting the expiratory outlet of the former's gas mask to the inlet of the latter's mask. The outlet valve of the casualty's mask permits passive expiration (ELAM et al. 1956). The attendant's hands are free to elevate the casualty's jaw to keep the upper airway open.

In mouth-to-nose, mouth-to-mouth, or mask-to-mask respiration the rescuer doubles his normal inflation volume of 600 ml and breathes at a normal rate or slightly faster, 12 to 20 times a minute, so that mild hyperventilation overcomes the slight hypoxia of expired air and maintains normal exchange of oxygen and carbon dioxide in the casualty (GREEN et al. 1957, 1959; ELAM et al. 1958). The rescuer can maintain sufficient ventilation for himself and the casualty for over an hour without fatigue, although mild giddiness and paresthesias attributable to hyperventilation occasionally occur.

2. Other manual methods of artificial respiration

The manual methods of artificial respiration which produce both active inspiration and active expiration, the so-called "push-pull" methods, result in more than twice as much pulmonary ventilation as methods which produce only active expiration (e.g., SCHAEFER prone-pressure) or active inspiration (e.g., EMERSON hip-lift). The push-pull methods include the back-pressure, arm-lift (modified HOLGER-NEILSEN), hip-lift, back-pressure (SCHAEFER-EMERSON-IVY), and arm-lift, chest-pressure (SYLVESTER) methods. All the push-pull methods are capable of maintaining arterial oxygen saturation at near normal levels (GORDON et al. 1955), provided that the upper airway does not become obstructed as a result of flaccid paralysis of the pharynx and tongue. With a paralyzed or unconscious patient, one attendant would have to elevate the jaw and hyperextend the head while another applied any of these methods of artificial respiration.

3. Hand-operated breathing bag or bellows

Artificial respiration can be effectively maintained by means of a rubber bag, kept inflated by an oxygen tank and rhythmically deflated by one hand while the other hand applies a face mask and supports the mandible. A bellows can be used for the same purpose, provided that it is attached to a mask which can be held to the face by the hand supporting the mandible while the opposite hand compresses the bellows. The latter can also be used in a contaminated atmosphere if it is equipped with a canister at the intake valve and with an expiratory valve.

4. Mechanical artificial respiration

This may be carried out by either the negative pressure body (tank) respirator or the positive pressure-cycled resuscitator, preferably with an endotracheal tube in place to maintain patency of the upper airway. The body respirator has proved to be effective and has the advantage of permitting more efficient suction of secretions from the pharynx or endotracheal tube (GROB 1956a). The pressure-cycled resuscitator should have a higher pressure range of operation ($+27$ and -15 mm of mercury) than is commonly employed, in order to permit adequate inspiratory pressure to overcome airway resistance (ELAM et al. 1956). It should also be equipped with a manually controlled override with which the inflating pressure can be temporarily increased to $+35$ mm of mercury when necessary. If an endotracheal tube has not been inserted, the mandible should be elevated manually and the head hyperextended, as in other forms of artificial respiration.

VII. Management of convulsions and of apprehension; rest; prevention of pulmonary infection

1. Management of convulsions

If convulsions occur, tonic and clonic spasm of the respiratory muscles and of the glottis may greatly increase the difficulties of artificial respiration (GROB 1956a). While the seizures are diminished following the administration of large doses of atropine, and possibly of oxime, and are likely to be followed by flaccid paralysis during which ventilation can be better performed, they are occasionally so severe and prolonged as to interfere seriously with respiration and to threaten life. In this situation, an anticonvulsant or muscle-relaxant drug may be administered intravenously, but excessive doses must be avoided lest respiration be depressed. Facilities must be available for intubation and artificial respiration. Trimethadione (Tridione), which is administered in doses of 1 g every 15 minutes up to a maximum of 5 g, has less depressant effect on respiration than the barbiturates. If trimethadione is not available or proves ineffective, sodium thiopental (Pentothal) (in 2.5% solution) may be administered, or d-tubocurarine may be injected in doses of 40 units every five or more minutes up to a maximum of 200 units (GROB et al. 1950).

2. Rest and relief of apprehension

Since physical activity tends to increase weakness in patients with anti-ChE intoxication, and may be followed by exacerbation of generalized symptoms, rest is desirable. If the casualty is apprehensive, he may be given a barbiturate by mouth in doses sufficient to allay apprehension and to produce mild sedation but not sufficient to produce marked drowsiness. This may be achieved by 0.1 gram of sodium pentobarbital by mouth, repeated in one-half hour and then every six hours, if necessary. Morphine should not administered, as its respiratory depressant action may be enhanced by anti-ChE compounds.

3. Prevention of pulmonary infection

In casualties who have had severe respiratory depression or increased bronchial secretion, and for whom the absence of hypersensitivity can be ascertained, penicillin or a broad spectrum antibiotic may be administered intramuscularly to prevent or treat pneumonia. The occurrence of atelectasis may necessitate tracheal and bronchial aspiration.

VIII. Summary of treatment of anti-ChE intoxication

1. Termination of exposure

Removal of casualty or use of gas mask if atmosphere is contaminated; removal of contaminated clothing; washing of contaminated skin or eyes with copious amounts of water; gastric lavage if ingestion has occurred; application of tourniquet if exposure is by percutaneous or parenteral routes of entry.

2. Atropine administration

In severe intoxication, particularly by organophosphorus compounds, 2 to 4 mg intravenously, followed by 2 mg every three to ten minutes until muscarinic symptoms and signs disappear, and whenever they reappear; a total of 24 to 48 mg may be required during the first day; in less severe intoxication, 2 mg intravenously or intramuscularly, repeated at ten to thirty-minute intervals until muscarinic symptoms are relieved; maintenance of a mild degree of atropinization for twenty-four to forty-eight hours.

3. Oxime administration

In severe intoxication 2,000 mg of P-2-AM (500 mg/min) or DAM (200 mg/min) or 250 mg TMB-4 (25 mg/min) intravenously; repetition of dose after 20 minutes if weakness is not relieved, or recurs; in moderate intoxication, one-half the above doses, repeated if weakness is not relieved or recurs.

4. Removal of secretions and maintenance of patent airway

Prone position with head down and to one side, mandible elevated, and tongue pulled forward; clearing of mouth and pharynx with finger or by suction; in unconscious or flaccid patients, oropharyngeal or nasopharyngeal airway, or endotracheal intubation if airway obstruction persists.

5. Artificial respiration when necessary

Mouth-to-nose, mouth-to-mouth, mask-to-mask, bellows, or mechanical.

6. Alleviation of convulsions if these interfere with respiration and are not relieved by atropine

Trimethadion (Tridione), 1 g intravenously every fifteen minutes up to a maximum of 5 g, or sodium thiopental (2.5% solution) intravenously.

Literature

ANNIS, J. W., and J. W. WILLIAMS: Change in electrolytes in case of parathion poisoning. J. Amer. med. Ass. 152, 594—596 (1953).

ARANOW, H. jr., P. F. A. HOEFER and L. P. ROWLAND: The long-acting anticholinesterase drugs in the management of myasthenia gravis. J. chron. Dis. 6, 113—115 (1958).

ASKEW, B. M.: Oximes and hydroxamic acids as antidotes in anticholinesterase poisoning. Brit. J. Pharmacol. 11, 417—423 (1956).

— D. R. DAVIES, A. L. GREEN and R. HOLMES: The nature of the toxicity of 2-oxo-oximes. Brit. J. Pharmacol. 11, 424—427 (1956).

AUGUSTINSSON, K. B.: The normal variation of human blood cholinesterase activity. Acta physiol. scand. 35, 40—52 (1955).

BAETJER, A. M., and R. SMITH: Effect of environmental temperature on reaction of mice to Parathion, an anticholinesterase agent. Amer. J. Physiol. 86, 39—46 (1956).

BAKER, J. P., and J. D. FARLEY: Toxic psychosis following atropine eye-drops. Brit. med. J. 1958 II, 1390—1391.

BARNES, J. M.: Toxic hazards of certain pesticides to man. Wld. Hlth. Org. Monogr. Ser. (1953).

—, and F. A. DENZ: Experimental demyelination with organo-phosphorus compounds. J. Path. Bact. 65, 597—605 (1953).

—, and J. I. DUFF: The role of cholinesterase at the myoneural junction. Brit. J. Pharmacol. 8, 334—339 (1953).

BARSTAD, J. A. B.: The effect of d-tubocurarine on the neuromuscular blocks caused by diisopropylfluorophosphate and acetylcholine. Arch. int. Pharmacodyn. 107, 4—20 (1956).

BECK, I. T.: Pharmacological study of injected cholinesterase. Brit. J. Pharmacol. 6, 144—154 (1951).

BERGNER, D. H., and S. H. DURLACHER: Histochemical detection of fatal anticholinesterase poisoning Amer. J. Path. 27, 1011—1021 (1951).

BERRY, W. K., and E. C. LOVETT: Cholinesterase and neuromuscular block. J. Physiol. (Lond.) 115, 46 (1951).

BIDSTRUP, P. L., J. A. BONNELL, A. G. BECKETT: Paralysis following poisoning by a new organic phosphorus insecticide (Mipafox). Brit. Med. J. 1953 I, 1068.

BIDSTRUP, L. P.: Anticholinesterase paralysis in man following poisoning by cholinesterase inhibitors. Chem. and Ind. 1954, 675—676.

BLANK, I. H., R. D. GRIESEMER and E. GOULD: The penetration of an anticholinesterase agent (sarin) into skin. Rate of penetration into excised human skin. J. invest. Derm. 29, 299 to 309 (1957).

BROWN, R. V., A. M. KUNKEL, L. M. SOMERS and J. H. WILLS: Pyridine-2-aldoxime methiodide in the treatment of poisoning by sarin or tabun, with notes on its pharmacology. J. Pharmacol. exp. Ther. 120, 276—284 (1957).

BURGEN, A. S. V., and F. HOBBIGER: The inhibition of cholinesterases by alkylphosphates and alkylphenolphosphates. Brit. J. Pharmacol. 6, 593—605 (1951).

BURNS, B. D., and W. D. M. PATON: Depolarization of the motor end-plate by decamethonium and acetylcholine. J. Physiol. (Lond.) 115, 41 (1951).

CALLAWAY, S., and D. R. DAVIES: The association of blood cholinesterase levels with the susceptibility of animals to Sarin and Ethyl Pyrophosphate poisoning. Brit. J. Pharmacol. 12, 382 (1957).

CHAMBERLIN, H. R., and R. E. COOKE: Organic phosphate anticholinesterase insecticide poisoning. Amer. J. Dis. Child. 85, 164—172 (1953).

CHILDS, A. F., D. R. DAVIES, A. L. GREEN and J. P. RUTLAND: The reactivation by oximes and hydroxamic acids of cholinesterase inhibited by organo-phosphorus compounds. Brit. J. Pharmacol. 10, 462—465 (1955).

CONLEY, B. E.: Health problems of vaporizing and fumigating devices for insecticides. J. Amer. med. Ass. 152, 1232—1234 (1953).

CRAIG, A. B., and G. S. WOODSON: Observations on the effects of exposure to nerve gas. Clinical observations and cholinesterase depression. Amer. J. med. Sci. 238, 13—17 (1959).

CULLUMBINE, H., and P. DIRNHUBER: Oral and bronchial fluids in poisoning with anti-cholinesterase. J. Pharm. (Lond.) 7, 580—585 (1955).

DAVIES, D. R.: Cholinesterases and the mode of action of some anticholinesterases. J. Pharm. (Lond.) 6, 1—26 (1954).

—, and A. L. GREEN: The chemotherapy of poisoning by organophosphate anticholinesterases. Brit. J. industr. Med. 16, 128—134 (1959).

— — and G. L. WILLEY: 2-Hydroxyiminomethyl-N-methylpyridinium methanesulphonate and atropine in the treatment of severe organophosphate poisoning. Brit. J. Pharmacol. 14, 1—5 (1959).

— P. HOLLAND and M. J. RUMENS: The relationship between the chemical structure and neurotoxicity of alkyl organophosphorus compounds. Brit.J.Pharmacol.15, 271—278(1960).

—, and G. L. WILLEY: The toxicity of 2-hydroxyiminomethyl-N-methylpyridinium methane-sulphonate (p2S). Brit. J. Pharmacol. 13, 202 (1958).

DEBURGH, DALY, M., and P. G. WRIGHT: The effects of anticholinesterases upon peripheral vascular resistance in the dog. J. Physiol. (Lond.) 133, 475—497 (1956).

DECANDOLE, C. A., W. W. DOUGLAS, E. C. LOVATT, R. HOLMES, K. E. V. SPENCER, R. W. TORRANCE and K. M. WILSON: The failure of respiration in death by anticholinesterase poisoning. Brit. J. Pharmacol. 8, 466—475 (1953).

DEICHMANN, W. B., P. BROWN and C. DOWNING: Unusual protective action of a new emulsifier for the handling of organic phosphates. Science 116, 221 (1952).

—, and R. RAKOCZY: Buscopan in treatment of experimental poisoning by parathion, methyl parathion and systox. A.M.A. Arch. industr. Hyg. 7, 152—156 (1953).

DEL CASTILLO, J., and B. KATZ: Biophysical aspects of neuromuscular transmission. Progr. Biophys. 6, 121—170 (1956).

DELGA, J.: Les anticholinestérasiques organophosphores. Actualités Pharmacol. 10, 47—87 (1957).

DEPIERRE, F., and MARTIN: Anticholinestérasiques. Protection in vitro par les ammonium quaterinaires. C. R. Acad. Sci. (Paris) 246, 1 183—186 (1958).

DIRNHUBER, P., and H. CULLUMBINE: The effect of anticholinesterase agents on the rat's blood pressure. Brit. J. Pharmacol. 10, 12—15 (1955).

DIXON, E. M.: Dilatation of the pupils in parathion poisoning. J. Amer. med. Ass. 163, 444 to 445 (1957).

DOUGLAS, W. W., and P. B. V. MATTHEWS: Acute tetraethylpyrophosphate poisoning in cats and its modification by atropine or hyoscine. J. Physiol. (Lond.) 116, 202—218 (1952).

1022   Literature

DuBois, K. P., J. Doull and J. M. Coon: Studies on the toxicity and pharmacological action
    of octamethyl pyrophosphoramide (OMPA: Pestox III) J. Pharmacol. exp. Ther. **99**, 376
    to 393 (1950).
Dultz, L., M. A. Epstein, G. Freeman, E. H. Gray and W. B. Weil: Studies on a group
    of oximes as therapeutic compounds in Sarin poisoning. J. Pharmacol. exp. Ther. **119**,
    522—531 (1957).
Durham, W. F., T. B. Gaines and W. J. Hayes jr.: Paralytic and related effects of certain
    organic phosphorus compounds. A.M.A. Arch. industr. Hlth **13**, 326—330 (1956).
Durlacher, S. H., W. G. Banfield and A. D. Bergner: Post-mortem pulmonary edema.
    Yale J. Biol. Med. **22**, 565—572 (1949/50).
Elam, J. O., E. S. Brown and J. D. Elder jr.: Artificial respiration by mouth to mask
    methods. A study of the respiratory gas exchange of paralyzed patients ventilated by
    operator's expired air. New Engl. J. Med. **250**, 749—754 (1954).
— J. A. Clements, E. S. Brown and N. W. Elton: Artificial respiration for the nerve gas
    casualty. U. S. armed Forces med. J. **7**, 797—810 (1956).
— D. G. Green, M. A. Schneider, H. M. Ruben, A. S. Gordon, R. F. Hustead, D. W.
    Benson, J. A. Clements and A. Ruben: Head-tilt method of oral resuscitation. J. Amer.
    med. Ass. **172**, 812—815 (1960).
— — E. S. Brown and J. A. Clements: Oxygen and carbon dioxide exchange and energy
    cost of expired air resuscitation. J. Amer. med. Ass. **167**, 328—334 (1958).
Erdmann, W. D., u. D. Heye: Analyse der erregenden und lähmenden Wirkung von Alkyl-
    phosphaten (Parathion, Paraoxon, Systox) am isolierten Kaninchendarm. Naunyn-
    Schmiedeberg's Arch. exp. Path. Pharmak. **232**, 507—521 (1958).
—, u. L. Lendle: Vergiftungen mit esteraseblockierenden Insecticiden aus der Gruppe der
    organischen Phosphosaure-Ester (E 605 und Verwandte). Ergebn. inn. Med. Kinderheilk.
    10, 104—184 (1958).
Fatt, P.: Biophysics of junctional transmission. Physiol. Rev. **34**, 674 (1954).
Faust, J.: Poisoning due to tetraethylpyrophosphate. J. Amer. med. Ass. **141**, 192—193 (1949).
Fleisher, J. H., J. P. Corrigan and J. W. Howard: Potentiation of the response of frog
    rectus muscle to acetylcholine by isopropyl methyl phosphonofluoridate and its modifica-
    tion by pyridine-2-aldoxime methiodide. Brit. J. Pharmacol. **13**, 291—295 (1958a).
— J. W. Howard and J. P. Corrigan: Effect of pyridine aldoximes on response of frog rectus
    muscle to acetylcholine. Brit. J. Pharmacol. **13**, 288—290 (1958b).
Fredriksson, T.: Pharmacological properties of methyl-fluorophosphorylcholines. Two syn-
    thetic cholinergic drugs. Arch. int. Pharmacodyn. **113**, 101—113 (1957).
— Further studies on fluoro-phosphorylcholines. Pharmacological properties of two new
    analogues. Arch. int. Pharmacodyn. **115**, 474—482 (1958).
Freeman, G., and M. A. Epstein: Therapeutic factors in survival after lethal cholinesterase
    inhibition by phosphorus insecticides. New Engl. J. Med. **253**, 266—271 (1955).
Friedman, A. M., and H. E. Himwich: Effect of age on lethality of di-isopropyl fluoro-
    phosphate. Amer. J. Physiol. **153**, 121—126 (1948).
Funke, A., F. Depierre and M. W. Krucker: Exaltation de l'activité anticholinestérasique
    des sels d'ammonium quaternaires des phenoxyacanes par l'introduction de groupements
    uréthanes. C. R. Acad. Sci. (Paris) **234**, 762—764 (1952).
Glasson, J., and F. H. Stelling: An unusual cause for paralysis of the extremities. Report
    of prolonged paralysis due to anticholinesterase agent. Sth. Med. J. (Bgham, Ala.) **49**, 1325
    (1956).
Gold, A. J., J. M. Weller and G. Freeman: Metabolic and acid base changes following acute
    cholinesterase inhibition. Amer. J. Physiol. **188**, 321—326 (1957).
Goldman, H., and M. Teitel: Malathion poisoning in a 34 month old child following accidental
    ingestion. J. Pediat. **52**, 76—81 (1958).
Gordon, A. S., and C. W. Frye: Large doses of atropine. Low toxicity and effectiveness in
    anticholinesterase intoxication. J. Amer. med. Ass. **159**, 1181—1184 (1955).
— — R. D. Miller and G. M. Wyant: Comparative methods of artificial respiration. U.S.
    armed Forces med. J. **6**, 781—793 (1955).
— — L. Gittelson, M. S. Sadove and E. J. Beattie jr.: Mouth-to-mouth versus manual
    artificial respiration for children and adults. J. Amer. med. Ass. **167**, 320—328 (1958).
Green, A. L., and H. J. Smith: The reactivation of cholinesterase inhibited with organo-
    phosphorus compounds. I. Reactivation by 2-oxoaldoximes. Biochem. J. **68**, 28—31 (1958a).
— The reactivation of cholinesterase inhibited with organophosphorus compounds.
    2. Reactivation by pyridinealdoxime methiodides. Biochem. J. **68**, 32—35 (1958b).
— R. O. Bauer, C. D. Janney and J. O. Elam: Expired air resuscitation in paralyzed human
    subjects. J. appl. Physiol. **11**, 313—318 (1957).
— J. O. Elam, I. L. Bunnell and J. L. Evers: The expired air ventilator. Amer. J. Surg.
    97, 407—413 (1959).

GRIESEMER, R. D.: The penetration of an anticholinesterase agent (Sarin) into skin. III. A method for studying the rate of penetration into the skin of a living rabbit. J. invest. Derm. **31**, 255—258 (1958).

GROB, D.: Uses and hazards of the organic phosphate anticholinesterase compounds. Ann. intern. Med. **32**, 1229—1234 (1950a).

— The toxic effects in man of the organic phosphate insecticides (Report of the Committee on Pesticides of the Council on Pharmacy and Chemistry of the Amer. Med. Assoc.). J. Amer. med. Ass. **144**, 105—107 (1950b).

— The anticholinesterase activity in vitro of the insecticide, parathion (p-nitrophenyl diethyl thionophosphate). Bull. Johns Hopk. Hosp. **87**, 95—105 (1950c).

— The manifestations and treatment of poisoning due to nerve gas and other organic phosphate anticholinesterase compounds. A.M.A. Arch. intern. Med. **98**, 221—239 (1956a).

— Manifestations and treatment of nerve gas poisoning in man. U.S. armed Forces med. J. **7**, 781—789 (1956b).

— The neuromuscular system. Chapter 30 in Clinical Physiology, 725—756, ed. by ARTHUR GROLLMAN. New York: McGraw-Hill Inc. 1957.

— Myasthenia gravis, current status of pathogenesis, clinical manifestations and management. J. chron. Dis. 8, 536—566 (1958).

— J. L. LILIENTHAL, A. M. HARVEY and B. F. JONES: The administration of diisopropyl fluorophosphate (DFP) to man. I. Effect on cholinesterase; general systemic effects; use in study of hepatic function and erythropoiesis; properties of plasma cholinesterase. Bull. Johns Hopk. Hosp. **81**, 217—244 (1947a).

— — and A. M. HARVEY: The administration of di-isopropyl fluorophosphate to man. II. Effect on intestinal motility and use in the treatment of abdominal distention. Bull. Johns Hopk. Hosp. **81**, 245—256 (1947b).

— A. M. HARVEY, O. R. LANGWORTHY and J. L. LILIENTHAL jr.: The administration of di-isopropyl fluorophosphate to man. III. Effect on the central nervous system, with special reference to the electrical activity of the brain. Bull. Johns Hopk. Hosp. **81**, 257—266 (1947c).

— W. L. GARLICK, G. G. MERRILL and H. C. FREIMUTH: Death due to parathion, an anticholinesterase insecticide. Ann. intern. Med. **31**, 899—904 (1949).

—, and A. M. HARVEY: Observations on the effects of tetraethyl pyrophosphate (TEPP) in man, and on its use in the treatment of myasthenia gravis. Bull. Johns Hopk. Hosp. **84**, 532—567 (1949).

— W. L. GARLICK and A. M. HARVEY: The toxic effects in man of the anticholinesterase insecticide, parathion. Bull. Johns Hopk. Hosp. **87**, 107—129 (1950).

—, and A. M. HARVEY: The effects and treatment of nerve gas poisoning. Amer. J. Med. **14**, 52—63 (1953).

— R. J. JOHNS and A. M. HARVEY: Studies in neuromuscular function. I. Introduction and Methods. Bull. Johns Hopk. Hosp. **99**, 115—124 (1956a).

— — — Studies in neuromuscular function. III. Stimulating and depressant effects of acetylcholine and choline in normal subjects. Bull. Johns Hopk. Hosp. **99**, 136—152 (1956b).

— — — Studies in neuromuscular function. V. Effects of anticholinesterase compounds, d-tubocurarine, and decamethonium in normal subjects. Bull. Johns Hopk. Hosp. **99**, 195—218 (1956c).

—, and J. C. HARVEY: Effects in man of the anticholinesterase compound sarin (isopropyl methyl phosphonofluoridate). J. clin. Invest. **37**, 350—368 (1958).

—, and R. J. JOHNS: Use of oximes in the treatment of intoxication by anticholinesterase compounds in normal subjects. Amer. J. Med. **24**, 497—511 (1958a).

— — Use of oximes in the treatment of intoxication by anticholinesterase compounds in patients with myasthenia gravis. Amer. J. Med. **24**, 512—518 (1958b).

— — Treatment of anticholinesterase intoxication in normal subjects and myasthenic patients with oximes. J. Amer. med. Ass. **166**, 1855—1858 (1958c).

— — Treatment of anticholinesterase intoxication with oximes. Neurology 8, 897—902 (1958d).

— — Use of the oxime 1,1'-trimethylene bis (4-formylpyridinium bromide) dioxime (EA 1814, TMB-4) in the management of intoxication by anticholinesterase compounds. Contractor's Progress Report to U.S. Army Chemical Corps. Medical Laboratories, Army Chemical Center, Md., August (1958e).

HAMBLIN, D. O., and H. H. GOLZ: Parathion poisoning — A brief review. Industr. Med. Surg. **24**, 65—72 (1955).

HARVEY, A. M., J. L. LILIENTHAL jr., D. GROB, B. F. JONES and S. A. TALBOT: The administration of di-isopropyl fluorophosphate to man. IV. The effects on neuromuscular function in normal subjects and in myasthenia gravis. Bull. Johns Hopk. Hosp. **81**, 267—292 (1947).

HEYMANS, C., A. POCHET and H. VAN HOUTTE: Contributions à la pharmacologie due Sarin et due Tabun. Arch. int. Pharmacodyn. **104**, 293—332 (1956).

HIMWICH, H. E., C. F. ESSIG, J. L. HAMPSON, P. D. BALES and A. M. FREEDMAN: Effect of trimethadione (Tridione) and other drugs on convulsions caused by di-isopropyl fluorophosphate (DFP). Amer. J. Psychiat. **106**, 816—820 (1950).

HOBBIGER, F., D. G. O'SULLIVAN and P. W. SADLER: New potent reactivators of acetylcholinesterase inhibited by tetraethyl pyrophosphate. Nature (Lond.) **182**, 1498—1499 (1958).

HOLMES, J. H.: Effect of exposure to Sarin or Parathion on blood coagulation. Progress report to U.S. Army Chemical Corps. Med. Laboratories, Army Chem. Center, Md. (1956).

HOLMES, R., and E. L. ROBINS: The reversal by oximes of neuromuscular block produced by anticholinesterases. Brit. J. Pharmacol. **10**, 490—495 (1955).

HOLMSTEDT, B.: Synthesis and pharmacology of dimethylamido-ethoxy-phosphoryl cyanide (Tabun) together with a description of some allied anticholinesterase compounds containing the N—P bond. Acta physiol. scand. **25**, 1—120 (1951).

— Pharmocology of organophosphorus cholinesterase inhibitors. Pharmacol. Rev. **11**, 567 to 688 (1959).

— L. KROOK and J. R. ROONEY: The pathology of experimental cholinesterase-inhibitor poisoning. Acta pharmacol. (Kbh.) **13**, 337—344 (1957).

HOTTINGER, A., and H. BLOCH: Über die Spezifität der Cholinesterase-Hemmung durch Tri-o-kresylphosphat. Helv. chim. Acta **26**, 142—155 (1943).

JAGER, B. V., G. N. STAGG, N. GREEN and L. JAGER: Studies on distribution and disappearance of pyridine-2-aldoxime methiodide (PAM) and of diacetyl monoxime (DAM) in man and in experimental animals. Bull. Johns Hopk. Hosp. **102**, 225—234 (1958).

— — Toxicity of diacetyl monoxime and of pyridine-2-aldoxime methiodide in man. Bull. Johns Hopk. Hosp. **102**, 203—211 (1958).

JACQUES, R.: Entstehung von Magenulcera unter dem Einfluß von Cholinesterasegiften. Helv. physiol. pharmacol. Acta **12**, C 24 (1954).

JEWELL, H. A., and R. A. LEHMAN: Pharmacology of phospholine iodide—an alkyl phosphothiocholine. Fed. Proc. **17**, 381 (1958).

JOHNSON, R. P., A. J. GOLD and G. FREEMAN: Comparative lung-airway resistance and cardiovascular effects in dogs and monkeys following Parathion and Sarin intoxication. Amer. J. Physiol. **192**, 581—584 (1958).

KARCZMAR, A. G., and J. P. LONG: Relationship between peripheral cholinolytic potency and tetraethylpyrophosphate antagonism of a series of atropine substitutes. J. Pharmacol. exp. Ther. **123**, 230—237 (1958).

KARLOG, O., M. NIMB and E. POULSON: Parathion (bladan) forgiftning, behandlet med 2-PAM (pyridyl-2-aldoxim-N-methyliodid). Ugeskr. Laeg. **120**, 177—193 (1958).

KATZ, B., and S. THESLEFF: A study of the "desensitization" produced by acetylcholine at the motor end-plate. J. Physiol. (Lond.) **138**, 63 (1957).

KAY, K., L. MONKMAN, J. P. WINDISCH, T. DOHERTY, J. PARE and C. RACICOT: Parathion exposure and cholinesterase response of Quebec apple growers. A.M.A. Arch. industr. Hyg. **6**, 252—262 (1952).

KELENSKY, N. C., W. G. MORAN, M. FELDSTEIN and N. E. FIDLER: Poisoning from TEPP. J. Amer. med. Ass. **149**, 1015 (1952).

KEWITZ, H., I. B. WILSON and D. NACHMANSOHN: A specific antidote against lethal alkyl phosphate intoxication. II. Antidotal properties. Arch. Biochem. **64**, 456 (1956).

—, and D. NACHMANSOHN: A specific antidote against lethal alkyl phosphate intoxication. IV. Effects in brain. Arch. Biochem. **66**, 271 (1957).

KOELLE, G. B.: Protection of cholinesterase against irreversible inactivation by di-isopropylfluorophosphate *in vitro*. J. Pharmacol. exp. Ther. **88**, 232—237 (1946).

— Histochemical demonstration of reactivation of acetylcholinesterase in vivo. Science **125**, 1195—1196 (1957a).

— Histochemical demonstration of reversible anticholinesterase action at selective cellular sites in vivo. J. Pharmacol. exp. Ther. **120**, 488—503 (1957b).

—, and A. GILMAN: The chronic toxicity of di-isopropyl fluorophosphate (DFP) in dogs, monkey and rats. J. Pharmacol. exp. Ther. **87**, 435—448 (1946).

— — Anticholinesterase drugs. J. Pharmacol. exp. Ther. **95** (Part 2, Pharmacol. Rev.), 166—216 (1949).

—. and E. C. STEINER: The cerebral distribution of a tertiary and a quaternary anticholinesterase agent following intravenous and intraventricular injection. J. Pharmacol. exp. Ther. **118**, 420—434 (1956).

KONDRITZER, A. A.: Chemistry, detection and decontamination of nerve gases. U.S. armed Forces med. J. **7**, 765—771 (1956).

Kosolapoff, G. M.: Organophosphorus compounds. New York: John Wiley & Sons, Inc., and New York: Chapman & Hall, Ltd. 1959.

Koster, R.: Synergisms and antagonisms between physostigmine and di-isopropyl fluorophosphate in cats. J. Pharmacol. exp. Ther. 88, 39—46 (1946).

Krivoy, W. A., E. R. Hart and A. S. Marrazzi: Further analysis of the actions of DFP and curare on the respiratory center. J. Pharmacol. exp. Ther. 103, 361 (1951).

Krop, S., and A. M. Kunkel: Observations on the pharmacology of the anticholinesterases sarin and tabun. Proc. Soc. exp. Biol. (N. Y.) 85, 530—533 (1954).

Ladell, W. S. S.: Treatment of anticholinesterase poisoning. Brit. Med. J. 1958, 141—142.

Lancaster, M. C.: A note on the demyelination produced in hens by dialkylfluoridates. Brit. J. Pharmacol. 15, 279—281 (1960).

Lehman, R. A., H. M. Fitch, L. P. Bloch, H. A. Jewell and M. E. Nicholls: Antidotes and potentiating agents for phospholine iodide. J. Pharmacol. exp. Ther. 128, 307—317 (1960).

Mark, W. G., and D. Grob: Some ocular effects of a new anticholinesterase agent, tetraethyl pyrophosphate (TEPP) and its use in the treatment of chronic glaucoma. Amer. J. Ophthal. 33, 904—908 (1950).

March, R. B., T. R. Fukuto, R. L. Metcalf and M. G. Maxon: Fate of P^{32} labeled malathion in the laying hen, white mouse and American cockroach. J. econ. Entom. 49, 185—195 (1956).

Maresch, W.: Die Vergiftung durch Phosphorsäureester (E 605, Parathion, Thophos). Arch. Toxikol. 16, 285—319 (1957).

Merrill, G. G.: Neostigmine toxicity. Report of fatality following diagnostic test for myasthenia. J. Amer. med. Ass. 137, 362 (1948).

Metcalf, R. L.: Organic insecticides. Their chemistry and mode of action. New York and London: Interscience Publishers 1955.

— Advances in pest control research. I. New York and London: Interscience Publishers 1957.

Michel, H. O.: An electrometric method for the determination of red blood cell and plasma cholinesterase activity. J. Lab. clin. Med. 34, 1564—1568 (1949).

Milles, H. L., and H. B. Salt: Parathion poisoning. Brit. Med. J. 1950 II, 444.

Moore, W. K. S.: Two cases of poisoning with di-isopropylfluorophosphate (DFP). Brit. J. industr. Med. 13, 214—216 (1956).

Murtha, E. F., B. P. McNamara, G. E. Gorblewski and J. H. Wills: Site of action of magnesium in treatment of some toxic effects produced by TEPP. Proc. Soc. exp. Biol. (N. Y.) 90, 505—507 (1955).

Namba, T., and K. Hiraki: PAM (pyridine-2-aldoxime methiodide) therapy for alkylphosphate poisoning. J. Amer. med. Ass. 166, 1834—1839 (1958).

Nolan, K., and F. Wilcoxon: Method of bioassay for traces of parathion. Reprint from Agricultural Chemicals (1950).

Oberst, F. W., and M. K. Christensen: Regeneration of erythrocyte and brain cholinesterase activity in rats after sublethal exposures to GB vapor. J. Pharmacol. exp. Ther. 116, 216—219 (1956).

— R. S. Ross, M. K. Christensen, J. W. Crook, P. Cresthull and C. W. Unland: The use of atropine and artificial respiration in the resuscitation of dogs exposed by inhalation to lethal concentrations of GB vapor. J. Pharmacol. exp. Ther. 116, 44—45 (1956).

O'Leary, J. F., J. H. Wills and L. A. Carlstrom: Relative efficacy of various prophylactic adjuncts to atropine in Sarin poisoning. Fed. Proc. 17, 401 (1958).

Osserman, K. E., P. Teng and L. I. Kaplan: Studies in myasthenia gravis. Preliminary report on therapy with Mestinon bromide. J. Amer. med. Ass. 155, 961 (1954).

Parkes, M. W., and P. Sacra: Protection against the toxicity of cholinesterase inhibitors by acetylcholine antagonists. Brit. J. Pharmacol. 9, 299—305 (1954).

Patzisky, K., E. Herzfelt and C. Stumpf: Der Effekt von Polymethylen-bis-(N-methyl-carbaminolyl-m-trimethylammoniumphenolen) BC40, BC47, BC48 auf Cholinesterase-aktivität und Muskeltätigkeit bei Myasthenia gravis pseudoparalytica. Wien. klin. Wschr. 69, 2—7 (1957).

— O. Kraupp and C. Stumpf: Klinische Erfahrungen mit Hexamethylen-bis-(N-methyl-carbaminoyl-m-trimethylammoniumphenol) (BC40) bei Myasthenia gravis pseudoparalytica. Wien. klin. Wschr. 67, 578 (1955).

Petry, H.: Polyneuritis durch E 605. Zentralblatt für Arbeitsmedizin und Arbeitschutz 1, 86—89 (1951).

Petty, C. S.: Organic phosphate insecticide poisoning. Amer. J. Med. 24, 467—470 (1958).

Polet, H.: Effect of Sarin on the cardio-inhibitory, vasomotor and respiratory centers of the isolated head in dogs. Arch. int. Pharmacodyn. 118, 231—247 (1959).

Poziomek, E. J., B. E. Hackley jr., and G. M. Steinberg: Pyridinium aldoximes. J. org. Chem. 23, 714—717 (1958).

1026   Literature

QUINBY, G. E., and A. B. LEMMON: Parathion residues as a cause of poisoning in crop workers
    pesticidal spray. J. Amer. med. Ass. **166**, 740—746 (1958).
RAJAPURKAR, M. V., and G. B. KOELLE: Reactivation of DFP-inactivated acetylcholinesterase
    by monoisonitrosoacetone (MINA) and diacetylmonoxime (DAM) in vivo. J. Pharmacol.
    exp. Ther. **123**, 247—253 (1958).
RIDER, J. A., S. SCHULMAN, R. B. RICHTER, H. C. MOELLER and K. P. DUBOIS: Treatment
    of myasthenia gravis with octamethyl pyrophosphoramide. J. Amer. med. Ass. **145**, 967
    to 972 (1951).
RIKER, W. F. jr., and W. C. WESCOE: The relationship between cholinesterase inhibition and
    function in a neuro-effector system. J. Pharmacol. exp. Ther. **95**, 515—527 (1949).
— — The direct action of prostigmine on skeletal muscle; its relationship to the choline
    esters. J. Pharmacol. exp. Ther. **88**, 58—77 (1946).
RUBIN, L. S., and M. N. GOLDBERG: Effect of Sarin on dark adaption in man: threshold
    changes. J. appl. Physiol. **11**, 439—444 (1957).
— — Effect of tertiary and quaternary atropine salts on absolute scotopic threshold changes
    produced by an anticholinesterase (Sarin). J. appl. Physiol. **12**, 305—310 (1958).
— S. KROP and M. N. GOLDBERG: Effect of Sarin on dark adaptation in man. Mechanism
    of action. J. appl. Physiol. **11**, 445—449 (1957).
RUTLAND, J. P.: The effect of some oximes in sarin poisoning. Brit. J. Pharmacol. **13**, 399—403
    (1958).
SAFAR, P.: Mouth-to-mouth airway. Anesthesiology 18, 904 (1957).
— Ventilatory efficacy of mouth-to-mouth artificial respiration. J. Amer. med. Ass. **167**, 335
    to 341 (1958).
— L. A. ESCARRAGO and J. O. ELAM: A comparison of the mouth-to-mouth and mouth-to-
    airway methods of artificial respiration with the chest-pressure arm-lift methods. New Engl.
    J. Med. **258**, 671—677 (1958).
SANDERSON, D. M.: Assessment of direct cholinesterase inhibitory activity of pupillary miosis.
    J. Pharm. (Lond.) **9**, 600—604 (1957).
SCHAUMANN, W., and C. JOB: Differential effects of quaternary cholinesterase inhibitor, phos-
    pholine, and its tertiary analogue, compound 217-AO, on central control of respiration and
    on neuromuscular transmission. The antagonism by 217-AO of the respiratory arrest caused
    by morphine. J. Pharmacol. exp. Ther. **123**, 114—120 (1958).
SCHWAB, R. S., C. K. MARSHALL and W. H. TIMBERLAKE: WIN 8077 in treatment of myasthe-
    nia gravis, use of N,N′bis (2-diethyl-aminoethyl) oxamide bis-2-chlorobenzyl chloride in
    50 patients. J. Amer. med. Ass. **158**, 625—628 (1955).
SHELLEY, H.: A correlation between cholinesterase inhibition and increase in muscle tone in
    rabbit duodenum. Brit. J. Pharmacol. **10**, 26—35 (1955).
SLEISENGER, M. H., C. M. LEWIS, J. H. PERT, D. R. ROSEMAN, W. F. NICHEM and T. P. ALMY:
    Use of parasympathetic stimulation in the production of bloody diarrhea in dogs, with
    reference to the role of red cell and colon cholinesterase. Gastroenterology **34**, 582—594
    (1958).
SMITH, H. V., and M. J. SPALDING: Outbreak of paralysis in Morocco due to ortho-cresyl
    phosphate poisoning. Lancet **1959 II**, 1019—1021.
SNYDER, G. H.: Encephalopathy in a child following exposure to Malathion. Ochsner Clin.
    Rep. **37** (1956).
SPRAGUE, F., R. J. JOHNS and D. GROB: Unpublished observations (1958).
SUMMERSON, W. H.: Progress in the biochemical treatment of nerve gas poisoning. U.S.
    Armed forces chem. J. 24—26 (1955).
SUMERFORD, W. H., J. WAYLAND, M. J. JOHNSTON and K. J. WALKER: Cholinesterase re-
    sponse and symptomatology from exposure to organic phosphorus insecticides. A.M.A.
    Arch. Hyg. Occup. Med. **7**, 383—398 (1953).
SUSSER, M., and Z. STEIN: An outbreak of tri-ortho-cresyl phosphate (T.O.C.P.) poisoning in
    Durban. Brit. J. industr. Med. **14**, 111—120 (1957).
THOMPSON, J. H.: Cholinesterase inhibiting insecticides (Parathion). Calif. Med. **82**, 91—95
    (1955).
UPHOLT, W. M., G. E. QUINBY, G. S. BATCHELOR and J. P. THOMPSON: Visual effects ac-
    companying TEPP-induced miosis. A.M.A. Arch. Ophthal. **56**, 128—134 (1956).
VARAGIC, V.: The action of eserine on the blood pressure of the rat. Brit. J. Pharmacol.
    10, 349—353 (1955).
WALKER, M. B.: Treatment of myasthenia gravis with physostigmine. Lancet **1934 I**, 1200
    to 1201.
WALTERS, M. N. I.: Malathion intoxication. Med. J. Aust. **44**, 876—880 (1957).
WELLER, J. M., T. J. MIRANDA, M. LEVINE and G. FREEMAN: Effect of cholinesterase inhibitors
    on electrolyte distribution in vivo. Proc. Soc. exp. Biol. (N. Y.) **90**, 699—702 (1955).

WESCOE, W. C., R. E. GREEN, B. P. McNAMARA and S. KROP: The influence of atropine and scopolamine on the central effects of DFP. J. Pharmacol. exp. Ther. **92**, 63—72 (1948).

WILHELMI, G., u. R. DOMENJOZ: Therapeutische Möglichkeiten bei der Parathion-Vergiftung. Arch. int. Pharmacodyn. **86**, 321—334 (1951).

WILLIAMS, J. W., and J. T. GRIFFITHS jr.: Parathion poisoning in Florida Citrus. J. Fla. med. Ass. **37**, 707—709 (1951).

WILLS, J. H., and R. V. BROWN: The pharmacology of nerve gas poisoning. U.S. Armed forces chem. J. **11**, 24—26 (1957).

— A. M. KUNKEL, R. V. BROWN and G. E. GROBLEWSKI: Pyridine-2-aldoxime methiodide and poisoning by anticholinesterases. Science **125**, 743—744 (1957).

WILSON, I. B.: Acetylcholinesterase. XI. Reversibility of tetraethyl pyrophosphate inhibition. J. biol. Chem. **190**, 111—117 (1951).

— Designing of a new drug with antidotal properties against the nerve gas Sarin. Biochem. biophys. Acta **27**, 196—199 (1958).

—, and E. K. MEISLICH: Reactivation of acetylcholinesterase inhibited by alkylphosphates. J. Amer. chem. Soc. **75**, 4, 528 (1953).

— S. GINSBURG and E. K. MEISLICH: The reactivation of acetylcholinesterase inhibited by tetraethyl pyrophosphate and diisopropyl fluorophosphate. J. Amer. chem. Soc. **77**, 4286 to 4291 (1955).

WIRTH, W.: Zur Wirkung system-insecticider Phosphorsäure-ester im Warmbluter-Stoffwechsel. Naunyn-Schmiedeberg's Arch. exp. Path. Pharmak. **234**, 352—363 (1958).

WISHAHI, A.: Parathion (phosphorus compound) poisoning. Arch. Pediat. **75**, 387 (1958).

WRIGHT, P. G.: An analysis of the central and peripheral components of respiratory failure produced by anticholinesterase poisoning in the rabbit. J. Physiol. (Lond.) **125**, 52—70 (1954).

YAMADA, M.: Alkyl phosphate poisoning. III. Effect of 2-pyridinealdoxime methiodide in the therapy of parathion poisoning. Okayama Igakkai Zasshi **69**, 525—539 (1957).

Chapter 23

Therapy of Myasthenia Gravis

By

DAVID GROB

With 5 Figures

Contents

Myasthenia gravis is a chronic disease characterized by weakness and abnormal fatigability of skeletal muscle. The muscles innervated by the cranial nerves are particularly affected, and usually those of the neck, trunk, and extremities. In severe cases, weakness of the muscles of respiration occurs. Smooth and cardiac muscles are not involved. The disease usually becomes generalized, but in a minority of cases it remains localized to the extraocular muscles. The symptoms are commonly ameliorated, although to a variable degree, by anticholinesterase (anti-ChE) compounds. This response serves as the basis for diagnosis and management of the disease.

A. Mechanism of neuromuscular block in myasthenia gravis

I. Normal neuromuscular transmission

Resting skeletal muscle fibers normally have a potential difference of approximately 90 mV between the two sides of the surface membrane, the inner surface being negative with respect to the outer. They are, therefore, said to be in a state of polarization. When a nerve impulse reaches the motor nerve endings, acetylcholine (ACh), the normal mediator of neuromuscular transmission, is released. This compound causes a localized disappearance of the potential difference across the muscle membrane in the motor endplate (MEP) region adjacent to the motor nerve ending (the endplate potential, EPP) (FATT 1954). The localized EPP in turn initiates a wave of depolarization (actually a reversed polarization), which is propagated along the muscle membrane as a wave of increased negativity, preceded by a spike, termed the muscle action potential (MAP). This in turn initiates contraction of the muscle fiber. Shortly after ACh has initiated depolarization of the endplate, it is hydrolyzed into acetate and choline by acetylcholinesterase (AChE) which is concentrated in the muscle at the endplate region. The potential difference across the entire muscle membrane is then restored, i.e., repolarization occurs, and the muscle membrane is thereby made ready to be depolarized again.

II. Pharmacological and other types of neuromuscular block

Disturbance of neuromuscular transmission may result from interruption of the foregoing normal sequence of events at any step. In most instances, neuromuscular block occurs as a result of either deficient or excessive action of ACh on the motor endplates, or as a result of drugs or diseases which simulate these effects (GROB et al. 1956a, GROB 1957).

1. Deficient action of ACh

a) *Deficient release of ACh from the motor nerve endings* is believed to be responsible for the weakness of botulinus poisoning (BROOKS 1954).

b) *Antagonism of the depolarizing action of ACh on the motor endplate ("ACh-inhibitory block")* occurs in at least three situations:

α) *Block occurring without change in the resting potential of the muscle membrane, and reversible by excess ACh or by anty-ChE compounds.* The block produced by d-tubocurarine is of this type (KUFFLER 1943, GROB et al. 1956d). This drug is believed to exert its effect by competing with ACh for receptor sites at the endplate, so that the resulting block has been termed "competitive." This type of block is characterized by its inhibition of the depolarizing action of injected ACh, and by its reversal following the injection of sufficient ACh or anti-ChE compound.

β) *Block not associated with any change in membrane potential, but not reversible by ACh.* This type of block occurs several minutes after the beginning of exposure of frog muscle to ACh, and persists even after recovery of the muscle membrane from the initial depolarization. It is attributable to the development of refractoriness of the motor endplate to ACh, and has been termed "desensitization" block (KATZ and THESLEFF 1957).

γ) *Block associated with hyperpolarization of the muscle membrane.* The weakness of hypokalemia is probably due in part to this mechanism, resulting from an increase in the ratio of intracellular to extracellular concentration of potassium (GROB et al. 1957).

2. Abnormally prolonged depolarization in the region of the endplate

When the endplate region is in the depolarized state, and for a period of time after the return of normal polarity, it is inexcitable (KATZ and THESLEFF 1957). This type of block is produced by an excessive concentration of ACh, by anti-ChE compounds, by choline, and in most animal species by decamethonium (C-10) and succinylcholine (Burns and Paton 1951, Hutter 1952, Grob et al. 1956b, d). During the period of depolarization there is characteristically no inhibition of the depolarizing action of injected ACh or anti-ChE compound; in fact, these agents intensify the block by their additive effect. Neuromuscular block which is not antagonized or reversed by ACh (i.e., which is non-competitive) is frequently presumed to be of the depolarizing type, but confirmation of such a mechanism requires measurement of the membrane potential in the region of the endplates. This measurement has only recently been made in man (Johns 1958), and has not yet been applied to the study of disease or drug action.

Following prolonged depolarization, and persisting even after the return of normal membrane polarity, the block may change to the "desensitization" type (1, b, β), in which the motor endplates are refractory to the depolarizing action of injected ACh (Katz and Thesleff 1957).

3. Mixed types of block

The effect of some chemical agents, such as decamethonium, on neuromuscular transmission varies in different species, and even in different muscles. In some instances, a neuromuscular block results which has some properties of both the competitive and depolarizing types (Zaimis 1953).

III. Mechanism of neuromuscular block in myasthenia gravis

1. General characteristics

A single supramaximal stimulation of the nerve to affected muscle evokes a muscle action potential (MAP) and twitch that are below the normal range only in muscles that are severely affected by myasthenia gravis (Johns et al. 1955, 1956). However, in all muscles affected by the disease, repetitive stimulation at frequencies that normally produce responses of consistent amplitude results in progressive decline of these responses (Fig. 1). The degree and rate of decline vary with the frequency of nerve stimulation and with the degree of involvement of the muscle by the disease. In an occasional patient, the response to the first few stimuli increases progressively, a phenomenon that has been termed neuromuscular facilitation. Both the facilitation and depression (Fig. 1) are restored toward normal by the administration of ACh (Grob et al. 1955, 1956c), neostigmine (Harvey and Masland 1941), or one of the other anti-ChE compounds. Similar alterations in neuromuscular transmission occur in normal subjects following the administration of d-tubocurarine (Grob et al. 1956d).

Since there is no known abnormality of central or peripheral neural function in myasthenia gravis, and since the evidence for a defect in muscle contractility (Botelho 1955a, b) does not appear to be conclusive, the manifestations of this disease are believed to be due primarily to impairment of neuromuscular transmission. At present the evidence suggests that the defect in neuromuscular transmission is due to some alteration in the ACh mechanism. This could result from (1) an excessive concentration of AChE at the neuromuscular junction, (2) failure of each nerve impulse to release a normal quantum of ACh, or (3) elevation of the excitatory threshold of the motor endplate to the ACh released by each nerve impulse. There is no evidence for excessive AChE activity in the muscle of myasthenic patients (Wilson et al. 1951), and no data are available in support of the second possibility, deficiency of released ACh. Recent studies are consistent with the third possibility, and indicate that the defect in neuromuscular transmission in myasthenia is due to a competitive (ACh-inhibitory) block, produced by ACh released in a normal manner during neuromuscular transmission, or by choline or a closely related compound formed following hydrolysis of the naturally released ACh (GROB et al. 1956c). (See, however, section A III 3.)

When ACh is administered to normal subjects or myathenic patients intra-arterially, there occurs a transient prompt depression of muscle action potentials evoked by nerve stimulation, lasting several seconds, followed by temporary recovery and then by a more prolonged "late" depression lasting one-half to one hour (Fig. 1). In both groups the prompt depression is enhanced and prolonged by the prior injection of anti-ChE compound, and is probably due to excessive depolarization caused by the injected ACh. The properties of the late depression

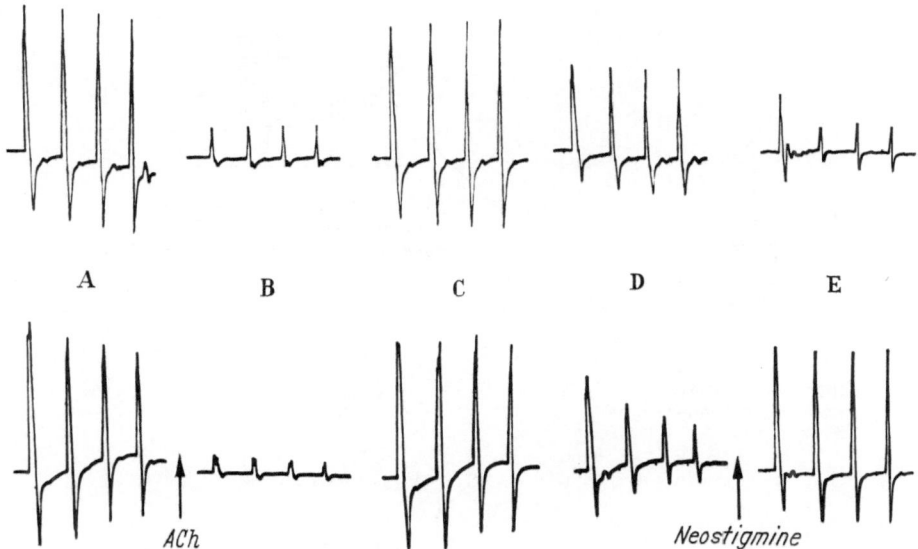

Fig. 1. Effect of acetylcholine and neostigmine on the muscle action potential response to nerve stimulation in a normal subject (upper row) and a patient with myasthenia gravis (lower row). All injections intra-arterial. A, control response to four supramaximal nerve stimuli at 40 millisecond intervals; B, prompt depression 7 seconds after 5 mg ACh; C, recovery 15 seconds after injection; D, late depression one hour after injection; E, effect of 0.5 mg neostigmine. (From GROB 1958a)

differ in the two groups, as indicated by the effect of injection of a second dose of ACh, or of anti-ChE compound. In normal subjects the late block is not reversed by these compounds, and it does not prevent them from producing a prompt depression of evoked potentials attributable to depolarization (Fig. 1, E). Since the late block produced by ACh in normal subjects neither inhibits the depolarizing action of ACh, nor is reversed by ACh, it may be described as a non-ACh-inhibitory, non-ACh-reversible, and non-competitive type of block. It is not yet known whether this late block, which has many of the properties of a depolarizing block, is caused by persistence of excessive depolarization, or by some other change in the muscle membrane or endplate. In the great majority of myasthenic patients, the late block produced by ACh is reversed by the injection of ACh, or of an anti-ChE compound, and it prevents these compounds from producing a prompt depression of evoked potentials (Fig. 1, E). Since the late block produced by ACh in these myasthenic patients inhibits the depolarizing action of ACh and is re-versed by ACh, it may be described an ACh-inhibitory, ACh-reversible, and com-petitive type of block (Fig. 2). Choline, in moderate doses, also produces a non-competitive block in normal subjects and a competitive block in myasthenic patients. Since injected ACh or choline reproduces, or enhances, in myasthenic patients the defect in neuromuscular transmission characteristic of the disease, it is likely that the endogenous transmitter, or its products of hydrolysis, plays an important part in bringing about the defect.

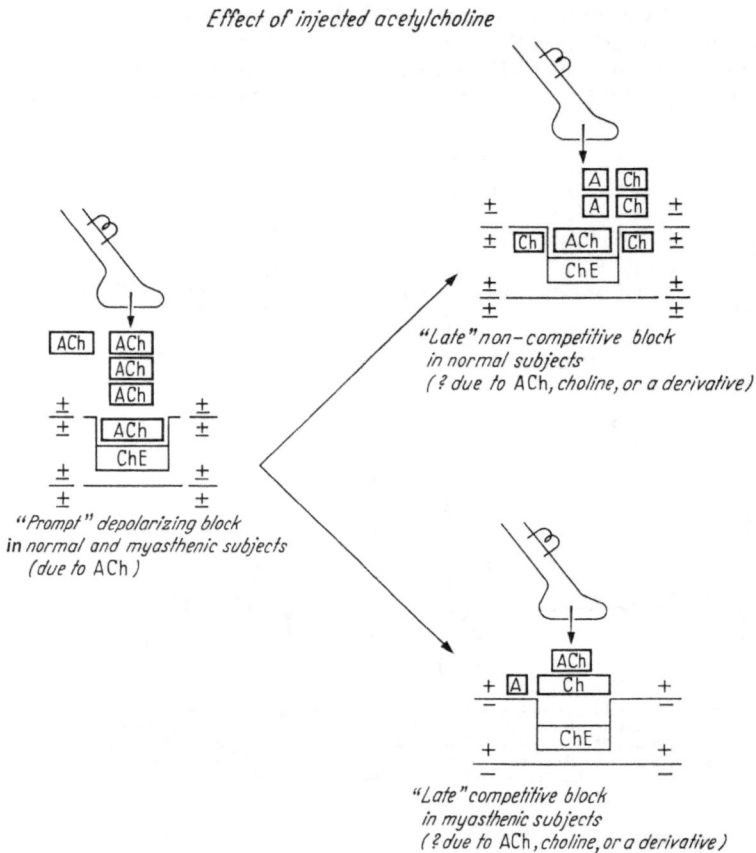

Fig. 2. Effect of acetylcholine in normal subjects and patients with myasthenia gravis. Prompt depolarizing block occurred in both (left). This was followed by a late non-competitive block in normal subjects and a competitive block in myasthenic patients (right). (From GROB 1958a)

It is not clear whether the myasthenic block is the result of an abnormal response of the endplate to substances normally released from the motor nerve endings, or to the formation of an abnormal product of ACh or choline which has competitive blocking action. The former seems more likely, since the myasthenic patient reacts abnormally not only to ACh and choline, but also to many other quaternary ammonium compounds, including decamethonium and succinylcholine (CHURCHILL-DAVIDSON and RICHARDSON 1953, GROB et al. 1956e). In normal subjects, decamethonium block of moderate degree, like that produced by choline, is intensified by ACh or anti-ChE agents, while block of marked degree is reversed by these compounds within certain definite limits (GROB et al. 1956d). In myasthenic patients, decamethonium block, like that produced by choline, is reversed by ACh or anti-ChE compounds at all levels.

2. Different types of neuromuscular block in myasthenia gravis; the acetylcholine-insensitive state

In the majority of myasthenic patients the late block produced by the intra-arterial injection of ACh or choline inhibits the depolarizing (promptly depressant) effect of ACh and is reversed by ACh or anti-ChE compounds; i.e., it is both ACh-inhibitory and ACh-reversible (Table 1). However, in some myasthenic patients this late block inhibits the depolarizing effect of ACh but is not reversed by ACh or anti-ChE compounds; i.e., it is ACh-inhibitory but not ACh-reversible (GROB and JOHNS 1959). Such a block, which resembles one stage of the block produced by ACh in the frog (KATZ and THESLEFF 1957), may be termed ACh-insensitive. Patients who manifest this type of block respond poorly or not at all to anti-ChE medication; they are clinically insensitive to ACh and to anti-ChE compounds. Patients in whom ACh produces the more usual ACh-reversible block may become ACh-insensitive during an exacerbation of their disease, or they may be rendered ACh-insensitive by the repeated intra-arterial administration of ACh or choline, or by prolonged repetitive nerve stimulation, which probably causes the local accumulation of endogenous ACh or choline.

This ACh-insensitive state is probably responsible for the well known clinical observation that while increasing doses of anti-ChE medication result in an increase in strength in muscles affected by the disease, the maximal strength attained is frequently far below normal. The maximal strength and amplitude of evoked potentials attained in any muscle are approximately the same following the administration of ACh or of any of the anti-ChE compounds (GROB 1958). Further increase in dose of anti-ChE compound does not result in any further increase in strength, and excessive dosage may result in weakness, without passing through a stage of normal strength. While weakness due to overdose of anti-ChE medication may be reversed by the careful administration of an oxime, such as pyridine-2-aldoxime methiodide (P-2-AM), which probably reverses the combination of AChE and anti-ChE compound, the strength never exceeds the peak level attained following optimal doses of anti-ChE compound (GROB and JOHNS 1958a). The maximal level of strength attained following optimal doses of anti-ChE compounds is lowered during exacerbations of the disease, and it may be lowered experimentally by the repeated intra-arterial administration of ACh or choline, or by prolonged repetitive nerve stimulation (GROB and JOHNS 1959). At these times the patient is insensitive to ACh or anti-ChE medication, the block having changed from one that is ACh-inhibitory and ACh-reversible to one that is ACh-inhibitory but non-ACh-reversible. It is this insensitive state that constitutes the main problem in management of the disease, and often leads to the administration of large doses of anti-ChE medication and confusion as to whether the patient is overdosed (in "cholinergic crisis") or underdosed (in "myasthenic weakness"). Many patients who are thought to be overdosed are really in an insensitive state, and large doses of anti-ChE compound often render the patient more insensitive.

It seems likely that in man, as in the frog (KATZ and THESLEFF 1957), de-polarizing agents, including ACh released from the motor nerve endings, may combine with any of several forms of receptor substance in the motor endplate, and that these combinations may result in at least three different types of block; alternatively, the combination of ACh with receptor substance may be altered, resulting in different types of block. On the basis of the observed effects of injected ACh in normal subjects and myasthenic patients, these types of block may be characterized as: 1. non-ACh-inhibitory, non-ACh-reversible (probably depolarizing); 2. ACh-inhibitory, ACh-reversible (competitive); and 3. ACh-inhibitory, non-ACh-reversible (ACh-insensitive) (Table 1). It is likely that mixtures of these types of block may occur, and that the predominance of one or the other may explain the clinical state of the myasthenic patient and his response to anti-ChE medication. The disease may be due to the presence of abnormal forms of receptor substance, or to alterations occurring in receptor substance or in the combination of ACh with receptor substance.

Table 1. *Possible events at the neuromuscular junction following combination of acetylcholine with various forms of receptor substance* (R, R', and R'')

	Inhibition of depo-larizing action of ACh (ACh-Inhibitory)	Reversibility by ACh (ACh-Reversible)
ACh + R $\rightleftharpoons$ ACh R $\rightarrow$ Depolarizing Block	—	—
ACh + R' $\rightleftharpoons$ ACh R' $\rightarrow$ Competitive Block	+	+
ACh + R'' $\rightleftharpoons$ ACh R'' $\rightarrow$ ACh-Insensitive Block	+	—

3. Other possible causes of neuromuscular block in myasthenia gravis

Reports of demonstration in the blood of myasthenic patients of a substance capable of producing neuromuscular block in experimental animals (WILSON and STONER 1944, TSUKIYAMA et al. 1959), and of a substance in serum capable of inhibiting the synthesis of ACh (TORDA and WOLF 1945), have not been confirmed (LAMMERS and MOST VAN SPYK 1954, ROE et al. 1955). In this regard, it is of interest that curare itself is rapidly removed from the blood stream and fixed in the tissues (VAN MAANEN 1955). Exchange transfusions between myasthenic and non-myasthenic subjects have no effect on the strength of either (SCHWARZ 1952). The thymus glands of myasthenic patients, normal subjects, and animals contain quaternary ammonium compounds having neuromuscular blocking action (MCSWEYN and SCHWARTZ 1954, NOWELL and WILSON 1960), but the role of these compounds, or of the gland, in the disease is not clear.

It has been suggested that myasthenia gravis may be due to an "auto-immune" response in which an antibody to endplate receptor protein is produced by the reticulo-endothelial system, including the thymus (SIMPSON 1960). The antibody would then combine with endplate protein and produce an alteration in the response of the endplate to endogenous ACh. This theory has been lent support by the recent observation that the serum of myasthenic patients contains, in the globulin fraction, a substance which combines with normal or myasthenic muscle in the presence of complement (STRAUSS et al. 1960).

It has also been suggested that myasthenia gravis may be due to impaired release of ACh from motor nerve endings, as indicated by the resemblence between the post-tetanic exhaustion of myasthenic muscle and of normal muscle treated with hemicholinium, which inhibitis the synthesis of ACh (DESMEDT 1959). The relationship of any of these functional changes to abnormalities which have been described in the distal nerve endings and motor endplates of myasthenic muscle is not clear (COERS and DESMEDT 1959, MACDERMOT 1960, BICKERSTAFF 1960).

B. Anticholinesterase compounds used in the diagnosis of myasthenia gravis: neostigmine and edrophonium

A presumptive diagnosis can generally be made on the basis of the history, distribution, and usual fluctuating nature of the weakness, and by the usual increase in weakness that occurs on repeated effort of involved muscles. The diagnosis is confirmed by the improvement in strength which characteristically occurs following the administration of an anti-ChE compound, such as neostigmine (Prostigmin) (VIETS and SCHWAB 1935, HARVEY and WHITEHILL 1937) or edrophonium (Tensilon) (WESTERBERG et al. 1951, OSSERMAN and KAPLAN 1952), when the patient is in a "basal" state at least 6 hours after the last medication. The improvement is often incomplete even after maximum doses, but careful measurement and recording of the level of strength reveals a significant change in all except a few patients with localized ocular myasthenia and the rare patient with generalized myasthenia. In these patients a response can sometimes be elicited later in the course of the disease. Unequivocal increase in strength of more than slight degree following neostigmine or edrophonium does not occur in patients who are not considered to have myasthenia gravis, with the exception of a few patients with polymyositis, disseminated lupus erythematosus, or carcinomatous neuropathy or myopathy (ANDERSON et al. 1953), and with the exception of the extraocular muscles of a few patients with disseminated sclerosis or arteriosclerotic cerebral vascular disease (GROB and HARVEY 1953). However, these responses are sufficiently unusual to detract little from the diagnosic value of the test.

The width of the palpebral fissures is noted with the eyes at rest and after one minute of continuous upward deviation, and the movement of each eye is recorded in the four directions (normal ranges: up 40 degrees, down 60 degrees, out 45 degrees, and in 45 degrees). Measurement is made of the length of time that the head and each extended leg can be elevated when the patient is in a supine position, and the length of time the arms can be held above the horizontal position when the patient is sitting. Grip strength is recorded by means of a dynamometer or ergometer. Dysphagia may be evaluated by the use of the fluoroscope with barium swallow (VIETS 1947). In patients with a mild degree of weakness, and in those in whom emotional factors are thought to contribute to the subjective complaint, the effect of placebo administration on the level of strength should be determined. Atropine sulfate may be administered prior to the anti-ChE compound, to prevent its muscarinic effects, and the influence on strength regarded as a placebo effect. An improvement in performance indicates that emotional factors are contributing to the patient's complaint, since atropine does not alleviate weakness due to other causes.

The most widely used anti-ChE compound for the diagnostic test has been neostigmine, administered intramuscularly in a dose of 1 mg per 100 pounds body weight. Atropine sulfate (0.5 mg per 100 pounds) should be injected intramuscularly before or with the neostigmine to prevent the stimulating effect of the latter drug on smooth and cardiac muscle and secretory glands. Improvement in strength of involved muscles begins within 10 minutes, is maximal in 30 minutes, and lasts 3 to 4 hours.

When the response is equivocal, the test should be repeated on another day in a dose of 1.4 mg neostigmine and 0.7 mg atropine per 100 pounds. Non-myasthenic subjects experience either no change in strength or mild weakness, and usually develop fasciculation in the muscles of the face, neck, and to a lesser extent trunk and extremities, although occasionally there is no fasciculation. In patients with generalized myasthenia, fasciculation is usually absent except in the least involved muscles, particularly in the lower extremities. In patients with localized ocular or oculobulbar myasthenia, fasciculation frequently occurs but is usually less pronounced than in non-myasthenic subjects. The latter are also more likely to experience gastrointestinal symptoms, and occasionally reduction in blood pressure (MERRILL 1948). Neostigmine may also be administered intravenously in a dose of 0.5 mg following 0.5 mg atropine (TETHER 1948). This produces a more dramatic response within a few minutes.

Another intravenous diagnostic test employs edrophonium (WESTERBERG et al. 1951, OSSERMAN and KAPLAN 1953), which has both anti-ChE and a direct depolarizing action on muscle (GROB et al. 1956e). This drug is injected in an initial dose of 2 mg, followed in 30 seconds by an additional 8 mg if the first injection does not produce an increase in strength. Atropine need not be administered. For this reason, and because of its rapidity of action, edrophonium is now widely used as a diagnostic agent. However, the brief duration of its effect (1 to 3 minutes) necessitates speed in carrying out a detailed evaluation of muscle strength.

In the majority of patients the diagnosis of myasthenia gravis can be established or excluded with the help of the response to intramuscular neostigmine. In a few patients with predominantly ocular manifestations, and in a rare patient with generalized myasthenia, the response to neostigmine and edrophonium is so meager that the diagnosis cannot be established. When the upper extremity is involved by the disease, the intra-arterial injection of neostigmine in doses of 0.05 to 1 mg can be employed to elicit a local improvement in strength and in muscle response to nerve stimulation (HARVEY and LILIENTHAL 1941, GROB et al. 1956e). In half the patients with localized ocular or oculobulbar myasthenia, a latent myasthenic defect in the upper extremity can be brought out by the intra-arterial injection of ACh or choline, and identified by the reparative effect of neostigmine (GROB et al. 1956c). It is rarely necessary to administer oral quinine (0.3 g, repeated in 3 hours) (HARVEY and WHITEHILL 1937), or intravenous (PELIKAN et al. 1953) or intra-arterial (GROB et al. 1956e) d-tubocurarine (0.1 to 0.5 mg) to bring about an aggravation of symptoms. d-Tubocurarine must be used with care and muscle function promptly restored by intravenous neostigmine, to avoid a critical exacerbation of symptoms, with respiratory dysfunction.

C. Anticholinesterase compounds used in the management of myasthenia gravis

The management of myasthenia gravis relies mainly on anti-ChE compounds, which are administered for the amelioration of weakness. The most useful of these are the quaternary ammonium compounds, neostigmine, pyridostigmin (Mestinon) (SEIBERT 1953, OSSERMAN et al. 1954, TETHER 1956, SCHWAB et al. 1957), and ambenomium (Mytelase) (SCHWAB 1955, SCHWAB et al. 1955, WESTERBERG 1956). *Bis*-neostigmine (BC-40) (PATEISKY et al. 1955, 1957) and *bis*-pyridostigmin (BC-51, Hexamarium) (HERZFELD et al. 1957, GROB and OSSERMAN 1958) are longer acting quaternary ammonium anti-ChE compounds which require less frequent administration, but are less suitable for general use because of the danger of cumulation and overdose. Several organophosphorus anti-ChE compounds have also had clinical trials in the management of myasthenia gravis. These have included di*iso*propyl phosphorofluoridate (DFP) (COMROE et al. 1946, HARVEY et al. 1947), tetraethylpyrophosphate (TEPP) (GROB and HARVEY 1949, WESTERBERG and MAGEE 1955), hexaethyltetraphosphate (HETP) (WESTERBERG and LURES 1948), octamethylpyrophosphortetramide (OMPA) (RIDER et al. 1951, OSSERMAN and KAPLAN 1954, ARANOW et al. 1958), 0,0-diethyl-S-2-trimethylammonium-ethyl phosphonothiolate iodide (echothiophate, Phospholine) (FOLDES 1959, SCHAUMANN and JOB 1958), and *iso*propyl methylphosphorofluoridate (Sarin) (GROB 1955). While these compounds are more prolonged in their action than the quaternary ammonium compounds, and produce a more even and sustained increase in strength, particularly in limb and girdle muscles, following the administration of only one or two doses a day, the danger of cumulation and overdose of drug has precluded their general clinical use except under carefully controlled circumstances.

The maximal strength obtained after optimal doses of any of these quaternary ammonium or organophosphorus anti-ChE compounds is approximately the same (GROB 1958). The compounds differ mainly in their duration of action (organophosphorus compounds > *bis*-neostigmine and *bis*-pyridostigmin > pyridostigmin and ambenomium > neostigmin), and in the severity of their parasympathomimetic side-effects (organophosphorus compounds > *bis*-neostigmine and *bis*-pyridostigmin > neostigmine > pyridostigmin and ambenomium). The administration of graded doses of any of these compounds results in an increase in strength in muscles affected by the disease, but in patients with severe myasthenia the maximal strength attained is frequently far below normal. Before regulation of a patient is attempted, the maximal strength should be determined by the response to the intramuscular injection of 1.5 mg neostigmine per 100 lbs. body weight. The optimal oral dose of any of the anti-ChE compounds may then be determined by gradually increasing the dose until the same degree of maximal improvement is attained. Further increase in dose seldom results in a further increase in maximal strength, and excessive dosage, particularly of the longer acting compounds, is likely to produce generalized weakness — the so-called "cholinergic crisis."

The longer the duration of action of the anti-ChE compound, the more prolonged and even is the increase in strength which is produced, and the longer may be the interval between doses, but the likelihood of cumulative effect of repeated doses and of administration of overdose is also greater. Pyridostigmin and ambenomium are intermediate in their duration of action and danger of overdose,

Table 2. *Drugs useful in myasthenia gravis*

Drug	Purpose	Average Dose (mg)		
		Oral	I. M.	I. V.
Diagnosis				
Neostigmine (Prostigmin) with atropine (0.6 mg) . . .			1.5—2	0.5
Edrophonium (Tensilon)				10.0
Management of weakness				
Neostigmine		30 q 3 h	2 q 2 h	1 q 2 h
Pyridostigmin (Mestinon)		240 q 4 h		
Ambenomium (Mytelase)		20 q 4 h		
Potassium chloride (occasionally useful)		2000 q 4 h		
Ephedrine sulfate (occasionally useful)		25 q 4 h		
Management of overtreatment ("cholinergic crisis")				
Pyridine-2-aldoxime methiodide (P-2-AM)				1000
Diacetyl monoxime (DAM)				1000
1,1′trimethylene-*bis*-(4-formylpyridinium bromide)-dioxime (TMB-4)				125
Atropine sulfate			1—2	1

and generally produce more satisfactory regulation than the other compounds when oral administration is feasible. Most patients are satisfactorily regulated on 120 to 300 mg of pyridostigmin or 10 to 30 mg of ambenomium administered orally at 3- to 4-hour intervals when the patient is awake (Table 2). The initial dose can generally be near the lower limit of these ranges. The dose is then increased every 1 to 2 days until no further increase in strength occurs. Further increase in dose should be avoided unless there appears to be a decrease in the patient's response to the drug. Pyridostigmin and ambenomium produce the same peak strength as neostigmine, but their longer duration of action results in (1) more even strength, (2) better endurance, and (3) greater residual effect during the night and on awakening, and generally permits the patient to omit medication during sleeping hours. They also produce less severe gastrointestinal symptoms than neo-stigmine, although higher doses are more likely to cause headache. Pyridostigmin is less likely to produce weakness following an overdose than ambenomium, and is therefore usually the drug of choice.

Some patients with mild myasthenia can be satisfactorily regulated with neostigmine alone administered in doses of 15 to 45 mg orally at 2 to 4 hour intervals. Some patients with severe myasthenia obtain more even strength when a small dose of neostigmine (15 mg) is administered one hour after each dose of pyridostigmin, ambenomium, or organophosphorus compound. Slow-release tablets of neostigmine and pyridostigmin, having a duration of action of 4 and 6 hours, respectively, are of occasional use at bed-time for eliminating the necessity of interrupting sleep, but regular pyridostigmin taken at bed-time usually achieves the same purpose. A few patients develop exacerbation of acne vulgaris while receiving the bromide salt of pyridostigmin or neostigmine, and prefer the chloride salt of the former.

When the patient is unable to swallow, intramuscular neostigmine (1 to 2 mg every 1 to 3 hours) generally produces the most satisfactory regulation, since adjustment in dose and effect of drug can be made more rapidly than in the case of the other anti-ChE compounds, and overdose avoided. In emergencies, 1 mg neostigmine may be injected intravenously with 0.4 mg atropine. The patient and his family should be instructed in the intramuscular ad-ministration of neostigmine for the management of dysphagia or respiratory distress due to insufficient anti-ChE medication.

D. Use of atropine to control side-effects of anticholinesterase compounds

Atropine sulfate is administered orally or intramuscularly as needed to prevent or suppress the muscarinic effects of anti-ChE compounds, such as excessive saliva-tion and sweating, nausea, vomiting, abdominal cramps, diarrhea, bradycardia, and rarely hypotension. Myasthenic patients generally have a much higher threshold for the development of these effects of anti-ChE compounds than non-myasthenic subjects. During the initial period of drug regulation, atropine is best administered only as needed to ameliorate these side-effects, so that the occurrence of cumulation and overdose of anti-ChE compound may be more easily detected. A sudden increase in side-effects alerts the physician to the more serious effects of overdose on neuromuscular transmission: weakness, frequently accompanied by muscular fasciculation and subjective "tightness." After satisfactory regulation has been attained, atropine is administered if needed to prevent side-effects, usually in a dose of 0.6 mg orally or intramuscularly every 4 to 8 hours. A few patients prefer propantheline (Pro-Banthine), administered in a dose of 15 mg orally or intramuscularly every 6 hours, for the same purpose.

E. Other drugs

Approximately one-third of myasthenic patients experience a slight increase in strength following the oral administration of ephedrine sulfate (25 mg 3 times a day) as an adjuvant to anti-ChE medication, and a smaller number have a similar response to potassium chloride (2 g four times a day). The use of guanidine has been virtually abandoned. Cortisone, adreno-corticotropin, and thyroid hormone have been recommended by some, but were found to produce either no change or a decrease in strength (GROB and HARVEY 1952 and 1953). Reports of a beneficial effect following the administration of post-partum serum (GRANIRER 1953), urecholine (SCHWARZ 1955), and glutamic acid (DULCE 1954) have not been substantiated. A group of alkaloids of plant origin, including galanthamine and lycoramine, have been found to have anticholinesterase activity (IRWIN and SMITH 1960) and are undergoing clinical trial.

There are certain drugs that must be avoided in myasthenic patients, lest they produce a critical exacerbation of weakness. The most important of these are the competitive muscle-relaxing agents, such as curare (or d-tubocurarine) and flaxedil (BERGH 1953). While decamethonium, and particularly succinylcholine, are better tolerated, it is best to avoid the use of muscle relaxants during anesthesia, if possible, since even these drugs may aggravate weakness (BERGH 1953, ANDERSON et al. 1953). Quinine, quinidine, and neomycin should also be avoided, as they may increase neuromuscular block. Since morphine may depress respiration, and since its effects may be potentiated by anti-ChE compounds, it must be used with caution. There have been a few instances of myasthenic patients who succumbed a few hours after the injection of 8 or 16 mg of morphine sulfate. Meperidine (Demerol) is generally well tolerated, although it is best to begin with half the usual dose. Mild sedatives may be used in most patients, but those who are having difficulty swallowing or breathing may develop serious difficulty if they are too heavily sedated.

Although procaine and its derivatives have neuromuscular blocking action, these compounds can be used for local anesthesia, particularly if large doses are avoided and injection is made with adrenaline to delay absorption. Ether is usually well tolerated, although most myasthenic patients require smaller amounts to induce and maintain general anesthesia than normal subjects. Cyclopropane is also well tolerated.

F. Thymectomy

The results following the first successful thymectomies in myasthenia gravis, carried out in 1941 at the Johns Hopkins Hospital, were sufficiently encouraging to warrant continued trial of this procedure (BLALOCK et al. 1941). Since that time, 53 patients have had a thymectomy there and have been observed for 2 to 17 years (average 10 years) (GROB 1953, GROB and HARVEY 1953).

The avarage severity in these cases was greater than in the patients who were not operated upon. The average duration of the disease at the time of surgery was 3 years, but one-third of the patients were operated upon during the first year of their illness. Within a few days after operation many patients experienced an increase in responsiveness to, and a decrease in requirement for anti-ChE medication (HARVEY et al. 1942). Failure to reduce the dose sometimes resulted in the appearance of muscular fasciculation and occasionally weakness. This change was persistent in some patients but lasted only a few days or weeks in most. While 4 patients had a dramatic and lasting remission following thymectomy, the course of the disease in other patients has been only slightly better than in those who have not been operated on. At the time of writing, of the thymectomized patients, 17% are in remission, 27% have improved, 22% are unchanged, 4% are worse, and 30% have died, compared to 14, 21, 16, 11, and 37% respectively in the control group. The course of female and younger patients following thymectomy has been slightly better than that of male and older patients, but this has also been true of patients who were not operated upon. Of 13 patients who had operative removal of a thymoma, 3 have had a dramatic and lasting remission (which had begun prior to operation in one), but the remainder were not improved and in most instances died of the disease within several months after operation.

Thymectomy has now been carried out over a number of years in several large clinics. It is the general consensus that while patients who have a thymoma occasionally develop a remission after thymectomy, most have a poor prognosis which is seldom altered by the operation (GROB and HARVEY 1953, SCHWAB and LELAND 1953, EATON et al. 1953). Nevertheless it is felt by most that a thymoma should be removed because it may extend locally and may occasionally produce symptoms. Irradiation prior to excision has been recommended (KEYNES 1955). There is more difference of opinion concerning removal of the gland when a tumor is not present. The largest number of thymectomies (258) has been carried out by KEYNES (SIMPSON 1956). Twelve per cent of these patients had a thymoma. Omitting these patients, who generally did poorly, 55% improved following the operation, 19% were unchanged or became worse, and 19% died. In a control group, only one-third as large, followed for the same period of time, 33% improved, 19% were unchanged or became worse, and 30% died. The difference between the two groups was greater for female patients than for males, and was significant only for the former. Results were better in those with short preoperative duration of symptoms. Irradiation of the thymic region was usually performed prior to thymectomy. SCHWAB and LELAND (1953) compared the effect of thymectomy in 78 patients with 289 who were not subjected to operation. They reported a significant increase in remission rate following operation only in female patients under 30 years who did not have a thymoma. Of these, 63% improved significantly, compared to 34% of the control group. In men and older female patients there was no difference between the operated and nonoperated groups; in fact, only 24% of the males who had thymectomy improved, compared to 56% in the control group. EATON et al. (1953) have also reported a higher rate of improvement following thymectomy in 44 female patients who did not have a thymoma: 53% compared to 20% of a control group of 48. Other investigators (HOEFER et al. 1953, DUNLOP 1953, JORGENSEN and THERKELSEN 1954, FERGUSON et al. 1955) have not found a significant effect of thymectomy on the course of the disease, although the number of patients studied was small.

The value of thymectomy has not been conclusively demonstrated, and there are still no definite criteria which may serve as a guide in individual patients. In a disease in which there is such a pronounced tendency toward spontaneous variability, it is extremely difficult to know whether favorable results are due to the therapeutic procedure or to an unrelated change in the course of the disease, to increased encouragement of the patient, or to exacerbation of the myasthenia, which is sometimes followed by improvement. VIETS (1953) has recommended that the operation be performed only in young female patients who are not doing well on medical management. He does not recommend thymectomy, except in rare instances, in patients over 50 or under 5 years of age, or in those who are in remission or are well adjusted on medication. It would seem best at this time to limit the procedure to those patients who are becoming progressively worse despite careful medical management and in whom the chance for spontaneous remission appears to be small.

Reports of a beneficial effect following carotid sinus denervation, (THEVENARD 1954, MERTENS 1955) and parathyroidectomy (AKAO and KAWAISHI 1952) have not been substantiated.

G. Management of exacerbation of myasthenia gravis

I. Description of the patient

The patient with the typical features of generalized myasthenia gravis has ptosis, resulting in a characteristic sleepy appearance, sometimes accompanied by compensatory wrinkling of the forehead. Facial weakness causes an apathetic, "myasthenic" expression, and weakness of the orbicularis oris a smirk or "snarl" when smiling or laughing is attempted. When the frontalis is severely affected, it is impossible to wrinkle the forehead, and when the orbicularis oculi are very weak, the eyes cannot be shut. Weakness of the masseters causes sagging of the jaw, which often has to be supported by the hand. As the disease progresses, there ensues difficulty in swallowing, with nasal regurgitation and choking spells, and difficulty in speaking, with nasal slurred speech. Weakness of the neck muscles may make it difficult to hold up the head. The upper extremities are usually affected before the lower, and the proximal muscles before the distal ones. The muscles of the trunk and abdomen and of respiration are among the last involved after the disease has become severe. There then occurs shortness of breath and weakness of cough, which may become extremely troublesome during respiratory infections, resulting in pooling of secretions in the respiratory tract, bronchitis, atelectasis, and pneumonitis. Thirty per cent of patients die of the disease, with 70% of deaths occurring within one year after onset and 85% within three years (GROB 1958). Death is usually due to failure of the muscles of respiration, or less often to respiratory obstruction following aspiration of food.

Exacerbation of the disease is characterized not only by increased weakness, but also by increased requirement for, and diminished response to, anti-ChE medication. The factors most commonly associated with exacerbation are upper respiratory infection, other infectious illness, emotional tension, and the post-partum period. In addition, most women feel weakest for several days before each menstrual period. Sometimes, however, exacerbation of the disease occurs without evident cause. When the exacerbation is severe, with difficulty in swallowing and breathing, it has been termed by some a "myasthenic crisis."

II. Administration of anticholinesterase compound

Exacerbation of myasthenia gravis is managed by increasing the dose of anti-ChE medication and employing mechanical measures when needed to maintain the respiration and remove secretions. When dysphagia or respiratory weakness is severe, oral medication should be discontinued and the patient managed with intramuscular neostigmine, supplemented by atropine and suction to diminish and remove secretions (Table 3). The longer acting drugs, pyridostigmin and ambenomium, may also be administered parenterally, but while they produce less salivation and bronchial secretion than neostigmine, their longer action makes adjustment of dose and avoidance of overdose more difficult.

Table 3. *Management of weakness of muscles of swallowing and respiration*

1. *Due to exacerbation or under-treatment of myasthenia gravis*
   ("myasthenic weakness or crisis")

   Mechanical Aids: Respiratory tract: suction, artificial respiration (mouth-to-nose, mouth-to-mouth, mechanical), endotracheal intubation, tracheotomy, bronchial aspiration, exsufflation, oxygen
   Nutrition: intravenous feeding, stomach tube

   Drugs: *Anti-ChE:* neostigmine, 1 to 2 mg intramuscularly or intravenously, q 1 to 3 hr; reduce dose when patient is in respirator
   Anticholinergic: atropine, 0.2 to 0.6 mg intramuscularly q 3 to 6 hr
   Others: KCl, antibiotics

2. *Due to overdose of anti-ChE drug ("cholinergic crisis")*
   (Management is similar in myasthenic and nonmyasthenic patients)

   Mechanical Aids: Same as in "myasthenic crisis"

   Drugs: *Anticholinergic:* atropine, 1 to 2 mg intravenously or intramuscularly q 1/2 to 2 hr
   Anti-anti-ChE: P-2-AM or DAM, 1000 to 2000 mg, or TMB-4, 125 to 250 mg, intravenously

III. Maintenance of airway and artificial respiration

Severe dysphagia and weakness of the pharyngeal and tongue muscles may result in upper airway obstruction and choking spells. If this is severe enough to cause cyanosis, an endotracheal catheter should be inserted, as described in the preceding chapter. The patient at this stage is usually too weak to resist effectively attempts at intubation. The endotracheal tube should not be left in place more than 48 hours, as this produces edema of the larynx, which may result in airway obstruction when the tube is removed. Since most myasthenic patients continue to have severe dysphagia after withdrawal of the tube, it is usually best to perform a tracheotomy under local procaine anesthesia while the tube is still in place. The tracheotomy can be utilized as long as dysphagia persists or recurs, for years if necessary. The overlying skin may be allowed to close whenever the patient's condition permits, but the sinus tract of the trachectomy persists and can be utilized again if necessary. Since respiratory weakness usually develops concomitantly with pharyngeal weakness, most patients who are intubated or tracheotomized require artificial respiration. Conversely, patients who are unable to breathe usually have obstruction of the upper airway, and artificial respiration is greatly facilitated, and aspiration of secretions prevented, by intubation or tracheotomy.

If facilities for intubation and mechanical artificial respiration are not immediately available, manual artificial respiration may be instituted by mouth-to-nose, or mouth-to-mouth means (SAFAR 1957, 1958, SAFAR et al. 1958, ELAM et al. 1958, 1960). During this procedure, the hands are placed at the angle of the patient's mandibles, which are pulled up and forward and the head tilted back as far as possible, in order to prevent the base of the tongue from blocking the airway. As soon as possible, however, mechanical artificial respiration should be instituted. While the patient is being moved, or is awaiting a respirator, breathing can be maintained by means of a rubber bag, kept inflated by an oxygen tank and rhythmically deflated by one hand while the other hand applies a face mask and supports the mandible. Since artificial respiration must be maintained for hours or days, it should be continued by means of a motor driven negative-pressure body (tank) respirator or positive-pressure-cycled resuscitator. The former is most satisfactory for prolonged use, as it permits more efficient suction of secretions from the pharynx, endotracheal tube, or tracheotomy. The chest respirator is less suitable for patients with severe weakness, as it often does not cause sufficient exchange of air.

Regardless of the means of artificial respiration employed, endotracheal intubation or tracheotomy and periodic suction should be performed as soon as possible to reduce upper airway obstruction, pooling of secretions in the pharynx, aspiration, and pneumonitis. Oxygen may be administered, with nebulized moisture to prevent drying of mucus membranes and with a detergent such as Alevare or Turgomist to assist in the removal of secretions. The foot of the respirator can be elevated when needed to promote drainage. It is sometimes helpful to make the patient "cough" by periodically decreasing rapidly the negative pressure within the respirator by means of an attached exsufflator. Although the value of prophylactic administration of antibiotics to patients in respirators has been questioned, it is probably helpful to administer penicillin and streptomycin parenterally, since the dysphagia and impairment of cough and respiration that precede institution of artificial respiration predispose to atelectesis and pneumonia. The occurrence of atelectasis necessitates bronchial suction, which can usually be carried out through a catheter passed into the trachea and bronchi, with the help of proper positioning of the patient. Bronchoscopy is seldom required.

While the patient is in the respirator, the dose of neostigmine should be reduced to 0.5 to 1 mg, or less, every 2 to 3 hours, as this is frequently followed by some improvement in response to the drug. Precipitous withdrawal of anti-ChE medication has been recommended by some (RANDT 1953), but has the disadvantage of leaving the patient more susceptible to deficiencies in the mechanical respirator. Fluid and electrolyte balance are maintained by intravenous administation of glucose (dextrose), sodium chloride, and 1 to 2 g of potassium chloride daily. Protein hydrolysate (Amigen) may be added. If the patient is unable to swallow by the third day, a stomach tube should be inserted, and feeding begun to maintain an adequate nutritional state. Improvement and even remission of myasthenia gravis has occurred in some patients after as long as 6 months of continual respirator care (GROB 1958).

H. Management of overdose of anticholinesterase compound

I. Occurrence and detection of overdose

Intoxication by anti-ChE compounds may occur in patients with myasthenia gravis following the administration of excessive doses. In the management of this disease graded doses of an anti-ChE compound are administered until a maximal level of strength is attained in the affected muscles. Unfortunately, in patients with severe myasthenia the maximal strength attained may be far below normal. Increasing doses may result in no further increase in strength, and excessive drug may produce generalized weakness, attributable to the accumulation of an excessive concentration of ACh at the motor endplates and prolonged depolarization of this region, followed by refractoriness of the endplates to the action of ACh (GROB and JOHNS 1959). This state has been termed "cholinergic crisis" by some, to distinguish it from weakness due to the disease itself ("myasthenic weakness, or crisis"). If the cholinergic crisis is severe, death may occur as a result of paralysis of the muscles of respiration and of the pharynx and tongue unless artificial respiration and an open airway are maintained until recovery occurs.

The long-acting organophosphorus anti-ChE compounds such as tetraethylpyrophosphate (TEPP) (GROB and HARVEY 1949) and octamethyl pyrophosphortetramide (OMPA) (SCHULMAN et al. 1953), and long-acting quaternary ammonium compounds such as bis-neostigmine (BC-40) and bis-pyridostigmin (Hexamarium, BC-51), are most likely to produce cumulation and overdose. Short-acting quaternary ammonium compounds such as neostigmine are least likely to have this effect, unless administered in conjunction with one of the longer acting drugs. While neostigmine is safest in this regard, its short action results in less even strength and requires more frequent administration. If excessive doses are given, even neostigmine may produce weakness (ROWLAND et al. 1955). Quaternary ammonium compounds with an intermediate duration of action, such as pyridostigmin (OSSERMAN et al. 1954) and ambenomium (SCHWAB et al. 1955), usually produce more satisfactory regulation because they afford a more sustained increase in strength than does neostigmine, but they are also intermediate with regard to danger of overdose.

The weakness that occurs in myasthenic patients following excessive doses of anti-ChE compounds is in many ways similar to that produced by smaller doses of these compounds in normal subjects. However, whereas generalized muscular fasciculation and muscarinic symptoms (nausea, vomiting, abdominal cramps, diarrhea, sweating) almost invariably develop in normal subjects (Grob 1956), fasciculation is frequently absent or minimal in patients with severe myasthenia, and muscarinic symptoms may be either pronounced, mild, or absent. Furthermore, the prior administration of atropine may suppress the muscarinic symptoms. In the absence of these collateral signs of anti-ChE intoxication, it is sometimes difficult to determine whether an increase in weakness in a myasthenic patient is due to an overdose of anti-ChE drug or to progression of the myasthenia and the need for more drug.

If overdose is suspected, the simplest procedure is to withhold medication for several hours and carefully observe whether the strength increases or decreases. It is frequently helpful to observe the effect on the weakness of administration of an oxime such as pyridine-2-aldoxime methiodide (P-2-AM) or diacetyl

Table 4. *Differentiation between underdose and overdose of anticholinesterase drug in myasthenia gravis*

	Underdose ("Myasthenic Crisis")	Overdose ("Cholinergic Crisis")
Muscle fasciculation and "tightness"	0	0 to $+++++$
Nausea, vomiting, cramps, diarrhea, sweating	0	0 to $++++$
Effect on strength of:		
Discontinuation of anti-ChE drug	↓	↑
P-2-AM or DAM (500 mg) or TMB-4 (60 mg) intravenously .	↓	↑
Edrophonium (2 mg, intravenously) or other anti-ChE drug	↑	↓

monoxime (DAM), or 1,1′trimethylene-*bis*-(4-formylpyridinium bromide)-dioxime (TMB-4, EA 1814), which is capable of reversing cholinesterase inhibition and neuromuscular block produced by anti-ChE compounds in myasthenic patients as well as in normal subjects (Grob and Johns 1958a to c). Following the intravenous injection of 500 mg of P-2-AM or DAM, or 60 mg TMB-4, an increase in strength indicates that the patient was weak because of an excess of anti-ChE drug, while a decrease indicates that he was either at his maximal level of strength or had not received enough anti-ChE medication (Table 4). The converse of this is seen following the intravenous injection of 2 mg of edrophonium, when an increase in strength indicates that the patient was weak due to insufficient anti-ChE medication, and a decrease in strength indicates that he was weak due to excess of medication (Osserman and Kaplan 1953). If the patient is very weak, administration of oxime or edrophonium should be carried out only if the patient is in or near a respirator, and facilities are available for endotracheal intubation, since exacerbation of weakness may require these aids. Unfortunately, many patients with severe myasthenia who are responding poorly to anti-ChE medication fail to improve following either expectant management or administration of oxime or edrophonium, and they may become worse after any of these measures. The main difficulty in these patients is probably neither insufficient nor excessive anti-ChE medication, but a refractory or "insensitive" state of the motor endplates to the normal depolarizing action of ACh. The only therapeutic measure available for this condition is to maintain respiration and reduce the dosage of anti-ChE medication until the response to this medication improves.

II. Administration of oxime

If the myasthenic patient is weak due to overdose of anti-ChE medication, strength will be improved by the intravenous administration of oxime, such as

66*

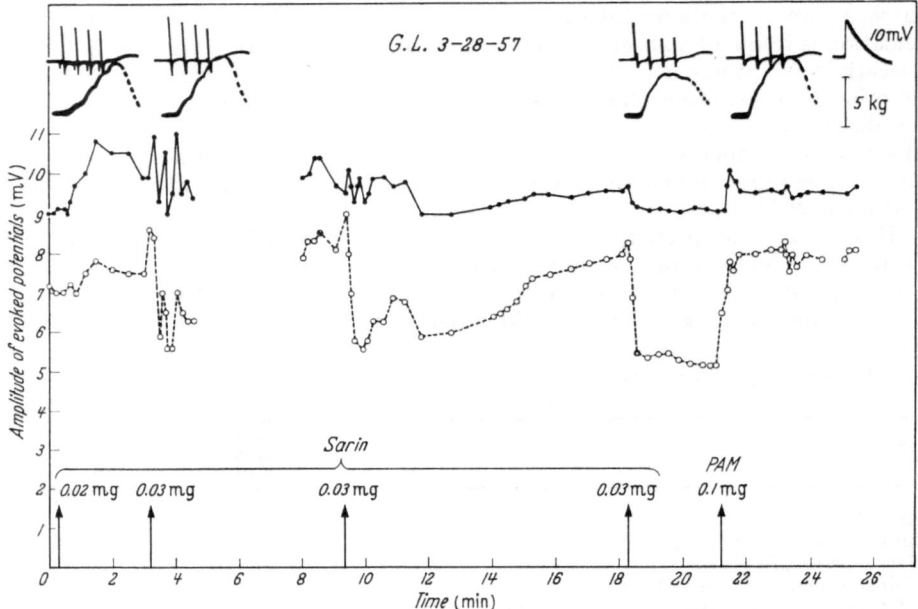

Fig. 3. Reversal by P-2-AM of the depressant effect of excessive Sarin on evoked muscle action potentials and tension of a myasthenic patient. The latter had been preceded by the reparative effect of prior injections of Sarin. The amplitude of the first (●———●) and fourth (○-----○) potentials in response to a train of four nerve stimuli (40 msec apart) evoked every 5 seconds has been plotted, and illustrative potentials (mV) and tension (kg) recorded above. Injections were intra-arterial. (From GROB and JOHNS 1958)

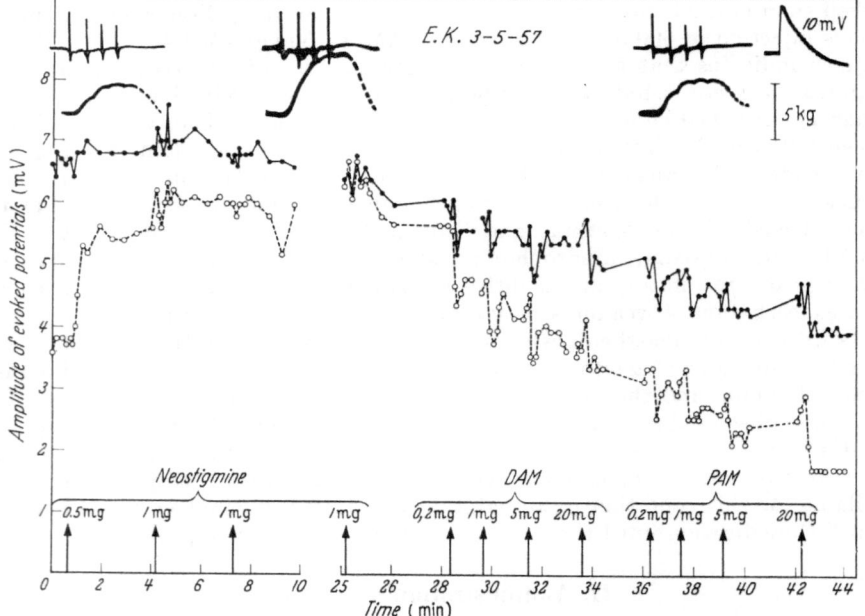

Fig. 4. Reversal by DAM and P-2-AM of reparative effect of neostigmine on evoked muscle action potentials and tension of a myasthenic patient. Amplitude of first (●———●) and fourth (○-----○) potentials in response to a train of four nerve stimuli (40 msec apart) evoked every 5 seconds has been plotted, and illustrative potentials (mV) and tension (kg) recorded above. Injections were intra-arterial. (From GROB and JOHNS 1958)

P-2-AM, DAM, or TMB-4 (GROB and JOHNS 1958a to c). The neuromuscular actions of anti-ChE compounds are reversed by these oximes. The effect of this reversal depends on the prior action of the anti-ChE compound, since neuromuscular function is restored toward its initial state. Whereas in normal subjects neuromuscular function and strength are returned toward normal, in myasthenic patients the effect depends on the status of the patient at the time of oxime administration. If sufficient anti-ChE compound has been administered to depress function, this is restored to a more optimal level (Fig. 3), but if function was optimal at the time of oxime administration, it is restored toward the basal level present prior to the administration of anti-ChE compound; i.e. it is depressed (Fig. 4).

While the oximes are equally effective in the management of anti-ChE intoxication in myasthenic patients and normal subjects, more cautious administration is necessary in the former. Following the amelioration of weakness due to this intoxication by the administration of 1,000 mg of P-2-AM or DAM, or 125 mg of TMB-4, repetition of this dose has no effect on strength in normal subjects, but produces weakness in some patients with severe myasthenia. In these patients, over-treatment with oxime may convert a cholinergic crisis into a myasthenic

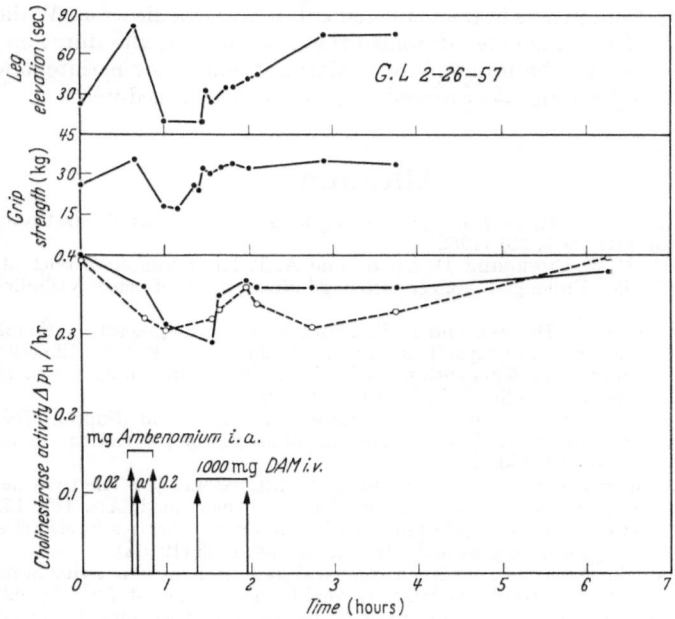

Fig. 5. Reversal by DAM of generalized weakness and plasma (●——●) and red blood cell (○-----○) cholinesterase inhibition produced by excess ambenomium in a myasthenic patient. The weakness was preceded by an increase in strength resulting from the prior injection of smaller doses of ambenomium. (From GROB and JOHNS 1958)

crisis. It is therefore recommended that myasthenic patients suffering from anti-ChE intoxication be titrated with successive 500 mg doses of P-2-AM or DAM, or 60 mg of TMB-4, at five-to-ten minute intervals until strength is restored to the maximal level attained following the administration of optimal doses of anti-ChE compound (Fig. 5). Availability of these oximes should enable potent and long-acting anti-ChE compounds to be employed in the management of myasthenia gravis with less danger from the effects of drug cumulation and overdose.

Systemic weakness produced by the oximes in myasthenic patients is due to reversal of the action of previously administered anti-ChE compound. The local neuromuscular block produced by large doses of P-2-AM injected intra-arterially is no greater in these patients than in normal subjects. This block therefore does not appear to be due to competitive inhibition of the action of ACh on the motor endplate, since such inhibition would be more marked in myasthenic patients (GROB et al. 1956).

III. Administration of atropine

If the muscarinic manifestations of anti-ChE intoxication are present, atropine should be administered in a dose of 1 to 2 mg intravenously or intramuscularly, and repeated if necessary, since these manifestations are not affected by the oximes. Inasmuch as salivary and bronchial secretions are usually profuse, frequent suction should also be employed. As in normal subjects, atropine has no effect on weakness due to anti-ChE compounds.

IV. Maintenance of airway and artificial respiration

Upper airway obstruction due to weakness of the pharyngeal and tongue muscles, and respiratory weakness are managed by endotracheal intubation and artificial respiration, just as in the management of myasthenic crisis. While prompt administration of an oxime may diminish the necessity for, and duration of, these measures, there should be no delay in initiating them, since maintenance of the airway and of respiration takes precedence over other procedures.

Literature

AKAO, S., and H. KAWAISHI: Case of myasthenia gravis cured by partial parathyroidectomy. Rinshô-Naika Shônika 7, 281 (1952).

ANDERSON, H. J., C. H. CHURCHILL-DAVIDSON and A. T. RICHARDSON: Bronchial neoplasm with myasthenia: Prolonged apnoea after administration of succinylcholine. Lancet 1953 II, 1291.

ARANOW, H. jr., P. F. A. HOEFER and L. P. ROWLAND: The long-acting anticholinesterase drugs in the management of myasthenia gravis. J. chron. Dis. 6, 113—125 (1958).

BERGH, N. P.: Reaction of patients with myasthenia gravis to different agents causing neuromuscular block. Scand. J. clin. Lab. Invest. 5, 11 (1953).

— Thymectomy in Treatment of myasthenia gravis. Acta chir. scand. (Suppl.) 1753, 1 (1953).

BICKERSTAFF, E. R., and A. L. WOOLF: The intramuscular nerve endings in myasthenia gravis. Brain 83, 10—23 (1960).

BLALOCK, A., A. M. HARVEY, F. R. FORD and J. L. LILIENTHAL jr.: The treatment of myasthenia gravis by removal of the thymus gland. J. Amer. med. Ass. 117, 1529 (1941).

BOTELHO, S. Y.: Alterations in muscle tension without similar changes in electrical activity in patients with myasthenia gravis. J. clin. Invest. 34, 1403 (1955a).

— Comparison of simultaneously recorded electrical and mechanical activity in myasthenia gravis patients and in partially curarized normal humans. Amer. J. Med. 19, 693 (1955b).

BROOKS, V. B.: The action of botulinum toxin on motor nerve filaments. J. Physiol. (Lond.) 123, 501 (1954).

BURNS, B. D., and W. D. M. PATON: Depolarization of the motor end-plate by decamethonium and acetylcholine. J. Physiol. (Lond.) 115, 41 (1951).

CHURCHILL-DAVIDSON, H. C., and A. T. RICHARDSON: Neuromuscular transmission in myasthenia gravis. J. Physiol. (Lond.) 122, 252—263 (1953).

COËRS, C., and J. E. DESMEDT: Evidence for characteristic malformation of the neuromuscular junction in myasthenia gravis. Acta neurol. belg. 59, 539—561 (1959).

COMROE, J. H. Jr., J. TODD, G. D. GAMMON, I. H. LEOPOLD, G. B. KOELLE, O. BODANSKY and A. GILMAN: The effect of di-isopropyl-fluorophosphate (DFP) upon patients with myasthenia gravis. Amer. J. med. Sci. 212, 641—651 (1946).

DESMEDT, J. E.: Neurochemical lesion in myasthenia gravis. Fed. Proc. 18, 36 (1959).

DULCE, N. J.: Behandlung der myasthenia gravis und psychischer Störungen bei der Chorea minor mit Glutaminsäure. Münch. med. Wschr. 96, 1235 (1954).

DUNLOP, D. M.: Thymectomy in myasthenia gravis. Trans. med. chir. Soc. Edinb. **132**, 59 (1953).

EATON, L. M., O. P. CLAGETT and J. A. BASTRON: Thymus and its relationship to diseases of nervous system. Study of 374 cases of myasthenia gravis and comparison of 87 patients undergoing thymectomy with 225 controls. A. Res. Nerv. a. Ment. Dis., Proc. **32**, 107 (1953).

ELAM, J. O., D. G. GREEN, M. A. SCHNEIDER, H. M. RUBEN, A. S. GORDON, R. F. HUSTEAD, D. W. BENSON, J. A. CLEMENTS and A. RUBEN: Head-tilt method of oral resuscitation. J. Amer. med. Ass. **173**, 812—815 (1960).

— E. S. BROWN and J. A. CLEMENTS: Oxygen and carbon dioxide exchange and energy cost of expired air resuscitation. J. Amer. med. Ass. **167**, 328—334 (1958).

FATT, P.: Biophysics of junctional transmission. Physiol. Rev. **34**, 674 (1954).

FERGUSON, F. R., E. C. HUTCHINSON and L. A. LIVERSEDGE: Myasthenia gravis; Results of medical management. Lancet **1955 II**, 636.

GRANIRER, L. W.: Beneficial effect of postpartum plasma in a case of myasthenia gravis. Conn. med. J. **172**, 934 (1953).

GROB, D.: Course and management of myasthenia gravis. J. Amer. med. Ass. **153**, 529 (1953).

— Effect of Sarin in patients with myasthenia gravis. Progress Report to U.S. Army Chemical Corps Medical Laboratories, Army Chemical Center, Med. (1955).

— The manifestations and treatment of poisoning due to nerve gas and other organic phosphorus anticholinesterase compounds. Arch. intern. Med. **98**, 221—239 (1956).

— The neuromuscular system. Chapter 30 in Clinical Physiology. 725—756. Ed. by ARTHUR GROLLMAN. New York: McGraw-Hill Inc. 1957.

— Myasthenia gravis: Current status of pathogenesis, clinical manifestations and management. J. chron. Dis. 8, 536—566 (1958).

—, and A. M. HARVEY: Observations on the effects of tetraethyl pyrophosphate (TEPP) in man and on its use in the treatment of myasthenia gravis. Bull. Johns Hopk. Hosp. **84**, 533—567 (1949).

— — Effect of adrenocorticotropic hormone (ACTH) and cortisone administration in patients with myasthenia gravis and report of onset of myasthenia gravis during prolonged cortisone administration. Bull. Johns Hopk. Hosp. **91**, 124—136 (1952).

— — Abnormalities in neuromuscular transmission, with special reference to myasthenia gravis. Amer. J. Med. **15**, 695—709 (1953).

—, and R. J. JOHNS: Use of oximes in the treatment of intoxication by anticholinesterase compounds in patients with myasthenia gravis. Amer. J. Med. **24**, 512—518 (1958a).

— — Treatment of anticholinesterase intoxication in normal subjects and myasthenia patients with oximes. J. Amer. med. Ass. **166**, 1855—1858 (1958b).

— — Use of the oxime 1,1'-trimethylene bis-(4-formylpyridinium bromide) dioxime (EA 1814, TMB-4) in the management of intoxication by anticholinesterase compounds. Contractor's Progress Report to U.S. Army Chemical Corps. Medical Laboratories, Army Chemical Center, Md., August (1958c).

— — Further studies on the mechanism of the defect in neuromuscular transmission in myasthenia gravis, with particular reference to the acetylcholine-insensitive block. In H. R. VIETS, ed., Myasthenia Gravis: Second Internat. Sympos. Proc. 127—149. Springfield, Ill.: Chas. C. Thomas 1961.

— and A. M. HARVEY: Studies in neuromuscular function. I. Introduction and methods. Bull. Johns Hop. Hosp. **99**, 115—124 (1956a).

— — — Studies in neuromuscular function. III. Stimulating and depressant effects of acetylcholine and choline in normal subjects. Bull. Johns Hopk. Hosp. **99**, 136—152 (1956b).

— — — Studies in neuromuscular function. IV. Stimulating and depressant effects of acetylcholine and choline in patients with myasthenia gravis, and their relationship to the defect in neuromuscular transmission. Bull. Johns Hopk. Hosp. **99**, 153—181 (1956c).

— — — Studies in neuromuscular function. V. Effects of anticholinesterase compounds, d-tubocurarine, and decamethonium in normal subjects. Bull. Johns Hopk. Hosp. **99**, 195 (1956d).

— — — Studies in neuromuscular function. VI: Effects of anticholinesterase compounds, d-tubocurarine, and decamethonium in patients with myasthenia gravis. Bull. Johns Hopk. Hosp. **99**, 219—238 (1956e).

— — — Alterations in neuromuscular transmission in myasthenia gravis, as determined by studies of drug action. Amer. J. Med. **19**, 684—690 (1955).

— A. LILJESTRAND and R. J. JOHNS: Potassium movement in normal subjects and in patients with familial periodic paralysis. Amer. J. Med. **23**, 340—375 (1957).

—, and K. E. OSSERMAN: Unpublished observations (1958).

HARVEY, A. M., and J. L. LILIENTHAL: Observations on the nature of myasthenia gravis. The intra-arterial injection of acetylcholine, prostigmine and adrenaline. Bull. Johns Hopk. Hosp. **69**, 566 (1941).

HARVAY, A. M., J. L. LILIENTHAL Jr., D. GROB, B. F. JONES and S. A. TALBOT: The administration of di-isopropyl fluorophosphate to man: IV. The effects on neuromuscular function in normal subjects and in myasthenia gravis. Bull. Johns Hopk. Hosp. 81, 267—292 (1947).

— — and S. A. TALBOT: Observations on the nature of myasthenia gravis. The effect of thymectomy on neuromuscular transmission. J. clin. Invest. 21, 579 (1942).

—, and R. L. MASLAND: The electromyogram in myasthenia gravis. Bull. Johns Hopk. Hosp. 69, 1 (1941).

—, and M. R. WHITEHILL: Prostigmine as aid in diagnosis of myasthenia gravis. J. Amer. med. Ass. 108, 1329 (1937).

— — Quinine as adjuvant to prostigmine in diagnosis of myasthenia gravis. Preliminary report. Bull. Johns Hopk. Hosp. 61, 216 (1937).

HERZFELD, E., O. KRAUPP, K. PATEISKY u. C. STUMPF: Pharmakologische und klinische Wirkungen des Cholinesterashemmkörpers Hexamethylen-bis-(N-methyl-carbaminoyl-1-methyl-3-oxypyridiniumbromid) (BC 51) (Pharmacological and clinical effects of the cholinesterase inhibitor hexamethylene-bis-(N-methylcarbaminoyl-1-methyl-3-oxypyridinium bromide) (BC 51). Wien. kin. Wschr. 69, 245—248 (1957).

HOEFER, P. F. A., H. ARONOW and L. P. ROWLAND: Therapy of myasthenia gravis. Neurology 3, 691 (1953).

HUTTER, O. F.: Effect of choline on neuromuscular transmission in the cat. J. Physiol. (Lond.) 117, 241 (1952).

IRWIN, R. U., and M. J. SMITH III: Cholinesterase inhibition by galanthamine and lycoramine. Biochem. Pharmacol. 3, 147—148 (1960).

JOHNS, R. J.: Factors influencing muscle membrane potential in man, as recorded with intracellular microelectrodes. J. Pharmacol. exp. Ther. 122, 36a (1958).

— D. GROB and A. M. HARVEY: Electromyographic changes in myasthenia gravis. Amer. J. Med. 19, 679—683 (1955).

— — — Studies in neuromuscular function. II. Effects of nerve stimulation in normal subjects and in patients with myasthenia gravis. Bull. Johns Hopk. Hosp. 99, 125—135 (1956).

JORGENSEN, J. B., and F. THERKELSEN: Thymectomy in the treatment of myasthenia gravis. Acta chir. scand. 107, 414 (1954).

KATZ, B., and S. THESLEFF: A study of the "desensitization" produced by acetylcholine at the motor endplate. J. Physiol. (Lond.) 138, 63 (1957).

KEYNES, G.: Investigation into thymic disease and tumor formation. Brit. J. Surg. 42, 449 (1955).

KUFFLER, S. W.: Specific excitability of the endplate region in normal and denervated muscle. J. Neurophysiol. 6, 99—110 (1943).

LAMMERS, W., and D. MOST VAN SPIJK: Unsuccessful attempt to demonstrate a paralytic factor in serum of myasthenia gravis patients. Nature (Lond.) 173, 1192 (1954).

MacDERMOT, V.: The changes in the motor endplate in myasthenia gravis. Brain 83, 24—35 (1960).

McSWEYN, N. F., and H. SCHWARTZ: Thymectomy in myasthenia gravis. Canad. med. Ass. J. 70, 311 (1954).

MERRILL, G. G.: Neostigmine toxicity: Report of fatality following diagnostic test for myasthenia. J. Amer. med. Ass. 137, 362 (1948).

MERTENS, H. G.: Über den Verlauf der Myasthenie nach Carotissinus-denervierung. Nervenarzt 26, 150 (1955).

NOWELL, P. T., and A. WILSON: Isolation of quaternary ammonium compounds from the extracts of thymus glands. In H. R. VIETS, ed., Myasthenia Gravis: Second Internat. Sympos. Proc., 238—256. Springfield, Ill.: Chas. C. Thomas 1961.

OSSERMAN, K. E., E. S. COHEN and G. GENKINS: Phospholine iodide: An anticholinesterase drug of new structure. Preliminary report in the treatment of myasthenia gravis. In H. R. VIETS, ed., Myasthenia Gravis: Second Internat. Sympos. Proc., 581—594. Springfield, Ill.: Chas. C. Thomas 1961.

—, and L. I. KAPLAN: Studies in myasthenia gravis. Present status of therapy with octamethyl pyrophosphoramide (OMPA). Ann. intern. Med. 41, 108 (1954).

— — Studies in myasthenia gravis: Use of edrophonium chloride (Tensilon) in differentiating myasthenic from cholinergic weakness. Arch. Neurol. Psychiat. (Chicago) 70, 385 (1953).

— — Rapid diagnostic test for myasthenia gravis: Increased muscle strength, without fasciculation, after intravenous administration of edrophonium (tensilon) chloride. J. Amer. med. Ass. 150, 265 (1952).

— P. TENG and L. I. KAPLAN: Studies in myasthenia gravis. Preliminary report on therapy with Mestinon bromide. J. Amer. med. Ass. 155, 961 (1954).

PATEISKY, K., E. HERZFELT and C. STUMPF: Der Effekt von Polymethylen-bis (N-methyl-carbaminolyl-m-Trimethylammoniumphenolen) BC 40, BC 47, BC 48 auf Cholinesterase-aktivat und Muskeltätigkeit bei Myasthenia gravis pseudoparalytica. Wien. klin. Wschr. **69**, 2—7 (1957).
— O. KRAUPP u. C. STUMPF: Klinische Erfahrungen mit Hexamethylen-bis-(N-methyl-carbaminoyl-m-trimethylammoniumphenol) (BC 40) bei Myasthenia gravis pseudopara-lytica. Wien. klin. Wschr. **67**, 578 (1955).
PELIKAN, E. W., J. E. TETHER and K. R. UNNA: Sensitivity of myasthenia gravis patients to tubocurarine and decamethonium. Neurology **3**, 284 (1953).
RANDT, C. T.: Myasthenia gravis. Med. Clin. N. Amer. **37**, 535 (1953).
RIDER, J. A., S. SCHULMAN, R. B. RICHTER, H. D. MOELLER and K. P. DuBois: Treatment of myasthenia gravis with octamethyl pyrophosphoramide. J. Amer. med. Ass. **145**, 967 to 972 (1951).
ROWLAND, L. P., M. C. KORENGOLD, I. A. JAFFE, L. BERG and G. M. SHY: Prostigmine induced muscle weakness in myasthenia gravis patients. Neurology **5**, 89 (1955).
ROE, J. H., R. J. JOHNS and D. GROB: Unpublished observations (1955).
SAFAR, P.: Mouth-to-mouth airway. Anesthesiology **18**, 904 (1957).
— Ventilatory efficacy of mouth-to-mouth artificial respiration. J. Amer. med. Ass. **167**, 335—341 (1958).
— L. A. ESCARRAGO and J. O. ELAM: A comparison of the mouth-to-mouth and mouth-to-airway methods of artificial respiration with the chest-pressure arm-lift methods. New Engl. J. Med. **258**, 671—677 (1958).
SCHAUMANN, W., and C. JOB: Differential effects of quaternary cholinesterase inhibitor, phos-pholine, and its tertiary analogue, compound 217-AO, on central control of respiration and on neuromuscular transmission. The antagonism by 217-AO of the respiratory arrest caused by morphine. J. Pharmacol. exp. Ther. **123**, 114—120 (1958).
SCHULMAN, S., J. A. RIDER and R. B. RICHTER: Use of octamethyl pyrophosphoramide in the treatment of myasthenia gravis. J. Amer. med. Ass. **152**, 1707 (1953).
SCHWAB, R. S.: WIN-8077 in the treatment of sixty myasthenia gravis patients. A twelve month report. Amer. J. Med. **19**, 734 (1955).
—, and C. LELAND: Sex and age in myasthenia gravis as critical factors in incidence and remission. J. Amer. med. Ass. **153**, 1270 (1953).
— C. K. MARSHALL and W. T. TIMBERLAKE: WIN 8077 in treatment of myasthenia gravis, use of N,N'-bis (2-diethyl-aminoethyl) oxamide bis-2-chlorobenzyl chloride in 50 patients. J. Amer. med. Ass. **158**, 625—628 (1955).
— K. E. OSSERMAN and J. E. TETHER: Treatment of myasthenia gravis. J. Amer. med. Ass. **165**, 671—674 (1957).
SCHWARZ, H.: Urecholine in myasthenia gravis. Canad. med. Ass. J. **72**, 346 (1955).
— Curare-like factor in serum of myasthenia gravis patients. Canad. med. Ass. J. **67**, 238 (1952).
SEIBERT, P.: Zur Behandlung der Myasthenia gravis. Klinische Erfahrungen über die Be-handlung der Myasthenia gravis pseudoparalytica mit Pyridostigmin. Dtsch. med. Wschr. **78**, 805 (1953).
SIMPSON, J. A.: Discussion on myasthenia. The value of thymectomy. Proc. roy. Soc. Med. **49**, 795 (1956).
— Myasthenia gravis: A new hypothesis. Scot. med. J. **5**, 419—436 (1960).
STRAUSS, A. J. L., B. C. SEEGAL, K. S. HSU, P. M. BURKHOLDER, W. L. NASTUK and K. E. OSSERMAN: Immunofluorescence demonstration of a muscle binding complement-fixing serum globulin fraction in myasthenia gravis. Proc. Soc. exp. Biol. (N. Y.) **105**, 184—191 (1960).
TETHER, J. R.: Treatment of myasthenia gravis with mestinon bromide. J. Amer. med. Ass. **160**, 156 (1956).
TETHER, J. E.: Intravenous neostigmine in diagnosis of myasthenia gravis. Ann. intern. Med. **29**, 1132 (1948).
THEVENARD, A.: Les effets de l'énervation sin-carotidienne sur la myasthenia bulbospinal essai d'interprétation. Rev. neurol. **90**, 107 (1954).
TORDA, C., and H. G. WOLF: Depression of acetylcholine synthesis by serum from working muscle, healthy subjects and myasthenia gravis patients. Proc. Soc. exp. Biol. (N. Y.) **59**, 13 (1945).
TSUKIYAMA, K., A. NAKAI, R. MINE and T. KITANI: Studies on a myasthenic substance present in the serum of patient with myasthenic gravis. Med. J. Osaka Univ. **10**, 159—170 (1959).
VAN MAANEN, E. F.: Neuromuscular blocking agents. Amer. J. Med. **19**, 669 (1955).
VIETS, H. R.: Thymectomy for myasthenia gravis. J. Amer. med. Ass. **151**, 1248 (1953).

1050   Literature

VIETS, H. R.: Diagnosis of myasthenia gravis in patients with dysphagia. J. Amer. med.
    Ass. **134**, 988 (1947).
—, and R. S. SCHWAB: Prostigmin in the diagnosis of myasthenia gravis. New Engl. J. Med.
    213, 1280 (1935).
WESTERBERG, M. R.: Clinical evaluation of ambenomium (Mysuran) chloride. Arch. Neurol.
    Psychiat. (Chicago) **75**, 91 (1956).
—, and K. R. MAGEE: Treatment review. Myasthenia gravis. Neurology **5**, 729 (1955).
— — and F. E. SHIDEMAN: Effect of 3-hydroxy phenyldimethylethylammonium chloride
    (Tensilon) in myasthenia gravis. Univ. Mich. med. Bull. **17**, 311 (1951).
—, and J. T. LURES: The clinical use of hexaethyltetraphosphate in myasthenia gravis. Univ.
    Mich. med. Bull. **14**, 15 (1948).
WILSON, A., G. A. MAN and H. GEORHEGAN: Cholinesterase activity of blood and muscle in
    myasthenia gravis. Quart. J. Med. **20**, 13 (1951).
—, and H. B. STONER: Myasthenia gravis. A consideration of its causation in a study of 14
    cases. Quart. J. Med. **13**, 1 (1944).
ZAIMIS, E. J.: Motor endplate differences as a determining factor in the mode of action of
    neuromuscular blocking substances. J. Physiol. (Lond.) **122**, 238 (1953).

Chapter 24

Local Use of Anticholinesterase Agents in Ocular Therapy

By

IRVING H. LEOPOLD and NARENDRA KRISHNA

Contents

Anticholinesterase (Anti-ChE) agents occupy a prominent place in ocular therapy. They are employed locally in the eye mainly to induce miosis, increase the power of accommodation, and lower the intraocular pressure. Occasionally they have been employed as local insecticides.

A. Sites of cholinesterase activity in the ocular tissues and fluids

If the mechanism of action of anti-ChE agents in the eye is to be explained in terms of inhibition of the cholinesterase (ChE) enzymes, one has to furnish evidence of the existence of ChE activity in the ocular tissues and fluids. Cholinesterases may be inherent at these sites or brought from other sources via the circulating blood. The presence of ChE's in the motor neurons of the cranial motor nuclei, the neurons giving rise to preganglionic autonomic fibers, the neurons of the autonomic ganglia (especially the ciliary and superior cervical), and the neuro-muscular and autonomic effector cells is important from the ocular viewpoint.

Until recently, studies of the presence of ChE's in the ocular tissues and fluids have been far from satisfactory. The principal reasons for this have been 1) limitations of the biologic methods employed for determining ChE-activity; 2) ChE-activity determinations made with very little information concerning the characteristics of the enzymes, such as stability and optimum pH, temperature, and substrate concentrations; 3) attempts made to find ChE's in the ocular fluids, whereas, as will be shown subsequently, they contain little, if any; 4) the non-availability of sufficient normal human material; 5) failure to distinguish, in most cases, between the types of ChE's.

The methods available at present for determining ChE-activities are 1) biochemical analysis, 2) histochemical localization, 3) improved Cartesian diver technique, 4) centrifugal fractionation.

I. Biochemical analysis of ocular ChE's

So far, distribution of ChE's in the body tissues has usually been studied manometrically with slices or homogenates (AUGUSTINSSON 1948); for a critical and comprehensive evaluation of the methods of biochemical analysis, the reader is referred to AUGUSTINSSON's (1957) recent monograph and Chapter 4 in the present volume. While the methods based on biochemical assay provide quantitative data on concentrations of ChE's in the various tissues, the techniques employed generally necessitate determining ChE activities on larger quantities of tissues than are available from the ocular structures of a single animal. Consequently these tissues have to be pooled from a number of animals of the same species to do single ChE determinations. Furthermore a serious drawback of this type of study is that it does not show in which cells or parts of cells the ChE-activity is located.

In an excellent study published in 1950, DE ROETTH reviewed the literature to date and presented in addition quantitative data of his own on ChE's (types not distinguished) of the ocular tissues and fluids of several species of animals (Table 1) and normal humans (Table 2), using HESTRIN's colorimetric technique,

Table 1. *Cholinesterase activity in tissues and fluids of normal experimental animal eyes expressed in mg of ACh hydrolyzed per g of tissue or per ml of fluid per hour.*

Animal	Number of eyes	Iris	Ciliary Body	Retina	Aqueous	Vitreous
Rabbit	50	28	28	130	0	0
Cat	15	55	227	160	0	—
Kitten	4	38	50	—	—	—
Dog	4	28	124	125	—	—
Pigeon	4	—	55	—	—	—
Rooster	4	115	72	183	—	—
Ox	10	44	24	—	0.56	5.6
Horse	10	20	10	—	0.16	0.2
Pig	6	56	45	—	—	—

(From: DE ROETTH 1950)

a method of biochemical analysis for residual acetylcholine (ACh) (DE ROETTH 1950). On the basis of the relative rates of hydrolysis of ACh, propionylcholine, and butyrylcholine, it was assumed that acetylcholinesterase (AChE) or specific-cholinesterase (specific-ChE) was predominant in the iris of rabbit, ox, horse, and cat; ciliary body of rabbit, ox, and cat; retina of rabbit, ox, horse, cat, and dog; and aqueous and vitreous of ox. Butyrocholinesterase (BuChE) or non-specific-cholinesterase (non-specific-ChE) similarly was identified in the ciliary body of horse and the secondary aqueous of cat, the BuChE in the latter being derived from the blood serum.

Histologic studies carried out to correlate the ChE-activity demonstrated that the highest concentrations of ChE were present in the muscle- and nerve-containing tissues, namely the iris, ciliary body, retina and extraocular muscles. The aqueous and vitreous contained only traces of ChE, which were probably derived, during the process of cell degradation, from the broken-up cell particles of the neighboring structures, i.e., the iris, ciliary body, and retina, or from the plasma. The latter may be the chief source of aqueous ChE, as an increase of BuChE occurs in the secondary aqueous following paracentesis, which is associated with increased permeability of the blood-aqueous barrier. Thus, the aqueous is not normally a site of significant ChE-activity. This point needs to be stressed, as numerous reports continue to appear in which ChE-activity of the aqueous is still considered a measure of the effectiveness and ocular penetration of anti-ChE agents, instead of direct determination of the concentration of these drugs in the aqueous. Studies based on the former concept can be grossly misleading.

Low ChE-activity was demonstrated by DE ROETTH (1950) in the ciliary body of the rabbit and ox. Histologically, these species have been shown to have poorly developed ciliary muscle. High ChE-activity in the ciliary body of the cat, dog, and pig could be associated with well developed ciliary muscle. The iris followed a somewhat similar pattern. The retina of all these animals exhibited approximately the same degree of ChE-activity. Unusually high ChE content

Table 2. *Cholinesterase activity of tissues of the normal human eye, expressed in mg of ACh hydrolyzed per g of tissue per hour.* (From: DE ROETTH 1950)

Extraocular Muscle	Iris	Ciliary Body
56	15	587
43	41	...
43	28	257
54	45	...
38	26	...
44	39	...
34	23	384
43	39	...
..	23	379
..	26	368
Average 44	30	355

was noted in the rooster iris; in birds, the iris contains skeletal muscle, which possesses high ChE concentration elsewhere in the body. In normal human eyes, the iris contained nearly the same amount of ChE as in most of the experimental animals; the ciliary body showed invariably a high content, which again could be correlated histologically to the large amount of muscular tissue. The extraocular muscles showed high ChE-activity, probably related to the great number of motor endplates and high innervation ratio of the extraocular muscles.

Most of these findings have been substantiated by others (FELDBERG et al. 1951; MINAMI 1952; HARUTA et al. 1953; DARDENNE et al. 1957). In addition, indirect confirmation exists in numerous studies primarily performed for other purposes (KOELLE and FRIEDENWALD 1949, 1950b; KOELLE 1950a, 1951, 1954; KOELLE et al. 1952; SCHOFIELD 1952a, 1952b).

II. Histochemical localization of ocular ChE's

The histochemical methods of determination of ChE-activity *in situ* in tissue sections are of interest from the point of cholinergic function. Knowledge regarding the types of ChE's may be far more important to explain the transmission processes than the mere demonstration of the enzymes at the cellular and subcellular levels. FRIEDENWALD (1955) has discussed very ably the advantages and limitations of the histochemical methods, and has pointed out that with well controlled studies it is possible to minimize diffusion artifacts.

The thiocholine method, one of the histochemical methods, as developed by KOELLE and subsequently modified by him (KOELLE and FRIEDENWALD 1949; KOELLE 1950a, 1951) has been used to distinguish between the two types of ChE, AChE and BuChE, in ocular tissues of the rabbit, cat, horse, ox, and pig (KOELLE and FRIEDENWALD 1950b; KOELLE et al. 1952; HEBB et al. 1953; FRANCIS 1953; HEBB 1954; KOELLE 1954; EICHNER 1955; LEPLAT and GEREBTZOFF 1956). This method involves the use of fresh frozen sections, and thus has certain disadvantages as summed up by PEARSE (1953). These are of minor consideration compared to the uncertainties regarding the effects of fixatives on enzymatic activity. The pH, substrate concentration, time of incubation, and temperature all influence the enzymatic activity and must be controlled rigidly. Biochemical controls are also necessary. It may be assumed that at present the thiocholine method, involving the use of fresh frozen sections, and employing selective substrates and inhibitors along with biochemical controls, is adequate for qualitative determination of the sites of AChE and BuChE in ocular tissues. Mention should be made in this connection of the latest modifications of this method of simultaneous histochemical localization and manometric determination, which could be successfully employed for demonstrating ChE-activities in ocular tissues (KOELLE 1955; HOLMSTEDT 1957a, 1957b).

Using diisopropyl phosphorofluoridate (DFP) as the selective inhibitor, and acetylthiocholine and butyrylthiocholine as the substrates for AChE and BuChE, respectively, deep staining was demonstrated for AChE in the ciliary and iris sphincter muscle fibers and their associated nerve fibers, with practically no evidence of BuChE (KOELLE et al. 1952). This is in contrast to the smooth muscle fibers at other sites, which show predominance of BuChE. The optic nerve showed practically no AChE in the visual nerve fiber bundles, but definite staining was visible in the nerve fibers in the trabeculae between the visual nerve fiber bundles, which were presumed to be autonomic; BuChE was found in the glial cells and septa of the optic nerve.

With regard to ChE in the retina there is some difference of opinion. Cholinesterase has been found in the inner plexiform layer of the retina, but the interpretation differs as to the exact cytologic localization. HEBB et al. (1953) noticed AChE in the cells of the bipolar layer, the tissue of the inner synaptic layer and in the region of the ganglion cells; small amounts of BuChE were noticed in the ganglion and bipolar layer cells, as well as in the supporting network and cells of the retina. KOELLE et al. (1952) found a more limited distribution. They were unable to demonstrate any BuChE, and the AChE was confined only to the amacrine cells in the bipolar layer. FRANCIS (1953) found nearly the same distribution in the inner synaptic layer but interpreted it as being associated with the bipolar layer and ganglion cells. HEBB (1954), commenting on this discrepancy, stated that while the modified method of KOELLE (1951) intended to prevent intercellular diffusion of ChE, it also seemed to reduce the penetration of the tissues by the substrate, and thus she preferred the original method of KOELLE and FRIEDENWALD (1949). KOELLE (1954) maintained that diffusion of the ChE's occurred with the original procedure, and in order to apply the modified procedure with a degree of accuracy one should make simultaneous manometric determinations with the concentrations of sodium sulfate and DFP employed with homogenates of the tissues, which he did in his experiments. The question is by no means settled. EICHNER (1955) suggested that the localization of the enzyme resided at the site of the synapse at the border between the inner fiber and inner nuclear layers, on the basis of enzyme staining at this site, while LEPLAT and GEREBTZOFF (1956) demonstrated AChE in the inner plexiform layer and regarded the ganglion cells to be cholinergic.

Unfortunately no such studies are available on normal human intraocular tissues; a study of this nature employing simultaneously the most recent modifications of the histochemical localization and manometric determination could be highly rewarding.

It would be equally interesting to determine ChE-activities of the ocular tissues by the improved Cartesian diver technique (ZAJICEK and ZEUTHEN 1956; GIACOBINI and ZAJICEK 1956; ZAJICEK 1957; GIACOBINI 1959) and by the centrifugal fractionation methods (SCHNEIDER and HOGEBOOM 1956), both of which have provided valuable information concerning ChE-activity in other body tissues.

The concept of a dual localization of AChE, i.e., located both outside and inside the cell membrane, elaborated recently on the basis of comparisons of the effects of tertiary and quaternary amine anti-ChE agents (BURGEN and CHIPMAN 1952; KOELLE and STEINER 1956), may also be important to explain the pharmacological actions of anti-ChE agents on the ocular tissues.

It is generally agreed that the erythrocytes contain AChE and the serum BuChE. Acetylcholinesterase has been demonstrated in motor neurons of cranial motor nuclei, neurons giving rise to preganglionic autonomic fibers, peripheral cholinergic neurons, occasional peripheral sympathetic neurons (of superior cervical ganglia, with species variations), and motor endplates (KOELLE 1955).

B. Anticholinesterase (anti-ChE) agents employed in ophthalmology

The conjunctival cul-de-sac has been a favorite site for studying the action of drugs from times immemorial. Thus, nearly all anti-ChE agents have been subjected to this mode of study from time to time. In addition, anti-ChE agents occupy a place of unusual interest in ocular therapy. The miosis, lacrimation, painful sensation in the supraorbital and ciliary regions, and blurred vision induced on local instillation of the calabar bean extract (*Physostigma venenosum* Balfour) in the eye were described (FRASER 1863) long before the ChE-inhibiting action of its alkaloid, physostigmine (eserine), was known (ENGLEHART and LOEWI 1930). Physostigmine was the first substance to be used as a miotic, particularly to counteract the mydriatic and cycloplegic actions of atropine (ARGYLL ROBERTSON 1863). The first medical treatment of glaucoma started with the use of physostigmine to bring about the lowering of ocular tension (LAQUEUR 1876, 1877). An attempt to elucidate the miotic action of physostigmine led to the synthesis of neostigmine (Prostigmin), another anti-ChE agent of ophthalmological interest (STEDMAN 1926, 1929a, b; AESCHLIMANN and REINERT 1931). The same approach has led to the synthesis of innumerable compounds in the same and other series. During the initial studies of the pharmacological actions of the organophosphates (ADRIAN et al. 1947), the prolonged miosis following exposure to DFP was explained as due to inhibition of ChE rather than a direct action on the effector cells; since then, the organophosphorus cholinesterase inhibitors have continued to interest the ophthalmologist.

It would be to no particular advantage to mention the numerous anti-ChE agents which have been tested ocularly at one time or the other. Instead, only those ChE inhibitors are listed which have found eventually a place in ocular therapy, or are of unusual interest to the ocular physiologist (Table 3).

Table 3. *Anticholinesterase agents in ocular therapy*

Reversible inhibitors:

 *1. Physostigmine (Eserine; tertiary amine with urethane group).
 *2. Neostigmine (Prostigmin; quaternary compound with urethane group; Eustigmine).
  3. Pyridostigmin (Mestinon; dimethyl-carbo-amino acid ester of 1-methyl-3-oxypyridine bromide).
 *4. Demecarium (Humorsol, BC-48, quaternary compound with two neostigmine molecules joined with polymethylene chain).

Irreversible inhibitors:

 *1. Diisopropyl phosphorofluoridate (Isofluorophate, Floropryl, DFP).
  2. Tetraethyl pyrophosphate (TEPP).
  3. Tetraethyl monothiono-pyrophosphate (A_2).
 *4. Mintacol (Paraoxon, diethyl-4-nitrophenyl phosphate, Bayer E 600).
 *5. Echothiophate (Phospholine, Diethoxyphosphoryl-thiocholine iodide, 217-MI).
  6. Diethyl tetrachlor-ethyl phosphate.

 * Anticholinesterase agents commonly employed in ocular therapy.

C. Ocular effects of locally used anti-ChE agents

We are primarily concerned here with the ocular effects induced by anti-ChE agents when used locally in the eye, but it must not be forgotten that ocular effects are noted sometimes after systemic administration of the ChE inhibitors. The ocular effects are produced by exposure of the eye to the vapor of the anti-ChE agents, by the application of these agents in the form of drops of aqueous and oily solutions or ointments, and by iontophoresis and injection, i.e., subconjunctival and retrobulbar. Anticholinesterase agents are no exception to the rule that each drug probably has more than one mode of action.

The degrees of ocular effects are dependent on the intraocular concentration of the drug and the ability of the individual eye to respond. The ocular penetration of the drug is affected by its physical properties, chemical structure, quantity, method of administration, the vehicle employed, the relative affinity for water and lipid, and the permeability of corneal epithelium and blood-aqueous barrier. The eyes of usual laboratory animals differ in significant anatomical details from human eyes, and within human eyes there are marked individual variations. Thus, with so many variable factors operating, it is obvious that direct comparisons of one anti-ChE agent with another have to be controlled very carefully in order to be meaningful.

Errors in evaluating the influence of drugs on the ocular tissues arise also from the methods and tools employed to study these effects. With a better understanding of the physiological concepts, and the improved techniques and appliances made available within recent years, it is now possible to study the ocular effects of drugs with a degree of accuracy and precision not known before.

The anterior segment of the eye lends itself ideally to examination by slit lamp biomicroscopy (BERLINER 1949). Under very high magnifications, it is now possible to study the effects of drugs on the conjunctiva, episclera, sclera, cornea, iris, lens, and pupil of the living eye. The behavior of conjunctival blood vessels, both superficial and deep, and the blood vessels of the iris in response to these drugs can be observed in the living eye under direct visualization. No longer has one to resort to histological examination of the ocular tissues with its shortcomings and attendant artifacts.

While the anterior segment of the eye can be examined conveniently with slit lamp biomicroscopy, no such method has so far been evolved for examination of the posterior segment.

The heat-drying of sclera (LEOPOLD 1951; GREAVES and PERKINS 1952) and the scleral-window (WUDKA and LEOPOLD 1956) techniques alter normal physiology and are not feasible in man, although they have yielded data of considerable significance on the choroidal circulation in animals. The extreme miosis induced by the anti-ChE agents acts as a further deterrant in the study of the posterior segment, because through an otherwise normal or dilated pupil it is possible to examine all details of the fundus with both direct and indirect ophthalmoscopy. Other ingenious devices, like the insertion of a small mirror into the vitreous to study the effects of drugs on the ciliary body (MATSUDA 1959), are still in the experimental stages.

With the help of a gonioscopic contact lens, a well focussed small light, and a binocular microscope, it is now possible to study the structural details of the angle of the anterior chamber or the filtration angle of the living eye, i.e., one can inspect the posterior surface of the cornea in the periphery, the trabecular meshwork through which the aqueous humor must pass to gain access to SCHLEMM's canal, the scleral spur to which the ciliary body is attached, a narrow portion of the ciliary body to which the iris is attached, and the iris itself (GORIN and POSNER 1957). The changes produced by the drugs on the various structures that constitute the angle of the anterior chamber can thus be studied very easily and in great detail with the help of gonioscopy.

It is also possible now to study the effects of drugs on the extraocular muscles in both animals and man by recording the electrical activity (BROWN and HARVEY 1941) and mechanical activity (KRISHNA 1960c) of these muscles.

Measurements of intraocular pressure still present a challenging problem. Exact measurement of intraocular pressure requires complete relaxation on the part of the subject, which in the case of animals involves the use of general anesthesia. All general anesthetics in use today are known to affect the intraocular pressure, and it therefore becomes very difficult to evaluate whether a certain change in intraocular pressure is due to the general anesthetic employed or to the drug under trial. Diurnal variations in the intraocular pressure further complicate the picture. Additional errors in evaluating the influence of drugs on the intraocular pressure arise from ignoring certain physiological factors, like the pressure readjustments due to compensatory changes of aqueous volume. Sometimes the observations are over too brief a period, and certain methods of measurement in themselves disturb the normal processes.

The most direct method for measuring the intraocular pressure is certainly the manometry of cannulated eyes (GUERRY 1951). However, cannulization of the anterior chamber may irritate the eye or otherwise impair the blood-aqueous barrier, and thus the normal compensatory mechanism of the intact eye is lost in such eyes. A further limitation of this method is its inapplicability to human eyes; even in animal eyes, the observations have to be confined to short periods of time.

In human eyes, and for prolonged observations in animal eyes, intraocular pressure is measured by tonometry, which really measures the tension of the eye, i.e., the measurement of the state of tension of the tissues of the eye. The tension depends on the intraocular pressure, the thickness and rigidity of the tissues, the surface area, and probably several other factors. Therefore, tension is not an exact and accurate measurement of intraocular pressure. Attempts continue to be made to bring tonometry more in line with accurate measurements of intraocular pressure. The impression tonometer of SCHIOTZ, of which both mechanical (SCHIOTZ 1924, 1927) and electronic (FRIEDENWALD 1948) models, along with the improved calibrations (FRIEDENWALD 1954, 1957; KRONFELD 1957) are now available, measures the depth of the impression produced by a given free-acting force on the tissues of the eye. The degree of indentation produced depends not only on the intraocular pressure present before the application of the tonometer, but on the increase in pressure resulting from the weight of the tonometer itself, plus the high degree of resistance of the tissues of the eye to deformation and stretching, and the resistance of the intraocular fluids to displacement. The applanation tonometer of MAURICE (MAURICE 1951) and the slit lamp applanation tonometer of GOLDMANN (GOLDMANN 1954) are designed to overcome these difficulties, and with these tonometers it is now possible to measure very approximately the intraocular pressures. Attempts have been made to improve the SCHIOTZ tonometer, and a friction-free SCHIOTZ tonometer is now available (SCHMIDT 1958a, 1958b).

Increasing interest has been shown in recent years in assessing the rate of flow of the aqueous humor and resistance to its outflow, and how these are influenced by various drugs.

Measurements by direct cannulization and perfusion of animal eyes can be rightly criticized, as the procedures interfere with the permeability of the blood-aqueous barrier. The rate of flow of aqueous humor in animal eyes has been determined on the assumption that if a lipid-insoluble molecule of relatively larger molecular size could be introduced into the aqueous humor without modifying the eye, its rate of decay would be determined almost completely by aqueous flow. Rayopake, Diodrast, and para-aminohippuric acid are the substances employed in these studies (BARANY and KINSEY 1949; KINSEY and BARANY 1949; BARANY and WIRTH 1954) and glucose, galactose, and insulin in a somewhat analogous study (ROSS 1952). Such studies, however, may have to take into account active transfer from the eye of these substances and not simply outflow. The aqueous outflow has been determined in animal eyes by the perfusion method (BECKER and CONSTANT 1956). Fluorescein has been employed as the test substance to measure the rate of flow and aqueous outflow in human eyes by GOLDMANN (1950, 1951), and in animal eyes by LANGHAM and WYBAR (1954) and LANGHAM and WOOD (1956). This fluorometric method has the great advantage of an undisturbed eye, but has the disadvantage of requiring expensive and complicated equipment with a cumbersome, time-consuming procedure. Thus, the tonographic method, in spite of its limitations, has become the standard method for evaluating the rate of flow of aqueous humor and outflow resistance in man (MOSES and BRUNO 1950; GRANT 1950a, 1951), although for studies on animals, with a few exceptions this enthusiasm is generally not shared. Tonography is based on the hydrodynamic principle that the rate of outflow of the aqueous humor is proportional to the outflow pressure and inversely proportional to the resistance in the outflow mechanism. The use of an electronic SCHIOTZ tonometer, connected to a recording device, for a period of four to six minutes over the anesthetized cornea, enables the outflow resistance to be measured, from which the rate of flow can be easily calculated.

An attempt has been made recently to record ocular tension continuously in both animals and man under the normal working conditions of daily life by means of a continuous recording tonometer (MAURICE 1958). This method when perfected may truly reflect the intraocular pressure measurements under normal physiological conditions.

I. Effects on extraocular muscles — Electrical and mechanical activity

It is surprising that no studies have been reported on the effects of anti-ChE agents on the extraocular muscles either *in vitro* or *in vivo*, when applied locally, in spite of the fact that the extraocular muscles present such peculiar anatomical, physiological, and pharmacological characteristics. BROWN and HARVEY (1941) are the only ones who have studied the effects of intravenous and intraarterial injections of eserine on the extraocular muscles of decerebrated cats.

After eserine had been injected, the extraocular muscles sometimes showed spontaneous contraction. The contraction produced by maximal single shocks, applied to the motor nerve supplying the muscle, was enhanced. Single nerve volleys produced a regular series of repetitive spikes, which produced greater tension. Double nerve volleys had more complex effects, the eserine prolonging the refractory period of the muscle and interfering with the transmission by the nerve of the second succeeding volley. Eserine lowered the threshold of the curarized muscle to direct electrical stimulation. After eserine, both ACh and repetitive nerve stimuli evoked a contracture which blocked the propagation of excitation along the muscle fiber.

II. Effects on ocular blood vessels — Permeability of blood-aqueous barrier

All anti-ChE agents produce engorgement of the vascular supply of the anterior segment of the eye in both animals and man. This manifests itself in the form of conjunctival hyperemia, circumcorneal injection, and dilatation of iridic blood vessels, all of which can be observed in the living eye with the slit lamp biomicroscope. Engorgement of the ciliary body, and swelling and edema of the ciliary processes have been observed in the living eye (MATSUDA 1959) following aministration of physiostigmine locally, and histologically following administration of DFP (SCHOLZ 1946; VON SALLMANN and DILLON 1947), echothiophate (Phospholine) (KRISHNA and LEOPOLD, unpublished data) and demecarium (Humorsol, BC-48) (KRISHNA and LEOPOLD 1960a). The dilatation of capillaries profoundly affects the blood-aqueous barrier and the osmotic pressure of the aqueous (BARANY 1947).

The dilatation of blood vessels results in increased permeability to protein and causes a slight rise in intraocular pressure in the normal eye. The increase in turbidity of the aqueous humor induced by increased protein content can be detected in the aqueous on slit lamp biomicroscopic examination. Instillation of physiostigmine causes significant increase of protein content of the aqueous of rabbit eyes (WESSELY 1913; SWAN and HART 1940). Increased permeability and definite increase of protein in the aqueous has been demonstrated in rabbit eyes following instillation of DFP (LEOPOLD and COMROE 1946b; SCHOLZ, 1946; VON SALLMANN and DILLON 1947). CASELLI (1953) showed that diethyl 4-nitrophenyl phosphate (Mintacol, Paraoxon) produced a marked increase in permeability of the blood-aqueous barrier 30 minutes after instillation in the rabbit eye.

III. Effects on iris and ciliary body — Pupillary reaction and accommodation

The effects on the iris and ciliary body of the locally used anti-ChE agents have been investigated in great detail both in animals and man. As a matter of fact no work on the ocular use of these agents can be regarded as complete without some reference to the state of the pupil and accommodation of such treated eyes.

Much information in the past has been gained on the iris and ciliary body by *in vitro* studies. In these experiments fresh isolated pieces of these tissues are obtained and the effects of various anti-ChE agents studied by means of various mechanical, electrical, and photographic devices. Such experiments can be rightly criticized as unphysiological when one considers that these tissues have been deprived of their vascular and nervous supply. We therefore shall not go into the details of these *in vitro* studies, but shall proceed with a consideration of the effects *in vivo* of the ocularly employed ChE inhibitors.

Ever since the first studies of FRASER (1863) on the effects of physostigmine (eserine) on the eye when applied locally, and its use as a miotic to counteract the cycloplegic action of atropine by ARGYLL ROBERTSON (1863), numerous reports have appeared concerning its miotic action and induced accommodative spasm. Instillation of physostigmine into the conjunctival cul-de-sac of the human eye in the strengths of 0.1 to 1 % causes pupillary constriction and spasm of accommodation.

Miosis begins in a few minutes and is maximal in about thirty minutes; intense miosis persists for nearly twelve hours and some degree of miosis may last as long as several days. The spasm of accommodation, starting at nearly the same time as miosis, is of a shorter duration; the intense accommodative spasm tends to disappear in about two hours, but the ciliary muscle tends to remain irritable so that the slightest effort on accommodation for looking at a near object results in ciliary spasm. The minimum concentration necessary to produce detectable pupillary constriction is of the order of one drop of 0.01% in humans (MARUI 1922), and in rabbits (MOLITOR 1936). In rabbits, physostigmine can be demonstrated in the iris and ciliary body for seven to eight hours after instillation into the conjunctival sac, and the duration of miosis corresponds to the duration of the presence of eserine in the iris (SCHUMACHER 1956).

It was at first believed that the miotic action of physostigmine was due to the urethane group which it contains (STEDMAN and BARGER 1925). Later, on the basis of synthesis of several compounds which are as potent miotics as physostigmine and in addition to being urethanes also possess the common property of being phenyl esters, it was concluded that the miotic action of physostigmine was due to the latter moiety (STEDMAN 1926, 1929a, 1929b). It was only after the ChE-inhibiting nature of physostigmine was identified (ENGLEHART and LOEWI 1930) that attention was paid to this mode of action to explain the mechanism of miosis.

Neostigmine (Prostigmin), a synthetic quaternary urethane compound (AESCHLIMANN and REINERT 1931) which in some respects resembles the tertiary urethane compound physostigmine, is somewhat less effective as a miotic agent than physostigmine.

A concentration of 3 to 5% is necessary to produce maximal miosis and spasm of accommodation, beginning within a few minutes and persisting for a number of hours after its instillation into the conjunctival sac of human subjects. While ROSSI (1935) indicated that several instillations of 0.05% are effective in inducing minimal miosis in human eyes, MYERSON and THAU (1937) considered 1% to be the minimal concentration necessary to induce detectable miosis. In rabbits, ROSSI believed 0.5% of neostigmine to be approximately equivalent to 0.5% of physostigmine as far as the miotic effect is concerned.

Of the new series of synthetic ChE inhibitors belonging to the group polymethylene-*bis*(N-methylcarbaminoyl-*m*-trimethylammonium phenol) characterized by two neostigmine molecules connected by a polymethylene chain (KRAUPP et al. 1955a, b), the quaternary compound demecarium has been investigated by KRISHNA and LEOPOLD (1960a) with regard to its ocular effects in rabbits and human eyes.

Single instillation of 0.1, 0.25, and 0.5% solutions into the conjunctival sac of normal human subjects produces miosis which is distinctly noticeable within forty-five to sixty minutes. The maximum miosis is achieved between 2 to 4 hours, the pupils becoming pinpoint. Miosis persists on an average between 3 to 10 days. One percent atropine or 4% homatropine abolishes this miosis readily; the effect is noticeable within ten minutes. Miosis is also induced in atropinized and homatropinized eyes, which becomes noticeable in those markedly dilated eyes within one to three hours and reaches a maximum in about twenty-four hours. Miosis is accompanied by accommodative spasm which is directly proportional to the concentration of drug employed. Accommodative spasm however tends to disappear sooner than the miotic effect. In rabbit eyes miosis is noticeable within ten minutes and complete recovery ensues in 24 hours.

Diisopropyl phosphorofluoridate (DFP) produces intense and prolonged miosis in rabbits, cats, dogs, and man (LEOPOLD and COMROE 1946b; SCHOLZ 1946), following instillation into the conjunctival sac. Following instillation of 0.1% DFP in peanut oil in human eyes, miosis begins within five to ten minutes, is maximal within fifteen to twenty minutes and gradually disappears within 4 to 7 days, although in a few instances it may persist as long as 4 weeks. One-hundredth per cent produces no observable pupillary effect, and 0.05% is the lowest concentration which produces maximum pupillary constriction. The speed and intensity of action of 0.1% DFP is greater than that of 1% physostigmine, or 5% neostigmine, and the duration of its action much longer than that of physostigmine or neostigmine. Maximal miosis is noticeable in rabbit eyes in about four minutes, but complete recovery occurs within 24 hours. Diisopropyl phosphorofluoridate produces ciliary spasm in human eyes which is maximal within one hour and gradually disappears in forty-eight hours. Miosis is induced by DFP in previously atropinized and homatropinized eyes within 1 hour.

The miosis and accommodation produced by TEPP have been investigated in normal human eyes by GRANT (1948) and by UPHOLT et al. (1956). According to GRANT, 0.1% TEPP in peanut oil in normal human eyes produces rapid miosis in about 7 minutes, and spasm of accommodation. The accommodation returns to normal after 4 days, but a relative miosis may persist for 2 to 3 weeks. According to UPHOLT et al. 0.05% produced only slight miosis and spasm of accommodation.

Mintacol, 1:5000 (0.02%), induces miosis in the normal human eye in about 11 minutes, and the miosis persists from 3 to 10 days (HUERKAMP and WAGNER 1950). It is capable of overcoming the pupillary effects of atropine. Its intensity and duration of action are shorter than those of DFP, and more like those of physostigmine.

Echothiophate produces marked and prolonged miosis. In normal human eyes instillation of 0.05 cc. of 0.25 to 0.5% aqueous solutions induces miosis noticeable within 10 to 45 minutes and lasting seven to twenty-seven days (LEOPOLD et al. 1957). In normal rabbit eyes miosis is maximal within 5 to 10 minutes but disappears within 24 hours (KRISHNA and LEOPOLD, unpublished data). Partial miosis is induced in previously atropinized and homatropinized eyes within ten minutes after two to three instillations of echothiophate.

While the anti-ChE agents have been shown to exert a powerful miotic effect on normal eyes, they fail to induce miosis in denervated pupils. Thus, ANDERSON (1904, 1905a, b) showed that physostigmine failed to constrict the pupils in cats after the ciliary ganglia had been removed. LEOPOLD and COMROE (1945) have confirmed this observation and shown it to be true for neostigmine as well; DFP also acts in the same way (LEOPOLD and COMROE 1946b). It is assumed that after degeneration following postganglionic denervation, there is no ACh liberated at the nerve terminals to excite effector organs. Thus, the anti-ChE agents have no effect when instilled into such eyes. On the other hand, the ineffectiveness of anti-ChE agents on the denervated pupil might be explained on the basis that after denervation there is marked decrease in the ChE of the denervated structures, as has been demonstrated in irises of cats after ciliary ganglionectomies (SCHOFIELD 1952a, 1952b). Thus, very little ChE is available for inhibition by anti-ChE agents which exert their principal action by inhibition of the enzyme.

IV. Effects on intraocular pressure — Aqueous outflow

Local application of anti-ChE agents into normal animal and human eyes generally causes decrease in intraocular pressure, usually of the order of a few millimeters of mercury. In the vast majority of cases, there is a transient increase of intraocular pressure before the eyes show evidence of decrease. The degree of intraocular pressure lowering effect and its duration are directly proportional to the concentrations of the anti-ChE agents, apart from the individual potency possessed by each drug. The transient increase appears to be related to the ability of these agents to produce hyperemia and vasodilatation, especially of the iris and ciliary body. The dilatation of capillaries results in a temporary increase in permeability of the blood-aqueous barrier, with the appearance of protein in the aqueous and increase in intraocular pressure, as has been demonstrated in both animal and human eyes in numerous studies (WESSELY 1913; SZASZ 1931; SWAN and HART 1940; LEOPOLD and COMROE 1946b; BARANY 1947; VON SALLMANN and DILLON 1947; CASELLI 1953; KRISHNA and LEOPOLD unpublished data, KRISHNA and LEOPOLD 1960a). The elevation of pressure in eyes with narrow angles of the anterior chamber may be secondary to a pupillary block due to the intense miosis, i.e., the small pupillary border rests firmly against the lens and allows the posterior aqueous humor to push the iris plane forward, crowding and occluding the angle.

Although the decrease in intraocular pressure by the anti-ChE agents has also been suggested on the basis of increased blood-aqueous barrier, resulting in diminution in the formation of aqueous humor (BARANY 1947), this is not borne out by numerous other studies. It is now generally agreed that all anti-ChE agents lower the intraocular pressure by lowering the resistance to aqueous outflow, or by improving the facility of aqueous outflow. The exact mechanism is, however, not clear. Two different views have been expressed to explain this mechanism of action. According to one, improvement in the facility of aqueous outflow is due to the mechanical action on the trabecular meshwork exerted by the anti-ChE agents, due to pull of the scleral spur by the contracting iris and ciliary body. This results in opening of the channels in the trabecular meshwork, through which the aqueous then has ready exit. According to the other viewpoint, the collector channels and aqueous veins peripheral to SCHLEMM's canal are dilated, and thus the resistance to outflow is lowered.

D. Systemic effects of ocularly administered anti-ChE agents

In general, anti-ChE agents dropped into the conjunctival sac diffuse through the cornea and are distributed to various ocular tissues and fluids, and thus mostly the ocular effects are noticeable in local administration of these agents. However, it is reasonable to assume that some absorption of these drugs takes place into the general blood stream via the conjunctival sac, the nasal and pharyngeal mucosae, and even the gastrointestinal tract. The undesirable effects resulting from this absorption can be eliminated to a certain extent, if care is taken to apply pressure on the corresponding nasolacrimal canaliculus for a very short period during and immediately following the instillation, to prevent the passage of tears into the nasopharyngeal passages. In spite of this precaution. enough general absorption may occur to produce remote effects in other parts of the body. This is particularly apt to occur after repeated instillation of these agents over prolonged periods of time. Subconjunctival and retrobulbar modes of administration lead to more rapid and profound absorption of these agents, both in the ocular tissues as well as in the systemic circulation. Fortunately these routes are resorted to rarely for the administration of these drugs. In addition, increased susceptibility of certain individuals to the drugs is responsible for some of the remote systemic effects.

Systemic absorption of the various anti-ChE agents, when applied locally in the eyes, has been demonstrated in a carefully controlled study by determining the blood ChE levels both before and after their instillation (LEOPOLD et al. 1959). Blood plasma BuChE and red blood cell AChE levels of normal human subjects were determined prior to any medication. One-tenth cc of a 0.5% aqueous solution of physostigmine, 5% aqueous solution of neostigmine, 0.25 and 0.5% aqueous solutions of demecarium, 0.1% DFP in peanut oil, and 0.25% aqueous solution of echothiophate were instilled into each eye of these subjects, using only one drug in each patient. Cholinesterase levels were again determined at intervals of one, three and five hours after the instillation. Apart from minor variations of the blood ChE levels in the majority of these cases, significant depression of red blood cells ChE levels was demonstrated only in some patients following single instillations of demecarium. Significant depression of the blood ChE levels occurs in a fairly large number of cases on prolonged therapy with the various anti-ChE agents. This will be discussed in greater detail subsequently. This study has given unequivocal evidence that significant depression of blood ChE levels is to be expected following repeated instillation into the conjunctival sac of some of the commonly employed ChE inhibitors.

It is generally accepted that systemic toxic symptoms, following acute administration of an anti-ChE agent, manifest themselves when the red blood cell AChE level falls below 20 to 30 percent of normal, and severe toxicity does not appear until the AChE of brain or other nervous tissue is depressed to below 10% of normal. In man, however, the relationship between symptomatology and red blood cell AChE depression also depends to a large extent on the route and rate of administration. Repeated small doses can produce considerable depression of red blood cell AChE without apparent discomfort. This is of particular importance in ocular therapy, since the anti-ChE agents are employed in small doses repeatedly, over prolonged periods, and sometimes even indefinitely.

The systemic manifestations following exposure of the eye to the vapor or liquid of the anti-ChE agents are similar to those following other routes of administration. Nearly all of these systemic effects have been reported following the instillation into the conjunctival sac of these agents. However, as is to be

Table 4. *Local and systemic manifestations of ocularly administered anticholinesterase agents*

Site	Symptoms and Signs
Local effects:	
Eye Lids	Swollen and red (contact dermatitis)
Lacrimal glands	Increased lacrimation
Conjunctivae	Hyperemia, both superficial and deep. Follicular conjunctivitis (chemical irritation), usually on prolonged use
Cornea	Edema (?)
Pupil	Marked to maximal miosis (pin-point). Pupillary block (resulting in increase in intraocular pressure). Pupil border shows epithelial cysts on prolonged use
Iris	Hyperemia of iris vessels. Peripheral anterior synechiae (goniosynechiae) embarrassing the filteration angle (resulting in increase in intraocular pressure). Posterior synechiae (adhesions between the posterior surface of iris and anterior surface of lens) occasionally
Ciliary body	Frontal headache, dimness of vision, increase in myopia, pain in the eye on focussing at near objects, and occasional nausea and vomiting (spasm of accommodation). Uveitis varying from mild iritis and transient aqueous flare to acute fibrinous uveitis with marked persistent aqueous flare occasionally. Hyperemia and swelling of the ciliary body with occasional embarrassment of the filteration angle (resulting in increase in intraocular pressure)
Retina	Retinal detachment occasionally
Intraocular pressure . . .	Increase in capillary permeability and vasodilatation; increase in permeability of blood-aqueous barrier; pulling effect of ciliary body on scleral spur, causing the opening of Schlemm's canal (resulting in increased facility of aqueous outflow and decrease in intraocular pressure). Occasional dilatation of blood vessels of the iris and ciliary body near the angle of anterior chamber and increased permeability, resulting in increased protein content in the aqueous, causing mechanical obstruction to the filteration angle (resulting in decreased facility of aqueous outflow and increase in intraocular pressure)
Systemic effects:	
Respiratory system . . .	Rhinorrhea and hyperemia of nasal mucosa. Dyspnea, cough, pain in the chest, feeling of tightness and constriction in the chest, audible wheezing sounds (bronchoconstriction or increased secretion). Death resulting from poor ventilation and weakness of respiratory muscles in spite of forceful respiratory movements
Cardiovascular system . .	Bradycardia, elevation of blood pressure
Gastrointestinal system . .	Nausea, vomiting, abdominal cramps, anorexia, and diarrhea
Excretory system	Increased sweating
Urogenital system	Frequency of micturition
Musculoskeletal system . .	Generalized weakness and easy fatigability, muscular twitchings, fasciculations, and cramps
Nervous system	Tension, anxiety, restlessness, headache, giddiness, sleep disturbances and impairment of memory, ataxia and slurred speech, convulsions, and coma

expected, marked ocular effects are manifested in addition to systemic reactions. On the other hand, the characteristic ocular effects may be minimal or not occur at all following administration by other routes. The local and systemic effects to be expected on local administration of the anti-ChE agents are summarized in Table 4.

Fortunately, systemic toxic reactions are not common following ocular administration of anti-ChE agents. Most of the reactions which manifest themselves in an acute form following single instillation of the drug are easily detected, and can be eliminated easily by discontinuing the drug. In a few instances more definitive measures, in the form of artificial respiration and pharmacological treatment of anti-ChE poisoning, may have to be employed. However, subacute and chronic toxicity is to be expected in some instances on repeated instillation over prolonged periods of time. This assumes greater importance when one realizes that new, powerful, long-acting ChE inhibitors, such as demecarium and echothiophate, which cause significant depression of red blood cell AChE levels, are being used with increasing frequency in ocular therapy and in most cases are used indefinitely. It may therefore be worthwhile in such instances to follow their course by periodic checks of the blood ChE levels, and in the event of significant depression of these levels the drug should be temporarily discontinued, and time allowed for return of the red blood cell AChE. Besides, it should be mandatory on the part of the ophthalmologist to look for signs of systemic toxicity, and on the part of the internist to be aware when the patient is using anti-ChE agents as ocular therapy, so that some of the bizarre symptoms manifested by such patients may be attributed to the agents.

E. Synergism and antagonism between ocularly employed anti-ChE agents

An important practical consideration from the point of view of ocular therapy is the synergism and antagonism exhibited by the various anti-ChE agents used in the eye. KOSTER (1946) demonstrated that a small dose of physostigmine given to cats protects against the fatal action of a subsequent dose of DFP, whereas a small dose of DFP given first results in a long lasting increase in the susceptibility of cats to the lethal action of physostigmine.

Table 5. *Synergism and antagonism between cholinesterase inhibitors in rabbits*

| Cholinesterase Inhibitor and concentration (%) | | No. of Rabbits | Average time of death after 2nd injection (min.) |
1st Injection [1]	2nd Injection [2]		
Demecarium 0.5	Physostigmine 1.0	6	3.5
Physostigmine 1.0	Demecarium 0.5	6	4.5
Echothiophate 0.5	Physostigmine 1.0	6	4.5
Physostigmine 1.0	Echothiophate 0.5	6	34
DFP 0.1	Physostigmine 1.0	6	4.5
Physostigmine 1.0	DFP 0.1	6	105

[1] 0.05 cc./lb. body weight, subconjunctival injection.
[2] Five minutes after 1st injection 0.05 cc./lb. body weight subconjunctival injection.
(From KRISHNA and LEOPOLD 1960a).

Synergisms and antagonisms between physostigmine, demecarium, DFP, and echothiophate have been studied in rabbits by KRISHNA and LEOPOLD (1960a). Using the subconjunctival route and pharmacologically equivalent concentrations of these anti-ChE agents, an attempt was made to determine the time interval required to cause the death of rabbits following their administration. If physostigmine was injected first, followed very shortly by demecarium, DFP or echothiophate, it was found that the survival period was shortened in rabbits receiving subsequent doses of demecarium, and prolonged in the cases of DFP and echothiophate. If, however, the order of injections was reversed, the survival period was shortened in all rabbits (Table 5). From this it may be concluded that physostigmine and demecarium are additive, regardless of the order in which the drugs are administered. In the case of physostigmine and DFP, or physostigmine and echothiophate, the drugs are antagonistic if physostigmine is administered first, but additive if physostigmine is administered second. The blocking mechanism of physostigmine to subsequent instillation of DFP for miosis in normal human eyes has been shown by LEOPOLD and McDONALD (1948). Clinically, the blocking action of physostigmine against DFP has been demonstrated by COMROE et al. (1946), and of neostigmine against DFP by HARVEY et al. (1947) in patients with myasthenia gravis. The blocking mechanism on intraocular pressure forms the subject matter of numerous studies on glaucoma; however, here the evidence presented is equivocal as it is difficult to say whether the failure to bring down the intraocular pressure to normal is due to this blocking action or due to the refractoriness of the patient to the drug.

An attempt has been made to explain this strange phenomenon of blocking action. There is evidence to suggest that physostigmine, neostigmine, and demecarium react reversibly with the same moiety of the AChE molecule as do DFP, TEPP, Mintacol, and echothiophate irreversibly. KOELLE (1946) reacted rat brain homogenate first with various reversible inhibitors, then added DFP, and after an interval dialyzed the mixtures. In the presence of physostigmine or neostigmine, the ChE was protected from inactivation by DFP. Perhaps *in vivo* this phenomenon may be explained in the following manner. When physostigmine is given first, it occupies most of the AChE reversibly and thereby protects it against DFP; during the time required to reverse completely the physostigmine-AChE complex, most of the excess DFP is hydrolysed, but a small, "physiologically sufficient" amount of AChE is liberated almost immediately. On the other hand, when DFP is given first it forms an irreversible combination with some of the AChE, leaving a reduced concentration particularly vulnerable to near complete inhibition by physostigmine. The relationship between physostigmine and echothiophate may be explained on the same basis. It may be important that compounds like physostigmine react equally well with both AChE and BuChE, while DFP, echothiophate, TEPP, and other organophosphorous anti-ChE compounds show a preference for BuChE, while demecarium appears to react selectively with AChE. The importance of this in ophthalmology has not been evaluated fully.

Thus, from a practical point, if an organophosphorus ChE inhibitor like DFP, TEPP, Mintacol, or echothiophate is to be given to a subject who has already received physostigmine, neostigmine, or demecarium, its administration should be delayed until the reversible inhibitor has been excreted. If an additive effect is desired, it is recommended that the order be reversed, *i. e.*, the organophosphorus irreversible inhibitor be given prior to the reversible ChE inhibitor. Another way of obtaining an additive effect, of course, is the use of a combination of only reversible or irreversible anti-ChE agents.

F. Properties, concentrations employed, and stability in vehicles of ocularly used anti-ChE agents

1. Physostigmine (Eserine)

Physostigmine is an alkaloid obtained from the calabar bean dried ripe seeds, and is available also in synthetic form (JULIAN and PIKL 1935). Physostigmine base itself is unstable, insoluble in water and sensitive to light, moisture, and alkali; it may be used as a solution in olive or castor oil. It is used as physostigmine salicylate in concentrations of 0.1 to 1 per cent in aqueous solutions or ointments. Physostigmine salicylate should be prepared in acid vehicles with a pH adjusted to 4 to 5 and a reducing agent incorporated. HIND and GOYAN (1947) recommended metabisulfite as the reducing agent, while FEINSTEIN favored sodium bisulfite because of its ready availability (FEINSTEIN as quoted by POSNER 1950). FEINSTEIN favored the following vehicle: boric acid 2.2%, sodium bisulfite 0.3%, and phenylmercuric nitrate 0.001%. The solutions prepared this way are stable for years if kept under refrigeration. Solutions, if not properly prepared or stored, undergo decomposition and the degradation products eseroline and methylamine are formed. Eseroline undergoes further deterioration to rubrescerine, pink crystals which cause mechanical irritation in the conjunctival sac. Methylamine by itself produces ocular irritation. Furthermore, these degradation products possess very little or no anti-ChE activity. Thus, it is imperative that physostigmine solutions should be prepared in an acidic pH of 4 to 5, be dispensed in colored bottles and preferably kept in a dark place, and stored under refrigeration. If stored at ordinary room temperatures, the solutions must be renewed every two to three months, although it has been reported that they maintain their potency as long as six months. If the solutions change to pink color, they should be immediately discarded.

2. Neostigmine (Prostigmin, Eustigmine)

Neostigmine is a synthetic alkaloid chemically related to physostigmine (AESCHLIMANN and REINERT 1931); it is a white crystalline powder, freely soluble in water and stable in aqueous solutions at room temperature, particularly if buffered at a pH of 3 to 4. It is used as neostigmine bromide or neostigmine methylsulfate in 3 to 5% aqueous solutions. The solutions should be renewed preferably every two to three months, although potency is maintained as long as six months.

3. Pyridostigmin (Mestinon)

Pyridostigmin is chemically the dimethyl carbamate of 3-hydroxy-1-methylpyridinium bromide. It may be used in a concentration of 5% in aqueous solution, but has been employed rarely in ophthalmology.

4. Demecarium (Humorsol, BC-48)

Demecarium is a synthetic quaternary compound composed of two neostigmine molecules connected by a polymethylene chain (KRAUPP et al. 1955a, b). It is a white or slightly colored crystalline powder, readily soluble in water, forming a neutral solution, and is stable at neutral pH indefinitely at ordinary room temperatures. It is rapidly decomposed on heating in an alkaline solution. It is used as demecarium bromide in concentrations of 0.1 to 1% aqueous solutions. It can be dispensed in ointment form.

5. Diisopropyl phosphorofluoridate (Isofluorophate, Floropryl, DFP)

This is a synthetic organophosphorus compound belonging to the series of dialkoxy-phosphoryl fluorides (McCOMBIE and SAUNDERS 1946). It is a colorless liquid of high volatility and is rapidly hydrolysed in water to form hydrofluoric acid. However, DFP is stable in peanut or sesame oil or in the form of H_2O-free ointment for as long as three months. It is used as 0.005 to 0.2% solutions in anhydrous peanut oil or sesame oil. Sensitivity to peanut oil and sesame oil exists in some persons (THEODORE 1953). Acute drug irritation may possibly result from the hydrolysis of DFP when it comes in contact with the tears. Some persons are sensitive to DFP itself. It is important that moisture be excluded from all preparations to prevent deterioration. This may be achieved by prescribing only small quantities at a time, and warning the patient against contacting the bottle-dropper or ointment tube-tip with the tears during the process of application.

6. Tetraethylpyrophosphate (TEPP)

Tetraethylpyrophosphate is an organophosphorus compound which is the active ingredient of the insecticide HETP (DE CLERMONT 1854). It is colorless liquid of low volatility which is rapidly hydrolysed in water, but it is stable in peanut oil in which it is used in concentrations of 0.05 to 0.1%. It offers no particular advantage over DFP, and more eyes develop sensitivity to it.

7. Tetraethylmonothiono-pyrophosphate (A$_2$)

This is a sulfur analogue of TEPP, which is poorly soluble and unstable in water.

8. Mintacol (Paraoxon, Bayer E 600, diethyl 4-nitrophenyl phosphate)

Mintacol is a synthetic organophosphorus compound (SCHRADER 1952). It is used in concentrations of 1:10,000 to 1:5000 in aqueous solution.

9. Echothiophate (Phospholine, 217-MI)

Echothiophate is a synthetic organophosphorus compound, and is chemically 2-diethoxy-phosphinyl thioethyltrimethylammonium iodide. It is a white, crystalline, water-soluble compound and is stable at 5° C in aqueous solutions for indefinite periods. At ordinary room temperature it gradually loses its potency over a period of weeks, the solutions retaining approximately 75% activity at the end of 5 weeks, and 50% activity at the end of 30 weeks.

It is used in 0.1 to 0.25% aqueous solutions, using physiological saline with 0.5% chlorobutanol as the preservative. It is usually supplied in the form of powder in one bottle and an accompanying vial of diluent and dropper assembly. In this way the solutions can be prepared freshly to the desired strengths, and if kept at ordinary room temperature can be safely used for at least 3 weeks without significant loss of potency. If use of the same solution over a prolonged period is desired, it should be stored under refrigeration.

10. Diethyl-tetrachlorethylphosphate

Diethyl-tetrachlorethylphosphate is an ester of phosphorus acid, and is used in concentrations of 1:3000 in aqueous solution.

G. Reversal of ocular effects of locally applied anti-ChE agents

The use of pharmacological agents to reverse the systemic effects of anti-ChE agents is well known. The two principal groups of agents employed for such purposes are the cholinergic blocking agents (e. g., atropine), and the reactivators of ChE, i. e., the oximes and hydroxomic acids, such as pyridine-2-aldoxime methiodide (P-2-AM). The efficacy of these modes of treatment has been proven in both animal and clinical studies. Atropine is given in doses higher than used generally. Pyridine-2-aldoxime methiodide can be given either in repeated injections or by slow intravenous drip; 1000 mg of P-2-AM may be given without untoward side effects. Systemic administration of these agents is indicated in systemic toxicity resulting from ocular use of anti-ChE agents.

It is well known that the miosis resulting from systemic administration of anti-ChE agents responds only to local administration of cholinergic blocking agents, such as atropine and homatropine, and is not affected by systemic administration of massive doses of atropine. Apart from this, there may be occasions when it may be desired to reverse the ocular effects of locally administered anti-ChE agents. In nearly all instances, miosis can be counteracted by repeated and frequent instillation of 1% atropine plus 4% homatropine solution. In the case of reversible inhibitors, like physostigmine, the result may be achieved in a shorter period than with irreversible inhibitors like DFP. Oximes and hydroxamic acids, administered locally into the eyes have been investigated from the point of view of counteracting the miosis induced by locally applied anti-ChE agents (Mamo and Leopold 1958). Pyridine-2-aldoxime methiodide or methanesulphonate (P-2-AM, P2S), diacetyl monoxime (DAM, DAMO), 1,3-bis-(pyridinium-4-aldoxime)-propane dibromide, or 1,1-trimethylene bis (4-formylpyridinium oxime bromide) (TMB-4), and monoisonitroso acetone (MINA) were the reactivators employed against the anti-ChE agents physostigmine, DFP, and echothiophate. Administration into the eyes of the oximes and hydroxamic acids alone does not produce any change in the pupillary size of rabbits and normal humans. Administration of these agents locally after miosis has been induced by anti-ChE agents results in dilatation of the pupils. Local instillation or application of ointments is not very effective. Subconjunctival injection of 5% P-2-AM is effective in counteracting the miosis induced by these anti-ChE agents. The oximes are not quite as effective in reversing the miotic effects of eserine as they are after the use of DFP or echothiophate.

Reversal of the tonographic effects of topical echothiophate by P-2-AM has been studied (Becker et al. 1959a). Subconjunctival administration of 4% P-2-AM solution in normal and untreated glaucomatous eyes produces no change in pupillary size, intraocular pressure, or facility of aqueous outflow. In glaucomatous eyes previously treated with echothiophate, the miosis is counteracted and the pupils are dilated, and there is increase in intraocular pressure and decrease in facility of aqueous outflow, reaching approximately the same levels as prior to echothiophate administration. Thus, oximes like P-2-AM, when administered subconjunctivally, counteract the actions of locally administered anti-ChE agents, including miosis, decrease in intraocular pressure, and increase in aqueous outflow facility. Solutions of 25% P-2-AM chloride will occasionally penetrate sufficiently when instilled locally into the *cul de sac* to overcome pupillary effects of echothiophate. Ten percent solutions of TMB_4 in a vehicle containing a detergent such as sodium lauryl sulfonate will also penetrate when applied locally. The detergent must be present in the vehicle to break temporarily the epithelial barrier to penetration. Systemically administered TMB_4 at 25 mg/kg (which is close to the lethal dose) will overcome the pupillary effects of locally instilled echothiophate. The structure of these oximes, when used topically or administered systemically, apparently interferes with their arrival at the site of union of anti-ChE agent with ChE. The local administration of oximes and hydroxamic acids to counteract local effects of anti-ChE agents presents interesting possibilities, but at present their value is limited because their effectiveness is marked only via the subconjunctival route.

H. Ocular use of anti-ChE agents in glaucoma

The exact etiology and pathogenesis of glaucoma still remain unknown. One of the cardinal features of this symptom and sign complex is the increase in intraocular pressure. Failure to control the increase in intraocular pressure results in irreparable damage to the eyes and eventual blindness. Anticholinesterase agents have been found to be very effective in lowering the increase in intraocular pressure in glaucomatous eyes, and in bringing it within normal limits. Because of the beneficial effects exerted by the anti-ChE agents, attempts have been made from time to time to associate glaucoma with some sort of disturbance of the ACh-ChE mechanism.

One such attempt has been to find out if there is any difference between the blood ChE levels of normal and glaucomatous subjects. RADOS (1943) failed to find a change in whole blood ChE levels in glaucomatous subjects, but these results are not surprising since the enzyme of the plasma would obscure any changes occurring in the erythrocytes. Blood ChE activity has been shown to be increased (GALLOIS and HERSCHBERG 1947; VANYSEK 1948) and serum BuChE activity decreased (ARATO and ARATO 1952) in glaucomatous patients. Recent well controlled studies employing newer standard techniques are equally conflicting (DIENSTBIER 1958; LEOPOLD et al. 1959). DIENSTBIER could not demonstrate any appreciable difference between the red blood cell AChE activity of normal and glaucomatous subjects. LEOPOLD et al. found the red blood cell AChE levels to be slightly but significantly lower in glaucomatous subjects as compared to normals; however, further studies in progress at present, employing a different technique, seem to fall more in line with DIENSTBIER's findings. The reasons for such a discrepancy in the results of various workers have been discussed by LEOPOLD et al. It may be concluded that at present there is no convincing evidence of a systemic disturbance of ACh-ChE mechanisms in glaucoma. Further studies are needed to clarify this point.

Apart from attempts to incriminate systemic ChE's in glaucoma, studies have been carried out to find whether any disturbances exist in the ACh-ChE mechanism of the ocular tissues and fluids of glaucomatous patients.

As has already been pointed out, conclusions based on any determination of ChE activity of the aqueous humor are misleading. Manometric determinations of ChE in glaucomatous eyes have been attempted by DE ROETTH (1950). All the eyes utilized in this study were absolute glaucomatous eyes, representing the terminal phase of the disease accompanied by secondary changes. In both glaucomatous eyes and degenerated eyes, ChE contents were found to be diminished. If any conclusions are to be drawn from such a study, numerous glaucomatous eyes in various stages of the disease would have to be studied; this would be extremely difficult because of lack of material. Attempts at histochemical localization of ChE in such eyes may prove more rewarding. Thus, there is no established evidence at present of any local disturbance of ACh or AChE in glaucomatous eyes.

There is no doubt that the various anti-ChE agents effectively lower the intraocular pressure in glaucomatous eyes for several hours, and this decrease of pressure may be maintained for long periods, even for many years, if these agents are applied to the eyes regularly. How this decrease is brought about is not quite clear. These drugs are used in primary glaucoma, and for the same reason in some forms of secondary glaucoma, for their effects on the iris, ciliary body, trabecular meshwork, and blood vessels of the eye including SCHLEMM's canal. The sustained effect of these agents on intraocular pressure cannot be explained fully on the basis of volume changes of the intraocular vascular bed, although some influence may be exerted this way. The principal action of these drugs is a lowering of the resistance to aqueous outflow, as mentioned previously. This has been confirmed amply by tonography. In angle-closure glaucoma the beneficial effect is exerted by freeing the entrance to the trabecular space from the obstructive effect of iris block. This is brought about by contraction of the *sphincter iridis*, which withdraws the iris from contact with the trabecular meshwork and thus frees the angle from the mechanical block, so that the aqueous can now escape freely through it. It is, however, another matter to account for the pressure-lowering effect of these agents in open angle glaucoma, which obviously is not due to obstruction of the angle of the anterior chamber by the iris. It may be postulated that the increased resistance to aqueous outflow which is so definite in these cases is lowered by the anti-ChE agents by their changing the anatomical disposition of the trabecular meshwork as a result of marked contraction of the iris and ciliary muscles, or by their vasomotor effect on the canal of Schlemm or scleral plexuses of vessels.

A different mode of action of the anti-ChE agents, less common than the action on resistance to outflow, is suggested under special circumstances. A temporary lowering of pressure is brought about by intensive local administration of the anti-ChE agents in patients having a high intraocular pressure as a result of permanent obstruction of outflow channels; tonographic studies in such cases have shown decreased flow of aqueous humor. Possibly, intensive therapy results in temporary increase in permeability of the blood-aqueous barrier, and decrease of the osmotic effectiveness of the aqueous barrier, resulting in diminished flow and lowered intraocular pressure.

A paradoxical rise of intraocular pressure may occur in certain glaucomatous eyes after instillation of anti-ChE agents. This is more liable to occur in eyes with the angle closure type of glaucoma. The pupillary block resulting from intense miosis induced by anti-ChE agents results in iris bombé due to accumulation of aqueous in the posterior chamber, and thus causes a mechanical obstruction to the angle of the anterior chamber. Again, the hyperemia and vasodilation resulting from the use of these drugs causes swelling and edema of the iris and ciliary body, and increase in the caliber of the blood vessels near the angle of the anterior chamber, all of which may embarrass the filteration angle mechanically. By the same token, dilatation of the capillaries causes an increase of protein in the aqueous content and a rise in intraocular pressure in spite of the increased permeability of the blood-aqueous barrier.

Physostigmine was the first anti-ChE agent used in glaucoma by LAQUER (1876, 1877) to bring down the intraocular pressure. As such it represents the first medical treatment of glaucoma. The beneficial effect was attributed to miosis, although it was not known at that time that miosis was due to the anti-ChE action of physostigmine. Physostigmine, alone or in conjunction with pilocarpine, was the mainstay of medical treatment for nearly half a century from the days of LAQUER, and even today remains one of the most popular forms of antiglaucomatous therapy. Thus, the first anti-ChE agent known to mankind, the first anti-ChE agent to be used in ophthalmology, and the first anti-ChE agent to be used in the medical treatment of glaucoma has proved its efficacy beyond doubt and holds an honored place in the armamentarium for glaucoma therapy.

After the anti-ChE nature of physostigmine was known (ENGLEHART and LOEWI 1930), other anti-ChE agents were employed to determine their effectiveness in lowering the intraocular pressure in glaucomatous eyes. Neostigmine was introduced in glaucoma therapy by Rossi (1935), DFP by LEOPOLD and COMROE (1946a), Mintacol by THIEL (1949) and by GLEES and WUSTENBERG (1949), demecarium by GITTLER and PILLAT (1956), and echothiophate by LEOPOLD, GOLD and GOLD (1957). Others have evaluated neostigmine (Rossi 1935; CLARKE 1939; MONTALVAN 1943; SIMONELLI 1947; dela FUENTE 1948; MYKALYAN 1952; JUNGHANNSS 1954). Further reports have been made on DFP (McDONALD 1946; DUNPHY 1947; ALDRIDGE et al. 1947; MARR 1947; QUILLIAM 1947; WEEKERS 1947; HAAS 1948; LEOPOLD and McDONALD 1948; DOLLFUS 1948; CHLOUSER 1949; WEINSTEIN 1949; HERAIN 1949; RAIFORD 1949; VANYSCK 1949; GALLINO and BOTTINI 1949; GOEDBLOED 1949; MERCIER 1949; BOCK and VEITL 1949; HAUCK and BIGGENS 1949; BOND 1949; QUINN 1949; STONE 1950; EHLERS 1950; FERRER 1950; BAYO and DELA PENA 1950; STAJDUHAR 1950; ANTONIBON 1950; OURGAUD 1951; THOMAS et al. 1951; HOORENS and PHILIPS 1951; LaRocca 1952; TICHOMIROV and DMITRIEVA 1952; BUTLER 1952; LEOPOLD and CLEVELAND 1953; NISBET 1953; ZEKMAN and SNYDAEKER 1953; ANDREANI 1954, SWAN 1954; WESTSMITH and ABERNETHY 1954; WEEKERS and LAVERGNE 1955; OURGAUD and BERARD 1955; ABBOND 1955; CENTANNI 1956; CALLAHAN 1957). Mintacol has been studied by several (THIEL 1949; GLEES and WUSTENBERG 1949; BUNING 1949; WIRTH 1949; NEUENSCHWANDER 1950; HUERKAMP and WAGNER 1950; GITTLER 1950; PUR 1951; ISERLE and REZEK 1951; FAGERLIND et al. 1952; LEHRINGER 1952; HOORENS and PIETTE 1952; MORAX and FOREST 1953; POLYCHRONAKOS et al. 1953; BAYO and DELA PENA 1954; KAHAN and KNOLL 1954; QUINTIERI 1955; PALICH-SZANTO 1957). Demecarium has been used in many clinics (GITTLER and PILLAT 1956; MILLER et al. 1957; GOUGNARD 1957; GERHARD and KETTER 1958; KRISHNA 1959a; GITTLER 1959; DRANCE and CARR 1959; BECKER et al. 1959b, 1959c; KRISHNA and LEOPOLD 1960b; BECKER and GAGE 1960), and so has echothiophate (LEOPOLD et al. 1957; KRISHNA and LEOPOLD 1959b; BECKER et al. 1959a, b, c; BECKER and GAGE 1960). Other anti-ChE agents like Pyridostigmin (NIEDERMEIER 1952; HECKENHAHM 1955), Phosphacol (structure unavailable to reviewers) (CHLOUSER 1955), A_2 (OUSTINMENKO 1956), and TEPP (GRANT 1948, 1950b) have been employed with less success and less frequently in the control of glaucoma.

For the proper management of glaucoma, it is imperative to know the type of glaucoma that is to be treated. Generally we distinguish between three types of glaucoma: primary, secondary, and congenital. Congenital glaucoma is due to developmental anomalies, mainly of the angle of the anterior chamber. Any form of medical therapy in such cases is rarely successful, and surgery, perhaps in the form of goniotomy or goniopuncture, offers the best prognosis. The secondary type, as its name implies, is secondary to some other diseases of the eye. The treatment in such cases is essentially the treatment of the primary disease. The use of anti-ChE agents may be indicated or contraindicated, depending solely on the nature of the disease. Thus we are mainly concerned here with primary glaucoma which is characterized by a persistently elevated intraocular pressure. Primary glaucoma may be further differentiated into angle-closure (closed angle; narrow angle; acute obstructed angle; acute congestive) and open angle (wide angle; chronic simple) types depending upon the gonioscopic configuration of the angle of the anterior chamber.

In the obstructed angle type of glaucoma, the eye has usually a narrow angle and is thus anatomically disposed to obstruction of the filteration angle, which occurs usually suddenly. There is marked resistance to aqueous outflow, and the rise of pressure is swift and severe, the disease occurring suddenly and with devastating severity. The obstruction of the angle is brought about by pupillary dilatation or vasomotor factors which cause engorgement of the blood vessels of the ciliary body, resulting in rolling in or pushing of the iris against the filteration angle. The same type of obstruction may also be induced as a result of pupillary block, particularly in the case of strong miotics. Acute obstructed angle glaucoma is a medical emergency, and measures have to be taken to relieve the abnormally high intraocular pressure.

Open angle glaucoma is a slow insidious disease and hence the term chronic simple. There is obstruction to outflow of the aqueous in the vast majority of cases, although excessive aqueous formation has been suggested by some; if the later occurs at all, it must be extremely rare. The site of this obstruction to outflow is not known. The filteration angle gonioscopically is open. Therefore, the obstruction must be in one or more of the following structures: the trabecular meshwork, SCHLEMM's canal, the collector channels, the deep scleral plexus, the connecting vessels between the deep scleral plexus and the episcleral plexus, the connecting vessels between the deep scleral plexus and the episcleral veins, or the aqueous veins. Nearly all of these structures have been suggested as the site of obstruction at one time or the other.

Acute obstructed angle glaucoma, as pointed out earlier, is an emergency situation. There is obstruction to the aqueous outflow, elevation of intraocular pressure, and severe frontal and temporal headache with associated nausea and vomiting. Anticholinesterase agents play a very definite role in this disease. In addition to the measure which may be adopted to decrease the aqueous formation, such as administration of intraveneous carbonic anhydrase inhibitors (e. g., acetazoleamide) or the osmotic agents (e.g., urea) to produce dehydration, the main therapy is directed towards relieving the obstruction to the angle of the anterior chamber, and thus improving the facility of aqueous outflow. This is brought about by miotics acting directly on the effector cells, or by inhibiting the AChE, or by a combination of both. Methacholine chloride (Mecholyl chloride), 20%, plus neostigmine bromide (Prostigmin bromide), 5%, every ten minutes for six doses, and then every 30 minutes for the next three doses, is generally used to abort an acute attack. An equally favorite combination is pilocarpine nitrate, 4%, plus physostigmine salicylate, 1%, every 10 minutes for six doses, and then every thirty minutes for the next three doses. It has been suggested that the combined use of methacholine and neostigmine is no more effective than the use of methacholine alone by iontophoresis (SWAN 1948), but iontophoresis is not a very pleasant mode of administration of drugs in the eye. Although an additive effect of small doses of pilocarpine and physostigmine has been demonstrated (LOWEN-STEIN and LOEWENFELD 1951), it has been suggested that in maximum doses the effect is competitive and pilocarpine blocks the action of physostigmine (SWAN and GEHRSITZ 1951). This later view is, however, not generally shared. Another drawback of this form of therapy may be the aggravation of nausea and vomiting due to systemic parasympathomimetic action. Other powerful anti-ChE agents, like DFP, 0.2% in peanut oil, echothiophate, 0.25%, and demecarium, 0.5 to 1%, may be employed. But the use of these agents must be very judicious, as all anti-ChE agents can cause a further elevation of intraocular pressure due to vasodilatation, particularly in eyes with narrow angles. Also, when one of the anti-ChE agents fails to lower the intraocular pressure, and the use of another anti-ChE agent is desired, the choice of this agent must be guided by the synergism or antagonism between these agents. Thus, the use of DFP or echothiophate may be of no avail in a patient who has already received physostigmine, but the use of neostigmine or demecarium in such a patient may prove of real value. Again, sometimes in addition to other measures, retrobulbar injection of procaine is given to lower the intraocular pressure in such cases. In such a case the ciliary ganglion is blocked, and thus anti-ChE agents administered subsequently are of no avail, as any ACh present is not released to the effector cells. Thus, if such a measure is adopted, drugs like pilocarpine which act directly on the effector cells will have to be administered. It may be pointed out that in acute obstructed angle glaucoma, all these measures are temporary and are employed to get relief from the acute attack. The angle is narrow and predisposed to elevation of intraocular pressure, and therefore surgical procedures aimed at making the angle permanently open are extremely gratifying.

In chronic simple or open angle glaucoma, the situation is altogether different. Here the angle is already open, and most of the surgical procedures are generally disappointing. The main treatment is medical, and the anti-ChE agents are one of the chief lines of defense. One should be reminded again that open angle glaucoma is a slow insidious disease, persisting through the rest of the life of the patient. Thus, any therapy decided upon will have to be continued indefinitely. The choice of local application of the drug to the eye is obvious because of the ease of administration, the small quantities of drug required, and lower incidence of systemic reactions. Systemic reactions may occur via this route especially when more potent agents are administered in high concentrations and at frequent intervals. For the same reason the weakest effective concentration of the drug, used as infrequently as possible, is desirable. The drug should be able to take care of the diurnal fluctuations of intraocular pressure, so that the administration of the drug during the sleeping hours is not required. The agent should produce minimal local reactions. Physostigmine, 0.1 to 1 %, is the most commonly employed anti-ChE agent. Usually it has to be repeated two to four times a day. Diurnal fluctuations with elevated pressure are liable to occur. On prolonged use it may give rise to follicular conjunctivitis, and pupillary border epithelial cysts. Retinal detachments have also been reported as well as provocative rises in intraocular pressure.

Diisopropyl phosphorofluoridate (DFP), in 0.005 to 0.2% concentration in peanut oil or sesame oil, has been found to be quite effective. It may be administered less frequently. Cases which are not controlled on other forms of therapy may be controlled by it. The frequency of drug reactions, reactions to the vehicle, iris cysts, rises in intraocular pressure, and retinal detachment are probably higher with DFP.

The latest anti-ChE agents, demecarium and echothiophate, seem to be promising. These are potent, long-acting ChE inhibitors. Demecarium, in a strength of 0.1 to 0.5% in aqueous solution, and echothiophate, 0.1 to 0.25% in aqueous solution, can effectively keep the intraocular pressure within normal limits when administered once or twice a week. They probably will replace DFP, as they are relatively stable in aqueous solution. They also produce the reactions attributed to other anti-ChE agents, such as cysts, retinal detachment, etc.

The anti-ChE agents may be combined with drugs like epinephrine in the control of open angle glaucoma. The use of epinephrine may prove of great benefit, as in addition to its tension-lowering effect it may counteract some of the miosis induced by the anti-ChE agents.

I. Ocular use of anti-ChE agents in accommodative esotropia

Esotropia, or convergent strabismus, may be accommodative, nonaccommodative, or a combination of the two. The nonaccommodative type and the nonaccommodative element of the combined type, as the name implies, are not influenced by accommodation and their treatment therefore is mainly surgical, supplemented by orthoptics when indicated. The accommodative type and the accommodative element of the combined type are caused by accommodative effort and are amenable to measures other than surgery. Miotics are indicated in addition to other usual measures in the type of esotropia characterized by abnormal accommodation-convergence ratio, especially if the esotropia is markedly greater for near vision than for distance. The use of miotics alone or in combination with bifocal lenses is necessary. The principle on which the use of miotics is based is as follows. Accommodative effort is initiated by the central nervous system and this is accompanied by convergence. If there is less central effort, there is less convergence. By the use of miotics in the eyes, accommodation is achieved peripherally without any effort on the part of the central nervous system and consequently no convergence occurs. Thus, the aim is to increase peripheral accommodation and decrease central accommodation which is accompanied by a greater amount of convergence.

Di*iso*propyl phosphorofluoridate is the most commonly used anti-ChE agent for this purpose, although others, like physostigmine and Mintacol, have been used (ABRAHAM 1949, 1952; COSTENBADER 1953, 1954; SCHLOSSMAN 1954, MALBRAN and NORBIS 1955; KNAPP and CAPOBIANCO 1956; STEPHEN 1958; STERNBERG and RAAB 1959). The newer anti-ChE agents, demecarium and echothiophate, are at present under trial in various clinics and seem to compare favorably with DFP. The use of DFP has been found most encouraging in suitably selected cases; strengths of 0.01, 0.025, 0.05, and 0.1 % in peanut or sesame oil, or ointments have been employed. A drop is put in the eye each day for about two weeks. If a beneficial effect is noted, the drug is continued at reduced frequency of administration, at the widest interval of time compatible with therapeutic response, from once every other day to once a week. In several instances the treatment has been continued over a period of two years. Pupillary or iris cysts occur with greater frequency in children (ABRAHAM 1954), but their incidence can be reduced by less frequent instillation. Nearly all anti-ChE agents have been found more effective than pilocarpine, which was previously employed, because of the greater degree of accommodative spasm induced by the others.

J. Ocular use of anti-ChE agents in myasthenia gravis

Myasthenia gravis, a disease characterized by weakness and paralysis of skeletal muscle, is of particular interest to the ophthalmologist, as in nearly one-half of the patients, the initial symptoms are referable to the muscles of the eye and eyelids. These symptoms are ptosis and diplopia (MATTIS 1941; WALSH 1945). Later, in practically all patients symptoms are referable to the extraocular muscles. Again there is a type of myasthenia gravis termed ocular myasthenia in which only muscles of the eyes and eyelid are involved (WALSH 1948; LISMAN 1949).

The pathogenesis of myasthenia gravis still remains obscure, although it is referable to a disturbance in the ACh-AChE mechanism, resulting in deficiency of transmission at the myoneural junction. While the unusual susceptibility of the extraocular musles in this disease is difficult to explain with certainty, it may be postulated that it is due to a cholinergic disturbance, as the normal extraocular muscles are unusually excitable by ACh and physostigmine (FENG and LI 1940; BROWN and HARVEY 1941).

The use of physostigmine as a likely drug for treating myasthenia gravis was suggested by JOLLY (1895). But it was left to WALKER to try not only physostigmine (WALKER 1934) but also neostigmine (WALKER 1935) in the treatment of myasthenia gravis. Systemic administration of these and several other newer anti-ChE agents since then has become the standard procedure for the management of such patients. Neostigmine intramuscularly and edrophonium intravenously are also used as diagnostic tests for myasthenia gravis, where a positive response, characterized by improvement in ptosis and ophthalmoplegia, confirms the diagnosis. (See Chapter 23 for full account.)

While the majority of cases are well controlled by systemic administration of anti-ChE agents, there are patients who still complain of symptoms referable to their eyes in spite of the fact that they are free from symptoms in the rest of the body. This may be ascribed to the fact that either there is not enough penetration of the anti-ChE agents to these muscles, or there is an abnormally high accumulation of AChE which the administered drugs are unable to inhibit. Recently AChE has been demonstrated by histochemical technique in the motor endplates of the extraocular muscles of both normal subjects and myasthenia gravis patients (COHEN and ZACKS 1959) whose ocular symptoms remained uncontrolled on systemic administration of neostigmine; the presence of AChE in these patients suggests either that there is not enough penetration of neostigmine in the extraocular muscles to inactivate the enzyme, or the unusually high concentration of the enzyme, if such is the case, or that inhibition is reversed during the histochemical procedure. Apart from the failure of the anti-ChE agents to control the symptoms referable to the extraocular muscles, there are cases whose symptoms are confined only to the eyes, the so-called ocular myasthenia. It is logical that this latter group of patients be treated by means other than systemic administration of anti-ChE agents with their accompanying undesirable systemic side effects.

Recently, the local use of anti-ChE agents in the form of instillation of drops or by iontophoresis in the conjunctival sacs has been advocated in patients with ocular myasthenia, and in conjunction with systemically administered anti-ChE agents in patients whose ocular symptoms are not relieved by the systemically administered drugs alone (DAMIANI 1957; LEOPOLD et al. 1960). Cases have been reported in which marked subjective and objective improvement has been noted following instillation of neostigmine, 5% aqueous solution, and demecarium, 0.25, 0.5, and 1.0% aqueous solution, into the conjunctival sac from twice a day to every second day. Electromyographic studies on the muscles of the eye and eyelids, both before and after instillation of these agents, confirm their efficacy and the value of this mode of administration, as indicated by the improved and persistent firing of motor unit potentials on maximum and sustained effort following instillation, in contrast to the early disappearance of motor unit potentials on maximum and sustained effort before instillation. The local use of these anti-ChE agents in conjunction with electromyographic studies of these muscles presents an attractive possibility for its being used as a diagnostic test for myasthenia gravis.

Literature

ABBOND, I.: Retinal detachment after DFP. Bull. ophthal. Soc. Egypt 48, (Session 52) 167—168 (1955).

ABRAHAM, S. V.: The use of miotics in the treatment of convergent strabismus and anisometropia: a preliminary report. Amer. J. Ophthal. 32, 233—240 (1949).

— The use of miotics in the treatment of non-paralytic convergent strabismus: a progress report. Amer. J. Ophthal. 35, 1191—1195 (1952).

— Intra-epithelial cysts of the iris: their production in young persons and possible significance. Amer. J. Ophthal. 37, 327—331 (1954).

ADRIAN, E. D., W. FELDBERG and B. A. KILBY: Cholinesterase inhibiting action of fluorophosphates. Brit. J. Pharmacol. 2, 56—58 (1947).

AESCHLIMANN, J. A., and M. REINERT: The pharmacological action of some analogues of physostigmine. J. Pharmacol. exp. Ther. 43, 413—444 (1931).

ALDRIDGE, W. H., H. DAVSON, E. B. DUNPHY and G. I. UHDE: The effect of diisopropyl fluorophosphate vapour on the eye. Amer. J. Ophthal. 30, 1405—1412 (1947).

AMBROSIA, A., A. BARONE e C. SERRA: Prime osservazioni sull'attività elettrica dei muscoli oculari estrinse durante la stimolazione luminosa intermittente. Boll. Soc. ital. Biol. sper. 33, 1218—1221 (1957).

ANDERSON, H. K.: The action of eserine and atropine upon the denervated sphincter iridis. (Preliminary communication). J. Physiol. (Lond.) 31, XXII—XXIV (1904).

— The paralysis of involuntary muscle. Part II. On the paralysis of the sphincter of the pupil with special reference to paradoxical constriction and the functions of the ciliary ganglion. J. Physiol. (Lond.) 33, 156—174 (1905a).

— The paralysis of involuntary muscle. Part III. On the action of pilocarpine, physostigmine, and atropine upon the paralyzed iris. J. Physiol. (Lond.) 33, 414—438 (1905b).

1074 Literature

ANDREANI, D.: Sull'aumento secondario della tensione oculare, prodotto dal D.F.P., in soggetti glaucomatosi. Osservazationi in rapporto alle condizioni dell angolo irido-corneale. Ann. Ottal. **80**, 341—348 (1954).

ANTONIBON, A.: Il D.F.P. nel glaucoma. Atti 38 Cong. Soc. oftal. ital. **11**, 519 (1950).

ARATO, S., and M. ARATO: Cholinesterase activity of the serum and the aqueous humor in glaucoma (In Hungarian). Ophthalmologica (Basel) **123**, 374—382 (1952).

ARGYLL ROBERTSON, D.: The Calabar bean as a new agent in ophthalmic medicine. Edinb. med. J. **8**, pt. 2, 815—820 (1863).

AUGUSTINSSON, K. B.: Cholinesterases. A study in comparative enzymology. Acta physiol. scand. **15**, Suppl. 52, 1—182 (1948).

— Assay methods for cholinesterases. In: D. GLICK, Ed., Methods of biochemical analysis, Vol. V, 1—64. New York: Interscience Publishers, Inc. 1957.

BARANY, E.: Action of atropine, homatropine, eserine and prostigmine on osmotic pressure of aqueous humor. Acta physiol. scand. **13**, 95—102 (1947).

—, and V. E. KINSEY: Rate of flow of aqueous humor. I. The rate of disappearance of para-aminohippuric acid, radioactive Rayopake, and radioactive Diodrast from the aqueous humor of rabbits. Amer. J. Ophthal. **32**, 177—188 (1949).

—, and A. WIRTH: An improved method for estimating rate of flow of aqueous humor in individual animals. Acta ophthal. (Kbh.) **32**, 95—108 (1954).

BARONE, A., e C. SERRA: Risposta dell'effettore muscolare alla stimulazione luminosa inter-mittente. Boll. Soc. ital. Biol. sper. **33**, 1216—1218 (1957).

BAYO, J. M., y A. DELA PENA: Parasimpaticomimetics de sintesis de acción periferica indirecta (estudio previo experimental sobre la miosis, tono ocular y permeabilidad uveal del diiso-propilfluorofosfato, dietilparanitrofenilfosfato y diisopropylparanitrofenilfosfato. Arch. Soc. oftal. hisp.-amer. **10**, 1310—1333 (1950).

— — Acción del diisopropilparanitrofenilfosfato (Mioticol) sobre el glaucoma. Arch. Soc. oftal. hisp.-amer. **14**, 415—424 (1954).

BECKER, B., and M. A. CONSTANT: The facility of aqueous outflow. A.M.A. Arch. Ophthal. **55**, 305—312 (1956).

— G. C. PYLE and R. C. DREWS: The tonographic effects of echothiophate (phospholine) iodide. Reversal by pyridine-2-aldoxime methiodide (P_2AM). Amer. J. Ophthal. **47**, (Pt. I) 635—640 (1959a).

— T. GAGE and A. E. KOLKER: The effect of phenylepherine hydrochloride on the miotic treated eye. Amer. J. Ophthal. **48**, 313—321 (1959b).

— A. J. GAY and C. S. GASSIN: Applanation tonometry in the diagnosis and treatment of glaucoma. A.M.A. Arch. Ophthal. **62**, 211—215 (1959c).

—, and T. GAGE: Demecarium bromide and echothiophate iodide in chronic glaucoma. A.M.A. Arch. Ophthal. **63**, 102—107 (1960).

BERLINER, M. L.: Biomicroscopy of the eye. Slit lamp microscopy of the living eye. Vol. I and II. New York: Paul B. Hoeber, Inc. 1949.

BOCK, K., u. W. VEITL: Über Erfahrungen mit Di-isopropyl Fluorophosphate bei normalen und glaukomatosen Augen. Ber. dtsch. ophthal. Ges. **55**, 185—191 (1949).

BOND, F. M.: Di-isopropyl fluorophosphate in glaucoma. Trans. Pacif. Cst. Oto-ophthal. Soc. **30**, 115—120 (1949).

BROWN, G. L., and A. M. HARVEY: Neuromuscular transmission in the extrinsic muscles of the eye. J. Physiol. (Lond.) **99**, 379—399 (1941).

BUNING, K.: Erfahrungen mit Mintacol. Klin. Mbl. Augenheilk. **115**, 534—538 (1949).

BURGEN, A. S. V., and L. M. CHIPMAN: The location of cholinesterase in the central nervous system. Quart. J. exp. Physiol. **37**, 61—74 (1952).

BUTLER, W. E.: Acute glaucoma precipitated by DFP. Report of a case. Amer. J. Ophthal. **35**, 1031—1033 (1952).

CALLAHAN, A.: Use of di-isopropyl fluorophosphate in 0.01 per cent and 0.025 per cent con-centrations. Amer. J. Ophthal. **43**, 281—283 (1957).

CASELLI, F.: L'azione del Mintacol sulla permeabilità della barriera emato-oftalmica. Arch. Ottal. **57**, 413—424 (1953).

CENTANNI, L.: Osservazioni cliniche sull'impiego del DFP. Ann. Ottal. **82**, 89—98 (1956).

CHLOUSER, G. R.: Di-isopropylfluorophosphate in the treatment of glaucoma (in Russian). Vestn. Oftal. **28**, No. 2, 13—16 (1949).

— Phosphacol in glaucoma (in Russian). Vestn. Oftal. **34**, 30—33 (1955).

CLARKE, S. T.: Mecholyl and prostigmine in the treatment of glaucoma. Amer. J. Ophthal. **22**, 249—257 (1939).

CLERMONT, P. DE: Chimie organique — Note sur la préparation de quelques éthers. C. R. Acad. Sci. (Paris) **39**, 338—341 (1854).

COHEN, R. B., and S. I. ZACKS: Myasthenia gravis. II. Histochemical demonstration of acetyl-cholinesterase activity in motor end-plates of extraocular muscle in patients with myasthenia gravis. A postmortem study. Amer. J. Path. **35**, 399—405 (1959).

COMROE, J. H. Jr., J. TODD, I. H. LEOPOLD, G. B. KOELLE, O. BODENSKY and A. GILMAN: The effect of di-isopropyl-fluorophosphate (DFP) upon patients with myasthenia gravis. Amer. J. med. Sci. **212**, 641—651 (1946).

COSTENBADER, F. D.: Symposium: Strabismus, principles of treatment. Trans. Amer. Acad. Ophthal. **57**, 163—169 (1953).

— Symposium: Accommodative esotropia, clinical course and management. Amer. Orthop. J. **4**, 12—16 (1954).

DAMIANI, A.: La prostigmina locale nelle manifestazioni oculari della miastenia. Ann. Neurol. Psychiat. **50**, 31—45 (1957).

DARDENNE, U., W. LEYDHECKER u. E. HELFERICH: Die Cholinesterase in der Iris von Mensch und Rind. Albrecht v. Graefes Arch. Ophthal. **158**, 434—438 (1957).

DIENSTBIER, E.: The cholinesterase activity of erythrocytes in patients with glaucoma (in Czech). Čsl. Oftal. **14**, 321—326 (1958).

DOLLFUS, M. A.: Nos premiers essais thérapeutiques par le DFP (Diisopropylfluorophosphonate) dans la glaucoma et la mydriase paralytique. Bull. Soc. Ophtal. Paris **10**, 749—757 (1948).

DRANCE, S. M., and F. CARR: Effect of demecarium bromide (BC-48) on intraocular pressure in man. A.M.A. Arch. Ophthal. **62**, 673—678 (1959).

DUNPHY, E. B.: Di-isopropyl fluorophosphate in glaucoma. Bull. New Engl. med. Cent. **9**, 102—106 (1947).

EHLERS, H.: Experiences with DFP (in Danish). Ugeskr. Laeg. **112**, 82—83 (1950).

EICHNER, D. v.: Frage der Fermentlokalisation in der Netzhaut des Rindes. Z. Zellforsch. **41**, 493—508 (1955).

ENGLEHART, E., u. O. LOEWI: Fermentative Azetylcholinspaltung im Blut und ihre Hemmung durch Physostigmine. Naunyn-Schmiedeberg's Arch. exp. Path. Pharmak. **150**, 1—13 (1930).

FAGERLIND, L., B. HOLMSTEDT and O. WALLEN: Preparation and determination of diethyl p-nitrophenyl phosphate (E 600), a drug used in the treatment of glaucoma. Svensk farm. T. **56**, 303—308 (1952).

FELDBERG, W., G. W. HARRIS and R. C. Y. LIN: Observations on the presence of cholinergic and noncholinergic neurones in the central nervous system. J. Physiol. (Lond.) **112**, 400—404 (1951).

FENG, T. P., and T. LI: Studies on the neuro-muscular function. Acetylcholine sensitivity of a muscle and its aptitude to give contracture of the eserine type. Chin. J. Physiol. **15**, 197—212 (1940).

FERRER, O.: Results in a series of cases treated with DFP. Ophthal. ib.-amer. **12**, 123—124 (1950).

FRANCIS, C. M.: Cholinesterase in the retina. J. Physiol. (Lond.) **120**, 435—439 (1953).

FRASER, T. R.: On the characters, actions, and therapeutical uses of the ordeal bean of calabar (Physostigma venenosum, Balfour). Edinb. med. J. **9**, 36—56, 123—132, 235—248 (1863).

FRIEDENWALD, J. S.: Recent advances in tonometer construction. Trans. Amer. Acad. Ophthal. **52**, 543—547 (1948).

— Committee on standardization of tonometers. Amer. Acad. Ophthal. Otolaryng. Decennial Report. (1954).

— Histochemistry — a review. Pharmacol. Rev. **7**, 83—96 (1955).

— Tonometer calibration. Trans. Amer. Acad. Ophthal. Otolaryng. **61**, 108—123 (1957).

DE LA FUENTE, G. L.: La prostigmina en el glaucoma. Arch. Soc. oftal. hisp.-amer. **8**, 130—133 (1948).

GALLINO, J. A., y. E. E. BOTTINI: Observaciones clinicos con el empleo de D.F.P. (Di-isopropilfluorofosfate). Arch. Oftal. B. Aires **24**, 195—208 (1949).

GALLOIS, J., et A. D. HERSCHBERG: Glaucoma et cholinestérase sérique. Bull. Soc. franç. ophtal. **59**, 228—230 (1947).

GERHARD, J. P., et N. KETTER: Nos expériences avec le bromure de décamethyléne (BC-48). Bull. Soc. franç. Ophtal. **7**—**8**, 549—555 (1958).

GIACOBINI, E., and J. ZAJICEK: Quantitative determination of acetylcholinesterase in individual nerve cells. Nature (Lond.) **177**, 185—186 (1956).

— The distribution and localization of cholinesterases in nerve cells. Acta physiol. scand. **45**, Suppl. 156, 1—45 (1959).

GITTLER, R.: Erfahrungen mit Mintacol. Wien. klin. Wschr. **62**, 379 (1950).

—, u. B. PILLAT: Die Verwendung von Dekamethylen-bis-(N-methylcarbaminoyl-m-trimethylammoniumphenol) (BC-48) bei der Therapie des Glaukoms. Albrecht v. Graefes Arch. Ophthal. **157**, 473—494 (1956).

— Die klinische Erprobung von Dekamethylen-bis-(N-methylcarbaminoyl-m-trimethylammoniumphenol) (BC-48) beim Glaucoma acutum, chronicum und secundarium. Ost. ophthal. Ges. 2nd Ann. Meeting June 1956, 26—32 (1959).

GLEES, M., u. W. WUSTENBERG: Über Erfahrungen mit Mintacol am normalen und glaukomkranken Augen. Klin. Mbl. Augenheilk. **114**, 455—458 (1949).

GOEDBLOED, J.: Enkele ervaringen met di-isopropylfluorphosphaat. Ned. T. Geneesk. **2**,
1634—1636 (1949).

GOLDMANN, H.: Über Fluorescein in der menschlichen Vorderkammer. Das Kammerwasser-
Minutenvolumen des Menschen. Ophthalmologica (Basel) **119**, 65—95 (1950).

— Abflußdruck, Minutenvolumen und Widerstand der Kammerwasserströmung des Menschen. Docum. ophthal. (s'-Grav.) **5—6**, 278—356 (1951).

— Un nouveau tonométre à aplanation. Bull. Soc. franç. Ophtal. **67**, 474—478 (1954).

GORIN, G., and A. POSNER: Slit lamp gonioscopy. Baltimore: The Williams and Wilkins
Company 1957.

GOUGNARD, L.: Le traitement de l'hypertension oculaire par le bromure de decamethylene-bis-
N-methyl-carbaminoyl-4-trimethylammoniumphenol (BC-48). Ann. oculist., Paris 190, 874
(1957). Bull. Soc. belge Ophtal. **116**, 411—415 (1957).

GRANT, W. M.: Miotic and antiglaucomatous activity of tetraethyl pyrophosphate in human
eyes. Arch. Ophthal. (Chicago) **39**, 579—586 (1948).

— Tonographic method for measuring the facility and rate of aqueous flow in human eyes.
A.M.A. Arch. Ophthal. **44**, 204—214 (1950a).

— Additonal experiences with tetraethyl pyrophosphate in treatment of glaucoma. Arch.
Ophthal. (Chicago) **44**, 362—364 (1950b).

— Clinical measurements of aqueous outflow. A.M.A. Arch. Ophthal. **46**, 113—131 (1951).

GREAVES, D. P., and E. S. PERKINS: Influence of the sympathetic nervous system on the
intraocular pressure and vascular circulation of the eye. Brit. J. Ophthal. **36**, 258—264
(1952).

GUERRY, D.: The use of the Sanborn electromanometer in the study of pharmacological
effects upon the intraocular pressure. Trans. Amer. ophthal. Soc. **49**, 525—555 (1951).

HAAS, J. S.: Response to DFP. Amer. J. Ophthal. **31**, 227—228 (1948).

HARUTA, CH., M. MINAMI and K. TOSHIMA: Cholinesterase and acetylcholine in the iris (in
Japanese). Acta Soc. Ophthal. jap. **57**, 219—221 (1953).

HARVEY, A. M., J. L. LILIENTHAL Jr., D. GROB, B. F. JONES and S. A. TALBOT: The administration of DFP to man. IV. The effects on neuromuscular function in normal subjects and
in myasthenia gravis. Bull. Johns Hopk. Hosp. **81**, 267—292 (1947).

HAUCK, E. L., and C. H. BIGGINS: The use of DFP in treatment of refractory glaucoma. Med.
Arts Sci. **3**, 53—55 (1949).

HEBB, C. O., A. SILVER, A. A. B. SWAN and E. G. WALSH: A histochemical study of cholinesterases of rabbit retina and optic nerve. Quart. J. exp. Physiol. **38**, 185—191 (1953).

— Acetylcholine metabolism of nervous tissue. Pharmacol. Rev. **6**, 39—43 (1954).

HECKENHAHN, K.: Erfahrungen bei der Behandlung von Glaukomkranken mit Pyridostigmin.
Klin. Mbl. Augenheilk. **126**, 334—335 (1955).

HERAIN, V. J.: Neoglaucet-nove miotikum. Čsl. oftal. **5**, 14—30 (1949).

HIND, H. W., and F. M. GOYAN: A new concept of the role of hydrogen in concentration and
buffer system in the preparation of ophthalmic solutions. J. Amer. Pharm. Ass. **36**, 33—41
(1947).

HOLMSTEDT, B.: A modification of the thiocholine method for the determination of cholinesterase. I. Biochemical evaluation of selective inhibitors. Acta physiol. scand. **40**, 322—
330 (1957a).

— A modification of the thiocholine method for the determination of cholinesterase. II.
Histochemical application. Acta physiol. scand. **40**, 331—337 (1957b).

HOORENS, A., and PHILIPS: Contribution à l'étude de l'action mystique du diisopropylfluorophosphonate (DFP). Bull. Soc. belge Ophtal. **99**, 415—419 (1951).

—, et PIETTE: Contribution à l'étude d'un nouveau myotique: le Mintacol. Bull. Soc. belge.
Ophtal. **102**, 558—561 (1952).

HUERKAMP, B., u. O. WAGNER: Über die Wirkung des Mintacols auf die Pupille und den
Augenbinnendruck. Klin. Mbl. Augenheilk. **117**, 586—597 (1950).

ISERLE, i V. REZEK: Syntheticke miotikum TS 219. Čsl. Ofthal. **7**, 174—180 (1951).

JOLLY, F.: Über Myasthenia gravis pseudoparlaytica. Berl. klin. Wschr. **32**, 1—7 (1895).

JULIAN, P. L., and J. PIKL: Studies in the indole series: III. On the synthesis of physostigmine.
J. Amer. chem. Soc. **57**, 539—544 (1935).

JUNGHANNSS, K.: Die Behandlung des Glaucoms mit Eustigmin. Dtsch. Gesundh.wes. **9**,
629—631 (1954).

KAHAN, A., and A. KNOLL: Ophthalmological application of ortho (In Hungarian). Szemeszet
91, 71—77 (1954).

KINSEY, V. E., and E. BARANY: Rate of flow of aqueous humor. II. Derivation of rate of flow
and its physiologic significance. Amer. J. Ophthal. **32**, 189—202 (1949).

KNAPP, P., and N. M. CAPOBIANCO: Use of miotics in esotropia. Amer. orthopt. J. **6**, 40—46 (1956).
KOELLE, G. B.: Protection of cholinesterase against irreversible inactivation by DFP in vitro. J. Pharmacol. exp. Ther. **88**, 232—237 (1946).
—, and J. S. FRIEDENWALD: A histochemical method of localizing cholinesterase activity. Proc. Soc. exp. Biol. (N. Y.) **70**, 617—622 (1949).
— The histochemical differentiation of types of cholinesterases and their localizations in tissues of the cat. J. Pharmacol. exp. Ther. **100**, 158—179 (1950a).
—, and J. S. FRIEDENWALD: The histochemical localization of cholinesterase in ocular tissues. Amer. J. Ophthal. **33**, 253—256 (1950b).
— The elimination of enzymatic diffusion artifacts in the histochemical localization of cholinesterases and a survey of their cellular distribution. J. Pharmacol. exp. Ther. **103**, 153—171 (1951).
— L. WOLFAND, J. S. FRIEDENWALD and R. A. ALLEN: Localization of specific cholinesterase in ocular tissues of the cat. Amer. J. Ophthal. **35**, 1580—1584 (1952).
— The localization of specific cholinesterase in the retina. Pharmacol. Rev. **6**, 47—48 (1954).
— The histochemical identification of acetylcholinesterase in cholinergic, adrenergic and sensory neurones. J. Pharmacol. exp. Ther. **114**, 167—184 (1955).
—, and E. C. STEINER: The cerebral distribution of a tertiary and a quaternary anticholinesterase agent following intravenous and intraventricular injection. J. Pharmacol. exp. Ther. **118**, 420—434 (1956).
KOSTER, R.: Synergisms and antagonisms between physostigmine and di-isopropyl fluorophosphate in cats. J. Pharmacol. exp. Ther. **88**, 39—46 (1946).
KRAUPP, O., H. G. SCHWARZACHER and C. STUMPF: Über die pharmakologischen Eigenschaften einiger polymethylene-bis-carbaminoyl-m-trimethylammoniumphenole. Naunyn-Schmiedebergs Arch. exp. Path. Pharmak. **225**, 117—119 (1955a).
— C. STUMPF, E. HERZFELD u. B. PILLAT: Pharmakologische Eigenschaften einiger langwirksamer Cholinesterase-Hemmkörper aus der Reihe der Polymethylen-bis-carbaminoyl-m-trimethylammoniumphenole. Arch. int. Pharmacodyn. **102**, 281—303 (1955b).
KRISHNA, N.: Demecarium Bromide (BC-48): A new anticholinesterase agent in the treatment of glaucoma. Amer. J. Ophthal. **47**, (pt. I) 98 (1959a).
—, and I. H. LEOPOLD: Echothiophate (phospholine) iodide (217-MI) in treatment of glaucoma: Further observations. A.M.A. Arch. Ophthal. **62**, 300—313 (1959b).
— — The effect of BC-48 (Demecarium Bromide) on normal rabbit and human eyes. Amer. J. Ophthal. **49**, 270—277 (1960a).
— — Use of BC-48 (Demecarium Bromide) in treatment of glaucoma. Amer. J. Ophthal. **49**, 554—560 (1960b).
— Effects of lateral rectus muscle contraction upon intraocular pressure. Fed. Proc. **10**, 299 (1960c).
—, and I. H. LEOPOLD: The effect of echothiophate (phospholine) iodide (217-MI) on normal rabbit and human eyes. Unpublished data.
KRONFELD, P. C.: Tonometer calibration, empirical validation. Trans. Amer. Acad. Ophthal. Otolaryng. **61**, 123—126 (1957).
KUBOKI, T.: Studies on discharge intervals of a single motor unit in the human extraocular muscles. Part I. During fixation of the gaze. Part II. During horizontal movement of the eye. Tôhuku J. exp. Med. **66**, 91—105 (1957a).
— I. SEKINO and K. FUKUSHI: Periodicity in the electromyograph of human extraocular muscles. I. (In Japanese with English summary). Acta Soc. Ophth. Jap. **61**, 1565—1569 (1957b).
LANGHAM, M. E., and P. WOOD: The transfer of fluorescein across the blood-aqueous barrier. J. Physiol. (Lond.) **132**, 55—56 (1956).
LAQUEUR, L.: Über eine neue therapeutische Verwendung des Physostigmin. Zbl. med. Wiss. **14**, 421—422 (1876).
— Über Atropin und Physostigmin und ihre Wirkung auf den intraocularen Druck. (Ein Beitrag zur Therapie des Glaucoms.) Albrecht v. Graefes Arch. Ophthal. **23**, pt. 3, 149—176 (1877).
LEHRINGER, F. E.: Über Erfahrungen mit dem Mioticum Miotisal. Dtsch. Gesundh.-Wes. **7**, 430—433 (1952).
LEOPOLD, I. H., and J. H. COMROE JR.: Effect of neostigmine (prostigmine) and physostigmine upon the denervated iris of the cat. Proc. Soc. exp. Biol. (N. Y.) **60**, 382—384 (1945).
— and J. H. COMROE JR.: Use of di-isopropylfluorophosphate (DFP) in treatment of glaucoma. Arch. Ophthal. (Chicago) **36**, 1—16 (1946a).
—, and J. H. COMROE: Effect of di-isopropyl fluorophosphate (DFP) on the normal eye. Arch. Ophthal. (Chicago) **36**, 17—32 (1946b).
—, and P. R. McDONALD: Di-isoprolpy fluorophosphate (DFP) in treatment of glaucoma. Further observations. Arch. Ophthal. (Chicago) **40**, 176—186 (1948).

LEOPOLD, I. H.: Autonomic drugs and their influence on choroidal vessel caliber. Trans. Amer.
    ophthal. Soc. **49**, 625—672 (1951).
—, and A. F. CLEVELAND: Di-isopropyl fluorophosphate (DFP) (0.01 per cent) in chronic
    wide angle glaucoma. Amer. J. Ophthal. **36**, 226—231 (1953).
— P. GOLD and D. GOLD: Use of a Thiophosphinyl quaternary compound (217-MI) in treat-
    ment of glaucoma. A.M.A. Arch. Ophthal. 58, 363—366 (1957).
— N. KRISHNA and R. A. LEHMAN- The effects of anticholinesterase agents on the blood
    cholinesterase levels of normal and glaucoma subjects. Trans. Amer. Ophth. Soc. **57**,
    63—85 (1959).
— T. R. HEDGES JR., J. MONTANA, N. KRISHNA and S. BECKETT: Local administration of
    anticholinesterase agents in ocular myasthenia gravis. A.M.A. Arch. Ophthal. **63**, 544 to
    547 (1960).
LEPLAT, G., et M. A. GEREBTZOFF: Localisation de l'acetylcholinesterase et des médicateurs
    diphénoliques dans la rétine. Ann. Oculist. (Paris) **189**, 121—128 (1956).
LISMAN, J. V.: Ocular myasthenia gravis. Amer. J. Ophthal. **32**, 565—571 (1949).
LOWENSTEIN, O., and I. E. LOEWENFELD: Effect of physostigmine and pilocarpine on iris
    sphincter of normal man. A.M.A. Arch. Ophthal. **50**, 311—318 (1953).
MALBRAN, E. S., and A. L. NORBIS: Le D.F.P. dans le traitement du strabisme convergent.
    Ann. Oculist. (Paris) **188**, 720—733 (1955).
MAMO, J. G., and I. H. LEOPOLD: Evaluation and use of oximes in ophthalmology. Amer. J.
    Ophthal. **46**, (Pt. I) 724—731 (1958).
MARR, W. G.: The clinical use of di-isopropyl fluorophosphate (D.F.P.) in chronic glaucoma.
    Amer. J. Ophthal. **30**, 1423 (1947).
MARUI, S.: Über Kombinationswirkung von Physostigmin (Eserin) und Pilokarpin am mensch-
    lichen Auge. Klin. Mbl. Augenheilk. **68**, 145—152 (1922).
MATSUDA, T.: Studies of the ciliary body. (In Japanese). Acta Soc. ophthal. jap. **63**, 155—168
    (1959).
MATTIS, R. D.: Ocular manifestations in myasthenia gravis. Arch. Ophthal. (Chicago) **26**,
    969—982 (1941).
MAURICE, D. M.: An applanation tonometer of new principle. Brit. J. Ophthal. **35**, 178—182
    (1951).
— A recording tonometer. Brit. J. Ophthal. **42**, 321—335 (1958).
McCOMBIE, H., and P. C. SAUNDERS: Alkyl fluorophosphonates: Preparation and physiological
    properties. Nature (Lond.) **157**, 287—289 (1946).
McDONALD, P. R.: Treatment of glaucoma with DFP. Amer. J. Ophthal. **29**, 1071—1081
    (1946).
MERCIER, A.: Indications du DFP dans le glaucome. Bull. Soc. franç. Ophtal. **62**, 320—324
    (1949).
MERTENS, H. G., E. ESSLEN and W. PAPST: Die oligosymptomatische Oculare Myositis
    (Pseudomyasthenia). Nervenarzt **29**, 213—226 (1958).
MILLER, H. A., J. DIVERT and J. GROUZET: Le bromure de dècamethylène bis neostigmine
    (BC-48) dans le traitement des hypertonies oculaires. Bull. Soc. franç. ophtal. **70**, 518—539
    (1957).
MINAMI, M.: The location of cholinesterase in the retina. (In Japanese). Acta Soc. ophthal. jap.
    56, 604—613 (1952).
MOLITOR, H.: A comparative study of the effects of five choline compounds used in therapeutics.
    J. Pharmacol. exp. Ther. **58**, 337—360 (1936).
MONTALVAN, P.: Prostigmine in the treatment of glaucoma: its effect on intraocular pressure.
    Amer. J. Ophthal. **26**, 57—62 (1943).
MORAX, P. V., et A. FOREST: Essais cliniques d'un nouveau myotique et hypotenseur oculaire:
    le Mintacol. Bull. Soc. franç. Ophtal. **4**, 370—374 (1953).
MOSES, R. A., and M. BRUNO: Rate of outflow of fluid from the eye under increased pressure.
    Amer. J. Ophthal. **33**, Pt. I., 389—397 (1950).
MYERSON, A., and W. THAU: Human autonomic pharmacology: IX. Effect of cholinergic and
    adrenergic drugs on the eye. Arch. Ophthal. (Chicago) **18**, 78—90 (1937).
MYKALYAN, A. N.: The action of prostigmine and proserine in glaucoma. (In Russian). Vestn.
    oftal. **31**, No. 1, 24—26 (1952).
NEUENSCHWANDER, M.: Mintacol „Bayer", Ein neues Glaucom-Mittel. Ophthalmologica
    (Basel) **120**, 104—105 (1950).
NIEDERMEIER, S.: Ein neues Mioticum: Pyridostigmin. Klin. Mbl. Augenheilk. **120**, 410—411
    (1952).
NISBET, A. A.: Glaucoma in aphakia. Tex. St. J. Med. **49**, 134—137 (1953).
OURGAUD, A. G.: Traitement du glaucome par la di-isopropyl fluorophosphate (DFP) Ann.
    thér. **2**, 248—259 (1951).

OURGAUD, A. G., and P. V. BERARD: Décollement rétinien et hypertonie oculaire. Bull. Soc. franç. Ophtal. **68**, 384—391 (1955).

OUSTINMENKO, L. L.: A new soviet miotic tetra-ethyl-monothio-pyrophosphate (2) in glaucoma. (In Russian). Vestn. oftal. **2**, 11—18 (1956).

PALICH-SZANTO, O.: Über die Wirkung des Mioticums „Ortho" in der augenärztlichen Praxis. Ophthalmologica (Basel) **133**, 414—418 (1957).

PAPST, W., H. G. MERTENS u. E. ESSLEN: Die chronische okulare Myositis. I. Mitteilung: Die exophthalmische okulare Myositis. Klin. Mbl. Augenheilk. **133**, 673—694 (1958).

PEARSE, A. G. E.: Histochemistry, theoretical and applied. London: J. A. Churchill 1953.

POLYCHRONAKOS, D., D. LEANIS and A. ANASTASSIADIS: Mintacol in glaucoma (In Greek). Arch. Soc. Ophtal. Grèce Nord. **2**, 7—11 (1953).

POSNER, A.: Notes on ophthalmology; comments on mydriatic and miotic alkaloids as told by R. FEINSTEIN. Eye, Ear, Nose, Thr. Monthly **29**, 632 (1950).

PUR, S.: Klinicke Zkusenosti STS 219. Čsl. Oftal. **7**, 169—174 (1951).

QUILLIAM, J. P.: Di-isopropylfluorophosphate (DFP): its pharmacology and its therapeutic uses in glaucoma and myasthenia gravis. Postgrad. med. J. **23**, 280—282 (1947).

QUINN, L. H.: Treatment of glaucoma. Tex. St. med. J. **45**, 142—145 (1949).

QUINTIERI, C.: Ulteriori osservazioni sull'impiego del Mintacol: ricerche cliniche. Boll. Oculist. **34**, 478—483 (1955).

RADOS, A.: Blood cholinesterase levels of patients with glaucoma. Arch. Ophthal. (Chicago) **30**, 371—375 (1943).

RAIFORD, M. B.: Clinical evaluation of DFP in glaucoma therapy. Amer. J. Ophthal. **32**, 1399—1403 (1949).

LA ROCCA, V.: Retinal detachment from di-isopropyl fluorophosphate in an aphakic eye. N. Y. St. J. Med. **52**, 1329—1330 (1952).

DE ROETTH, A. JR.: Cholinesterase activity in ocular tissues and fluids. Arch. Ophthal. (Chicago) **43**, 1004—1025 (1950).

ROSS, E. J.: Circulation of the aqueous humor and the experimental determination of its rate of flow. Brit. J. Ophthal. **36**, 41—51 (1952).

ROSSI, G.: Azione sull'occhio di un nuovo farmaco sintetico exerino-simile: la prostigmina. (Ricerche spermiimentali e cliniche) Arch. Ottal. **42**, 341—360 (1935).

SALLMANN, L. V., and B. DILLON: The effect of di-isopropyl fluorophosphate on the capillaries of the anterior segment of the eye in rabbits. Amer. J. Ophthal. **30**, 1244—1262 (1947).

SCHMIDT, T.: Ein Standard-Schiotz-Tonometer. Klin. Mbl. Augenheilk. **132**, 428 (1958 a).

— Ein Standard-Schiotz-Tonometer. Ophthalmologica (Basel) **135**, 645—648 (1958 b).

SCHIOTZ, H.: Tonometrie. Acta ophthal. (Kbh.) **2**, 1—14 (1924).

— Tonometer mit konvexem Zapfen. Acta ophthal (Kbh.) **4**, 1—11 (1927).

SCHLOSSMANN, A.: Strabismus and refraction: Miotics in the treatment of strabismus. Eye, Ear, Nose. Thr. Monthly **33**, 538 (1954).

SCHNEIDER, W. C., and G. H. HOGEBOOM: Biochemistry of cellular particles. Ann. Rev. Biochem. **25**, 201—224 (1956).

SCHOFIELD, B. M.: Cholinesterase in the iris after removal of the ciliary ganglion. Brit. J. Pharmacol. **7**, 670—673 (1952 a).

— The cholinesterase content of the cats' iris after removal of the ciliary ganglion. J. Physiol. (Lond.) **118**, 32 P (1952 b).

SCHOLZ, R. O.: Studies on the ocular reactions of rabbits to di-isopropyl fluorophosphate. J. Pharmacol. exp. Ther. **88**, 23—26 (1946).

SCHRADER, G.: Die Entwicklung neuer Insektizide auf der Grundlage von organischen Fluor- und Phosphorverbindungen. Monographie No. 62, 2. Aufl. Weinheim: Verlag Chemie 1952.

SCHUMACHER, H.: Experimentelle Untersuchungen über die Wirkungsweise von Eserin im Auge. Ophthalmologica (Basel) **131**, 173—178 (1956).

SIMONELLI, M.: L'uso della prostigmina nella terapia del glaucoma. Riv. oto-neuro-oftal. **2**, 119—124 (1947).

STAJDUHAR, J.: Nasa isknostva sa diisopropylfluorofosfatom (DFP Kod glaukome. Lijecn. Vijesn. **72**, 293—296 (1950).

STEDMAN, E., and G. BARGER: Physostigmine (eserine). Part. III. J. chem. Soc. **127**, 247—258 (1925).

— Studies on the relationship between chemical constitution and physiological action. I. Position isomerism in relation to miotic activity of synthetic urethanes. Biochem. J. **20**, 719—734 (1926).

— Studies on the relationship between chemical constitution and physiological action. II. The miotic activity of urethanes derived from the isomeric hydroxybenzyldimethylamines (HBDM). Biochem. J. **23**, 17—24 (1929 a).

— Chemical constitution and miotic action. Amer. J. Physiol. **90**, 528—529 (1929 b).

STEPHEN, R. W.: Use of drugs in treatment of strabismus. Brit. orthopt. J. **15**, 73—76 (1958).

STERNBERG, A. R., and K. RAAB: Application of a cholinesterase inhibitor in the treatment of esophoric asthenopia. (In Hungarian). Szemészet **96**, 20—23 (1959).

STONE, W. C.: Use of di-isopropyl fluorophosphate (DFP) in treatment of glaucoma. Arch. Ophthal. (Chicago) **43**, 36—42 (1950).

SWAN, K. C., and W. HART: A comparative study of the effects of mecholyl, doryl, eserine, pilocarpine, atropine, and epinephrine on the blood-aqueous barrier. Amer. J. Ophthal. **23**, 1311—1319 (1940).

— Ocular effects of the choline esters. Trans. Amer. ophthal. Soc. **46**, 651—672 (1948).

—, and L. GEHRSITZ: Competitive action of miotics on the iris sphincter. A. M. A. Arch. Ophthal. **46**, 477—481 (1951).

— Iris pigment nodules complicating miotic therapy. Amer. J. Ophthal. **37**, 886—889 (1954).

SZASZ, A.: Die medikamentöse Beeinflussung der reaktiven Hypertonie. Arch. Augenheilk. **104**, 155—166 (1931).

THEODORE, F. H.: Drug sensitivities and irritations of the conjunctiva. J. Amer. med. Ass. **151**, 25—30 (1953).

THIEL, H. L.: Über Versuche mit einem neuen synthetischem Miotikum „Mintacol“ bei Glaukom. Klin. Mbl. Augenheilk. **114**, 454—455 (1949).

THOMAS, C., J. CORDIER and B. ALGAN: Utilisation du DFP dans certaines formes d'hypertonie oculaire. Bull. Soc. franç. Ophtal. **8**, 847—850 (1951).

TICHOMIROV, P. E., and N. N. DMITRIEVA: The action of di-isopropyl fluorophosphate on the intraocular tension in glaucoma. (In Russian). Vestn. Oftal. **31**, No. 1, 27—31 (1952).

UPHOLT, W. M., G. E. QUIMBY, G. S. BATCHELOR and J. P. THOMPSON: Visual effects accompanying TEPP-induced miosis. A. M. A. Arch. Ophthal. **56**, 128—134 (1956).

VANYSCK, J.: Cholinesterase and glaucoma. (In Czech.) Čsl. Oftal. **4**, 259—261 (1948).

— Di-isopropyl-fluorofosfat-Nove miotikum. Čsl. Ofthal. **5**, 8—14 (1949).

WALKER, M. B.: Treatment of myasthenia gravis with physostigmine. Lancet **1934**, 1200—1201.

— Case showing the effect of prostigmine on myasthenia gravis. Proc. roy. Soc., B **28**, 759—761 (1935).

WALSH, F. B.: Myasthenia gravis and its ocular signs: A review. Amer. J. Ophthal. **28**, 13—33 (1945).

— Myasthenia gravis: brief notes regarding diagnosis and treatment. Trans. ophthal. Soc. Aust. **8**, 39—56 (1948).

WEEKERS, R.: Le traitement médicamentaux de l'hypertension intraoculaire. Indications et mode d'action du diisopropylfluorophosphonate. Bull. Soc. belge Ophtal. **86**, 38—58 (1947).

—, et G. LAVERGNE: Decollement de la rétine provoqué par le diisopropylfluorophosphonate (DFP). Bull. Soc. belge Ophtal. **110**, 273—276 (1955).

WEINSTEIN, P.: Glaucoma treatment by Furmethide and Di-isopropylfluorophosphonate (DFP). Ophthalmologica (Basel) **118**, 76—79 (1949).

WESSELY, K.: Zur Wirkungsweise des Eserins. Klin. Mbl. Augenheilk. **37**, 303—310 (1913).

WESTSMITH, R. A., and R. E. ABERNETHY: Detachment of retina with use of diisopropyl fluorophosphate (Floropryl) in treatment of glaucoma. A. M. A. Arch. Ophthal. **52**, 779 to 780 (1954).

WIRTH, W.: Zur Pharmakologie des Mintacol, eines neuen synthetischen Glaukommittels. Dtsch. med. Wschr. **74**, 1243—1245 (1949).

WUDKA, E., and I. H. LEOPOLD: Experimental studies of the choroidal vessels: I. Historical survey. A. M. A. Arch. Ophthal. **55**, 605—607 (1956).

ZAJICEK, J., and E. ZEUTHEN: Quantitative determination of cholinesterase activity in individual cells. Exp. cell. Res. **11**, 568—579 (1956).

— Studies on the histogenesis of blood platelets and megakaryocytes. Acta physiol. scand. **40**, Suppl. 138 (1957).

ZEKMAN, T. N., and D. SNYDAEKER: Increased intraocular pressure produced by di-isopropyl fluorophosphate (DFP). Amer. J. Ophthal. **36**, 1709—1715 (1953).

Author Index

Page numbers in *italics* refer to the bibliography

Subject Index

(Compiled by the Editor with the collaboration of the individual contributors)

The following abbreviations are used, excepting as primary headings, throughout:
ACh: acetylcholine; AChE: acetylcholinesterase; AliE: aliesterase; anti-ChE: anticholinesterase, anticholinesterase agent; ArE: arylesterase; ATP: adenosine triphosphate; BuChE: butyrocholinesterase; ChAc: choline acetylase; ChE(s): cholinesterase(s); CNS: central nervous system; CoA: coenzyme A.

72*

Handb. d. exp. Pharmakol. Erg. W. Bd. XV

74

1208   Subject Index

Pyrolan (1-Phenyl-3-methyl-pyrazolyl-(5)- dimethyl carbamate), actions of, on insects 777
Pyrophosphonates 875
Pyrophosphoric acid derivatives, toxicology of, experimental animals 838—839
Pyrrole-2-aldoxime, reactivation of phosphorylated AChE by, *in vitro* 939
Pyrrolocaine, anti-ChE action of 419
Pyruvylcholine, actions of, on rectus abdominis, frog 574

Q

Quantum content, of transmitter, at neuromuscular junction 641
Quaternary ammonium anti-ChE agents (see also Anti-Cholinesterase agents, Reversible, quaternary compounds, and other subheadings; Quaternary ammonium ions) absorption of, in man 993
anti-ChE action of 93, 101—102, 104—105
human AChE and BuChE 992
intoxication, that have produced, in man 992
lipoid solubility of 992
toxic doses of, in man 994
Quaternary ammonium ions
actions of (at, in, on)
depolarizing 718
electric organ, teleost 658
endplate potentials, spontaneous 643
nerve afterpotentials 654
anti-ChE action of 93, 101—102, 104—105
binding forces with AChE 330, 333
depolarizing action of 718
effects of (at, in, on)
ion transport 652—653, 781
teratogenic, chick embryo 802—805
inhibition of ChAc by 51, 52
mechanism of action of, endplate membrane 645
potentiation of muscle contraction by, mammalian 628—629
Quaternary ammonium ions, lipid-soluble reversible effects on conduction, nerve and muscle fibers, electroplax 724
physostigmine, competitive action with 725
Quaternary anticholinergic compounds, antagonism of anti-ChE poisoning by 899—902, 904
Quaternary compounds (see Quaternary ammonium anti-ChE agents; Quaternary ammonium ions; Anticholinesterase agents, Reversible, quaternary compounds, and other subheadings)
Quaternary pyridine aldoximes (see P-2-AM; other individual compounds)
Quinacrine, anti-ChE action of 416
Quinidine
actions of, on heart, rabbit 516
anti-ChE action of 416
Quinine
actions of, on neuromuscular transmission, mammalian 623
anti-ChE action of 416

Quinoline aldoximes, reactivation of phosphorylated AChE by, *in vitro* 935
Quinone derivatives, anti-ChE action of 408 to 411

R

R-6199 (Amiton) 459
Rabbit, ACh in tissues of 3
Racemorphan, anti-ChE action of 415
Rachiglossa, choline esters in 6
Raia, ChE's of 220, 273
Rana pipiens (see Frog)
Rana sphenocephala (see (Frog)
Ranvier nodes
effect of AChE inhibitors on 708
effect of neostigmine on, frog sciatic nerve 726
effects of PAD and nor-ACh-12 on electrical activity of 725
effect of D-tubocurarine on, frog sciatic nerve 726
fine structure of, frog sciatic nerve 707
Rape *(Draba nemorosa),* sinapylcholine in 4
Rat liver, palmitylcholine in 5
Reactivation, phosphorylated AChE, of induced 342—346
pH-dependence 340, 342
spontaneous 340—341, 345
therapeutic value in anti-ChE intoxication 910—911
Reactivators of AChE (see Acetylcholinesterase, reactivation of; Acetylcholinesterase, reactivators of)
Receptor activators, block by, with depolarization 718—720
Receptor inhibitors, block by, without depolarization 718—720
Receptors, ACh (see also Acetylcholine receptor protein) 189, 443—445, 643—645, 717 to 724, 886, 894
A-groups 444
B-groups 445
C-groups 445
molecular patterns 444
non-specific 256
pre- and postjunctional 265
Red blood cells (see Erythrocytes)
Reflexes,
echinoderms, in 133
medullary, effects of anti-ChE agents on 884, 906
spinal, effects of anti-ChE agents on 689 to 693, 884
Regeneration
AChE, of 228—229
Amphibia, in 148—149
Reineckates, of choline esters 13, 17
Renshaw cells
AChE and 203, 258
effects on, by anti-ChE agents and other drugs 693—694
Reserve and functional AChE 224—229
Resistance to alkylphosphates, in insects 743, 770, 774